COMPLICATIONS of DIALYSIS

COMPLICATIONS
of
DIALYSIS

EDITED BY

Norbert Lameire

University Hospital and University of Gent
Gent, Belgium

Ravindra L. Mehta

University of California, San Diego
San Diego, California

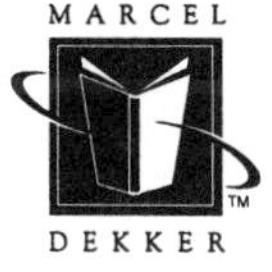

MARCEL DEKKER, INC. NEW YORK • BASEL

ISBN: 0-8247-8871-0

This book is printed on acid-free paper.

Headquarters
Marcel Dekker, Inc.
270 Madison Avenue, New York, NY 10016
tel: 212-696-9000; fax: 212-685-4540

Eastern Hemisphere Distribution
Marcel Dekker AG
Hutgasse 4, Postfach 812, CH-4001 Basel, Switzerland
tel: 41-61-261-8482; fax: 41-61-261-8896

World Wide Web
http://www.dekker.com

The publisher offers discounts on this book when ordered in bulk quantities. For more information, write to Special Sales/Professional Marketing at the headquarters address above.

Current printing (last digit):
10 9 8 7 6 5 4 3 2 1

PRINTED IN THE UNITED STATES OF AMERICA

To Cecile, Ingeborg, Els, and Hendrik
—*N. Lameire*

To my parents Raj and Rajindra L. Mehta; my mentor Prof. K. S. Chugh; my wife, Gita; my children, Isha and Sachin, and to my patients, from whom I continue to learn
—*R. Mehta*

Preface

The worldwide incidence of end-stage renal disease (ESRD) is increasing, with the current total number of cases estimated at 3 million cases. Over the last three decades, advances in the management of this chronic disease have focused primarily on renal replacement therapy with dialysis on renal transplantation. Of the 600,000 people worldwide who will be treated with renal replacement therapy, fewer than 40,000 patients will receive a renal transplant. The large numbers of patients supported with dialysis has spurred several advances in dialysis technology that have allowed nephrologists to offer patients a choice of therapeutic modalities. However, as new applications of dialysis have emerged, new complications have also been identified that are often not well reported. The availability of several books covering dialytic techniques and their applications raises the question: Whey another book on dialysis? We believe the answer lies in the focus of this book on recognition and management of complications of dialysis.

This book is a comprehensive multidisciplinary resource for the nephrologist and caregiver providing dialysis, covering all aspects of dialysis therapies. We have developed the book on the premise that complications result from the interaction of the patient, the technique, and the environment in which dialysis is provided. As a consequence, the complications have been discussed from three angles: patient-related, technique-related, and those contributed to by the organization of care reflecting the changing relationship between providers and beneficiaries of dialysis. We have integrated the knowledge gained from experience with each technique with clinical outcomes, and have explored the emerging role of the economics of these therapies in contributing to adverse outcomes. New and original material has been added rather than known material duplicated. The result is a book that not only is comprehensive and resourceful but also offers details on management of each major complication and practical advice to the dialysis team on several topics that are only covered as exceptions in other books.

Another unique feature of this book is that it is truly international. It was our ambition to cover the problems globally and not to limit coverage to North America and Western Europe. Both our contributors and the topics reflect this theme. We believe that in the immediate future the strategic context of ESRD therapy will make it necessary to maximize clinical and economic outcomes in a rapidly changing healthcare environment. Therefore, attention has also been given to the economic, public health, and environmental problems involved in dialysis. We hope therefore that this book will be useful beyond the need for continuing postgraduate education of the nephrologists and that it will also be of interest to health care providers ranging from government to hospital administrators, health care economists, and all who are directly and indirectly involved in the care of patients with ESRD.

Some degree of overlap among chapters in a multiauthored book, whose writers hail from several countries cannot be avoided. As it should be in a book at the postgraduate academic level, some differences of opinion among authors have not been discarded. We are extremely grateful to all contributors for their time and their efforts in making this book a reality. We are indebted to several people at Marcel Dekker, Inc., for their patience and support as this book has developed.

We sincerely appreciate the enormous work by our secretaries Mrs. I. Verslycken and Ms. I. Van Dorpe in Gent for Dr. Lameire and Ms. Rachel Manaster in San Diego for Dr. Mehta.

Norbert Lameire
Ravindra L. Mehta

Contents

Contributors

Konrad Andrassy, M.D. Department of Medicine, Renal Section, University Hospital, Heidelberg, Germany

C. H. Barton, M.D. Department of Medicine, Division of Nephrology, University of California, Irvine, Irvine, California

Gerald A. Beathard, M.D., Ph.D., F.A.C.P. Capital Nephrology, U.S. Vascular Access Centers, Inc., Austin, Texas; LSU Medical School, Shreveport, Louisiana; University of Texas Health Science Center, Houston, Texas; University of Texas Medical Branch, Galveston, Texas

Hilde Beele, M.D., Ph.D. Department of Dermatology, University Hospital of Gent, Gent, Belgium

Stefano Biasioli, M.D. Legnago Hospital, Legnago, Italy

Peter George Blain, Ph.D., F.R.C.P., F.F.O.M., Fl.Biol. Medical School, University of Newcastle-upon-Tyne, United Kingdom

Peter G. Blake, M.B., F.R.C.P.S., F.R.C.P.C. Division of Nephrology, Department of Medicine, University of Western Ontario, Ontario, Canada

Paola Boccardo, Biol. Sci.D. Mario Negri Institute for Pharmacological Research, Bergamo, Italy

Jacques J. Bourgoignie, M.D. Division of Nephrology, University of Miami School of Medicine, Miami, Florida

Timothy E. Bunchman, M.D. Department of Pediatrics, The University of Michigan, Ann Arbor, Michigan

Alfred K. Cheung, M.D. Division of Nephrology and Hypertension, University of Utah School of Medicine, Veterans Affairs Medical Center, Salt Lake City, Utah

Kirpal S. Chugh, M.D., F.A.C.P. Department of Nephrology, Postgraduate Institute of Medical Education and Research, Chandigarh, India

Sumant Chugh, M.D. Department of Medicine, Renal Section, Boston Medical Center, Boston, Massachusetts

William R. Clark, M.D. Department of Scientific Affairs, Renal Division, Baxter Healthcare Corp., and Department of Medicine, Indiana University School of Medicine, Indianapolis, Indiana

Gerald Anthony Coles, M.D., M.R.C.P. Institute of Nephrology, University of Wales College of Medicine, Cardiff, United Kingdom

Frank Comhaire, M.D., Ph.D. Department of Internal Medicine—Endocrinology, University Hospital of Gent, Gent, Belgium

Margarita Craen, M.D. Department of Pediatric and Adolescent Endocrinology, University Hospital of Gent, Gent, Belgium

Ronald Daelemans, M.D., Ph.D. Nephrology, Hypertension, and Medical Intensive Care Unit, General Hospital Stuivenberg, Antwerp, Belgium

Andrew Davenport, M.D., F.R.C.P. Center for Nephrology, The Royal Free Hospital, London, United Kingdom

Simon J. Davies, M.D., F.R.C.P. Department of Nephrology, North Staffordshire Hospital Trust, Stoke-on-Trent, United Kingdom

Marc E. De Broe, M.D., Ph.D. Department of Nephrology, University Hospital Antwerp, Antwerp, Belgium

Jean-Jacques De Laey, M.D., Ph.D. Department of Ophthalmology, University Hospital of Gent, Gent, Belgium

Thomas A. Depner, M.D. Department of Internal Medicine/Division of Nephrology, University of California, Davis, Sacramento, California

Rita De Smet, Lic. Eng. Department of Nephrology, University Hospital of Gent, Gent, Belgium

Annemieke Dhondt, M.D., Ph.D. Department of Internal Medicine, Renal Division, University Hospital of Gent, Gent, Belgium

Jorge Diego, M.D. Department of Nephrology, University of Miami School of Medicine, Miami, Florida

Joel E. Dimsdale, M.D. Department of Psychiatry, University of California, San Diego, San Diego, California

Wilfred Druml, M.D. Division of Nephrology, University of Vienna, Vienna, Austria

Aldo Fabris, M.D. Nephrology and Dialysis Service, City Hospital, Bassano del Grappa, Italy

Bernadette Faller, M.D. Hospital Louis Pasteur, Colmar, France

Mariano Feriani, M.D. Department of Nephrology, S. Bartolo Hospital, Vicenza, Italy

Steven Fishbane, M.D. Department of Medicine, Winthrop-University Hospital, Mineola, New York

Jürgen Floege, M.D. Department of Medicine, University of Aachen, Aachen, Germany

Norbert Fraeyman, Ph.D. Department of Pharmacology, Heyman Institute, Gent, Belgium

Eli A. Friedman, M.D. Department of Medicine, Renal Division, SUNY Health Science Center at Brooklyn, Brooklyn, New York

F. John Gennari, M.D. Department of Medicine, University of Vermont College of Medicine, Burlington, Vermont

Eric E. O. Gheuens, M.D., Ph.D. Nephrology, Hypertension, and Medical Intensive Care Unit, General Hospital Stuivenberg, Antwerp, Belgium

Ram Gokal, M.D., F.R.C.P. Department of Renal Medicine, Manchester Royal Infirmary, Manchester, United Kingdom

Thomas A. Golper, M.D. Department of Nephrology/Medicine, University of Arkansas for Medical Sciences, Little Rock, Arkansas, and Renal Disease Management, Inc., Youngstown, Ohio

Muhammed A. Goreja, M.D. Department of Medicine, Winthrop-University Hospital, Mineola, New York

Susan Grossman, M.D. Residency Program Director, St. Vincent's Medical Center of Richmond, Staten Island, New York

Steven Guest, M.D. Department of Medicine, Stanford University Medical Center, Stanford, California

Johathan Himmelfarb, M.D. Maine Medical Center, Portland, Maine

Nicholas Andrew Hoenich, Ph.D. Medical School, University of Newcastle-upon-Tyne, United Kingdom

Walter H. Hörl, M.D., Ph.D., F.R.C.P. Division of Nephrology and Dialysis, University of Vienna, Vienna, Austria

Susan S. Hou, M.D., F.A.C.P. Loyola University School of Medicine, Maywood, Illinois

T. Alp Ikizler, M.D. Department of Medicine, Division of Nephrology, Vanderbilt University Medical Center, Nashville, Tennessee

Alkesh Jani, M.D. Department of Medicine, Stanford University Medical Center, Stanford, California

V. Jha, M.D., F.A.C.P. Department of Nephrology, Postgraduate Institute of Medical Education and Research, Chandigarh, India

André A. Kaplan, M.D., F.A.C.P. Division of Nephrology, University of Connecticut Health Center, Farmington, Connecticut

Jean Marc Kaufman, M.D., Ph.D. Department of Internal Medicine—Endocrinology, University Hospital of Gent, Gent, Belgium

Ramesh Khanna, M.D., F.A.C.P. Department of Medicine, University of Missouri–Columbia, Columbia, Missouri

J. P. Kooman, M.D., Ph.D. Department of Internal Medicine, Academic Hospital Maastricht, Maastricht, The Netherlands

Edward A. Kowalski, M.D. Department of Nephrology, Winthrop-University Hospital, Mineola, New York

Michael A. Kraus, M.D. Department of Medicine, Indiana University School of Medicine, Indianapolis, Indiana

Raymond T. Krediet, M.D., Ph.D. Division of Nephrology, Department of Medicine, Academic Medical Center, Amsterdam, The Netherlands

Richard A. Lafayette Department of Medicine, Stanford University Medical Center, Stanford, California

Norbert Lameire, M.D., Ph.D. Renal Division, University Hospital of Gent and University of Gent, Gent, Belgium

Bart Lafaut, M.D., Ph.D. Department of Ophthalmology, University Hospital of Gent, Gent, Belgium

Geert Leroux-Roels, M.D., Ph.D. Department of Clinical Chemistry, Microbiology, and Immunology, University Hospital of Gent, Gent, Belgium

K. M. L. Leunissen, M.D., Ph.D. Department of Nephrology, Academic Hospital Maastricht, Maastricht, The Netherlands

A. Leys, M.D., Ph.D. Department of Ophthalmology, University Hospital St.-Rafaël, Leuven, Belgium

Gerhard Lonnemann, M.D. Department of Nephrology, Medicinische Hochschule, Hannover, Germany

Iain C. Macdougall, B.Sc., M.B., Ch.B., M.D., F.R.C.P. Department of Renal Medicine, King's College Hospital, London, United Kingdom

John K. Maesaka, M.D. Department of Medicine, Winthrop-University Hospital, Mineola, New York

Ahmed Mahmoud, M.D. Medical Centre for Andrology, University Hospital of Gent, Gent, Belgium

Rosario Maiorca, M.D. Institute and Division of Nephrology, University and Civil Hospital, Brescia, Italy

Norma J. Maxvold, M.D. Pediatric Critical Care Medicine, The University of Michigan Health System, Ann Arbor, Michigan

Ravindra L. Mehta, M.B.B.S., M.D., F.A.C.P. Department of Medicine, Division of Nephrology, University of California, San Diego, San Diego, California

David L. Mendelssohn, M.D., F.R.C.P. Department of Medicine, St. Michael's Hospital and University of Toronto, Toronto, Ontario, Canada

Maruschka Patricia Merkus, Ph.D. Clinical Epidemology and Biostatistics, Academic Medical Center, Amsterdam, The Netherlands

Anne Marie Miles, M.D. Department of Medicine, Renal Division, SUNY Health Science Center at Brooklyn, Brooklyn, New York

Madhukar Misra, M.D., M.R.C.P.(UK) Division of Nephrology, University of Missouri–Columbia, Columbia, Missouri

Bruce A. Mueller, Pharm.D. School of Pharmacy and Pharmacological Sciences, Purdue University, West Lafayette, Indiana

Jean Marie Naeyaert, M.D., Ph.D. Department of Dermatology, University Hospital of Gent, Gent, Belgium

Patrick S. Parfrey, M.D., F.R.C.P. Department of Medicine, Health Sciences Centre, Memorial University, St. John's, Newfoundland, Canada

Renaat Peleman, M.D., Ph.D. Department of Internal Medicine, Division of Infectious Diseases, University Hospital of Gent, Gent, Belgium

Mariavalentina Pellanda, M.D. Nephrology and Dialysis Service, City Hospital, Bassano del Grappa, Italy

Brian J. G. Pereira, M.D., D.M. Department of Medicine, Tufts University School of Medicine, New England Medical Center, Boston, Massachusetts

Pradeep Ramamirtham, M.D. Department of Medicine, Division of Gastroenterology, University of California, San Diego, San Diego, California

Giuseppe Remuzzi, M.D. Azienda Ospedaliera, Ospedali Riuniti di Bergamo, and Mario Negri Institute for Pharmacological Research, Bergamo, Italy

Claudio Ronco, M.D. Division of Nephrology, St. Bortolo Hospital, Vicenza, Italy

Thomas J. Savides, M.D. Department of Medicine, Division of Gastroenterology, University of California, San Diego, San Diego, California

Theodore I. Steinman, M.D. Dialysis Unit Renal Division, Beth Israel Deaconess Medical Center and Harvard Medical School, Boston, Massachusetts

Nicholas Topley, B.Sc., Ph.D. Institute of Nephrology, University of Wales College of Medicine, Cardiff, United Kingdom

Zbylut J. Twardowski, M.D., Ph.D., F.A.C.P. Department of Medicine, University of Missouri–Columbia, Columbia, Missouri

Antonios H. Tzamaloukas, M.D., F.A.C.P. Department of Medicine, University of New Mexico School of Medicine, and Veterans Affairs Medical Center, Albuquerque, New Mexico

Wim Van Biesen, M.D. Department of Internal Medicine, University Hospital of Gent, Gent, Belgium

F. M. van der Sande, M.D., Ph.D. Department of Internal Medicine, Academic Hospital Maastricht, Maastricht, The Netherlands

Raymond C. Vanholder, M.D., Ph.D. Department of Internal Medicine, University Hospital of Gent, Gent, Belgium

N. D. Vaziri, M.D., M.A.C.P. Department of Medicine, Division of Nephrology, University of California, Irvine, Irvine, California

Maria E. Wiedemann, M.A., M.B.A. Public Affairs, Baxter Deutschland GmbH, Unterschleissheim, Germany

William C. Wilson, M.D. Department of Anesthesiology, University of California, San Diego, San Diego, California

James F. Winchester, M.D., F.R.C.P. (Glas.), F.A.C.P. Georgetown University Medical Center, Washington, D.C.

Jane Y. Yeun, M.D., F.A.C.P. Department of Internal Medicine, University of California, Davis, Sacramento, California

Bum-Hee Yu, M.D., Ph.D. Department of Psychiatry, Samsung Medical Center, Sungkyunkwan University, Seoul, Korea

COMPLICATIONS
of
DIALYSIS

1

Complications of Vascular Access

Gerald A. Beathard
Capital Nephrology, U.S. Vascular Access Centers, Inc., Austin, Texas
LSU Medical School, Shreveport, Louisiana
University of Texas Health Science Center, Houston, Texas
University of Texas Medical Branch, Galveston, Texas

Nowhere in clinical medicine is there a better example of the benefits of biomedical engineering to patient care than that offered by chronic hemodialysis. This technology, using a machine to maintain and preserve the life of the patient, has been and continues to be successful. Unfortunately, the interface between the two is defective. The vascular access is associated with complications. These complications result in patient morbidity and mortality and add considerably to the cost of managing chronic renal failure. The annual cost of maintaining vascular access in the United States is approaching one billion dollars (1). This represents only the tip of the iceberg, however. Problems that derive both directly and secondarily from these complications result in a major proportion of the hospitalizations required in this frequently hospitalized population of patients (2).

Vascular access can be divided into three types: tunneled-cuffed catheters (TCCs), prosthetic bridge grafts (PBGs), and autologous native fistulas (AVFs). Each of these has an important role to play in hemodialysis, but each has the potential for complications.

I. TUNNELED-CUFF CATHETERS

Since their introduction in the 1980s (3–5), TCCs have come to play an increasingly important role in the delivery of hemodialysis to patients with chronic renal failure. Data collected by the United States Renal Data System indicates that in 1996, 18.9% of all new hemodialysis patients were being dialyzed with a TCC 60 days after starting dialysis (2). These catheters are used for a variety of reasons, as shown in Table 1. Unfortunately as we have learned all too well, the TCC is a double-edged sword. The tremendous advantages that it brings can also carry a tremendous cost.

A. Complications of Initial Placement

As listed in Table 2, a variety of complications can occur at the time of catheter placement. The major determinant for problems at the time of insertion is the experience of the operator (6). Even in the hands of experienced surgeons in the operating room, blind insertion results in complication rates as high as 5.9% (7,8). These complications include (3–5,7–14): pneumothorax (0–1.8%), hemothorax (0–0.6%), hemomediastinum (0–1.2%), recurrent laryngeal nerve palsy (0–1.6%), and bleeding that required reexploration and/or transfusion (0–4.7%). This contrasts with the series reported by Trerotola et al. (15) using real-time ultrasound guidance. Their complication rate was limited to 2 cases (0.8%) of clinically silent air embolism in 250 catheter placements. The use of ultrasound has resulted in a substantial decrease in procedural complications (16,17) and is strongly recommended (18).

B. Catheter Thrombosis

In general, flow problems that occur early are related to catheter position, while those that occur late are re-

Table 1 Uses of the Tunneled-Cuffed Catheter

As a temporary vascular access (more than a few days of dialysis required)
Acute renal failure
Immediate transplantation
Immediate peritoneal dialysis
As a back up vascular access
Failure of vascular access
Dialysis access graft revision or replacement
Removal of peritoneal catheter
Bridge access to allow time for maturation of permanent access
Native fistula
PTFE graft
Permanent vascular access
Severe peripheral vascular disease
Morbid obesity?
AIDS?

lated to thrombosis. Thrombosis is a common problem; the mean patency rate for these catheters has been reported to range from 73 to 84 days (19,20). The specific factors leading to catheter thrombosis in an individual case are seldom obvious. Rarely one encounters a patient with a definable hypercoagulability state. From a study of central venous catheters, Francis et al. (21) reported evidence to indicate that thrombin is locally deposited on catheter surfaces in vivo. Although this phenomenon was not correlated with identifiable thrombosis, under favorable conditions it could predispose to thrombus formation. Catheter-associated thrombosis can be classified as extrinsic and intrinsic (Table 3).

Table 2 Complications of Tunneled-Cuffed Catheters

Limited ability to provide sufficient blood flow
Complications of initial placement
Pneumothorax
Bleeding
Hematoma formation
Arterial puncture
Hemothorax
Air embolism
Hemomediastinum
Recurrent laryngeal nerve palsy
Thrombosis
Infectious complications
Bacteremia, sepsis
Tunnel infection
Exit site infection
Central vein stenosis

1. Extrinsic Thrombosis

The magnitude of the problem presented by this category of thrombosis is not as great as that of the intrinsic category.

a. Central Vein Thrombosis

The presence of a catheter within the central veins can precipitate thrombosis of the vein. How often this occurs is not clear. Agraharkar et al. (22) suggested that it is not common. They reported an incidence of only 2% in a series of 101 percutaneously inserted catheters. Karnik et al. (23), in a study of 63 patients with central venous catheters (not dialysis), found an incidence of 63.5%. It is certainly clear that symptomatic central vein thrombosis is not common, but when it does occur the symptoms can be dramatic. Diagnosis is based primarily upon the clinical picture presented by the patient. The patient presents with swelling of the ipsilateral extremity, which may also be tender and painful. The presence of central vein thrombosis may be con-

Table 3 Classification of Catheter Thrombosis

Extrinsic
Mural thrombus
Central vein thrombosis
Atrial thrombus
Intrinsic
Intraluminal
Catheter tip thrombus
Fibrin sheath

firmed by the use of ultrasound evaluation. Treatment consists of catheter removal and anticoagulation. In cases in which the potential sites for vascular access are depleted or extremely limited, it may be possible to preserve the catheter. These patients must be systemically anticoagulated and observed very closely, however.

b. Mural Thrombus

This refers to a thrombus that is attached to the wall of the vessel or the atrium at the point of contact by the tip of the catheter. It is presumed that catheter tip movement causes damage, which results in thrombus formation. The tip of the catheter is frequently attached to this mural thrombus. When this occurs, it can interfere with catheter function. Most of these thrombi are not recognized unless there is catheter malfunction, at which time they may be recognized at the time of angiographic evaluation. When recognized, removal of the catheter is indicated and represents adequate treatment.

c. Atrial Thrombus

Rarely a large intra-atrial thrombus may develop in association with a dialysis catheter and present as a mass within the right atrium as seen angiographically or with an echocardiogram (24). This probably represents a variant of the mural thrombus. Removal of the catheter, anticoagulation, and echocardiographic follow-up have been used in these cases.

2. Intrinsic Thrombosis

This type of thrombosis represents the major complication associated with these catheters.

a. Intraluminal Thrombus

Intraluminal thrombosis occurs when a thrombus forms within the catheter lumen. It results from either an inadequate volume of heparin being placed within the catheter lumen, heparin being lost from the catheter between dialysis treatments, or the presence of blood within the catheter. When this occurs, the catheter becomes totally occluded. This type of thrombus is not very common because routine catheter maintenance techniques are generally sufficient to prevent the problem.

b. Catheter Tip Thrombus

Many catheters have side holes at the tip of the arterial limb. Unfortunately, that portion of the catheter from the side holes to the tip will not retain heparin and a thrombus can form. A tip thrombus may be occlusive, or it may act as a ball valve. Preventative measures that are commonly used to avoid intraluminal thrombosis are largely subverted by the presence of the side holes. It is probable that forcible flushing before and after dialysis does aid in clearing poorly attached catheter tip thrombi.

c. Fibrin Sheath Thrombus

This is the most common type of thrombus that forms in association with the TCC. The term fibrin sheath refers to a sleeve of fibrin that surrounds the catheter starting at the point where it enters the vein. This sheath is only loosely attached to the catheter. It is probable that all central venous catheters become encased in a layer of fibrin within a few days of insertion. Hoshal et al. (25) reported a fibrin sheath in 100% of 55 patients with central venous catheters at autopsy. These are not always symptomatic. The incidence of catheter dysfunction secondary to fibrin sheath has been reported to be 13–57% (19). When a catheter is removed, gentle angiography of the catheter can demonstrate a ''wind sock'' of residual fibrin sleeve (Fig. 1) in approximately 40% of cases (26).

As the sheath extends downwards, it eventually closes over the tip of the catheter. In this position, it can be disrupted by inward pressure to create a flap valve that will allow injection but prevents withdrawal of blood and fluid. The TCC moves up and down within the vein and in and out at the point where the catheter enters the vein. This occurs to a greater degree in patients that have large breasts or a thick layer of fat on their chest at the point of the exit site. Whether this plays any role in promoting the formation of a fibrin sheath is not clear.

Fibrin sheath formation generally causes catheter dysfunction weeks or months after catheter placement. However, it has been seen as early as 48 hours. It is not clear whether or not prevention of the formation of a fibrin sheath is possible. There is considerable anecdotal experience to suggest that chronic systemic anticoagulation with warfarin is beneficial, at least in selected patients.

3. Treatment of Catheter Thrombosis

The first step in the management of catheter malfunction is the recognition of the problem. Early malfunction is usually due to improper placement with poor tip positioning or subcutaneous kinking of the catheter. Although it is possible for a catheter to become displaced

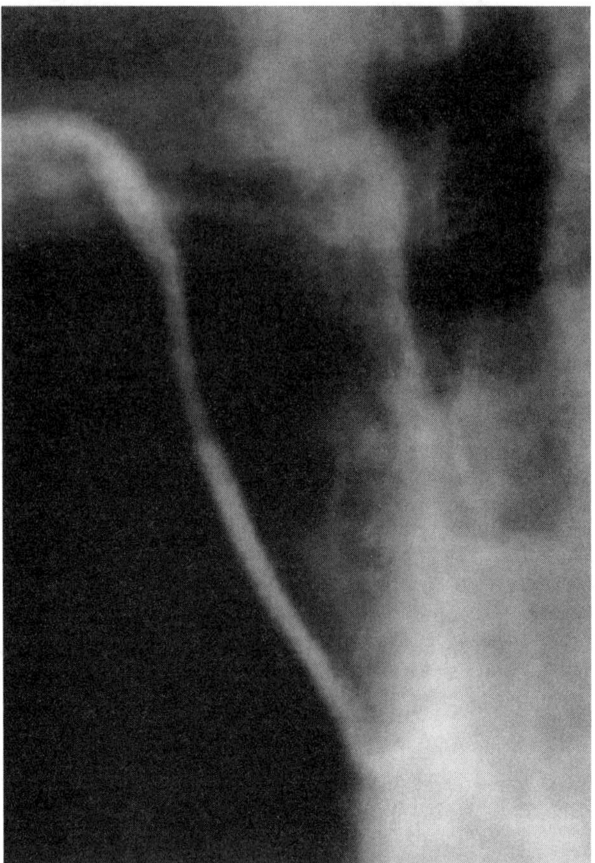

Fig. 1 Fibrin sheath thrombus: The catheter (narrow portion) has been partially removed, leaving the sheath (broader portion) hanging below its tip having the appearance of a "windsock."

Table 4 Protocol for Urokinase Administration

1. Attempt to aspirate the occluded catheter lumen to remove heparin.
2. Inject 1 mL of urokinase (5000 IU/mL) into the occluded catheter lumen.
3. Fill the remainder of the catheter lumen with saline (e.g., for a 1.9 catheter lumen use 1 mL urokinase and 0.9 mL saline).
4. Wait 10 minutes, then add 0.3 mL saline every 10 min × 2 to move active urokinase to the distal catheter.
5. Ten minutes after the final 0.3 mL of saline is added, aspirate the catheter.
6. Repeat procedure if necessary.

after it has been in satisfactory use for a period of time, later cases of malfunction are generally due to thrombosis (5,10,19).

Catheter malfunction is defined as failure to attain and maintain an extracorporeal blood flow sufficient to perform hemodialysis without significantly lengthening the hemodialysis treatment. Sufficient extracorporeal blood flow is considered to be 300 mL/min (27). Once catheter malfunction is recognized, it should be immediately treated. Treatment can be categorized as primary and secondary.

a. Primary Treatment of Catheter Malfunction

Primary treatment of catheter malfunction refers to the treatment that can be immediately applied in the hemodialysis facility.

Urokinase Numerous protocols for urokinase administration are in use, an effective example of which is given in Table 4. Proper use of intraluminal urokinase has been shown to be successful in restoring catheter function in 74–95% of cases (3,19). The advantages of the urokinase technique are that it has a high rate of success, produces no systemic effect and is therefore safe, and can be performed by the nurse in the hemodialysis facility.

Urokinase is not a good solution for the treatment of a fibrin sheath. Thrombolysis only occurs within the catheter and at its tip. There is no systemic effect and no mechanism by which the enzyme can come into contact with the major portion of the sheath.

Mechanical Mechanical treatment to remove the occluding thrombus has been reported. Shrivastava et al. (28) reported an 88% success rate using a 25 cm wire. The same basic procedure can be followed using a Fogarty catheter if the TCC will permit its passage. The advantages of the mechanical technique are that it has a high rate of success, produces no systemic effect, and is therefore safe and is relatively inexpensive. It has the disadvantages of not being a permanent solution to the problem, and in general, a physician must perform the procedure. If a fibrin sheath is the cause of catheter dysfunction, mechanical removal of the occlusion will not provide a long-term solution.

b. Secondary Treatment of Catheter Malfunction

If the primary treatments are unsuccessful or if the problem quickly recurs, a radiographic study using contrast should be performed. Further secondary treatment should be performed based upon the radiographic findings.

Fibrin Sheath Stripping The fibrin sheath can be stripped using a snare catheter. The snare is introduced through the femoral vein, from where it is advanced up to the level of the dialysis catheter. The reported success of this procedure ranges from 92 to 98% (19,26,29). The reported duration of patency has varied from a mean of 20 days to a mean of 90 days. Fibrin sheath stripping generally results in asymptomatic embolization of the fibrin sheath.

Advantages of this technique are its (1) high success rate, (2) safety, (3) preserving of the catheter and (4) reasonable duration patency. Disadvantages of the procedure include the cost of the snare and the procedure and the fact that it is not a permanent solution to the problem.

Catheter Exchange Over Guidewire This technique can be effectively used to eliminate the problem of catheter thrombosis (20,30,31). This can be done using a technique that preserves both the exit site and the venotomy site. It is important that the patient be checked for a fibrin sheath prior to inserting the new catheter. It is possible to place the new catheter back into the retained sheath and have the same problem within a short time.

Advantages of this procedure are that (1) it preserves the exit and venotomy site and it is safe, (2) it is less expensive than fibrin sheath stripping, and (3) it has a high rate of success. A disadvantage of this technique is that you create a new catheter exit wound with its associated risks of bleeding and infection.

Urokinase Infusion Treatment of catheter thrombosis by prolonged administration of urokinase has been used (20). This involved the administration of 20,000 units of urokinase per hour for 6 hours. Lund et al. (20) reported a success rate of 79.5% with this technique. This dose of urokinase is not large enough to result in systemic effects and does not require hospital admission.

Advantages of this technique are that (1) it is safe, (2) it preserves the catheter, and (3) it is less expensive than either fibrin sheath stripping or catheter exchange. The primary disadvantage lies in the fact that it has a lower success rate. Since there is no systemic thrombolytic effect, a fibrin sheath would not be exposed to the enzyme.

4. Catheter-Related Infection

Infection is a very common complication in hemodialysis patients using a catheter. Infection rates ranging from 14 to 54% have been reported (9,10,19,20). Secondary complications of hemodialysis catheter-related bacteremia (CRB) and sepsis such as septic arthritis, endocarditis, and epidural abscess have dire consequences and can result in death (10,32).

a. Nature of Infections

In a series of 488 catheters, we observed a 28.5% CRB rate with new catheter insertions and a 15.6% rate with catheter replacements. The overall incidence of infection was 0.51 per 100 catheter days (1.87 per catheter year). Within the cases of CRB, 26% had an associated exit site infection and 2% had a tunnel infection.

The most commonly reported isolate in cases of CRB has been *Staphylococcus aureus* (10,33). In a series of 101 cases of CRB, we observed gram-negative organisms in 29%. Multiple organisms were isolated in 17% of these cases.

b. Risk Factors

In addition to the foreign body effect of the TCC, a number of factors have been identified as risk factors for the development of CRB (34–36). These include skin and nasal colonization with *Staphylococcus*, catheter hub colonization, duration of catheterization, thrombosis, frequency of catheter manipulation, diabetes mellitus, iron overload, immunoincompetency, use of a transparent dressing, and the conditions of catheter placement.

c. Prevention of Infection

Prevention of catheter-associated infection involves three areas: technique of catheter placement, daily cathether exit site care, and catheter management in the hemodialysis facility. First, it is critically important that maximal barrier precautions be used when a catheter is placed (17). If not done in an operating room, the environment should simulate an operating room.

Care given to the catheter after placement is of equal importance. The use of either mupirocin or povidone-iodine ointment at the exit site until it is healed has been advocated (37). The use of a transparent dressing occlusive dressing has been indicated as a risk factor for CRB (35) since it promotes skin colonization. Nevertheless, the question as to whether it is best to use gauze or a plastic dressing remains unresolved and controversial (38).

Most cases of catheter associated infection occur at a point in time distant from the time of insertion. This suggests that factors related to pathogenesis are most likely to be located within the hemodialysis facility. It appears that bacterial colonization plays an important role. Colonization of the patient's nares, the patient's skin, and the catheter hub have been examined. Zimakoff et al. (39) found that catheter-related staphylococcal infection occurred most often in patients who had nasal colonization, and in more than half of the cases it was with the same strain. Nasal carriage can be eliminated (40), but it is not permanent. Continuous treatment is necessary. Additionally, there is very little evidence to suggest that elimination of nasal colonization has a beneficial effect on the incidence of catheter infection.

Skin colonization was found by Moro et al. (36) to be present in 16.2% of patients undergoing central venous catheterization. They concluded that this was the source of infection in 56% of their cases, but most of these were localized to the exit site. Catheter hub colonization was less frequent (3.5%) but was responsible for systemic infections more frequently. When systemic infection was considered, the risk associated with hub colonization was substantially higher than that associated with skin colonization.

The strategy applied in the hemodialysis facility should be to minimize the effects of bacterial colonization by minimizing the chances of exposure to these sources of potential contamination. The catheter hub must be protected. Table 5 lists a suggested protocol for the prevention of catheter-related infection. When this protocol was instituted in our hemodialysis facility, we observed a decrease in the CRB rate from 1 every 123 catheter days to 1 every 345 catheter days (unpublished data).

d. *Treatment of Infection*

Infection associated with TCCs can be classified into three categories: exit site infection, tunnel infection, and catheter-related bacteremia (CRB). The therapeutic approach to each of these is somewhat different.

Exit Site Infection This is defined as infection localized to the catheter exit site. It is characterized by localized redness, crusting, and exudate. If the patient has systemic symptoms and a positive blood culture, the case should be managed as for CRB below. An exit site infection is a local infection and should be treated with local measures (41). Since the great majority of these are staphylococcal, mupirocin (Bactraban, SmithKline Beecham, Inc.) generally works well. Systemic antibiotics are necessary only in more severe cases characterized by worsening of the local signs of inflammation and the appearance of increasing amounts of drainage. Cases that fail to respond quickly to local measures may necessitate catheter removal. Patients with exit site infection should be monitored for the development of tunnel infection or systemic symptoms suggesting the appearance of a CRB.

Table 5 Protocol for Catheter Care in the Hemodialysis Facility

1. Wrap the catheter caps with povidone-iodine solution soaked gauze for 5 min prior to removal of caps.
2. Patient and nurse must weak a mask.
3. Nurse handling hubs of catheter must wear a fresh pair of disposable gloves.
4. After removing caps, wipe the hubs with a fresh povidone-iodine pledget.
5. Connect the catheter immediately.
6. Repeat this procedure when the catheter is disconnected from the blood lines at the end of the dialysis treatment or any time that catheter manipulation is necessary.
7. Never permit catheter hubs to remain open to the air.

Tunnel Infection A tunnel infection is defined as infection within the catheter tunnel above the Dacron cuff. Involvement of the tunnel below the cuff is commonly seen as part of the exit site infection. When the tunnel is infected above the cuff, it is a serious problem because the catheter moves back and forth within this portion of the tunnel and there is direct communication with the blood stream. Appropriate treatment consists of parenteral antibiotics according to culture results and catheter removal. The catheter should not be immediately replaced at this site.

Catheter-Related Bacteremia When a TCC patient presents with a positive blood culture, immediate and prolonged antibiotic treatment is essential. The antibiotic used must be based upon culture and sensitivity data. The empiric use of vancomycin should be avoided because of the risk of inducing vancomycin-resistant *Enterococcus*. Antibiotic therapy should be continued for a minimum of 3 weeks. Blood cultures should be repeated a week following therapy to assure that the infection has been eradicated. Routine evaluation for valvular vegetations by echocardiography should be considered. Appropriate management of the catheter must also be addressed. There are several choices: leave the catheter in, change the catheter over a guidewire, change the catheter over a guidewire with a new tunnel and exit site, remove the catheter and delay replacement until the infection has been treated. There are several issues that affect this choice.

The presence of a biofilm on the surface of the catheter may play an important role in catheter-related sepsis (42,43). Bacteria adhere and become embedded in the glycocalyx of the biofilm making them more resistant to antibiotics than those floating in the circulation (42,44). Passerini et al. (43) demonstrated the presence of a biofilm on the surface of 100% of the central venous catheters removed from 26 ICU patients. Some of these catheters had been in place for only 1 day. Bacteria were demonstrated within 88% of these biofilms.

From a purely infectious disease viewpoint, removal of the catheter appears to be important (45,46), and where possible this course of action should be followed. However, in the dialysis patient the issue is complicated by the fact that patient must continue to receive dialysis treatments. Removal of the catheter creates a requirement for the use of temporary catheters and the risk of their associated complications. It mandates multiple procedures, a period of hospitalization, and increased costs. Additionally, removal of the catheter may be associated with a loss of the central venous entry site. Saltissi and Macfarlane (47) suggested treating the patient with the catheter in place. However, in an attempt to treat catheter-related bacteremia with the catheter in place, Marr et al. (48) observed a failure rate of 68% even with prolonged antimicrobial therapy. Their study suggests that this approach should not be considered as a therapeutic option.

Unfortunately, when the catheter is removed, the entry site may be permanently lost. Replacement may necessitate using an alternative venous site that is less desirable.

Central venous stenosis, an occurrence that can render the extremity virtually unusable for a permanent vascular access, is well known (49). Many patients with catheter-related sepsis have no external evidence of infection or inflammation. In these patients, there is no local indication for risking the loss of the site. Several studies have recommended treating infection associated with short-term, nontunneled central venous catheters by changing the catheter over a guidewire under antibiotic coverage (50–53). Carlisle et al. (54) and Shaffer (31) demonstrated that hemodialysis catheter-related sepsis in the absence of exit site or tunnel infection could be managed successfully by guidewire catheter exchange and antimicrobial coverage. In a series of 46 patients with minimal symptoms and no exit site infection, we have observed an 86% cure rate for CRB treated by catheter exchange over a guidewire 24–48 hours after initiation of antibiotics followed by 3 weeks of continued antibiotic treatment.

In patients who have exit site infections, the catheter must be removed and a new tunnel and exit site must be created when it is replaced. In patients who are ill with severe symptoms of sepsis, there is no choice but to remove the catheter and leave it out until the patient has been treated. To do otherwise exposes the patient to unacceptable risks.

5. Central Venous Stenosis Complicating Catheter Usage

For over a decade the relationship between central catheters, particularly subclavian catheters, and central venous stenosis has been recognized (49,55–57). This has been a serious problem with the use of temporary catheters. The incidence of subclavian stenosis following catheter placement has been reported to be in the range of 42 to 50%. In contrast, the rate of innominate stenosis following use of the internal jugular vein has been reported to be 0–10% (58,59). In these reports, the catheters were not tunneled and were placed without imaging guidance.

The right internal jugular is the preferred initial access site for catheter placement. The second choice for placement of a catheter is not at all clear. It appears that the left internal jugular is a very poor access site. For the catheter to reach the right atrium it must traverse two curves, in contrast to the single curve required of the subclavian catheter. Not only does a catheter in this position risk stenosis, it also has a higher malfunction rate (4). If the epsilateral arm is to never be used for a permanent vascular access, the subclavian is a better choice for catheter placement than the left internal jugular.

6. Tunneled Cuffed Catheters Versus Temporary Catheters

Noncuffed, double-lumen catheters are frequently used by nephrologists as a temporary vascular access. These catheters are suitable for bedside insertion and provide marginally acceptable blood flow rates (250 mL/min) for short-term dialysis. When compared to TCCs, these catheters have a higher incidence of infection, higher incidence of loss of function, and higher incidence of dislodgement. It is recommended that their use be limited to no more than 3 weeks and if placed in the femoral vein, their use should be limited to no more than 5 days (60). When everything is taken into account, the only advantage that the noncuffed temporary catheter possesses is that it can be inserted at the bedside.

7. Tunneled Cuffed Catheters Versus Peripheral Vascular Access

Tunneled cuffed catheters are relatively high-resistance devices and therefore have a restricted ability to provide adequate flow for efficient dialysis in comparison to when peripheral vascular access is used (PBG or AVF). Resistance to flow is inversely proportional to catheter diameter raised to the fourth power and directly related to its length. For this reason catheters should be selected that have the greatest available diameter and the shortest length compatible with proper tip placement. In this regard, it is interesting to note that a 19% increase in catheter diameter will compensate for a doubling of length.

Because resistance to pumped blood flow is generally higher, prepump pressures are likely to be lower when catheters are used for access. Low prepump pressures can cause partial collapse of the blood line pump segment, rendering the pump flow meter of the dialysis machine highly inaccurate as a measure of dialyzer blood flow. To prevent this from creating an error in the dialysis prescription, prepump pressures should not be allowed to fall below −200 to −250 mmHg.

Under ordinary circumstances, there is little or no recirculation when arterial and venous catheter ports are connected normally and the catheter tip is positioned correctly. If the catheter tip is located in the superior vena cava or higher, it is possible to get some recirculation (5–10%) since the blood flow is not continuous in the central veins in many patients. When radiographic contrast media is injected into the subclavian, it is frequently seen to move forward very slowly in a back-and-forth fashion synchronous with the cardiac cycle. This pattern of flow is conducive to some degree of recirculation if the catheter tip is in this location. When arterial and venous lines are reversed, recirculation may vary from 4 to 10%. Femoral catheters frequently recirculate. This is especially true with shorter catheters. A femoral catheter should be more than 19 cm in length (60).

Cardiopulmonary recirculation occurs when a peripheral vascular access is used (PBG or AVF). This is caused by dialyzed blood recirculating through the path of least resistance back to the dialyzer. Cardiopulmonary recirculation accounts for approximately 30% of postdialysis BUN rebound in patients dialyzed with peripheral A-V access devices and can reduce urea clearance up to 10%. This phenomenon is absent when catheters are used for access unless a peripheral vascular access is also present. Clearance is therefore slightly enhanced with a catheter, and blood flow need not be as high to achieve the same clearance in a comparable patient. Adjustments for cardiopulmonary recirculation are not required for catheters.

II. PROSTHETIC BRIDGE GRAFT

The development of the polytetrafluoroethylene (PTFE) prosthetic bridge graft (PBG) 21 years ago (61) made it possible to provide chronic hemodialysis to virtually any patient. Unfortunately, these grafts are particularly prone to problems, especially venous stenosis and thrombosis. These problems occur at a rate of approximately 1–1.5 times per patient per year (62). Cumulative patency rates for PBGs in most centers are only 55–75% as one year and 50–60% at 2 years (62–67). The major complications seen in association with the PBG are shown in Table 6.

Table 6 Complications of Prosthetic Bridge Grafts

Venous stenosis
Thrombosis
Infection
Pseudoaneurysm
Ischemia

A. Venous Stenosis

The most common complications associated with the PBG are venous stenosis and thrombosis. In most cases these two problems share the relationship of disease and symptom. Venous stenosis results in problems that have the net effect of inadequate dialysis, loss of PBGs, and frustration for patients, nephrologist, and the staff of the dialysis unit. For all of these reasons, it has been recommended that venous stenosis be actively screened for and treated prospectively (68).

1. Nature of Venous Stenosis Lesion

Stenosis occurs most frequently at the venous anastamosis but may occur anywhere within the system composed of the PBG, the anastamosis, and its draining veins, both peripheral and central. In a review of 536 cases of venous stenosis (69), the following distribution of lesions was reported: venous anastamosis 58.4%, peripheral veins 48.2%, central veins 5%, within the graft 27.8%, and multiple locations 33.2%.

2. Screening for Venous Stenosis

It is important that all hemodialysis facilities have in place a system designed to detect venous stenosis so that it can be diagnosed and treated prospectively (68). Monitoring should be performed at intervals of 1 month or less. The best method to assess the PBG for venous stenosis is an angiogram. However, this is not practical as a screening test. The nephrologist must rely upon less direct techniques for this purpose. Several

Table 7 Screening Techniques for Venous Stenosis

Primary techniques
Dynamic venous pressure
Static venous pressure
Intra-access flow
Supplemental techniques
Physical examination
Character of pulse
Presence and location of thrills
Character of bruit
Clinical parameters
Swelling of arm
Frequent clotting
Prolonged bleeding post-treatment
Difficulty with needle placement
Pain in access arm or hand
Recirculation
Unexplained decreases in URR or Kt/V
Doppler ultrasound imaging

approaches to the screening for venous stenosis have been advocated. As shown in Table 7, these techniques have been divided into primary and supplemental categories.

a. Monitoring Venous Pressure on Dialysis

For many years it has been recognized that an elevation of the venous pressure measured on dialysis (VPm) was indicative of venous outflow stenosis (70). Schwab et al. (71) and Beathard (69) demonstrated that VPm could be utilized as a diagnostic test if it was standardized by measurement early in dialysis at a low blood flow (200 mL/min). This measurement is referred to as the dynamic venous pressure (dynamic VPm). An elevation of 150 mmHg or greater is considered to be significant. Because there are other factors that can affect this measurement, single measurements are not reliable. The pattern observed over time is important, and it is essential that elevation be persistent for it to be of predictive value (69). These measurements are not reliable in cases of stenosis within the graft. Measuring dynamic VPm is the easiest method for monitoring venous pressure.

Approximately 75% of the pressure measured under dynamic conditions is related to factors external to the graft, i.e., the needle and tubing. Even when measured under standardized conditions, dynamic VPm is higher than the actual intra-access pressure as measured by an external pressure transducer at zero blood flow (72,73). Besarab et al. (73) have shown that, although more difficult to do, the measurement of static VPm is superior to the dynamic measurement as a screening tool for the diagnosis of venous stenosis. For this measurement, the blood pump is turned off and the blood line between the blood pump and the prepump pressure monitor is clamped. The pressure is then read from the prepump pressure monitor. An offset factor to compensate for the difference in heights of the access and pressure transducer is added. The value obtained is divided by the patient's systolic pressure to obtain a ratio. A ratio greater than 0.5 is considered to be abnormal.

b. Monitoring Intra-access Flow

Venous stenosis causes increased resistance that results in decreased flow leading to thrombosis. The measurement of intra-access blood flow appears to be the best predictor of incipient thrombosis. All of the other techniques used for screening represent attempts to determine decreased flow secondary to increased resistance by indirect means. A direct measurement of flow obviates the need for other modalities. May et al. (74) measured flow prospectively in a cohort of 172 patients with PTFE grafts and found an average flow of 1134 mL/min. Using this as the reference access blood flow, they observed a relative risk for graft thrombosis of 1.23 at a blood flow of 950 mL/min, 1.67 at 650 mL/min, and 2.39 at 300 mL/min. Intra-access flow can be performed by either Doppler ultrasound (75,76) or ultrasound (77,78). Doppler ultrasound is operator dependent and is prohibitively expensive for routine screening assessments. Currently, ultrasound measurement requires specialized devices that are cumbersome to operate and require excessive time. Although the measurement of intra-access blood flow looks very promising, it is not yet suitable for routine screening in most dialysis facilities (68). As the technology improves this will change.

c. Measurement of Recirculation

Percent recirculation refers to the amount of dialyzed blood that is rewithdrawn from the access for repeated dialysis without entering the central pool. This occurs when there is retrograde flow from the venous needle to the arterial needle during dialysis. It results when the access inflow is not sufficient to meet the demands of the blood pump. The measurement of dialysis access recirculation has been advocated as a guide to detecting venous stenosis (79,80). There are three methods for measuring recirculation: the three-needle method, the stop flow or slow flow method, and the dilution method. Each of these gives a different answer. The three-needle technique using arterial, venous, and systemic samples with peripheral venous blood used for the systemic sample is grossly inaccurate and should be abandoned (81). The peripheral venous BUN exceeds that in arterial blood as a result of arteriovenous disequilibrium due to cardiopulmonary recirculation (82–85) and venovenous disequilibrium secondary to regional blood flow inequalities (86–88).

The stop flow or slow flow technique (89), in which arterial, venous, and a second arterial sample obtained 30 seconds after the blood pump has been slowed or stopped, also gives erroneous results. This is due to the variability in urea measurement (90) and to the 30-second delay in sampling after slowing or stopping the blood pump. The BUN in the arterial line blood will begin to rebound within about 15 seconds of slowing or stopping dialysis. If the third blood sample (systemic) is drawn from the arterial ports exactly 10 seconds after the blood flow is abruptly reduced to 120 mL/min (Table 8), a valid test can be obtained (81). The normal values obtained with this technique are −5 to +5%, with an average of 0%. Recirculation values that are 10% or greater should be investigated.

The dilutional method for measuring recirculation avoids the problem of cardiopulmonary recirculation and is the most accurate of the three approaches. When this method is applied, recirculation should be 0% in a properly cannulated, well-functioning PBG. Recirculation values that are 5% or greater should be investigated (81). Although it is more accurate, its utility is compromised by the fact that special devices are required.

Actually, recirculation measurement has poor predictive power for the diagnosis of venous stenosis in PBGs (73,74). It is much better in AVFs. The reason for this relate to the fact when the flow in a PBG drops below 600–700 mL/min, it is at a substantial risk for thrombosis (74,91–95). Recirculation does not occur until flow is less than the blood pump rate. In other words, as venous stenosis causes a decrease in flow, thrombosis generally occurs before recirculation.

Table 8 Protocol for Urea-Based Measurement of Recirculation

1. Draw arterial (A) and venous (V) line samples.
2. Immediately reduce blood flow rate (BFR) to 120 mL/min.
3. Turn blood pump off exactly 10 sec after reducing BFR.
4. Clamp arterial line immediately above sampling port.
5. Draw systemic arterial sample (S) from arterial line port.
6. Unclamp line and resume dialysis.
7. Measure BUN in A, V, and S samples and calculate percent recirculation (R).

d. Clinical Parameters

Rather than rely on a single screening test, some have felt that a more broad-based approach to screening of dialysis patients for venous stenosis was appropriate. This has involved using the combination of a group of clinical indicators and a physical examination of the PBG to determine the need for an angiogram (96–99). These clinical indicators have included swelling of the access arm (central vein stenosis), frequent clotting of the access, prolonged bleeding from the needle sites posttreatment (high venous pressure), difficulty with needle placement (intra-access stenosis), and pain in the access arm or hand (with heparin injection—retrograde flow into artery). In examining the PBG and arm above the PBG, careful attention should be paid to the presence and location of thrills, the characteristics of bruit, and the nature of the pulse. In a retrospective study of 328 angiograms performed after screening the patients using these criteria (96), Beathard found a 91.7% incidence of significant venous stenosis (>50%). In their study Safa et al. (99) found abnormal physical examination findings to be the most common sole indicator of graft dysfunction. This approach is inexpensive, easily performed, noninvasive, and reliable.

3. Selection of Cases for Treatment

Because of the frequency and the recurrent nature of venous stenosis, some standard must be applied to determine when a case should be treated. It seems reasonable at this point in our knowledge to use 50% or greater stenosis plus evidence of a clinical or physiological abnormality, e.g., elevated venous pressure or decreased flow this standard (100). An exception to this principle might be applied in the case of the thrombosed PBG. Any stenosis found at the time of thrombosis should be considered as a candidate for treatment.

4. Treatment of Venous Stenosis

The preferred method of treatment has not been established. There are two choices: surgical revision and percutaneous angioplasty. The choice of therapeutic modality should depend upon the expertise of the treatment facility (100).

a. Surgical Therapy

There are no good reports concerning the systematic, prospective treatment of venous stenosis by surgical means. Evaluation of 84 cases of surgical graft revision in the absence of thrombosis at our institution revealed a primary (unassisted) patency of 81% at 1 month, 56% at 3 months, 41% at 6 months, and 23% at 1 year by life table analysis (unpublished data).

There are certain problems that are intrinsic to surgical therapy. It is invasive, creates a risk of infection, and the blood loss associated with the procedure may be significant (101). Temporary vascular access with all of its associated complications is frequently required. This may be because of postoperative swelling of the arm or the need to replace the PBG and the necessity of avoiding its use during a maturation period (102).

Many patients require hospitalization in association with surgical therapy for access dysfunction (103). Surgical therapy of venous stenosis also results in the loss of potential vascular access sites. Nevertheless, surgery offers the most definitive treatment for this problem.

b. Percutaneous Angioplasty

In recent years, angioplasty has developed into a reasonable alternative to surgical therapy for venous stenosis affecting PBGs. This is undoubtedly due to an increased awareness of the problem and its consequences, but also due to the fact that it has been shown to be a safe, effective, and easily performed procedure (69,104–106). Percutaneous angioplasty treatment of venous stenosis affecting the PBG is an outpatient procedure that does not prohibit the immediate use of the access for dialysis. Lesions in all locations within the PBG and its draining veins, both peripheral (Figs. 2, 3) and central, can be easily, effectively, and safely treated (69).

Initial success rates for angioplasty therapy of venous stenosis in this setting have ranged from 80 to 94% (69,105–107). The highest rate of technical failure has occurred in the treatment of central lesions. Long-term success rates have ranged from 41 to 76% at 6 months and 31 to 45% at one year (69,105–109). Treatment of central lesions has been met with poor long-term success. In a series of 50 cases of central vein stenosis, a 6-month patency of only 25.4% was reported (96). Lumsden et al. (110) attempted to do a prospective randomized study comparing the results of angioplasty with no treatment in a group of 64 patients with 50% or greater stenosis. They reported no differences in patency rates between the two groups, however, 53% of their treatment group had central vein in contrast to only a 22% incidence in the control group. This divergence between the two groups makes their results impossible to interpret. Since venous stenosis lesions tend to recur, repeat therapy plays an important role in their management. Initial and long-term success rates for repeat treatments have been identical to those with the primary treatment (69).

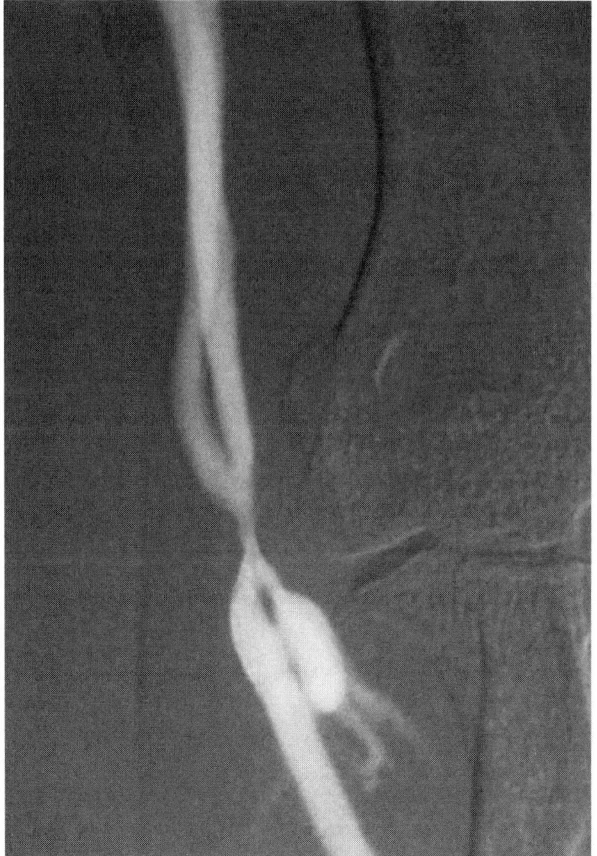

Fig. 2 Venous stenosis: The venous anastomosis is markedly narrowed.

5. Benefits of Prospective Treatment of Venous Stenosis

The prospective treatment of venous stenosis has proven to be cost effective because it decreases the incidence of thrombosis and preserves the life of the PBG (71–73,108,109). In one facility, a program to prospectively identify and treat venous stenosis resulted in a fall in thrombosis rate from 0.58 per patient per year to 0.19 per patient per year (73) and in another from 0.48 to 0.17 (99). Since all of the methods for screening are aimed at the early detection of access-

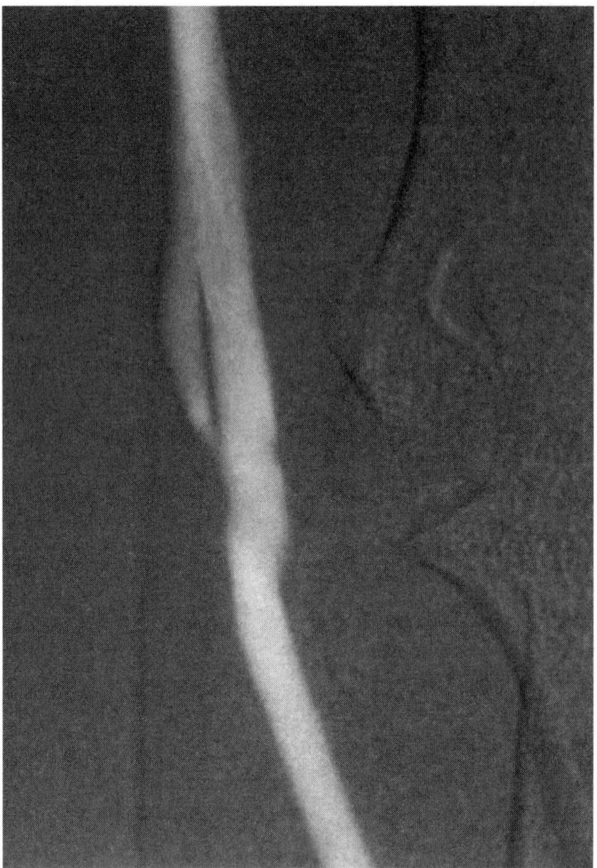

Fig. 3 Postangioplasty: This is the graft as shown in Fig. 2; the stenotic lesion has been treated with angioplasty.

related stenoses, prospective detection and treatment will not prevent thrombosis that is not related to stenosis.

B. Graft Thrombosis

An inescapable relationship exists between the use of a PBG as a dialysis access and thrombosis. When this occurs there are two choices for therapy—surgical and percutaneous. Two prospective randomized trials have been reported in which thrombolysis was compared with surgical therapy (111,112), both of which concluded that surgical therapy was superior to thrombolysis. However, in one the initial success rate for thrombolysis was only 67% and in the other it was 72%. Reports in which such low initial success rates for thrombolysis were obtained must raise questions concerning the performance of the procedure. At this time no conclusions concerning the superiority of either of these therapeutic modalities can be made. The choice of therapy should be based on the expertise of the local facility (113). Regardless of the choice of therapeutic modality, it is essential that treatment be provided as quickly as possible in order to avoid the use of temporary catheters. Every attempt should be made to provide treatment as an outpatient under local anesthesia. Venous stenosis must be treated and the access must be evaluated angiographically for residual stenosis posttreatment. It is important, regardless of the treatment modality used, that any abnormal monitoring tests used to screen for venous stenosis return to normal following the treatment of a thrombosed PBG (113).

1. Surgical Therapy

Until recently surgical therapy has been the standard treatment for a patient with a thrombosed PBG. This therapy consists of either thrombectomy alone, thrombectomy with graft revision, or graft replacement. In most cases thrombectomy alone is inadequate therapy because it ignores venous stenosis, which is generally present (114).

Long-term patency rates for thrombectomy alone without revision are not well defined. In one report (115) the values obtained were: one month—64%; 2 months—37%; 3 months—29%; 6 months—15%; and one year—5%. In the same series long-term patency rates for thrombectomy with revision were: 68% at one month; 56% at 2 months; 51% at 3 months; 33% at 6 months; and 14% at one year. The values for graft replacement performed following thrombosis were: one month—69%; 2 months—55%; 3 months—45%; 6 months—34%; and one year—17%.

The type of surgical revision performed varies according to the location and character of the stenotic lesion. If the stenosis is at the anastamosis and short, a patch angioplasty using an oval-shaped piece of PTFE is affected. If the lesion is longer, extending up the vein, a jump graft to an area beyond the stenosis or to an alternative vein is performed. The same type of procedure is done if the lesion is more proximally (upstream) located (101). Graft revision always results in the loss of at least a small portion of vein. Central venous lesions are difficult to treat surgically (49). A bypass across the shoulder from the access graft or the cephalic vein to the ipsilateral internal jugular has been used successfully (116).

2. Percutaneous Therapy

Although several mechanical devices are available, the term percutaneous therapy is generally used to refer to thrombolysis. Three lytic agents have been used for thrombolysis in association with PBGs: streptokinase, urokinase, and tissue plasminogen activator. Streptokinase is an unsatisfactory agent for this purpose because it is associated with an erratic response, drug resistance, and allergic reactions (117,118). Even though tissue plasminogen has been used with success (119,120), its high cost and the fact that better results have been reported using less expensive alternatives (119,121) should eliminate it from consideration. Urokinase is the agent of choice.

Thrombolysis as applied to PBGs can be divided into three types: pharmacological, pharmacomechanical, and mechanical.

a. *Pharmacological Thrombolysis*

Pharmacological thrombolysis (PT) refers to thrombus dissolution using only the effects of a fibrinolytic enzyme. Lytic enzymes that have been used include streptokinase (117,122,124,125), tissue plasminogen activator (119,120), and urokinase (123,126–128). The lytic agent has been given as a continuous infusion (117,126,128), an initial bolus injection followed by a continuous infusion (123,124), and as intermittent injections (125,127). Treatment times have ranged from 2 to 72 hours. The patients have generally been admitted to the intensive care unit. The rate of success has varied from a low of 14.3% (124) to a high of 100% (126). Complication rates have ranged from none to 85.7%. Although most of these complications have been local due to bleeding at needle puncture sites, some have been more serious. In one report, 6.3% of the patients experienced an embolus to the peripheral artery (122), and in another 12% of the cases required blood transfusions (128). Because of the large doses of enzyme used, systemic fibrinogen depletion has been routinely seen. PT is unsatisfactory as a treatment for thrombosed PBGs and should not be used.

b. *Pharmacomechanical Thrombolysis*

Pharmacomechanical thrombolysis (PTA) is composed of two phases. The first is pharmacological, consisting of enzymatic lysis. The second phase involves mechanical maceration and removal of the residual clot. In the initial attempts at PMT, referred to as lacing-maceration (129,130), highly concentrated urokinase was injected through two hook-shaped catheters as they were rotated and withdrawn through the clotted graft. This was combined with angiographic evaluation of the graft-vein circuit and angioplasty of any stenotic lesion that was found. Using this method, Valji et al. (129) reported 96% success with only a 3% rate of minor complications. They were able to accomplish lysis within a mean time of 86 minutes.

Subsequently these investigators adopted a modification of their technique that they referred to as the pulse-spray method of PMT (119,129,131). This utilizes a catheter design that produces a penetrating spray of concentrated enzyme. The spray produced by this catheter macerates the clot and increases its contact area with the lytic agent while simultaneously treating the entire length of the graft. The proponents of PMT use a combined approach consisting of angiography to visualize the graft and draining veins, thrombolysis by pulse-spraying concentrated urokinase, and angioplasty to macerate residual thrombus and dilate any venous stenosis that is present. In this manner diagnosis and treatment of the stenosis and treatment of the thrombosis are combined into a single procedure. Valji et al. (132) reported a series of 284 cases treated using this technique with a success rate of 92%. A mean time of 67 minutes was required for the procedure in this series. Long-term primary patency following PMT has been in the range of 68% at one month and 26% at one year (129). The quickness, safety, and effectiveness of PMT make it attractive as a nonsurgical means of restoring function to a PBG.

c. *Mechanical Thrombolysis*

Several investigators (121,133,134) have questioned whether the pharmacological component of pharmacomechanical thrombolysis is necessary to safely reestablish flow in a thrombosed PBG. This gave rise to a technique that has come to be referred to as mechanical thrombolysis (MT). The technique is actually more accurately referred to as percutaneous endovascular thrombectomy. No lytic enzyme is used with this technique; only mechanical means are applied to restore flow to the thrombosed PBG.

In a prospective randomized trial comparing MT and PMT (121), the initial success rate, complication rate, and long-term patency of treated PBGs were statistically the same for the two techniques and were comparable to those reported by others for PMT (119,129). The type of MT used in this study consists of angiography to visualize the PBG and draining veins, clot maceration by pulse-spraying heparinized saline, followed by endovascular thrombectomy with an embolectomy catheter and angioplasty to macerate residual thrombus and dilate any venous stenosis that is present. In this manner diagnosis and treatment of the stenosis and treatment of the thrombosis are combined into a single procedure as with PMT.

When compared with surgical treatment of the thrombosed PBG (25), the initial failure rates for MT and surgery were the same. Long-term primary patency for grafts treated by MT was superior to that for surgical thrombectomy and comparable to those for thrombectomy-revision and graft replacement. In a series of 1176 cases treated with mechanical thrombolysis (114), an initial success rate of 96% was obtained. The primary patency at 3 months was 52% and was 39% at 6 months. Other investigators (133–135) have applied their own variations of mechanical thrombolysis to the problem of the thrombosed PBG with equally satisfactory results.

d. Mechanical Devices

A number of mechanical devices that macerate or remove thrombus have been developed and are currently being investigated (136–138). While these devices in general are effective, their cost is a major detraction since the simpler methods have such a high success rate and have proven to be safe.

e. Pulmonary Embolization with Thrombolysis

Concern has been expressed that pulmonary emboli, even though relatively small, could represent a risk to the patient undergoing MT (139). Even though the long-term effects of recurrent treatment are not known, this immediate fear has not been realized. No instance in which clinical signs or symptoms suggest acute pulmonary embolization has been encountered in MT studies (114,121,133–135). Beathard et al. (114) reported finding multiple small perfusion defects in five of six patients undergoing lung scans. These cleared by 2 weeks with no adverse sequelae. The occurrence of small emboli is not unique to MT. These occur with removal of central venous catheters, percutaneous catheter stripping (26,29), surgical thrombectomy of dialysis access (133), and pharmacological thrombolysis (123,127). Two fatalities have been described in a cohort of 31 patients treated by Swan et al. (140) using the PMT technique. The intervals between the procedures and the death of the patients were 2 and 4 days. Both patients had co-morbid conditions. These occurrences are difficult to explain in view of the nature and volume of clot associated with a thrombosed PBG. The occluded PBG contains two types of thrombus, a firm arterial plug, and soft, friable thrombus that disintegrates easily. Most of the thrombus is of the latter type. The arterial plug consists of firm, laminated, organizing thrombus. It is resistant to enzyme lysis and embolizes to the lung regardless of the technique used for percutaneous therapy. The total thrombus volume removed from an occluded PBG at the time of surgical thrombectomy has been shown to average only 3.2 mL (141,142).

3. Comparison Between Percutaneous Therapy and Surgery

In comparing these two approaches—percutaneous and surgical—several parameters should be considered. These include risk to the patient (e.g., pain, infection, blood loss), complications of therapy, timeliness (e.g., how quickly the patient can be returned to dialysis), effectiveness (e.g., initial success rate and duration of patency posttherapy), and economic factors. Since it is a percutaneous technique, thrombolysis is associated with less patient discomfort, risk of infection, and blood loss than is involved with a surgical thrombectomy. Surgical therapy is associated with very few complications during the procedure, however, this is also true for thrombolysis—both are relatively safe.

Basically the timeliness with which any procedure can be accomplished is dependent upon the availability of the operator and the facility (143). For this reason there is great value in having a dedicated laboratory for managing vascular access problems. Unfortunately, when dialysis patients with clotted grafts are forced to compete for facility space and operator time in either surgery or radiology, treatments are frequently delayed and missed unless central venous catheters are used. In some centers delay and hospitalization are routine.

The effectiveness of endovascular procedures must be evaluated from two viewpoints: immediate and long term. Immediate effectiveness relates to both the operators' ability to remove the thrombus and their ability to deal with any anatomical lesions that are present. Long-term effectiveness, or long-term patency, relates to the management of anatomy lesions (i.e., venous stenosis). The various thrombolysis techniques are associated with immediate success rates in order of 90–95%. Immediate surgical failure rates, defined as the need to replace the graft, have been reported to be 6.9% (121) and 18% (112). In a study that compared the immediate success rate for 537 cases of thrombosed access graft treated surgically with the results obtained in 473 cases treated by MT, no statistically significant difference was seen (115).

Data on long-term patency following surgical thrombectomy are difficult to find. In one study (115) sequential data were collected comparing surgical therapy with MT therapy. In 380 cases treated with only surgical thrombectomy, primary (unassisted) patency rates of 64% at one month, 29% at 3 months, 15% at

6 months, and 5% at 1 year were reported. Primary (unassisted) patency rates for MT were 66% at 1 month, 44% at 3 months, 31% at 6 months, and 10% at one year. The differences between surgery and thrombolysis were highly significant statistically. In the same study, when long-term primary patency rates for graft revision or for graft replacement used to treat thrombosed grafts were compared to that for MT, no statistically significant difference was seen.

The surgical treatment of venous stenosis always results in a loss of vein to some degree. Since venous stenosis is a recurrent condition, this loss leads to a progressive depletion of potential access sites. The type of surgical revision performed varies according to the location and character of the stenotic lesion. Regardless of the procedure used there is always some loss of vein.

In reviewing a series of 282 episodes of graft thrombosis, Raju (144) reported that some type of revision was performed in two thirds of the cases. In another series (115), 21.8% of the cases required a graft revision and in 6.8% of the access was replaced with a new graft. All of these resulted in venous losses. It must be noted that when a thrombosed access graft is treated surgically by simple thrombectomy, without graft revision or replacement, it has a 90–95% chance of being inadequate therapy since that is the frequency of venous stenosis.

Economic factors are important in any therapeutic consideration. Reliable cost figures for surgery and endovascular therapy are difficult to obtain, and there are significant regional differences. Sands et al. (145) reported charge figures of $6,802 ($n$ = 71) for thrombolysis compared to $12,740 ($n$ = 75) for surgical thrombectomy. Vesely et al. (146) discovered charges of $6,062 ($n$ = 10) for thrombolysis and $5,580 ($n$ = 10) for surgery in their institution. When Marston et al. (112) reviewed their cost data, they found that thrombolysis charges ranged from $3,104 to $11,646 ($n$ = 15) and surgical treatment ranged from $6,711 to $11,430 ($n$ = 15). They concluded that there were no significant differences between the two, but their data suggest at least the potential for performing thrombolysis more economically than surgery. Additionally, thrombolysis is an outpatient procedure. It is rare for the patient to require admission. In many centers, patients having surgical treatment for a thrombosed graft are routinely admitted. This adds considerably to the cost of management. Delayed and missed treatments also have an economic effect on the dialysis facility. Any procedure that will minimize this problem will have a positive economic effect. The costs of large quantities of urokinase and the price of a mechanical device must also be added to the equation when a comparison is made between techniques that utilize these items and surgery.

C. Graft Infection

Infection of the PBG is a serious complication. It has been reported to account for 20% of all dialysis access complications (147) and to be the second leading cause of graft loss. Infection has been reported to occur at a frequency of 1.3 episodes per 100 dialysis-months and to be associated with bacteremia at a rate of 0.7 cases per 100 dialysis-months (148). *S. aureus* is the most common organism involved. The personal hygiene of the patient appears to be the most important risk factor for the development of access-related infection (149). Therefore, hemodialysis patients with poor personal hygiene habits should be given special attention.

Cannulation of an access site places the hemodialysis patient at risk for infection via bacterial contamination. At times an episode of infection can be traced to an individual member of the dialysis facility staff and to be related to poor needle-insertion technique (150). This underscores the importance of staff training in infection-control measures. Dialysis staff should comply with OSHA regulations, including hand washing and use of clean gloves during needle cannulation. Washing the access site with soap and water will decrease the skin microflora that can be introduced inadvertently into the blood stream during needle cannulation (148,149). The skin should be further cleansed with either 70% alcohol or 10% povidone iodine immediately prior to cannulation (151).

When infected, a PBG must be treated aggressively. An untreated access infection can lead to bacteremia, sepsis, hemorrhage, and even death (152,153). Although a superficial infection that does not involve the graft directly may respond to antibiotic therapy alone, effective treatment generally requires both antibiotic and surgical therapy (154,155).

Localized infection should be treated with appropriate antibiotics based on culture results and by localized resection of the infected portion of the PBG. Extensive infection may require total resection of the graft. Infection of a newly placed PBG should be treated with antibiotics and removal of the PBG, regardless of the extent of the infection (155).

D. Pseudoaneurysm Formation

When inserted into a PBG, the dialysis needle creates a defect that will seal but does not heal (156,157). Degenerative changes occur within the PBG and the overlying skin with long-term use or, more often, with repetitive use in the same spot. This can result in pseudoaneurysm formation, a situation in which there is an enlarged area overlying a defect in the PBG. Insertion of dialysis needles into a pseudoaneurysm may result in prolonged bleeding following needle withdrawal and should be avoided. With progressive enlargement, a pseudoaneurysm can eventually compromise circulation to the skin covering the PBG and may ultimately lead to rupture and severe hemorrhage. Large pseudoaneurysms can also prevent access to the adjacent areas of the PBG for needle placement, thereby limiting potential puncture sites.

A pseudoaneurysm is most effectively treated by graft revision and segment interposition. Delorme et al. (157) report that pseudoaneurysm formation is the primary cause of surgical removal of a PBG more than 2 years after implantation. A pseudoaneurysm should be treated surgically when (1) it exceeds twice the diameter of the graft, (2) it is rapidly increasing in size, (3) severe degenerative changes of overlying skin are present, (4) there is risk of graft rupture due to poor eschar formation, (5) there is evidence of spontaneous bleeding, or (6) puncture sites are limited due to its size (158,159).

E. PBG-Related Ischemia

1. General

When a vascular access is created in the arm, it offers a low resistance route for blood to bypass the higher resistance circuit of the hand. This anomaly can lead to ischemia, a serious and occasionally devastating complication. Ischemia may take one of two forms: primary ischemia and vascular steal syndrome. Primary ischemia refers to the process that occurs secondary to inadequate distal extremity blood flow. Vascular steal syndrome occurs when blood destined for the hand is shunted through the graft, depriving the hand of perfusion. Both of these problems are more likely to occur when the radial artery is used for the graft construction. Diabetics, elderly individuals, patients with severe peripheral vascular disease, and those who have had multiple access attempts are at high risk for these complications. Ischemia is most often seen early after access construction, but it can occur at any time. If not treated promptly it can result in loss of digits, the hand, or the extremity. Severe ischemia can cause irreparable injury to nerves within hours and should be considered a surgical emergency.

2. Diagnosis

For the first 24 hours the patient with a newly created access should be monitored for subjective complaints of sensations of coldness, numbness, tingling, and impairment of motor function (not limited by postoperative pain). Skin temperature, gross sensation, movement, and distal arterial pulses in comparison to the contralateral side should also be assessed. Patients with an established PBG should be assessed monthly. An interval history of distal pain or coldness during dialysis, decreased sensation, reduction in function, or skin changes should be obtained. Patients demonstrating abnormalities should be further evaluated immediately (160).

Lin et al. (161) reported that comparing digital oxygen saturation (SaO_2) in the normal arm and the access arm was helpful in identifying patients that developed ischemia of their hand on dialysis. After studying the SaO_2 before and 20 minutes after the initiation of dialysis using the normal arm as a control, they found that a predialysis SaO_2 difference of 4% or more between the arms predicted decreased SaO_2 of the arm with the access during hemodialysis. A high percentage of the patients with decreased SaO_2 on dialysis were symptomatic.

Electrophysiological detection of a conduction block shortly after the onset of symptoms of neuropathy has been reported to be early indicator of reversible ischemic nerve injury associated with a vascular access (162). Plethysmography has been used to evaluate patients for vascular steal syndrome (163). A positive finding consists of showing a flat waveform converting to pulsatile waveform when the proximal PBG is compressed. Arteriography of the access arm will generally identify the nature and the extent of the vascular problem and may be indicative of the appropriate therapy in some cases (164).

3. Treatment

Mild ischemia manifested by subjective coldness and paresthesias and objective reduction in skin temperature but with no loss of sensation or motion generally improves with time. Patients with mild ischemia should undergo symptom-specific therapy (e.g., wearing a glove) and frequent physical examination, with special attention to subtle neurological changes and muscle wasting. Failure to improve may require surgical intervention.

Surgical intervention consists of either graft ligation, banding, or an arterial ligation-bypass procedure. With ligation the access is sacrificed. Banding represents an attempt to increase the resistance in the vascular access in order to force blood to circulate into the hand (165). The arterial ligation-bypass procedure consists of two parts: ligation of the radial artery below the origin of the PBG and creating a bypass from the artery proximal to the point of origin to a site distal to the point of the ligation (166–168).

Haimov et al. (168) reported a series of hemodialysis patients with severe ischemia in their access extremity secondary to vascular steal syndrome. In this series of patients they compared ligation, banding, and the arterial ligation-bypass procedure. Of seven patients who underwent ligation, five had complete resolution of symptoms, one had persistent pain, and one patient had residual ischemic neuropathy. Of four patients who underwent banding, three lost their access due to thrombosis shortly after the banding procedure, and in one patient partial resolution of symptoms was achieved. Of 23 patients who underwent arterial ligation-bypass procedure, all showed immediate signs of improvement. They concluded that the arterial ligation-bypass procedure gave results superior to either ligation or banding.

In instances in which stenotic lesions are found in the vessel proximal to the origin of the access by arteriography, either surgical treatment or percutaneous angioplasty (164) may result in amelioration of the problem and permit salvage of the access.

III. AUTOLOGOUS ARTERIOVENOUS FISTULA

Either a wrist (radial-cephalic) or elbow (brachial-cephalic) autologous arteriovenous fistula (AVF) created using the patient's native vein provides the best possible vascular access for hemodialysis (62,66,67,150,169–174). Compared to the PBG, the AVF has better long-term patency and fewer complications, including lower incidence of venous stenosis, infection, and vascular steal syndrome. Additionally, there is lower morbidity associated with creation, and performance (i.e.,flow) improves over time.

An AVF provides superior access survival relative to a PBG (175,176). This is true even after adjusting for the effect of age, race, sex, diabetes, and peripheral vascular disease on access survival. The magnitude of the benefit of the AVF is greatest among younger patients, but the advantage of an AVF persisted for patients older than 65 years. The relative risk of access failure for a patient with an AVF, compared with a patient of the same age with a PBG, has been shown to be 67% lower at the age of 40 years, 54% lower at the age of 50 years, and 24% lower at the age of 65 years (176).

Table 9 Complications of Native Fistulae

Poor inflow
Poor development
Ischemia
Venous stenosis
Thrombosis
Aneurysm formation
Infection

Unfortunately the AVF does have some disadvantages; the vein may fail to mature, a period of 1–4 months must elapse following creation before the AVF can be used, some AVFs are difficult to cannulate, and the enlarged vein may be cosmetically unattractive (177). Taking all of this into account, however, the AVF is far superior to any other type of vascular access. In spite of its obvious advantage, the relative number of AVFs being created has been decreasing. Patients starting dialysis had a 70% greater chance of receiving a PBG instead of an AVF in 1990 than they did in 1986 (178). In 1996 only 17.9% of hemodialysis patients were using an AVF 60 days after the intiation of therapy (2).

The complications associated with an AVF (Table 9) are somewhat the same as for the PBG (see Table 6), however; there are several distinct differences. These complications are seen with less frequency and, in general, less severity. The overall complication rate for PBGs is twice as high as that for AVFs. Specifically, PBGs have 6 times the rate of thrombosis and 10 times the rate of infection as AVFs (179).

A. Poor Flow and Inadequate Development

Both blood flow and fistula development are essential for a successful AVF access. These are separate problems in one sense, but they are so closely linked that they must be discussed together. An AVF can remain patent in the face of relatively low blood flow (93). For effective dialysis, the AVF only has to deliver a blood flow that is marginally greater than the pump rate. Unfortunately, dialysis may not be technically possible in these cases with lower flow because the pulsatile pressure that is applied to the vein wall is not sufficient for it to dilate to a size adequate for cannulation. The pressure necessary for fistula development is dependent upon the inflow pressure and the upstream resistance of the draining vein. For any given flow rate, vein enlargement will depend upon resistance. In ideal circumstances, inflow pressure is great enough for fistula development to occur, although the upstream resistance is very low. In less than ideal circumstances fistula development may fail either because of low inflow pressure, decreased upstream resistance caused by a branching vein, or a combination of the two.

Most cases of primary nonfunction are the result of arterial abnormalities causing low flow into the vein used to create the AVF (174). Arteries that are either anatomically small or atherosclerotic can cause this. These problems can usually be diagnosed before surgery is performed through physical examination and other noninvasive procedures. Of the two major types of AVF, the radiocephalic and the brachiocephalic, the former is more often associated with poor inflow (177).

The optimum venous anatomy for AVF development is a single cephalic vein stretching from the wrist to the antecubital space. In many instances, however, this is not the case. The cephalic vein has one or several side branches. Each of these accessory veins diverts blood flow from the main channel. This has the effect of reducing resistance and reducing blood flow to the vein above the branch(es). This in turn reduces the pressure on the vein wall that is essential for expansion, dilation, and arterialization to occur. Ligation of these accessory veins will redirect flow and may promote the development of a usable AVF (187). Retrograde flow into distal veins of the hand can also prevent adequate AVF maturation. It can also be a harbinger of upstream venous lesions eventually resulting in late AVF loss. This phenomenon often causes hand pain, edema, and limitation of motion. Retrograde venous flow can be corrected by distal vein ligation (174).

Inadequate development of an AVF can also be caused by venous abnormalities. Small vein caliber may result from poor vascular development or from deeply imbedded vessels, especially in obesity. This situation can restrict the necessary expansion, dilation, and arterialization of the veins once the AVF is created. Vein caliber can be easily assessed before surgery by performing a physical examination of the arm with a tourniquet. In selected cases venography (180) or Doppler ultrasound (91,181–185) will allow the identification of veins suitable for attempted access creation and can be used to exclude unsuitable sites. Doppler studies may be preferred to venography in patients with residual renal function in whom contrast agents should be avoided.

A situation more difficult to diagnose is the presence of fibrotic veins. Fibrosis can result from prior intravenous catheter placement as well as venipuncture or intravenous drug use. Since venous fibrosis is generally focal, this condition may not become apparent until after the AVF has been created. All patients who are likely to develop end-stage renal failure should be examined early in the course of their disease to determine the presence of veins suitable for AVF creation. Arm veins suitable for placement of vascular access should be preserved, regardless of arm dominance, by making that arm off-limits for venipuncture or intravenous catheters (186).

B. Ischemia

Ischemia is not as frequent with AVFs as it is with PBGs. Susceptibility to the development of ischemia can usually be diagnosed before surgery is performed through physical examination and other noninvasive procedures. Absent distal pulses, a positive Allen test result, or vascular calcifications shown on plain radiographs increase the risk of the steal phenomenon. Use of vascular Doppler can increase the effectiveness of the Allen test in predicting collateral arterial perfusion of the hand. If collateral flow is adequate, the Doppler should detect augmented pulsation in the palmar arch during occlusion of either the radial or ulnar artery. Failure to do so suggests inadequate collateral circulation in the hand and predicts a higher risk for vascular steal if the dominant artery is used for AVF formation (174). Once ischemia occurs, immediate treatment is important. The treatment principles discussed for dialysis access PBGs also hold for AVFs.

C. Venous Stenosis

As with other complications, venous stenosis is not a common phenomenon. However, when it does occur it may be more problematic than with a PBG. Romero et al. (188), in evaluating all causes of late (beyond 6 weeks) AVF loss in a large dialysis patient population, found that 87% had some type of stenosis. The great majority of these lesions were in the vein at or just beyond the anastomosis (Figs 4, 5). The success rate of percutaneous angioplasty in the treatment of venous stenosis associated with an AVF is significantly lower than that obtained in PBGs. Hunter et al. (189) were able to obtain only a 43% patency for more than 24 hours in treating 28 cases of AVF occlusion. They found that stenoses associated with occlusion were frequently difficult to cross with a wire and were ex-

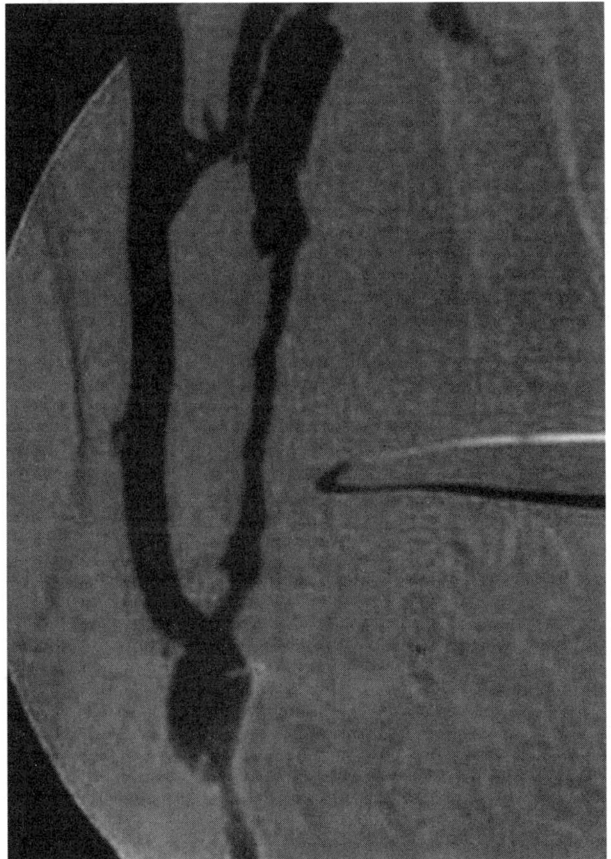

Fig. 4 Stenosis of arteriovenous fistula: This is a radiocephalic fistula. The vessel on the right is the radial artery. On the left is the cephalic vein. At the apex of the V is the anastomosis. The vein immediately above the anastomosis is stenotic.

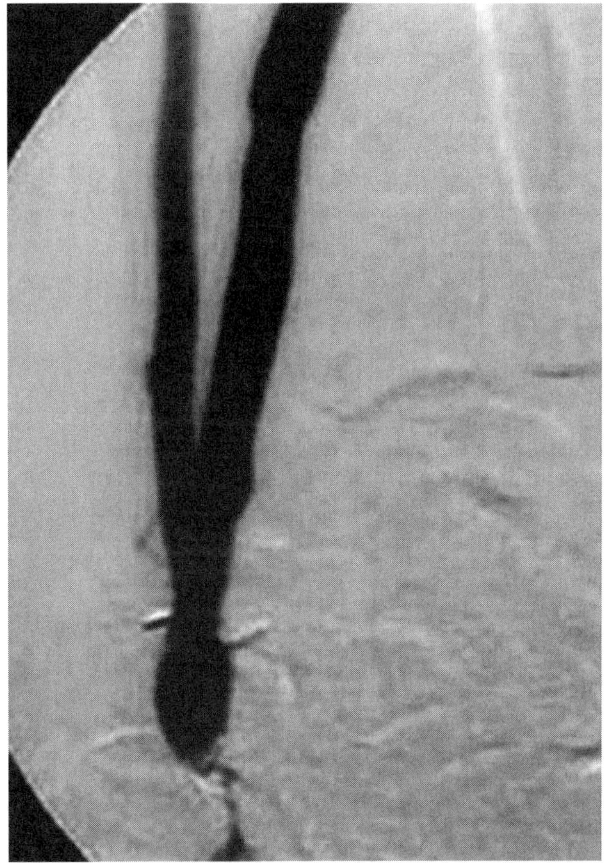

Fig. 5 The same fistula as shown in Fig. 4: The stenotic lesion has been treated with angioplasty.

tremely resistant to dilation. An AVF should be surgically revised when its blood flow is inadequate to sustain adequate dialysis. Treatment of hemodynamically significant venous stenosis can prolong the uselife of the AVF.

Unlike the situation for dialysis PBGs, pressure and flow measurements are not very sensitive for the detection of stenosis associated with AVFs (190). Blood entering the venous system of the AVF can return through multiple collateral veins originating peripheral to a stenosis. This can decrease the degree of pressure elevation despite the presence of significant stenosis. Detection of recirculation, on the other hand, is valuable for screening because most AVFs can maintain patency at very low flow rates, less than those needed for dialysis. When the flow in the AVF is less than that of the blood pump, recirculation occurs.

D. Thrombosis

Even though AVFs have one sixth the thrombosis rate of PBGs, once the access is successfully established, thrombosis is the most common mechanism of loss. The causes of this complication can be divided into temporally related groups: early thromboses—occurring within the first 4–6 weeks—and late thromboses. Early thrombosis is generally related to poor inflow, proximal venous stenotic lesions, and venous fibrosis caused by prior episodes of phlebitis. In addition, early cannulation of the AVF before it has had the opportunity to mature can lead to access loss. Repetitive attempts to cannulate an infiltrated AVF carries a high risk of inaccurate cannulation, which may further exacerbate the existing swelling and possibly lead to permanent loss of the access. An infiltrated AVF should be rested until the swelling has subsided and the vessel is sufficiently mature to allow successful cannulation (187).

Late AVF thromboses are generally associated with some type of anatomical lesion. The great majority of these are in the vein at or just beyond the anastamosis. Problems in the arterial side of the AVF account for 17% of AVF thrombosis (188).

Thrombosis of an AVF is associated with a poor prognosis. As with the treatment of stenosis, the success rate for AVF thrombosis treated percutaneously is poor (188). Surgical thrombectomy and revision should be attempted.

E. Aneurysm Formation

Blood flow in the AVF increases with time (177). As a consequence of this, it has a tendency to continue to increase in size. Over a period of years the AVF can dilate to aneurysmal proportions. Generally this is not a problem. In addition, localized aneurysm formation can occur along the arterialized vein after repeated needle punctures at the same site. In general, this is not a problem unless it is associated with stenosis or thinning of the overlying skin. Progressive enlargement of an aneurysm can eventually compromise the skin above the AVF, leading to possible rupture. This can result in severe hemorrhage, exsanguination, and death (191). Large aneurysms can prevent access to the adjacent AVF for needle placement, thereby limiting potential puncture sites. Eventually, aneurysm formation may require ligation of the AVF. Usually this is necessary only after years of use (188).

F. Infection

Infection is an uncommon occurrence in AVFs (174). It occurs at a rate of about one-tenth that seen in PBGs. The most common organism found in association with infection is *S. aureus*. AVF infections can be treated with systemic antibiotic therapy alone and do not generally require excision. The exception to this rule occurs in AVFs that have associated anatomical abnormalities such as aneurysms, perigraft hematomas, or associated abscesses from infected needle puncture sites. These lesions require surgical drainage or excision with access revision. There is no need to abandon the access entirely unless the associated lesion causes complete loss of vascular integrity (174).

IV. SUMMARY

Vascular access is essential for hemodialysis; without effective access dialysis can not be done. However, access also accounts for many of the complications seen in hemodialysis patients. The hemodialysis community has a great need for a better solution for the management of vascular access and an organized strategy to decrease the incidence of complications and to handle them appropriately when they occur. At a minimum, this strategy must include a plan to maximize the use of native fistulae, a policy for appropriate use of dialysis catheters, a quality-assurance program to detect the access at risk, implementation of procedures to increase access longevity, and a system to manage graft thrombosis effectively and efficiently. In addition, the nephrologist involved with hemodialysis should become an expert on vascular access, develop the strategy, and oversee its operation.

REFERENCES

1. Excerpts from the USRDS 1997 Annual Report. X. the economic cost of ESRD, vascular access procedures, and Medicare spending for alternative modalities of treatment. Am J Kidney Dis 1997; 30(suppl 1): S160–S177.
2. Excerpts from the USRDS 1997 Annual Report. IV. the USRDS dialysis morbidity and mortality study. Wave 2. Am J Kidney Dis 1997; 30(suppl 1):S67–S85.
3. Schwab SJ, Buller GL, McCann RL, Bollinger RR, Stickel DL. Prospective evaluation of a Dacron cuffed hemodialysis catheter for prolonged use. Am J Kidney Dis 1988; 11:166–169.
4. Moss AH, McLaughlin MM, Lampert KD, Holley JI. Use of a silicon catheter with a Dacron cuff for dialysis short term access. Am J Kidney Dis 1988; 12: 492–498.
5. Moss AH, Vasilakis C, Holley JL, Foulks CJ, Pillai K, McDowell DE. Use of a silicon dual-lumen catheter with a Dacron cuff as a long-term vascular access for hemodialysis patients. Am J Kidney Dis 1990; 16: 211–215.
6. Sznajder JI, Zveibil FR, Bitterman H, Weiner P, Bursztein S. Central vein catheterization: failure and complication rates by three percutaneous approaches. Arch Intern Med 1986; 146:259–261.
7. Bour ES, Weaver AS, Yang HC, Gifford RRM. Experience with the double lumen silastic catheter for hemoaccess. Surg Gynecol Obstet 1990; 171:33–39.
8. McDowell DE, Moss AH, Vasilakis C, Bell R, Pillai L. Percutaneously placed dual lumen silicon catheters for long-term hemodialysis. Am Surg 1993; 59:569–573.
9. Gibson SP, Mosquera D. Five years experience with the Quinton Permcath for vascular access. Nephrol Dial Transplant 1991; 6:269–274.

10. Tesio F, De Baz H, Panarello G, Calianno G, Quaia P, Raimondi A, Schinella D. Double catheterization of the internal jugular vein for hemodialysis: indications, techniques, and clinical results. Artif Organs 1994; 18: 301–304.
11. Uldall R, Debruyne M, Besley M, Mcmillan J, Simons M, Francoeur R. A new vascular access catheter for hemodialysis. Am J Kidney Dis 1993; 21:270–277.
12. Mosquera DA, Gibson SP, Goldman MD. Vascular access surgery: a 2-year study and comparison with the Permcath. Nephrol Dial Transplant 1992; 7:1111–1115.
13. Shusterman NH, Kloss K, Mullen JL. Successful use of double-lumen, silicon rubber catheters for permanent hemodialysis access. Kidney Int 1989; 35:887–890.
14. Blake PG, Huraib S, Wu G, Uldall PR. The use of dual lumen jugular venous catheters as definitive long term access for hemodialysis. Int J Artif Organs 1990; 13:26–31.
15. Trerotola SO, Johnson MS, Harris VJ, Shah H, Ambrosius WT, McKusky MA, Kraus MA. Outcome of tunneled hemodialysis catheters placed via the right internal jugular vein by interventional radiologists. Radiology 1997; 203:489–495.
16. Lameris JS, Post PJM, Zonderland HM, Gerritsen PG, Kappers-Klunne MC, Schutte HE. Percutaneous placement of Hickman catheters: comparison of sonographically guided and blind techniques. Am J Roentgenol 1990; 155:1097–1099.
17. Mallory DL, McGee WT, Shawker TH, Brenner M, Bailey KR, Evans RG, Parker MM, Farmer JC, Parillo JE. Ultrasound guidance improves the success rate of internal jugular vein cannulation. Chest 1990; 98:157–160.
18. NKF-DOQI Clinical Practice Guidelines for Vascular Access. Guideline 5: type and location of tunneled cuffed catheter placement. Am J Kidney Dis 1997; 30(suppl 3):S157–S158.
19. Suhocki PV, Conion PJ, Knelson MH, Harland R, Schwab SJ. Silastic cuffed catheters for hemodialysis vascular access: thrombolytic and mechanical correction of malfunction. Amer J Kidney Dis 1996; 28: 379–386.
20. Lund GB, Trerotola SO, Scheel PF, Savader SJ, Mitchell SE, Venbrux AC, Osterman FA. Outcome of tunneled hemodialysis catheters placed by radiologists. Radiology 1996; 198:467–472.
21. Francis CW, Felcher AH, White J, Braaten JV, Goss R. Thrombin activity associated with indwelling central venous catheters. Thromb Haemost 1997; 77:48–52.
22. Agraharkar M, Isaacson S, Mendelssohn D, Muralidharan J, Mustata S, Zevallos G, Beseley M, Uldall R. Percutaneously inserted silastic jugular hemodialysis catheters seldom cause jugular vein thrombosis. ASAIO J 1995; 41:169–172.
23. Karnik R, Valentin A, Winkler WB, Donath P, Slany J. Duplex sonographic detection of internal jugular venous thrombosis after removal of central venous catheters. Clin Cardiol 1993; 16:26–29.
24. Rotellar C, Sims SC, Freeland J, Korba J, Jessen M, Taylor A. Right atrium thrombosis in patients on hemodialysis. Amer J Kidney Dis 1996; 27:726–728.
25. Hoshal VJ, Ause RG, Hoskins PA. Fibrin sleeve formation on indwelling subclavian central venous catheters. Arch Surg 1971; 102:253–258.
26. Crain MR, Mewisseen MW, Ostrowski GJ, Paz-Fumagalli R, Beres RA, Wertz RA. Fibrin sleeve stripping for salvage of failing hemodialysis catheters: technique and initial results. Radiology 1996; 198:41–44.
27. NKF-DOQI Clinical Practice Guidelines For Vascular Access. Guideline 23: treatment of tunneled cuffed catheter dysfunction. Am J Kidney Dis 1997; 30(suppl 3):S175–S176.
28. Shrivastava D, Lundin AP, Dosunmu B, Rao TKS, Beyer MM, Friedman EA. Salvage of clotted jugular vein hemodialysis catheters. Nephron 1994; 68:77–79.
29. Haskal ZJ, Leen VH, Thomas-Hawkins C, Shlansky-Goldberg RD, Baum RA, Soulen MC. Transvenous removal of fibrin sheaths from tunneled hemodialysis. JVIR 1996; 7:513–517.
30. Duszak RL, Haskal SJ, Hawkins C, Soulen M, Cope C, Denno M. Replacement of failing hemodialysis catheters using the preexisting subcutaneous tunnel (abstr). Radiology 1995; 197:284.
31. Shaffer D. Catheter related sepsis complicating long term tunneled central venous catheters: management by guidewire exchange. Am J Kidney Dis 1995; 25: 593–596.
32. Kovalik E, Schwab SJ, Albers F, Raymond J, Conlon P. A clustering of cases of spinal epidural abscess in hemodialysis patients. J Am S Nephrol 1996; 7:2264–2267.
33. Schwartz RD, Messana JM, Biyer CJ, Lunde NM, Weitzel WF, Hartman TL. Successful use of cuffed central venous hemodialysis catheters inserted percutaneously. J Am Soc Nephrol 1994; 4:1719–1725.
34. Howell PB, Walters PE, Donowitz GR, Farr BM. Risk factors for infection of adult patients with cancer who have tunneled central venous catheters. Cancer 1995; 75:1367–1375.
35. Raad II. The pathogenesis and prevention of central venous catheter-related infections. Middle East J Anesthesiol 1994; 12:381–403.
36. Moro ML, Vigano EF, Cozzi Lepri, A. Risk factors for central venous catheter-related infections in surgical and intensive care units. Infect Control Hosp Epidemiol 1994; 15:253–264.
37. Hospital Infection Control Practices Advisory Committee: guideline for prevention of intravascular device-related infections. Part II. Recommendations for

the prevention of nosocomial intravascular device-related infections. Am J Infect Control 1996; 24:277–293.

38. Lau CE. Transparent and gauze dressings and their effect on infection rates of central venous catheters: a review of past and current literature. J Intraven Nurs 1996; 19:240–245.
39. Zimakoff J, Bangsgaard Pedersen F, Bergen L, Baago-Nielsen J, Daldorph B, Espersen F, Gahrn Hansen B, Hoiby N, Jepsen OB, Joffe P, Kolmos HJ, Klausen M, Kristoffersen K, Ladefoged J, Olesen-Larsen S, Rosdahl VT, Scheibel J, Storm B, Tofte-Jensen, PJ. Staphylococcus aureus carriage and infections among patients in four haemo- and peritoneal-dialysis centres in Denmark. The Danish Study Group of Peritonitis in Dialysis (DASPID). Hosp Infect 1996; 33:289–300.
40. Boelaert JR, Van Landuyt HW, Gordts BZ, De Baere YA, Messer SA, Herwaldt LA. Nasal and cutaneous carriage of Staphylococcus aureus in hemodialysis patients: the effect of nasal mupirocin. Infect Control Hosp Epidemiol 1996; 17:809–811.
41. NKF-DOQI Clinical Practice Guidelines for Vascular Access. Guideline 26: treatment of infection of tunneled cuffed catheters. Am J Kidney Dis 1997; 30:(suppl 3):S176–S177.
42. Hoyle BD, Costerton JW. Bacterial resistance to antibiotics: the role of biofilms. Prog Drug Res 1991; 37:91–105.
43. Passerini L, Lam K, Costerton JW, King EG. Biofilms on indwelling vascular catheters. Crit Care Med 1992; 20:665–673.
44. Richards GK, Gagnon RF, Prentis J. Comparative rates of antibiotic action against Staphylococcus epidermidis biofilms. Trans Am Soc Artif Intern Organs 1991; 37:M160–162.
45. Lowell JA, Bothe A Jr. Venous access: preoperative, operative and postoperative dilemmas. Surg Clin North Am 1991; 71:1231–1247.
46. Reed CR, Sessler CN, Glauser FL, Phelan BA. Central venous catheter infections: concepts and controversies. Intensive Care Med 1995; 21:177–183.
47. Saltissi D, Macfarlane DJ. Successful treatment of *Pseudomaonas paucimobilis* haemodialysis catheter-related sepsis without catheter removal. Postgrad Med J 1994; 70:47–48.
48. Marr KA, Sexton D, Conlon P, Corey R, Schwab SJ, Kirkland K. Catheter-related bacteremia and outcome of attempted catheter salvage in patients undergoing hemodialysis. Ann Int Med 1997; 127:275–280.
49. Schwab SJ, Quarles LD, Middleton JP, Cohan RH, Saeed M, Dennis VW. Hemodialysis associated subclavian vein stenosis. Kidney Int 1988; 33:1156–1159.
50. Bozzetti F, Terno G, Bonfanti G, Scarpa D, Scotti A, Ammatuna M, Bonalumi MG. Prevention and treatment of central venous catheter sepsis by exchange via a guidewire: a prospective controlled trial. Ann Surg 1983; 198:48–52.
51. Porter KA, Bistrian BR, Blackburn GL. Guidewire catheter exchange with triple culture technique in management of catheter sepsis. J Parenter Enteral Nutr 1988; 12:628–632.
52. Norwood S, Jenkins G. An evaluation of triple lumen catheter infections using a guidewire exchange technique. J Trauma 1990; 30:706–712.
53. Badley AD, Steckelberg JM, Wollan PC, Thompson RI. Infection rates of central venous pressure catheters: comparison between newly placed catheters and those that have been changed. Mayo Clin Proc 1996; 71:838–846.
54. Carlisle EJF, Blake P, McCarthy F, Vas S, Uldall R. Septicemia in long-term jugular hemodialysis catheters: eradicating infection by changing the catheter over a guidewire. Int J Artif Organs 1991; 14:150–153.
55. Vanherweghem JL, Yassine T, Goldman M, Vandenbosch G, Delcour C, Struyven J, Kinnaert P. Subclavian vein thrombosis: a frequent complication of subclavian vein cannulation for hemodialysis. Clin Nephrol 1986; 26:235–238.
56. Clark DD, Albina JE, Chazan JA. Subclavian vein stenosis and thrombosis: a potential serious complication in chronic hemodialysis patients. Am J Kid Dis 1990; 15:265–268.
57. Barrett N, Spencer S, McIvor J, Brown EA. Subclavian stenosis: a major complication of subclavian dialysis catheters. Nephrol Dial Transplant 1988; 3:423–425.
58. Cimochowski GE, Worley E, Rutherford WE, Sartain J, Blondin J, Harter H. Superiority of the internal jugular over the subclavian access for temporary hemodialysis. Nephron 1990; 54:154–161.
59. Schillinger F, Schillinger D, Montagnac R, Milcent T. Post catheterization vein stenosis in haemodialysis: comparative angiographic study of 50 subclavian and 50 internal jugular accesses. Nephrol Dial Transplant 1991; 6:722–724.
60. NKF-DOQI Clinical Practice Guidelines for Vascular Access. Guideline 6: acute hemodialysis vascular access—noncuffed catheters. Am J Kidney Dis 1997; 30(suppl 3):S158–S159.
61. Baker LD Jr, Johnson JM, Goldfarb D. Expanded polytetrafluoroethylene (PTFE) subcutaneous arteriovenous conduit: an improved vascular access for chronic hemodialysis. Trans Am Soc Artif Intern Organs 1976; 22:382–387.
62. Glanz S. What can be done to preserve vascular access for dialysis? Semin Dial 1991; 4:157–158.
63. Palder SB, Kirkman RL, Whittemore AD, Hakim RM, Lazarus JM, Tilney NL. Vascular access for hemodialysis: patency rates and results of revision. Ann Surg 1985; 202:235–239.

64. Tellis VA, Kohlberg WI, Bhat DJ, Driscoll B, Veith FJ. Expanded polytetrafluoroethylene graft fistula for chronic hemodialysis. Ann Surg 1979; 189:101–105.
65. Sabanayagam P, Schwartz AB, Soricelli RR, Chinitz J, Lyons P. Experience with one hundred reinforced expanded PTFE grafts for angio-access in hemodialysis. Trans Am Soc Artif Intern Organs 1980; 26:582–586.
66. Munda R, First MR, Alexander JW, Linnemann CC, Fidler JP, Kittur D. Polytetrafluoroethylene graft survival in hemodialysis. JAMA 1983; 249:219–222.
67. Kherlakian GM, Roedersheimer LR, Arbough JJ, Newmark KJ, King LR. Comparison of autogenous fistula versus expanded polytetrafluoroethylene graft fistula for angioaccess in hemodialysis. Am J Surg 1986; 152:238–243.
68. NKF-DOQI Clinical Practice Guidelines for Vascular Access. Guideline 10: monitoring dialysis AV grafts for stenosis. Am J Kidney Dis 1997; 30(suppl 3): S162–S164.
69. Beathard GA. Percutaneous transvenous angioplasty in the treatment of vascular access stenosis. Kidney Int 1992; 42:1390–1397.
70. Mennes PA, Gilula LA, Anderson CB, Etheredge EE, Weerts C, Harter HR. Complications associated with arteriovenous fistulas in patients undergoing chronic hemodialysis. Arch Int Med 1978; 138:1117–1121.
71. Schwab SJ, Raymond JR, Saeed M, Newman GE, Dennis PA, Bollinger RR. Prevention of hemodialysis fistula thrombosis. Early detection of venous stenosis. Kidney Int 1989; 36:707–711.
72. Besarab A, Dorrell S, Moritz M, Michael H, Sullivan K. Determinants of measured dialysis venous pressure and its relationship to true intra-access venous pressure. ASAIO J 1991; 37:M270–M271.
73. Besarab A, Sullivan KL, Ross RP, Moritz MJ. Utility of intra-access pressure monitoring in detecting and correcting venous outlet stenoses prior to thrombosis. Kidney Int 1995; 47:1364–1373.
74. May RE, Himelfarb J, Yenicesu M, Knights S, Ikizler TA, Schulman G, Hernanz-Schulman M, Shyr Y, Hakim RM. Predictive measures of vascular access thrombosis: a prospective study. Kidney Int 1997; 52: 656–662.
75. Finlay DE, Longley DG, Foshager MC, Letourneau JG. Duplex and color Doppler sonography of hemodialysis arteriovenous fistulas and grafts. Radiographics 1993; 13:983–989.
76. Safa AA, Valji K, Roberts AC, Ziegler TW, Hye RJ, Oglevie SB. Detection and treatment of dysfunctional hemodialysis access grafts: effects of a surveillance program on graft patency and the incidence of thrombosis. Radiology 1996; 199:653–657.
77. Krivitsky NM. Theory and validation of access flow measurement by dilution technique during hemodialysis. Kidney Int 1995; 48:244–250.
78. Depner TA, Krivitsky NM. Clinical measurement of blood flow in hemodialysis access fistulae and grafts by ultrasound dilution. ASAIO J 1995; 41:M745–M749.
79. Windus DW, Audrain J, Vanderson R, Jendrisak MD, Picus D, Delmez JA. Optimization of high-efficiency hemodialysis by detection and correction of fistula dysfunction. Kidney Int 1990; 38:337–341.
80. Collins DM, Lambert MB, Middleton JP, Proctor RK, Davidson CJ, Newman GE, Schwab ST. Fistula dysfunction: effect on rapid hemodialysis. Kidney Int 1992; 41:1292–1296.
81. NKF-DOQI Clinical Practice Guidelines for Vascular Access. Guideline 12: recirculation methodology, limits, evaluation and follow-up. Am J Kidney Dis 1997; 30(suppl 3):S165–S166.
82. Depner TA, Rizwan S, Cheer AY, Waner JM, Eder LA. High venous urea concentrations in the opposite arm. ASAIO J 1991; 37:M141–M143.
83. Tattersall JE, Farrington K, Raniga PD, Thompson H, Tomlinson C, Aldridge C, Greenwood RN. Haemodialysis recirculation detected by the three-sample method is an artifact. Nephrol Dial Transplant 1993; 8:60–63.
84. Buur T, Will EJ. Haemodialysis recirculation measured using a femoral artery sample. Nephrol Dial Transplant 1994; 9:395–398.
85. Van Stone JC. Peripheral venous blood is not the appropriate specimen to determine the amount of recirculation during hemodialysis. ASAIO J 1996; 42:41–45.
86. Schneditz D, Kaufman AM, Polaschegg H, Levin N, Daugirdas J. Cardiopulmonary recirculation during hemodialysis. Kidney Int 1993; 42:1450–1456.
87. Schneditz D, Van Stone JC, Daugirdas JT. A regional blood circulation alternative to in-series two compartment urea kinetic modeling. ASAIO J 1993; 39: M573–M577.
88. Sherman RA. The regional blood flow model: a revisitation. Semin Dial 1995; 8:12–14.
89. Sherman RA. The measurement of dialysis access recirculation. Am J Kidney Dis 1993; 22:616–621.
90. Hester RL, Curry E, Bower J. The determination of hemodialysis blood recirculation using blood urea nitrogen measurements. Am J Kidney Dis 1992; 20: 598–602.
91. Sands JJ, Young S, Miranda CL. The effect of Doppler flow screening studies and elective revisions on dialysis access failure. ASAIO J 1992; 38:M524–M527.
92. Strauch BS, O'Connell RS, Geoly KL. Forecasting thromboses of vascular access with Doppler color flow imaging. Am J Kidney Dis 1992; 554–557.
93. Besarab A, Ross R, El-Ajel E, Deane C, Frinak S, Zasuwa G. The relation of intra-access pressure to intra-access flow (abstr). J Am Soc Nephrol 1995; 6: 483.

94. Kosoy C, Kuzu A, Erden I, Turkcaper AG, Duzgun I, Anadol E. Predictive value of colour Doppler ultrasonography in detecting failure of vascular access grafts. Br J Surg 1995; 82:50–52.
95. Sands JJ, Miranda CL. Prolongation of hemodialysis access survival with elective revision. Clin Nephrol 1995; 44:334–337.
96. Beathard GA. The treatment of vascular access graft dysfunction: a nephrologist's view and experience. Adv Renal Replace Therapy 1994; 1:131–147.
97. Beathard GA. Physical examination of AV grafts. Semin Dial 1992; 5:74.
98. Trerotola SO, Scheel PJ, Powe NR, Prescott C, Feeley N, He J, Watson A. Screening for access graft malfunction: comparison of physical examination with ultrasound. J Vasc Interv Radiol 1996; 7:15–20.
99. Safa AA, Valji K, Roberts AC, Ziegler TW, Hye RJ, Ogletree SB. Detection and treatment of dysfunctional hemodialysis access grafts: effect of a surveillance program on graft patency and incidence of thrombosis. Radiology 1996; 199:653–657.
100. NKF-DOQI Clinical Practice Guidelines for Vascular Access. Guideline 19: treatment of stenosis without thrombosis in dialysis AV grafts and primary AV fistulae. Am J Kidney Dis 1997; 30(suppl 3):S173–S174.
101. Kirkman RL. A prophylactic approach to graft thrombosis is not yet justifiable. Semin Dial 1993; 6:203–205.
102. Connally JE, Brownell DA, Levine EF, McCart PM. Complications of renal dialysis access procedures. Arch Surg 1984; 119:1325–1328.
103. Etheredge EE, Haid SD, Maeser MN, Sicard GA, Anderson CB. Salvage operations for malfunctioning polytetrafluoroethylene hemodialysis grafts. Surgery 1983; 94:464–470.
104. Schwab SJ, Saeed M, Sussman SK, McCann RL, Stickel DL. Transluminal angioplasty of venous stenoses in polytetrafluoroethylene vascular access grafts. Kidney Int 1987; 32:395–398.
105. Glanz S, Gordon DH, Butt KHM, Hong J, Lipowitz GS. The role of percutaneous angioplasty in the management of chronic hemodialysis fistulas. Ann Surg 1987; 206:777–781.
106. Hunter DW, So SK. Dialysis access: radiographic evaluation and management. Radiol Clin North Am 1987; 25:249–260.
107. Gmelin E, Winterhoff R, Rinast E. Insufficient hemodialysis access fistulas: late results of treatment with percutaneous balloon angioplasty. Radiology 1989; 171:657–660.
108. Beathard GA. Percutaneous angioplasty for the treatment of venous stenosis: a nephrologist's view. Sem Dial 1995; 8:166–170.
109. Burger H, Zijlstra JJ, Kluchert SA, Scholten AP, Kootstra G. Percutaneous transluminal angioplasty improves longevity in fistulae and shunts for hemodialysis. Nephrol Dial Transplant 1990; 5:608–611.
110. Lumsden AB, MacDonald MJ, Kikeri D, Cotsonis GA, Harker LA, Martin LG. Prophylactic balloon angioplasty fails to prolong the patency of expanded polytetrafluoroethylene arteriovenous grafts: results of a prospective randomized study. J Vasc Surg 1997; 26:382–392.
111. Schuman E, Quinn S, Standage B, Gross G. Thrombolysis versus thrombectomy for occluded hemodialysis grafts. Am J Surg 1994; 167:473–476.
112. Marston WA, Criado E, Jaques PF, Mauro MA, Burnham SJ, Keagy BA. Prospective randomized comparison of surgical versus endovascular management of thrombosed dialysis access grafts. J Vasc Surg 1997; 26:378–381.
113. NKF-DOQI Clinical Practice Guidelines for Vascular Access. Guideline 21: treatment of thrombosis and associated stenosis in dialysis AV grafts. Am J Kidney Dis 1997; 30(suppl 3):S174–S175.
114. Beathard GA, Welch BR, Maidment HJ. Mechanical thrombolysis for the treatment of thromobosed dialysis access grafts: report of a series. Radiology 1996; 200:711–716.
115. Beathard GA. Thrombolysis versus surgery for the treatment of thrombosed dialysis access grafts. J Am Soc Neph 1995; 6:1619–1624.
116. Piotrowski JJ, Rutherford RB. Proximal vein thrombosis secondary to hemodialysis catheterization complicated by arteriovenous fistula. Ann Vasc Surg 1987; 5:876–878.
117. Klimas VA, Denny KM, Paganini EP, Graor RA, Nakamoto S, Risus B, Young J. Low dose streptokinase therapy for thrombosed arteriovenous fistulas. Trans Am Soc Artif Intern Organs 1984; 30:511–513.
118. McNamara TO, Fischer JR. Thrombolysis of peripheral arterial and graft occlusions: improved results using high-dose urokinase. AJR 1985; 144:769–775.
119. Roberts AC, Valji K, Bookstein JJ, Hye RJ. Pulse-spray pharmacomechanical thrombolysis for the treatment of thrombosed dialysis access grafts. Am J Surg 1993; 166:221–226.
120. Ahmed A, Shapiro WB, Porush JG. The use of tissue plasminogen activator to declot arteriovenous accesses in hemodialysis patients. Am J Kidney Dis 1993; 21:38–43.
121. Beathard GA. Mechanical versus pharmacomechanical thrombolysis for the treatment of thrombosed dialysis access grafts. Kidney Int 1994; 45:1401–1406.
122. Zeit RM. Clearing of clotted dialysis shunts by streptokinase injection at multiple sites. Am J Roentgenol 1983; 141:1053–1054.
123. Mangiarotti G, Canavese C, Thea A, Segoloni P, Stratta P, Salomone M, Vercellone A. Urokinase treatment for arteriovenous fistulae declotting in dialyzed patients. Nephron 1984; 36:60–64.
124. Young AT, Hunter DW, Castaneda-Zuniga WR, So SK, Mercado S, Cardella JF, Amplatz K. Thrombosed

synthetic hemodialysis fistulas: failure of fibrinolytic therapy. Radiology 1985; 154:639–642.
125. Zeit RM. Arterial and venous embolization: declotting of dialysis shunts by direct injection of streptokinase. Radiology 1986; 159:639–641.
126. Docci D, Turci F, Baldrati L. Successful declotting of arteriovenous grafts with local infusion of urokinase in hemodialysed patients. Artif Organs 1986; 10:494–486.
127. Schilling JJ, Eiser AR, Slifkin RF, Whitnet JT, Neff MS. The role of thrombolysis in hemodialysis access occlusion. Am J Kidney Dis 1987; 10:92–97.
128. Cohen MAH, Kumpe DA, Durham JD, Zwerdlininger SC. Efficacy of thrombolysis of thrombosed dialysis accesses with urokinase (abstr). Am J Kidney Dis 1989; 15:A5.
129. Valji K, Bookstein JJ, Roberts AC, Davis GB. Pharmacomechanical thrombolysis and angioplasty in the management of clotted hemodialysis grafts: early and late results. Radiology 1991; 178:243–247.
130. Davis GB, Dowd CF, Bookstein JJ, Maroney TP, Lang EV, Halasz N. Thrombosed dialysis grafts: efficacy of intrathrombic deposition of concentrated urokinase, clot maceration and angioplasty. AJR 1987; 149:177–181.
131. Bookstein JJ, Valji K. "How I do it": pulse-spray pharmacomechanical thrombolysis. Cardiovasc Intervent Radiol 1992; 15:228–233.
132. Valji K, Bookstein JJ, Roberts AC, Oglevie SB, Pittman C, O'Neill MP. Pulse-spray pharmacomechanical thrombolysis of thrombosed hemodialysis access grafts: long-term experience and comparison of original and current techniques. AJR 1995; 164:1495–1500.
133. Trerotola SO, Lund GB, Scheel PJ Jr, Savader SJ, Venbrux AC, Osterman FA Jr. Thrombosed dialysis access grafts: percutaneous mechanical declotting without urokinase. Radiology 1994; 191:721–726.
134. Middlebrook MR, Amygdalos MA, Soulen MC, Haskal ZJ, Shlansky-Goldberg RD, Cope C, Pentecost MJ. Thrombosed hemodialysis grafts: percutaneous mechanical balloon declotting versus thrombolysis. Radiology 1995; 196:73–77.
135. Sharafuddin MJA, Kadir S, Joshi SJ, Parr D. Percutaneous balloon-assisted aspiration thrombectomy of clotted hemodialysis access grafts. J Vasc Interv Radiol 1996; 7:177–183.
136. Uflacker R, Rajagopalan PR, Vujic I, Stutley JE. Treatment of thrombosed dialysis access grafts: randomized trial of surgical thrombectomy versus mechanical thrombectomy with the Amplatz device. J Vasc Interv Radiol 1996; 7:185–192.
137. Vorwerk D, Sohn M, Schurmann K, Hoogeveen Y, Gladziwa U, Guenther RW. Hydrodynamic thrombectomy of hemodialysis fistulas: first clinical results. J Vasc Interv Radiol 1994; 5:813–821.
138. Schmitz-Rode T, Gunther RW. Percutaneous mechanical thrombolysis: a comparative study of various rotational catheter systems. Invest Radiol 1991; 26:557–563.
139. Dolmatch BL, Gray RJ, Horton KM. Will iatrogenic pulmonary embolization be our pulmonary embarrassment? Radiology 1994; 191:615–617.
140. Swan TL, Smyth SH, Ruffenach SH, Berman SS, Pond GD. Pulmonary embolism following hemodialysis access thrombolysis/thrombectomy. J Vasc Interv Radiol 1995; 6:683–686.
141. Trerotola SO. Pulse spray thrombolysis of hemodialysis grafts: not the final word. Am J Roentgenol 1995; 164:1501–1503.
142. Winkler TA, Trerotola SO, Davidson DD, Milgrom ML. Study of thrombus from thrombosed hemodialysis access grafts. Radiology 1995; 197:461–465.
143. Didlake R, Curry E, Rigdon EE, Raju S, Bower J. Outpatient vascular access surgery: impact of a dialysis unit-based surgical facility. Am J Kidney Dis 1992; 19:39–44.
144. Raju S. PTFE grafts for hemodialysis access: techniques for insertion and management of complications. Ann Surg 1987; 206:666–673.
145. Sands JJ, Patel S, Plaviak DJ, Miranda C. Pharmacomechanical thrombolysis with urokinase for treatment of thrombosed hemodialysis access grafts. A comparison with surgical thrombectomy. ASAIO J 1994; 40:M886–888.
146. Vesely TM, Idso MC, Audrain J, Windus DW, Lowell JA. Thrombolysis versus surgical thrombectomy for the treatment of dialysis graft thrombosis: pilot study comparing costs. J Vasc Interv Radiol 1996; 7:507–512.
147. Butterly DW. A quality improvement program for hemodialysis vascular access. Adv Renal Replace Ther 1994; 1:163–166.
148. Kaplowitz LG, Comstock JA, Landwehr DM, Dalton HP, Mayhall CG. A prospective study of infections in hemodialysis patients: patient hygiene and other risk factors for infection. Infect Control Hosp Epidemiol 1988; 9:534–541.
149. Kaplowitz LG, Comstock JA, Landwehr DM, Dalton HP, Mayhall CG. Prospective study of microbial colonization of the nose and skin and infection of the vascular access site in hemodialysis patients. J Clin Microbiol 1988; 26:1257–1262.
150. Fan PY, Schwab S. Vascular access: concepts for the 1990's. J Am Soc Nephrol 1992; 3:1–11.
151. NKF-DOQI Clinical Practice Guidelines for Vascular Access. Guideline 14: skin preparation technique for permanent AV access. Am J Kidney Dis 1997; 30(suppl 3):S167.
152. Francioli P, Masur H. Complications of Staphylococcus aureus bacteremia: occurrence in patients undergoing long-term hemodialysis. Arch Intern Med 1982; 142:1655–1658.

153. Ballard JL, Bunt TJ, Malone JM. Major complications of angioaccess surgery. Am J Surg 1992; 164:229–232.
154. Bhat DJ, Tellis VA, Kohlberg WI, Driscoll B, Veith FJ. Management of sepsis involving expanded polytetrafluoroethylene grafts for hemodialysis access. Surgery 1980; 87:445–450.
155. NKF-DOQI Clinical Practice Guideline For Vascular Access. Guideline 24: treatment of infection of dialysis AV grafts. Am J Kidney Dis 1997; 30(suppl 3): S176.
156. Charara J, Guidoin R, Gill F, Guzman R. Morphologic assessment of ePTFE graft wall damage following hemodialysis needle punctures. J Appl Biomaterials 1990; 1:279–287.
157. Delorme JM, Guidoin R, Canizales S, Charara J, How T, Marois Y, Batt M, Hallade P, Ricci M, Picetti C. Vascular access for hemodialysis: pathologic features of surgically excised ePTFE grafts. Ann Vasc Surg 1992; 6:517–524.
158. NKF-DOQI Clinical Practice Guidelines For Vascular Access. Guideline 17: when to intervene—dialysis AV grafts for venous stenosis, infection, graft degeneration and pseudoaneurysm formation. Am J Kidney Dis 1997; 30(suppl 3):S170–S171.
159. NKF-DOQI Clinical Practice Guidelines For Vascular Access. Guideline 27: treatment of pseudoaneurysm of dialysis AV grafts. Am J Kidney Dis 1997; 30(suppl 3):S177.
160. NKF-DOQI Clinical Practice Guidelines For Vascular Access. Guideline 16: managing potential ischemia in a limb bearing an AV access. Am J Kidney Dis 1997; 30(suppl 3):S170.
161. Lin G, Kais H, Halpern Z, Chayen D, Weissgarten J, Negri M, Cohn M, Averbukh J, Halevy A. Pulse oxymetry evaluation of oxygen saturation in the upper extremity with an arteriovenous fistula before and during hemodialysis. Am J Kidney Dis 1997; 29:230–232.
162. Kaku DA, Malamut RI, Frey DJ, Parry GJ. Conduction block as an early sign of reversible injury in ischemic monomelic neuropathy. Neurology 1993; 43: 1126–1130.
163. Mattson WJ. Recognition and treatment of vascular steal secondary to hemodialysis prostheses. Am J Surg 1987; 154:198–201.
164. Valji K, Hye RJ, Roberts AC, Oglevie SB, Ziegler T, Bookstein JJ. Hand ischemia in patients with hemodialysis access grafts: angiographic diagnosis and treatment. Radiology 1995; 196:697–701.
165. Odland MD, Kelly PH, Ney AL, Andersen RC, Bubrick MP. Management of dialysis-associated steal syndrome complicating upper extremity arteriovenous fistulas: use of intraoperative digital photoplethysmography. Surgery 1991; 110:664–669.
166. Schanzer H, Schwartz M, Harrington E, Haimov M. Treatment of ischemia due to "steal" by arteriovenous fistula with distal artery ligation and revascularization. J Vasc Surg 1988; 7:770–773.
167. Schanzer H, Skladany M, Haimov M. Treatment of angioaccess-induced ischemia by revascularization. J Vasc Surg 1992; 16:861–864.
168. Haimov M, Schanzer H, Skladani M. Pathogenesis and management of upper-extremity ischemia following angioaccess surgery. Blood Purif 1996; 14:350–354.
169. Harland RC. Placement of permanent vascular access devices: surgical considerations. Adv Ren Replace Ther 1994; 1:99–106.
170. Windus DW. Permanent vascular access: a nephrologist's view. Am J Kidney Dis 1993; 21:457–471.
171. Kinnaert P, Vereerstraeten P, Toussaint C, Van Geertruyden J. Nine years' experience with internal arteriovenous fistulas for hemodialysis: study of some factors influencing results. Br J Surg 1977; 64:242–246.
172. Dunlop MG, Mackinlay JY, Jenkins AM. Vascular access: experience with the brachiocephalic fistula. Ann R Coll Surg Engl 1986; 68:203–206.
173. Ryan JJ, Dennis MJS. Radiocephalic fistula in vascular access. Br J Surg 1990; 77:1321–1322.
174. Albers F. Causes of hemodialysis access failure. Adv Ren Replace Ther 1994; 1:107–118.
175. Churchill DN, Taylor DW, Cook RJ, LaPlante P, Barre P, Cartier P, Fay WP, Goldstein MB, Jindal K, Mandin H, McKenzie JK, Muirhead N, Parfrey PS, Posen GA, Slaughter D, Ulan RA, Werb R. Canadian Hemodialysis Morbidity Study. Am J Kidney Dis 1992; 19:214–234.
176. Woods JD, Turenne MN, Strawderman RL, Young EW, Hirth RA, Port FK. Vascular access survival among incident hemodialysis patients in the United States. Am J Kidney Dis 1997; 30:50–57.
177. NKF-DOQI Clinical Practice Guidelines For Vascular Access. Guideline 3: selection of permanent vascular access and order of preference for placement of AV fistulae. Am J Kidney Dis 1997; 30(suppl 3):S156–S157.
178. Hirth RA, Turenne MN, Woods JD, Young EW, Greer JW, Pauly MV, Held PJ. Predictors of type of vascular access in patients starting hemodialysis. JAMA 1996; 276:1303–1308.
179. Zibari GB, Rohr MS, Landreneau MD, Bridges RM, DeVault GA, Petty FH, Costley KJ, Brown ST, McDonald JC. Complications from permanent hemodialysis vascular access. Surgery 1988; 104:681–686.
180. NKF-DOQI Clinical Practice Guidelines For Vascular Access. Guideline 2: diagnostic evaluation prior to permanent access selection. Am J Kidney Dis 1997; 30(suppl 3):S154–S156.
181. Tordoir JHM, Hoeneveld H, Eikelboom BC, Kitslaar PJEHM. The correlation between clinical and duplex ultrasound parameters and the development of complications in arterio-venous fistulae for hemodialysis. Eur J Vasc Surg 1990; 4:1979–1984.

182. Tordoir JHM, De Bruin HG, Hoeneveld H, Eikelboom BC, Kitslaar PJEHM. Duplex ultrasound scanning in the assessment of arteriovenous fistulas created for hemodialysis access: comparison with digital subtraction angiography. J Vasc Surg 1989; 10:122–128.
183. Nonnast-Daniel B, Martin RP, Lindert O, Mugge A, Schaeffer J, vdLieth H, Sochtig E, Galanski M, Koch KM, Daniel WG. Colour doppler ultrasound assessment of arteriovenous haemodialysis fistulas. Lancet 1992; 339:143–145.
184. Middleton WD, Picus DD, Marx MV, Melson GL. Color doppler sonography of hemodialysis vascular access: comparison with angiography. Am J Roentgenol 1989; 152:633–639.
185. Scheible W, Skram C, Leopold GR. High resolution real-time sonography of hemodialysis vascular access complications. Am J Roentgenol 1980; 134:1173–1176.
186. NKF-DOQI Clinical Practice Guidelines For Vascular Access. Guideline 7: preservation of veins for AV access. Am J Kidney Dis 1997; 30(suppl 3):S159–S160.
187. NKF-DOQI Clinical Practice Guidelines For Vascular Access. Guideline 9: access maturation. Am J Kidney Dis 1997; 30(suppl 3):S160–S161.
188. Romero A, Polo JR, Morato EG, Garcia Sabrido JL, Quintans A, Ferreiroa JP. Salvage of angioaccess after late thrombosis of radiocephalic fistulas for hemodialysis. Int Surg 1986; 71:122–124.
189. Hunter DW, Castaneda-Zuniga WR, Coleman CC, Young AT, Salomonowitz E, Mercado S, Amplatz K. Failing Arteriovenous dialysis fistulas: evaluation and treatment. Radiology 1984; 152:631–635.
190. Sullivan KL, Besarab A. Hemodynamic screening and early percutaneous intervention reduce hemodialysis access thrombosis and increase graft longevity. J Vasc Interv Radiol 1997; 8:163–170.
191. NKF-DOQI Clinical Practice Guidelines For Vascular Access. Guideline 18: when to intervene—primary AV fistula. Am J Kidney Dis 1997; 30(suppl 3):S171–S172.

2

Complications Related to Water Treatment, Substitution Fluids, and Dialysate Composition

Jürgen Floege
University of Aachen, Aachen, Germany

Gerhard Lonnemann
Medicinische Hochschule, Hannover, Germany

I. WATER TREATMENT FOR USE IN DIALYSIS AND PREPARATION OF DIALYSATE—AN OVERVIEW

Prior to its use in hemodialysis, water has to be treated to remove particles, to reduce hardness, and to remove inorganic ions from municipal water. The most commonly used water-purification systems in hemodialysis units consist of several components, which are connected in line in order to improve water quality step by step (Fig. 1). The first device is usually a large surface filter to remove large particles (5–500 μm) from incoming tap water preventing fouling of equipment downstream. In most systems the next unit is an activated carbon filter, which removes dissolved organic contaminants, chlorine, and chloramines from the water supply. After a second filtration through microfilters (1.0–0.45 μm), the water is pumped through a softener. Water softeners are ion exchangers necessary to reduce total hardness of the incoming water to <1 ppm. The resin of the ion exchanger is a cationic form that exchanges two Na^+ ions for Ca^{2+} and Mg^{2+} as well as other cations such as iron and manganese. The ion exchange resin promotes bacterial growth. Thus, softened water may be highly contaminated by bacterial products because the municipal water used to feed the softener is allowed to contain up to 100 colony-forming units of microorganisms per milliliter.

Filtered and softened water is finally pumped through a reverse osmosis (RO) unit. Reverse osmosis is a pressure-driven membrane filtration process resulting in ionic exclusion with 90–99% rejection. Osmosis occurs if two solutions with different ionic concentrations are separated by a semi-permeable membrane. The osmotic pressure is responsible for solvent flowing from the less concentrated to the more concentrated side of the membrane. In RO, the applied hydraulic pressure on the concentrated side is higher than the osmotic pressure, resulting in a solvent flow from the more concentrated to the less concentrated side. The more concentrated solution (retentate) is drained. The RO unit is connected to a recirculating loop pipe in which the RO water (permeate) is distributed to the hemodialysis machines in the hemodialysis unit. RO is the most effective method to purify water from dissolved organic and inorganic particles, including bacteria and endotoxins (1).

Hemodialysis machines are connected to the distribution loop using polyvinyl chloride (PVC) tubes. These tubes should be as short as possible to reduce dead space and water stagnation. The connection site between the tubing and the loop is the most common source of bacterial contamination of the loop. Long tubes and water stagnation promote bacterial growth and the formation of a biofilm on the inner surface of the tubing and the distribution loop. The biofilm is gen-

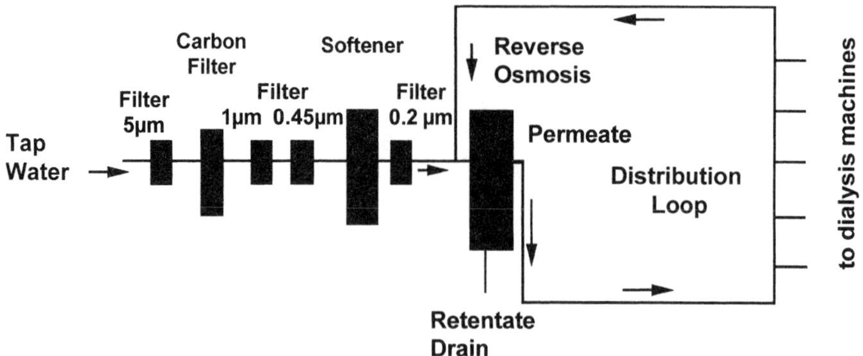

Fig. 1 Schematic outline of a typical water-purification system.

erated by waterborne microorganisms (predominantly gram-negative *Pseudomonas* species) and their products and is a constant source of endotoxins and other pyrogenic bacterial products in the water. Because the RO water-distribution loops and the dialysis machines are used intermittently, water stagnation cannot be prevented and bacterial growth in the loop and tubing is evident.

The dialysis machines use the RO water provided by the loop to prepare dialysate from treated water and concentrated salts. Salt concentrates, in particular liquid bicarbonate concentrates, may be heavily contaminated with microorganisms such as *Pseudomonas*. Furthermore, bicarbonate promotes growth of bacteria present in RO water. The recent introduction of solid bicarbonate cartouches for dialysate preparation is an important step in reducing this latter problem. Taken together, preparation of dialysate in the dialysis machine from RO water and concentrated salts is an important source of bacterial and pyrogen contamination of dialysate.

The problem of dialysate contamination is particularly important if on-line–produced dialysate is intended to be used as substitution fluid in hemofiltration or hemodiafiltration. In order to remove bacteria and pyrogens such as endotoxins from ready-to-use dialysate, ultrafiltration of dialysate across pyrogen-adsorbing membranes has been successfully introduced. The intactness of these ultrafilters must be monitored using pressure tests, bacterial cultures, and pyrogen tests. Microorganisms are completely rejected by intact ultrafilter membranes, but the adsorbing capacity for small-sized pyrogenic bacterial products can be saturated and breakthrough of pyrogens can occur. To decrease the risk of pyrogen breakthrough, it is recommended to perform double filtration of dialysate using two ultrafilters in line before dialysate is infused intravenously. In addition, since the degree of dialysate contamination depends on the bacteriological quality of the RO water provided by the loop and the presence or absence of a biofilm in the tubing outside and inside the dialysis machine, additional procedures to ensure high quality of dialysate in hemodiafiltration are recommended. These procedures include routine chemical and/or heat disinfection of the dialysis machines including all tubing on a daily basis and frequent replacement (once a month) of the tubing outside the machine.

If reuse of dialyzers is performed using RO water to rinse the blood compartment of the dialyzers, the same precautions described for on-line–produced substitution fluid in hemodiafiltration must be followed. In other words, cold sterilization of RO water by double ultrafiltration through pyrogen-adsorbing membranes is recommended to prevent direct contamination of the blood compartment during the rinsing procedure.

II. COMPLICATIONS RELATED TO WATER TREATMENT, SUBSTITUTION FLUIDS, AND DIALYSATE COMPOSITION

As summarized in Table 1, failure of the water-treatment system for dialysis may expose the patient to incorrect electrolyte levels, in particular inadequately high calcium concentrations (leading to hard water syndrome), increased water levels of some other chemical compounds (e.g., nitrates, fluorides, or chloramines derived from municipal water plants) in the dialysate, as well as contamination of the water with microorganisms and their products. Failure of the subsequent dialysate-preparation system may also result in erroneous electrolyte composition or expose the patient to dialysate with an inadequate temperature (Table 1). Because

Table 1 Overview of Complications Related to Dialysate and Substitution Fluids

Complication related to:		Potential clinical consequence(s)
Electrolyte composition	Low sodium	Hypotension Muscle cramps Hemolysis (if very hypotonic dialysate) Dysequilibrium-like syndrome[a]
	High sodium	Thirst Dysequilibrium-like syndrome[a]
	Low potassium	Cardiac arrhythmias
	High potassium	Cardiac arrhythmias
	Low calcium	Mild hypotension Hyperparathyroidism Twitching, tetany, petechiae
	High calcium	Hypertension, cardiac arrhythmias Hypercalcemia, soft tissue calcification Hard water syndrome[b] if very high calcium
	Low magnesium	?Hyperparathyroidism
	High magnesium	?Contribution to osteoporosis and osteomalacia Nausea, blurred vision, muscular weakness, ataxia, hypotension Cardiac arrhythmias if very high
Glucose content	No glucose	Hypoglycemia (rare)
Buffer	Usage of acetate	Hypotension Cardiac arrhythmias Headache Hypoventilation Hypocapnia, hypoxia
	Usage of bicarbonate	Metabolic alkalosis (nausea, vomiting, lethargy, increased soft tissue calcification) and hypoventilation Bacterial overgrowth of dialysate
Temperature	Low	Chills, patient discomfort
	High	Sweating, sensation of warmth, hypotension, hyperventilation, tachykardia, vomiting Hemolysis and hyperkalemia if >55°C
Dialysate contamination	Hydrogen peroxide, formaldehyde, hypochlorite, chloramine, nitrate, copper[c]	Hemolysis and subsequent hyperkalemia Methemoglobinemia (nitrate, chloramine) resulting in cyanosis, brownish discoloration of venous blood; fatigue, malaise, coma
	Fluoride[d]	Early: nausea, vomiting, pruritus, headache, syncope, back or abdominal pain, diarrhea, cardiac arrhythmias Late: symptoms related to precipitation of calcium (see above), respiratory failure, hypotension, seizure, coma, cardiac arrest.
	Microorganisms, pyrogens	Fever, hypotension, shock ?Nutritional status ?Arthropathies, amyloidosis Liver failure (microcystins from cyanobacteria)

[a]Dysequilibrium [sic] syndrome, early manifestations: tiredness, severe headache, nausea, vomiting, pulse rate increased, blood pressure increased, restlessness. Late, serious manifestations: seizures, obtundation, coma.

[b]Hard water syndrome: mild blood pressure increase (rarely decrease), pulse rate normal or slow, sweating, retrosternal pain, nausea, vomiting, progressive lethargy and weakness, headache, dysarthria, seizures, hallucinations, confusion.

[c]See also Refs. 42–48.

[d]See also Refs. 49–51.

most of the potential complications and causes are dealt with in other chapters, the reader is referred to them for further detail. In the following, we will confine ourselves to the acute and chronic consequences of dialysate or substitution fluids contaminated with microorganisms and microbial products. We will first discuss data of multicenter studies on the bacteriological quality of water and dialysate. We will continue with the description of various pyrogenic substances derived from microorganisms in dialysate and discuss the frequency of pyrogenic reactions and other acute consequences related to contaminated dialysate as well as possible clinical long-term consequences possibly related to contaminated dialysate and substitution fluids. Finally, we will briefly discuss the topic of dialysate contamination with disinfectants such as hydrogen peroxide, formaldehyde, hypochlorite, and chloramine as well as with nitrates, copper, and fluoride as these substances are not covered in other chapters (Table 1).

A. Bacterial Growth in Dialysate

The microbiological quality of drinking water is controlled in the United States and most European countries. In general it should not contain more than 100 colony-forming units (CFU) of microorganisms per milliliter. Because of the experience of severe pyrogenic reactions due to heavily contaminated dialysate in the beginning of hemodialysis therapy, the American Association of Medical Instrumentation (AAMI) proposed standards for the microbiological quality of water for dialysis. These standards were set for water and dialysate at 200 CFU/mL and 2000 CFU/mL, respectively. Klein et al. (2) reported that in a 1990 multicenter study in the United States, 35% of water samples and 19% of dialysate samples exceeded these AAMI standards. These data were confirmed in a multicenter study in Germany in which 18% of water samples and 12% of dialysate samples were not in compliance with the AAMI standards (3). In a 7-year multicenter study in Canada, the percentage of water samples containing more than 200 CFU/mL was 36–49% in the years 1987–1989 and improved to 15% in 1993 (4). This improvement was associated with the general use of reverse osmosis to purify water. The degree of bacterial contamination of dialysate in the United States, Canada, as well as Europe was very variable (10^2–10^5 CFU/mL) between hemodialysis centers but also within the same centers over time (4–6). Thus, even with improved water treatment for hemodialysis, approximately 15–20% of water and dialysate samples today must be considered to be highly contaminated.

Several studies were performed to characterize the microorganisms growing in dialysate. Klein et al. (2) reported that bacteria grown from dialysate were almost exclusively gram-negative, with *Pseudomonas* species being most commonly found. The predominance of *Peudomonas* species in water and dialysate has recently been confirmed by several studies (3,4). In addition, fungi are occasionally found. Gram-positive microorganisms rarely occur in dialysate. The groups of Harding and Pass showed that adequate culture conditions are required to correctly determine bacterial numbers in dialysate (7,8). Gram-negative bacteria isolated from dialysate grow better in nutrient-poor culture media such as R2A or tryptone glucose extract (TGE) agar as compared to standard media such as tryptic soy agar (TSA) (8). Furthermore, growth of these microorganisms was enhanced when cultures were incubated at room temperature as compared to 37°C. In order to improve the sensitivity of the bacterial cultures, incubations were prolonged to 96 hours (7). Because these special culture conditions have not been used in the above-mentioned multicenter studies (3,4), it is conceivable that the true degree of bacterial contamination in those studies might have been underestimated. We therefore used optimized culture conditions to test the dialysate quality in our center. Dialysate samples were taken under sterile conditions at the end of a dialysis session from the dialysate outlet port of the dialyzer. Samples were cultured on TGE agar for 5 days at 28°C (9). Out of 277 dialysate samples, bacterial growth was <100 CFU/mL in 87.3% and 101–1000 CFU/mL in 12.7%. In agreement with other studies, *Pseudomonas* species were predominantly found. The good dialysate quality in our center was maintained over 4 years due to routine monthly controls of bacterial growth in dialysate. In cases in which more than 100 CFU/mL were determined, chemical disinfection of water tubing and the dialysis machine was performed.

B. Pyrogenic Bacterial Substances

Microorganisms are unable to cross intact dialyzer membranes. The risk of pyrogenic reactions during hemodialysis relates to the fact that contaminated dialysate contains cell wall components derived from debris of dead microorganisms. In contrast to gram-positive bacteria in which the cell wall is abundant in peptidoglycans, gram-negative bacteria have an additional outer membrane consisting of lipoproteins and lipopolysaccharides (LPS), which are highly pyrogenic. Peptidoglycans and LPS are large molecules (Table 2) and therefore unlikely to pass across intact dialyzer membranes in sufficient amounts to cause fever in patients. However, subunits such as muramyl dipeptides derived from peptidoglycans as well as lipid A and polysaccharide fragments derived from LPS may be as small as 1–5 kDa (Table 2), may retain pyrogenic activity, and may penetrate even low-flux dialyzer membranes to induce fever during hemodialysis. In addition to pyrogenic cell wall components, *Pseudomonas aeruginosa*, growing in dialysate, actively secrete peptides such as exotoxin A (10). The intact exotoxin A is a relatively large molecule with a molecular weight of 71 kDa. Two subunits of exotoxin A have been described: a 45 kDa N-terminal binding domain, which binds to the α_2-macroglobulin receptor on target cells, and a 26 kDa C-terminal subunit with cytotoxic activity (11). The N-terminal subunit is cytotoxic by inhibiting peptide prolongation and prevents protein synthesis, including the production of pyrogenic cytokines. In contrast, small exotoxin A fragments derived from the N-terminal subunit may retain pyrogenic activity as indicated by the induction of cytokines in peripheral blood mononuclear cells (PBMC). Such pyrogenic exotoxin A fragments have been identified in bicarbonate dialysate contaminated with *P. aeruginosa* and are able to cross intact dialyzer membranes (12). However, compared to purified LPS, the pyrogenic activity of purified exotoxin A is weak and does not contribute significantly to the total pyrogenic activity of contaminated dialysate. In addition to these identified substances, several unknown bacterial products of small size are present in contaminated dialysate (Table 2). These products are not related to endotoxins or exotoxin A but induce cytokines and are able to penetrate intact dialyzer membranes (13,14).

Table 2 Bacteria-Derived Pyrogens

	Molecular weight (daltons)
Cell Wall Components	
Lipopolysaccharide (LPS)	>100,000
Lipid A–related LPS fragments	2–4000
Other LPS fragments	<8000
Peptidoglycans	1000–20,000
Muramylpeptides	400–1000
Actively Secreted Toxins	
Exotoxin A	71,000
Exotoxin A fragments	<5000
Unknown Pyrogens	<20,000

C. Pyrogen Permeability of Dialyzer Membranes

As the molecular size exclusion of dialyzer membranes is between 5 kDa for low-flux and 25–30 kDa for high-flux membranes, one may speculate that low-flux membranes might be less permeable to small pyrogens than high-flux membranes. This question was addressed by several in vitro studies investigating the permeability of dialyzer membranes to bacterial substances. Bacterial products were measured by the Limulus amebocyte lysate (LAL) assay, which detects only LPS and lipid A–containing subunits of LPS. Other studies used the in vitro incubation of human PBMC to measure the cytokine-inducing activity of purposefully contaminated dialysate samples. After an overnight incubation of such stimulated PBMC, pyrogenic cytokines, including interleukin-1 (IL-1β) and tumor necrosis factor (TNF-α), were quantified in their culture supernatants in order to assess the net pyrogenic activity of all bacterial substances present in the challenge material.

Using purified LPS to contaminate the dialysate and the LAL test to measure LPS penetration into the blood compartment, studies failed to show any LPS permeability of low-flux regenerated cellulosic as well as high-flux polysulfone dialyzer membranes (15,16). In contrast, when the in vitro incubation of PBMC was used to determine the cytokine-inducing activity, pyrogens were readily detected in the blood side of low-flux regenerated cellulosic membranes after the dialysate was challenged with purified LPS (15). In confirmation of these latter findings, subsequent studies using radiolabeled low molecular weight fragments of LPS demonstrated that low-flux regenerated cellulose, high-flux AN69, and polysulfone membranes were permeable to these compounds as assessed both by the determination of radioactivity and by the cytokine-inducing activity in the blood compartment (17,18). In these studies, the LAL assay again failed to detect the LPS-derived fragments in the blood side.

Thus, LAL test–negative LPS fragments apparently are released from purified LPS during in vitro dialysis, cross dialyzer membranes, and are highly active in inducing blood side cytokine production. Reasons for the failure of the LAL test to detect these LPS-derived subunits remain speculative. It has been suggested that the fragments are either too small (<4000 daltons) to be detected by the LAL assay (18) or do not contain the LAL-reactive lipid A subunit of LPS.

Further studies were performed using culture filtrates from dialysate-born bacteria such as *Pseudomonas maltophilia, P. aeruginosa, Pseudomonas testosteroni, Alcaligenes,* and other species (13,18,19). All studies used the PBMC assay to measure the cytokine-inducing activity of the bacterial filtrates. In spite of differences in experimental designs of the in vitro studies, it can be concluded that all dialyzer membranes, high flux as well as low flux, are in principle permeable to pyrogenic substances of bacterial origin. However, considerable quantitative differences in the pyrogen permeability of the various dialyzer membranes were noted. In contrast to cellulosic membranes, synthetic dialyzer membranes such as polysulfone, polyamide, and acrylonitrile adsorb plasma proteins as well as bacterial products due to hydrophobic interactions between these factors and hydrophobic domains in the membrane polymer. The adsorptive capacity for pyrogens of the specific dialyzer membrane material itself (20,21), as well as the formation of a pyrogen-adsorbing protein layer on the dialyzer membrane, may reduce the permeability of dialyzer membranes to bacterial products (17,22). Because of the high adsorptive capacity for pyrogens, high-flux polysulfone and polyamide membranes have indeed been successfully used as ultra-filters to reduce the pyrogen content of contaminated dialysate (20,21).

Due to the presence of small pyrogens (molecular weight below the cutoff of low-flux membranes) in contaminated dialysate, low-flux dialyzer membranes also cannot prevent permeation of pyrogens into the patient's blood. To the contrary, low-flux cellulosic membranes are very thin (6–8 μm) and hydrophilic, characteristics that facilitate diffusive transport of small molecular substances across the membrane and reduce adsorption of pyrogens to the membrane surface.

D. Pyrogenic and Other Reactions to Bacterial Products During Hemodialysis and Hemofiltration

Dialysate (or substitution fluid) contamination with microorganisms and their products is the most plausible explanation of fever occurring 2–3 hours after the start of hemofiltration or hemodialysis if no other origin can be identified. Over the last 20 years, the pathogenesis of fever has been clarified predominantly by the work of Dinarello and Wolff (23). Invading microorganisms and microbial products are recognized by circulating macrophages, which are activated either by phagocytosis of the whole bacteria or by binding of bacterial products such as endotoxin to their CD14 receptor via specific binding proteins (e.g., LPS-binding protein) (24). Both routes of macrophage activation result in de novo production of endogenous pyrogens such as IL-1, IL-6, and TNF-α. IL-1 and TNF-α induce the release of PGE_2 in the hypothalamus, which in turn upregulates the set point of body temperature with fever as consequence (25). Because of the essential role of cytokines in the induction of pyrogenic reactions, measurement of cytokine plasma levels and cytokine production by isolated mononuclear cells is a useful tool to determine the pyrogenic activity of bacterial products and contaminated fluids.

In order to illustrate the association between contaminated substitution fluid, cytokine induction, and fever, we present the following case report (26): a 21-year-old woman with end-stage renal disease was on intermittent postdilution hemofiltration (HF) for 5 years. At the start of a new session the patient felt fine and the oral temperature was 36.4°C. One hour after start of treatment she felt cold and ill. After 2 hours, HF was terminated because her condition worsened, her temperature rose to 37.8°C, and her blood pressure dropped to shock-like hypotension. Blood samples showed a drop in WBC to 600/μL with no detectable neutrophils and revealed a very high level of the proinflammatory cytokine TNF-α at 5000 pg/mL (normal value in ESRD patients is approximately 50–100 pg/mL in the assay used). The patient remained ill during the next 6 hours with body temperature reaching 39.5°C. The remaining substitution fluid was assayed for endotoxin using the LAL assay. The LAL test detected 100 pg/mL of endotoxin in the substitution fluid, although the bags were undamaged and the fluid was clear. This concentration of endotoxin is sufficient to account for the pyrogenic reaction because 150 mL/min of substitution fluid were infused containing a total of 15 ng of endotoxin/min. After HF was terminated, the patient recovered during the following 24 hours, and the hemofiltration 2 days later was uneventful.

It is easily accepted that i.v. infusion of endotoxin during hemofiltration may cause a pyrogenic reaction. In hemodialysis where pyrogenic factors such as endotoxin in dialysate need to penetrate the dialyzer membrane to get into the patient's blood, it is much more difficult to prove that treatment-associated fever is in fact due to contaminated dialysate fluid. In the beginning of hemodialysis therapy, pyrogenic reactions were the most frequent complications. In the 1960s, dialysate was prepared in a tank using softened water, acetate as a buffer, and salt. Bacterial contamination was obvious when dialysate turned foamy and began to smell like a bacterial culture. In those days shivering patients were a regular feature in dialysis units. This pyrogen fever was explained by ruptures in the dialyzer membranes, which were very common during that time when coil or Kiil dialyzers were built by hand (27). Today, artificial membranes and dialyzers are manufactured by the dialysis industry and membrane ruptures are rare. In addition, water treatment using reverse osmosis significantly reduces bacterial contamination of dialysate. The question is therefore whether pyrogenic reactions do still occur in today's hemodialysis therapy.

To answer this question, data obtained from the national surveillance of hemodialysis-associated diseases of the Centers for Disease Control (CDC) in the United States should be discussed. In their reports, the influence of bicarbonate dialysate versus acetate dialysate, the use of high-flux dialyzers versus low-flux dialyzers, performance of single use versus reuse of dialyzers, and combinations of all these factors on the frequency of pyrogenic reactions in hemodialysis were analyzed. Dialysis centers using high-flux dialyzers in combination with bicarbonate dialysate were more likely to report pyrogenic reactions, particularly when dialyzers were reused. In centers performing only single use of dialyzers, the frequency of pyrogenic reactions in patients treated with high-flux dialyzers was not significantly different from that found in patients treated with low-flux dialyzers (28). In 1991, the number of pyrogenic reactions in dialysis centers performing reuse was higher compared to centers performing only single use (15% vs. 7%, $p < 0.05$) (29). It is important to mention that rinsing of the used dialyzers is done with reverse osmosis water, which may be contaminated with more than 200 CFU/mL as outlined below. During reprocessing of the dialyzer, water is used to rinse the blood compartment and may easily contaminate the blood-side surface of the dialyzer membrane. Bacterial toxins such as endotoxins are not inactivated by the reprocessing procedure and may induce a pyrogenic fever during the following dialysis session.

In 1994, 538 out of 2449 (22%) hemodialysis centers in the United States reported more than one hemodialysis-associated pyrogenic reaction per year. This number had remained stable since 1989 (30). Centers reporting more pyrogenic reactions also had a higher risk for clusters of pyrogenic reactions. Similar to the reports of previous years, fever reactions were significantly associated with the use of high-flux membranes and reuse of dialyzers (30). Although the survey data did not include measurements of bacterial contamination in dialysate and water for dialyzer reprocessing, one may speculate that bacterial contamination of dialysate in combination with reuse of high-flux dialyzers increases the risk of pyrogenic reactions.

The frequency of fever reactions during hemodialysis adjusted for total number of treatments is difficult to determine because of limited data. The best estimate is that approximately 1–10 pyrogenic reactions occur per 10,000 hemodialysis sessions, as reported in several studies conducted in the United States (31). These data indicate that a dialysis center with 100 patients may have one pyrogenic reaction in a time period of 4 weeks to 8 months.

As mentioned above, a pyrogenic reaction induced by bacterial products is mediated by endogenous pyrogens, i.e., proinflammatory cytokines such as IL-1β and TNF-α. Besides the induction of fever, cytokines express multiple biological activities contributing to chronic inflammatory processes including the catabolic loss of lean body mass, fibrosis, and secondary (AA-)amyloidosis (25). Cytokines are not detectable in normal plasma and are not spontaneously produced by healthy human donor PBMC in culture. In patients on hemodialysis, cytokine production may be detectable even in the absence of a significant rise in body temperature. The measurement of cytokines in isolated PBMC has therefore been proposed as a sensitive method to detect pyrogen transfer from contaminated dialysate or substitution fluid into the blood stream of ESRD patients (32).

Despite good bacteriological dialysate quality in our center (see above), we still observed dialysate-induced cytokine (IL-1) production in whole blood in 75% of the samples (9). Also, we noted no correlation between CFU/mL and the amount of IL-1 induced. This is in agreement with studies by Klein et al. (2), who failed to demonstrate a correlation between bacterial growth in dialysate and its endotoxin content as measured by the LAL assay. A possible explanation of this discrepancy is provided by the observation that bacterial growth takes place predominantly on the surfaces of water pipes, dialysate tubing and the dialyzer membrane forming a biofilm. Microorganisms grow on these surfaces and may release pyrogens into the water and dialysate after they die. Living bacteria may only periodically appear in the fluid phase if clusters disrupt from the biofilm. In order to monitor the bacteriological quality of dialysate, bacterial growth using adequate culture conditions should therefore be determined frequently, at least once a month. Ideally, these tests should be supplemented with a determination of dialysate pyrogenicity in terms of cytokine-inducing activity using one of the assays discussed in this review.

Apart from inducing fever, other acute responses to bacterial products are rarely encountered during dialysis. Recently, an outbreak of acute liver injury, hepatic failure, and death in a considerable number of patients has been related to dialysate contamination with microcystins (i.e., cyclic peptides with potent hepatotoxicity) derived from several strains of cyanobacteria (33). In this case inadequate water treatment at both the municipal water plant as well as at the dialysis center resulted in the parenteral exposure of hemodialysis patients to microcystins. Cyanobacteria have been detected in water worldwide but are particularly common in Brazil.

E. Effect of Ultra-Pure Dialysate on Cytokine Release in ESRD Patients

We studied the cytokine content in PBMC isolated from the blood of ESRD patients under the conditions of low-flux hemodialysis with Cuprophan® membranes and either regular bicarbonate dialysate or ultra-pure bicarbonate dialysate. Whereas in standard dialysate the median of the bacterial count was 148 CFU/mL (range 61–400 CFU/mL), there were no CFU detectable in polysulfone-ultrafiltered dialysate. To determine cytokine induction in these patients, we measured the PBMC production of IL-1 receptor antagonist (IL-1Ra). IL-1Ra is a functional antagonist of IL-1, is easily detected since its production by PBMC is one log higher than that of IL-1 itself, parallels IL-1 production, and is the most sensitive marker of PBMC activation (25). In our study the IL-1Ra content of PBMC fell significantly from an average value of 1467 ng/2.5 $\times$ 10^6 PBMC to 1166 ng/2.5 $\times$ 10^6 PBMC ($p = 0.016$) in the patients on clean dialysate (32).

In a similar study we tested the effect of ultra-pure versus standard dialysate on the spontaneous production of IL-1β in whole blood samples taken from ESRD patients on low-flux Hemophan® dialyzers. Six ESRD patients were studied following an A-B-A′ protocol in which ultra-pure (A) or standard (B) bicarbonate dialysate was used. Ultra-pure dialysate was prepared by the Genius® system, in which 75 L of dialysate are freshly prepared in a tank for a single dialysis session using UV-radiated reverse osmosis water and prepacked salt concentrates. Dialysate samples for the determination of bacterial growth were taken at the end of a dialysate session from the dialysate outlet port of the dialyzer twice during study periods of 4 weeks each. Bacterial cultures were done on nutrient-poor tryptone glucose extract agars for 5 days at room temperature in order to achieve optimal conditions. Blood samples were taken three times per study period always after the long interdialytic interval at the start of the next hemodialysis session. Whole blood samples were incubated with equal volumes of pyrogen-free tissue culture medium at 37°C for 18 hours. After incubation, the spontaneous release of IL-1β was measured in whole blood culture supernatants by radioimmunoassay (34). The results are shown in Fig. 2. Bacterial growth (median, range) increased from 2 (0–25) CFU/mL in period A to 385 (130–1000) CFU/mL in period B and decreased to 0 (0–1) CFU/mL in period A′. This significant change in dialysate contamination was accompanied by significant changes in spontaneous whole blood IL-1β release from 70 (20–105) pg/mL to 110 (28–150) pg/mL and back to 50 (20–85) pg/mL. These data demonstrate that in the presence of even moderately contaminated dialysate (which would be acceptable by AAMI standards; see above), cytokine production is enhanced in ESRD patients when thin low-flux dialyzer membranes without pyrogen-adsorbing capacity are used. The fact that a switch to ultra-pure dialysate significantly reduces whole blood IL-1β release in these patients supports the concept that the tested low-flux membranes are permeable to pyrogens from contaminated dialysate (see above). If low-grade contamination of dialysate under these conditions causes detectable cytokine induction in ESRD patients, one may extrapolate that high-grade contamination of dialysate results in hemodialysis-associated fever. The threshold is, of course, patient dependent. At first glance, our data seem to be in conflict with a study recently published by Grooteman et al. (35), who measured plasma levels of TNF-α and IL-1β after hemodialysis with a high-flux cellulose triacetate membrane, using either standard dialysate or ultra-filtered dialysate. Although no statistically significant differences were detected, a trend towards lower TNF-α levels after dialysis with ultrafiltered dialysate was apparent (35). Taking into account that the measurement of plasma cytokine levels is less sensitive than the measurement of whole blood cytokine production, the results of this study (35) seem compatible with our data, showing that the use of ultra-pure dialysate reduces cytokine induction in ESRD patients. In conclusion, in order to reduce the risk of pyrogenic reactions during hemodialysis, the quality of dialysate should be improved to less than 100 CFU/mL and as little as possible cytokine induction. Ultrafiltration of dialysate through pyrogen-adsorbing membranes or special pro-

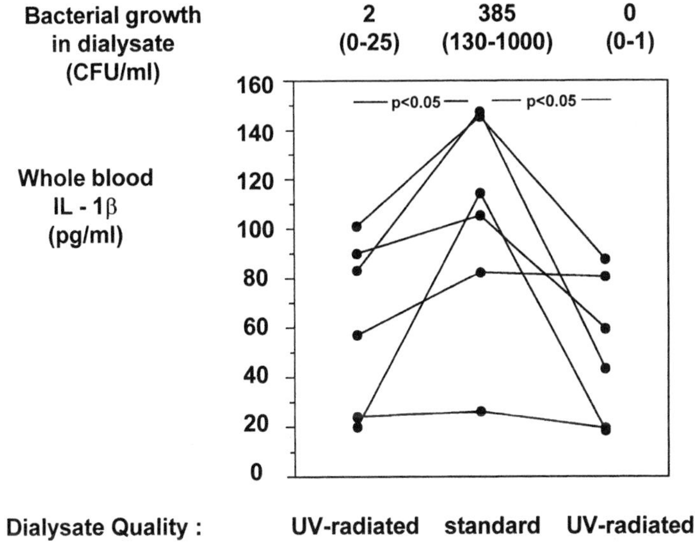

Fig. 2 Effect of dialysate quality on whole blood IL-1β release in ESRD patients on low-flux Hemophan® dialysis. Six ESRD patients were studied in study periods of 4 weeks each with either UV-radiated dialysate (A) or standard dialysate (B) following an A-B-A protocol. Bacterial growth is given in CFU/mL; numbers represent the median (range) of 12 samples per study period. Heparinized whole blood samples were taken from the arterio-venous fistula before start of the hemodialysis session after the long interdialytic interval. Whole blood samples were incubated with equal volumes of pyrogen-free tissue culture medium for 18 hours at 37°C. IL-1β was measured in whole blood culture supernatants. The data points represent the means of three determinations per study period.

cedures such as UV radiation of dialysate have successfully been used to achieve these goals.

F. Clinical Long-Term Consequences of Dialysate and Substitution Fluid Contamination with Microorganisms and Pyrogens

In spite of a wealth of data on the acute effects of biocompatibility of the dialysis circuit, little evidence is available to implicate these phenomena in clinical long-term sequelae of chronic dialysis treatment. Most studies investigating these issues were focused at the importance of the dialyzer membrane. These studies have suggested, but usually not proven, that the choice of a so-called biocompatible dialyzer membrane may lead to improved survival and lower infection rates (reviewed in Refs. 36,37). Several large studies on the clinical impact of dialyzer choice are ongoing in Italy and the United States and may potentially shed further light on these issues. In contrast to the aforementioned studies, the role of the dialysate, in particular contamination of dialysate with microbial products, for the development of long-term complications of hemodialysis treatment has received little attention. This may in large part be due to the facts that microbial dialysate contamination is not constant and therefore difficult to quantify (see above) and that the availability of ultrapure dialysate is still limited. However, given the variable permeability of dialyzer membranes to microbial products in the dialysate, it is conceivable that some of the clinical observations in the above studies may relate to the dialysate rather than the dialyzer membranes. One of the few areas where at least some evidence for a role of dialysate contamination in contributing to clinical long-term sequelae is available is the development of β_2-microglobulin–derived amyloidosis (Aß2M amyloidosis, also known as dialysis amyloidosis).

Baz et al. (38) reported that carpal tunnel syndrome, one of the manifestations of Aß2M amyloidosis, was significantly less common in patients treated with ultrapure dialysate as opposed to those receiving conventional dialysate. In various other studies on factors influencing the occurrence of Aß2M amyloidosis in hemodialysis patients, the investigators exclusively focused on the influence of the dialyzer membrane (39,40). Some but not all of these studies suggested that the use of a high-flux synthetic membrane as opposed to low-flux membranes made from regenerated cellulose led to a decreasing prevalence of the amyloidosis (39,40). Again, given the considerable influence of the dialyzer membrane on the permeation of bacterial products into the blood stream, these studies do not rule out the possibility that the effects only indirectly relate to the dialyzer membrane.

In a recent case-control study, we noted that between 1988 and 1996 clinical signs of Aß2M amyloidosis decreased by about 80% in our dialysis unit (41). During the same period, the use of both high-flux synthetic dialyzer membranes increased by only 7% of the total time spent on dialysis. Highly significant changes, however, were noted for dialysate parameters: home hemodialysis markedly decreased, demineralized water for dialysate preparation was replaced by reverse osmosis water, and acetate was replaced by bicarbonate (41). Although no systematic data were available, spot checks suggest that at least home hemodialysis and the use of demineralized water were associated with significantly higher bacterial burdens in the dialysate than in-center hemodialysis with reverse osmosis water. These data lend further support to the notion that dialysate-related factors may contribute to the development of Aß2M amyloidosis.

G. Dialysate Contamination with Disinfectants and Other Rare Substances

Contamination of the dialysate with disinfectants such as hydrogen peroxide or formaldehyde as well as accidental hypochlorite infusion can all be associated with marked hemolysis (Table 1) (42–45). Clinical signs include malaise, nausea, headache, and severe abdominal pain. Death may result from hyperkalemia (Table 1). Another rare cause of hemolysis is copper, which may leak from heating coils or copper pipes if used in dialysate-delivery systems (Table 1) (46).

Chloramines, which are widely used instead of free chlorine to sanitize public drinking water, may cause oxidative injury to red cells and thereby also induce hemolysis. Hemolysis is observed if dialysate concentrations exceed 0.25 mg/L. AAMI standards have been set at a maximum concentration of 0.1 mg/L (47). Chloramine concentrations in drinking water usually range from 1 to 2.5 mg/L but may fluctuate widely. Because chloramines, unlike many other water contaminants, are small and nonionic, removal by water softeners, reverse osmosis systems, and deoinization systems is insufficient (47). Current recommendations therefore include the usage of granular activated charcoal filters, preferentially two in series, and regular testing of the dialysate using DPD (*N,N*-diethyl-*o*-phenylenediamine) tests, preferentially at each shift (47).

In addition to causing hemolysis, chloramines as well as high levels of nitrate in dialysate can cause methemoglobinemia (Table 1). Dialysate nitrate contamination, similar to chloramine contamination, results from high levels in the water supply combined with insufficient or defective water purification (48). Treatment in mild cases of methemoglobinemia is not necessary, while in severe cases 1–2 mg/kg of a 1% solution of methylene blue in saline should be administered i.v. over 10 minutes (48).

Fluoride intoxication generally results from the combination of high fluoride levels in municipal water and failure or exhaustion of the reverse osmosis and/or deionization system (49–51). Signs of fluoride intoxication relate to its ability to interfere with various intracellular metabolic processes and the precipitation of calcium and magnesium (Table 1). Laboratory investigations reveal metabolic acidosis (high anion gap) and/or primary respiratory acidosis, hypocalcemia, hyperkalemia (49–51). Upon recognition, fluoride intoxication should be treated by prompt hemodialysis with fluoride-free, bicarbonate-based dialysate containing low potassium (or other standard measures for the treatment of acute hyperkalemia) and high calcium (or i.v. substitution of calcium). Alternatively, peritoneal dialysis should be instituted.

III. SUMMARY

Following an overview of water treatment and dialysate preparation, the present chapter focuses on acute and chronic consequences of dialysate or substitution fluids contaminated with microorganisms and microbial products. American Association of Medical Instrumentation (AAMI) standards for water and dialysate currently are set at 200 and 2000 CFU/mL, respectively. Despite improved modes of water purification, they are still frequently exceeded, contributing to acute pyrogenic reactions during dialysis. Low- as well as high-flux membranes may, to a variable extent, permit the permeation of pyrogenic bacterial products, in particular low molecular weight bacterial wall fragments, into the blood. Several of these fragments are not detected using the Limulus amebocyte lysate assay. Additional biological tests, such as the induction of inflammatory mediator release (e.g., cytokine release) from mononuclear cells, are therefore proposed as other means to monitor the purity of the dialysate as well as to assess the biological responses of patients to contaminated dialysate. Apart from the induction of acute pyrogenic reactions, the long-term consequences of dialysate contaminated with bacterial products are largely speculative. However, recent evidence suggests that highly purified dialysate might delay the onset of β_2-microglobulin–derived amyloidosis in chronic hemodialysis patients.

In the second part of the chapter, the various consequences of dialysate contamination with disinfectants and some chemical water contaminants (hydrogen peroxide, formaldehyde, hypochlorite, copper, chloramines, nitrate, and fluoride) are discussed.

REFERENCES

1. Canaud BJM, Mion CM. Water treatment for contemporary hemodialysis. In: Jacobs C, Kjellstrand CN, Koch KM, Winchester FJ, eds. Replacement of Kidney Function by Dialysis. Dordrecht: Kluwer Academic Publishers, 1996:231–255.
2. Klein E, Pass T, Harding GB, Wright R, Million C. Microbial and endotoxin contamination in water and dialysate in the central United States. Artif Organs 1990; 14:85–94.
3. Bambauer R, Schauer M, Jung WK, Daum V, Vienken J. Contamination of dialysis water and dialysate: a survey of 30 centers. ASAIO J 1994; 40:1012–1016.
4. Laurence RA, Lapierre ST. Quality of hemodialysis water: a 7-year multicenter study. Am J Kidney Dis 1995; 25:738–750.
5. Bambauer R, Meyer S, Jung H, Goehl H, Nystrand R. Sterile versus non-sterile dialysis fluid in chronic hemodialysis treatment. ASAIO Trans 1990; 36:317–320.
6. Pegues DA, Oettinger CW, Bland LA, Oliver JC, Arduino MJ, Aguero SM, McAllister SK, Gordon SM, Favero MS, Jarvis WR. A prospective study of pyrogenic reactions in hemodialysis patients using bicarbonate dialysis fluids filtered to remove bacteria and endotoxin. J Am Soc Nephrol 1992; 3:1002–1007.
7. Pass T, Wright R, Sharp B, Harding GB. Culture of dialysis fluids on nutrient-rich media for short periods at elevated temperatures underestimate microbial contamination. Blood Purif 1996; 14:136–145.
8. Harding GB, Klein E, Pass T, Wright R, Million C. Endotoxin and bacterial contamination of dialysis center water and dialysate; a cross sectional survey. Int J Artif Organs 1990; 13:39–43.
9. Lonnemann G. Assessment of quality of dialysate. Nephrol Dial Transplant 1998; 13(suppl. 5):17–20.
10. Misfeldt ML, Legaard PK, Howell SE, Fornella MH, Le Grand RD. Induction of interleukin-1 from murine peritoneal macrophages by *Pseudomonas aeruginosa* exotoxin A. Infect Immun 1990; 58:978–982.
11. Fitzgerald D, Pastan I. Pseudomonas exotoxin and recombinant immunotoxins derived from it. Ann NY Acad Sci 1993; 685:740–745.
12. Krautzig S, Lonnemann G, Koch KM. Penetration of exotoxin A related cytokine-inducing substances through dialyzer membranes (abstract). Blood Purif 1995; 13:S61.
13. Lonnemann G, Behme TC, Lenzner B, Floege J, Schulze M, Colton CK, Koch KM, Shaldon S. Permeability of dialyzer membranes to TNF alpha-inducing substances derived from water bacteria. Kidney Int 1992; 42:61–68.
14. Schindler R, Krautzig S, Lufft V, Lonnemann G, Mahiout A, Marra MN, Shaldon S, Koch KM. Induction of interleukin-1 and interleukin-1 receptor antagonist during contaminated in vitro dialysis with whole blood. Nephrol Dial Transplant 1996; 11:101–108.
15. Lonnemann G, Bingel M, Floege J, Koch KM, Shaldon S, Dinarello CA. Detection of endotoxin-like interleukin-1-inducing activity during in vitro dialysis. Kidney Int 1988; 33:29–35.
16. Bommer J, Becker KP, Urbaschek R, Ritz E, Urbaschek B. No evidence for endotoxin transfer across high flux polysulfone membranes. Clin Nephrol 1987; 27:278–282.
17. Urena P, Herbelin A, Zingraff J, Lair M, Man NK, Descamps LB, Drueke T. Permeability of cellulosic and non-cellulosic membranes to endotoxin subunits and cytokine production during in-vitro haemodialysis. Nephrol Dial Transplant 1992; 7:16–28.
18. Laude-Sharp M, Caroff M, Simard L, Pusineri C, Kazatchkine MD, Haeffner-Cavaillon N. Induction of IL-1 during hemodialysis: transmembrane passage of intact endotoxins (LPS). Kidney Int 1990; 38:1089–1094.
19. Evans RC, Holmes CJ. In vitro study of the transfer of cytokine-inducing substances across selected high-flux hemodialysis membranes. Blood Purif 1991; 9:92–101.
20. Dinarello CA, Lonnemann G, Maxwell R, Shaldon S. Ultrafiltration to reject human interleukin-1-inducing substances derived from bacterial cultures. J Clin Microbiol 1987; 25:1233–1238.
21. Schindler R, Dinarello CA. Ultrafiltration to remove endotoxins and other cytokine-inducing materials from tissue culture media and parenteral fluids. Bio Techniques 1990; 8:408–413.
22. Lonnemann G, Schindler R, Lufft V, Mahiout A, Shaldon S, Koch KM. The role of plasma coating on the permeation of cytokine-inducing substances through dialyzer membranes. Nephrol Dial Transplant 1995; 10: 207–211.
23. Dinarello CA, Wolff SM. The role of interleukin-1 in disease. N Engl J Med 1993; 328:106–113.
24. Wright SD, Ramos RA, Tobias PS, Ulevitch RJ, Mathison JC. CD14, a receptor for complexes of lipopolysaccharide (LPS) and LPS binding protein. Science 1990; 249:1431–1433.
25. Dinarello CA. Biologic basis for interleukin-1 in disease. Blood 1996; 87:2095–2147.
26. Lonnemann G, van der Meer JWM, Cannon JG, Dinarello CA, Koch KM, Granolleras C, Deschodt G,

Shaldon S. Induction of tumor necrosis factor during extracorporeal blood purification [letter]. N Engl J Med 1987; 317:963–964.
27. Favero MD, Petersen NJ, Boyer KM, Carson LA, Bond WW. Microbial contamination of renal dialysis and associated health risk. Trans Am Soc Artif Internal Organs 1974; 20:175–183.
28. Tokars JI, Alter MJ, Favero MS, Moyer LA, Bland LA. National surveillance of hemodialysis associated diseases in the United States, 1990. ASAIO J 1993; 39: 71–80.
29. Tokars JI, Alter MJ, Favero MS, Moyer LA, Bland LA. National surveillance of dialysis associated diseases in the United States, 1991. ASAIO J 1993; 39:966–975.
30. Tokars JI, Alter MJ, Miller E, Moyer LA, Favero MS. National surveillance of dialysis associated diseases in the United States—1994. ASAIO J 1997; 43:108–119.
31. Gordon SM, Oettinger CW, Bland LA, Oliver JC, Arduino MJ, Aguero SM, McAllister SK, Favero MS, Jarvis WR. Pyrogenic reactions in patients receiving conventional, high-efficiency, or high-flux hemodialysis treatments with bicarbonate dialysate containing high concentrations of bacteria and endotoxin. J Am Soc Nephrol 1992; 2:1436–1444.
32. Schindler R, Lonnemann G, Schäffer J, Shaldon S, Koch KM, Krautzig S. The effect of ultrafiltered dialysate on the cellular content of interleukin-1 receptor antagonist in patients on chronic hemodialysis. Nephron 1994; 68:229–233.
33. Jochimsen EM, Carmichael WW, An J, Cardo DM, Cookson ST, Holmes CEM, De C. Antunes MB, De Melo Filho DA, Lyra TM, Barreto VST, Azevedo SMFO, Jarvis WR. Liver failure and death after exposure to microcystins at a hemodialysis center in Brazil. N Engl J Med 1998; 338:873–878.
34. Lonnemann G, Dumann H, Schmidt-Gürtler H. Improved dialysate quality is associated with decreased whole blood cytokine production in ESRD patients on the Genius hemodialysis system (abstract). Blood Purif 1997; 15S2:6.
35. Grooteman MPC, Nubé MJ, Daha MR, van Limbeek J, van Deuren M, Schoorl M, Bet PM, van Houte AJ. Cytokine profiles during clinical high-flux dialysis: no evidence for cytokine generation by circulating monocytes. J Am Soc Nephrol 1997; 8:1745–1754.
36. Churchill DN. Clinical impact of biocompatible dialysis membranes on patient morbidity and mortality: an appraisal of the evidence. Nephrol Dial Transplant 1995; 10(suppl):52–56.
37. Locatelli F. Influence of membranes on morbidity. Nephrol Dial Transplant 1996; 11(suppl. 2):116–120.
38. Baz M, Durand C, Ragon A, Jaber K. Andrieu D, Merzouk T, Purugs R, Olmer M, Reynier JP, Berland Y. Using ultrapure water in hemodialysis delays carpal tunnel syndrome. Int J Artif Organs 1991; 14:681–685.
39. Floege J, Koch KM. Beta-2-microglobulin associated amyloidosis and therapy with high flux hemodialysis membranes. Clin Nephrol 1994; 42(suppl. 1):S52–S56.
40. Koda Y, Nishi S, Miyazaki S, Haginoshita S, Sakurabayashi T, Suzuki M, Sakai S, Yuasa Y, Hirasawa Y, Nishi T. Switch from conventional to high flux membrane reduces the risk of carpal tunnel syndrome and mortality of hemodialysis. Kidney Int 1997; 52:1096–1101.
41. Schwalbe S, Holzhauer M, Schaeffer J, Galanski M, Koch KM, Floege J. β_2-Microglobulin associated amyloidosis: a vanishing complication of hemodialysis? Kidney Int 1997; 52:1077–1083.
42. Klein E. Effects of disinfectants in renal dialysis patients. Environ Health Perspect 1986; 69:45.
43. Gordon SM, Bland LA, Alexander SR, Newman HF, Arduino MJ, Jarvis WR. Hemolysis associated with hydrogen peroxide at a pediatric dialysis center. Am J Nephrol 1990; 10:123.
44. Ng YY, Chow MP, Lyou JY, Huh Y, Yung CH, Fan CD, Huang TP. Resistance to erythropoietin: immuno-hemolytic anemia induced by residual formaldehyde in dialyzers. Am J Kidney Dis 1993; 21:213.
45. Orringer EP, Mattern WD. Formaldehyde-induced hemolysis during chronic hemodialysis. N Engl J Med 1976; 294:1416.
46. Klein WJ, Metz EN, Price AR. Acute copper intoxication. A hazard of hemodialysis. Arch Intern Med 1972; 129:578.
47. Ward DM. Chloramine removal from water used in hemodialysis. Adv Renal Replace Ther 1996; 3:337.
48. Carlson DJ, Shapiro FI. Methemoglobinemia from well water nitrates: a complication of home dialysis. Ann Intern Med 1970; 73:757.
49. Arnow PM, Bland LA, Garcia-Houchins S, Fridkin S, Fellner SK. An outbreak of fatal fluoride intoxication in a long-term hemodialysis unit. Ann Intern Med 1994; 131:339.
50. McIvor M, Baltazar RF, Beltran J, Mower MM, Wend R, Lustgarten J, Salomon J. Hyperkalemia and cardiac arrest from fluoride exposure during hemodialysis. Am J Cardiol 1983; 51:901.
51. Wathen RL, Burcham CW. Understanding the dangers of fluoride during dialysis. Nephrol News Issues 1993; (Sept.):32–36.

3

Complications of Bioincompatibility of Hemodialysis Membranes

Brian J. G. Pereira
Tufts University School of Medicine, New England Medical Center, Boston, Massachusetts

Alfred K. Cheung
University of Utah School of Medicine, Veterans Affairs Medical Center, Salt Lake City, Utah

I. INTRODUCTION

During hemodialysis, blood comes into contact with several components of the extracorporeal circuit (Table 1). These include the dialyzer itself (dialysis membrane, sterilants used during the manufacturing process, and substances that leach from the dialyzer), extracorporeal circuit (temporary vascular access, blood lines, and cannulas), chemicals used for reprocessing (germicides and cleansing agents), and contaminants in the dialysate. While exposure to each of the above can result in perturbations of cellular or plasma components of blood, this chapter will restrict its focus to the dialyzer membrane.

II. BIOMATERIALS USED FOR ARTIFICIAL KIDNEY MEMBRANES

Biomaterials for hemodialysis membranes are broadly classified into unsubstituted cellulose, substituted (modified) cellulose, and synthetic (Table 2).

A. Unsubstituted Cellulose Membranes

These membranes are composed of regenerated cellulose in which the basic structure is a linear chain of glucosan rings with free surface hydroxyl groups. Cuprophan membranes were developed by regeneration of cellulose using the cuprammonium process (a modification of the process for preparing cellophane). These cuprammonium membranes have been used extensively for hemodialysis since they can be made thin, are mechanically strong, and provide good diffusive transport properties for small solutes. Although the name Cuprophan is often used to describe all cuprammonium membranes, the fact that cuprammonium membranes are manufactured by several other companies, and are not identical, should be remembered. All regenerated cellulose membranes are highly hydrophilic because of the large number of free hydroxyl groups on the cellulose monomer and are homogeneous in structure—their porosity is similar throughout the entire membrane thickness. While the original cellulose membranes had low permeability to solutes larger than urea, cellulose membranes with high permeability to larger solutes are currently available.

B. Substituted (Modified) Cellulose

The substitution of the free surface hydroxyl groups on cellulose membranes results in "substituted" or "modified" cellulose membranes. Accordingly, substitution of an increasing fraction of the surface free hydroxyl groups with acetyl residues leads to cellulose acetate, cellulose diacetate, and cellulose triacetate membranes, respectively. Cellulose acetate and cellulose triacetate

Table 1 Components of the Extracorporeal Circuit that Play a Role in Biocompatibility

Dialysis component	Determinants of biocompatibility
Dialyzer	Membrane material
	Geometry of blood path
	Sieving coefficient
Dialysis components	Blood lines
	Vascular access devices
Sterilant	Ethylene oxide/Steam/Gamma ray
Residual material	Phthalate
Reuse	Automatic/Manual
	Number of reuses
	Germicide/Physical agent
	Cleansing agent
Dialysate	Acetate/Bicarbonate
	Water treatment
	Bacterial contamination

membranes are more hydrophobic than regenerated cellulose membranes because of acetylation of the hydroxyl moieties on the cellulose monomer. Substitution of the hydroxyl radicals on cellulose with the tertiary amino residue diethylaminoethyl (DEAE) is the principle behind the manufacture of Hemophan® membranes (1–3). In general, substituted/modified cellulose membranes have substantially less complement-activating potential than unsubstituted cellulose membranes. A new-generation cellulose membrane, Excebrane, has recently been developed by covalent binding of synthetic block polymers to the hydroxyl groups on cellulose. In addition to the reduced complement-activating potential, the oleyl alcohol and vitamin E incorporated into the synthetic surface reduce thrombosis and provide antioxidant reserves, respectively (4).

C. Synthetic (Noncellulose)

Synthetic membranes were developed during the 1970s, primarily for use as hemofilters. AN69 was originally prepared from a copolymer of acrylonitrile and methallyl sulfonate. The latter polymer contains negatively charged ionizable groups. This property was originally deemed desirable for a dialysis membrane because a negatively charged membrane might mimic the glomerular basement membrane (5). However, recent studies demonstrate that such negative charges may impart a specific bioincompatible characteristic. The AN69 membrane is also morphologically homogeneous (6). Polysulfone and polyamide membranes were originally developed for use as hemofilters and were highly asymmetrical and hydrophobic. Such membranes required a thick supporting layer to impart mechanical strength to the thin and highly porous inner skin of the hollow fiber. Diffusion rates for small solutes across these membranes were therefore low. Addition of polyvinylpyrolidone into the manufacturing process (7,8) led to membranes that exhibited high diffusive as well as high convective permeability properties. Such membranes are asymmetrical (6,9) but exhibit a sponge- or foam-like structure, not the large finger-like pores of the original membranes. Polysulfone membranes are now commercially available with

Table 2 Classification of Hemodialysis Membranes

Group	Membrane	Structure
Cellulose	Cellulose	Glucosan rings with free hydroxyl (OH^-) groups
	Cuprophan	Dissolution of purified cellulose in ammonia solution of cupric oxide
Substituted or modified cellulose	Cellulose acetate (CA)	Substitution of increasing proportion of OH^- with acetate results in CA, CDA, and CTA, respectively
	Cellulose diacetate (CDA)	
	Cellulose triacetate (CTA)	
	Hemophan	Substitution of OH^- with diethylaminoethyl
	Excebrane	Synthetic block polymers covalently bound to OH^-. Additional synthetic surface containing oleyl alcohol and vitamin E
Synthetic	Polyacrilonitrile (PAN)	
	Polysulfone (PS)	
	Polyamide (PA)	
	Polymethylmethacrylate (PMMA)	
	Polycarbonate	

a wide range of pore sizes. Other synthetic membranes in clinical use include polyacrylonitrile (PAN), polymethylmethacrylate (PMMA), and polycarbonate. With the exception of polycarbonate, all these synthetic membranes are hydrophobic and tend to adsorb cells and plasma proteins. In contrast, hydrophilic membranes such as polycarbonate activate cells and proteins. However, the manufacturing methods for a given biomaterial can vary between manufacturers and, consequently, the biocompatibility of a given membrane.

"High flux" refers to membranes with larger pore size that possess high ultrafiltration coefficients and permit clearances of larger solutes (middle molecules). Although high-flux dialyzers were originally manufactured with synthetic membranes, cellulose membranes can also be configured to have larger pore sizes by altering the manufacturing process. Conversely, synthetic membranes can be manufactured as low-flux dialyzers. Dialyzers with cellulose membranes are often termed "conventional" dialyzers because of the modest urea clearances and relatively small pores. However, urea clearance can be significantly enhanced by increasing the surface area, and such dialyzers are termed "high-efficiency" dialyzers.

III. BIOCOMPATIBILITY OF DIALYSIS MEMBRANES

During dialysis, the blood-membrane interactions can lead to activation of the complement, kinin, coagulation, and fibrinolytic pathways, as well as cellular elements such as neutrophils, monocytes, and lymphocytes. In general, a biocompatible dialysis membrane refers to one that elicits little or no reaction from the patient as the result of blood contact with the biomaterials. Reactions resulting from ultrafiltration of fluid or exchanges of electrolytes through the semipermeable membrane are usually excluded from these discussions.

A. Complement Activation

Since the early 1980s, complement activation has been the "gold standard" for assessment of dialysis membrane biocompatibility. Consequently, membranes are often classified as biocompatible or bioincompatible, based on their ability to activate complement. The complement system is comprised of two cascades of plasma proteins that can be sequentially activated by proteolytic enzymes (10). Activation of either the classical pathway or the alternative pathway leads to activation of C3 and, under conducive conditions, activation of the terminal components (C5, C6, C7, C8, C9). Complement activation by cuprophan and cellulose acetate membranes occurs primarily via the alternative pathway (Fig. 1) (11–14), although the classical pathway may also contribute. The mechanism by which complement activation occurs on other membranes is less certain. Nonetheless, complement activation leads to activation of multiple cell systems, which in turn can have significant clinical implications (Table 3).

1. Complement Activation Associated with Different Hemodialysis Membranes

Based on plasma $C3a_{desArg}$ concentrations, cuprophan and unsubstituted cellulose membranes are the most potent complement activators among dialysis membranes (Fig. 2) (11,15). Plasma $C3a_{desArg}$ concentrations usually peak 10–20 minutes after starting dialysis and decline to almost baseline values by the end of the treatment. On a molar basis, plasma $C5a_{desArg}$ and

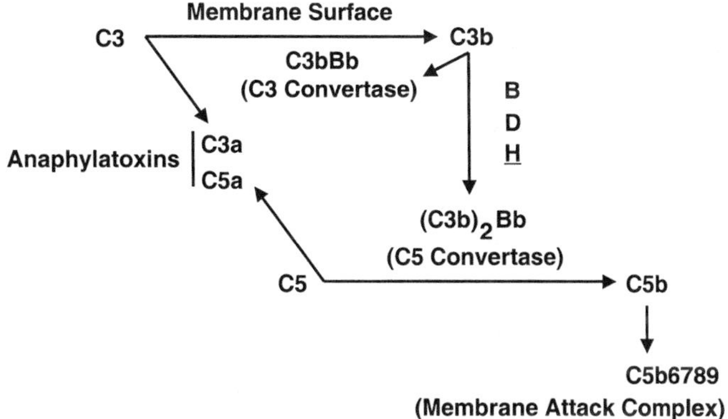

Fig. 1 Schematic diagram of complement activation via the alternative pathway on the membrane surface. Underlined text inhibits reaction.

Table 3 Cellular and Clinical Consequences of Complement Activation

Target cells	Mediator(s)	Actions	Potential clinical consequences
Mast cells Basophils	Histamine Leukotrienes	Increase vascular permeability Smooth muscle contraction	First-use syndrome Pulmonary edema Peripheral edema Hypoxemia
Neutrophils	Leukotrienes Reactive oxygen species Proteases Platelet-activating factor	Release of β_2-microglobulin Polymerization of β_2-microglobulin Upregulation adhesion molecules Platelet activation Phagocytic abnormalities Endothelial damage	Neutropenia Altered immunity Tissue damage
Platelets	Thromboxanes Prostaglandins	Aggregation Degranulation Adhesion to endothelial cells Coagulation	Thrombocytopenia Bleeding abnormalities Clotting abnormalities
Monocytes	Cytokines	See Table 4	See Table 4

SC5b-9 levels are usually lower than those of $C3a_{desArg}$ (11,15,16), because activation of the late components of complement is usually less efficient than that of C3 (17). Binding of C5a to its receptor on neutrophil surfaces may also lower its plasma levels to a modest extent (18). Substituted cellulose membranes such as cellulose acetate and Hemophan® are associated with lower C3a levels than cuprophan (19). Cellulose triacetate membranes and the synthetic polymer membranes are associated with lower plasma C3a levels than cuprophan or cellulose acetate (11,16,20,21).

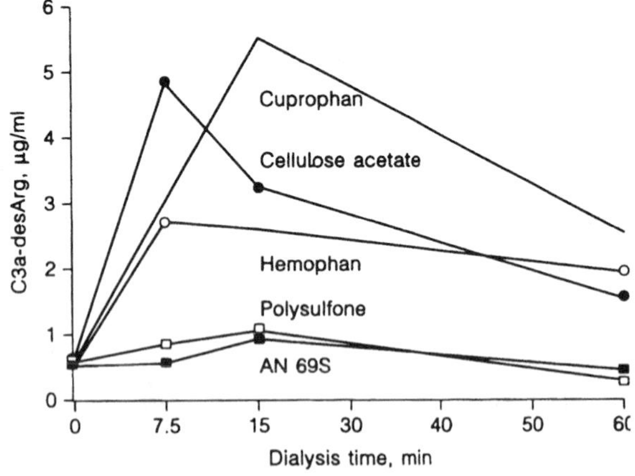

Fig. 2 C3a generation using different dialysis membranes. Cuprophan: GFS Gambro 12H (1.3 m^2); cellulose acetate: CD4000. CD-Medical (1.4 m^2): Hemophan: GFS Gambro 120 Plus (1.3 m^2); Polysulfone: Fresenius F 60 (1.25 m^2); AN 69S: Filtral 12 (1.3 m^2), Hospal. (From Ref. 233.)

Nonetheless, all dialysis membranes in clinical use, without exception, are associated with complement activation, albeit to differing degrees.

Complement activation by cuprophan membrane can be attenuated by cooling the extracorporeal blood (22), chelation of Mg^{2+} in the plasma during citrate hemodialysis (23), or increasing the amount of heparin in the circuit (24). Cuprophan membranes reprocessed with formaldehyde or peracetic acid are also associated with less complement activation and leukopenia than new dialyzers (15,20,25). This reduction is presumably because of the presence of inactive C3 fragments (13) or other proteins on the used membrane surface, which inhibit amplification of the alternative pathway. Cleansing of reprocessed cuprophan membranes with sodium hypochlorite restores complement activation and leukopenia to levels similar to those with new dialyzers (25). This is presumably because sodium hypochlorite effectively removes the proteins on the membrane surfaces (13).

2. Clinical Dialysis

The acute effects of intradialytic complement activation on patients are controversial. These effects are primarily inferred from the known biological activities of complement activation products and the fact that the complement system is activated during dialysis. Dialysis-induced peripheral leukopenia has traditionally been attributed to C5a and its ability to modulate neutrophil surface adhesion molecules, although there is evidence that noncomplement factors, such as platelet-activating factors, are also involved. Anaphylatoxins may also cause acute pulmonary hypertension [demonstrated during sham hemodialysis in uremic patients using cuprophan membrane (26)] and contribute to the development of hypoxemia. Because of their ability to release histamine from mast cells, anaphylatoxins may be responsible for some of the allergy-like symptoms on dialysis. Since the spasmogenic properties of anaphylatoxins are markedly diminished when they are degraded to their desarginine derivatives by serum carboxypeptidase, the ability of these peptides to induce acute intradialytic symptoms would not be as great as their plasma levels (as determined by immunoassays) may indicate. However, during hemodialysis, carboxypeptidase activity has been shown to be diminished (27). Depending on the magnitude of generation, the rate at which they are inactivated and catabolized, as well as the sensitivity of the end organs, anaphylatoxins may rarely cause anaphylactoid reactions in susceptible individuals. However, some investigators dispute this association.

More recent investigations have concentrated on the potential subacute and chronic effects of complement activation during hemodialysis. Both C5a and iC3b are well known to have neutrophil-modulating properties. Stimulation of neutrophils by these complement proteins promotes the release of oxygen radicals (28) and intragranular proteases (18,29,30) from the cells, which may result in catabolism of plasma proteins and injury of other tissues such as the kidneys. C5a has also been shown to promote the production of cytokines from monocytes (31) and the release of β_2-microglobulin from peripheral blood monocytes (32), which may contribute to the development of amyloidosis. Definitive demonstration of the roles of complement in clinical problems associated with hemodialysis may require the ability to inhibit its activation. Inhibition of complement activation during hemodialysis using specific inhibitors, such as soluble complement receptor type 1 (sCR1), has only been studied in vitro (33). Chelation of divalent cations and the administration of protease inhibitors can also inhibit complement activation, but their effects are relatively nonspecific.

B. Neutrophil Activation

1. Hemodialysis-Induced Leukopenia

Leukopenia during hemodialysis has been one of the earliest indices of membrane bioincompatibility. The onset is usually rapid, occurring within the first 2–3 minutes, and is maximum at 10–15 minutes (11,34). Leukocyte counts usually return to normal by the end of dialysis and sometimes exceed the predialysis values. Neutrophils and other granulocytes are primarily affected. Although granulocytes are readily seen on the dialyzer membrane surface under microscopy (35,36), the disappearance of these cells from the circulation is primarily due to sequestration in the pulmonary vasculature. Pulmonary leukosequestration has been demonstrated using radiolabeled cells in clinical studies (37). Binding of C5a and $C5a_{desArg}$ to their specific receptors has been considered to be the primary mechanism behind dialysis-induced neutropenia. In general, the degree of complement activation correlates closely with the degree of leukopenia (2,3,15,19,20,22,23,38). More recently, alterations in several other receptors on the neutrophil surface, which may or may not be related to C5a, have also been incriminated in the development and resolution of dialysis-induced leukopenia. Platelet-activating factor and leukotriene B_4 released from the activated neutrophils can further promote cell aggregation. Transient neutropenia during hemodialysis by itself may be of less significance than the accompanying events, such as the release of reactive oxygen species from stimulated neutrophils and dysfunction of circulating neutrophils. However, the degree of neutropenia may, under some but not all circumstances, serve as a marker of these other events.

2. Degranulation

Several proteins stored in the azurophilic and specific granules of neutrophils possess proteolytic, antimicrobial, and/or cell-modulating properties. Release of these intracellular constituents (degranulation) in response to specific inflammatory stimuli is essential for host defense (39). Although neutrophil degranulation during hemodialysis has been well documented (40–42), the mechanisms that mediate this process have not been elucidated. Based on in vitro degranulating activities of C3a and C5a (29,30,43), these anaphylatoxins have been postulated to participate in dialysis-induced neutrophil degranulation. However, plasma concentrations of the granular proteins during clinical dialysis do not correlate closely with plasma C3a levels. For example, dialysis with PMMA membranes is associated with lower plasma C3a levels but higher plasma elastase levels than with cuprophan (40–42). Additional evidence suggests that noncomplement plasma factor/s also contribute to neutrophil degranulation induced by cuprophan membranes (18) and perhaps other membranes as well. Mechanical shearing of the cells possibly plays a role in this phenomenon. In support of this hypothesis is the observation that clinical dialysis using cuprophan plate dialyzers induced higher plasma levels of elastase and lactoferrin than with hollow fiber dialyzers (44). Proteolytic enzymes that are released into plasma as a result of neutrophil degranulation may contribute to the protein catabolic state that is observed during clinical dialysis (45,46).

3. Release of Reactive Oxygen Species

The release of reactive oxygen species (ROS) is an important mechanism by which neutrophils injure foreign tissues. Clinical studies have shown that cuprophan membranes induced substantially greater ROS production than PMMA membranes (47). One of the mediators in this process is likely to be C5a. The release of ROS by activated neutrophils during dialysis may alter surrounding tissues, such as plasma proteins and lipids (48). Endothelium that is exposed to activated neutrophils sequestered in the lungs (49) and the kidneys (50) may potentially be affected as well.

4. Dysfunction

When neutrophils are activated by hemodialysis membrane, they temporarily lose their ability to respond to subsequent stimuli. The resultant abnormalities include alterations in cell surface receptors, decrease in aggregation and adherence (51,52), and defective oxidative metabolism and chemiluminescence (53,54). These abnormalities are often above and beyond those observed with uremia per se. An early study by Henderson and colleagues showed that while cellulose acetate membranes adversely affected phagocytosis and random motility of neutrophils in vitro, polysulfone membranes did not (55). In a subsequent study, Vanholder and colleagues randomly assigned 15 new patients with end-stage renal disease to dialysis using low-flux cuprophan or low-flux polysulfone membranes (56). Although both groups experienced deterioration in neutrophil function upon initiation of chronic hemodialysis, the deterioration with cuprophan was greater than that with polysulfone (Fig. 3). Neutrophil dysfunction following exposure to dialysis membrane impairs host defense mechanisms when infectious microorganisms are subsequently encountered. Therefore, dialysis membrane bioincompatibility probably contributes to impaired immunity in hemodialysis patients.

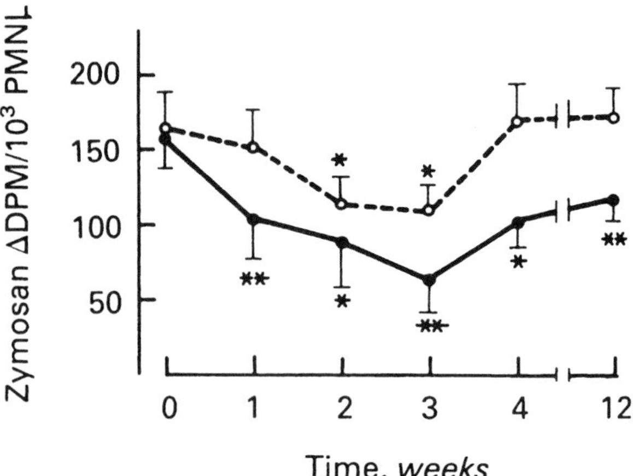

Fig. 3 Glucose-1-C^{14} utilization by polymorphonuclear leukocytes (PMNL) expressed as Δ disintegration per minutes (DPM) per 10^3 PMNL in response to zymosan for patients maintained on hemodialysis with cuprophan membrane dialyzers (---) and polysulfone (——) dialyzers for 12 weeks after initiation of hemodialysis. $*p < 0.05$. $**p < 0.01$ from initiation of dialysis. The difference between both groups was statistically significant at all time points (except 2nd week). (From Ref. 56.)

C. Lymphocytes and Natural Killer Cells

Limited data are available on the effects of dialysis membranes on lymphocytes, probably because significant intradialytic lymphopenia is not a common event, the effects of complement on lymphocytes is less prominent (57,58), and the methods of studying lymphocytes are often more complicated. Activation of T lymphocytes during hemodialysis has been detected by changes in cell surface markers such as interleukin-2 receptor (IL-2R). In the presence of interleukin-1 (IL-1), stimulation of T lymphocytes by antigens leads to the release of interleukin-2 (IL-2) and the expression of its receptor (IL-2R) on the cell surface. Binding of IL-2 to IL-2R is important in T-cell proliferation and the development of functionally active effector T cells (59). Expression of IL-2R is increased when T lymphocytes are activated. The high-affinity IL-2R receptor is comprised of an α and a β chain. Under certain conditions, the α chain (Tac or p55) is released into the plasma and is known as soluble IL-2R. Plasma soluble IL-2R retains the ability to bind IL-2, thereby reducing the availability of the cytokine to interact with cell surface IL-2R. Elevated plasma level of soluble IL-2R therefore reflects both a state of T-lymphocyte activation and a downregulation of IL-2 effects.

Different dialysis membranes affect T cells differently. Zaoui and colleagues observed that dialysis with cuprophan membranes was associated with greater expression of IL-2R on T lymphocytes compared to with

PMMA membrane (60). When the cells were stimulated in vitro using phytohemagglutinin, those that had been exposed to cuprophan responded poorly. Others have shown that in vitro proliferation of T lymphocytes obtained from patients on chronic dialysis with polysulfone membrane was normal but was impaired among patients on cuprophan membranes. These data suggest that T lymphocytes are activated during hemodialysis with cuprophan membranes and subsequently become dysfunctional. The mechanism(s) by which T cells are activated by cuprophan membranes is unclear, but they may be related to its ability to activate complement (60) and monocytes (61). Abnormal T-cell function may predispose dialysis patients to various infections.

Natural killer (NK) cells are normal peripheral leukocytes with cytotoxic activity against tumor cells, microorganism, infected cells, and transplanted tissues. NK cell counts have been shown to increase during chronic clinical dialysis using cuprophan membranes, but their in vitro cytotoxic function (against K562 cells) was impaired (62). In vitro studies suggest that different types of dialysis membranes have different effects on NK cell function, with cuprophan faring worse than cellulose acetate or polycarbonate membranes (63,64). Whether the higher incidence of malignancy among ESRD patients (65,66) is related to NK cell dysfunction has not been determined.

B lymphocytes have also been found to be activated during clinical dialysis using cuprophan, cellulose acetate, or polysulfone membranes, but not with AN69 (67). The mechanisms behind intradialytic B-cell activation are unknown.

D. Monocyte Activation

Cytokines are polypeptides with molecular weights of 10–45 kDa. These are highly potent molecules, active at picomolar and femtomolar concentrations, and synthesized by cells in response to infection, inflammation, or trauma (68–70). There are currently more than a dozen cytokines that have been designated as interleukins (71). In addition, cytokines such as tumor necrosis factor, interferon, transforming growth factor, and colony-stimulating factors continue to be known by their original names (71). In 1983, the "interleukin hypothesis" was proposed, incriminating IL-1 produced during dialysis as the cause of hypotension, fever, and other acute phase responses observed in patients on hemodialysis (72). Indeed, both studies using in vitro models of hemodialysis as well as clinical studies in patients on hemodialysis have demonstrated increased production of a variety of pro-inflammatory cytokines such as interleukin-1 (IL-1) and tumor necrosis factor (TNF) during hemodialysis (69,70,73). Over the decade since this hypothesis, a better understanding of the biological effects of pro-inflammatory cytokines, and the close similarities between dialysis-related morbidity and the biological effects of these cytokines, have further strengthened the possibility that cytokines could be involved in dialysis-related symptoms (Table 4) (69,70,73).

1. Plasma Cytokine Levels

Predialysis plasma levels of IL1 and TNF have been shown to be elevated in patients on chronic hemodi-

Table 4 Cellular and Clinical Consequences of Cytokine Production

Biological actions of interleukin-1 in human volunteers/experimental models	Potential clinical consequences
Fever, sleepiness, anorexia, myalgia, arthralgia, headache, gastrointestinal disturbances, hypotension	Fever, sleepiness, anorexia, myalgia, arthralgia, headache, gastrointestinal disturbances, hypotension
Proliferation of vascular smooth muscle cells Stimulation of platelet-derived growth factor Atherosclerotic plaques	Accelerated atherosclerosis
Synthesis of collagenases Osteoblast activation mRNA for phospholipase A_2 and cyclooxygenase	Bone and joint disease
Suppression of albumin gene expression	Hypoalbuminemia
Muscle proteolysis Negative nitrogen balance	Muscle wasting

alysis using cellulose membranes (74–79). Interestingly, undialyzed patients with ESRD did not show evidence of elevated IL-1 levels (78), leading to the conclusion that the hemodialysis procedure itself rather than that renal failure leads to increased IL-1 production. This hypothesis was further strengthened by the observation that hemodialysis with these "bioincompatible" cellulose membranes leads to a further rise in plasma levels of TNF-α (78,80,81). In contrast, dialysis with "biocompatible" membranes such as PAN was not associated with a further rise in plasma levels of TNF-α (80,81). In fact, in some studies, plasma levels of TNF-α declined during dialysis with PAN membranes (81). However, others have failed to show elevated plasma levels of IL-1β or TNF-α either before, during, or after a hemodialysis treatment (82–84).

More recently, using specific radioimmunoassays, predialysis plasma levels of IL-1β and TNF-α in hemodialysis patients were shown to be higher than those in healthy controls (85). However, plasma levels of IL-1β and TNF-α were also elevated in undialyzed patients with chronic renal failure (CRF) and patients on continuous ambulatory peritoneal dialysis (CAPD), and there were no significant differences in the plasma levels of these cytokines between CRF, CAPD, or HD patients. Similar results have been reported by Herbelin and colleagues who found elevated plasma levels of TNF-α and IL-6 in both undialyzed patients with ESRD as well as patients on HD (78,86). Elevated plasma cytokine levels among patients with renal insufficiency could be due to increased production and/or decreased clearance. Indeed, several investigators have demonstrated a strong linear correlation between plasma cytokine levels and serum creatinine (85,87). This correlation suggests that the kidney has an important role in the metabolism and/or clearance of these molecules. Further, the fact that the plasma levels of IL-1β and TNF-α were not significantly different between undialyzed CRF, CAPD, and HD patients suggests that these dialysis modalities may not significantly affect the clearance of these proteins. Interestingly, studies in septic patients on continuous arteriovenous hemofiltration with polyacrylonitrile membranes have shown that TNF-α is removed from the circulation by adsorption to the membrane and to a lesser extent by ultrafiltration (88). This suggests that although these proteins may be to some extent be cleared by dialysis, the clearance may not match the natural excretion by the kidney.

2. Cytokine Production by Peripheral Blood Mononuclear Cells

Peripheral blood mononuclear cells (PBMC) from patients on chronic hemodialysis show signs of mononuclear cell activation. Interleukin-1 is present in the mononuclear cells of patients on dialysis (75,89–91). In contrast, mononuclear cells isolated from healthy subjects do not contain IL-1 protein nor mRNA for IL-1 using Northern hybridization or polymerase chain reaction. Even after 24 hours of incubation, there is no evidence of IL-1 synthesis in the mononuclear cells of healthy donors (92,93). However, incubation of mononuclear cells from patients undergoing chronic hemodialysis in the absence of exogenous stimuli results in spontaneous IL-1 production (89,91). When these cells are stimulated with LPS, they produce as much as fivefold more IL-1 compared to mononuclear cells from normal subjects (75,89–91). Similar results have been reported for the production of TNF and IL-6 (94–96).

In vitro studies have shown that when human blood is circulated through a hollow fiber cuprophan membrane, transcription of mRNA for IL-1 is apparent within 2 hours. However, in the absence of endotoxin in the dialysate, there is no translation into IL-1 protein (Fig. 4) (97). Similarly, mononuclear cells drawn from the arterial limb of the dialysis circuit in patients on chronic HD contain a small but significant amount of IL-1β and TNF-α (98,99). However, within 5 minutes of dialysis with a new cuprophan membrane, the mononuclear cells in the blood from the venous limb demonstrate abundant messenger RNA for IL-1β and TNF-α. Interestingly, the mononuclear cells returning to the dialyzer from the arterial side do not show evidence of IL-1 gene expression (99). A single pass through a cuprophan membrane is apparently sufficient to trigger transcription, and once activated, the mononuclear cells do not return into the circulation during the course of the dialysis session. In contrast to cuprophan membranes, cytokine genes are not activated by membranes that are weak complement activators during either in vitro or clinical dialysis (97,99).

Thus, among patients on hemodialysis with cellulose membranes, cytokine gene expression takes place in the absence of contaminated dialysate. These cells can either degrade their mRNA without translation into cytokine protein or receive a second signal from ongoing infection or illness, leading to rapid and efficient translation into cytokine protein. However, the most likely source of a second signal is the dialysate (Fig. 4) (100).

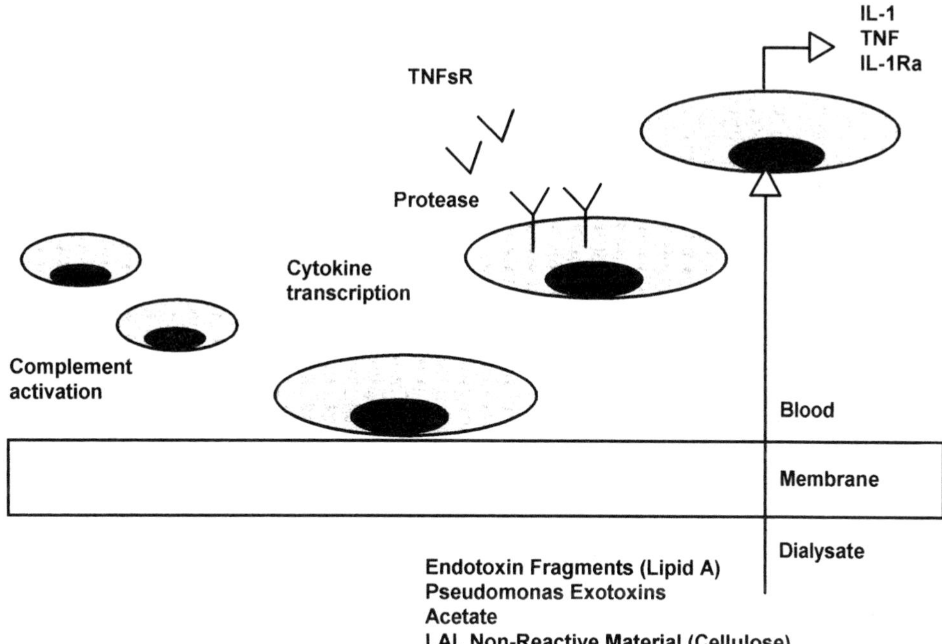

Fig. 4 Potential mechanisms for cytokine production during dialysis. Complement activation by dialysis membranes leads to transcription of mRNA for interleukin-1 (IL-1) and tumor necrosis factor (TNF) in monocytes. In the absence of a "second signal," the mRNA for those cytokines is not translated into protein. The second signal could potentially come from the dialysate, leading to synthesis of IL-1, TNF, as well as interleukin-1 receptor antagonist (IL-1Ra). Concurrently, proteases cleave the extracellular fragment of the TNF receptors resulting in soluble TNF receptors (TNFsR). Thus, the hemodialysis procedure serves as a stimulus for cytokines such as IL-1 and TNF, as well as their specific antagonists. (From Ref. 100.)

In the absence of a second stimulus, it is unclear where the mRNA-primed mononuclear cells exit the circulation during the 5 hours of HD. Certainly, a large pool of cells could be adhering to endothelium, particularly in the lung. Further, receptors on monocytes and adhesion molecules on endothelial cells may attract activated monocytes to the synovium or into other tissues.

3. Cytokine Production by Peripheral Blood Mononuclear Cells—An Index of the Transmembrane Passage of Bacterial Products from the Dialysate

The increasing popularity of high-flux as well as high-efficiency membranes and the associated risk for backfiltration (101) have raised concerns that patients dialyzed with these membranes may be at a high risk of being exposed to bacterial contaminants in the dialysate (102). Further, the risk of passage of bacterial products from the dialysate to the blood compartment could potentially be exacerbated by reprocessing of high-flux dialyzers, which has been shown to increase the permeability of the membranes (103,104). Indeed, the U.S. Centers for Disease Control and Prevention has reported a significant correlation between pyrogen reactions during dialysis and the use of high-flux as well as reprocessed dialyzers (105). In contrast, others have not found an increased incidence of pyrogen reactions among patients dialyzed with high-flux dialyzers compared to conventional or high-efficiency dialyzers (106).

The molecular weight of endotoxins is estimated to be $\sim 1 \times 10^6$ daltons. On the basis of their sizes, endotoxins are not expected to traverse intact dialysis membranes, including high-flux membranes. However, cytokine-inducing products derived from bacteria are not limited to the whole endotoxin particles. The lipid A portion of endotoxins and other fragments of bacteria such as muramyl peptides also possess monocyte-stimulating activities. Indeed, cytokine production by PBMC is a sensitive indicator of the presence of endotoxin (68). Consequently, several authors have designed in vitro models of hemodialysis in which the reverse transfer of cytokine-inducing substances from intentionally contaminated dialysate was used to assess the permeability of different hemodialysis (HD) membranes to bacterial products (107–111). Using cytokine production as an index of the reverse transfer of bacterial products from the dialysate to blood compartment, several studies have demonstrated that high-flux synthetic membranes such as polyamide or polysulfone are less likely to permit the transfer of bacterial products from the dialysate than low-flux cellulose membrane such as cuprophan or Hemophan (107,110). Further, transmembrane passage of bacterial products has been shown to occur in the absence of backfiltration, suggesting an important role for diffusive transfer of these toxins across dialysis membranes (107). Synthetic membranes such as polysulfone and polyacrylonitrile bind significantly higher amounts of I^{125}-labeled lipopolysaccharide than cuprophan membranes (112). Hence, it is postulated that the interaction between hydrophobic domains on the synthetic membranes and hydrophobic domains on the bacterial toxins leads to avid adsorption of these toxins on the dialysate side of the membrane and prevents the transfer into the blood compartment (113). This characteristic could be considered to be another index of biocompatibility.

4. Clinical Effects of Dialysis-Induced Monocyte Activation

The hypothesis that cytokine production is a contributing cause of several of the acute and chronic metabolic and inflammatory changes associated with hemodialysis is based on the fact that similar signs and symptoms are also observed in (1) healthy volunteers or experimental animals administered cytokines, and (2) diseases such as rheumatoid arthritis, inflammatory bowel disease, some chronic infections and cancers, and various collagen vascular diseases where the pathophysiology is largely attributed to enhanced cytokine production (68–70). Healthy human volunteers administered IL-1 in doses of 10–100 ng/kg develop fever, sleepiness, anorexia, myalgia, arthralgia, headache, and gastrointestinal disturbances and in larger doses (>300 ng/kg), hypotension (68–70). Likewise, when injected into humans at low concentrations (<1 μg/kg), TNF produces hypotension and leukopenia as well as metabolic dysfunction. Indeed, IL-1 and TNF are highly synergistic in both animal and in vitro studies and act synergistically in the production of hemodynamic shock (114). IL-1 and TNF also induce a rapid increase in slow wave sleep (68–70). The similarity between these signs and symptoms observed during experimental administration of pro-inflammatory cytokines and the fever, hypotension, fatigue, somnolence, and other acute phase responses observed during hemodialysis was the basis of the "interleukin hypothesis" (72). However, the further understanding of the biological actions of these cytokines has expanded the scope of the role of cytokines in dialysis-related morbidity. In experimental models, cytokines lead to proliferation of vascular smooth muscle cells, stimulation of platelet-derived growth factor, and atherosclerotic plaques (68–70). Consequently, cytokines may have a role in the accelerated atherosclerosis and cardiovascular morbidity observed in hemodialysis patients. Further, IL-1 and TNF induce osteoblast activation and increase gene expression for phospholipase A_2 and cyclooxygenase (115). In isolated tissues perfused with IL-1, prostaglandin E_2 increases rapidly in the perfusate (116,117). Consequently, cytokines may contribute to various bone, articular, and periarticular diseases. In addition, IL-1 increases the hepatic production of amyloid A, which may contribute to the development of AA amyloidosis. Although amyloid deposits in hemodialysis patients are often composed of β_2-microglobulin, AA amyloid is also seen. The presence of macrophages stained positive for IL-1 and TNF-α in chronic renal failure patients' bones that are afflicted with severe β_2-microglobulin amyloidosis (118) suggests the possibility that these cytokines also participate in the pathogenesis of this disease as well. IL-1 and TNF are also appetite suppressants, but their mechanism of action as anorectic agents is thought to be due to peripheral effects on hepatic metabolism rather than in the central nervous system. Further IL-1, TNF, and IL-6 stimulate hepatic acute phase proteins and suppress albumin synthesis, induce muscle proteolysis and a negative nitrogen balance. Taken together, these actions could contribute to the malnutrition observed in dialysis patients. However, to date, a definitive link between dialysis-induced cytokine production and clinical symptoms, signs, or outcomes has not been demonstrated.

As in the case of neutrophils and T lymphocytes, chronic low-grade activation of monocytes induced by hemodialysis leads to dysfunction of these cells. Monocytes obtained from patients dialyzed with cuprophan membranes for 2 weeks released less IL-1β and TNF-α when stimulated by phytohemagglutinin in vitro than cells from patients who were dialyzed using low-flux PMMA membranes (119). Presumably, this subnormal response would represent a diminished ability of the host to respond appropriately to foreign materials such as infectious microorganisms.

IV. CLINICAL IMPLICATIONS OF DIALYSIS MEMBRANE BIOCOMPATIBILITY

A. Hemodialysis-Induced Hypoxemia and Pulmonary Hypertension

A decrease of 10–15 mmHg in systemic arterial partial oxygen tension (pO_2) commonly occurs during hemodialysis using cuprophan membrane and acetate dialysate (120–122). This hypoxemia is obviously undesirable for patients with underlying cardiopulmonary diseases. There is little question that acetate dialysate is the major contributor to dialysis-induced hypoxemia, presumably because of the loss of carbon dioxide from blood into dialysate (123) and the metabolism of acetate by the body (124). Both mechanisms lead to hypoventilation and a decrease in the respiratory quotient. However, there is substantial evidence to support the contribution of membrane bioincompatibility:

1. Patients on mechanical ventilators with constant minute volume and constant inspired oxygen concentration can still develop hypoxemia during hemodialysis (125).
2. Decrease in pulmonary diffusion capacity (120,126–128) and transthoracic impedance (127), widening of alveolar-arterial oxygen tension gradient (121,128), as well as increase in closing volume (120) and dead space to tidal volume ratio (123) have all been demonstrated during hemodialysis. These aberrations are suggestive of impairment in intrapulmonary gas exchange and cannot be explained by hypoventilation alone.
3. The degree of peripheral leukopenia has been correlated with the degree of hypoxemia (129).
4. Dialysis using cuprophan membranes has been associated with a larger decrease in diffusion capacity compared to PAN membranes (130).
5. Replacement of unsubstituted cellulose membranes with PMMA (122) or PAN (121,131) membranes can ameliorate the hypoxemia.
6. During dialysis with cuprophan membranes, replacement of acetate with bicarbonate dialysate does not necessarily abolish the hypoxemia (129,130), but dialysis using the combination of reused cuprophan membrane and bicarbonate dialysate does (132).
7. Infusion of cuprophan-activated plasma into humans (127) or experimental animals (127,133) causes hypoxemia.
8. Sham hemodialysis without dialysate in normal human volunteers produces hypoxemia (134).

Therefore, it appears that membrane bioincompatibility does play a role in the development of dialysis-induced hypoxemia. This effect is probably more prominent during the early phase of the treatment, when complement activation and leaching of noxious substances is most intense.

Invasive monitoring of pulmonary arterial pressure has documented the development of pulmonary hypertension during dialysis with cuprophan membranes, but not with polycarbonate membranes (26). In some instances, this hemodynamic derangement can lead to clinical symptoms (135). In vitro and animal studies described above suggest that the mechanisms by which dialysis membrane bioincompatibility causes pulmonary hypertension and hypoxemia involve the activation of complement and other humoral factors. Anaphylatoxins cause smooth muscle contraction (136) and in vivo activation of C3 and/or C5 results in pulmonary hypertension in animals (137). Anaphylatoxins stimulate the production of thromboxane and leukotrienes, which are potent airway constrictors (138). In addition, anaphylatoxins increase vascular permeability (139) and may thus cause transient pulmonary interstitial edema. Pulmonary leukosequestration (leukocyte thromboemboli) is likely to be a result of intradialytic complement activation but is unlikely to be the cause of pulmonary hypertension or hypoxemia.

B. Dialyzer Reactions

Occasionally, severe reactions during hemodialysis can be life-threatening to the patient. These reactions, by definition, cannot be attributed to the acute loss of fluid, changes in electrolytes, improper composition of dialysate, and malfunctioning of the dialysis machine. The severity and time of onset are variable. The manifestations include various combinations of hypertension or hypotension, dyspnea, coughing, sneezing, wheezing, choking, rhinorrhea, conjunctival injection, headache, muscle cramps, back pain, abdominal pain, chest pain, nausea, vomiting, fever, chills, flushing, urticaria, and pruritus. Death occasionally occurs (140–152). The term "hypersensitivity reaction" has been used to describe these signs and symptoms. Whether some of these patients are indeed hypersensitive to the offending agents is unclear since the nature and amount of the agents are frequently unknown. Consequently, a more appropriate term is "dialyzer reaction." The etiologies of dialyzer reactions are diverse and have been reviewed elsewhere. Only those relevant to biocompatibility will be discussed here.

1. Ethylene Oxide

Ethylene oxide (ETO) is a sterilant commonly used in the manufacturing process of dialyzers and other equipment. Residual ETO in the dialyzer usually requires days or months to dissipate during storage. Hollow-fiber dialyzers, in particular, retain a substantial amount of ETO because the polyurethane potting materials (used to hold the fibers together at the ends of the dialyzers) are large reservoirs for ETO (153). The dissipation process is therefore slow. Part of this residual ETO is leached into the patient's blood stream during hemodialysis. ETO presumably exerts a toxic effect through the generation of a derivative, 2-chloroethanol, which has been isolated from a patient suffering a severe reaction. Cuprophan membrane was reported to potentiate the generation of this compound (148). More commonly, ETO induces anaphylactic reactions probably by eliciting an allergic response. In this case, it functions as a hapten and combines with albumin or other particles to form antigens. During reexposure in a subsequent dialysis session, the antigens stimulate the presensitized lymphocytes to release IgE, which in turn causes the release of histamine from mast cells and basophils to cause allergic reactions.

There is evidence supporting the role of ETO in dialysis-induced anaphylactoid reactions:

1. Hollow-fiber dialyzers, which trap more ETO (153,154), were associated with a higher incidence of reactions than plate dialyzers in the U.S. survey in the 1980s (149). On an individual basis, some patients experience symptoms with cuprophan hollow fiber but not with cuprophan plate dialyzers (150). In contrast, one European study showed that these reactions were associated primarily with plate dialyzers (151).
2. Some patients with anaphylactic reactions have specific IgE antibodies directed against ETO in their sera, as detected by a standard radioadsorbant test (RAST), even though their serum total IgE levels may not be elevated (151,155). It should be noted that some dialysis patients without anaphylactic reactions and even some dialysis staff also have ETO-specific IgE (155). Conceivably, these individuals also have blocking IgG that is protective. Alternatively, the doses of ETO that they receive during their dialysis treatments may not be large enough to elicit clinical responses.
3. A longitudinal study showed that when ETO-sterilized equipment was withheld from the patients, antibodies to ETO and anaphylactoid reactions decreased (156).

2. Complement Activation

All commercially used dialysis membranes activate complement. Furthermore, uremic plasma is more susceptible than normal plasma to complement activation because it contains substantially more factor D (157), an essential catalytic enzyme in the alternative pathway of complement activation. The potent biological activities of anaphylatoxins in vitro and in animals suggest that they play a role in dialyzer reactions during hemodialysis. The spasmogenic activities of these polypeptides, however, are substantially diminished when they are converted by a serum carboxypeptidase to $C3a_{desArg}$ and $C5a_{desArg}$ (158–160). Since the commonly used immunoassays do not distinguish between the anaphylatoxins and their desarginine derivatives, the plasma concentrations of the uncleaved anaphylatoxins are usually unknown although they are assumed to be small. Conceivably, patients who have unusually active C3 conversion, impaired degradation of anaphylatoxins because of carboxypeptidase deficiency, or enhanced end organ sensitivity would be more likely to suffer from complement-induced reactions. In support of the first possibility is the observation that patients who developed recurrent reactions (respiratory symptoms, chest and back pain, flushing, and/or angioedema) to new cuprophan membrane dialyzers during the initial 15–30 minutes of treatment had higher peak intradialytic plasma $C3a_{(desArg)}$ levels than those who did not have reactions (147). The second possibility, carboxypeptidase deficiency (161), is an uncommon familial disorder, but carboxypeptidase activity has been shown to decrease during hemodialysis (27). Whether the third possibility, enhanced end organ sensitivity, occurs in certain ESRD patients has not been tested. Data on the relationship between complement activation and mild to moderate intradialytic symptoms are conflicting. Some have observed that, compared to cellulose acetate, clinical dialysis using cuprophan was associated with higher plasma $C3a_{(desArg)}$ levels and higher intradialytic symptom scores (19). Using cellulose dialyzers processed with various reuse methods (formaldehyde, peracetic acid, and/or bleach), some investigators have found a linear correlation between symptom scores and plasma $C3a_{(desArg)}$ levels (25). In contrast, a more recent multicenter trial on acute intradialytic symptoms did not demonstrate significant differences between cuprophan and polysulfone membranes (162). Similarly, another recent clinical study failed to find differences in symptoms between cuprophan and AN69 membrane (163).

3. Kinins

Activation of the contact proteins by the membrane surface leads to conversion of high molecular weight kininogen to kinins (Fig. 5) (164). The kinins, such as bradykinin, are potent peptides that increase vascular permeability, diminish arterial resistance, and mediate a variety of inflammatory responses. Intradialytic anaphylactoid reactions have been associated with the use of AN69 membrane and the generation of kinins (165,166). In the anaphylactoid reactions associated with AN69 membrane and angiotensin-converting enzyme inhibitors (ACEI), kinins appear to be the mediators. As discussed earlier, the anionic sulfonate domains of AN69 favors the binding and activation of factor XII, which lead to the subsequent conversion of high molecular weight kininogen to kinins (164,165,167,168). Besides catalyzing the formation of angiotensin II, ACE also functions as a kininase, which inactivates bradykinin. The presence of ACEI therefore allows the accumulation of bradykinin that is generated as a result of blood contact with the AN69 membrane. Conversion of kininogen to bradykinin by AN69 membrane has been demonstrated in vitro (169). Clinical studies showed that intradialytic plasma kinin levels in patients dialyzed with this membrane were significantly elevated and the levels during reactions (170). In the case of reused dialyzers, the sterilants and/or the procedures for reuse processing may be responsible for dialyzer reactions. In sufficient quantities, all sterilants, such as sodium hypochlorite, formaldehyde, and peracetic acid, are toxic. In a recent cluster of anaphylactoid reactions reported with polysulfone membrane, the reactions disappeared after reused was stopped (171).

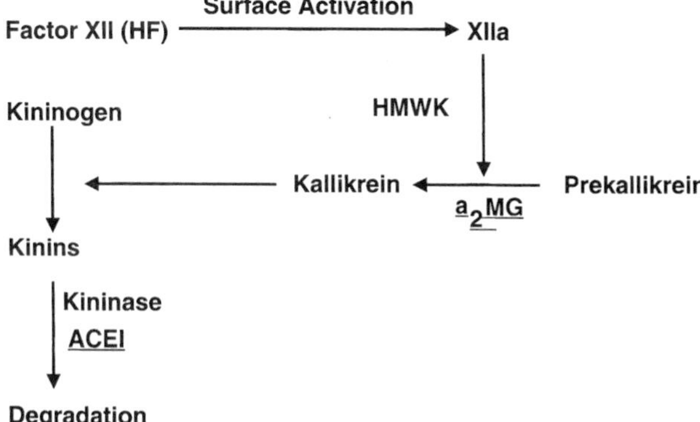

Fig. 5 Schematic diagram of kinin generation on a negatively charged membrane surface. HF, Hageman factor; HMWK, high molecular weight kininogen; a_2MG, alpha$_2$-macroglobulin; ACEI, angiotensin-converting enzyme inhibitor. Underlined text inhibits reaction.

4. Dialysate Contaminants

Dialysate contaminated with bacteria and endotoxins is probably responsible for some of the intradialytic and postdialytic reactions that are characterized by fever and rigors. In these cases, the mediators may be cytokines released from activated monocytes. The incidence of these pyrogenic reactions are relatively rare considering the frequency with which dialysate is contaminated with bacteria in many dialysis units (83,172). Furthermore, the incidence associated with high-flux membranes and conventional membranes are equivalent (172), even though the former have larger pores that potentially allow easier passage of bacterial products. One possible explanation is that some synthetic high-flux membranes also have high capacities to bind endotoxins, thus preventing their entry into the blood compartment (110,173–175). On the other hand, many low-flux cellulose membranes have higher potentials to activate complement and generate anaphylatoxins, which promote the generation of fever-producing cytokines (31,176–178).

5. Management of Dialyzer Reactions

Identification of the etiology of a specific case of dialyzer reaction is often difficult. Careful consideration of all known possibilities, including those related or unrelated to dialysis membranes, and epidemiological investigations are helpful. Direct toxic effects of sterilants should be suspected for reactions that occur immediately (1–2 min) after starting dialysis. Because of the temporal profile of complement activation during hemodialysis, anaphylatoxin-mediated reactions are more likely to occur at 15–30 minutes or later rather than within the first 1–2 minutes of the treatment. Plasma anti-ETO IgE and $C3a_{desArg}$ levels are nonspecific. The clinical picture of fever and rigors raise the possibility of bacterial or endotoxin contamination. When anaphylactoid reactions occur in patients who are taking ACEI and dialyzed with AN69 membrane, this combination should obviously be suspected as the possible offender. Although they are rarely incriminated, dialysis tubing and the type of heparin employed should also be considered.

If the etiology of a specific case cannot be identified, prevention of further episodes is empirical. The strategies include:

1. Vigorous rinsing of the blood and dialysate compartments of the new dialyzer with saline prior to use. Preferably 2 L of saline should be used for the blood side. This removes some ETO and other potentially pathogenic contaminants. Subjecting a new dialyzer to the reuse process prior to first use has been found to decrease allergic symptoms. The effect of this maneuver may be related to the rinsing as part of the process.
2. Increasing the storage time of new dialyzers prior to use would allow more residual ETO to dissipate.
3. Replacement of hollow fiber with plate dialyzers would exclude the potting compounds.
4. Replacement of ETO-treated dialyzers with dialyzers sterilized by other methods (such as heat or irradiation).
5. Meticulous processing of dialyzers and removal of sterilants for reuse.
6. Replacement of strong complement activating membranes with weak complement-activating membranes.
7. Avoid the combination of AN69 membrane and ACEI and, if suspicious in that particular patient, avoid AN69 membrane altogether.
8. Switching dialysis tubing and type of heparin.
9. Prophylactic administration of antihistamine has been successful in ameliorating mild allergic symptoms in some patients.
10. If frequent pyrogenic reactions are encountered, measures that decrease bacterial counts and/or endotoxins in the dialysate should be considered. These include decreasing the storage time of the bicarbonate dialysate or purifying the dialysate by passing it through a hemofilter (110,173,175).

A subset of dialysis patients seems to be more susceptible to anaphylactoid reactions and is likely to experience recurrent symptoms. Special attention should be paid to these patients, especially when some aspects of the dialysis, reuse, or water purification procedures are changed.

Acute treatments for dialysis-induced anaphylactoid reactions are largely symptomatic. Treatment may not be necessary for minor symptoms; some of them disappear spontaneously even if the dialysis treatment is continued. Sneezing and rhinorrhea may be treated with an antihistamine. If the reaction is severe, the dialysis must be stopped immediately. The blood remaining in the extracorporeal circuit probably contains the offending agents and should be discarded. Epinephrine, corticosteroid, and antihistamine all have theoretical basis for treating these reactions, depending on the specific etiology. Hemodynamic support using volume expansion and sympathomimetic agents as well as respiratory therapies should be instituted as necessary.

C. β_2-Microglobulin and Amyloidosis

Amyloid deposit containing β_2-microglobulin (β_2MG) is well recognized as a complication of long-term dialysis (Fig. 6) (179,180). The pathogenesis of this disease is unclear, although recent data suggest that some alterations of the β_2MG peptide [e.g., by glycosylation (181) or proteolytic cleavage (182,183)] favor its deposition into tissues. Plasma β_2MG levels in ESRD patients are in general markedly elevated to 30–60 μg/mL (184–189), compared to those in normal subjects of ~1 μg/mL. It is likely that the high plasma concentrations in these patients also promote its deposition. To this end, efforts have been directed to decreasing the plasma β_2MG levels in ESRD patients.

In vitro incubation of peripheral mononuclear cells with various types of dialysis membranes in the presence of plasma showed that cuprophan membrane induced the release of more β_2MG than did PMMA or AN69 membrane. Stimulation of mononuclear cells with C5a or IL-1 also enhanced β_2MG release (32), suggesting that the effect of cuprophan on β_2MG release is mediated both by its ability to activate complement and indirectly by inducing cytokine generation. In contrast, incubation studies performed in the absence of plasma showed that β_2MG release was inhibited to a greater extent by cuprophan (rather than enhanced) compared to Hemophan or PAN membranes (190). β_2MG is also a constituent of neutrophil granules (191). Theoretically, dialysis membrane induced neutrophil degranulation may also increase plasma β_2MG levels. However, the intragranular content of β_2MG is small, and therefore the contribution of this mechanism to plasma β_2MG increase during dialysis is modest at most. Nonetheless, these experiments indicate that there is a cellular basis for dialysis-induced

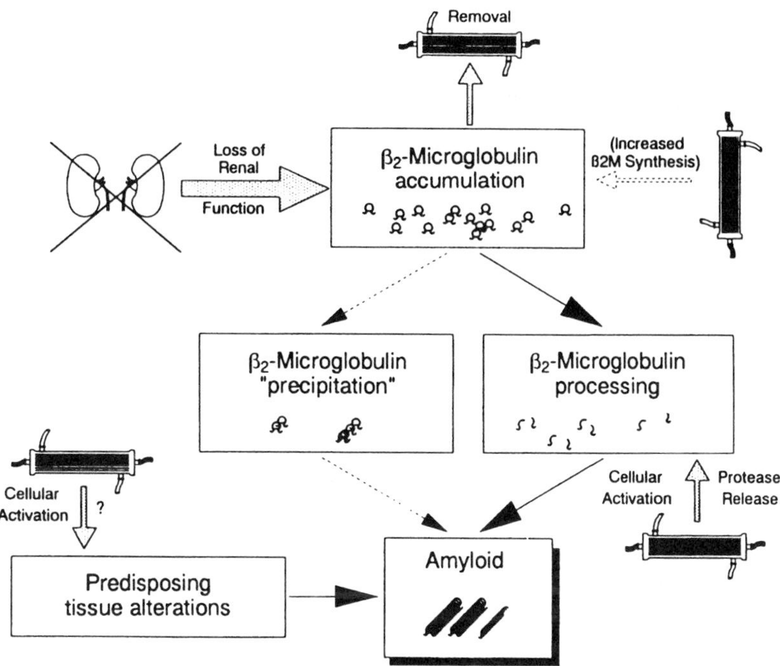

Fig. 6 Effect of membrane bioincompatibility on β_2-microglobulin. Bioincompatible membranes increase transcription, synthesis, and release of β_2-microglobulin (β_2MG) by mononuclear cells. Bioincompatible membranes also induce release of proteases and oxygen free radicals resulting in β_2MG polymerization. Bioincompatible low-flux membranes neither adsorb β_2MG nor do they clear it by filtration. Biocompatible membranes favor maintenance of residual renal function and hence endogenous excretion of β_2MG. (From Ref. 234.)

release of β_2MG. The presence of macrophages in bone tissues afflicted by β_2MG deposits also suggests the possibility that dialysis membrane-induced activated monocytes contribute to the local inflammatory or destructive process (118).

Whether there is a real increase in total extracellular β_2MG during dialysis using cuprophan membrane has been debated. Some investigators have argued that the apparent increase in plasma β_2MG concentration is due to a hemoconcentration effect as a result of ultrafiltration (192,193), while others have reported a 3–15% increase in plasma β_2MG levels despite correction for hemoconcentration (184,185). Some investigators have failed to demonstrate an increase in plasma β_2MG levels during sham hemodialysis in renal failure patients using cuprophan membrane (193). In contrast, when whole blood was circulated through cuprammonium rayon hemofilters in vitro, a 70% increase in plasma β_2MG levels was seen in 15 minutes (194). Abolishment of the increment by leukocyte depletion in this study further suggested that these cells were the source of the additional β_2MG. The plasma appearance rate of β_2MG has been estimated using radiolabeled β_2MG turnover techniques. A higher plasma appearance rate in the patient would suggest that the enhanced release of this protein by activated leukocytes. Clinical data on this issue have been inconclusive. β_2MG appearance rates in patients dialyzed with cuprophan membrane were 30–50% higher than those in normal subjects, but the differences did not reach statistical significance (186,187). The β_2MG appearance rates in patients dialyzed with AN69 membrane were normal and lower than the values for patients dialyzed with cuprophan membrane. However, the differences between AN69 and cuprophan were not statistically significant (187).

Clinical dialysis with high-flux synthetic membranes decreases plasma B_2MG levels, probably by both membrane adsorption and transfer to the dialysate (189). Cuprophan membrane induces an increase, whereas high-flux synthetic membranes induce a decrease in plasma β_2MG levels. Hence, one may postulate that patients dialyzed with the latter would suffer from less β_2MG amyloid disease. Studies have shown that patients dialyzed with AN69 membrane had less bone cysts and required less decompression surgery for carpal tunnel syndrome than those dialyzed with cuprophan membrane (195–197). These data are suggestive, but not definitive, since they are retrospective, there was overlap between the study groups, and histological confirmation for β_2MG was not uniformly obtained.

If β_2MG amyloidosis in the ESRD patients results only from high plasma β_2MG levels as a result of renal failure, it should not be considered a biocompatibility issue. Decreasing the plasma levels by using high-flux membranes, if it partially prevents β_2MG disease, is an issue of dialysis efficiency and not biocompatibility. However, to the extent that dialysis membrane may increase the release of the peptide from circulating leukocytes (32) and may activate leukocytes such that they promote β_2MG deposition by altering its structural properties (182,183) or potentiate the local inflammatory process in the tissues (118), β_2MG is a biocompatibility issue. To what extent bioincompatibility contributes to clinical β_2MG amyloid disease is difficult to determine.

D. Susceptibility to Infection

Deactivation of neutrophils, T lymphocytes, monocytes, and natural killer cells after exposure to the dialysis membrane has been discussed above. Hypothetically, this would impair the ability of the leukocytes to subsequently combat infections and malignant cells. Indeed, chronic hemodialysis patients are prone to infections and have a higher incidence of malignancy than the general population (65,66). Bacterial infections are common, but many of them are at least partially related to anatomical abnormalities, such as vascular access. Nonetheless, dialysis-related immunodeficiency exaggerates the problem. Chronic hemodialysis patients have frequent viral infections, abnormal antibody response to vaccines and hepatitis B infection, cutaneous anergy, prolonged graft survival, and altered response to and perhaps increased incidence of tuberculosis. These are disorders that are probably due to T-cell dysfunction. Whether this propensity to infections and perhaps malignancy is related to dialysis membrane bioincompatibility is, however, unclear. In a prospective study in which new ESRD patients were started on chronic hemodialysis using either cuprophan or polysulfone membrane, the cuprophan group had more significant deterioration of their neutrophil metabolism in response to phagocytic stimuli (56). In addition, three out of the eight patients in the cuprophan group, and none of the seven patients in the polysulfone group, developed an episode of sepsis during a follow-up period of 20 weeks. However, the sample size in this study was small, precluding definitive conclusions.

E. Protein Catabolism

Membrane bioincompatibility has been incriminated as a cause of protein catabolism in dialysis patients. There are two potential cellular mechanisms by which this may occur: neutrophil degranulation and release of cytokines from monocytes. Intragranular proteins, such as elastase, are known to be proteolytic enzymes (39). Elastase released into plasma is usually complexed to plasma α_1-proteinase inhibitor, which limits its functional activity. However, it has been shown that ROS potentiate the effect of elastase on protein degradation, even in the presence of the plasma inhibitor (198). The simultaneous release of ROS (47) and proteases (40–42) from neutrophils during hemodialysis could therefore damage plasma proteins (45,46). Another candidate is IL-1β, which is known to induce protein breakdown by releasing prostaglandin E_2 (199).

Using plasma free amino acids as an indicator of protein catabolism, sham hemodialysis without dialysate using cuprophan membranes in normal humans has been shown to induce more protein catabolism than sham dialysis using AN69 membranes (200). The enhanced release occurred almost 3 hours after the completion of the dialysis treatments and could be partially inhibited by a cyclooxygenase inhibitor. Based on this latter observation, it would be reasonable to postulate that AN69 membrane induces less monocyte activation and therefore it causes less protein catabolism. In vitro (201) and clinical (91) data on monokine release by AN69 membrane, however, do not support this hypothesis. A more recent clinical study using a radiolabeled amino acid turnover technique did not suggest an increase in protein catabolism associated with cuprophan membranes (202). The issue of protein catabolism induced by membrane bioincompatibility is unsettled at present.

V. OUTCOMES AMONG PATIENTS WITH ACUTE RENAL FAILURE

Activated neutrophils release oxygen radicals and proteolytic enzymes that can injure surrounding cells. Indeed, neutrophils stimulated by C5a release oxygen radicals, which damage endothelial cells (28,49). Since neutrophils are activated to release oxygen radicals (47) and proteolytic enzymes (40–42) during hemodialysis, it is possible that they could cause injury to various organs, including the kidneys. In support of this hypothesis is the fact that rats with ischemic ARF and exposed to cuprophan-activated plasma recover renal function at a slower rate compared to those exposed to PAN membrane-treated plasma (50). Infiltration of the glomeruli by neutrophils could be further demonstrated in the cuprophan group. Zymosan-activated plasma produced similar results as cuprophan-activated plasma, suggesting that the effect of cuprophan was mediated by complement activation products.

Several recent studies have prospectively examined the effect of biocompatibility on clinical outcomes in patients with ARF requiring dialysis. Schiffl and colleagues (203) randomly assigned 52 patients with ARF following surgical procedures to dialysis with either a biocompatible (PAN) or a bioincompatible dialyzer (cuprophan). Compared to patients in the PAN group, patients in the cuprophan group had a higher mortality (35% vs. 62%) and required more dialysis treatments (9 vs. 12 treatments) (Fig. 7). Dialysis with cuprophan dialyzers was associated with greater activation of the complement system (C3a) and lipooxygenase pathway (leukotriene B4), resulting in alterations of neutrophil kinetics and function (203). An extension of this study revealed a survival benefit for patients with medical or surgical ARF (204). However, a higher proportion of patients in the cuprophan group had gram-negative sepsis. Although the authors speculated that the use of biocompatible dialyzers may have resulted in a predisposition to sepsis, an alternate possibility that there may have been an imbalance between groups should be considered. Hakim and colleagues prospectively assigned 72 patients with ARF to HD with a biocompatible dialyzer (PMMA) or cuprophan in alternate order (205). The two groups were similar with respect to

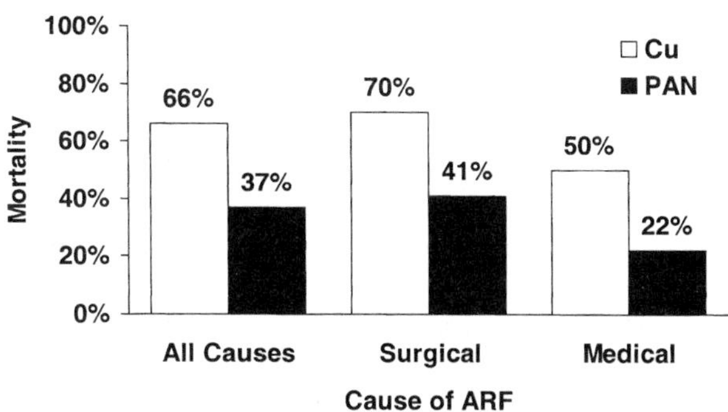

Fig. 7 Effect of dialysis membrane on mortality rates among patients with acute renal failure. Seventy two patients with acute renal failure randomized to dialysis with cuprophan (Cu) or polyacrylonitrile (PAN) membranes. (From Ref. 234.)

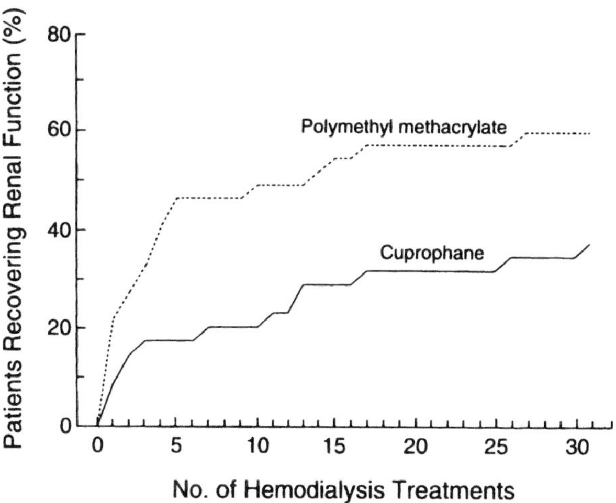

Fig. 8 Effect of dialysis membrane on recovery of renal function among patients with acute renal failure. Seventy two patients were assigned in alternating order to dialysis with polymethylmethacrylate or cuprophane membranes. Not shown on the graph are the results of one patient in the group undergoing dialysis with the polymethylmethacrylate membrane, who recovered renal function after 72 treatments. (From Ref. 205.)

Acute Physiological and Chronic Health Evaluation (APACHE-II) scores, age, gender, and cause of ARF. Compared to PMMA, the cuprophan group had a higher mortality (43% vs. 63%) and were less likely to recover renal function (62% vs. 37%) (Fig. 8) (205). The biocompatibility benefit was more apparent among patients with nonoliguric ARF. However, as many as 30% of patients in the PMMA group recovered renal function after a single dialysis, again raising the possibility that there may have been an imbalance between groups. Kurtal and colleagues (206) prospectively assigned patients with ARF to dialysis with a biocompatible dialyzer (polyamide, 25 patients) or cuprophan (32 patients). Survival rate was similar in among the polyamide and cuprophan groups (64% vs. 72%) and so was the recovery of renal function. Likewise, among 748 cases of ARF at 13 tertiary care centers in Madrid over a period of 9 months, 270 patients (36%) required dialysis (207). Among 134 patients who received HD, the membrane was recorded and was cellulose in 84 and synthetic in 50. The overall mortality among patients dialyzed with cellulose dialyzers (58%) was not significantly different from that among patients dialyzed with synthetic dialyzers (66%). Also, the number of dialysis treatments required was similar between the two groups (207). Consequently, although some studies suggest that the use of biocompatible dialyzers could improve clinical outcomes among ARF patients requiring dialysis, definitive proof is lacking. Further, the mechanisms behind this possible benefit have not been clearly elucidated.

VI. OUTCOMES AMONG PATIENTS WITH CHRONIC RENAL FAILURE

Several retrospective studies have examined the association between the type of dialyzer used and clinical outcomes among patients on chronic dialysis. Levin and colleagues compared clinical outcomes among noncontemporaneous cohorts—438 patients on cellulose dialyzers and 548 on high-flux polysulfone dialyzers (208). Patients on polysulfone dialyzers have a 0.19 relative risk (RR) of death, 0.17 RR of death due to cardiovascular disease, and 0.14 RR of death due to infection (208). Although these risks were adjusted for age, gender, race, and cause of ESRD, dose of dialysis and flux may have confounded the analysis. Likewise, in an comparison of noncontemporaneous cohorts, Hornberger and colleagues observed a 0.24 RR of death among 107 patients on high-flux polysulfone dialyzers treated during the years 1989–91 compared to 146 patients on cellulose dialyzers treated during the years 1987–89 (209). However, differences in the dose of dialysis, flux and albumin levels in the polysulfone group might have influenced these results. Likewise, in a historical prospective study by the U.S. Renal Data System (USRDS), prevalent patients on chronic dialysis as of December 31, 1990, were randomly selected from 523 dialysis units (210). Patients on dialysis for less than one year, those using acetate dialysate, those in whom the dialyzer was not specified, and those in whom data on the dose of dialysis was not available were excluded. The remaining 2410 patients were followed from December 30, 1990, until death, transplantation, switch to peritoneal dialysis, or end of study (median 1.4 years). Dialyzers were classified as unsubstituted cellulose, modified cellulose, and synthetic and were used by 65.8, 16.1, and 18.1% of patients, respectively. In a Cox proportional hazards model, compared to patients on unsubstituted cellulose dialyzers, the relative risk of death for patients on modified cellulose and synthetic dialyzers was 0.72 and 0.72, respectively (210). When adjusted for Kt/V, the relative risk of death for patients on modified cellulose and synthetic dialyzers was 0.74 and 0.75, respectively (Fig. 9) (210). These studies suggest that use of more biocompatible synthetic dialyzers may be associated with a decreased mortality in patients on chronic hemodialysis. However, for several reasons these conclusions need to be viewed with caution. The fact that the majority of biocompatible dialyzers were also high-flux dialyzers raises the possibility that flux rather than biocompatibility may be the factor that caused better outcomes. Also, the possibility that the use of biocompatible dialyzers (which are more expensive) may reflect greater attention to improvements in dialysis technology, and commitment of greater resources to patient care, which in turn leads to better outcomes needs to be considered. Ongoing multicenter studies may resolve some of these issues.

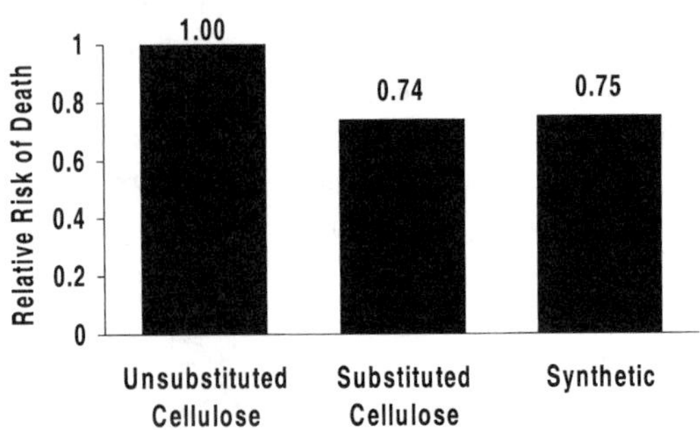

Fig. 9 Effect of dialysis membrane on mortality rates among patients with chronic renal failure. A historical prospective study of 2,410 patients from United States Renal Data System (USRDS) Case-Mix Adequacy Study. Prevalent patients on chronic dialysis as of December 31, 1990 were randomly selected from 523 dialysis units. (From Ref. 210.)

VII. IMPACT OF BIOCOMPATIBILITY ON PRESERVATION OF RESIDUAL RENAL FUNCTION

It has also been suggested that inflammatory mediators such as interleukin 1 generated by the extracorporeal circulation of hemodialysis may be nephrotoxic in their repeated exposure to native kidneys; consequently hemodialysis with so-called bioincompatible membranes compared to more biocompatible membranes should be associated with a more rapid deterioration in residual renal function (RRF) (211–213).

A study by Van Stone (213) prospectively compared the effects of four different dialysis membranes on GFR. Three types of membrane (polysulfone, polymethylmethacrylate, and cellulose acetate) were considered biocompatible, while the cuprophane membrane was considered bioincompatible. Within one year, GFR decreased to negligible amounts in the majority of the patients, although a considerable minority maintained RRF for more than 3 years. Renal function deteriorated less rapidly in patients treated with dialyzers with biocompatible membranes.

Other studies (211,212) found similar results. However, results have been conflicting, with some studies reporting that the choice of membrane does not influence RRF. Patients dialyzed with biocompatible membranes as polysulfone or polyacrylonitrite were observed to lose residual creatinine clearance at a rate similar to patients dialyzed with bioincompatible cuprophane membranes (214).

VIII. BIO(IN)COMPATIBILITY OF REUSE

Reuse of hemodialyzers is applied to enable the repeated application of the same dialyzer in one and the same patient, which is made possible by the repeated sterilization of the filter. The main purpose of this technique is the reduction of expenses because the purchase of dialyzers is of course drastically reduced. The repeated sterilization of dialyzers has, however, an impact on various aspects of biocompatibility.

A. Complement and Leukocyte Activation

The well-known characteristic of dialyzers in unmodified cellulose to activate complement and leukocytes is dramatically reduced with any reuse method that applies sterilants that fix plasma proteins to the dialyzer membrane (215) (e.g., formaldehyde, glutaraldehyde, peracetic acid). The reason for this is that the chemical structures inducing complement activation (mainly hydroxyl groups) are hidden by the covering protein layer for the complement cascade. A similar effect is not observed for sterilization with bleach, which is known to destroy the protein layer and thereby restore the original capacity of the membrane to activate complement.

Together with the mitigation of complement and leukocyte activation, all subsequent reactions and clinical consequences, such as pulmonary dysfunction or the lack of leukocyte response upon stimulation, are also reduced in intensity (215,216).

B. Susceptibility to Infection

One of the problems with dialyzer reuse is that germs may enter the blood stream each time sterilization is inadequate. Even if bacteria are destroyed, reused dialyzers may contain pyrogens or endotoxins, inducing systemic reactions in the patients. In an extensive study by the CDC, the number of pyrogenic reactions was clearly higher in dialysis units applying reuse (217). A potential confounding factor was, however, the dialyzer pore size, because the centers applying reuse at the same time also applied more high-flux dialysis and hemodiafiltration (217). Nevertheless, in other studies, reuse has been held responsible for pyrogenic reactions, even with conventional dialysis, and discontinuation of reuse was associated with the disappearance of the pyrogenic reactions (218). Clusters of bacteremia with pseudomonads have been observed when the sterilization procedure failed without eliciting an appropriate alarm (219). More exceptional germs, such as atypical mycobacteria, have also been found to provoke infection in association with reuse (220). The odds ratio for transmission of hepatitis C was higher in units where reuse of dialyzers of hepatitis C positive and negative patients was done on the same reuse machine, even if hepatitis C dialyzers were sterilized last during the day's routine (221).

C. Surface Adhesion and Surface Modification

If adsorption occurs on dialyzer membranes, this process is prevented by those reuse procedures that fix the protein layer to the dialyzer membrane during the sterilization. A typical example is AN69, which currently adsorbs β_2-microglobulin when first-use dialyzers are applied. This capacity is lost when AN69 is reused with peracetic acid, which fixes the protein layer, but not with bleach, which removes the protein layer (222). For polysulfone, however, removal of β_2-microglobulin becomes progressively more important when dialyzers are reused with bleach, which is attributed to modifications of the membrane structure and possible increase in pore size (223). Similarly, transdialyzer protein losses gradually increase with the number of bleach reuse procedures, with losses up to 20 g/dialysis once dialyzers are reused more than 20 times (224). Substantial protein losses, however, tend to start only from the tenth reuse on. If membranes are more permeable for proteins from blood to dialysate, a similar shift of large molecules can occur from dialysate to blood; it has been demonstrated that cytokine-inducing substances cross the membrane more easily when polysulfone dialyzers are reprocessed 20 times (225).

D. Allergic Reactions

Due to the repeated rinsing of dialyzers, leachable compounds with an allergenic potential are removed more readily by the reuse procedure. Hence, hypersensitivity reactions from the first-use type have been observed more rarely when reuse was applied (226), but a similar tendency can be expected with thorough rinsing of first-use dialyzers. In a recent study, no major differences in intradialyic symptoms could be observed between first-use and reuse dialyzers (227). Anaphylactoid reactions, currently occurring in patients on first-use AN69 membranes treated by ACE inhibitors, are attributed to blocking of bradykinin degradation by the ACE inhibitors in combination with a strong bradykinin production due to the negative charge of the membrane. Such reactions have equally been observed when polysulfone or cellulosic dialyzers were reused with peracetic acid (228). Probably, the reuse procedure induces changes in the membrane structure or electric charge so that similar reactions are induced as with genuine AN69 membranes.

E. Leaching

Sterilants are released from reused dialyzers. Although release into the patient's circulation can be reduced by thorough predialysis rinsing, rebound release has been described for several sterilants, especially formaldehyde and peracetic acid (229). This might be responsible, in the case of formaldehyde reuse, for the development of anti-N–like antibodies, which are held responsible for hemolytic reactions, even with adequate prerinsing (230).

F. Conclusions

Reuse might reduce bioincompatibility, but at the same time it can induce new bioincompatibility reactions as well. Whether the outcome will be positive or negative depends both on the membrane and the sterilant. It should be stressed that many of the negative reactions have been depicted with the hardware applied in the early 1990s and that the newer technology might offer a possibility to avoid these reactions. Convincing scientific evidence of this is to our knowledge not yet available.

IX. OUTCOMES IN RENAL TRANSPLANT RECIPIENTS

Use of biocompatible dialyzers has also been demonstrated to protect against postrenal transplant allograft dysfunction and to hasten renal recovery among patients with postrenal transplant. A recent study by Van Loo and colleagues examined outcomes among 44 hemodialysis patients who underwent renal transplantation (231). Of these, 24 were on cuprophan and 20 on polysulfone dialyzers prior to transplantation. Compared to patients dialyzed with cuprophan dialyzers, patients on polysulfone dialyzers decreased their serum creatinine levels to 50% of pretransplant levels earlier (7.4 vs. 3.1 days), were less likely to develop delayed graft function (46% vs. 25%), and were less likely to develop posttransplant ARF (40% vs. 5%) (Fig. 10). In contrast, Valeri prospectively studied 46 patients with ARF following cadaveric renal transplantation (232). Sixteen patients were excluded due to biopsy-proven rejection, primary graft nonfunction, or other causes. Of the remaining 30 patients, 16 were randomized to cuprophan and 14 polymethylmethacrylate. There were no differences in pretransplant characteristics or immunosuppressive regimen. The time to recovery of ARF and the number of dialysis treatments required were similar between the two groups.

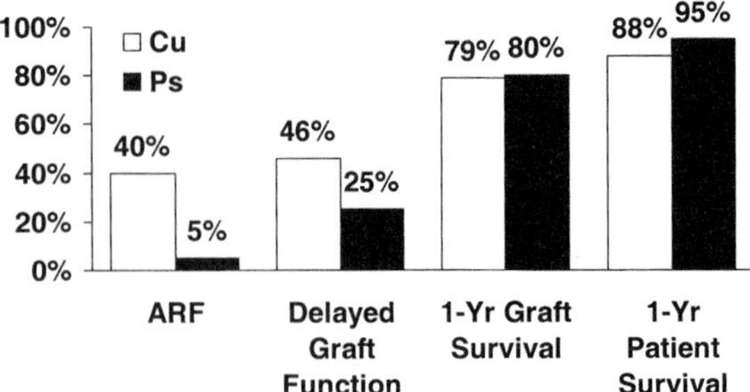

Fig. 10 Effect of pretransplant dialysis membrane use on posttransplant outcomes. An observational study of the effect of the dialysis membrane in use prior to transplantation on posttransplant outcomes. Forty-four patients were dialyzed pretransplant with cuprophan (Cu) or polysulfone (Ps) membranes. (From Ref. 231.)

ACKNOWLEDGMENTS

The authors acknowledge the support from the Research Service of the U.S. Veterans Affairs, the National Institutes of Health (DK-45575 and 45609), Baxter Extramural Program, and the Departments of Medicine at the University of Utah School of Medicine, Salt Lake City, UT, and New England Medical Center, Boston, MA.

REFERENCES

1. Henne W, Duenweg G, Bandel W. A new cellulose membrane generation for hemodialysis and hemofiltration. Artif Organs 1979; 3:466–469.

2. Spencer P, Schmidt B, Samtleben W. Ex vivo model of hemodialysis membrane biocompatibility. Trans ASAIO 1985; 31:495–498.
3. Falkenhagen D, Bosch T, Brown GS, Schmidt B, Holtz M, Baurmeister U, Gurland H, Klinkmann H. A clinical study on different cellulosic dialysis membranes. Nephrol Dial Transplant 1987; 2:537–545.
4. Saito A, Ono M, Hisanaga S, Ogawa H, Saruhashi M, Sasaki M. Improved biocompatibility of modified regenerated cellulose (RC) dialyzer with vitamin E. J Am Soc Nephrol 1993; 4:380.
5. Anderson S, Garcia D, Brenner B. Renal and systemic manifestations of glomerular disease. In: Brenner B, Rector JF, eds. The Kidney. 4th ed. Philadelphia: WB Saunders, 1991:1831–1870.
6. Konstantin P. Newer membranes: cuprophane versus polysulfone versus polyacrylonitrile. In: Bosch J, Stein J, eds. Hemodialysis: High Efficiency Treatments. New York: Churchill Livingstone, 1993:63–77.
7. Streicher E, Schneider H. The development of a polysulfone membrane. Contrib Nephrol 1985; 46:1–13.
8. Göhl H, Buck R, Strathmann H. Basic features of the polyamide membranes. Contrib Nephrol 1992; 96:1–25.
9. Radovich J. Composition of polymer membranes for therapies of end-stage renal disease. In: Bonomini V, Berland Y, eds. Dialysis Membranes: Structure and Predictions. Vol. 113. Basel: Karger, 1995:11–24.
10. Muller-Eberhard H. Complement: chemistry and pathways. In: Gallin J, Goldstein I, Snyderman R, eds. Inflammation. New York: Raven Press, 1988:21–54.
11. Chenoweth DE, Cheung AK, Henderson LW. Anaphylatoxin formation during hemodialysis: effects of different dialyzer membranes. Kidney Int 1983; 24:764–769.
12. Craddock P, Fehr J, Dalmasso A. Hemodialysis leukopenia: pulmonary vascular leukostasis resulting from complement activation by dialyzer cellophane membranes. J Clin Invest 1977; 59:879–888.
13. Cheung A, Parker C, Janatova J. Analysis of the complement C3 fragments associated with hemodialysis membranes. Kidney Int 1989; 35:576–588.
14. Cheung A, Parker C, Wilcox L. Activation of the alternative pathway of complement by hemodialysis membranes. Kidney Int 1989; 36:257–265.
15. Chenoweth DE, Cheung AK, Ward DM, Henderson LW. Anaphylatoxin formation during hemodialysis: a comparison of new and re-used dialyzers. Kidney Int 1983; 24:770–774.
16. Deppisch R, Schmitt V, Bommer J, Hansch G, Ritz E, Rauterberg E. Fluid phase generation of terminal complement complex as a novel index of bioincompatibility. Kidney Int 1990; 37:696–706.
17. Bhakdi S, Fassbender W, Hugo F. Relative efficiency of terminal complement activation. J Immunol 1988; 141:3117–3122.
18. Cheung A, Paker C, Hohnholt M. B_2 integrins are required for neutrophil degranulation induced by hemodialysis membranes. Kidney Int 1993; 43:649–660.
19. Ivanovich P, Chenoweth D, Schmidt Rea. Symptoms and activation of granulocytes and complement with two dialysis membranes. Kidney Int 1983; 24:758–763.
20. Hakim R, Fearon D, Lazarus J. Biocompatibility of dialysis membranes: effects of chronic complement activation. Kidney Int 1984; 26:194–200.
21. Smeby L, Wideroe T, Balstad T, Jorstad S. Biocompatibility aspects of cellophane, cellulose acetate, polyacrylonitrile, polysulfone and polycarbonate hemodialyzers. Blood Purif 1986; 4:93–101.
22. Maggiore Q, Enia G, Catalano C. Effect of blood cooling on cucrophan-induced anaphylatoxin generation. Kidney Int 1987; 32:908–911.
23. MacDougall M, Diedrich D, Wiegmann T. Dissociation of hemodialysis leukopenia and hypoxemia from complement changes during citrate anticoagulation. Kidney Int 1985; 27:166(A).
24. Cheung A, Faezi-Jenkin B, Leypoldt J. Effect of thrombosis on complement activation and neutrophil degranulation during in vitro hemodialysis. J Am Soc Nephrol 1994; 5:110–115.
25. Dumler F, Zasuwa G, Levin N. Effect of dialyzer reprocessing methods on complement activation and hemodialyzer-related symptoms. Artif Organs 1987; 11: 128–131.
26. Schohn D, Jahn H, Eber M. Biocompatibility and hemodynamic studies during polycarbonate versus cuprophan membrane dialysis. Blood Purif 1986; 4:102–111.
27. McCormick J, Kreutzer D, Keating H. Alterations in activities of anaphylatoxin inactivator and chemotactic factor inactivator during hemodialysis. Am J Pathol 1982; 109:282–287.
28. Sacks T, Moldow C, Craddock P. Oxygen radicals mediate endothelial cell damage by complement-stimulated granulocytes. J Clin Invest 1978; 61:1161–1167.
29. Goldstein I, Brai M, Osler A. Lysosomal enzyme release from human leukocytes: mediation by the alternative pathway of complement activation. J Immunol 1973; 111:33–37.
30. Wright D, Gallin J. Secretory responses of human neutrophils: Exocytosis of specific (secondary) granules by human neutrophils during adherence in vitro and during exudation in vivo. J Immunol 1979; 123:285–294.
31. Schindler R, Gelfand J, Dinarello C. Recombitant C5a stimulates transcription rather than translation of IL-1 and TNF: priming of mononuclear cells with recombitant C5a enhances cytokine synthesis induced by LPS, IL-1 or PMA. Blood 1990; 76:1631–1635.
32. Zaoui P, Stone W, Hakim R. Effects of dialysis membranes on beta 2-microglobulin production and cellular expression. Kidney Int 1990; 38:962–968.

33. Cheung A, Parker C, Hohnholt M. Inhibition of complement activation on hemodialysis (HD) membranes by soluble complement receptor type I (sCR1). J Am Soc Nephrol 1993; 3:340(A).
34. Kaplow L, Goffinet J. Profound neutropenia during the early phase of hemodialysis. JAMA 1968; 203: 133–135.
35. Cheung AK, Hohnholt M, Gilson J. Adherence of neutrophils to hemodialysis membranes: role of complement receptors. Kidney Int 1991; 40:1123–1133.
36. Mason R, Zucker W, Bilinsky R. Blood components deposited on used and reused dialysis membranes. Biomat Med Dev Art Org 1976; 4:333–358.
37. Dodd N, Gordge M, Tarrant J. A demonstration of neutrophil accumulation in the pulmonary vasculature during hemodialysis. Proc EDTA 1983; 20:186–189.
38. Hakim R, Schafer A. Hemodialysis-associated platelet activation and thrombocytopenia. Am J Med 1985; 78: 575–580.
39. Silber R, Moldow C. Biochemistry and function of neutrophils, composition of neutrophils. In: Williams R, Brutler E, Erslev A, Lichtman, eds. Hematology. New York: McGraw-Hill, 1983:726–734.
40. Hörl W, Riegel W, Schollmeyer P. Different complement and granulocyte activation in patients dialyzed with PMMA dialyzers. Clin Nephrol 1986; 25:304–307.
41. Hörl W, Schaefer R, Heidland A. Effect of different dialyzers on proteinases and proteinase inhibitors during hemodialysis. Am J Nephrol 1985; 5:320–326.
42. Hörl W, Steinhauer H, Riegel W. Effect of different dialyzer membranes on plasma levels of granulocyte elastase. Kidney Int 1988; 33(suppl):S90–S91.
43. Showell H, Glovsky M, Ward P. Morphological changes in human polymorphonuclear leukocytes induced by Ca3 in the presence and absence of cytochalasin. Int Arch Allergy Appl Immunol 1982; 69: 62–67.
44. Schaefer R, Heidland A, Hörl W. Effect of dialyzer geometry on granulocyte and complement activation. Am J Nephrol 1987; 7:121–126.
45. Heidland A, Hörl W, Heller N. Proteolytic enzymes and catabolism: enhanced release of granulocyte proteinase in uremic intoxication and during hemodialysis. Kidney Int 1983; 24(suppl):S27–S36.
46. Hörl W, Heidland A. Evidence for the participation of granulocyte proteinases on intradialytic catabolism. Clin Nephrol 1984; 21:314–322.
47. Himmelfarb J, Ault K, Holbrook D. Intradialytic granulocyte reactive oxygen species production: a prospective, crossover trial. J Am Soc Nephrol 1993; 4: 178–186.
48. Maher E, Wickens D, Griffin J. Increased free-radical activity during hemodialysis. Nephrol Dial Transplant 1987; 2:169–171.
49. Till G, Johnson K, Kunke R. Intravascular activation of complement and acute lung injury. J Clin Invest 1982; 69:1126–1135.
50. Schulman G, Fogo A, Gung A, Badr K, Hakim R. Complement activation retards resolution of acute ischemic renal failure in the rat. Kidney Int 1991; 40: 1069–1074.
51. Klempner M, Gallin J, Balow J. The effect of hemodialysis and C5ades arg on neutrophil subpopulations. Blood 1980; 55:777–783.
52. Spagnuolo P, Bass J, Smith M. Neutrophil adhesiveness during prostacyclin and heparin hemodialysis. Blood 1982; 60:924–929.
53. Cohen MS, Elliott DM, Chaplinski T, Pike MM, Niedel JE. A defect in the oxidative metabolism of human polymorphonuclear leukocytes that remain in circulation early in hemodialysis. Blood 1982; 60:1283–1289.
54. Wissow L, Covenberg R, Burns R. Altered leukocyte chemiluminescence during dialysis. J Clin Immunol 1981; 1:262–265.
55. Henderson L, Miller ME, Hamilton RW, Norman ME. Hemodialysis leukopenia and polymorph random mobility—a possible correlation. J Lab Clin Med 1975; 85:191–197.
56. Vanholder R, Ringoir S, Dhondt A, Hakim R. Phagocytosis in uremic and hemodialysis patients: a prospective and cross sectional study. Kidney Int 1991; 39:320–327.
57. Needleman B, Weiler J, Feldbush T. The third component of complement inhibits human lymphocyte blastogenesis. J Immunol 1981; 126:1586–1591.
58. Hobbs M, Feldbush T, Needleman B. Inhibition of secondary in vitro antibody responses by the third component of complement. J Immunol 1981; 128: 1470–1475.
59. Greene W, Bohaleim E, Siekavitz M. Structure and regulation of the human IL-2 receptor. Adv Exp Med Biol 1989; 254:55–60.
60. Zaoui P, Green W, Hakim R. Hemodialysis with cuprophane membrane modulates interleukin-2 receptor expression. Kidney Int 1991; 39:1020–1026.
61. Meuer S, Hauer M, Purz P. Selective blockade of the antigen-receptor-mediated pathway of T cell activation in patients with impaired immune responses. Kidney Int 1987; 80:743–749.
62. Zaoui P, Hakim R. Natural killer-cell function in hemodialysis patients. Kidney Int 1993; 43:1298–1305.
63. Kay N, Raij L. Differential effect of hemodialysis membranes on human lymphocyte nautral killer function. Artif Organs 1987; 11:165–167.
64. Kay N, Raij L. Immune abnormalities in renal failure in hemodialysis. Blood Purif 1986; 4:120–129.
65. Port F, Ragheb N, Schwartz A. Neoplasms in dialysis patients: a population-based study. Am J Kidn Dis 1989; 14:119–123.

66. Lindner A, Farewell B, Sherrard D. High incidence of neoplasia in uremic patients receiving long term dialysis. Nephron 1981; 27:292–296.
67. Descamps-Latscha B, Herbelin A, Nguyen AT, et al. Soluble CD23 as an effector of immune dysregulation in chronic uremia and dialysis. Kidney Int 1993; 43: 878–884.
68. Dinarello CA. Interleukin-1 and interleukin-1 antagonism. Blood 1991; 77:1627–1652.
69. Dinarello C. Cytokines: agents provocateurs in hemodialysis? Kidney Int 1992; 41:683–694.
70. Dinarello C. Interleukin-1 and tumor necrosis factor and their naturally occurring antagonists during hemodialysis. Kidney International 1992; 42(suppl 38): S68–S77.
71. Vilcek J, Le J. Immunology of cytokines: an introduction. In: AT, ed. The Cytokine Handbook. San Diego: Academic Press, 1991:1–17.
72. Henderson LW, Koch KM, Dinarello CA, Shaldon S. Hemodialysis hypotension: the interleukin-1 hypothesis. Blood Purif 1983; 1:3–8.
73. Pereira BJ, Dinarello CA. Production of cytokines and cytokine inhibitory proteins in patients on dialysis. Nephrol Dial Transplant 1994; 9:60–71.
74. Lonnemann G, Bingel M, Koch KM, Shaldon S, Dinarello CA. Plasma interleukin-1 activity in humans undergoing hemodialysis with regenerated cellulosic membranes. Lymphokine Res 1987; 6:63–70.
75. Luger A, Kovarik J, Stummvoll HK, Urbanska A, Luger TA. Blood-membrane interaction in hemodialysis leads to increased cytokine production. Kidney Int 1987; 32:84–88.
76. Bingel M, Lonnemann G, Koch KM, Dinarello CA, Shaldon S. Plasma interleukin-1 activity during hemodialysis: the influence of dialysis membranes. Nephron 1988; 50:273–276.
77. Descamps-Latscha B, Herbelin A, Nguyen AT, Uzan M, Zingraff J. Haemodialysis-membrane-induced phagocyte oxidative metabolism activation and interleukin-1 production. Life Support Systems 1986; 4: 349–353.
78. Herbelin A, Nguyen AT, Zingraff J, Urena P, Descamps-Latscha B. Influence of uremia and hemodialysis on circulating interleukin-1 and tumor necrosis factor alpha. Kidney Int 1990; 37:116–125.
79. Pereira BJG, King AJ, Falagas ME, Shapiro L, Strom JA, Dinarello CA. Plasma levels of IL-1, TNF and their specific inhibitors in undialyzed chronic renal failure. Kidney Int 1994; 45:890–896.
80. Ghysen J, De Plaen JF, van Ypersele de Strihou C. The effect of membrane characteristics on tumour necrosis factor kinetics during haemodialysis. Nephrol Dial Transplant 1990; 5:270–274.
81. Canivet E, Lavaud S, Wong T, Guenounou M, Willemin JC, Potron G, Chanard J. Cuprophane but not synthetic membrane induces increases in serum tumor necrosis factor-alpha. Am J Kidney Dis 1994; 23:41–46.
82. Holmes C, Evans R, Ross D, Frankamp P. Plasma IL-1 and TNF levels during high-flux hemodialysis with cellulose triacetate membranes. Kidney Int 1990; 37: 301.
83. Powell A, Bland L, Oettinger C, McAllister SK, Oliver JC, Arduino MJ, Favero MS. Lack of plasma interleukin-1 beta or tumor necrosis factor-alpha elevation during unfavorable hemodialysis conditions. J Am Soc Nephrol 1991; 2:1007–1013.
84. Davenport A, Crabtree J, Androjna C, et al. Tumour necrosis factor does not increase during routine cuprophane haemodialysis in healthy. Nephrol Dialysis Transplant 1991; 6:435–429.
85. Pereira BJ, Shapiro L, King AJ, Falagas ME, Strom JA, Dinarello CA. Plasma levels of IL-1 beta, TNF alpha and their specific inhibitors in undialyzed chronic renal failure, CAPD and hemodialysis patients. Kidney Int 1994; 45:890–896.
86. Herbelin A, Urena P, Nguyen A, Zingraff J, Descamps-Latscha B. Elevated circulating levels of interleukin-6 in patients with chronic renal failure. Kidney Int 1991; 39:954–960.
87. Descamps-Latscha B, Herbelin A, Nguyen AT, et al. Imbalance between pro-inflammatory cytokines and their specific inhibitors in chronic renal. J Am Soc Nephrol 1993; 4:343.
88. Cottrell AC, Mehta RL. Cytokine kinetics in septic ARF patients on continuous veno-veno hemodialysis (CVVHD). J Am Soc Nephrol 1992; 3:361.
89. Lonnemann G, Haubitz M, Schindler R. Hemodialysis-associated induction of cytokines. Blood Purif 1990; 8:214–222.
90. Blumenstein M, Schmidt B, Ward RA. Altered interleukin-1 production in patients undergoing hemodialysis. Nephron 1988; 50:277–281.
91. Haeffner-Cavaillon N, Cavaillon JM, Ciancioni C. In vivo induction of interleukin-1 during hemodialysis. Kidney Int 1989; 35:1212–1218.
92. Endres S, Ghorbani R, Lonnemann G, van der Meer JWM, Dinarello CA. Measurement of immunoreactive interleukin-1 beta from human mononuclear cells: optimization of recovery, intrasubject consistency and comparison with interleukin-1 alpha and tumor necrosis factor. Clin Immunol Immunopathol 1988; 49: 424–438.
93. Endres S, Cannon JG, Ghorbani R, et al. In vitro production of IL-1beta, Il-1alpha, TNF, and IL-2 in healthy subjects: distribution, effect of cyclooxygenase inhibition and evidence of independent gene regulation. Eur J Immunol 1989; 19:2327–2333.
94. Memoli B, Rampino T, Libetta C, DalCanton A, Andreucci VE. Peripheral blood leukocytes interleukin-6 production in uremic hemodialyzed patients (abstr). J Am Soc Nephrol 1990; 1:369.

95. Ryan J, Beynon H, Rees AJ, Cassidy MJ. Evaluation of the in vitro production of tumour necrosis factor by monocytes in dialysis patients. Blood Purif 1991; 9: 142–147.
96. Oettinger CW, Powell AC, Bland LA, et al. Enhanced release of tumor necrosis factor alpha but not interleukin-1 beta by uremic blood stimulated with endotoxin (abstr). J Am Soc Nephrol 1990; 1:370.
97. Schindler R, Lonnemann G, Shaldon S, Koch K, Dinarello C. Transcription, not synthesis, of interleukin-1 and tumor necrosis factor by complement. Kidney Int 1990; 37:85–93.
98. Urena P, Gogusev J, Valdovinos R, Herbelin A, Drueke T. Transcriptional induction of TNF-alpha in uremic patients undergoing hemodialysis (abstr). J Am Soc Nephrol 1990; 1:380.
99. Schindler R, Linnenweber S, Shulze M, Opperman M, Dinarello CA, Shaldon S, Koch KM. Gene expression of interleukin-1β during hemodialysis. Kidney Int 1993; 43:712–721.
100. Pereira BJ, Dinarello CA. Role of cytokines in patients on dialysis [editorial]. Int J Artif Organs 1995; 18: 293–304.
101. Peterson J, Hyver S, Cajias J. Backfiltration during dialysis. Sem Dial 1992; 5:13–16.
102. Baurmeister U, Vienken J, Daum V. High-flux dialysis membranes: Endotoxin transfer by backfiltration can be a problem. Nephrol Dial Transplant 1989; 4(suppl 3):89–93.
103. Donahue PR. Dialyzer permeability alteration by reuse. J Am Soc Nephrol 1992; 3:363.
104. Graeber CW, Halley SE, Lapkin RA, Graeber CA, Kaplan AA. Protein Losses with Reused Dialyzers. J Am Soc Nephrol 1993; 4:349.
105. Tokars JI, Alter MJ, Favero MS, Moyer LA, Bland LA. National surveillance of hemodialysis associated diseases in the United States. ASAIO J 1990; 39:71–80.
106. Pegues D, Oettinger C, Bland L, Oliver CC, Arduino MJ, Aguero SM, McAllister SK, Gordon SM, Favero MS, Jarvis WR. A prospective study of pyrogenic reactions in hemodialysis patients using bicarbonate dialysis fluids filtered to remove bacteria and endotoxin. J Am Soc Nephrol 1992; 3:1002–1007.
107. Pereira BJG, Snodgrass BR, Hogan PJ, King AJ. Diffusive and convective transfer of cytokine-inducing bacterial products across hemodialysis membranes. Kidney Int 1995; 47:603–610.
108. Bingel M, Lonnemann G, Shaldon S, Koch KM, Dinarello CA. Human interleukin-1 production during hemodialysis. Nephron 1986; 43:161–163.
109. Lonnemann G, Binge M, Floege J, Koch KM, Shaldon S, Dinarello CA. Detection of endotoxin-like interleukin-1-inducing activity during in vitro dialysis. Kidney Int 1988; 33:29–35.
110. Lonnemann G, Behme TC, Lenzner B, Floege J, Schulze M, Colton CK, Koch KM, Shaldon S. Permeability of dialyzer membranes to TNF alpha-inducing substances derived from water bacteria. Kidney Int 1992; 42:61–68.
111. Evans RC, Holmes CJ. In vitro study of the transfer of cytokine-inducing substances across selected high-flux hemodialysis. Blood Purif 1991; 9:92–101.
112. Urena P, Herbelin A, Zingraff J, Lair M, Man K, Descamps-Latscha B, Druëke T. Permeability of cellulosic and non-cellulosic membranes to endotoxins and cytokine production. Nephrol Dial Transplant 1992; 7: 16–28.
113. Lonnemann G, Mahiout A, Schindler R, Colton CK. Pyrogen retention by the polyamide membranes. Contrib Nephrol 1992; 96:47–63.
114. Okusawa S, Gelfand JA, Ikejima T, Connolly RJ, Dinarello CA. Interleukin 1 induces a shock-like state in rabbits: synergism with tumor necrosis factor and the effect of cyclooxygenase inhibition. J Clin Invest 1988; 81:1162–1172.
115. Raz A, Wyche A, Siegel N, Needleman P. Regulation of fibroblast cyclooxygenase synthesis by interleukin-1. J Biol Chem 1988; 263:3022–3028.
116. Cominelli F, Nast CC, Dinarello CA, Gentilini P, Zipser RD. Regulation of eicosanoid production in rabbit colon by interleukin-1. Gastroenterology 1989; 97: 1400–1405.
117. Schweizer A, Feige U, Fontana A, Muller K, Dinarello CA. Interleukin-1 enhances pain reflexes. Mediation through increased prostaglandin E2 levels. Agents Actions 1988; 25:246–251.
118. Ohashi K, Hara M, Kawai R, et al. Cervical discs are most susceptible to beta 2-microglobulin amyloid deposition in the vertebral column. Kidney Int 1992; 41: 1646–1052.
119. Zaoui P, Hakim R. The effects of dialysis membrane on cytokine release. J Am Soc Nephrol 1994; 4:1711–1718.
120. Craddock P, Fehr J, Brigham K. Complement and leukocyte-mediated pulmonary dysfunction in hemodialysis. N Engl J Med 1977; 296:769–774.
121. De Backer W, Verpooten G, Borgonjon D, Van Waeleghem JP, Vermeire PA, De Broe ME. Hypoxemia during hemodialysis: effects of different membranes and dialysate compositions. Kidney Int 1983; 23:738–743.
122. Hakim R, Lowrie E. Hemodialysis-associated neutropenia and hypoxemia: the effect of dialyzer membrane materials. Nephron 1982; 32:32–39.
123. Dolan M, Whipp B, Davidson W. Hypopnea associated with acetate hemodialysis: carbon-dioxide-flow dependent ventilation. N Engl J Med 1981; 305:72–75.
124. Oh M, Uribarri J, Del Monte Mea. A mechanism of hypoxemia during hemodialysis. Am J Nephrol 1985; 5:366–371.
125. Jones R, Broadfield J, Parsons V. Arterial hypoxemia during hemodialysis for acute renal failure in mechan-

ically ventilated patients: observations and mechanisms. Clin Nephrol 1980; 14:18–22.
126. Mahajan S, Gardiner H, B DT. Relationship between pulmonary functions and hemodialysis induced leukopenia. Trans ASAIO 1977; 23:411–415.
127. Graf H, Stummvoll H, Haber P. Pathophysiology of dialysis related hypoxaemia. Proc EDTA 1980; 17: 155–161.
128. Morrison J, Wilson A, Vaziri N. Determination of pulmonary tissue volume, pulmonary capillary blood flow and diffusing capacity lung before and after hemodialysis. Int J Artif Organs 1980; 3:259–262.
129. Abu-Hamdan D, Desai S, Mahajan S, Muller BF, Briggs WA, Lynne-Davies P, McDonnald FD. Hypoxemia during hemodialysis using acetate versus bicarbonate dialysate. Am J Nephrol 1984; 4:248–253.
130. Fawcett S, Hoenich N, Laker M. Hemodialysis-induced respiratory changes. Nephrol Dial Transplant 1987; 2:161–168.
131. Vaziri N, Barton C, Warner A. Comparison of four dialyzer-dialysate combinations: effects on blood gases, cell counts, complement contact factors and fibrinolytic system. Contrib Nephrol 1984; 37:111–119.
132. Vanholder R, Pauwels R, Vandenbogaerde J, Lamont HH, Van Der Straeten ME, Ringoir SM. Cuprophan reuse and intradialytic changes of lung diffusion capacity and blood gasses. Kidney Int 1987; 32:117–122.
133. Cheung A, LeWinter M, Chenoweth D. Cardiopulmonary effects of cuprophan-activated plasma in the swine: role of complement activation products. Kidney Int 1986; 29:799–806.
134. Bergström J, Danielsson S, Freychuss U. Dialysis, ultrafiltration and shamdialysis in normal subjects. Kidney Int 1984; 27:157.
135. Agar J, Hull J, Kaplan M. Acute cardiopulmonary decompensation and complement activation during hemodialysis. Ann Int Med 1979; 90:792–793.
136. Cochrane C, Muller-Eberhard H. The derivation of two distinct anaphylatoxin activities from the third and fifth components of human complement. J Exp Med 1968; 127:371–386.
137. Cheung A, Parker C, Wilcox L. Effects of two types of cobra venom factor on porcine complement activation and pulmonary artery pressure. Clin & Exp Immunology 1989; 78:299–306.
138. Stimler-Gerard N. Immunopharmacology of anaphylatoxin-induced bronchoconstrictor responses. Complement 1986; 3:137–151.
139. Lepow I, Willms-Kretschmer K, Patrick R. Gross and ultrastructural observations on lesions produced by intradermal injection of human C3a in man. Am J Pathol 1970; 61:13–24.
140. Henderson L, Cheung A, Chenoweth D. Choosing a membrane. Am J Kidney Dis 1983; 3:5–20.
141. Foley R, Reeves W. Acute anaphylactoid reactions in hemodialysis. Am J Kid Dis 1985; 5:132–135.
142. Ogden D. New-dialyzer syndrome. N Engl J Med 1980; 302:262–1263.
143. Rault R, Silver M. Severe reactions during hemodialysis. Am J Kidney Dis 1985; 5:128–131.
144. Caruana R, Hamilton R, Pearson F. Dialyzer hypersensitivity syndrome: possible role of allergy to ethylene oxide. Am J Nephrol 1985; 5:271–274.
145. Key J, Nahmias M, Acchiardo S. Hypersensitivity reactions on first-time exposure to cucrophan hollow fiber dialyzer. Am J Kidney Dis 1983; 2:664–666.
146. Popli S, Ing T, Daugirdas J. Severe reactions to cucrophan capillary dialyzers. Artif Organs 1982; 6:312–315.
147. Hakim R, Breilatt J, Lazarus J. Complement activation and hypersensitivity reactions to dialysis membranes. N Engl J Med 1984; 311:878–882.
148. Gutch C, Eskelson C, Ziegler E. 2-chloroethanol as a toxic residue in dialysis supplies sterilized with ethylene oxide. Dial Transplant 1976; 5:21–25.
149. Villarroel F, Ciarkowski A. A survey on hypersensitivity reactions in hemodialysis. Artif Organs 1985; 9: 231–238.
150. Ing T, Daugirdas J, Popli S. First-use syndrome with cuprammonium cellulose dialyzers. Int J Artif Organs 1983; 6:235–239.
151. Nicholls A, Platts M. Anaphylactoid reactions during hemodialysis are due to ethylene oxide hypersensitivity. Proc EDTA 1984; 121:173–177.
152. Poothullil J, Shimizu A, Day R. Anaphylaxis from the product(s) of ethylene oxide gas. Ann Int Med 1975; 82:58–60.
153. Lee F, Durning C, Leonard E. Urethanes as ethelene oxide reservoirs in hollow-fiber dialyzers. Trans ASAIO 1985; 31:526–533.
154. Ansorge W, Pelger M, Dietrich W. Ethylene oxide in dialyzer rinsing fluid: effect of rinsing technique, dialyzer storage time, and potting compound. Artif Organs 1987; 11:118–122.
155. Pearson F, Bruszer G, Lee W. Ethylene oxide sensitivity in hemodialysis patients. Artif Organs 1987; 11: 100–103.
156. Bommer J, Wilhelms O, Barth H. Anaphylactoid reactions in dialysis patients: role of ethylene-oxide. Lancet 1985; 1985:1382–1385.
157. Pascual M, Paccaud J, Macon K. Complement activation by the alternative pathway is modified in renal failure: the role of factor D. Clin Nephrol 1989; 32: 185–193.
158. Bokisch V, Muller-Eberhard H. Anaphylatoxin inactivator of human plasma: its isolation and characterization as a carboxypeptidase. J Clin Invest 1970; 49: 2427–2436.
159. Gerard C, Hugli T. Identification of classical anaphylatoxin as the des-Arg form of the C5a molecule: evidence of a modulator role for the oligosaccharide unit in human des-Arg C5a. Proc Natl Acad Sci USA 1981; 78:1833–1837.

160. Hugli T. The structural basis for anaphylatoxin and chemotactic functions of C3a, C4a, and C5a. CRC Critical Reviews in Immunol 1981; 2:321–366.
161. Mathews K, Pan P, Gardner N. Familial carboxypeptidase N deficiency. Ann Int Med 1980; 93:443–445.
162. Bergamo Collaborative Dialysis Study Group. Acute intradialytic well-being: results of a clinical trial comparing polysulfone with cuprophan. Bergamo Collaborative Dialysis Study Group. Kidney International 1991; 40:714–719.
163. Collins D, Lambert M, Tannenbaum J. Tolerance of hemodialysis: a randomized prospective trial of high-flux versus conventional high-efficiency hemodialysis. J Am Soc Nephrol 1993; 4:148–154.
164. Kozin F, Cochrane C. The contact activation system of plasma: biochemistry and pathophysiology. In: Gallin J, Goldstein I, Snyderman R, eds. Inflammation: Basic Principles and Clinical Correlates. New York: Raven Press, 1988:101–120.
165. Colman R, Hirsh J, Marder V, Salzman E. Hemostasis and thrombosis: basic principles and clinical practice. In: Colman R, Hirsh J, Marder V, Salzman E, eds. Philadelphia: J.B. Lippincott, 1987.
166. Tielemans C, Goldman M, Vanherweghem J. Immediate hypersensitivity reactions and hemodialysis. Adv Nephrol 1993;22:401–416.
167. Vroman L, Adams A, Klings M. Interactions among human blood proteins at interfaces. Fed Proc 1971; 30:1494–1502.
168. Salzman E. Role of platelets in blood-surface interactions. Fed Proc 1971; 30:1503–1508.
169. Lemke H, Fink E. Accumulation of bradykinin generation formed by the AN69- or PAN 17DX-membrane is due to the presence of an ACE-inhibitor in vitro. J Am Soc Nephrol 1992; 3:376(A).
170. Verresen L, Fink E, Lemke H-D, Vanrenterghem Y. Bradykinin is a mediator of anaphylactoid reactions during hemodialysis with AN69 membranes. Kidney Int 1994; 45:1497–1503.
171. Pegues D, Beck-Sague C, Wollen S, et al. Anaphylactoid reactions associated with reuse of hollow-fiber hemodialyzers and ACE inhibitors. Kidney Int 1992; 42: 1232–1237.
172. Gordon S, Oettinger C, Bland L, Oliver JC, Arduino MJ, Aguero SM, McAllister SK, Favero MS, Jarvis WR. Pyrogenic reactions in patients receiving conventional, high-efficiency, or high-flux hemodialysis treatments with bicarbonate dialysate containing high concentrations of bacteria and endotoxin. J Am Soc Nephrol 1992; 2:1436–1444.
173. Henderson L, Beans E. Successful production of sterile pyrogen-free electrolyte solution by ultrafiltration. Kidney Int 1978; 14:522–525.
174. Dinarello C, Lonnemann G, Maxwell R. Ultrafiltration to reject human interleukin-1 indicating substances derived from bacterial cultures. J Clin Microbiol 1987; 25:1233–1238.
175. Schindler R, Dinarello C. A method for removing interleukin-1 and tumor necrosis factor inducing substances from bacterial cultures by ultrafiltration with polysulfone. J Immunol Methods 1989; 116:159–165.
176. Haeffner-Cavaillon N, Cavaillon J-M, Laude M, Kazatchkine M. C3a(C3adesArg) induces production and release of interleukin 1 by cultured human monocytes. J Immunol 1987; 139:794–799.
177. Schindler R, Lonnemann G, Shaldon S. Transcription, not synthesis, of interleukin-1 and tumor necrosis factor by complement. Kidney Int 1990; 37:85–93.
178. Goodman M, Chenoweth D, Weigle W. Induction of interleukin 1 secretion and enhancement of humoral immunity by binding of human C5a to macrophage surface C5a receptors. J Exp Med 1982; 1156:912–917.
179. Gorevic P, Casey T, Stone W. Beta-2 microglobulin is an amyloidogenic protein in man. J Clin Invest 1985; 76:2425–2429.
180. Gejyo F, Yamada T, Odani S, Nakagawa Y, Arakawa M, Kunimoto T, Kataoka H, Suzuki M, Hirasawa Y, Shirahama T, et al. A new form of amyloid protein associated with hemodialysis was identified as β2-microglobulin. Biochem Biophys Res Comm 1985; 129: 701–806.
181. Miyaya T, Oda O, Inagi R. β_2-Microglobulin modified with advanced glycation end products is a major component of hemodialysis-associated amyloidosis. J Clin Invest 1993; 92:1243–1252.
182. Ogawa H, Saito A, Ono M. Novel β_2-microglobulin and its amyloidogenic predisposition in patients on hemodialysis. Nephrol Dial Transplant 1989; 4(suppl): 14–18.
183. Linke R, Hampl H, Lobeck H. Lysine-specific cleavage of B2-microglobulin in amyloid deposits associated with hemodialysis. Kidney Int 1989; 36:675–681.
184. Floege J, Granolleras C, Koch K. Which membrane? Should beta-2 microglobulin decide on the choice of today's hemodialysis membrane? Nephron 1988; 50: 177–181.
185. Ritz E, Bommer J. Beta-2-microglobulin-derived amyloid-problems and perspectives. Blood Purif 1988; 6: 61–68.
186. Floege J, Bartsch A, Schulze M. Clearance and synthesis rates of B2-microglobulin in patients undergoing hemodialysis in normal subjects. J Lab Clin Med 1991; 118:153–165.
187. Vincent C, Chanard J, Caudwell V, Lavaud S, Wong T, Revillard J. Kinetics of 125I-beta 2-microglobulin turnover in dialyzed patients. Kidney Int 1992; 42: 1434–1443.
188. Floege J, Granolleras C, Bingel M, et al. B2-microglobulin kinetics during hemodialysis and hemofiltration. Nephrol Dial Transpl 1987; 1:223–228.
189. Jorstad S, Smeby L, Balstad T. Removal, generation and adsorption of beta-2-microglobulin during hemo-

filtration with five different membranes. Blood Purif 1988; 6:96–105.

190. Paczek L, Schaefer R, Heidland A. Dialysis membranes inhibit in vitro release of beta-2-microglobulin from human lymphocytes. Nephron 1990; 56:267–270.
191. Bjerrum O, Bjerrum O, Borregaard N. β_2-Microglobulin in neutrophils: an intragranular protein. J Immunol 1987; 138:3913–3917.
192. Bergstrom J, Wehle B. No change in corrected β_2-microglobulin concentration after cucrophane hemodialysis. Lancet 1987; 1:628–629.
193. Floege J, Granolleras C, Merscher S. Is the rise in plasma beta-2-microglobulin seen during hemodialysis meaningful? Nephron 1989; 51:6–12.
194. Klinke B, Rockel A, Perschel W. Beta-2-microglobulin adsorption and release in-vitro: influence of membrane material, osmolality and heparin. Int J Artif Organs 1988; 11:355–360.
195. Chanard J, Bindi P, Lavaud S. Carpal tunnel syndrome and type of dialysis membrane. Br Med J 1989:867–868.
196. van Ypersele de Strihou C, Jadoul M, Malghem J, Maldague B, Jamart J. Effect of dialysis membrane and patient's age on signs of dialysis-related amyloidosis. The Working Party on Dialysis Amyloidosis. Kidney Int 1991; 39:1012–1019.
197. Miura Y, Ishiyama T, Inomata A, et al. Radiolucent bone cysts and the type of dialysis membrane used in patients undergoing long-term hemodialysis. Nephron 1992; 60:268–273.
198. Weiss S, Regiani S. Neutrophils degrade subendothelial matrices in the present of alpha-1-proteinase inhibitor: cooperative use of lysosomal proteinases and oxygen metabolitews. J Clin Invest 1984; 73:1297–1303.
199. Baracos V, Rodemann HP, Dinarello CA, Goldberg AL. Stimulation of muscle protein degradation by leukocyte pyrogen (interleukin-1). N Engl J Med 1983; 308:553–558.
200. Gutierrez A, Alvestrand A, Wahren J, Bergstrom J. Effect of in vivo contact between blood and dialysis membranes on protein catabolism in humans. Kidney Int 1990; 38:487–494.
201. Lonnemann G, Koch KM, Shaldon S, Dinarello CA. Studies on the ability of hemodialysis membranes to induce, bind, and clear human interleukin-1. J Lab Clin Med 1988; 112:76–86.
202. Lim V, Bier D, Flanigan M. The effect of hemodialysis on protein metabolism: a leucine kinetic study. J Clin Invest 1993; 91:2419–2436.
203. Schiffl H, Lang SM, Konig A, Strasser T, Haider MC, Held E. Biocompatible membranes in acute renal failure: prospective case-controlled study. Lancet 1994; 344:570–572.
204. Schiffl H, Sitter T, Lang S, Konig A, Haider M, Held E. Bioincompatible membranes place patients with acute renal failure at increased risk of infection. ASAIO J 1995; 41:M709–M712.
205. Hakim RM, Wingard RL, Parker RA. Effect of the dialysis membrane in the treatment of patients with acute renal failure. N Engl J Med 1994; 331:1338–1342.
206. Kurtal H, von Herrath D, Schaefer K. Is the choice of membrane important for patients with acute renal failure requiring hemodialysis? Artif Organs 1995; 19:391–394.
207. Liano F, Pascual J and the Madrid Acute Renal Failure Study Group. Epidemiology of acute renal failure: a prospective, multi-center, community-based study. Kidney Int 1996; 50:811–818.
208. Levin NW, Zasuwa G, Dumler F. Effect of membrane type on causes of death in hemodialysis patients. J Am Soc Nephrol 1991; 2:335.
209. Hornberger J, Chernew M, Petersen J, Garber A. A multivariate analysis of mortality and hospital admissions with high-flux dialysis. J Am Soc Nephrol 1992; 3:1227–1237.
210. Hakim R, Held P, Stannard DC, Wolfe RA, Port FK, Daugirdas JT, Agodoa L. Effect of the dialysis membrane on mortality of chronic hemodialysis patients. Kidney Int 1996; 50:566–570.
211. Hartmann J, Fricke H, Schiffl H. Hemodialysis versus peritoneal dialysis: a comparison of adjusted mortality rates. Am J Kidney Dis 1997; 30:366–373.
212. McCarthy JT, Jenson BM, Squillace DP, et al. Improved preservation of residual renal function in chronic hemodialysis patients using polysulfone dialyzers. Am J Kidney Dis 1997; 29:576–583.
213. Van Stone JC. The effect of dialyzer membrane and etiology of kidney disease on the preservation of residual renal function in chronic hemodialysis patients. ASAIO J 1995; 41:M713–M716.
214. Caramelo C, Alcazar R, Gallar P, et al. Choice of dialysis membrane does not influence the outcome of residual renal function in hemodialysis patients. Nephrol Dial Transplant 1994; 9:675–677.
215. Vanholder RC, Pauwels RA, Vandenbogaerde JF, Lamont HH, Van Der Straeten ME, Ringoir SM. Cuprophan reuse and intradialytic changes of lung diffusion capacity and blood gasses. Kidney Int 1987; 32:117–122.
216. Vanholder R, Van Landschoot N, Waterloos MA, Delanghe J, Van Maele G, Ringoir S. Phagocyte metabolic activity during hemodialysis with different dialyzers not affecting the number of circulating phagocytes. Int J Artif Organs 1992; 15:89–92.
217. Tokars JI, Alter MJ, Favero MS, Moyer LA, Miller E, Bland L. National surveillance of dialysis associated diseases in the United States, 1992. ASAIO J 1994; 40:1020–1031.
218. Gordon SM, Tipple M, Bland LA, Jarvis WR. Pyrogenic reactions associated with the reuse of disposable

hollow-fiber hemodialyzers. JAMA 1988; 260:2077–2081.

219. Vanholder R, Vanhaecke E, Ringoir S. Pseudomonas septicemia due to deficient disinfectant mixing during reuse. Int J Artif Organs 1992; 15:19–24.
220. Bolan G, Reingold AL, Carson LA, Silcox VA, Woodley CL, Hayes PS, Hightower AW, MacFarland L, Brown JW, Petersen NJ, Favero MS, Good RC, Broome CV. Infections with *Mycobacterium chelonei* in patients receiving dialysis and using processed hemodialyzers. J Infect Dis 1985; 152:1013–1019.
221. Pinto dos Santos J, Loureiro A, Cendoroglo Neto M, Pereira BJG. Impact of dialysis room and reuse strategies on the incidence of hepatitis C virus infection in haemodialysis units. Nephrol Dial Transplant 1996; 11:2017–2022.
222. Goldman M, Lagmiche M, Dhaene M, Amraoui Z, Thayse C, Vanherweghem JL. Adsorption of β2-microglobulin on dialysis membranes: comparison of different dialyzers and effects of reuse procedures. Int J Artif Organs 1989; 12:373–378.
223. Diaz RJ, Washburn S, Cauble L, Siskind MS, Van Wyck D. The effect of dialyzer reprocessing on performance of β_2-microglobulin removal using polysulfone membranes. Am J Kidney Dis 1993; 21:405–410.
224. Kaplan AA, Halley SE, Lapkin RA, Graeber CW. Dialysate protein losses with bleach processed polysulphone dialyzers. Kidney Int 1995; 47:573–578.
225. Sundaram S, Barrett TW, Meyer KB, Perrella C, Cendoroglo Neto M, King AJ, Pereira BJG. Transmembrane passage of cytokine-inducing bacterial products across new and reprocessed polysulfone dialyzers. J Am Soc Nephrol 1996; 7:2183–2191.
226. Villaroel F, Ciarkowski AA. A survey on hypersensitivity reactions in hemodialysis. Artif Organs 1985; 9: 231–238.
227. Cheung AK, Dalpias D, Emmerson R, Leypoldt JK. A prospective study on intradialytic symptoms associated with reuse of hemodialyzers. Am J Nephrol 1991; 11:397–401.
228. Pegues DA, Beck-Sague CM, Woolen SW, Greenspan B, Burns SM, Bland LA, Arduino MJ, Favero MS, Mackow RC, Jarvis WR. Anaphylactoid reactions associated with reuse of hollow-fiber hemodialyzers and ACE inhibitors. Kidney Int 1992; 42:1232–1237.
229. Stragier A, Wenderickx D, Jadoul M. Rinsing time and disinfectant release of reused dialyzers: comparison of formaldehyde, hypochlorite, warexin and renalin. Am J Kidney Dis 1995; 26:549–553.
230. Vanholder R, Noens L, De Smet R, Ringoir S. Development of anti-N-like antibodies using formaldehyde reuse in spite of adequate predialysis rinsing. Am J Kidney Dis 1988; 11:477–480.
231. Van Loo A, Vanholder R, Bernaert P, Vermassen F, Van Der Vennet M, Lameire N. Pretransplantation hemodialysis strategy influences early renal graft function. J Am Soc Nephrol 1998; 9:473–481.
232. Valeri A. Bicompatible membranes (BCM) in acute renal failure (ARF): a study in post-cadaveric renal transplant acute tubular necrosis (ATN). J Am Soc Nephrol 1994; 5:481.
233. Falkenhagen D, Mitzner S, Stange J, Klinkmann H. Biocompatibility: methodology and evaluation. In: Bonomini V, ed. Evolution in Dialysis Adequacy. Basel: Karger, 1993:34–54.
234. Floege J, Smeby L. Dialysis-related amyloidosis and high-flux membranes. In: Shaldon S, Koch K, eds. Polyamide—The Evolution of a Synthetic Membrane for Renal Therapy. Basel: Karger, 1992:124–137.

4

Acute Dialysis Complications

K. M. L. Leunissen, J. P. Kooman, and F. M. van der Sande
Academic Hospital Maastricht, Maastricht, The Netherlands

I. INTRADIALYTIC HYPOTENSION

During intermittent hemodialysis, fluid that has accumulated during the inter-dialytic period has to be removed. Because this has to be achieved in a relatively short period of time, significant changes in the milieu interieur of the patient may occur, which can lead to symptomatic hypotensive periods, resulting in discomfort such as dizziness, nausea, and vomiting. Especially in elderly and cardiovascularly compromised patients, who are predominantly vulnerable to rapid changes in volume status, hypotension may have serious consequences, such as myocardial and cerebral ischemia.

Three major factors are responsible for the maintenance of hemodynamic stability during dialysis. First is the preservation of blood volume. During ultrafiltration, fluid is in first instance removed from the intravascular compartment. However, because of the decrease in intravascular pressure and the increase in colloid osmotic pressure, refill from the interstitium may partly compensate for the decline in blood volume.

Second, when blood volume declines, the structure and function of the heart is a major determinant in the hemodynamic response to hypovolemia. Under normal circumstances, the cardiac response to a decline in blood volume consists of an enhanced contractility and an increased pulse rate.

Third, a normal structure and function of the peripheral vasculature is of prime importance for the maintenace of hemodynamic stability. Under normal circumstances, both the resistance and capacitance vessels constrict during hypovolemia, which is primarily due to an increase in sympathetic tone. Constriction of the resistance vessels (small arteries and arterioles) maintains blood pressure at the precapillary level, whereas constriction of the capacitance vessels (venules and veins) means to centralize blood volume.

Both patient- and treatment-related factors may interfere with the normal response to fluid removal in hemodialysis patients. In this chapter, first the mechanisms responsible for hemodynamic instability will be discussed, followed by suggestions for treatment and prevention of symptomatic hypotension.

A. Pathophysiology: Blood Volume Preservation

Fluid that has accumulated during the inter-dialytic period is removed by ultrafiltration, realized by differences in hydrostatic pressure between the blood and dialysate compartment. This leads to convective transport of plasma water across the dialysis membrane, resulting in a decline in blood volume when refill from the interstitium is unable to compensate for the fluid lost from the intravascular compartment. Ultrafiltration can be performed with or without concomitant hemodialysis treatment ("isolated ultrafiltration").

The movement of fluid between the interstitial and intravascular spaces mainly depends on the hydrostatic and oncotic pressures in these two compartments and on the permeability of the capillary wall, as described by the Starling formula. During removal of plasma water, the hydrostatic pressure at the venular side of the capillary bed decreases, whereas plasma oncotic pressure increases, which promotes a shift of fluid from the interstitial to the intravascular compartment. However, both individual factors and the dialysis regimen itself may interfere with the refill of blood volume from the interstitium. Therefore, hypovolemia may occur even when the interstitial compartment is still fluid overloaded. Indeed, in one study the great majority of hypotensive periods occurred when the absolute blood volume of the patient was below 50 mL/kg (1).

1. Blood Volume Preservation

a. *Patient-Related Factors*

Fluid Status The fluid status of the patient has a profound influence on blood volume preservation. When the patient is hypervolemic before dialysis, the interstitial compartment is well hydrated and interstitial pressure is relatively high. Therefore, when fluid is removed during dialysis, refill of plasma volume from the interstitium will prevent a major decline in blood volume (2). However, when a patient is hypovolemic before dialysis, the interstitium is fluid depleted, which hampers the shift of fluid to the intravascular compartment. The difference in blood volume preservation between over- and underhydrated patients has been described by several authors and is also well recognized in daily clinical practice (1–4).

Venous Compliance In patients with a reduced compliance (volume:pressure ratio) of the venous system, refill of blood volume from the interstitium is hampered because of a disturbance in the capillary Starling equilibrium. Venous compliance is especially reduced in dialysis patients with preexistent hypertension, which appears to be due to structural abnormalities of the venous wall (5,6).

The effect of venous compliance on blood volume preservation can be explained by the fact that in patients with a reduced venous compliance (i.e., increased stiffness of the venous wall), the pressure in the postcapillary venules is higher for a given level of plasma volume, which impairs the fluid shift from the interstitial to the intravascular compartment (7). A steeper decline in blood volume was observed in patients with a reduced venous compliance during isolated ultrafiltration compared with patients with a normal venous compliance (8). Theoretically, this phenomenon will be most important in the first part of a dialysis session because refill of blood volume will increase after a fall in venous pressure. It has been observed that refill of plasma volume from the interstitium is relatively low immediately after the start of ultrafiltration, until after 60–120 minutes the rise in colloid osmotic pressure becomes high enough to result in a nearly steady state between refill of blood volume from the interstitial compartment and fluid removal (9,10).

b. *Treatment-Related Factors*

Ultrafiltration Rate The ultrafiltration rate is a major determinant for blood volume preservation. It has been shown that a major decline in plasma volume can be provoked by the use of excessive ultrafiltration rates (11–13) (Fig. 1). This can be explained by the quick removal of blood volume, which cannot be compensated for by refill from the interstitium.

Sodium Concentration of the Dialysate It is well known that blood volume preservation is impaired during low-sodium dialysis compared to dialysis with a sodium concentration of the dialysate equal to or higher than the sodium concentration in the plasma. It was at first believed that this phenomenon occurred because of diffusion of urea into the dialysate. Urea rapidly equilibrates between the intravascular and interstitial compartments, whereas the transport over the cellular membrane may lag behind. Especially with a low sodium concentration of the dialysate, the extracellular compartment becomes hypotonic to the intracellular space, which will promote the movement of fluid into the cell (13). A sodium shift from the dialysate into the patient would prevent the rapid fall in extracellular osmolality and therefore improve blood volume preservation. However, during dialysis with a variable sodium concentration of the dialysate, intracellular volume (assessed by bio-impedance spectroscopy) remained stable, whereas changes in extracellular volume were largely confined to the intravascular space. This can be explained by the fact that sodium transport accross the capillary wall is relatively slow. Therefore, the effect of higher dialysate sodium on blood volume preservation (14,15) is more likely explained by a fluid shift from the interstitial to the intravascular space due to an osmotic gradient over the capillary wall (16).

Choice of Dialysate Buffer The choice of dialysate buffer also influences blood volume preservation. Acetate induces arteriolar vasodilation, which increases precapillary hydrostatic pressure and provokes a shift from the intravascular into the interstitial space. Bicarbonate has less vasodilating properties and therefore exerts a more favorable effect on plasma volume preservation (17, 18).

Treatment Modality Few authors have studied differences in plasma volume preservation between various dialysis techniques. No differences in plasma volume preservation were observed between isolated

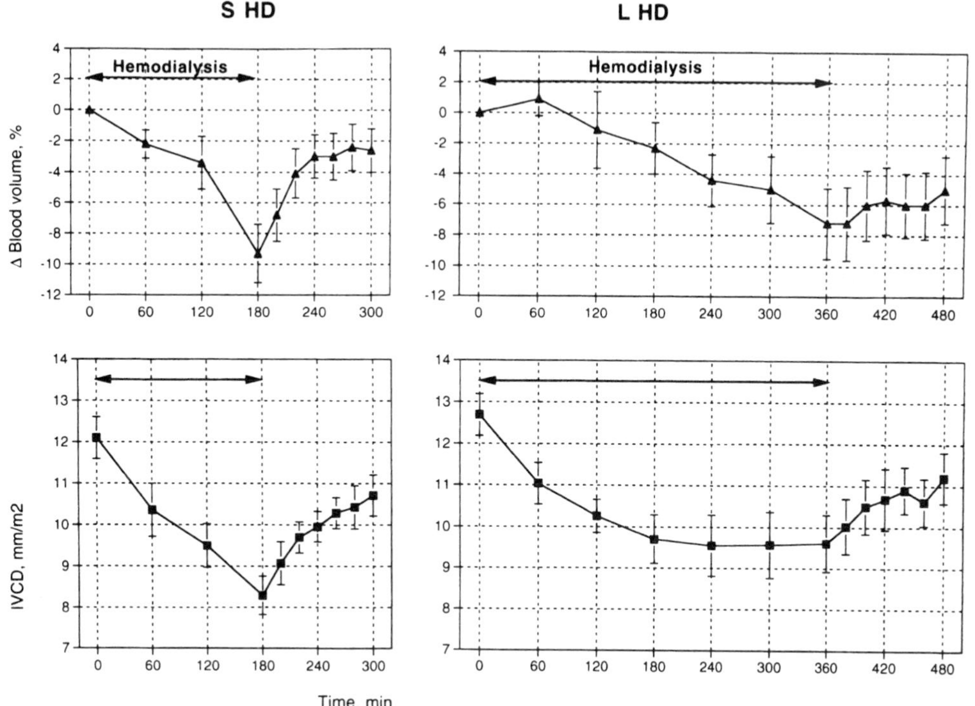

Fig. 1 Changes in blood volume during and after hemodialysis with high (S HD) and low (L HD) ultrafiltration rates. (From Ref. 11.)

ultrafiltration and ultrafiltration combined with bicarbonate hemodialysis (19).

It was found that, in contrast with hemodialysis, intracellular volume increased during hemodiafiltration, which can be explained by a more effective removal of solutes, leading to a reduced osmolality of the extracellular space. However, no difference in plasma volume preservation was observed between these two techniques (20). Also, a recent study did not show differences in plasma refilling between standard hemodialysis and high efficiency hemodiafiltration (21).

On the other hand, it was observed that the decrease in blood volume was less pronounced during hemofiltration compared with hemodialysis at an equivalent ultrafiltration rate, which can be explained by a decreased removal of low molecular weight substrates (22). However, other investigators did not observe a difference in blood volume preservation between bicarbonate dialysis and hemofiltration (23).

2. Cardiovascular Regulatory Mechanisms

When hypovolemia occurs in an otherwise healthy subject, compensatory mechanisms will initially prevent a fall in blood pressure. Blood pressure is determined by peripheral vascular resistance and cardiac output:

$$\text{Blood pressure} = \text{Systemic vascular resistance} \times \text{Cardiac output}$$

Therefore, during a decrease in blood volume, either peripheral vascular resistance has to rise or cardiac output has to remain stable to maintain hemodynamic stability. A decline in blood volume is primarily sensed by low-pressure receptors in the atria and pulmonary veins, whereas a decrease in blood pressure is primarily sensed by the high-pressure baroreceptors in the aorta. By a reduction in the amount of inhibitory impulses from these receptors to the vasomotor center in the medulla oblongata, peripheral vascular resistance increases because of an enhanced sympathetic activity and increased concentrations of vasopressor substances (24).

Cardiac output depends upon heart rate, myocardial contractility, and ventricular filling. During a decrease in blood volume, heart rate and myocardial contractility increase. Ventricular filling is mainly dependent upon venous return, which is determined by blood volume in combination with passive and active properties of the venous system.

The venous system can conceptually be regarded as a conductance system for the backflow of hemody-

Table 1 The Regulation of Blood Volume Preservation During Dialysis

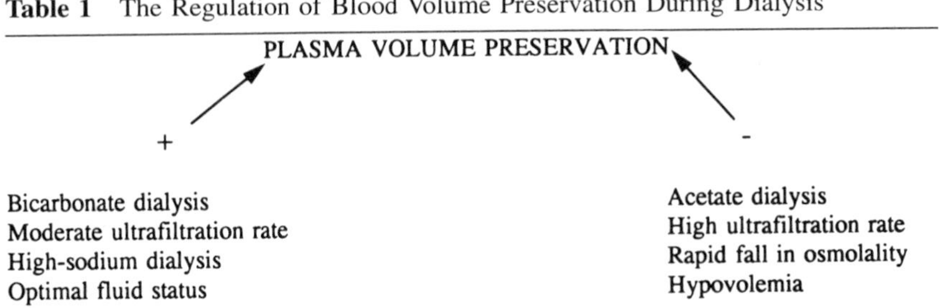

PLASMA VOLUME PRESERVATION

+	-
Bicarbonate dialysis	Acetate dialysis
Moderate ultrafiltration rate	High ultrafiltration rate
High-sodium dialysis	Rapid fall in osmolality
Optimal fluid status	Hypovolemia

namically active ("stressed") blood from the periphery to the heart and as a reservoir for hemodynamically inactive ("unstressed") blood volume (Table 1).

Approximately 60–80% of total blood volume resides in the venous system. With minimal sympathetic activity, a large amount of this blood volume is hemodynamically inactive. By shifting between the stressed and unstressed compartments, the venous system can rapidly provide the blood needed to maintain cardiac output at an optimum level. When blood volume declines hemodynamically inactive blood can become stressed by a sympathetically mediated increase in smooth muscle tone provoking venoconstriction in combination with passive recoil of the venous wall. Therefore, during a decrease in blood volume, the venous system can maintain ventricular filling by active and passive venoconstriction (25).

In addition, the structure of the venous wall, which determines the compliance (venous/pressure relationship) of the venous system, is also an important determinant of venous return. When venous compliance is reduced (i.e., the venous wall is stiffer), the venous system is more sensitive to changes in blood volume. Because of the reduced volume-pressure relationship, a small increase in blood volume will lead to a steep increase in venous pressure, whereas a small drop in blood volume may lead to a steep decline in venous pressure (25,26).

In hemodialysis patients, the regulation of the cardiovascular response may be disturbed, which may have deleterious effects, especially in patients with an impaired cardiovascular system. Both patient- and treatment-related factors contribute to the increased sensitivity of hemodialysis patients to changes in blood volume (Table 2).

a. *Patient-Related Factors*

Autonomous Neuropathy Many hemodialysis patients have signs of autonomous neuropathy, mainly

Table 2 Factors Influencing the Hemodynamic Response to a Decline in Blood Volume During Hemodialysis

Cardiac output	Heart rate	Myocardial contractility	Ventricular filling
Patient related	Autonomous neuropathy Bezold-Jarish reflex	Systolic dysfunction	Venous compliance Diastolic dysfunction
Treatment related		Dialysate calcium Acetate Extracorporeal blood temperature	*Venoconstriction*: Extracorporeal blood temperature
Systemic vascular resistance			
Patient related	Autonomous neuropathy (diabetics)		
Treatment related	Acetate Extracorporeal blood temperature Sympathetic activity Nitric oxide?		

characterized by a dysfunction of the baroreceptor reflex arc. The autonomous defect is primarily located in the afferent part of the baroreceptor reflex arc and in the efferent parasympathetic response, which may impair the heart rate response during hypovolemia (27,28).

Moreover, plasma catecholamines are generally increased in dialysis patients. This has been attributed to a reduced end-organ sensitivity for catecholamines (29). However, more likely a general state of sympathetic overactivity exists in the uremic state (30). Moreover, except in diabetic patients, the efferent sympathetic pathway appears to be generally intact; several authors found a normal vasoconstrictor response during a sympathetic stimulus (5,31).

Studies regarding the impact of autonomous neuropathy on intradialytic hemodynamics have shown conflicting results. Although in some studies a relationship was observed between disturbances in the baroreceptor reflex arc and intradialytic hypotension (32–34), the results are not confirmed by others (5,35,36). Also, the dialysis treatment itself may have some impact on the functioning of the autonomous nervous system, as will be discussed below.

Systolic Dysfunction Many dialysis patients have an abnormal systolic function of the heart, which is often related to a dilated cardiomyopathy. Pathogenetic factors in the development of a dilated cardiomyopathy of the heart include chronic volume overload, hypertension, anemia, hyperparathyroidism, coronary artery disease, the arteriovenous fistula, carnitine deficiency, and the uremic state itself. Systolic dysfunction of the heart predisposes the dialysis patient to symptomatic hypotension because the heart cannot respond well to changes in filling volume. Moreover, it is associated with significantly increased morbidity and mortality (37,38).

Diastolic Dysfunction of the Left Ventricle Diastolic dysfunction of the left ventricle can be defined as an impaired capacity of the ventricle to accept blood without a disproportionate change in ventricular pressure. In other words, the compliance (volume:pressure ratio) of the ventricle is reduced. Because of the increased sensitivity to changes in volume, a small increase in ventricular volume leads to a steep increase in ventricular pressure, whereas a small decrease in ventricular volume induces a steep decline in left ventricular pressure (39) (Fig. 2). Therefore, patients with a reduced left ventricular compliance have a very small margin between clinical under- and overhydration and are especially prone to symptomatic hypotension (40).

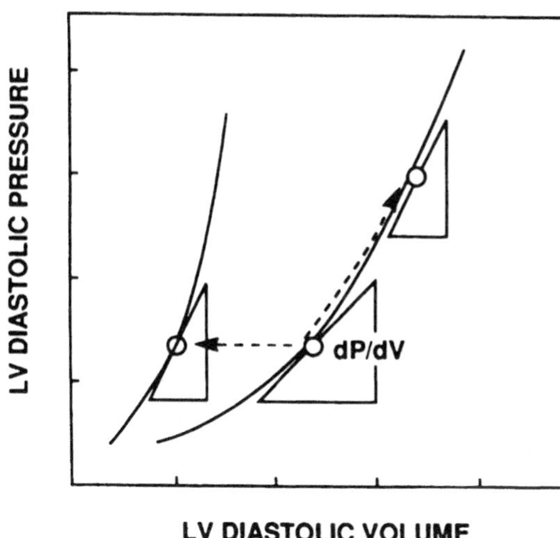

Fig. 2 Compliance characteristics of the left ventricle during diastolic filling. In end-stage renal disease, a leftward shift of the pressure-volume is common (decreased left ventricular compliance). (From Ref. 154.)

Patients with diastolic dysfunction of the left ventricle may have a completely normal or even supranormal systolic function. Diastolic dysfunction is primarily due to an abnormal structure of the ventricle and is often related to left ventricular concentric hypertrophy. The most important risk factor for diastolic dysfunction is hypertension, in combination with the uremic state itself. Moreover, an increased stiffness of the arterial tree may increase left ventricular hypertrophy by increasing the burden on the heart. Also, left ventricular concentric hypertrophy is associated with increased morbidity and mortality in the dialysis population (37–39).

Reduced Venous Compliance Independent from the effect on blood volume preservation (see above), we also found a larger fall in central venous pressure in patients with a reduced venous compliance. This can be explained by the steeper volume-pressure relationship of the venous system in these patients (7). Therefore, patients with a reduced venous compliance appear to be more sensitive to changes in volume status.

b. *Treatment-Related Factors*

Functioning of the Autonomous Nervous System In addition to preexistent autonomous neuropathy, the hemodialysis treatment itself may interfere with the normal heart rate response. Zuchelli et al. observed an acute dysfunction of the baroreceptors (assessed by the Valsalva maneuver) induced by the dialysis treatment itself (41), although this finding was not confirmed by others (36). In contrast, an improvement in baroreceptor function was observed after hemofiltration (41,42). More importantly, it was observed using microneurography that some episodes of acute hypotension during dialysis are related to an acute decrease in sympathetic activity, which is preceded by a large burst in sympathetic activity (43). This reduction in sympathetic activity was related to an acute decrease in peripheral vascular resistance and a reduction in heart rate. The acute reduction in sympathetic activity appears to be related to the Bezold-Jarisch reflex, which is evoked by a stimulation of left ventricular baroreceptors in response to severe left ventricular underfilling. However, this reflex is probably only elicited during severe hypovolemia, as many episodes of symptomatic hypotension are accompanied by an increased or unchanged heart rate (44,45) (Fig. 3).

Impaired Constriction of the Resistance and Capacitance Vessels The hemodialysis procedure itself has a strong impact on vascular reactivity. It is well known that vasoconstriction is impaired when fluid is removed during acetate dialysis, which is due to a direct vasodilating action (46,47). However, during bicarbonate dialysis the constriction of the capacitance and resistance vessels is also diminished, although to a lesser degree (46) (Fig. 4). The reduced vascular reactivity

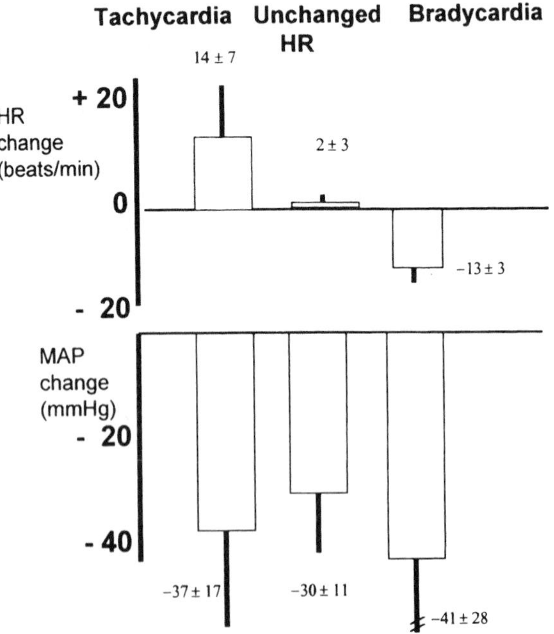

Fig. 3 Heart rate changes during tachycardic, bradycardic, and "fixed" heart-rate hypotensive crises. (From Ref. 45.)

may lead to hemodynamic instability, both by a reduced centralization of blood volume by the impaired venoconstriction and by a failure to maintain arterial blood pressure at the precapillary level by the reduced arteriolar constriction.

The reduced vascular response to hypovolemia observed during hemodialysis is in contrast with the physiological vascular reactivity during hemofiltration and isolated ultrafiltration (48). This probably explains the large difference in hemodynamic stability between hemodialysis on one hand and isolated ultrafiltration and hemofiltration on the other hand. How can this be explained?

Differences in plasma levels of vasoactive peptides have been observed between hemodialysis and isolated ultrafiltration. A fairly common finding is the larger increase in plasma levels of norepinephrine during isolated ultrafiltration and hemofiltration compared to (acetate and bicarbonate) hemodialysis (46,49–51). Moreover, a larger increase in plasma renin activity (46) and vasopressin (49) was observed during isolated ultrafiltration compared to hemodialysis. The mechanism behind these differences is not yet clear. Increased production of vasopressor substances during isolated ultrafiltration or increased removal by diffusion during hemodialysis may play a role, although the latter possibility is unlikely in view of the very rapid endogenous clearance of catecholamines (50).

Vasodilating agents have been less extensively investigated. Plasma levels of the strong vasodilator calcitonin gene related peptide (CGRP) did not differ between hemodialysis and isolated ultrafiltration (51). During severe dialysis hypotension, an increase in plasma levels of the vasodilating peptide adenosine has been observed, possibly due to release from ischemic tissue (52). Nevertheless, although vasoactive peptides will certainly contribute to the different hemodynamic response between the various treatment modalities, it is not yet clear whether they are primarily responsible for the difference in hemodynamic stability or represent more an epiphenomenon.

Other factors certainly play a role. It was hypothesized by Henderson et al. that hemodynamic instability during hemodialysis could be related to the release of cytokines like interleukin-1 and TNF-α by blood mononuclear cells after stimulation by complement (especially C5a) or endotoxin fragments (53). Interleukin-1 could induce hypotension by an increased production of nitric oxide by stimulation of mRNA in vascular smooth muscle cells. The better hemodynamic stability during isolated ultrafiltration and hemofiltration would reflect the absence of dialysate (with contaminants) in

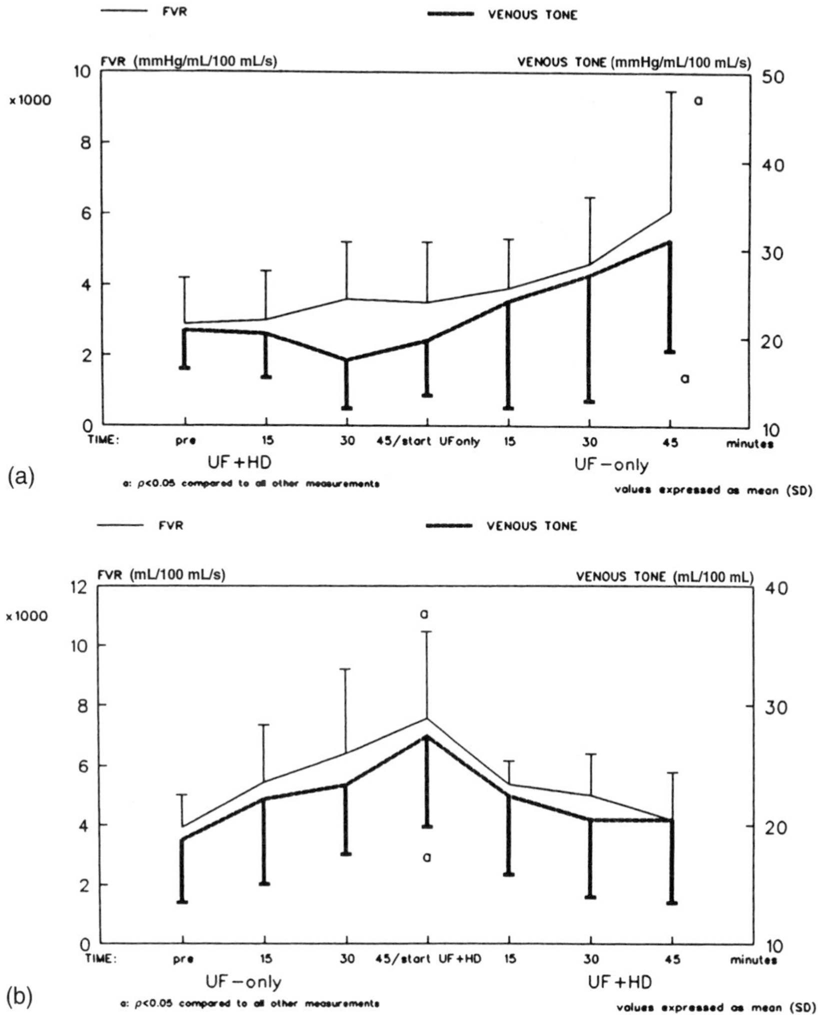

Fig. 4 Vascular response during sequential isolated ultrafiltration (UF only) hemodialysis combined with ultrafiltration (HD + UF) and during sequential HD + UF followed by UF only. FVR = Forearm vascular resistance.

both treatment modalities and the use of more biocompatible membranes during hemofiltration, leading to reduced complement stimulation.

It is well known that monocytes from hemodialysis patients are in an activated state, i.e., they have an elevated cytokine content and are "primed" to produce cytokines in larger amounts after in vitro stimulation by lipopolysaccharides compared to monocytes from healthy subjects (54). Moreover, nitric oxide was found to be increased in patients with symptomatic hypotension compared to patients without hemodynamic instability (55).

However, the relevance of the interleukin hypothesis in the pathogenesis of hemodynamic instability remains to be established. Although complement activation and nitric oxide production are more pronounced during dialysis with unsubstituted cuprophane membranes (54,56), four recent studies have failed to show any difference in hemodynamic stability or cardiovascular reactivity between dialysis treatment with biocompatible versus bioincompatible membranes (57–60). Moreover, vascular reactivity was not improved by the use of sterile dialysate in comparison to nonsterile dialysate (61). In addition, the difference in vascular reactivity between isolated ultrafiltration and hemodialysis is already evident after 15–30 minutes (7,44), whereas cytokine induction takes longer (62).

Therefore, there are other mechanisms involved in the impaired vascular response during hemodialysis. Although important for plasma volume preservation, changes in osmolality during dialysis do not appear to be of major importance in the reduced vascular response during hemodialysis, as addition of urea to the dialysate to prevent the fall in osmolality was still associated with a decrease in peripheral vascular resistance (63). Moreover, no difference in vascular reactivity was observed between hemodialysis with a low (134 mmol/L) and high (140 mmol/L) sodium concentration of the dialysate (64). Still, excessive lowering of the sodium concentration (126 mmol/L) might induce vasodilation due to prostaglandin E_2 production (65), although this phenomenon is probably not of major importance during standard hemodialysis. Changes in ionized calcium, although important for cardiac contractility during dialysis, do not appear to have a major impact on vascular reactivity during hemodialysis (66,67).

The differences in vascular reactivity between isolated ultrafiltration and hemofiltration on one hand and hemodialysis on the other appear to be related to differences in extracorporeal blood temperature between the various treatment modalities. Extracorporeal blood temperature decreases during isolated ultrafiltration, and hemofiltration because of the large extracorporeal circuit, the absence of heating during isolated ultrafiltration and the relatively low infusate flow during hemofiltration. Vascular reactivity was clearly increased during cold dialysis (dialysate temperature 35°C) compared to dialysis with a normal temperature of the dialysate (37.5°C) (68–70), whereas the constriction of the capacitance and resistance vessels was clearly diminished during hemofiltration with increased temperature of the infused substitution fluid (23). In this aspect, differences in heat balance are possibly of more importance than the extracorporeal blood temperature per se, as the effectivity of cold dialysis was found to be related to the core temperature of the patient (71). The mechanism behind the improved vascular response during cold dialysis has not been completely elucidated, although the differences in vascular reactivity have been related to sympathetic nervous activity (70,72).

Myocardial Contractility Myocardial contractility remains generally normal during standard hemodialysis and may even increase, possibly due to the reduction in afterload or the removal of cardiodepressant uremic toxins (73). However, especially in patients with impaired cardiac function, the use of acetate as dialysis buffer may have significant cardiodepressant effects (15,74). Moreover, because myocardial contractility is dependent upon the influx of ionized calcium (75,76), the use of low-calcium dialysate may impair the systolic function of the heart. Indeed, it was shown in patients with a reduced systolic function of the heart that cardiac contractility decreased during low-calcium dialysis but remained stable during high-calcium dialysis (77). Cardiac contractility can be improved with the use of cold dialysis, which will contribute to the improved hemodynamic stability with the use of this method (78).

B. Symptomatic Hypotension: Acute Treatment

During symptomatic hypotension, ultrafiltration is stopped and the legs of the patient elevated. If blood pressure does not rise, isotonic or hypertonic saline, mannitol, or a colloid solution can be administered. Few reports have compared the efficacy of these maneuvers during intradialytic hypotension. Gong et al. (79) assessed the effect of 30 mL 7.5% hypertonic saline (80 mOsm), 10 mL 23% saturated hypertonic saline (80 mOsm), and 7.5% saline with 6% dextran 70 (100 mOsm). The increase in blood pressure was greater with the two latter solutions compared with 7.5% hypertonic saline, whereas the effect of the dextran solution was most prolonged (79). Because during hemodialysis, a disequilibrium may exist between an underfilled intravascular compartment and a still overhydrated interstitium, the use of hyperoncotic solutions, such as 20% albumin, dextran, and hydroxyethyl starch (HES), may induce a fluid shift from the interstitium to the intravascular compartment because of an increase in plasma colloid somotic pressure. Indeed, we observed a more profound and longer-lasting effect on plasma volume after HES and hyperoncotic albumin compared with saline (80). Nevertheless, there is some concern regarding the elimination of dextran and HES in patients with end-stage renal failure (81). However, Steinhoff et al. (82) found only a very small amount of HES in the circulation of dialysis patients 48 hours after administration. Still, accumulation in the reticuloendothelial system must also be taken into account. Moreover, the risk of anaphylactoid reactions, although small, is present with the use of humane and synthetic colloids.

C. Symptomatic Hypotension: Prevention

1. Improving Plasma Volume Preservation

a. Preventing Excessive Interdialytic Weight Gain

Because a large amount of fluid has to be removed in a relatively short period of time, excessive interdialytic weight gain greatly increases the risk of hypotensive episodes. Dietary counseling and restriction of sodium and water intake may be of help.

b. *Determination of Dry Weight*

An adequate determination of dry weight is of utmost importance in dialysis patients, as this may prevent both symptomatic hypotension during dialysis and overhydration during the interdialytic period. Besides careful history and physical examination, the need for objective assessment of fluid status remains. Because pulmonary edema and redistribution occurs mainly in severely overhydrated patients, the use of chest x-rays is too imprecise to be of great value in this aspect. Biochemical markers, like -ANP and c-GMP, which are primarily released in response to atrial distension, may be of help especially in diagnosing overhydration (83). However, a disadvantage of biochemical markers is that they cannot be determined "on the spot." Moreover, their reliability in the assessment of fluid status is questionable (84). Bioimpedance analysis (BIA) has been proposed as a marker for body composition and fluid status in dialysis patients. With BIA, total body water (single-frequency BIA) and intra- and extracellular water (multifrequency BIA) can be estimated by measuring the impedance of the body to an alternating current (85,86). BIA is a reproducible and quick technique that is easily applied in the clinical setting. However, despite a generally good correlation between BIA and isotope dilution techniques, large differences were observed between these techniques in several patients (85,87). Furthermore, not all authors found total body BIA to be reliable in measuring changes in fluid status during dialysis (88,89). Promising results have been obtained with the use of regional impedance ("conductivity") measurements applied at the leg of the patient, which proved to be a fairly sensitive technique to detect changes in fluid status during dialysis (84).

Echography of the inferior caval vein has proven to be a useful technique in the assessment of postdialysis dry weight. A good correlation was found between the vena cava diameter (VCD) and right atrial pressure and blood volume in dialysis patients. Therefore, the VCD is a good marker of the intravascular fluid status (84,90). However, one should be careful with the use of vena cava measurements immediately after dialysis, because refill of plasma volume from the interstitium may extend after the end of a dialysis session (13). Measuring vena cava diameter 1–2 hours after dialysis will give more reliable results. In addition, in patients with severe left ventricular dysfunction, echography of the vena cava may not be reliable in the assessment of pulmonary filling pressures (91).

c. *Individualizing the Ultrafiltration Rate*

Many young and otherwise healthy dialysis patients tolerate rapid ultrafiltration rates without any problems. However, especially in patients with a compromised cardiovascular system, rapid ultrafiltration is not well tolerated (11). In these patients, we empirically adjust a maximal ultrafiltration rate to each individual patient (which is different for isolated ultrafiltration and ultrafiltration combined with dialysis). Increasing dialysis time may be an option in these patients (13,59,92), as this will lead to a more gradual decline in plasma volume.

d. *Dialysate Sodium and Sodium Profiling*

As discussed previously, a low sodium concentration of the dialysate (130–134 mmol/L) may lead to more rapid decline in plasma compared to dialysis with a higher dialysate sodium concentration (140–144 mmol/L). However, a positive sodium balance has been associated with increased interdialytic weight gain, thirst, and hypertension. Individualization of the dialysate sodium to the plasma sodium concentration of the patient might prevent too large an influx of sodium during dialysis without the detrimental effects of low-sodium dialysis.

Sodium profiling with a variable sodium concentration of the dialysate has been proposed as a tool to decrease morbidity without a concomitant increase in sodium load. Profiles with an increased sodium concentration throughout the dialysis reduce cramps in the last part of dialysis. However, they may aggravate the fall in osmolality and therefore increase the incidence of symptomatic hypotension at the start of dialysis (93,94). Decreasing sodium profiles reduce the fall in osmolality during the first part of dialysis and may, especially when used in combination with a decreasing ultrafiltration profile, reduce the incidence of symptomatic hypotension at the start of dialysis (93). Sodium profiling may lead to a decrease in hypotensive periods and allow greater individualization of dialysis therapy (93–96). Nevertheless, not all authors found a beneficial effect on hemodynamic stability (97,98), whereas there is also a risk of sodium retention with the use of some profiles (94). Moreover, due to the relative complexity of the method and technical limitations of various dialysis machines, the routine use of sodium profiling is still limited and the optimal sodium profile has until now not been elucidated. We think that an algorithm for sodium profiling should be based on the individual blood volume response of the patient, to be assessed with continuous blood volume monitoring.

e. Blood Volume Monitoring

It has recently become possible to monitor changes in blood volume continuously during dialysis. The principle of this technique lies in the continuous monitoring of hemoglobin from lysed erythrocytes or the hematocrit, from which the fall in blood volume can be estimated (99,100). With these methods, it becomes possible to detect a fall in plasma volume before it leads to symptomatic hypotension. If a steep fall in plasma volume occurs, one may prevent a further decline, for example, by slowing the ultrafiltration rate (10,12). It has been suggested that hypotensive periods occur at a patient-specific hematocrit (101). However, differences in ultrafiltration rate, changes in hydration state and changes in erythrocyte volume between various dialysis treatments by the use of erythropoietin may lead to errors when applying this method.

Despite these limitations, it will certainly be possible with the use of blood volume monitoring to individualize ultrafiltration better than previously possible. This may enable the physician to prevent symptomatic hypotension in a significant number of patients. However, the use of blood volume monitoring in all susceptible patients is still rather expensive. In the future, it may become possible to integrate blood volume monitoring within a "closed-loop" system, which automatically adjusts ultrafiltration rate or the sodium concentration of the dialysate according to the blood volume profile of the patient (102).

2. Improving Cardiovascular Regulatory Mechanisms

a. Vasoactive Medication

If possible, it is recommended to avoid vasoactive medication the morning before dialysis in patients susceptible to symptomatic hypotension, as this may influence the vascular response to hypovolemia.

b. Food and Caffeine

It has been observed that ingestion of a meal during dialysis leads to a more pronounced decrease in mean arterial pressure (103,104). The pathophysiological mechanisms could be an increased splanchnic vasodilation (105) or increased general vasodilation (104), possibly partly mediated by increased plasma levels of insulin (106). In contrast to studies in nonuremic patients, caffeine had no effect on postprandial hemodynamics during dialysis (103).

c. Isolated Ultrafiltration

When fluid removal is difficult during hemodialysis because of symptomatic hypotension, the use of isolated ultrafiltration before dialysis can be of great value because of the better vascular reactivity compared with dialysis (7,46), especially in case of excessive interdialytic weight gain. We use isolated ultrafiltration before dialysis when the amount of fluid that has to be removed during hemodialysis is in excess of the individualized maximal ultrafiltration rate.

d. Cold Dialysis

Hemodynamic stability can be improved by the use of cooled dialysate (35–36°C). This is mediated through an increase in venous tone, vascular resistance, and cardiac contractility, in association with enhanced sympathetic activity (22,68–70,72,78). We did not observe rebound hypotension after the use of cold dialysate (unpublished results). Except for chills, few side effects have been described with the use of this method. As the efficacy of cold dialysis appears to be related to the individual core temperature of the patient (70), adjustment of the dialysate temperature to the core temperature of the patient might be an option in the future.

e. Membranes

Although an earlier report suggested an improvement in hemodynamic stability with the use of cellulose acetate compared with cuprophane membranes (107), larger recent trials have failed to show a difference in the incidence of intradialytic hypotension between dialysis with biocompatible and bioincompatible membranes (57–59).

f. Dialysate Calcium

Calcium ions play a critical role in the contractility of cardiac and vascular smooth muscle cells and in the release of catecholamines from adrenergic nerves (108). A dialysate calcium concentration in the range of 1.5–1.75 mmol/L results in an increase in plasma ionized calcium of ±0.20 mmol/L, whereas plasma ionized calcium remains more or less unchanged with a dialysate calcium concentration of 1.25 mmol/L (109). The latter concentration has become a popular tool to prevent of secondary hyperparathyroidism. It has been shown that the change in ionized calcium can be an important determinant of the cardiac response during hemodialysis. Several studies found a difference in the blood pressure response between dialysis with low and normal dialysate calcium concentrations of the dialysate, which appears to be primarily related to an increase in left ventricular contractility (66,67,75–77,110). This phenomenon appears to be especially important in patients with an impaired left ventricular systolic function, in whom blood presure was found to decrease with the use of low dialysate calcium but remained stable with the use of higher dialysate calcium concentrations (110). However, as will be discussed later, one should be careful when inducing an excessive rise in serum calcium in patients with severe arrhythmias. Frequent control of serum calcium before and after dialysis is therefore warranted with the use of a high-calcium dialysate.

g. *Dialysate Buffer*

Because acetate leads to increased peripheral vasodilation and, especially in cardiac compromised patients, to a decrease in left ventricular function (46,74), acetate should not be used as dialysate buffer in hypotensive-prone patients.

h. *Hemofiltration*

Cardiovascular stability is better maintained during hemofiltration compared with hemodialysis. Although differences in blood volume preservation (22) and baroreceptor functioning (41,42) may play some role, the most important determinator of the improved blood pressure stability during hemofiltration appears to be the enhanced vascular reactivity compared to hemodialysis (23,46,69,111,112). Cardiac contractility does not differ to a great extent between these two techniques, and cardiac output may even be greater during hemodialysis due to the reduction in afterload and an increase in heart rate (46,111). The possible pathophysiological mechanisms behind the different vascular response between hemodialysis and hemofiltration have been addressed previously.

Surprisingly few hemodynamic studies have been performed during hemodiafiltration. In a study in patients with acute renal failure, vascular reactivity was reduced compared with hemofiltration but increased compared with hemodialysis (113). An improvement in blood pressure stability was noted with hemodiafiltration and acetate-free biofiltration compared to hemodialysis in elderly dialysis patients (114), although in another study, no difference in hemodynamic stability between hemodialysis and hemodiafiltration was observed (21).

i. *Pharmacological Maneuvers*

Attempts have been made to improve hemodynamic stability with the administration of vasoactive substances. Both sympathicomimetic agents like the norepinephrine precursor L-DOPS (115), amezinium methylsulphate (116) and midodrine (117), and other vasoactive agents like lysine vasopressin (118) have been succesfully used. However, the first agent is associated with significant side effects. As yet, experience with the use of antihypotensive agents is still limited in dialysis patients.

D. Intradialytic Hypotension: Summary

Symptomatic hypotension is a frequently occurring phenomenon in the dialysis population. Especially in elderly patients, who often suffer from cardiovascular disease, the incidence of symptomatic hypotension may be high, which puts these patients at risk for serious morbidity. Symptomatic hypotension may occur as a result of a fall in blood volume and a reduced cardiovascular reactivity during dialysis, in combination with structural abnormalities of the cardiovascular system. Of course, the relative importance of each of these factors may differ in the individual patient. In case of severe hypovolemia, cardiovascular collapse may ensue by an acute reduction in sympathetic activity (Bezold-Jarish reflex).

It is possible to reduce morbidity due to intradialytic hypotension by the use of relatively simple maneuvers (119). First, blood volume preservation can be improved by adequate estimation of the optimal dry weight of the patient, preferably with the help of objective methods. Furthermore, the ultrafiltration rate should be moderate and should be limited to a maximal value, to be defined empirically for each individual patient. The use of low-sodium dialysate should be avoided. A physiological sodium concentration of the dialysate is preferable because a higher sodium concentration may result in increased thirst and intradialytic weight gain. Continuous blood volume monitoring may be helpful but may not be available in each dialysis center. In the future, sodium profiling should be based on studies assessing plasma volume changes during dialysis in different patient groups.

Cardiovascular function during dialysis can be improved by the use of bicarbonate as dialysate buffer instead of acetate. The latter should never be used in patients prone to hypotensive periods because of its cardiodepressant and vasodilating properties. Moreover, in patients at risk for symptomatic hypotension, vasoactive medication should be withheld the morning before dialysis, if possible. One should be cautious with the use of low-calcium dialysate in patients with frequent hypotensive periods, as this may impair cardiac contractility. Because of its beneficial effect on vascular reactivity, isolated ultrafiltration can be used to remove fluid, especially in patients with excessive interdialytic weight gain. Also, an improved cardiovascular response may be obtained with a lowering of dialysate temperature.

If these maneuvers fail to control intradialytic hypotension, transferring the patient to hemofiltration or to other modalities such as continuous ambulatory peritoneal dialysis (CAPD) is another option.

II. CORONARY ISCHEMIA

Coronary ischemia frequently occurs in dialysis patients. It may lead to angina pectoris but can also be completely asymptomatic. Whereas coronary ischemia in dialysis patients is primary due to atherosclerosis, coronary angiography can also be completely negative (120). In this circumstance, ischemia is probably due to an increased cardiac wall stress in case of left ventricular hypertrophy (121).

The long-term management of coronary ischemia in dialysis patients, which does not differ to a great extent from patients without renal disease, is beyond the scope of this chapter. However, an important point in the prevention of coronary ischemia is the correction of anemia by rHu-erythropoietin (122,123), although it is not known whether an increase in hematocrit above 0.35 is beneficial. Preliminary data have shown that too high doses of erythropoietin might even be harmful in patients with cardiovascular disease (124), although this topic needs further investigation. Hypertension should be carefully controlled (122).

Coronary ischemia during hemodialysis may be due to hypovolemia, as this will decrease myocardial perfusion. When a patient complains of angina pectoris, ultrafiltration should be stopped and hypovolemia corrected. Arrhythmias should be excluded, as they are often associated with cardiac ischemia (123). Assuming blood pressure is not too low, sublingual nitroglycerin may be given. One should be careful with the administration of nitroglycerin in hypovolemic patients, as this may further induce hypotension due to venodilation.

On the other hand, severe overhydration may lead to cardiac ischemia, because the increased left ventricular pressure can compromise coronary perfusion (123). Under these circumstances, ultrafiltration of excess fluid is appropriate, preferably performed under cardiac rhythm monitoring. The difference between coronary ischemia due to under- and overhydration will usually be evident from clinical findings.

In hemodialysis patients with coronary artery disease, prevention of symptomatic hypotension is of utmost importance. This can be accomplished by the maneuvers discussed earlier. Careful estimation of dry weight, correction of anemia, avoidance of excessive ultrafiltration rates and of the use of acetate are recommended. In some patients, increasing dialysis time or transfer to CAPD or hemofiltration may be the only options. Overhydration may be prevented with a careful estimation of dry weight and meticulous dietary counseling, with special attention to the sodium and water intake.

III. ARRHYTHMIAS

Arrhythmias frequently occur in hemodialysis patients. In most cases, they are asymptomatic. In some studies using Holter electrocardiography, complex ventricular arrhythmias (multiform ventricular extrasystoles, couplets and runs) were observed in more than 50% of dialysis patients (125,126). While the clinical significance of these arrhythmias is uncertain (127), more severe symptomatic atrial and ventricular tachycardias may occur.

Although they may also occur in dialysis patients without cardiovascular disease, patient-related factors that may contribute to the occurrence of arrhythmias include left ventricular hypertrophy (125,128), coronary artery disease (129,130), patient age (127,131), fluid overload (132), and digoxin therapy (129,133). Arrthythmias in patients with renal failure have also been described with the use of cisapride (134). Antiarrhythmic drugs that accumulate in renal failure, such as sotalol, should only be prescribed with great caution. Another factor that has been related to arrhythmias in dialysis patients is an increased calcium-phosphate product. A role for parathormone as an arrhythmogenic factor remains, however, unproven (132).

It has been reported that most episodes of arrhythmias occur during or after a hemodialysis session (125,127,128,130,131,135), although not all authors agree (125,130). This discrepancy may well be explained by different patient characteristics.

Treatment-related factors that may contribute to arrhythmias include rapid changes in serum potassium (133), acid-base status (136), serum calcium (137), and rapid decreases in circulating blood volume (131). Hypokalemia increases the vulnerability of the heart for arrhythmias because of an increased ratio between intracellular and extracellular potassium, resulting in a negative membrane potential. Hemodialysis leads to rapid changes in serum potassium levels, especially when a low-potassium bath is used. Although in one study no difference in ventricular extrasystoles was observed between patients treated with a standard and a potassium-free bath (135), other studies did find an increase in ventricular ectopy in patients dialyzed against a low-potassium bath (128,133). The concomitant use of digoxin increases the sensitivity of the heart for rapid changes in serum potassium and is, especially in high doses, a known risk factor for potentially dangerous arrhythmias in dialysis patients (129,132).

The dialysate buffer may also influence the incidence of arrhythmias during dialysis. A study in dialysis patients including subjects with frequent and dangerous ventricular arrhythmias showed a clear reduction in these episodes with the use of bicarbonate versus acetate as dialysate buffer. This was explained by the more regular correction of acidosis with the use of bicarbonate dialysis (136). In another study, no difference in arrhythmias between acetate and bicarbonate dialysate was observed (130).

Dialysate calcium has also been involved in the pathogenesis of arrhythmias. A higher incidence of nonsymptomatic arrhythmias was observed in the group treated with higher-calcium dialysate (1.75 mmol/L) versus the group treated with 1.25 mmol/L calcium dialysate. The dialysate buffer in this study was acetate. This phenomenon was explained by an increase in reentry or triggered activity by an increased extra- or intracellular calcium concentration (137).

It has also been suggested that hemofiltration reduces the risk for arrhythmias. In an uncontrolled study, a reduced incidence in complex ventricular extrasystoles was observed in patients treated with hemofiltration compared to hemodialysis (138). Another study did not confirm these findings (130).

In patients prone for arrhythmias, preventive measures should be undertaken during a hemodialysis session. Special care should be given to the prevention of over- and underhydration. Excessive rises in serum calcium should be avoided. Although a dialysate calcium concentration of 1.75 mmol/L was found to be safe in cardiac-compromised patients and improved hemodynamic stability, postdialytic hypercalcemia is better avoided in patients at risk for severe arrhythmias. Acetate should preferably not be used because of its cardiodepressant and blood pressure–lowering effects.

An excessive and too rapid lowering of serum potassium should be avoided. During standard hemodialysis, approximately 50–80 mmol of potasssium is removed (139). Factors that influence potassium homeostasis during dialysis include the acid-base status of the patient and the glucose concentration in the dialysate. In acidemic patients, influx of bicarbonate may promote a shift of potassium from the extracellular to the intracellular space, which may lead to a more rapid decline in serum potassium. In severely acidemic patients, serum potassium decreased despite the use of a dialysate with a higher potassium concentration than the serum of the patient (140). The use of glucose-free dialysate may increase potassium removal because of an outward shift of potassium from the cell due to lower insulin levels (141).

In patients with predialysis serum potassium below 4.5 mmol/L, we give potassium suppletion over a sideline according to the following scheme (with a dialysate potassium concentration of 2.0 mmol/L).

K^+ 4.0–4.5 mmol/L: 5 mmol/h
K^+ 3.5–4.0 mmol/L: 10 mmol/h
K^+ 3.0–3.5 mmol/L: 15 mmol/h
K^+ <3.0 mmol/L: 20 mmol/h or more

However, an increase in the potassium concentration of the dialysate of 3.0 or 4.0 mmol/L can also be used. Digoxin should be used only in strict indications.

IV. DIALYSIS REACTIONS

During dialysis, blood is in contact with foreign material in the different components of the extracorporeal circuit, such as the tubing system, the dialysis membrane, and remnants of the sterilization procedure. Although infrequent, allergic reactions to these different parts of the extracorporeal system may occur. Two main types of allergic reactions have been distinguished: Type A (or I) anaphylactoid reactions and type B (II) reactions.

Type A reactions are anaphylactoid in nature and occur mainly during the first 5–10 (maximal 20) minutes of hemodialysis. These reactions are characterized by dyspnea, angioedema, urticaria, nausea, and diarrhea and may even result in cardiorespiratory arrest and death. Most type A reactions are IgE mediated. Primarily responsible for these IgE mediated reactions are hypersensitivity to ethylene oxide or to some disinfectants used with reuse procedures (142,143). Hypersensitivity reactions to AN-69 membranes appear to be primarily mediated through the release of bradykin via activation of factor XII (Hageman factor). This reaction may be enhanced by the use of angiotensin-converting enzyme (ACE) inhibitors, which inhibit the breakdown of bradykinin (142–144). Hypertensive reactions with AN-69 membranes occur rather heterogenously. This has been attributed to the fact that contact phase inhibition by AN-69 membranes is a pH-dependent mechanism and might therefore depend on the acid-base status of the patient (145). Intravenous infusion of iron dextran in iron-deficient dialysis patients may also lead to severe anaphylaxis (146).

When type A reactions occur during hemodialysis, dialysis must be terminated immediately and the blood should not be returned to the patient. Other catastrophes, like air embolism and massive hemolysis, have to be excluded. Antihistamines (H_1- and H_2-inhibitors) should be given (clemastine 2 mg i.v. and ranitidine 50 mg i.v). Steroids may prevent a delayed reaction. In severe cases, epinephrine (1 mL 1:1000 s.c. or 1 mL 1:10.000 i.v.) should be administered. Plasma expanders may be needed to maintain hemodynamic stability. In case of cardiopulmonary arrest, standard reanimation principles should be followed.

When a type A reaction has occurred, preventive measures include the rinsing of the dialyzer immediately before use, refraining from the use of ETO-sterilized membranes, and, if AN-69 membranes are implicated, changing to another membrane and stopping ACE inhibitor therapy. When an allergic reaction to iron dextran has occurred, iron saccharate or iron gluconate should be used instead (142,143).

Type B reactions occur later in dialysis (after 20–40 min) and are mainly characterized by chest or back pain. Usually these reactions are milder and can be easily distinguished from type A reactions, although the distinction may be difficult in case of severe chest pain and dyspnea.

The etiology of type B reactions is not entirely clear. It has been related to complement release, as these reactions were primarily observed after "first use" of unsubstituted cellulosic membranes and abated after reuse (147). However, a recent randomized study did not show a difference in dialysis reactions between treatment with biocompatible and bioincompatible membranes (57). In mild cases, dialysis must not be terminated and administration of oxygen may be sufficient. In more severe cases, dialysis may have to be stopped. (142,143).

V. INTRADIALYTIC HYPERTENSION

Severe hypertension occurring during or immediately after dialysis is an incompletely understood phenomenon. Hypovolemia, leading to increased stimulation of the renin-angiotensin and sympathetic nervous systems, has been implicated (148,149), although direct evidence for increased vasopressor activity during intradialytic hypertension is still lacking. Interesting was the finding of overhydration in patients presenting with intradialytic hypertension in one study (150). Other contributory factors may include hypercalcemia and hypokalemia, and increased blood viscosity by the use of high doses of rh-EPO may also play a role (148,149). Intradialytic hypertension may be treated with the use of antihypertensive agents (148). Although first overhydration should be excluded. We prefer ACE inhibitors to short-acting dihydropyridine calcium channel blockers (151), because the latter have been implicated in uncontrollable hypotension leading to coronary and myocardial ischemia (152).

VI. MUSCLE CRAMPS

Muscle cramps frequently occur during dialysis therapy, especially at the end of a session, after high ultrafiltration rates, and when the need occurs for excessive volume removal. Relative hypovolemia, an increase in vasopressor substances, tissue ischemia, and carnitine deficiency have been implicated in their pathogenesis. The role of relative hypovolemia is supported by the immediate relief of symptoms after the administration of a small amount of a hypertonic solution. Evidence for a pathogenetic role of local tissue ischemia and increased concentrations of vasopressor substances is indirect (153). Although supplementation with carnitine was found to reduce the incidence of muscle cramps (154), in nonuremic patients carnitine deficiency results in myopathy but not in cramps.

Muscle cramps can be alleviated by the infusion of small amounts of hyperosmolar solutions like hypertonic saline, dextrose, or mannitol. Increased interdialytic weight gain after infusion of small amounts of these agents was not observed (155).

Muscle cramps may be prevented by an adequate estimation of dry weight, although they may also occur in still overhydrated patients who require excessive ultrafiltration rates. Excessive interdialytic weight gain should be avoided, as this may necessitate the use of high ultrafiltration rates. Sodium profiling could also be of help in the prevention of muscle cramps in selected patients (93,94,96). Although pharmacological therapy with sympathicolytic agents like prazosin may reduce the incidence of muscle cramps, their use is restricted by an increase in episodes of symptomatic hypotension (156).

VII. DISEQUILIBRIUM

Especially in patients with high predialytic urea levels, a syndrome of mental and neurological abnormalities, nausea, and headache may occur, which may extend for hours after dialysis. This syndrome is possibly due to an osmotic disequilibrium between cerebral cells and plasma due to a rapid change in plasma osmolality with a lesser decrease in intracellular osmolality, although changes in intracerebral pH have also been implicated (157). Due to increased awareness, severe forms of disequilibrium are rarely observed nowadays.

The disequilibrium syndrome can be prevented by a shortening of dialysis time in patients with very high predialytic urea levels, which may prevent a large fall in osmolality. In these patients, one should refrain from the use of glucose-free dialysate, as this may increase the fall in osmolality during dialysis (158). A low sodium concentration of the dialysate should be avoided, except in patients with severe hyponatremia. The administration of osmotic agents like mannitol or hypertonic glucose may be of help (158). Once the disequilibrium syndrome occurs, the treatment is largely supportive.

REFERENCES

1. Kim KE, Neff M, Coen B, Somerstein M, Chinitz J, Swartz C. Blood volume changes and hypotension during hemodialysis. Trans Am Soc Artif Intern Organs 1970; 16:508–514.
2. Koomans HA, Geers AB, Dorhout Mees EJ. Plasma volume recovery after ultrafiltration in patients with chronic renal failure. Kidney Int 1984; 26:848–854.
3. Lopot F, Kotyk P, Blaha J, Forejt J. Use of continuous blood volume monitoring for detecting inadequately high dry weight. Int J Artif Organs 1996; 19:411–414.
4. Bogaard H, de Vries JPPM, de Vries PMJM. Assessment of refill and hypovolemia by continuous surveilance of blood volume and extracellular blood volume. Nephrol Dial Transpl 1994; 9:1283–1287.
5. Kooman JP, Wijnen JAG, Draaijer P, van Bortel L, Gladziwa U, Struyker Boudier HAJ, Peltenburg HG, van Hooff JP, Leunissen KML. Compliance and reactivity of the peripheral venous system in patients treated with chronic intermittent hemodialysis. Kidney Int 1992; 41:1041–1048.
6. Kooman JP, Daemen MJAP, Wijnen R, Verluyten-Goessens MJ, van Hooff JP, Leunissen KML. Morphological changes of the venous system in uremic patients. Nephron 1995; 69:454–458.
7. Kooman JP, Gladziwa U, Becker G, van Bortel LMAB, van Hooff JP, Leunissen KML. Role of the venous system in hemodynamics during ultrafiltration and bicarbonate dialysis. Kidney Int 1992; 42:718–726.
8. London GM, Safar ME, Levenson JA, Simon AC, Temmar MA. Renal filtration fraction, effective vascular compliance, and partition of fluid volumes in sustained essential hypertension. Kidney Int 1981; 20:97–103.
9. Fauchald P. Effect of ultrafiltration on body fluid volumes and transcapillary colloid osmotic gradient in hemodialysis patients. Contrib Nephrol 1989; 74:170–175.
10. Santoro A, Mancini E, Paolini F, Zuccheli P. Blood volume monitoring and control. Nephrol Dial Transpl 1996; 11(suppl 2):42–47.
11. van der Sande FM, Mulder AW, van Kuijk WHM, Leunissen KML. The hemodynamic effect of different ultrafiltration rates in patients with cardiac failure and patients without cardiac failure: comparison between isolated ultrafiltration and ultrafiltration with dialysis. Clin Nephrol 1998; 50:201–208.
12. Mann H, Ernst E, Gladziwa U, Schallenberg U, Stiller S. Changes in blood volume during dialysis are dependent upon the rate and amount of ultrafiltrate. Trans Am Soc Artif Organs 1989; 35:250–252.
13. Katzarski KS, Nisell J, Randmaa I, Danielsson A, Freyschuss U, Bergström J. A critical evaluation of ultrasound measurement of inferior vena cava diameter in assessing dry weight in normotensive and hypertensive dialysis patients. Am J Kidney Dis 1997; 30:459–465.
14. Fleming SJ, Wilkinson JS, Greenwood RN, Aldridge C, Baker LRI, Cattel WR. Effect of dialysate composition on intercompartimental fluid shift. Kidney Int 1984; 26:848–854.
15. van Stone JC, Bauer J, Carey J. The effect of dialysate sodium on body fluid distribution during dialysis. Trans ASAIO 1980; 26:383–386.
16. Kouw PM, Olthof CG, Gruteke P. Influence of high and low sodium dialysis on blood volume preservation. Nephrol Dial Transpl 1991; 6:876–880.
17. Leunissen KML, Cheriex EC, Janssen JHA, Teule GJJ, Mooy JMV, Ramentol M, van Hooff JP. Influence of left ventricular function on changes in plasma volume during acetate and bicarbonate dialysis. Nephrol Dial Transplant 1987; 2:99–103.
18. Hsu CH, Swartz RD, Somermeyer MG. Bicarbonate hemodialysis: influence on plasma refilling and hemodynamic stability. Nephron 1984; 38:202–208.

19. Rodriguez M, Pederson JA, Llach F. Effect of dialysis and ultrafiltration on osmolality, colloid osmotic pressure, and vascular refilling rate. Kidney Int 1985; 28: 808–813.
20. Kouw PM, van Es A, Olthof CG, Oe PL, de Vries PMJM, Donker AJM. High efficiency dialysis strategies: effects on fluid balance by means of conductivity measurements. In: Kouw PM. Determinants of Intra- and Extracellular Fluid Volume by Means of Non-invasive Conductivity Measurements. In Vivo Validation and Clinical Application (thesis). Amsterdam: Free University of Amsterdam Press, 1992.
21. Takenaka T, Tsuchiya Y, Suzuki H. High-performance hemodiafiltration and blood pressure stability. Nephron 1997; 73:30–35.
22. de Vries PMJM, Olthof CG, Solf A, Schuenemann B, Oe PL, Quellhorst E, Scheider H, Donker AJM. Fluid balance between haemodialysis and haemofiltration: the effect of dialysate sodium and a variable ultrafiltration rate. Nephrol Dial Transpl 1991; 6:257–263.
23. van Kuijk WA, Hillion D, Savoiu C, Leunissen KML. Critical role of the extracorporeal blood temperature in the hemodynamic response during hemofiltration. J Am Soc Nephrol 1997; 8:949–955.
24. Daugirdas JT. Dialysis hypotension; a hemodynamic analysis. Kidney Int 1991; 39:233–246.
25. Greenway CV, Wayne Lautt W. Blood volume, the venous system, preload and cardiac output. Can J Physiol Pharmacol 1986; 64:383–387.
26. Safar ME, London GM, Levenson JA, Simon AC, Chau NP. Rapid dextran infusion in essential hypertension. Hypertension 1979; 1:615–623.
27. Bondia A, Tabernero JM, Macias JF, Martin-Luengo C. Autonomic nervous system in hemodialysis. Nephrol Dial Transpl 1988; 2:174–180.
28. Nakashima Y, Fouad FM, Nakamoto S, Textor SC, Bravo EL, Tarazi RC. Localisation of autonomic nervous system dysfunction in dialysis patients. Am J Nephrol 1987; 7:375–381.
29. McGrath BP, Ledingham JGG, Benedict CR. Catecholamines in peripheral venous plasma in patients on chronic hemodialysis. Clin Sci Mol Med 1978; 55:89–96.
30. Converse RL, Jacobson TN, Jost CMT, Toto RD, Jost CMT, Cosentino F, Fouad-Tarazi F, Victor RG. Sympathetic overactivity in patients with chronic renal failure. N Engl J Med 1992; 327:1912–1918.
31. Naik MB, Mathis CJ, Wilson CA, Reid JL, Warren DJ. Cardiovascular and autonomous reflexes in hemodialysis patients. Clin Sci 1981; 60:165–170.
32. Heber ME, Lahiri A, Thompson D, Raftery EB. Baroreceptor, not left ventricular, dysfunction is the cause of hemodialysis hypotension. Clin Nephrol 1989; 32: 79–86.
33. Lin YF, Wang JY, Shum AY, Jiang HK, Lai WY, Lu KC, Diang LK, Shieh SD. Role of plasma catecholamines, autonomic, and left ventricular function in normotensive and hypotension prone dialysis patients. ASAIO J 1993; 39:946–953.
34. Stojceva-Taneva O, Masin G, Polenakovic M, Stojcev S, Stojkovski L. Autonomic nervous system dysfunction and volume nonresponsive hypotension in hemodialysis patients. Am J Nephrol 1991; 11: 123–126.
35. Nies AS, Robertson D, Stone WJ. Hemodialysis hypotension is not the result of uremic peripheral autonomous neuropathy. J Lab Clin Med 1979; 94:395–402.
36. Ligtenberg G, Blankestijn PJ, Boomsma F, Koomans HA. No change in automatic function tests during uncomplicated haemodialysis. Nephrol Dial Transplant 1996; 11:651–656.
37. Parfrey PS, Harnett Foley RN, Parfrey PS, Harnett JD. Left ventricular hypertrophy in dialysis patients. Sem Dial 1992; 5:34–41.
38. Kooman JP, Leunissen KML. Cardiovascular aspects in renal disease. Curr Opin Nephrol Hypert 1993; 2: 791–797.
39. Raine AE. The susceptible patient. Nephrol Dial Transplant 1996; 11(suppl 2):6–10.
40. Ritz E, Rambausek M, Mall G, Ruffman K, Mandelbaum A. Cardiac changes to uremia and their possible relation to cardiovascular instability on dialysis. Contrib Nephrol 1990; 78:221–229.
41. Zuchelli P, Santoro A, Sturani A, Degli Esposti E, Chiarini C, Zuccala A. Effects of hemodialysis and hemofiltration on the autonomic control of circulation. Trans Am Soc Artif Intern Organs 1984; 30:163–167.
42. Baldamus CA, Mantz P, Kachel HG, Koch KM, Schoeppe W. Baroreflex in patients undergoing hemodialysis and hemofiltration. Contrib Nephrol 1984; 41:409–414.
43. Converse RL, Jacobsen TN, Jost CMT, Toto RD, Grayburn PA, Obregon TM, Fouad-Tarazi F, Victor RG. Paradoxical withdrawal of reflex vasoconstriction as a cause of haemodialysis-induced hypotension. J Clin Invest 1992; 90:1657–1665.
44. Santoro A, Mancini E, Spongano M, Rossi M, Paolini F, Zucchelli P. A haemodynamic study of hypotension during haemodialysis using electrical bioimpedance cardiography. Nephrol Dial Transpl 1990; 5(suppl 1): 147–153.
45. Zoccali C, Tripepi G, Mallamaci F, Panuccio V. The heart rate response to dialysis hypotension in haemodialysis patients. Nephrol Dial Transpl 1997; 12:519–523.
46. Baldamus CA, Ernst W, Frei UW, Koch KM. Sympathetic and hemodynamic response to volume removal during different forms of renal replacement therapy. Nephron 1982; 31:324–332.
47. Nakamura Y, Ikeda T, Takata S, Yokoi H, Hirono M, Abe T, Takazakura F, Kobayashi K. The role of peripheral resistance and capacitance vessels in hypoten-

sion following hemodialysis. Am Heart J 1991; 121: 1170–1177.

48. Bradley JR, Evans DB, Gore SM, Cowley AJ. Is dialysis hypotension caused by an abnormality of venous tone? Br Med J 1988; 296:1634–1637.
49. Hegbrant J, Thysell H, Martensson L, Ekman R, Boberg U. Changes in plasma levels of vasoactive peptides during sequential bicarbonate dialysate. Nephron 1993; 63:309–313.
50. Bergstrom J. Catecholamines and control of blood pressure during hemodialysis and hemofiltration. Kidney Int 1988; 34:S110–S114.
51. Odar-Cederlof I, Theodorsson E, Eriksson CG. Hamberger B, Tidgren B, Kjellstrand CM. Vasoactive agents and blood pressure regulation in sequential ultrafiltration and hemodialysis. Int J Artif Organs. 1993; 16:662–669.
52. Shinzato T, Milwa M, Nakai S, Morita H, Odani H, Inove I, Maeda K. Role of adenosine in dialysis-induced hypotension. J Am Soc Nephrol 1994; 4:1987–1994.
53. Henderson LW, Koch KM, Dinarello CA, Shaldon S. Hemodialysis hypotension: the interleukin-1 hypothesis. Blood Purif 1983; 1:3–8.
54. Dinarello CA. Interleukin-1 and tumor necrosis factor and their naturally occurring antagonists during hemodialysis. Kidney Int 1992; 42(suppl 38):S68–S72.
55. Yokokawa K, Mankus R, Saklayen MG, Kohno M, Yasunari K, Minami M, Kano H, Horio T, Takeda T, Mandel AK. Increased nitric oxide production in patients with hypotension during hemodialysis. Ann Intern Med 1995; 123:35–37.
56. Rysz J, Luciak M, Kedziora J, Blaszczyk J, Sibinska E. Nitric oxide release in the peripheral blood during hemodialysis. Kidney Int 1997; 51:294–300.
57. Bergamo Collaborative Dialysis Study Group; Acute intradialytic well-being; results of a clinical trial comparing polysulfone with cuprophane. Kidney Int 1991; 40:714–719.
58. Collins DM, Kambert MB, Tannenbaum JS, Oliverio M, Schwab SJ. Tolerance of hemodialysis: A randomized prospective trial of high-flux versus conventional high-efficiency hemodialysis. J Am Soc Nephrol 1993; 4:148–154.
59. Skroeder NR, Jacobson SH, Lins LE, Kjellstrand-CM. Acute symptoms during and between hemodialysis: the relative role of speed, duration, and biocompatibility of dialysis. Artif-Organs 1994; 18:880–887.
60. Aakhus S, Bjoernstad K, Jorstad S. Systemic cardiovascular response in hemodialysis without and with ultrafiltration with membranes of high and low biocompatibility. Blood Purif 1995; 13:229–240.
61. van Kuijk WA, Buurman WA, Gerlag PGG, Leunissen KML. Vascular reactivity during combined ultrafiltration-hemodialysis: influence of dialysis derived contaminants. J Am Soc Nephrol 1996; 7:2664–2669.
62. Haeffner-Cavaillon N, Cavaillon JM, Ciancioni C, Bacle F, Delons S, Kazatchkine MD. In vivo induction of interleukin-1 during haemodialysis. Kidney Int 1989; 35:121–1218.
63. Wehle B, Asaba H, Castenfors J, Gunnarsson B, Bergstrom J. Influence of dialysate composition on cardiovascular function in isovolemic hemodialysis. Proc EDTA 1981; 18:153–159.
64. van Kuijk WHM, Wirtz JJJM, Grave W, de Heer F, Menheere PPCA, van Hooff JP, Leunissen KML. Vascular reactivity during combined ultrafiltration-haemodialysis. Influence of dialysate sodium. Nephrol Dial Transpl 1996; 11:323–328.
65. Schultze G, Maiga M, Neumayer HH, Wagner K, Keller F, Molzahn M, Nigam S. Prostaglandin E_2 promotes hypotension on low-sodium hemodialysis. Nephron 1984; 37:250–256.
66. van Kuijk WHM, Mulder WA, Hanff GA, Leunissen KML. The effect of changes in plasma ionized calcium on blood pressure and vascular reactivity during ultrafiltration and hemodialysis. Clin Nephrol 1997; 47:190–196.
67. Fellner SK, Lang RM, Neumann A, Spencer KT, Bushinsky DA, Borow KM. Physiological mechanisms for calcium-induced changes in systemic arterial pressure in stable dialysis patients. Hypertension 1989; 13:213–218.
68. Coli U, Landini S, Lucatello S, Fracasso A, Morachiello P Righetto F, Scanferla F, Onesti G, Bazzato G. Cold as cardiovascular stabilizing function in hemodialysis: hemodynamic evaluation. Trans Am Soc Artif Intern Organs 1983; 29:71–75.
69. van Kuijk WHM, Luik AJ, de Leeuw PW, van Hooff JP, Nieman FHM, Habets HML, Leunissen KML. Vascular reactivity during hemodialysis and isolated ultrafiltration: thermal influences. Nephrol Dial Transpl 1995; 16:1852–1858.
70. Jost CMT, Agrawal R, Khair-El-Din T, Grayburn PA, Victor RG, Henrich WL. Effects of cooler temperature dialysate on hemodynamic stability in Aproblem@ dialysis patients. Kidney Int 1993; 44:606–612.
71. Fine A, Penner B. The protective effect of cool dialysate is dependent on patients' predialysis temperature. Am J Kidney Dis 1996; 28:262–265.
72. Mahida BH, Dumler F, Zasuwa G, Fleig G, Levin NW. Effect of cooler dialysate on serum catecholamines and blood pressure stability. Trans Am Soc Artif Intern Organs 1983; 24:383–389.
73. Nixon JV, Mitchell JH, McPhaul JJ, Henrich WL. Effect of hemodialysis on left ventricular function. J Clin Invest 1983; 71:377–384.
74. Leunissen KML, Hoorntje SJ, Fiers HA. Acetate versus bicarbonate dialysis in critically ill patients. Nephron 1986; 42:146–151.
75. Henrich WL, Hunt JM, Nixon JV. Increased ionized calcium and left ventricular contractility during hemodialysis. N Engl J Med 1984; 310:19–23.

76. Lang RM, Fellner SK, Neumann A, Bushinsky DA, Borow KM. Left ventricular contractility varies directly with blood ionized calcium. Ann Intern Med 1988; 108:524–529.
77. Leunissen KML, van den Berg BW, van Hooff JP. Ionized calcium plays a pivotal role in controlling blood pressure during hemodialysis. Blood Purif 1989; 7:233–239.
78. Levy FL, Grayburn PA, Foulks CJ, Brickner ME, Henrich WL. Improved left ventricular contractility with cool temperature hemodialysis. Kidney Int 1992; 41:961–965.
79. Gong R, Lindberg J, Abrams J, Whitaker WR, Wade CE, Gouge S. Comparison of hypertonic saline solutions and dextran in dialysis-induced hypotension. J Am Soc Nephrol 1993; 3:1808–1812.
80. van der Sande FM, Kooman JP, Barendregt JNM, Nieman FHM, Leunissen KML. Effect of intravenous saline, albumin, or hydroxyethylstarch on blood volume during combined ultrafiltration and hemodialysis. J Am Soc Nephrol 1999; 10:1303–1308.
81. Köhler H. Einfluss der Nierenfunktion auf die Elimination und Wirkung von kolloidalen Plasma Ersatzmitteln. Fortschr Med 1979; 40:S1809–S1813.
82. Steinhoff J, Mansky T, Reitz M, Schulz E, Sack K. Pharmakokinetic von Hydroxyäthylstärke bei Patienten unter Hämodialyse und Hämofiltration. Nieren Hochdrückkrankheiten 1988; 17:S411–S414.
83. Lauster F, Gerzer R, Weil J, Fulle HJ, Schiffl H. Assessment of dry body weight in hemodialysis patients by the biochemical marker cGMP. Nephrol Dial Transpl 1990; 5:356–361.
84. Kouw PM, Kooman JP, Cheriex EC, Olthof CG, de Vries PMJM, Leunissen KML. Assessment of postdialysis dry weight: a comparison of techniques. J Am Soc Nephrol 1993; 4:98–104.
85. Kong CH, Thompson CM, Lewis CA, Hill PD, Thompson FD. Determination of total body water in uraemic patients by bioelectrical impedance. Nephrol Dial Transpl 1993; 8:716–719.
86. Segal KR, Burastero S, Chun A, Coronel P, Pierson RN, Wang J. Estimation of extracellular and total body water by multiple-frequency bioelectrical-impedance measurement. Am J Clin Nutr 1991; 54:26–29.
87. Chertow GM, Lowrie EG, Wilmore DW, Gonzalez J, Lew NL, Ling J, Leboff MS, Gottlieb MN, Huang W, Zebrowski B, College J, Lazarus JM. Nutritional assessment with bioelectrical impedance analysis in maintenance hemodialysis. J Am Soc Nephrol 1995; 6:75–81.
88. Formica C, Atkinson MG, Nyulasi I, McKay J, Heale W, Seeman E. Body composition following hemodialysis: studies using dual-energy x-ray absorptiometry and bioelectrical impedance analysis. Osteoporosis Int 1993; 3:192–197.
89. Mandolfo S, Farina M, Imbasciati E. Bioelectrical impedance and hemodialysis. Int J Artif Organs 1995; 18:700–704.
90. Leunissen KML, Kouw P, Kooman JP, Cheriex EC, de Vries PMJM, Donker AJM, van Hooff JP. New techniques to determine fluid status in hemodialyzed patients. Kidney Int 1993; 43:S50–S56.
91. Mandelbaum A, Ritz E. Vena cava diameter measurement for estimation of dry weight in haemodialysis patients. Nephrol Dial Transpl 1996; 11(suppl 2):24–27.
92. Brunet P, Saingra Y, Leonetti F, Vacher Coponat H, Ramananarivo P, Berland Y. Tolerance of haemodialysis: a randomized cross-over trial of 5-h versus 4-h treatment time. Nephrol Dial Transplant 1996; 11(Suppl 8):46–51.
93. Churchill DN. Sodium and water profiling in chronic uremia. Nephrol Dial Transpl 1996; 11(suppl 8):38–41.
94. Raja RM. Sodium profiling in elderly haemodialysis patients. Nephrol Dial Transpl 1996; 11(suppl 8):42–45.
95. Acchiardo SR, Hayden AJ. Is Na modeling necessary in high flux dialysis. Trans Am Soc Artif Intern Organs 1991; 37:M135–M137.
96. Sadowski RH, Allred EN, Jabs K. Sodium modeling ameliorates intradialytic and interdialytic symptoms in young hemodialysis patients. J Am Soc Nephrol 1993; 4:1192–1198.
97. Dialysate sodium delivery can alter chronic blood pressure management. Flanigan-MJ; Khairullah QT, Lim VS. Am J Kidney Dis 1997; 29:383–389.
98. Daugirdas JT, Al-Kudsi RR, Ing TS, Norusis MJ. A double-blind evaluation of sodium gradient dialysis. Am J Nephrol 1985; 5:163–168.
99. Steuer R, Leypoldt JK, Cheung A, Senekjan H, Connis J. Reducing symptoms during dialysis by continuously monitoring the hematocrit. Am J Kidney Dis 1996; 27: 525–532.
100. Schallenberg U, Stiller S, Mann H. A new method of continuous hemoglobinometric measurements of blood volume during dialysis. Life Support Syst 1987; 5:293–305.
101. Steuer R, Leypoldt JK, Cheung A, Senekjan H, Connis J. Hematocrit as an indicator of blood volume and a predictor of intradialytic morbid events. ASAIO J 1994; 40:M691–M696.
102. Ishihara T, Igarashi I, Kitano T, Shinzato T, Maeda K. Continuous hematocrit monitoring method in an extracorporeal circulation system and its application for automatic control of blood volume during artificial kidney treatment. Artif Organs 1993; 17:708–716.
103. Sherman RA, Torres F, Cody RP. Postprandial blood pressure changes during hemodialysis. Am J Kidney Dis 1988; 12:37–39.
104. Barakat MM, Nawab ZM, Yu AW, Lau AH, Ing TS, Daugirdas JT. Hemodynamic effects of intradialytic food ingestion and the effects of caffeine. J Am Soc Nephrol 1993; 3:1813–1818.
105. Brandt JL, Castleman L, Ruskin HD, Greenwald J, Kelly JJ. The effect of oral protein and glucose feed-

ing on splanchnic blood flow and oxygen utilization in normal and cirrhotic subjects. J Clin Invest 1955; 34:1017–1025.

106. Kahn AM, Husid A, Song T. Relationship between insulin and hemodialysis-associated hypotension.Curr Opin Nephrol Hypertens 1997; 6:1–5.

107. Branger B, Deschodt G, Oules R, Balducchi JP, Granolleras C, Alsadabani B, Fourcade J, Shaldon S. Biocompatible membranes and hemodynamic tolerance to hemodialysis. Kidney Int 1988; 33(suppl 24):S196–S197.

108. Rubin RP. Neurotransmitter substances and hormones. Pharmacol Rev 1970; 22:389–428.

109. Argilès A, Kerr PG, Canaud B, Flavier JL, Mion C. Calcium kinetics and the long-term effects of lowering dialysate calcium concentration. Kidney Int 1993; 43: 630–640.

110. van der Sande FM, Cheriex ET, van Kuijk WHM, Leunissen KML. The effect of low calcium (1.25 mmol/l) and high calcium dialysate (1.75 mmol/l) on haemodynamics during ultrafiltration and dialysis in cardiac compromised patients (abstr). Am J Kidney Dis.

111. Fox SD, Henderson LW. Cardiovascular response during hemodialysis and hemofiltration: thermal, membrane and catecholamine influences. Blood Purif 1993; 11:224–226.

112. Hampl H, Paeprer H, Unger V, Fischer C, Resa I, Kessel M. Hemodynamic changes during hemodialysis, sequential ultrafiltration, and hemofiltration. Kidney Int 1980; 18:S83–S88.

113. Wizemann V, Kramer W, Knopp G, Sychla M, Schmidt H, Rawer P, Schütterle G. Cardiovascular function during hemodialysis, hemofiltration, hemodiafiltration. In: Schütterle G, Wizemann V, Seyfart G, eds. Hemodiafiltration. Proceedings Symposium Giessen 1981:89–104.

114. Movilli E, Camerini C, Zein H, D'Avolio G, Sandrini M, Strada A, Maiorca R. A prospective comparison of bicarbonate dialysis, hemodiafiltration, and acetate-free biofiltration in the elderly. Am J Kidney Dis. 1996; 27:541–547.

115. Iida N, Tsubakihara Y, Shirai D, Imada A, Suzuki M. Treatment of dialysis induced hypotension with L-threo-3,4-dihydroxyphenylserine. Nephrol Dial Transpl 1994; 6:1130–1135.

116. Kanamura M, Nagashima S, Nakashima M. Clinical effect of amezinium methylsulfate (LU-1631) on hypotensive agents undergoing intermittent hemodialysis therapy. J Clin Therap Med 1988; 4:1311–1319.

117. Flynn JJ, Mitchell MC, Caruso FS, McElligott MA. Midodrine treatment for patients with hemodialysis hypotension. Clin Nephrol 1996; 45:261–267.

118. Lindberg JS, Copley JB, Melton K, Wade CE, Abrams J, Goode D. Lysine vasopressin in the treatment of refractory hemodialysis-induced hypotension. Am J Nephrol 1990; 10:269–275.

119. Leunissen KML, Kooman JP, van Kuijk W, Luik AJ, van der Sande F, van Hooff JP. Preventing haemodynamic instability in patients at risk for intra-dialytic hypotension. Nephrol Dial Transpl 1996; 11(suppl 2): 11–15.

120. Rostand SG, Kirk KA, Rutskey EA. The epidemiology of coronary artery disease in patients on maintenance hemodialysis: implications for management. Contr Nephrol 1986; 52:34–41.

121. Parfrey PS, Foley RN. Ischemic heart disease in chronic uremia. Blood Purif 1996; 14:321–326.

122. de Lemso JA, Hillis LD. Diagnosis and management of coronary artery disease in patients with end-stage renal disease on hemodialysis. J Am Soc Nephrol 1996; 7:2044–2054.

123. Wizemann V. Coronary artery disease in dialysis patients. Nephron 1996; 74:642–651.

124. Besarab A, Bolton WK, Browne JK, Egvie JC, Nissenson AR, Oleamoto DM, Schwab SJ, Goodkin DA. The effect of normal as compared with low hematocrit values in patients with cardiac disease who are receiving hemodialysis and epoietin. N Engl J Med 1998; 339:584–590.

125. de Lima JJG, Lopes HF, Grupi CJ, Abensur H, Clementina M, Giorgi P, Krieger EM, Pileggi F. Blood pressure influences the occurrence of complex ventricular arrhythmias in hemodialysis patients. Hypertension 1995; 26(part 2):1200–1203.

126. Shapira OM, Bar-Khayim Y. ECG changes and cardiac arrhythmias in chronic renal failure patients on hemodialysis. J Electrocardiol 1992; 53:273–279.

127. Sforzini S, Latini R, Mingardi G, Vincenti A, Redaelli B. Ventricular arrhythmias and four-year mortality in haemodialysis patients. Lancet 1892; 339:212–213.

128. Saragoca MA, Canziani E, Cassiolata JL, Gil MA, Andrade JL, Draibe SA, Martinez EE. Left ventricular hypertrophy as a risk factor for arrhythmias in hemodialysis patients. J Cardiovasc Pharamacol 1991; 17(suppl 2):S136–S138.

129. Blumberg A, Häusermann M, Strub B, Jenzer HR. Cardiac arrhythmias in patients on maintenance hemodialysis. Nephron 1983; 33:91–95.

130. Wizemann V, Kramer W, Funke T, Schütterle G. Dialysis-induced cardiac arrhythmias: fact or fiction? Nephron 1985; 39:356–360.

131. Abe S, Yoshizawa M, Nakanishi N, Yazawa T, Yokota K, Honda M, Sloman G. Electrocardiographic abnormalities in patients receiving hemodialysis. Am Heart J 1996; 131:1137–1144.

132. Kimura K-I, Tabei K, Asano Y, Hosoda S. Cardiac arrhythmias in hemodialysis patients. Nephron 1989; 53:201–207.

133. Ramirez G, Brueggemeyer CD, Newton JL. Cardiac arrhythmias on hemodialysis on chronic renal failure patients. Nephron 1984; 36:212–218.

134. Wysowski DK, Bacsanyi J. Cisapride and fatal arrhythmia. N Engl J Med 1996; 335:290–291.

135. Morrison G, Michelson EL, Brown S, Morganroth J. Mechanism and prevention of cardiac arrhythmias in chronic hemodialysis patients. Kidney Int 1980; 17: 811–819.
136. Fantuzzi S, Caico C, Amatruda O, Cervini P, Abu-Turky H, Baratelli L, Donati D, Gastaldi L. Hemodialysis-associated cardiac arrhythmias: a lower risk with bicarbonate? Nephron 1991; 58:196–200.
137. Nishimura M, Nakanishi T, Yasui A, Tsuji Y, Kunishige H, Hirabayashi M, Takahashi H, Yoshimura M. Serum calcium increases the risk of arrhythmias during acetate hemodialysis. Am J Kidney Dis 1992; 19: 149–155.
138. Quellhorst E, Schuenemann B, Mietzsch G. Long-term hemofiltration in 'poor-risk' patients. Trans Am Soc Artif Intern Organs 1987; 33:758–764.
139. Ketchersid TL, van Stone JC. Dialysate potassium. Semin Dial 1991; 4:46–51.
140. Wiegand CF, Davin TD, Raij L, Kjellstrand CM. Severe hypokalemia induced by hemodialysis. Arch Intern Med 11981; 141:167–170.
141. Ward RA, Wathen RL, Williams TE, Harding GB. Hemodialysate composition and intradialytic metabolic, acid-base and potassium changes. Kidney Int 1987; 32:129–135.
142. Jaber BJ, Pereira BJG. Dialysis reactions. Semin Dial 1997; 10:158–165.
143. Salem M, Ivanovich PT, Ing TS, Daugirdas JT. Adverse effect of dialyzers manifesting during the dialysis session. Nephrol Dial Transpl 1994; 9(suppl 2): 127–137.
144. Verresen L, Waer M, Vanrenterghem Y, Michielsen P. Angiotensin converting enzyme inhibitors and anafylactoid reactions to high flux membrane dialysis. Lancet 1990; 336:1360–1362.
145. Renaux JL, Crost T, Loughraieb N, Pereira M, Vantard G. Identification of plasma pH as cofactor involved in contact phase activation by polyacrylonitrile dialysis membranes (abstr). Blood Purif 1997; 15(suppl 2):7.
146. Novey HS, Pahl M, Haydik I, Vaziri ND. Immunologic studies of anaphylaxis to iron dextran in patients on renal dialysis. Ann Allergy 1994; 72:224–228.
147. Daugirdas JT, Ing TS. First use reactions during hemodialysis: a definition of subtypes. Kidney Int 1988; 24:S37–S43.
148. Levin NW. Intradialytic hypertension: I. Semin Dial 1993; 60:370–371.
149. Fellner SK. Intradialytic hypertension: II. Semin Dial 1993; 6:371–373.
150. Cirit M, Kakcicek F, Terzioglu E, Soydas C, Ok E, Özbasli CF, Basci A, Dorhout Mees EJ. Paradoxical rise in blood pressure during ultrafiltration in dialysis patients. Nephrol Dial Transpl 1995; 10:1417–1420.
151. Bazzato G, Coli U, Landini S. Prevention of intra- and post-dialytic hypertensive hypertensive crises by captopril. Contr Nephrol 1984; 41:292–298.
152. Grossman E, Messerli FH, Grodzicki T, Kowey P. Should a moratorium be placed on sublingual nifedipine capsules given for hypertensive emergencies and pseudo-emergencies? JAMA 1996; 276:1328–1331.
153. McGee SR. Muscle cramps. Ann Intern Med 1990; 150:511–518.
154. Ahmad S, Robertson HT, Golper TA, Wolfson M, Kurtin S, Katz LA, Hirschberg R, Nicora R, Ashbrook DW, Kopple JD. Multicenter trial of L-carnitine in maintenance hemodialysis patients II: Clinical and biochemical effects. Kidney Int 1990; 38:912–918.
155. Canzanello VJ, Hylander-Rossner B, Sands RE, Morgan TM, Jordan J, Burkart JM. Comparison of 50% dextrose water, 25% mannitol, and 23.5% saline for the treatment of hemodialysis-associated muscle cramps. Trans Am Soc Artif Intern Organs 1991; 37: 649–652.
156. Sidhom O, Odeh Y, Krumlovsky FA, Budris WA, Wang Z, Pospisil PA, Atkinson AJ. Low-dose prazosin in patients with muscle cramps during hemodialysis. Clin Pharmacol Ther 1994; 56:445–451.
157. Kleeman CR. Metabolic coma. Kidney Int 1989; 36: 1142–1158.
158. Rodrigo F, Shideman J, McHugh R, Buselmeier T, Kjellstrand C. Osmolality changes during dialysis. Ann Intern Med 1977; 86:554–559.
159. Palmer F, Henrich WL. The effect of dialysis on left ventricular function. In: Parfrey PS, Harnett JD, eds. Cardiac Dysfunction in Chronic Uremi. Dordrecht: Kluwer Academic, 1992:171–186.

5

Complications Related to Inadequate Delivered Dose: Recognition and Management in Acute and Chronic Dialysis

Jane Y. Yeun and Thomas A. Depner
University of California, Davis, Sacramento, California

Despite many improvements over the past three decades, hemodialysis fails to completely restore health in patients who have lost native kidney function, so debate continues about how much dialysis is enough. It is clear that uremic symptoms such as nausea, vomiting, pruritus, mental lethargy, and anorexia can appear in patients who are inadequately dialyzed and are certain to appear if dialysis is omitted. However, even in patients who have none of these overt symptoms, insufficient dialysis has been associated with an increase in the number and duration of hospitalizations and with a shortened life expectancy (1–4). Because these serious complications are potentially preventable, clinicians providing dialysis for patients with end-stage renal disease (ESRD) must have a practical understanding of dialysis adequacy, how to measure it, and the basis for currently acceptable minimum standards. This requires a working familiarity with the theoretical constructs of solute and membrane dynamics, the strategies to improve dialysis efficiency, and the pitfalls inherent in prescribing and supervising dialysis.

I. EFFECT OF DIALYSIS DOSE AND ADEQUACY ON MORTALITY

Mortality rates of dialysis patients in the United States are higher than in other countries for unclear reasons. Recent statistics show a mortality rate of 7% per year in Japan compared to >20% per year in the United States (4–6). The alarming U.S. statistics have focused attention on strategies for dialysis that differ in the United States compared to other countries, such as patient selection, dialysis techniques, and reimbursement policies that foster shorter dialysis treatments. Shorter treatments are often requested by patients but are also sought by dialysis administrators, who are influenced by current federal policies that provide reimbursement per treatment rather than per hour. Paradoxically, individual patients in the United States have been maintained on hemodialysis for over 25 years, suggesting that indefinite survival is possible and that the high mortality rate may be related to patient selection or center-related variables (7).

As noted in Fig. 1, mortality is strikingly correlated with age (6). Other significant factors that correlate either positively or negatively with mortality include the dose of dialysis expressed as *Kt/V*, urea reduction ratio (URR), or solute removal index (SRI); protein catabolism; body weight; and other measures of nutritional intake such as the serum concentrations of albumin, creatinine, and cholesterol (2,8–10). Since many of these are indicators of nutrition, concern has been raised that inadequate dialysis may suppress the appetite and lead to malnutrition (8,11,12). Whether inadequate dialysis, as currently defined, always causes malnutrition is debated, but examination of large hemodialysis populations suggests that it does in some patients (10,13,14). Regardless of the mechanism, numerous studies now show that mortality is strongly associated with dialysis adequacy, as summarized in Table 1 (1,8–10,15–18). Impressive data have been published from Tassin, France, where 445 hemodialysis

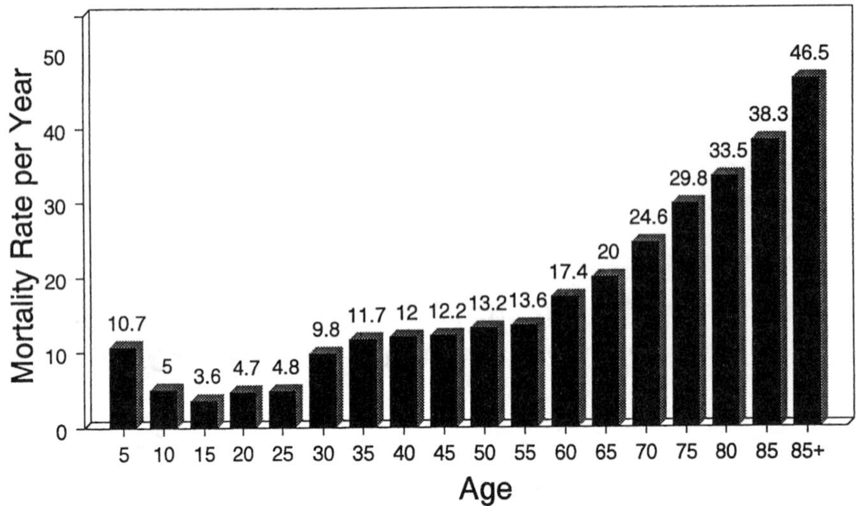

Fig. 1 One-year mortality rates for both hemodialysis and peritoneal dialysis patients from day 91 after starting treatment, by age. n = 193,995 patients. (From Ref. 6.)

patients receiving a mean *Kt/V* of 1.67 (current minimal standards are 1.2, see below for details concerning *Kt/V*) had an 87% survival rate at 5 years and 43% at 20 years (15). Several of the observational studies shown in Table 1 suggest that increasing the dose of dialysis above the current standard improves survival, but the data must be interpreted with caution because the studies were not prospective or randomized and may be confounded by mathematical artifacts and other factors that may influence mortality independent of the dose (8,9,16,19,20).

II. EFFECT OF DIALYSIS DOSE AND ADEQUACY ON MORBIDITY

Inadequate dialysis dose may also cause significant morbidity, as reported by the National Cooperative Dialysis Study (NCDS) (1). This project, the only prospective randomized examination of hemodialysis adequacy, showed that patients with high blood urea nitrogen (BUN) levels had higher rates of hospitalization and withdrawal from the study for medical reasons (42% vs. 7% withdrawal). The medical reasons for withdrawal included anorexia, nausea, pericarditis, pleuritis, anemia, gastrointestinal bleeding, neuropathy, and seizures (1,21). In a more recent study the number of hospital days per patient per year decreased from 15.2 to 10.3 when *Kt/V* increased from 0.82 ± 0.32 to 1.33 ± 0.23 (8). In other studies the relative risk of death from infections was 25% lower in patients receiving more dialysis (*Kt/V* of 1.2 vs. 0.9), and the risk of death from either coronary artery disease or infection was reduced by 9% for every 0.1 increase in *Kt/V* (22,23). Inadequate dialysis is also associated with a decreased response to erythropoietin (24–26).

III. UREMIC TOXICITY, THE TARGET OF DIALYSIS TREATMENTS

Hemodialysis was first successfully applied in the early 1940s as an empirical treatment for acute renal failure by a physician investigator, Willem Kolff (27). Although the equipment was crude, the initial trials were successful and quickly reversed uremic toxicity, to the surprise and delight of the inventor and his collaborators. Because of this early success and despite the complexities of maintaining an extracorporeal blood circuit, physicians soon began to apply hemodialysis widely, before theories were developed to explain how it worked and before a consensus was reached about the pathogenesis of uremia. Hemodialysis was thus born out of empiricism and in a setting where the disease it was designed to treat was incompletely understood.

IV. IDENTIFYING UREMIC TOXINS

Decades of research designed to define the precise cause of each of the multiple symptoms and signs of uremia preceded the first hemodialysis but were largely unsuccessful (28,29). Fluid and small molecular weight (dialyzable) solutes were assumed to accumulate due to failure of excretion by the native kidneys, but mea-

Table 1 Studies of the Relationship Between Mortality and Adequacy of Dialysis

Source (Ref.)	Study design	*N*	*Kt/V*	URR	Probability of failure (%)
Lowrie et al., 1981 (1)	Prospective, randomized	80	>0.9		13
		80	<0.8		57
					Patient survival (%)
					5 10 yr 15 yr 20 yr
Charra et al., 1992 (15)	Cross section	222	<1.6		85 71 50 33
		223	≥1.6		91 82 63 57
					Odds ratio of death
Owen et al., 1993 (10)	Cross section	13,473		≥70	1.04
				65–69	1.00 (Ref)
				60–64	1.15
				55–59	1.28
				50–54	1.39
				45–49	1.52
				<45	1.84
					Relative risk of death
					Diabetic Nondiabetic
Collins et al., 1994 (17)	Cross section	1,773	<1.00		1.06 1.14
			1.00–1.19		1.00 1.00 (Ref)
			1.20–1.39		0.70 0.65
			≥1.40		0.59 0.67
Held et al., 1996 (18)	Cross section	2,321	<0.91		1.20
			0.91–1.05		0.87
			1.06–1.16		1.00 (Ref)
			1.17–1.32		0.69
			≥1.33		0.71
					Crude mortality (%/yr)
Hakim et al., 1994 (8)	Observation	92	0.82 ± 0.32		22.8
		130	1.33 ± 0.23		9.1
Parker et al., 1994 (9)	Observation	809	1.18 ± 0.28		22.5
		764	1.46 ± 0.30		18.1
		24,561		57.1	21.8
		31,658		62.5	19.5
Yang 1996 (16)	Observation	97	1.3		16.1
		134	1.5		13.2
		108	1.7		8.0

sured levels of the various solutes known to accumulate were well below the levels necessary to evoke toxic responses in animals and in humans, even when overt signs of uremia such as pericarditis or uremic coma were present in patients (28,30). Urea, the most abundant organic substance to accumulate, had little demonstrable toxicity when added to the dialysate (31,32). Posttranslational modification of proteins by urea-induced carbamylation has been proposed more recently as an indirect toxic effect of urea, but this relatively slow non-enzymatic process cannot account for the immediate life-threatening syndrome that is quickly reversed by dialysis (33–35). Since dialysis does little more than remove fluid and dialyzable solutes, the uremic syndrome must result from the aggregate accumulation of toxins other than urea, perhaps each at subtoxic levels but with an additive and/or synergistic toxic effect (36). These retained solutes probably account for most if not all of the immediate life-threatening consequences of uremia such as uremic coma, pericarditis, and hemorrhage as well as the more indolent but also life-threatening manifestations such as malnutrition, susceptibility to infection, and peripheral neuropathy (37,38). Removal of toxins is essential, whereas removal of fluid, though viewed as a vital and intrinsic component of therapeutic dialysis, must be considered an adjunctive function that is not essential to dialysis because it can be accomplished independent of dialysis, because some uremic patients do not require removal of fluid, and because fluid removal alone does not prevent death from uremia. The fundamental observation that dialysis reverses uremia and prolongs life is the basis for contemporary concepts of uremia and for current guidelines designed to assure the adequacy of treatment.

Since investigators have not been successful in their efforts to identify and measure the most important solutes removed, clinicians have resorted to measuring the clearance of identified solutes as a substitute (39). At the current time, hemodialyzer urea clearance, expressed as a fraction of total body water cleared per dialysis (*Kt/V*), is the most popular quantitative expression of dialysis and the basis for current standards of dialysis adequacy (3). Measuring clearance avoids errors inherent in measuring concentrations of single solutes such as urea or creatinine that are also influenced by states of nutrition and tissue catabolism independent of dialysis. However, clearance is an indirect measure of the real goal of dialysis—that of lowering toxin levels in the patient. Recent evidence suggests that the performance of the dialyzer has been overemphasized and that evaluating the patient's response to dialysis must be included in the assessment of dialysis adequacy (20,40,41). This approach is especially important for the patient who is ill either because he is receiving less dialysis than suggested by the standards established for the average patient or because a superimposed disease has imparted a requirement for more dialysis than the standard.

Clinical Example: Dialysis Dosing

A patient recently began hemodialysis treatments three times weekly with an average *Kt/V* of 1.2 per dialysis. Over the past 3 months he has been eating poorly and losing weight, his serum albumin concentration fell from 4.0 to 3.0 g/dL, serum BUN concentration fell from 70 to 40 mg/dL, and he appears depressed. No specific cause for his clinical deterioration has been found. What recommendation regarding the dose of dialysis, if any, can be made at this time?

The symptoms are most compatible with psychological depression, which does not respond to more dialysis. However, the symptoms are also compatible with worsening uremia despite the decreased BUN. Therefore, assuming that this individual may have a poorly understood need for additional dialysis at this particular time, the dose of dialysis should be increased temporarily while waiting for antidepressant medications to take effect. Since the current standards for hemodialysis are derived more from consensus than firm data (see Sec. XVIII) and undiscovered factors may impose an increased need for dialysis, individualization of therapy takes precedence over established standards, as in other fields of medicine.

The above example illustrates the potential harm that may arise when obsessions with toxin levels target the concentration of a single substance as a surrogate for the real toxins. In the past, low BUN concentration due to poor nutrition has been misinterpreted as excessive dialysis, leading to further underdialysis, decreased appetite, and a potentially vicious cycle (Fig. 2) (42,43). Clinicians and designers of dialyzers and dialysis equipment should consider all potential toxins ranging from urea, an easily removed but relatively nontoxic compound, to phosphate, an easily dialyzed but poorly removed compound with devastating long-term toxicity.

Clinical Example: Potentially Toxic Solute Accumulation

A 30-year-old African American male with hypertensive renal disease has been hemodialyzed for 2 years with relative success. He tolerates dialysis well, maintains a constant postdialysis weight, and has acceptable levels of *Kt/V*, normalized protein catabolic rate (PCRn), and albumin. However, his serum creatinine levels are consistently above 20 mg/dL predialysis.

The predialysis level of creatinine is 15–20 times higher than the steady-state level in a person with normal renal function, so the concern is appropriate. However, creatinine is an end product of muscle creatine metabolism, one of several basic guanidino compounds that accumulate in renal failure, and has little demon-

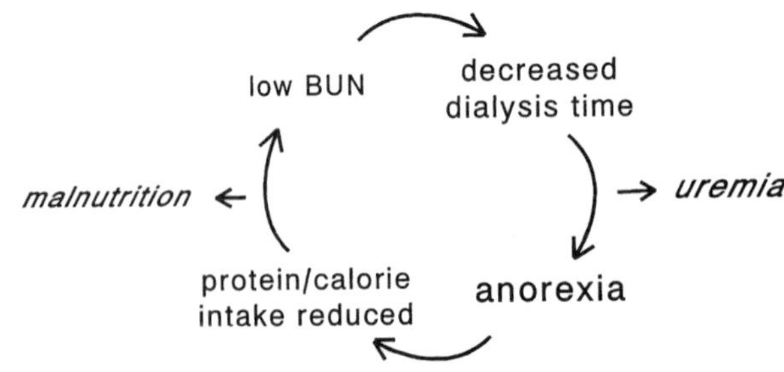

Fig. 2 If a low BUN is the primary indicator of dialysis quality, the patient becomes susceptible to this theoretical vicious cycle that is perpetuated by reducing time on dialysis when the BUN falls. Follow-up studies of the NCDS patients suggested that the cycle eventually becomes irreversible (126).

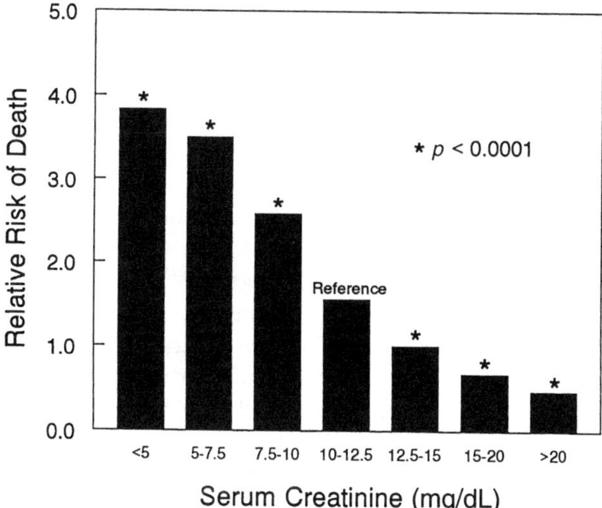

Fig. 3 In the ESRD population, serum creatinine is less an indicator of dialysis adequacy than of nutrition. This probably explains the inverse correlation with risk of death (n = 19,746; $*p < 0.0001$). p-values are for comparison of each group to the reference group of patients with serum creatinine of 12.5–15.0 mg/dL. (Adapted from Ref. 2.)

strable toxicity even at high blood levels (29,44). Furthermore, the high levels in this patient despite "adequate" dialysis reflect a high production rate caused by a relatively large muscle mass, which reflects good nutrition. As shown in Fig. 3, mortality in patients with ESRD correlates inversely with serum creatinine levels, indicating that the nutritional status takes precedence over any potential toxic effect of creatinine accumulation (2,10). This inverse correlation has prompted physicians to look elsewhere for indicators of toxicity and dialysis adequacy.

V. THE MEANING OF CLEARANCE

Clearance is an expression of solute removal that derives from the first-order nature of diffusion and filtration. First-order processes have an intrinsic auto-feedback property, wherein the product or result of the process is the driving force for the process itself. For dialysis, the driving force is the solute concentration gradient across the membrane, which varies directly with solute removal (the product). The progressive decline in this gradient during hemodialysis diminishes removal of solute. If the volume of the system is constant, then:

$$dC/dt = -k \cdot C \tag{1}$$

where C is the solute concentration, t is time, and k is a constant (fractional clearance). Stated another way, the change in concentration (dC/dt) is proportionate to the concentration (C). Factoring rate of concentration change by the concentration eliminates the variability in the removal rate. The resulting proportionality constant (k) is defined as a fractional clearance, a term that describes the process, in this case dialysis, independently of C. If k is converted to a volume clearance $K_d = k \cdot V$, then:

$$K_d = \frac{-d(C \cdot V)/dt}{C} = \frac{\text{immediate removal rate}}{\text{immediate concentration}} \tag{2}$$

Equation (2) is a more familiar expression of clearance (K_d) as a flow (mL/min) in terms of the removal rate divided by C. During intermittent hemodialysis, K_d remains constant despite the diminishing solute concentration. For continuous dialysis, both the removal rate (R) and C are constant, so Eq. (2) is simplified to:

$$K_d = R/C \tag{3}$$

Clearance of a dialyzer also depends on blood and dialysate flow rates, which for solutes like urea have predictable effects that can be included in the clearance equation. The resulting expression is a measure of dialysis called the dialyzer mass transfer area coefficient (K_0A), which is independent of the rates of blood and dialysate flow as well as solute concentration:

$$K_0A = \frac{Q_b \cdot Q_d}{Q_b - Q_d} \ln \left(\frac{1 - \dfrac{K_d}{Q_b}}{1 - \dfrac{K_d}{Q_d}} \right) \tag{4}$$

Q_b and Q_d are dialyzer blood and dialysate flow rates, respectively. K_0A can be considered a permeability constant for a particular dialyzer and solute combination. It can also be considered the maximum possible solute clearance achievable at infinite blood and dialysate flow rates. Recently, the K_0A for urea has been shown to increase slightly but significantly at higher dialysate flow rates, presumably due to better mixing and less channeling of dialysate flow (45).

Clinical Example: The Difference Between Solute Removal and Clearance

Two patients of similar height and weight undergo periodic dialysate monitoring to assess dialysis adequacy.

Despite use of the same dialyzer and similar blood and dialysate flows, a routine 3-hour dialysis in patient A removes twice as much urea as a similar 3-hour dialysis in patient B. Which patient is better dialyzed?

Although more solute was removed from patient A, the above data suggest that the delivered dose of dialysis is similar. If other factors are equal (including the dialyzer, blood flow, and dialysate flow), the adequacy is approximately equivalent because the clearances are the same as predicted by Eq. (19) below. However, the mean urea concentration in patient A would be twice that of patient B as predicted by Eq. (20) below. Note that the higher urea concentration in patient A, similar to the high creatinine concentration in a previous example, does not signify less adequate dialysis. Outcomes should be similar in the two patients despite the difference in concentration and removal rate. Taking into consideration the effect of protein catabolism on prognosis, one might predict a slightly better outcome in patient A with the higher urea concentration and generation rate (see Sec. VII.B) (2,21,46).

Additional expressions of clearance that have special applications are listed in Table 2. Residual native kidney clearance (K_r) is familiar to nephrologists who routinely measure it in patients with chronic renal failure prior to initiating dialysis. Unfortunately, K_r for urea cannot be simply added to K_d in the expression Kt/V because its effect is exerted primarily between dialyses when K_d is zero. Clearances at different time intervals, when solute levels are different, cannot be added. Methods are described below for adjusting the effect of K_r or K_d prior to adding the two clearances to give a more representative total K and Kt/V (see Sec. XIII).

Instant dialyzer clearance can be measured from dialyzer blood flow and urea concentrations obtained simultaneously at the inlet and outlet of the dialyzer or from dialysate concentrations and flow. To obtain the average or mean clearance during an entire dialysis, multiple measurements of instant clearance would be required throughout the treatment. Fortunately, this is not necessary because the modeled clearance derived from the predialysis and the immediate postdialysis BUN is the effective mean dialyzer clearance integrated over the entire dialysis. This automatic averaging illustrates both the simplicity and the power of single-pool urea kinetic modeling.

Patient clearance is discussed below (see Sec. VII). Note that the more complex two-compartment models also measure dialyzer clearance but allow determination of the equilibrated postdialysis BUN (C_e). Once C_e is determined, the simpler single-compartment model may be applied to the predialysis BUN and C_e to calculate the patient clearance, which, like the standard single pool dialyzer clearance, is also a mean clearance integrated over time on dialysis. Taking this a step further, one can calculate the continuous equivalent of re-

Table 2 Classification of Urea Clearances

Residual clearance

Clearance by the patient's native kidneys, often negligible or absent. Contributes little to total clearance during dialysis but exerts it major effect on total clearance between dialyses.

Dialyzer clearance

Instant dialyzer clearance: calculated from BUN values measured simultaneously at the dialyzer inlet and outlet: $K = Q_B(C_{in} - C_{out})/C_{in}$.

Integrated dialyzer clearance: determined by fitting the predialysis and immediate postdialysis BUN to the single-compartment model of urea kinetics. Integrated clearance may also be obtained from the more complicated two-compartment model using multiple intradialysis and postdialysis BUN values. Measured by either technique, this clearance is a mean dialyzer clearance averaged over the entire dialysis, ignoring urea disequilibrium.

Patient clearance

Also called whole body clearance or equilibrated clearance: a virtual integrated clearance derived, similar to the integrated dialyzer clearance, from the predialysis and equilibrated postdialysis BUN.

Always lower than dialyzer clearance due to urea disequilibrium and in some cases, recirculation.

Includes the usually small contribution of residual native kidney clearance (K_r).

Continuous equivalent of intermittent clearance (EKR)

Derived from G/TAC.

Always lower than patient clearance.

Allows comparisons among patients treated with different dialysis schedules including continuous dialysis.

nal clearance, or EKR, a more recent formulation of clearance that is discussed in more detail below (see Sec. XIX).

VI. DEFINITIONS OF THE "DOSE" OF DIALYSIS

The reasons for expressing the dose of hemodialysis as a clearance of urea (K) rather than as a solute level in the patient or as a rate of solute removal are outlined above. A clearance is essentially a rate of treatment analogous to a rate of medication dosing except that the dose is expressed as a volume of blood treated rather than a weight of medication given per unit of time. Because hemodialysis is not continuous (usually applied three times per week), this rate is further modified by expressing the time element as the duration of a single dialysis ($K \cdot t$) instead of traditional time elements like minutes or hours. Thus the duration for each treatment is deemphasized and more value is placed on the total dose, whether delivered over a short or a long period of time. As will be shown below (see Sec. XI), ignoring the rate of delivery creates a potential error that is partially corrected by a new expression of the dose (eKt/V) that incorporates the time element (47).

Because larger patients need more and smaller patients need less dialysis, the dose is adjusted to body size, analogous to dosing a medication proportionate to body weight or surface area. This adjustment is especially important for children, in whom relative body size varies over a greater range. The urea volume (V) is a convenient denominator for the size adjustment because it is readily derived from hemodialysis urea modeling and is closely related to lean body mass. V differs from body surface area, the usual denominator for clearance (e.g., urea, creatinine, and inulin clearances). Surface area is preferred because physiological functions scale to surface area better than to body mass (48–52). This potential source of error in smaller patients has only recently been addressed.

Combining the above adjustments, the complete expression of the dialysis dose is the volume of body water cleared per dialysis ($K \cdot t$) divided by the patient's water volume (V). This expression (Kt/V) has units of measurement best described as a fraction of body water volume cleared per dialysis. Expressing the dose in this somewhat unconventional fashion stems largely from mathematical considerations (see Sec. VII), but nevertheless it is roughly equivalent to our everyday prescription of drugs and other treatments. Kt/V is often expressed as an absolute number, ignoring the unit of time (per dialysis) and the frequency (three times per week), both of which are essential.

The prescribed dose, which is based on expected clearances and time on dialysis, must be distinguished from the delivered dose, which is the actual dose of dialysis the patient receives. Both are important quantitative expressions of hemodialysis, and a comparison of the two gives valuable insight regarding proper functioning of the dialyzer for quality assurance monitoring. The delivered dose, often lower than the prescribed dose, is more important because it reflects the effectiveness of the treatment, and fortunately it is easier to measure because it is derived primarily from predialysis and postdialysis BUN values. Further refinements have permitted distinctions among the delivered dose, the effective delivered dose, and the continuous equivalent of the delivered dose (53), each of which is lower than its preceding counterpart. The latter two expressions of dialysis dose have slightly different interpretations, and each has a different set of standards (see Secs. XI and XIX).

VII. MATHEMATICAL MODELS OF UREA KINETICS DURING HEMODIALYSIS

Intermittent hemodialysis perturbs the patient's urea concentration, which allows measurement of vital parameters such as V and the urea generation rate (G), neither of which is easily measured by other means (Table 3) (54). The changes in urea concentration must be evaluated by fitting them to a mathematical model of molecular kinetics, examples of which are shown in Figs. 4 and 5. The single-compartment mathematical model widely used today is built on a simple expression of urea mass balance that equates the change in urea content [$d(V \cdot C)dt$] to the difference between urea generation (G) and removal ($K \cdot C$) (Fig. 4):

$$d(V \cdot C)dt = G - K \cdot C \qquad (5)$$

The classic two-compartment model of urea kinetics adds another term (K_C) that limits diffusive movement of urea within the patient (Fig. 5):

$$d(V_1 \cdot C_1)dt = G - K \cdot C_1 - K_C(C_1 - C_2) \qquad (6)$$

and

$$dC_2/dt = K_C(C_1 - C_2) \qquad (7)$$

In the above equations, V is the urea distribution volume (total body water), C is urea concentration, G is the urea generation rate, K is the combined dialyzer

Table 3 Modeled Parameters Derived from Single Compartment Modeling

Parameter	Definition	Interpretation
K_d	Dialyzer clearance	Normally an entered (input) parameter. If V is the entered parameter, K_d will be slightly overestimated when Kt/V is low (below 1.3) and slightly underestimated when Kt/V is high (above 1.3/dialysis, 3×/week) (120).
V	Volume of urea distribution or total body water	Slightly underestimated when Kt/V is below 1.3 and overestimated when Kt/V is above 1.3/dialysis (120).
G	Generation rate or, more accurately, urea appearance rate	Always slightly overestimated by this model.

and native kidney clearance, t is time on dialysis, and the subscripts 1 and 2 refer to the two compartments. Solutions to these equations have been published in comprehensive mathematical treatises that are beyond the scope of this chapter (39,54–56). Fortunately, user-friendly computer programs are available that do not require intimate familiarity with the mathematics while allowing full use of these complex equations to assist with patient care (54).

The model is a mathematical description of the changes in urea concentration both during and between hemodialyses caused by predictable and relatively constant parameters such as the clearance, generation, and distribution volume of urea. Modeling is a process that applies a mathematical solution in reverse, that is, instead of calculating concentrations from the above physiological constants, the constants themselves are calculated by finding the most appropriate values that describe (or fit) a profile of measured urea concentrations. Each model includes certain physiological assumptions such as the number and size of compartments and the forces dictating movement of solute. The fitting of measured concentrations to a mathematical model requires a trial-and-error process called iteration to obtain the best fit. The goal of such an exercise is to find the parameters that cause a minimal deviation of the modeled concentrations from the actual measured concentrations.

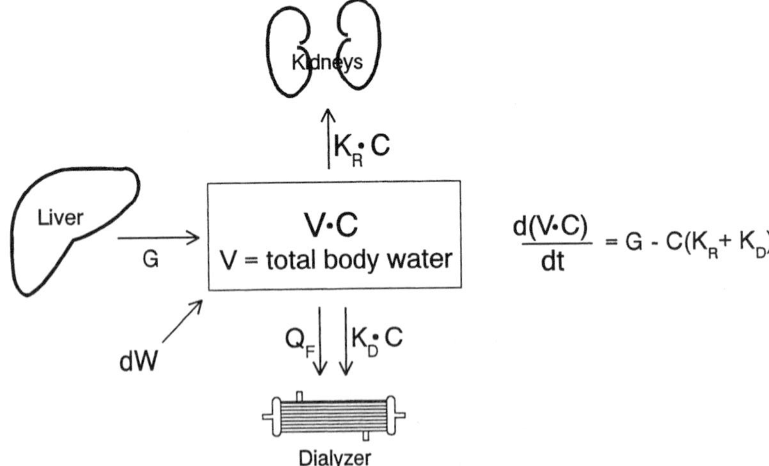

Fig. 4 Single-compartment, variable-volume model of urea mass balance. The equation to the right is the mathematical model shown in the diagram to the left. The model expresses an instant change in the patient's urea content, d(VC)/dt, as the sum of urea generation (G) and removal (K·C). K_R is the residual native kidney clearance, K_D is the dialyzer clearance, dW is the rate of fluid accumulation between dialyses, Q_F is the rate of fluid removal during dialysis, and V and C are the volume and concentration, respectively, of urea in the single pool. (Adapted from Ref. 65.)

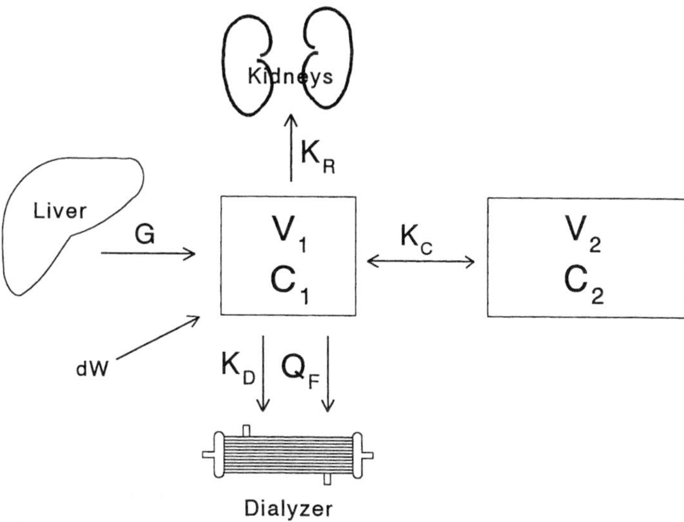

Fig. 5 A two-compartment, variable-volume model of urea mass balance. Symbols are similar to those defined in Fig. 3; subscripts 1 and 2 refer to compartments 1 and 2, respectively; V_2 is the volume of the second (remote) compartment, and K_C is the intercompartment mass transfer area coefficient. (From Ref. 54.)

A. How Many Compartments Are Required for the Model?

The original mathematical model of hemodialysis urea kinetics assumed that urea was distributed uniformly in a single well-mixed pool (Fig. 4), which is essentially equivalent to body water volume. It is now clear that such an assumption is incorrect, i.e., that urea distributes in multiple volumes with relatively rapid but finite rates of diffusion among them, as shown in Fig. 5. Furthermore, differences in blood flow to various regions of the body, as shown in Fig. 6, have been found recently to influence urea gradients among body compartments (57). As a result, even the classic two-compartment diffusional model shown in Fig. 5 does not completely describe the urea concentration gradients within the blood compartment during hemodialysis (58). Instead, a convective model incorporating blood flow to explain both the rapid early fall in BUN after starting dialysis and the rapid early rise in BUN postdialysis is required (Fig. 7) (55).

Despite these deviations from single pool predictions, the simpler single-compartment model continues to be used in most dialysis clinics to assess dialysis adequacy for several reasons (Table 4). First, although the model requires mathematical iteration, the equations are solvable without resorting to complicated numerical approximations required by the more complex multicompartment models. Second, only two parameters must be resolved (Kt/V and PCRn), which reduces the required number of blood samplings for BUN measurements (see Sec. VII.C). Third, the errors encountered by falsely assuming a single compartment tend to cancel one another, resulting in relatively accurate measurements of Kt/V (39,59,60). The single-compartment model became further entrenched when it was accepted as the gold standard for assessing dialysis adequacy in the United States (3,61,62). Formal two-compartment modeling has been restricted largely to research applications.

B. Measures of Nutrition: Urea Generation and Protein Catabolism

In addition to quantifying dialysis, formal urea modeling also provides a measure of urea generation (G) that can be translated to the patient's net protein catabolic rate (PCR), also known as the protein nitrogen appearance rate (63):

$$PCRn = 5420(G/V) + 0.17 \tag{8}$$

$PCRn$ is PCR normalized to V (much like $K \cdot t$ is normalized to V). In a steady state of nitrogen balance, protein intake must balance protein catabolism (PCRn). In the NCDS and subsequent larger population studies, patients with low G, and therefore low $PCRn$, had high

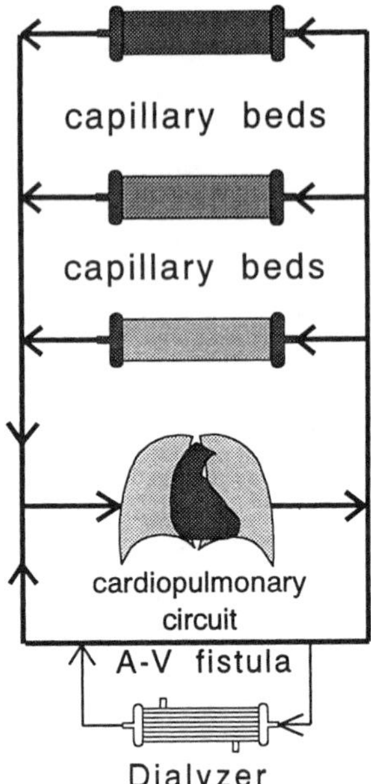

Fig. 6 Urea disequilibrium, evident from differing simultaneous concentrations throughout the body during dialysis, can develop solely as a consequence of differences in regional blood perfusion shown here as a parallel arrangement of dialyzers representing tissue compartments. Although the consequences are similar to that of the diffusion model shown in Fig. 5 and result in a concentration profile similar to that shown in Fig. 7, the mechanism is entirely different. Despite the absence of diffusion barriers, this model predicts a rapid fall in BUN at the beginning of dialysis and a sharp rebound following the end of the treatment. The proximal most rapidly flowing blood pathway is the cardiopulmonary circuit through the peripheral A/V access device.

morbidity and mortality rates, probably because of malnutrition (2,21). High mean BUN values (time-averaged concentration, or TAC) strongly predicted poor outcome, but low BUN values from low *PCRn* were associated with even higher morbidity. Since BUN levels are influenced by two separate processes, i.e., the dose of dialysis and nutritional intake, combining the two processes in the expression *Kt/V* establishes a constant ratio of PCRn to TAC and clarifies the net effect of these two opposing forces on patient morbidity and mortality (Fig. 8). Although *G* and *PCRn* vary widely from day to day and perhaps from hour to hour within a given patient, if formal urea modeling consistently reports low values for *PCRn*, a dietary evaluation should be undertaken and consideration given to both protein and calorie supplements. This recommendation is based on correlative evidence. Prospective studies are needed to determine if dietary intervention can definitively alter the patient's outcome.

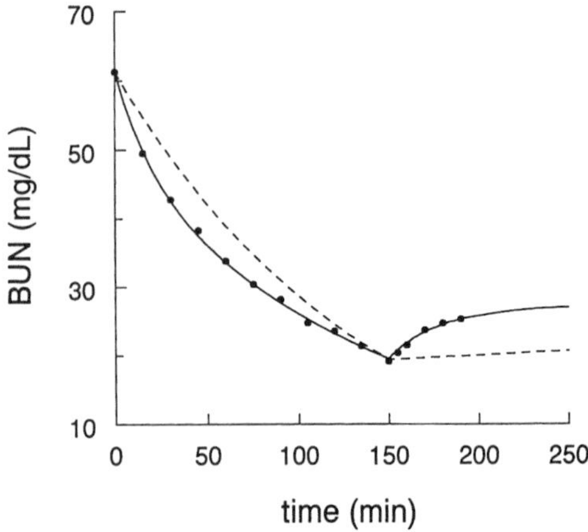

Fig. 7 Measured BUN levels during and immediately following dialysis fit best to a two-compartment variable-volume mathematical model (solid line). The single-compartment variable-volume model (dashed line) overestimates BUN levels during the dialysis and fails to predict the rebound.

VIII. TWO-BUN METHOD FOR DETERMINING G AND PCRn

As shown in Fig. 9, *Kt/V* is determined primarily from the fall in BUN during dialysis, while *G* is determined from the change in BUN levels between dialyses. The

Table 4 The Single-Compartment, Variable-Volume Model of Urea Kinetics

Advantages

1. Requires only two BUN measurements.
2. Converges quickly to a solution within a few milliseconds.
3. Includes the effects of ultrafiltration during dialysis.
4. Errors tend to cancel one another (see discussion).
5. The model is most accurate at spKt/V = 1.3 per dialysis, close to the consensus-derived target (3,120).
6. spKt/V is a measure of dialyzer clearance, a real measurable clearance.

Disadvantages

1. BUN levels are overestimated during dialysis.
2. The model fails to predict the rebound in serum urea concentration postdialysis.
3. Modeled values of G and nPCR are slightly overestimated.
4. As a measure of dialyzer urea clearance, spKt/V is slightly underestimated in the high range and slightly overestimated in the low range.
5. spKt/V is an inflated estimate of the real effect of dialysis in the patient.

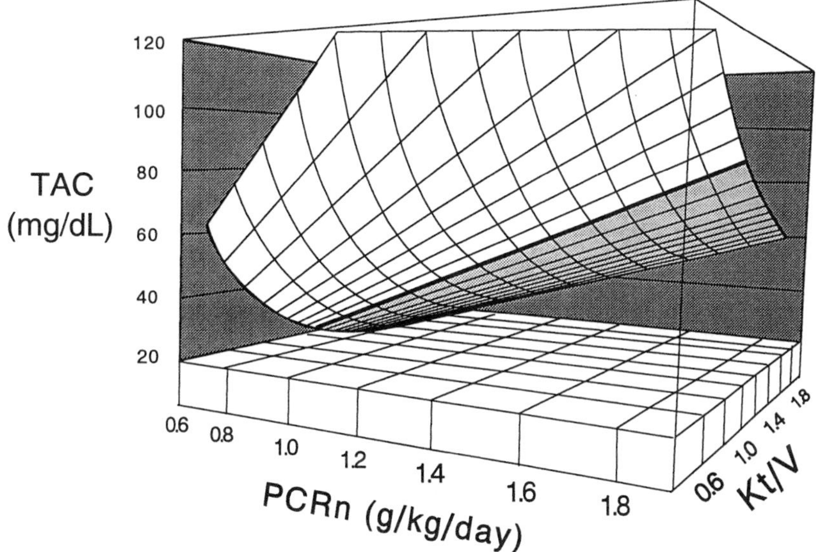

Fig. 8 The mathematical relationship among time-averaged BUN (TAC), normalized protein catabolic rate (PCRn), and Kt/V is shown as a curvilinear surface in this three-dimensional graph. The shaded area above the Kt/V isopleth of 1.2/dialysis represents the target for dialysis adequacy (see text). Data were derived from the single-compartment model; all three scales are linear. (From Ref. 127.)

latter suggests that a third blood sample is required to assess the interdialysis interval. However, several studies have shown that *G* can be determined just as reliably from the predialysis and postdialysis BUN measurements alone, using their ratio to determine *Kt/V* and their absolute values to determine *G* (64,65). This method requires a constant dietary protein intake, a constant dialysis prescription for at least a week (three dialyses), and a steady state of nitrogen balance. *G* is determined by an iterative computerized fitting of the weekly BUN profile (65).

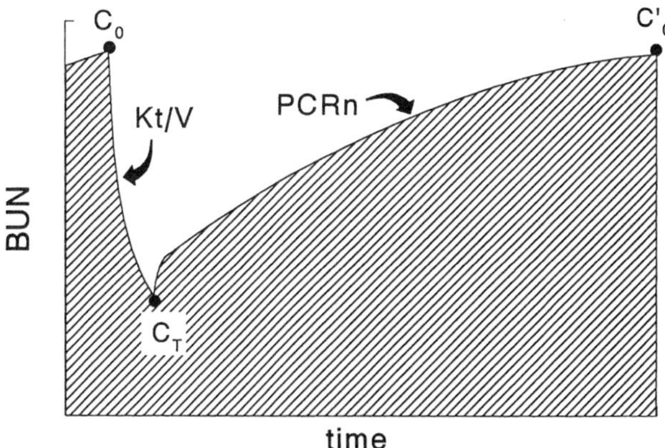

Fig. 9 Kt/V is derived from the fall in BUN during dialysis; PCRn from the rise between dialyses, and time-averaged BUN (TAC) from the shaded area under the curve that represents the patient's urea exposure. The rise from C_T to C'_0 is nonlinear in patients with significant weight (fluid) gain or residual native kidney function.

IX. METHOD FOR DRAWING THE POSTDIALYSIS BLOOD SAMPLE

The predialysis blood sample must be drawn before starting dialysis, but timing is otherwise not critical. In contrast, the postdialysis sample must be drawn within a relatively narrow window of time to avoid errors due to rebound and to access recirculation. Rebound causes a small to modest overestimation of the dose in all patients, and access recirculation causes a gross overestimation of *Kt/V* but only in a relatively small number of patients. Fig. 10 shows a magnified diagram of the upward rebound in serum BUN that begins soon after stopping dialysis (66). If recirculation is present and the sample is drawn immediately postdialysis at point A, the measured BUN will be lower than the actual BUN due to sample contamination with recirculated blood. The magnitude of error depends on the fractional recirculation rate. To avoid this error and to avoid errors in the opposite direction due to rebound, the sample should be taken within 10–20 seconds after slowing the blood pump (point B). Current recommendations by the Dialysis Outcomes Quality Initiative

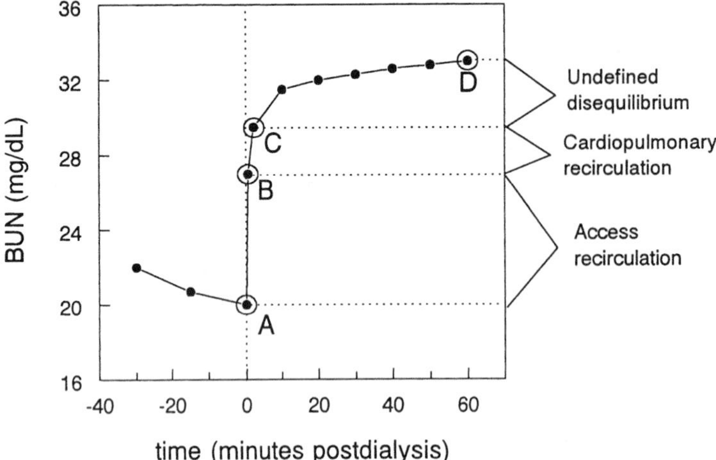

Fig. 10 Postdialysis BUN. The postdialysis BUN is a moving target, so attention to sampling time is needed for consistency and accuracy when measuring both Kt/V and PCRn. Point (A) is the immediate postdialysis sample obtained without taking precaution to prevent dilution artifacts from access recirculation. The sample at point (B) is taken from the arterial (inflow) port 10–20 seconds after slowing the blood pump at the end of dialysis to eliminate dilution from access recirculation. Point (C) is a sample taken 2 minutes postdialysis, which effectively eliminates the effects of cardiopulmonary recirculation. At point (D), one hour postdialysis, urea equilibration throughout the body is essentially complete. (From Ref. 66).

(DOQI) are to slow the pump to approximately 100 mL/min for 10 seconds (3). Stopping the pump at that point will allow ample time for sampling blood from the arterial port. More precise determination of the rate to which the pump should be slowed and the time to wait before stopping it requires measurement of the blood volume from the needle tip to the sampling port of the tubing. In general, at least one and one half times this volume of blood should pass by the sampling port after the blood pump is slowed and before the sample is drawn.

X. DIALYSATE METHODS

As discussed above, traditional blood-side monitoring of hemodialysis is subject to error because of disequilibrium and access recirculation. In addition, assumption of a constant, unchanging urea clearance during dialysis may distort the modeled value for V. For example, clotting within the dialyzer may lead to progressive loss of membrane area and clearance during a single treatment and falsely elevate V (67–69). Dialysate measurements of solute removal may eliminate these errors and provide a more direct measurement of V:

$$V = \frac{A - C_1 \cdot \Delta V - G \cdot t_d}{C_1 - C_E} \tag{9}$$

If residual clearance is included:

$$V = \frac{A - C_1 \cdot \Delta V - t_d(G - K_r \cdot C_{av})}{C_1 - C_E} \tag{10}$$

ΔV is the volume (weight) change during dialysis (mL); G is the urea generation rate (mg/min); t_d is the dialysis duration (min); V is postdialysis V; C_1 is the predialysis BUN; C_E is the rebounded BUN (mg/mL), K_r is residual urea clearance; C_{av} is the average BUN during dialysis. A is $C_d \cdot Q_d \cdot t_d$, but Q_d (the dialysate flow rate) must include the ultrafiltration rate.

In contrast to the dialyzer parameters K_d, Q_b, Q_d, Q_f, and K_0A, V is a physiological parameter that is constant within each patient. Once V is established within a narrow range of certainty, the measurement of the postdialysis BUN is no longer necessary, as it can be calculated from a rearrangement of Eq. (10):

$$C_E = \frac{C_1 \cdot V - A + C_1 \cdot \Delta V + t_d(G - K_r \cdot C_{av})}{V} \tag{11}$$

Because discarded dialysate is freely available during the treatment, continuous monitoring is possible and can provide real-time as well as a projection of dialysis adequacy (41,70,71). Current methods and technology include total dialysate collection for urea concentration, instruments that sample the dialysate intermittently to allow multiple measurements of dialysate urea concentrations throughout the treatment, and electrodes that monitor dialysate urea concentration continuously (41,71,72). The latter techniques are less cumbersome than total dialysate collection but require more technical support. Each of these methods provides measures of *Kt/V* and *nPCR* and, by equilibrating dialysate with blood prior to starting dialysis to obtain C_1, each can provide a totally bloodless analysis of dialysis adequacy (41).

Because solute removal is measured directly, the solute removal index (SRI) has been proposed as a more simplified expression of dialysis adequacy (73,74). SRI is defined as the amount of solute removed divided by the amount in the patient before starting the dialysis. This parameter is equivalent to *Kt/V* in continuously dialyzed patients and takes into consideration urea generation and fluid shifts during dialysis, but it is less subject to proportionate errors than *Kt/V* when direct dialysate measurements are used (75). Recently it has been shown that multiple or continuous measurements of dialysate concentration during hemodialysis sharpen the precision of *Kt/V* and *V* when determined by the dialysate method (75). It remains for the future to determine whether dialysate techniques will supersede current blood-side methods for quantifying hemodialysis.

XI. eKt/V: A SUBSTITUTE FOR TWO-COMPARTMENT MODELING

The single compartment model has an inherent error because it fails to predict the rebound in urea concentration, shown in Fig. 7, that invariably occurs immediately following termination of dialysis. The rebound phase lasts from 15 to 60 minutes as urea equilibrates among all body compartments. Following equilibration, the average urea concentration throughout the body is higher than predicted by the single-compartment model, so the effective clearance is overestimated. The effective clearance is often called the equilibrated clearance or the patient clearance and is always lower than the dialyzer clearance. The patient clearance can be conceptualized as the urea removal rate divided by the mean concentration of urea, averaged across all body compartments and integrated over time during dialysis (see Sec. V). Body compartments cannot be sampled during dialysis, so patient clearance must be considered a virtual clearance that is not directly measurable, in contrast to dialyzer clearance.

Patient clearance, however, is a more realistic measure of the dialysis effect on solute levels in the patient. Unfortunately, its measurement requires waiting for 30–60 minutes after dialysis to sample the fully equilibrated blood. To avoid this expensive and unacceptable delay and resorting to two-compartment modeling, efforts to estimate patient clearance have focused on the physiological variables that have been proven or conjectured to affect rebound listed in Table 5. Several patient studies have found that rebound and patient clearance are relatively predictable and that the most significant predictor is *K/V*, the fractional urea clearance (40,47,76–78):

Table 5 Potential Modulators of Disequilibrium and Rebound

Intensity of dialysis (K/V) (47)
Cardiac output (121,122)
Time on dialysis (3)
Body temperature (123)
Access blood flow (124,125)

$$eKt/V = spKt/V - 36K/V + 0.03 \qquad (12)$$

where *eKt/V* is the equilibrated clearance (patient clearance) and *spKt/V* is the single pool *Kt/V*. When access is a central venous catheter, Eq. (12) must be slightly altered to allow for the absence of cardiopulmonary recirculation:

$$eKt/V = spKt/V - 0.47spK/V + 0.02 \qquad (13)$$

Equations (12) and (13), termed rate equations, introduce time into the expression of dialysis dose as shown by rearranging Eq. (12):

$$eKt/V = spKt/V(1 - 36/t) + 0.03 \qquad (14)$$

where t is time in hours. Table 6 shows how *eKt/V* may vary from dialysis to dialysis or from patient to patient as a function of time on dialysis despite no change in *spKt/V*.

Table 6 Equilibrated *Kt/V* Values (*eKt/V*) as a Function of *spKt/V* and Treatment Time in Hours

spKt/V	2.0 h	3.0 h	4.0 h	5.0 h	6.0 h
1.00	0.73	0.83	0.88	0.91	0.93
1.10	0.80	0.91	0.97	1.00	1.02
1.20	0.87	0.99	1.05	1.09	1.11
1.30	0.94	1.07	1.14	1.17	1.20
1.40	1.01	1.15	1.22	1.26	1.29
1.50	1.08	1.23	1.31	1.35	1.38
1.60	1.15	1.31	1.39	1.44	1.47

Source: Ref. 3.

Equation 12 was developed empirically from observations of rebound in several sets of patients (40,47). An equation derived independently from theoretical considerations in patients with peripheral A-V access yields nearly identical results (76). The reproducibility of these equations in a wide variety of clinical settings reinforces the notion that rebound is predictable and therefore is more heavily influenced by diffusional disequilibrium. The latter is governed by cell membrane surface area and permeability, which are relatively constant from patient to patient, in contrast to regional blood flow, which is prone to greater changes.

A Clinical Example: When Is Dialysis Adequate?

A large patient requires 6 hours of dialysis to achieve a *spKt/V* of 1.1 per dialysis thrice weekly. Is this an adequate dose of dialysis?

Since the consensus-derived minimum adequate dose is 1.2 per dialysis, it would appear that the dose is insufficient. Table 6 shows that the *eKt/V* in this patient is 1.02, which is approximately equal to *eKt/V* in patients dialyzed for 4 hours but with a *spKt/V* of 1.20 and to patients dialyzed for 3 hours with a *spKt/V* of 1.25. The discrepancy among the *spKt/V* measurements for similar *eKt/V* values is the consequence of differences in dialysis time. By prolonging the treatment time to 6 hours, the magnitude of urea disequilibrium and rebound is reduced, and *spKt/V* approaches *eKt/V*. Since *eKt/V* is considered a better measure of the effective dose of dialysis, the above patient is adequately dialyzed. In addition, the patient's large size may be a favorable factor with respect to the denominator in the expression of *Kt/V*, because surface area–to–weight ratio decreases with increasing weight (48). Patients such as this have caused the dialysis community to reconsider time on dialysis as an important determinant of the dialysis effect on solute levels and possibly on outcome (79).

XII. COMPONENTS OF THE DIALYSIS PRESCRIPTION

Comparison of the prescribed dose of dialysis with the delivered dose allows both dialysis administrators and caregivers to focus on potential problems that can jeopardize the quality of care in the dialysis center. The prescribed dose is simply the product of expected dialyzer clearance and time on dialysis divided by the patient's urea volume. It is calculated from several measurable parameters including blood and dialysate flow rates and the dialyzer K_0A. The volume can be measured directly using indicator dilution techniques (80) or bioimpedance measurements, or indirectly from previous urea modelings. In many centers V is estimated using one of several anthropometric formulas (80–82), such as the most commonly used Watson formula (80), which is, for males:

$$V(\text{liters}) = 2.447 - 0.09516\cdot\text{age} + 0.1074\cdot\text{height} + 0.3362\cdot\text{weight} \tag{15}$$

and for females:

$$V(\text{liters}) = -2.097 + 0.1069\cdot\text{height} + 0.2466\cdot\text{weight} \tag{16}$$

Age is given in years, height in cm, and weight in kg. Note that these formulas and others apply to all people with widely differing anatomy independent of height and weight, so the variance is large. The coefficient of variation for the Watson formula is 10% (80). Use of the mean of several values for V determined from urea modeling can further refine and individualize this value. Note that urea modeling can be considered the inverse of the indicator dilution method for measuring volume, where the indicator is removed from rather than added to the patient.

XIII. INCORPORATION OF RESIDUAL NATIVE KIDNEY CLEARANCE

Renal creatinine clearance is a less ambiguous measure of native kidney function than urea clearance in healthy kidneys, but urea clearance becomes a more reliable index of glomerular filtration as renal function deteriorates. After hemodialysis is started, urea clearance is the preferred measure of dialyzer function because it is easier to measure and to interpret than dialyzer creatinine clearance. Therefore, after hemodialysis is started, urea replaces creatinine as the preferred solute for measuring residual clearance.

For patients beginning dialysis treatments, the dose required is often lower because native kidney function still contributes significantly to solute removal. Unfortunately, the contribution of residual urea clearance (K_r) cannot be added directly to dialyzer urea clearance (K_d), because K_r exerts most of its effect between dialysis when K_d is absent and because K_r is a continuous clearance. As will be discussed in more detail below (see Sec. XIX), a clearance applied continuously is always more effective than an equivalent time-averaged clearance applied intermittently. Two approaches can be used to combine dialyzer and native kidney urea clearances.

The first and oldest technique adjusts residual clearance to the equivalent of an intermittent clearance. This requires an upward adjustment in K_r since continuous K_r is more efficient than intermittent dialyzer clearance. Modeling programs can determine the equivalent dialyzer Kt/V that produces the same average BUN concentration when K_r is omitted from the model (83). Alternatively, finding the equivalent dialyzer Kt/V that produces the same peak BUN in the absence of K_r further increases the value of K_r, making the adjusted Kt/V even higher (39). The latter approach has merit because of the greater magnitude of disequilibrium observed for nearly all solutes compared to urea (84). Neither approach is readily available as part of formal urea modeling. Therefore, simplified formulas have been applied that approximate the effect of K_r in the average patient. For dialysis three times a week:

$$K't/V(\text{adjusted for } K_r) = Kt/V + f \cdot K_r/V \tag{17}$$

and for dialysis two times a week:

$$K't/V(\text{adjusted for } K_r) = Kt/V + f \cdot K_r/V \tag{18}$$

where values for f are approximately 4500 and 9500 minutes for Eqs. (17) and (18), respectively, if the goal is to equate the peak BUNs (39), and 4000 and 6500 minutes, respectively, if the goal is to equate mean BUNs (83).

The second approach to combining native kidney and dialyzer clearances adjusts the dialyzer clearance downward to the equivalent of a continuous clearance and then simply adds the two [K_d (adjusted) + K_r] (53). The adjustment of K_d to a continuous clearance equivalent is discussed in more detail below (see Sec. XIX).

Because of the mathematical complexity and the additional effort and expense required to measure it, most dialysis centers ignore residual clearance. In the past this was reasonable because residual function declined quickly (85). In addition, the patient is relatively protected since ignoring K_r will never lead to underdialysis. Today, K_r is better preserved, most likely from the elimination of acetate in the dialysate and from the use of more biocompatible membranes (86), so more patients have significant residual function for a longer time, sometimes for several years. Also, with increased emphasis on creating fistulas instead of grafts before initiating dialysis, access blood flow in an immature fistula may be insufficient to achieve the clearance required for an anephric patient but may be sufficient in a patient with significant K_r. In light of these developments and the push for earlier initiation of dialysis (87), continuing to ignore K_r seems unreasonable because the underestimation of dialysis adequacy early in the treatment course may lead to unnecessary access procedures and contribute to the cost of providing dialysis.

XIV. TECHNIQUES FOR PRESCRIBING HEMODIALYSIS

Because the dialysis equipment does not have a Kt/V adjustment knob, the target Kt/V must be broken down into its component parts to allow the dialysis technician to adjust the prescription. From the target Kt/V, the product $K \cdot t$ can be determined if the patient's V is known. The next task is to determine K based on achievable blood (Q_b) and dialysate (Q_d) flow rates and then to calculate the dialysis time (t). One ordinarily selects these flow rates based on the status of the patient's access device and then determines K from rearrangement of Eq. (4):

$$K_d = Q_b \left[\frac{e^{K_0A(Q_d - Q_b/Q_dQ_b)} - 1}{e^{K_0A(Q_d - Q_b/Q_dQ_b)} - \dfrac{Q_b}{Q_d}} \right] \tag{19}$$

Another approach is to select a set time (t), which determines K, and then calculate the required Q_b using an iterative solution of Eq. (19).

A less complicated approach, often used to initiate dialysis when formal modeling is available, applies common values for Q_b and Q_d and an average treatment time to an initial trial hemodialysis. Following the dialysis, these settings and the measured predialysis and postdialysis BUN values are entered into a formal modeling program that calculates K, V, and both the prescribed and delivered doses. The prescription is then modified by adjusting either K_d or t proportionate to the target/achieved Kt/V. Formal modeling programs can incorporate residual native kidney clearance and often give very specific recommendations for adjusting blood flow and/or time on dialysis or suggest selecting a different dialyzer.

If formal modeling is not available, the above approach can be applied using simplified formulas for Kt/V or URR (see Sec. XVII), but time on dialysis is the only easily adjusted parameter. For example, if the delivered Kt/V is 1.00 and the target is 1.30, the time on dialysis must be increased by 30%. If URR is the criterion for delivered dose, a trial-and-error method must be used. After adjusting the prescription, the predialysis and postdialysis BUN must be remeasured and calculations repeated to assure that the target has been reached. These simplified methods do not produce values for V, K_d, and G, which may be useful for other reasons, nor do they allow comparison of the prescribed Kt/V with the delivered Kt/V as a quality assurance monitor.

XV. PITFALLS THAT COMPLICATE THE HEMODIALYSIS PRESCRIPTION

Several pitfalls have already been described or mentioned: omission of K_r or failure to reduce the contribution of K_r as it declines with time, failure to recognize and prevent errors from access recirculation, use of V as a denominator for the prescription, and failure to incorporate ultrafiltration (Q_f) into the model. These and other pitfalls are described here in more detail.

Fluid accumulation attenuates the rise in BUN between hemodialyses much like the effect of K_r. The consequently required fluid removal during dialysis adds slightly to the dialyzer clearance and significantly enhances the efficiency of the dialysis (Fig. 11). The combined effect is significant and explains the relatively large error observed within patients when URR is used to measure dialysis (see Sec. XVII). Considering an extreme case, if enough fluid is gained between dialyses, the BUN will remain constant as in continuously dialyzed patients. URR will be zero despite adequate treatment which, in this extreme case, consists entirely of hemofiltration. Filtration during hemodialysis, therefore, tends to lower the URR while adding to the effectiveness of the treatment, invalidating URR as a true measure of dialysis (Fig. 12).

A poorly functioning vascular access may also distort urea modeling. When blood flow in the access is less than the prescribed blood flow through the dialyzer, recirculation in the access allows the blood pump to continue pumping at the higher flow rate. Dialyzer clearance in this state may be exemplary while patient clearance is severely reduced. To avoid this error, attention must be paid to the timing and method for drawing the postdialysis blood sample as diagrammed in Fig. 10 (see Sec. IX). If precautions are not taken to eliminate the effect of access recirculation, the postdialysis BUN will be falsely low, a false sense of security will likely prevail, and patient outcome will be jeopardized by underdialysis (88).

A distortion in V or K_d may occur if the blood pump is improperly calibrated or if prepump pressures fall below -200 mmHg (89,90). In the latter case, as shown in Figs. 13 and 14, the pump segment of the blood tubing collapses partially, reducing flow despite no change in the rpm (revolutions per minute) meter reading. Flow may fall significantly as a function of

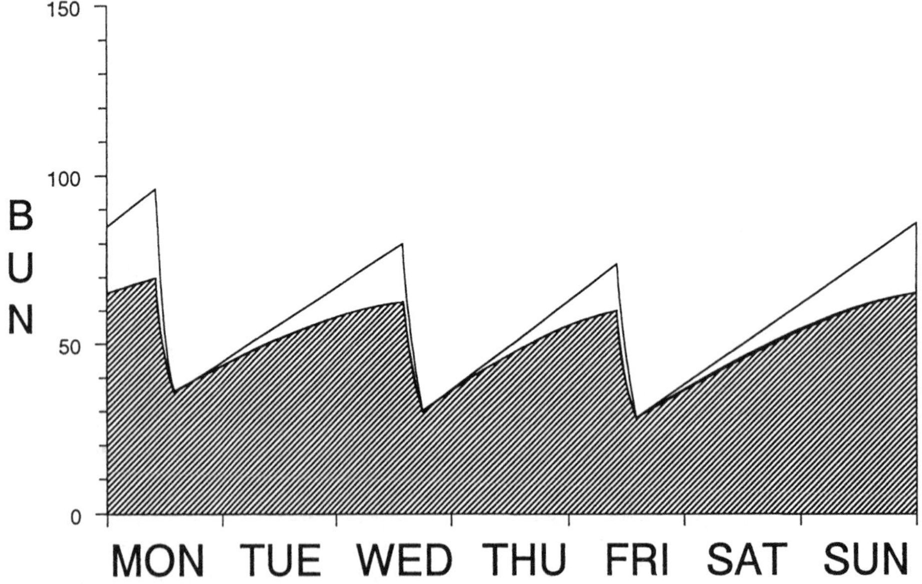

Fig. 11 Effect of fluid gain and removal. Weight gain between and loss during dialyses dampen the excursions in BUN. Despite the adverse effects on fluid balance and on hemodynamic stability, the effect on solute levels is beneficial. Upper profile: BUN levels when no fluid is gained or lost; shaded profile: effect of a 10% gain/loss. (From Ref. 83.)

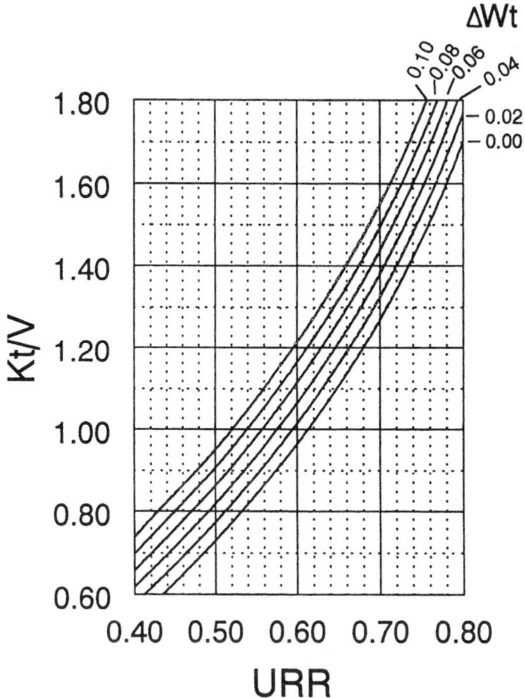

Fig. 12 When Kt/V is constant, the urea-reduction ratio varies with fluid removal. For example, if KT/V is 1.2 per dialysis, URR varies from 0.60 to 0.68 as the volume removed varies from 0 to 10% of body weight. ΔWt is the change in weight during dialysis expressed as a fraction of the postdialysis weight. (From Ref. 99.)

prepump subatmospheric pressure before the pump segment fully collapses. Readings from the blood pump rpm meter are reliable only if prepump pressures are monitored and limits are set to prevent excessive pump segment collapse.

A common cause of discrepancy between the prescribed and delivered dose is failure to accurately record time on dialysis. Access problems, the patient's need to temporarily discontinue dialysis, and other causes of "downtime" during the procedure often occur while the clock is running but no dialysis is provided. Inaccurate accounting of this downtime will result in a higher prescribed than delivered dose.

An unusual distortion of V may occur in patients who receive parenteral nutrition (IDPN) during hemodialysis. The standard IDPN formula calls for infusion of 20–40 g of amino acids in addition to a large glucose load over 3–4 hours of dialysis (91). Recent studies have shown that the amino acid nitrogen may be quantitatively converted to urea within a few minutes

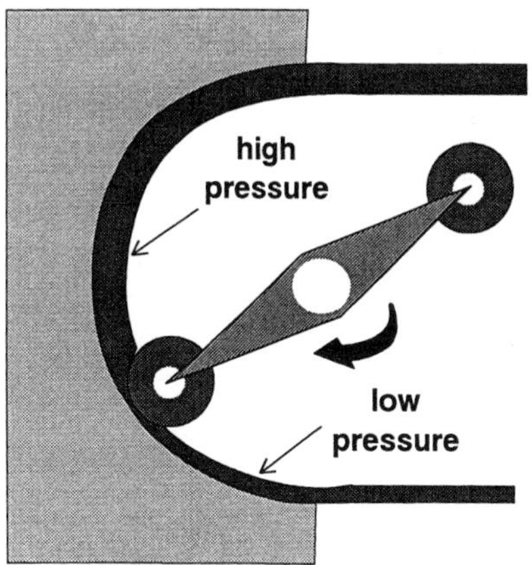

Fig. 13 Collapse of the prepump segment reduces blood flow. The rollers on the blood pump create a zone of high pressure in front and low pressure behind each roller. If the prepump pressure is too low, the blood line pump segment will not reexpand completely. This reduces the flow despite no change in the pump speed. (From Ref. 89.)

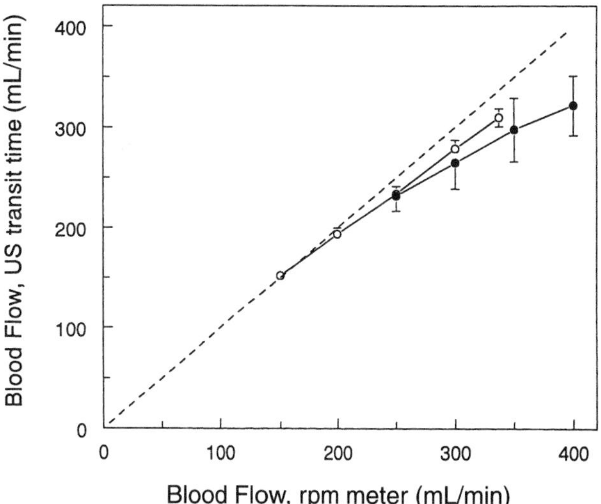

Fig. 14 Flow measured directly from an ultrasound (US) transit-time probe clamped onto the blood line differs from flow measured indirectly by the blood pump rpm meter. The dashed line is the line of identity. Open circles show pumped flow in 64 patients with peripheral A/V grafts (89). Solid circles show dialyzer blood flow in 28 patients with central venous cuffed catheters. (Adapted from Ref. 128.)

following intravenous infusion (92,93), falsely increasing *V*.

XVI. TROUBLESHOOTING COMPLICATIONS

When do prescribed and delivered doses differ sufficiently to warrant investigation? Since the coefficient of variation for *Kt/V* is 7–10% in most dialysis centers, a single difference of 15–20% deserves scrutiny, while smaller differences are likely due to random variation in the measurements. However, if a small difference is consistent from dialysis to dialysis, it should be investigated, starting with evaluation of the accuracy of the data, quickly moving on to the equipment and then to the patient. As discussed above, a significant source of error in data input is the duration of dialysis. Equipment errors include faulty or poorly calibrated blood and dialysate pumps, undetected low prepump pressures that compromise blood flow even in properly calibrated pumps, and faulty reuse practices (89,94). Patient problems include recirculation in the access device, improperly placed needles, reversal of arterial and venous ports, and clotting in the dialyzer. Inaccurate assessment of residual clearance also may contribute to errors as discussed above (see Sec. XIII).

Clinical Example: Troubleshooting

A dietitian mistakenly entered a clearance of 300 mL/min into a formal urea modeling program when the actual clearance achieve by the patient's dialyzer is 195 mL/min. The patient's *V* is 30 L (Watson formula) and dialysis duration is 3 hours during which 3 L of fluid were removed. Predialysis and postdialysis BUN values were 52 and 20 mg/dL, respectively. What effect will this enormous error in K_d have on calculated values for delivered *spKt/V* and PCRn; on modeled values for *V* and *G*?

To account for the fall in BUN when clearance is much higher than reality, the model must assume that the patient is larger than reality. Similarly, the rise in BUN between dialyses in a large patient produces a larger than real urea generation rate. The errors in modeled *V* and *G* are therefore proportionate to the error in K_d, which in this case is greater than 50%. However, since the delivered *Kt/V* is determined primarily by the change in predialysis to postdialysis BUN, the error in Kt/V is minor. The small error in *Kt/V* results from inaccurate assessment of the effect of ultrafiltration, which is 10% of body water in this patient, and from the falsely high estimation of *G*. The ultrafiltration effect normally adds to *Kt/V* but in this patient will diminish it because the program assumes that modeled *V* is approximately twice the real value. Similar to *Kt/V*, *PCRn* is proportionate to *G/V* [see Eq. (8)], both of which have errors that are similar in magnitude and direction, so the error in *PCRn* is minimized. The ultimate result is a falsely low value for *Kt/V* and for *PCRn*, but by only ~5% in each case.

This case illustrates the insensitivity of delivered *Kt/V* to errors in input parameters, provided the predialysis and postdialysis BUNs are sampled and measured accurately. Using a similar approach, one can show that delivered *Kt/V* is insensitive to errors in the entry of time on dialysis.

XVII. SIMPLIFIED METHODS FOR QUANTIFYING HEMODIALYSIS

Despite the availability of computers and programmable calculators, the complex mathematical expressions required to describe solute kinetics can be a challenge for the busy clinician seeking a simpler technique to quantify dialysis. Two methods, one in the form of algebraic formulas and the other in the form of nomograms, have been widely publicized (95–98). Such methods usually require a calculator or manual interpretation and a manual record of the result, though computers can be programmed to interpret simplified formulas and to generate a report. The computer may also be used for the more formal iterative solutions, which often require only a few additional milliseconds of computer time compared to the simplified formula. Recognizing that formal models offer a more accurate description of solute kinetics, the Dialysis Outcomes Quality Initiative (DOQI) committee assembled by the National Kidney Foundation (NKF) recommended the formal models for routine quantification of hemodialysis and the simplified formulas only if formal modeling is not available (3).

A highly simplified method for assessing the dose of intermittent dialysis is the URR, defined as the change in urea during dialysis divided by the predialysis urea. Although highly correlated with *Kt/V* in population studies, URR suffers from several sources of inaccuracy and was not recommended by the DOQI committee (3). The most prominent source of its inaccuracy is the effect of the inevitable loss of fluid during dialysis on URR, as shown in Fig. 12 (see Sec. XV) (99). Urea generation during dialysis, not accounted for by URR, also decreases its accuracy. Perhaps the most compelling reason to question the validity of URR as a measure of dialysis adequacy is the awareness that URR in continuously dialyzed people and in those with normal kidney function is zero.

XVIII. STANDARDS FOR DIALYSIS ADEQUACY

A. Standards before the NCDS

When hemodialysis was first applied to treat ESRD in the early 1960s, adequacy was less important than dialysis tolerance, a serious problem for many patients. The hydraulics of dialysis, dialysate electrolyte content, the vascular access device, acid-base balance, calcium balance, and anemia appropriately received more attention. The frequency and intensity of dialysis were often determined by the availability of and funding for dialysis, patient tolerance of dialysis, symptoms of uremia, fluid and potassium balance, and overall nutritional status. The severity of uremia was monitored by measuring serum urea concentration, a natural extension of clinical practice in the predialysis era. Accumulated experience soon suggested that the intensity of dialysis did not matter, only the size of the dialyzer and time on dialysis, a theory initially known as the square meter hour hypothesis that later evolved to the middle molecule hypothesis (100). The latter theory was based in part on the knowledge that hemodialysis membranes, in contrast to the native kidney, remove smaller molecular weight substances more efficiently than medium or larger molecular weight compounds. The more significant uremic toxins were presumed to be larger in size than urea, so removal was limited primarily by the size and permeability of the dialysis membrane and by the duration of dialysis.

B. Current Standards

It was therefore somewhat of a surprise when the NCDS showed in 1980 that time on dialysis was less important than control of urea (21) and that the patient's protein intake varied inversely with morbidity (1). It appeared that although control of urea was important, how it was controlled was equally important. If the serum urea concentration fell because of dialysis, outcome improved, but if it fell because of poor nutrition, outcome worsened. These observations shifted the focus from control of urea levels to measurement of dialyzer urea clearance as the index of adequacy. Serum urea measurements are vital to both urea concentration and clearance, but the change in urea concentration and not the absolute concentration is most important in calculating urea clearance.

The NCDS showed that dialysis provided maximum benefit when *Kt/V* was above 1.0 per dialysis administered three times per week (Table 1). Subsequent data from uncontrolled studies suggested that further improvements may be obtained by increasing *Kt/V* to 1.2 and above (8–10,15,16). Although nearly all of the studies are uncontrolled, the National Institutes of Health (NIH), the Renal Physicians Association, and the NKF recently established a minimum *spKt/V* at 1.2 per dialysis applied three times per week in their respective consensus conferences (3,61,62). The next logical question is whether there is an optimal amount of dialysis above which no further improvement in outcome is possible. Unfortunately, the answer to this question, which has far-reaching economic consequences as well as the potential for prolonging and improving the quality of life, is not available. A long-term prospective analysis designed to answer this and other important questions about dialysis adequacy (the NIH-sponsored Hemodialysis [HEMO] Study) is currently underway (101).

XIX. THE DIALYSIS SCHEDULE AND ITS EFFECT ON HEMODIALYSIS EFFICIENCY

Intermittent dialysis is less efficient than continuous dialysis. Attempts to reduce dialysis time by proportionately increasing *K/V* (to keep *Kt/V* constant) will result in diminishing solute removal rates and higher mean urea levels. Two explanations have been proposed for this decline in efficiency. First, although clearance is not compromised on the intermittent schedule, total solute removal is reduced because the decline in blood solute concentration during dialysis is logarithmic and not linear. The net effect over the course of a dialysis is a progressive reduction in the mean solute concentration, which is the net driving force for diffusion across the dialyzer membrane (Fig. 15). Since solute levels do not change during continuous dialysis, this effect is absent and solute removal is always maximal. This mechanism for inefficiency applies even in the absence of solute disequilibrium, the ideal premise for the single-compartment model. The second explanation applies to the more realistic situation where solute concentration in the blood compartment falls below that in other compartments during dialysis. Again, dialyzer clearance is unaffected, but solute access to the dialyzer is limited by solute disequilibrium, which is greater in

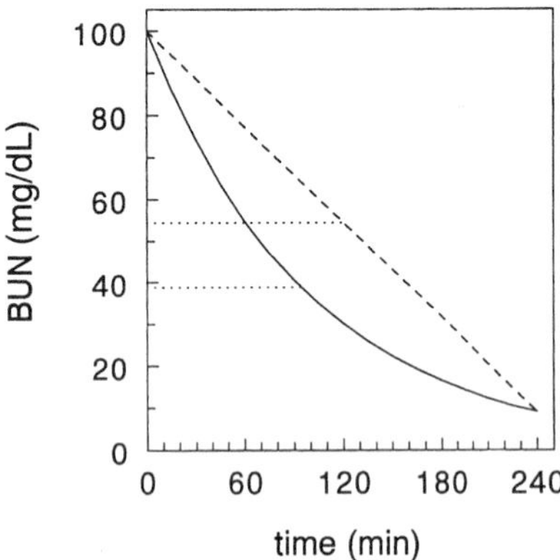

Fig. 15 During a 4-hour hemodialysis treatment the BUN falls in a curvilinear fashion. The more rapid early fall diminishes the trans-membrane concentration gradient that is the driving force for dialysis. The solid line represents the BUN predicted by the single compartment model. The upper horizontal line at 54.5 mg/dL is the simple arithmetic mean of the predialysis and the postdialysis BUN. The lower horizontal line at 38.9 mg/dL represents the integrated or time-averaged BUN during the treatment. (From Ref. 102.)

magnitude for less diffusible solutes but is significant even for urea, as shown in Fig. 16. For solutes that diffuse less readily across cell membranes than urea, the difference between weekly clearance requirements for intermittent and continuous dialysis is considerably greater (102). It is important to note that the solute diffusibility discussed here is the diffusibility within the patient, not the dialyzer. Reduced diffusibility across the dialyzer would diminish this effect, which is maximal for solutes that dialyze easily yet diffuse slowly within the patient.

These observations help to explain the difference between the minimum recommended doses for hemodialysis and continuous peritoneal dialysis. When expressed as a weekly clearance, the minimum Kt/V for hemodialysis is $1.2 \times 3 = 3.6$ per week. Despite recent upward adjustments in the minimum weekly Kt/V for peritoneal dialysis to 2.0–2.2 per week, these values remain far below the hemodialysis standard. It is important to note that the equivalency of these two values has been derived empirically but is based on the experience of many nephrologists treating large numbers of patients for many years.

On a practical scale, it is possible to extrapolate an intermittent clearance to the equivalent clearance for continuous treatment, to allow direct comparison of the Kt/V values regardless of the treatment modality. The previous comparison of hemodialysis with peritoneal dialysis is a prime example: the continuous equivalent of three times weekly hemodialysis at a Kt/V of 3.6 per week, based on accumulated experience, appears to be 2.0 per week.

Mathematical comparison of these two forms of dialysis yields slightly different equivalent values. In a steady state of urea nitrogen balance, the continuous equivalent of intermittent clearance, or EKR, is (53):

$$EKR_{mean} = \frac{\text{Removal rate}}{\text{Peak concentration}} = \frac{\text{Generation rate}}{\text{Mean concentration}} = \frac{G}{TAC} \quad (20)$$

$$EKR_{peak} = \frac{\text{Generation rate}}{\text{Peak concentration}} = \frac{G}{\text{AV Peak Bun}} \quad (21)$$

G and TAC are derived from formal urea modeling. Using Eq. (20) and after adjusting for time and patient volume, the quantity of hemodialysis necessary to keep a patient's time-averaged BUN constant falls from a weekly Kt/V of 3.6 for thrice-weekly treatments to an equivalent Kt/V (EKR) of 2.8 for continuous treatment (84). If one substitutes the mean peak BUN for TAC in Eq. (20), the equivalent Kt/V falls to approximately 2.0, consistent with the current clinically accepted equivalent for peritoneal dialysis (103). Although the continuous equivalent of Kt/V values calculated using the peak BUN [Eq. (21)] matches clinical experience better, the argument that peak urea levels mediate uremic toxicity does not naturally follow since urea is relatively nontoxic. Instead, the relationship likely reflects a fortuitous difference between the diffusibility of urea and the true uremic toxins, since urea has uniquely high diffusibility (104,105) compared with the candidates for uremic toxicity which are likely a variety of organic acids and bases with both size and charge restrictions (see Sec. IV). A noteworthy advantage of EKR is that it allows simple arithmetic summing of residual native kidney clearance and dialyzer clearance (see Sec. XIII).

Clinical Example: Prescribing for a Different Dialysis Schedule

A 70-kg female maintained on 3-hour hemodialysis thrice weekly wishes to take advantage of reported benefits afforded by daily hemodialysis. Formal urea modeling reveals that her current $spKt/V$ is 1.2 per dialysis (0.4 per hour of dialysis), V is 35 L, PCRn is 1.1 g/kg/day, and the average peak BUN is 70 mg/dL. Urine output is less than 50 mL/day. What dose of dialysis should be prescribed if dialysis is administered daily?

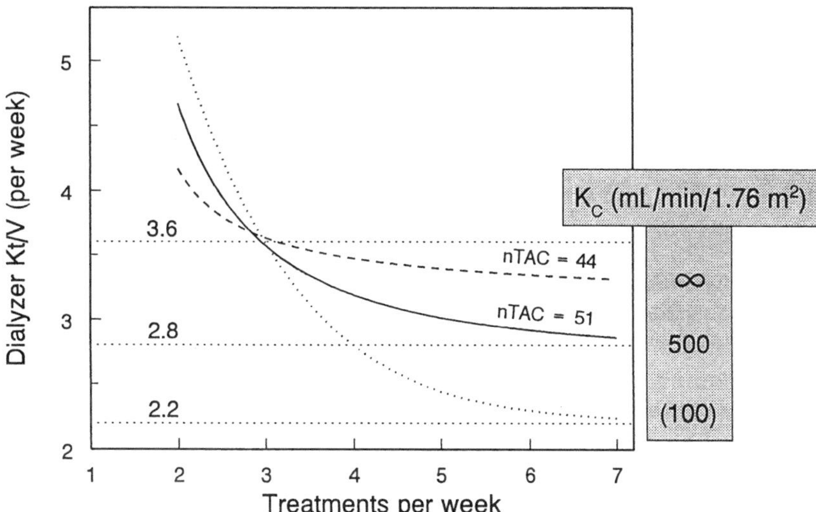

Fig. 16 Kt/V required to maintain the same TAC. To maintain the time averaged BUN constant, the dose of dialysis provided per week may be reduced as the frequency of dialysis increases. The solid line shows the required weekly Kt/V for urea based on an intercompartment mass transfer coefficient (K_C) of 500 mL/min. Even a simple single compartment model with no resistance to diffusion in the patient (dashed line = infinite K_C) shows a dependence of weekly Kt/V on dialysis frequency. The discrepancy in weekly Kt/V between intermittent and continuous dialysis is even greater for a theoretical substance that dialyzes as well as urea but exhibits greater disequilibrium within the patient (dotted line with K_C of 100 mL/min). (Adapted from Ref. 102.)

The urea generation rate derived from Eq. (8) is 6.0 mg/min. If the peak BUN is applied to Eq. (21), EKR is 8.6 mL/min. If daily hemodialysis can be considered the equivalent of continuous dialysis, the daily equivalent *Kt/V* would be (8.6 mL/min × 1440 min/day)/35000 mL = 0.35 per day. Note that the total weekly *Kt/V* is now only 2.45 (7 × 0.35), considerably lower than the 3.6 (3 × 1.2) on the thrice-weekly schedule. If the same dialyzer and flow rates are used, formal urea modeling shows that treatment time may be reduced to 0.9 hours daily and the BUN will fluctuate from 55 to 70 mg/dL. If the same treatment time is used, dialyzer clearance may be reduced from 233 to 72 mL/min and the BUN will fluctuate from 56 to 70 mg/dL. Note that the BUN profile for the two strategies is identical. Although daily hemodialysis, unless very slow and prolonged, is not the equivalent of continuous treatment, it approaches the efficiency of continuous dialysis with respect to urea removal. This improvement results from a marked attenuation of the effects of both solute disequilibrium and the logarithmic decline in BUN at the higher frequency, as illustrated by the above example.

Guidelines and standards have not been provided for hemodialysis schedules other than thrice weekly (3,61,62). Until these are available, those who attempt to increase the frequency would be well advised to take advantage of this more efficient form of dialysis and seek a higher total dose. Preliminary reports suggest that this approach may improve the quality of life and reduce mortality to a greater extent than can be achieved by increasing the dose of thrice-weekly dialysis (106–108).

XX. DOSING AND ADEQUACY OF HEMODIALYSIS FOR ACUTE RENAL FAILURE

It seems reasonable to apply the principles of dialysis measurement gained from experience with ESRD to patients with acute renal failure. However, it would be naïve to expect that the minimal need for dialysis in these critically ill patients is the same as in stable outpatients (109). Special considerations for measurement of dialysis and assessment of adequacy in patients with acute renal failure are listed in Table 7. Hormonal disturbances, bleeding disorders, activation of cytokines, inflammation, and the need for tissue healing are only a few of the differences encountered in these patients. Use of central vein catheters, parenteral nutrition, and vasopressors are common therapeutic options that are not standard treatment in stable outpatients. The BUN may be higher due to trauma and infection-induced hy-

Table 7 Special Considerations for Quantifying Hemodialysis in Patients with Acute Renal Failure

Protein catabolism
Tends to be higher, increased by parenteral nutrition
When high, causes a rapid rise in BUN between dialyses
Generation rate of other toxins is speculative but may be increased
A reason to consider more frequent or continuous hemofiltration/dialysis
Fluid balance
More critical, large fluid shifts
Parenteral nutrition adds an extra burden of fluid
Consider monitoring cardiac filling pressures
Another reason to consider daily dialysis or continuous hemofiltration/dialysis
Solute disequilibrium
Enhanced by low cardiac output (e.g., patients with heart failure or shock)
Diminished by central venous catheter access which eliminates cardiopulmonary recirculation
Intermittent dialysis may not be tolerated
Frequent hemodynamic instability
Another reason to consider daily dialysis or continuous hemofiltration/dialysis
Conditions other than "uremia" may determine need for dialysis
Hyperkalemia
Hyponatremia
Bleeding disorder
Acid-base disorder
Earlier initiation of dialysis than in ESRD

percatabolism, and volume control may be the more important indication for dialysis. Hyperkalemia, acidosis, and other electrolyte disturbances may dictate the need for dialysis more than the need to remove classic uremic toxins, the foundation for management of ESRD. Wound healing and the integrity of the immune system, both impaired by uremic toxicity, may require more intense dialysis to optimize the chance for survival. Many of these issues are explored in detail in a recent review (110). However, there are insufficient data to allow any evidence-based recommendations, with the possible exception that "standard" intermittent dialysis as performed in stable outpatients does not provide adequate solute removal in critically ill patients with acute renal failure (see below).

Because these relatively fragile patients may be more intolerant of dialysis and more easily harmed by the large fluctuations in solute and fluid balance that accompany intermittent treatments, efforts have been extended over the past decade to provide a continuous mode of treatment in the form of continuous hemofiltration or a combination of filtration and dialysis (111). In addition to smoother control of fluid balance and blood pressure, continuous therapies offer the added benefits of less solute disequilibrium, increased efficiency, and improved removal of other uremic toxins. Despite such potential benefits, an effect on mortality has been difficult to demonstrate, perhaps because other comorbid states are more important determinants of outcome (112–114).

Clinical Example: Prescribing Hemodialysis in Acute Renal Failure

A small, hypotensive, critically ill adult patient, requiring treatment with intermittent hemodialysis in the intensive care unit (ICU), has an unexpectedly high BUN that is consistently over 100 mg/dL predialysis. Is this patient suffering from severe urea disequilibrium, causing a large rebound postdialysis? How should this possibility be investigated?

Although solute disequilibrium between various body compartments is exacerbated by tissue hypoperfusion in the critically ill, this possibility is unlikely to cause the high BUN in this patient. Limited data from several centers have shown that urea rebound in ICU patients, as in stable outpatients, is predictable, although slightly higher on average than reflected by Eq. (12) (115–117). In one study, although cardiopulmonary recirculation was eliminated by the use of central vein catheters, the anticipated reduction in urea rebound was not seen, likely as a result of significant but only slightly enhanced solute disequilibrium (115). In the patient described above, a more likely explanation for the higher BUN is the combined effects of increased catabolism and inadequate dialysis. The standard prescription of 3–4 hours of treatment thrice weekly, at maximum blood flow rates of 200–300 mL/min limited by central vein catheters, is simply not enough to control the uremic state. This prescription usually delivers a dose of dialysis below the acceptable minimum standards in stable outpatients.

XXI. SUMMARY

Monitoring the delivery of dialysis in each patient is a vital function of dialysis care centers where life support is provided for patients who depend on substitute renal function. Awareness of the pitfalls will help ensure accurate measurement of the substitute renal function and further protect the patient from excessive morbidity and mortality. Excessive reliance on urea concentration as an indicator of dialysis adequacy is a pitfall that has been slow to be recognized but is now easily circumvented by focusing on dialyzer clearance. Since clearance has become the standard for determining adequacy, caregivers should have a clear understanding of this measurement as it applies to first-order processes such as diffusion, convection, and dialysis. The importance of the integrated average clearance achieved throughout the dialysis treatment is emphasized, as is the distinction between the mean patient clearance and the mean dialyzer clearance. When adjusted to body size, the average clearance per dialysis is expressed as *Kt/V*. Formal methods for measuring *Kt/V* have several advantages over simplified methods partly because the formal methods can be automated, easing the task of routine assessment of dialysis adequacy in each patient at frequent intervals. To assure accuracy of the measured dose, careful attention must be paid to timing of the postdialysis blood sampling, inclusion of residual clearance in the total effective clearance, and allowance for the gain and loss of fluid between and during dialysis treatments. Application of the two-BUN method reduces the opportunity for bias and error without reducing accuracy.

Current yardsticks for dialysis include *spKt/V*, *eKt/V*, SRI, URR, and EKR. Each has evolved from a different perspective, and each emphasizes a slightly different aspect of treatment. Current standards are based on *spKt/V*, but as dialysis schedules change in the future, this yardstick may require replacement. Solute disequilibrium, more significant for toxins other than urea, plays an important role in limiting the effectiveness of intermittent dialysis and makes direct comparisons among various dialysis schedules difficult. Efforts to normalize the effectiveness of various schedules, applying mathematical analysis of solute kinetics and two decades of clinical experience with continuous peritoneal dialysis, have resulted in an expression for the continuous equivalent of intermittent dialysis (EKR). Whether these measures of dialysis adequacy also apply in the acute renal failure setting is not clear and requires further study.

XXII. THE FUTURE

The future of hemodialysis as a principal modality for sustaining life in patients with ESRD is almost certain. Although renal transplantation currently offers more hope of improving the quality of life, the availability of organs remains a major impediment for the majority of ESRD patients. Peritoneal dialysis is limited intrinsically because it allows optimal treatment only in smaller people or in patients who have not yet lost residual renal function.

The future promises significant changes in the techniques, schedules, membranes, and methods for quantifying hemodialysis. On-line measurements of clearance and dialyzer fiber bundle volume and simplified measures of blood flow in the dialysis access device may become routine methods for assessing and assuring dialysis adequacy in the future (67,118). Application of dialysate monitoring, more frequent hemodialysis, measurement of cardiac output and central blood volume during dialysis, and continuous hemofiltration/dialysis for acutely ill patients are enhancements that have already begun to appear. Incorporation of residual clearance into hemodialysis adequacy will be required if the evidence for a benefit to starting dialysis earlier is confirmed (119). Better removal of phosphate and other uremic toxins, individualization of the dose based on removal of β_2-microglobulin or as-yet-undiscovered toxins, and a more universal expression of dialysis applicable to patients receiving more frequent treatments are desirable future developments. Additional factors for refining and individualizing dialysis may include increasing the dose for patients with acute renal failure or for patients with ESRD who develop an intercurrent illness.

REFERENCES

1. Lowrie EG, Laird NM, Parker TF, Sargent JA. Effect of the hemodialysis prescription on patient morbidity:

report from the National Cooperative Dialysis Study. N Engl J Med 1981; 305:1176–1181.
2. Lowrie EG, Lew NL. Death risk in hemodialysis patients: The predictive value of commonly measured variables and an evaluation of death rate differences between facilities. Am J Kidney Dis 1990; 15:458–482.
3. National Kidney Foundation—Dialysis Outcomes Quality Initiative: clinical practice guidelines for hemodialysis adequacy. Am J Kidney Dis 1997; 30:S22–S63.
4. Teraoka S, Toma H, Nihei H, Ota K, Babazono T, Ishikawa I, et al. Current status of renal replacement therapy in Japan. Am J Kidney Dis 1995; 25:151–164.
5. Hull AR, Parker TF. Proceedings from the morbidity, mortality and prescription of dialysis symposium: introduction and summary. Am J Kidney Dis 1990; 15: 375–383.
6. Agodoa LYC, Held PJ, Wolfe RA, Port FK. US Renal Data System 1998 Annual Data Report. 10th ed. Springfield VA: National Technical Information Service, 1998.
7. Lundin PA. Prolonged survival on hemodialysis. In: Maher JF, ed. Replacement of Renal Function by Dialysis. 3rd ed. Dordrecht: Kluwer Academic Publishers, 1989.
8. Hakim RM, Breyer J, Ismail N, Schulman G. Effects of dose of dialysis on morbidity and mortality. Am J Kidney Dis 1994; 23:661–669.
9. Parker TF, Husni L, Huang W, Lew N, Lowrie EG. Survival of hemodialysis patients in the United States is improved with a greater quantity of dialysis. Am J Kidney Dis 1994; 23:670–680.
10. Owen WF, Jr., Lew NL, Liu Y, Lowrie EG, Lazarus JM. The urea reduction ratio and serum albumin concentration as predictors of mortality in patients undergoing hemodialysis. N Engl J Med 1993; 329:1001–1006.
11. Lindsay RM, Spanner E. A hypothesis: the protein catabolic rate is dependent upon the type and amount of treatment in dialyzed uremic patients. Am J Kidney Dis 1989; 13:382–389.
12. Lindsay RM, Spanner E, Heidenheim RP, LeFebvre JM, Hodsman A, Baird J, et al. Which comes first, Kt/V or PCR—chicken or egg? Kidney Int Suppl 1992; 38:S32–S36.
13. Yeun JY, Kaysen GA. Factors influencing serum albumin in dialysis patients. Am J Kidney Dis. In press.
14. Kopple JD. Effect of nutrition on morbidity and mortality in maintenance dialysis patients. Am J Kidney Dis 1994; 24:1002–1009.
15. Charra B, Calemard E, Ruffet M, Chazot C, Terrat J-C, Vanel T, et al. Survival as an index of adequacy of dialysis. Kidney Int 1992; 41:1286–1291.
16. Yang C-S, Chen S-W, Chiang C-H, Wang M, Peng S-J, Kan Y-T. Effects of increasing dialysis dose on serum albumin and mortality in hemodialysis patients. Am J Kidney Dis 1996; 27:380–386.
17. Collins AJ, Ma JZ, Umen A, Keshaviah P. Urea index and other predictors of hemodialysis patient survival [published erratum appears in Am J Kidney Dis 1994; 24(1):157]. Am J Kidney Dis 1994; 23:272–282.
18. Held PJ, Port FK, Wolfe RA, Stannard DC, Carroll CE, Daugirdas JT, et al. The dose of hemodialysis and patient mortality. Kidney Int 1996; 50:550–556.
19. Gotch FA, Levin NW, Port FK, Wolfe RA, Uehlinger DE. Clinical outcome relative to the dose of dialysis is not what you think: the fallacy of the mean. Am J Kidney Dis 1997; 30:1–15.
20. Depner TA, Beck GJ, Daugirdas JT, Kusek JW, Eknoyan G. Lessons from the hemodialysis (HEMO) Study: An improved measure of the actual hemodialysis dose. Am J Kidney Dis. In press.
21. Laird NM, Berkey CS, Lowrie EG. Modeling success or failure of dialysis therapy: the National Cooperative Dialysis Study. Kidney Int 1983; 23(suppl 13):S101–S106.
22. Vanholder R, Ringoir S. Infectious morbidity and defects of phagocytic function in end-stage renal disease: a review. J Am Soc Nephrol 1993; 3:1541–1554.
23. Bloembergen WE, Stannard DC, Port FK, Wolfe RA, Pugh JA, Jones CA, et al. Relationship of dose of hemodialysis and cause-specific mortality. Kidney Int 1996; 50:557–565.
24. Ifudu O, Feldman J, Friedman EA. The intensity of hemodialysis and the response to erythropoietin in patients with end-stage renal disease. N Engl J Med 1996; 334:420–425.
25. Madore F, Lowrie EG, Brugnara C, Lew NL, Lazarus JM, Bridges K, et al. Anemia in hemodialysis patients: variables affecting this outcome predictor. J Am Soc Nephrol 1997; 8:1921–1929.
26. Depner TA, Rizwan S, James LA. Effectiveness of low dose erythropoietin: a possible advantage of high flux hemodialysis. ASAIO J 1990; 36:M223–M225.
27. Kolff WJ, Berk HTJ, ter Welle M, van der Ley AJW, van Dijk EC, van Noordwijk J. The artificial kidney, a dialyzer with a great area. Acta Med Scand 1944; 117:121–128.
28. Bergstrom J, Furst P. Uraemic toxins. In: Drukker W, Parsons FM, Maher JF, eds. Replacement of Renal Function by Dialysis. 2d ed. Boston: Martinus Nijhoff, 1983:354–390.
29. Vanholder R, Schoots A, Ringoir S. Uremic toxicity. In: Maher JF, ed. Replacement of Renal Function by Dialysis. 3rd ed. Dordrecht: Kluwer Academic Publishers, 1989:4–19.
30. Mason MF, Resnik H, Mino AS, Rainey J, Pilcher C, Harrison TR. Mechanism of experimental uremia. Arch Intern Med 1993; 60:312–1937.
31. Merrill JP, Legrain M, Hoigne R. Observations on the role of urea in uremia. Am J Med 1953; 14:519–520.

32. Johnson WJ, Hagge WW, Wagoner RD, Dinapoli RP, Rosevear JW. Effects of urea loading in patients with far-advanced renal failure. Mayo Clin Proc 1972; 47: 21–29.
33. Fluckiger R, Harmon W, Meier W, Loo S, Gabbay KH. Hemoglobin carbamylation in uremia. N Engl J Med 1981; 304:823–827.
34. Kwan JTC, Carr EC, Neal AD, Burdon J, Raferty MJ, Marsh FP, et al. Carbamylated haemoglobin, urea kinetic modelling and the adequacy of dialysis in haemodialysis patients. Nephrol Dial Transpl 1991; 6:38–43.
35. Davenport A, Jones S, Goel S, Astley JP, Feest TG. Carbamylated hemoglobin: a potential marker for the adequacy of hemodialysis therapy in end-stage renal failure. Kidney Int 1996; 50:1344–1351.
36. Smith HW. The Kidney. New York: Oxford University Press, 1951.
37. Schreiner GE, Maher JF. Uremia: Biochemistry, Pathogenesis and Treatment. Springfield IL: Charles C Thomas, 1961.
38. Depner TA. The uremic syndrome. In: Greenberg A, ed. NKF Primer on Kidney Diseases. San Diego: Academic Press, Inc., 1994:253–258.
39. Gotch FA. Kinetic modeling in hemodialysis. In: Nissenson AR, Fine RN, Gentile DE, eds. Clinical Dialysis. 3rd ed. Norwalk, CT: Appleton and Lange, 1995: 156–188.
40. Daugirdas JT, Depner TA, Gotch FA, Greene T, Keshaviah PR, Levin NW, et al. Comparison of methods to predict equilibrated Kt/V in the HEMO Pilot Study. Kidney Int 1997; 52:1395–1405.
41. Depner TA, Keshaviah PR, Ebben JP, Emerson PF, Collins AJ, Jindal KK, et al. Multicenter clinical validation of an on-line monitor of dialysis adequacy. J Am Soc Nephrol 1996; 7:464–471.
42. Bergstrom J. Nutrition and adequacy of dialysis in hemodialysis patients. Kidney Int Suppl 1993; 41:S261–267.
43. Depner TA. Quantifying hemodialysis. Am J Nephrol 1996; 16:17–28.
44. Giovannetti S, Balestri PL, Barsotti G. Methylguanidine in uremia. Arch Intern Med 1973; 131:709–713.
45. Leypoldt JK, Cheung AK, Agodoa LY, Daugirdas JT, Greene T, Keshaviah PR. Hemodialyzer mass transfer-area coefficients for urea increase at high dialysate flow rates. The Hemodialysis (HEMO) Study. Kidney Int 1997; 51:2013–2017.
46. Gotch FA, Sargent JA. A mechanistic analysis of the National Cooperative Dialysis Study (NCDS). Kidney Int 1985; 28:526–534.
47. Daugirdas JT, Schneditz D. Overestimation of hemodialysis dose depends on dialysis efficiency by regional blood flow but not by conventional two pool urea kinetic analysis. ASAIO J 1995; 41:M719–724.
48. Mahmood I, Balian JD. Interspecies scaling: predicting clearance of drugs in humans. Three different approaches. Xenobiotica 1998; 87:527–529.
49. Bachmann K, Pardoe D, White D. Scaling basic toxicokinetic parameters from rat to man. Environ Health Perspect 1996; 104:400–407.
50. West GB, Brown JH, Enquist BJ. A general model for the origin of allometric scaling laws in biology. Science 1997; 276:122–126.
51. Schmidt-Nielsen K. Scaling: Why is animal size so important? In: Calder WA, ed. Size, Function, and Life History. Cambridge, MA: Harvard University Press, 1984.
52. Edwards NA. Scaling of renal functions in mammals. Comp Biochem Physiol A 1975; 52:63–66.
53. Casino FG, Lopez T. The equivalent renal urea clearance: a new parameter to assess dialysis dose. Nephrol Dial Transpl 1996; 11:1574–1581.
54. Depner TA. Prescribing hemodialysis: A Guide to Urea Modeling. Boston: Kluwer Academic Publishers, 1991.
55. Smye SW, Will EJ. A mathematical analysis of a two-compartment model of urea kinetics. Phys Med Biol 1995; 40:2005–2014.
56. Schneditz D, Daugirdas JT. Formal analytical solution to a regional blood flow and diffusion based urea kinetic model. ASAIO J 1994; 40:M667–673.
57. Depner TA, Rizwan S, Cheer AY, Wagner JM, Eder LA. High venous urea concentrations in the opposite arm. A consequence of hemodialysis-induced compartment disequilibrium. ASAIO J 1991; 37:M141–143.
58. Schneditz D, Kaufman AM, Polaschegg HD, Levin NW, Daugirdas JT. Cardiopulmonary recirculation during hemodialysis. Kidney Int 1992; 42:1450–1456.
59. Depner TA. Multicompartment models. In: Prescribing Hemodialysis: A Guide to Urea Modeling. Boston: Kluwer Academic Publishers, 1991:91–126.
60. Daugirdas J, Greene T, Depner T, Gotch F, Keshaviah P, Star R. Estimation of double pool volume from single pool urea distribution volume (abstr). J Am Soc Nephrol 1996; 7:1510.
61. NIH Consensus Conference. Consensus development conference panel: morbidity and mortality of renal dialysis: an NIH consensus conference statement. Ann Intern Med 1994; 121:62–70.
62. Renal Physicians Association. Clinical Practice Guideline on Adequacy of Hemodialysis. Washington, DC: Renal Physicians Association, 1993.
63. Borah MF, Schoenfeld PY, Gotch FA, Sargent JA, Wolfson M, Humphreys MH. Nitrogen balance during intermittent dialysis therapy of uremia. Kidney Int 1978; 14:491–500.
64. Buur T. Two-sample hemodialysis urea kinetic modeling: validation of the method. Nephron 1995; 69: 49–53.

65. Depner TA. Single-compartment model. In: Prescribing Hemodialysis: A Guide to Urea Modeling. Boston: Kluwer Academic Publishers, 1991:65–89.
66. Depner TA. Assessing adequacy of hemodialysis: urea modeling. Kidney Int 1994; 45:1522–1535.
67. Krivitski NM, Kishlukhim V, Snyder J, MacGibbon D, Reasons AM, Depner T. A method for measuring dialyzer blood volume in vivo: theory and validation (abstr). J Am Soc Nephrol 1997; 8:770.
68. Dewanjee MK, Kapadvanjwala M, Cavagnaro CF, Panoutsopoulos GK, Suguihara CY, Elson R, et al. In vitro and in vivo evaluation of the comparative thrombogenicity of cellulose acetate hemodialyzers with radiolabeled platelets. ASAIO J 1994; 40:49–55.
69. Dewanjee MK, Kapadvanjwala M, Ruzius K, Serafini AN, Zilleruelo GE, Sfakianakis GN. Quantitation of thrombogenicity of hemodialyzer with technetium-99m and indium-111 labeled platelets. Nuclear Med Biol 1994; 40:49–55.
70. Keshaviah PR, Ebben JP, Emerson PF. On-line monitoring of the delivery of the hemodialysis prescription. Pediatr Nephrol 1995; 9:S2–S8.
71. Garred LJ, Rittau M, McCready W, Canaud B. Urea kinetic modelling by partial dialysate collection. Int J Artif Organs 1989; 12:96–102.
72. Garred LJ. Dialysate-based kinetic modeling. Adv Ren Replace Ther 1995; 2:305–318.
73. Keshaviah P. The solute removal index—a unified basis for comparing disparate therapies [editorial]. Perit Dial Int 1995; 15:101–104.
74. Keshaviah P, Star RA. A new approach to dialysis quantification: an adequacy index based on solute removal. Semin Dial 1994; 7:85–90.
75. Depner TA, Greene T, Gotch FA, Daugirdas JT, Keshaviah PR, Star RA. Imprecision of the hemodialysis dose when measured directly from urea removal. Kidney Int. In press.
76. Tattersall JE, DeTakats D, Chamney P, Greenwood RN, Farrington K. The post-hemodialysis rebound: predicting and quantifying its effect on Kt/V. Kidney Int 1996; 50:2094–2102.
77. Evans JH, Smye SW, Brocklebank JT. Mathematical modelling of haemodialysis in children. Pediatr Nephrol 1992; 6:349–353.
78. Leblanc M, Charbonneau R, Lalumière G, Cartier P, Déziel C. Postdialysis urea rebound: determinants and influence on dialysis delivery in chronic hemodialysis patients. Am J Kidney Dis 1996; 27:253–261.
79. Henderson LW. Of time, TACurea, and treatment schedules. Kidney Int 1988; 33(suppl 24):S105–S106.
80. Watson PE, Watson ID, Batt RD. Total body water volumes for adult males and females estimated from simple anthropometric measurements. Am J Clin Nutr 1980; 33:27–39.
81. Hume R, Weyers E. Relationship between total body water and surface area in normal and obese subjects. J Clin Pathol 1971; 24:234–238.
82. Chertow GM, Lazarus JM, Lew NL, Ma L, Lowrie EG. Development of a population-specific regression equation to estimate total body water in hemodialysis patients. Kidney Int 1997; 51:1578–1582.
83. Depner TA. Refinements and application of urea modeling. In: Prescribing Hemodialysis: A Guide to Urea Modeling. Boston: Kluwer Academic Publishers, 1991:168–194.
84. Depner TA. Benefits of more frequent dialysis: lower TAC at the same Kt/V. Nephrol Dial Transpl 1998; 13:20–24.
85. Lysaght MJ, Vonesh E, Gotch F, Ibels L, Keen M, Lindholm B, et al. The influence of dialysis treatment modality on the decline of remaining renal function. ASAIO J 1991; 37:598–604.
86. Van Stone JC. The effect of dialyzer membrane and etiology of kidney disease on the preservation of residual renal function in chronic hemodialysis patients. ASAIO J 1996; 41:M713–M716.
87. National Kidney Foundation—Dialysis Outcomes Quality Initiative: clinical practice guidelines for peritoneal dialysis adequacy. Am J Kidney Dis 1997; 30: S70–S136.
88. Mars DR, Doll MA. Uremic pericarditis in a chronic hemodialysis patient. Dial Transpl 1993; 22:23–26.
89. Depner TA, Rizwan S, Stasi TA. Pressure effects on roller pump blood flow during hemodialysis. ASAIO J 1990; 36:M456–M459.
90. Sands J, Glidden D, Jacavage W, Jones B. Difference between delivered and prescribed blood flow in hemodialysis. ASAIO J 1996; 42:M717–719.
91. Wolfson M. Use of nutritional supplements in dialysis patients. Semin Dial 1992; 5:285–290.
92. Kloppenburg WD, Wolthers BG, Tepper T, Stegeman CA, de Jong PE, Huisman RM. Fluctuations of urea generation rate following protein intake in hemodialysis patients measured using [13-C]urea (abstr). J Am Soc Nephrol 1995; 6:581.
93. McCann L, Feldman C, Hornberger J. Effect of intradialytic parenteral nutrition on delivered Kt/V (abstr). Am J Kidney Dis 1997; 29:11.
94. Depner TA. Pitfalls in quantitating hemodialysis. Semin Dial 1993; 6:127–133.
95. Daugirdas JT. Second generation logarithmic estimates of single-pool variable volume Kt/V: an analysis of error. J Am Soc Nephrol 1993; 4:1205–1213.
96. Daugirdas JT. Simplified equations for monitoring Kt/V, PCRn, eKt/V, and ePCRn. Adv Ren Replace Ther 1995; 2:295–304.
97. Depner TA, Daugirdas JT. Equations for normalized protein catabolic rate based on two-point modeling of hemodialysis urea kinetics. J Am Soc Nephrol 1996; 7:780–785.
98. Daugirdas JT, Depner TA. A nomogram approach to hemodialysis urea modeling. Am J Kidney Dis 1994; 23:33–40.

99. Depner TA. Estimation of Kt/V from URR for varying levels of weight loss: a bedside graphic aid. Semin Dial 1993; 6:242.
100. Scribner BH, Farrell PC, Milutinovic J, Babb AL. Evolution of the middle molecule hypothesis. In: Villarreal H, ed. Proceedings of the Fifth International Congress of Nephrology. Basel: Karger, 1974:190–199.
101. Eknoyan G, Levey AS, Beck GJ, Agodoa LY, Daugirdas JT, Kusek JW, et al. The hemodialysis (HEMO) study: rationale for selection of interventions. Semin Dial 1996; 9:24–33.
102. Depner TA. Quantifying hemodialysis and peritoneal dialysis: examination of the peak concentration hypothesis. Semin Dial 1994; 7:315–317.
103. Gotch FA. The current place of urea kinetic modeling with respect to different dialysis modalities. Nephrol Dial Transpl 1998; 13:10–14.
104. Kaplan MA, Hays L, Hays RM. Evolution of a facilitated diffusion pathway for amides in the erythrocyte. Am J Physiol 1974; 226:1327–1332.
105. Macey RI, Yousef LW. Osmotic stability of red cells in renal circulation requires rapid urea transport. Am J Physiol 1988; 254:C669–C674.
106. Buoncristiani U, Quintaliani G, Cozzari M, Giombini L, Ragaiolo M. Daily dialysis: long-term clinical metabolic results. Kidney Int 1988; 33:S137–S140.
107. Uldall R, Ouwendyk M, Francoeur R, Wallace L, Sit W, Vas S, et al. Slow nocturnal home hemodialysis at the Wellesley Hospital. Adv Ren Replace Ther 1996; 3:133–136.
108. Pierratos A, Ouwendyk M, Francoeur B, Wallace L, Sit W, Vas S, et al. Slow nocturnal home hemodialysis. Dial Transpl 1995; 24:557–576.
109. Leblanc M, Tapolyai M, Paganini EP. What dialysis dose should be provided in acute renal failure? A review. Adv Ren Replace Ther 1995; 26:910–917.
110. Clark WR, Mueller BA, Kraus MA, Macias WL. Dialysis prescription and kinetics in acute renal failure. Adv Ren Replace Ther 1997; 4:64–71.
111. Bellomo R, Mehta R. Acute renal replacement in the intensive care unit: now and tomorrow. N Horiz 1995; 3:760–767.
112. Mehta RL. Therapeutic alternatives to renal replacement for critically ill patients in acute renal failure. Semin Nephrol 1994; 14:64–82.
113. Ward DM, Mehta RL. Extracorporeal management of acute renal failure patients at high risk of bleeding. Kidney Int Suppl 1993; 41:S237–244.
114. Paganini EP, Halstenberg WK, Goormastic M. Risk modeling in acute renal failure requiring dialysis: the introduction of a new model. Clin Nephrol 1996; 46: 206–211.
115. Lo AJ, Depner TA, Chin ES, Craig MA. Urea disequilibrium contributes to underdialysis in the intensive care unit (abstr). J Am Soc Nephrol 1997; 8:287.
116. Jaber BL, King AJ, Cunniff PJ, Cendoroglo MN, Sundaram S, Pereira BJG. Prescribed versus delivered dose of intermittent hemodialysis in acute renal failure: a substantial discrepancy (abstr). J Am Soc Nephrol 1997; 8:284.
117. Mulhern JG, O'Shea MH, Germain MJ, Lipkowitz GS, Madden RL, Sweet SJ, et al. Reduced dialysis adequacy in hospitalized hemodialysis patients (abstr). J Am Soc Nephrol 1997; 8:289.
118. Depner TA, Krivitski NM. Clinical measurement of blood flow in hemodialysis access fistulae and grafts by ultrasound dilution. ASAIO J 1995; 41:745–749.
119. Mehrotra R, Nolph KD, Gotch F. Early initiation of chronic dialysis: role of incremental dialysis [editorial]. Perit Dial Int 1997; 17:426–430.
120. Daugirdas JT, Smye SW. Effect of a two compartment distribution on apparent urea distribution volume. Kidney Int 1997; 51:1270–1273.
121. Ronco C, Crepaldi C, Brendolan A, La Greca G. Intradialytic exercise increases effective dialysis efficiency and reduces rebound (abstr). J Am Soc Nephrol 1995; 6:612.
122. George TO, Priester CA, Dunea G, Schneditz D, Tarif N, Daugirdas JT. Cardiac output and urea kinetics in dialysis patients: evidence supporting the regional blood flow model. Kidney Int 1997; 52:1395–1405.
123. Depner T, Rizwan S, Cheer A, Wagner J. Peripheral urea disequilibrium during hemodialysis is temperature-dependent (abstr). J Am Soc Nephrol 1991; 2: 321.
124. Daugirdas JT, Schneditz D, Leehey DJ. Effect of access recirculation on the modeled urea distribution volume. Am J Kidney Dis 1996; 27:512–518.
125. Daugirdas JT, Burke MS, Balter P, Priester CA, Majka T. Screening for extreme postdialysis urea rebound using the Smye method: patients with access recirculation identified when a slow flow method is not used to draw the postdialysis blood. Am J Kidney Dis 1997; 51:1270–1273.
126. Parker TF, Laird NM, Lowrie EG. Comparison of the study groups in the National Cooperative Dialysis Study and a description of morbidity, mortality, and patient withdrawal. Kidney Int 1983; 23:S42–S49.
127. Depner TA. Approach to hemodialysis kinetic modeling. In: Henrich WL, ed. Principles and Practice of Dialysis. 2d ed. Baltimore: Williams & Wilkins, 1998.
128. Sands J, Jabayc P, Miranda C. Delivered blood flow in cuffed central venous dialysis catheters (abstr). ASAIO J 1997; 43:69.

6

Problems Related to Anticoagulation and Their Management on Intermittent Hemodialysis/Hemodiafiltration

Konrad Andrassy
University Hospital, Heidelberg, Germany

I. INTRODUCTION

A bleeding tendency in advanced renal failure was described as early as the nineteenth century (1). This tendency is mainly a consequence of a complex platelet dysfunction and a low hematocrit (2). No major alterations of plasmatic coagulation factors have been observed. A qualitative platelet defect is clinically documented by an increased bleeding time, which becomes manifest if creatinine clearance is less than 15 mL/min. A magnitude of platelet abnormalities has been described: impaired collagen-induced platelet aggregation correlates best with prolongation of bleeding time (3). The pathogenesis of these platelet abnormalities was recently resolved, and some therapeutic recommendations have been derived from these findings (see Chapter 17).

The introduction of dialysis has dramatically reduced the incidence of bleeding, particularly in chronic end-stage renal failure. Although biocompatibility of dialysis membranes has improved in the last few years they do not yet possess the antithrombogenic properties of endothelial surfaces. Therefore, anticoagulation is still needed to prevent clotting in the dialyzer, and unfractionated heparin (UFH) is and remains the drug of choice since the beginning of dialysis in 1960. A latent bleeding tendency persists during chronic hemodialysis/hemodiafiltration (HD/HF). Anticoagulation with heparin, the platelet dysfunction of uremia, functional platelet changes induced by dialysis procedures and drugs interfering with hemostasis are all responsible for this potential bleeding. New heparin preparations (low molecular weight heparins–LMWH) and the recent introduction of erythropoetin, however, have further reduced the bleeding episodes in the dialysis patients. As a consequence, particularly if the haemotocrit exceeds 40%, thrombotic complications, i.e., deep vein thrombosis and pulmonary embolism in high-risk patients and repeated clotting of the vascular access, are now seen more frequently than in the past. Thrombotic complications as a consequence of a hypersensitivity reaction against heparin are infrequent (heparin-associated thrombocytopenia and heparin-induced skin necrosis), but must be excluded in all cases with thrombocytopenia.

In the following, emphasis shall be placed on the clinical manifestation of spontaneous bleeding, mostly induced by heparin, on other side effects of chronic heparin application and on the therapeutic measures to prevent such complications.

II. SPONTANEOUS BLEEDING MANIFESTATIONS

An increased prevalence of spontaneous bleeding manifestation has been observed since the beginning of maintenance HD/HF. In dialysis patients on additional oral anticoagulant therapy the risk of spontaneous bleeding if further increased. An inexplicable pain with blood pressure drop, a falling hematocrit without external blood loss, a sudden enlargement of an organ or a sudden onset of headache, seizure, confusion or somnolence should make one think of such a complication.

A gastrointestinal bleeding is reportedly the most frequent bleeding site reported and is attributed to hypergastrinemia, gastroduodenal mucosa changes, the defective haemostasis and the use of ulcerogenic drugs (NSAIDS, steroids) (4). Dialysis-associated amyloid may be another cause of gastrointestinal bleeding in maintenance hemodialysis patients (5). Other bleeding episodes that occur at various times during chroinc hemodialysis and often in the absence of a trauma are subdural hematoma (6) (Fig. 1), haemopericardium (7), haemorrhagic pleural effusion (8) and retroperitoneal hematoma (9) (Fig. 2). Further bleeding sites are: hemorrhage in the anterior chamber of the eye (10), mediastinal haemorrhage (11), subcapsular liver hematoma (12), hemorrhage in a renal cyst or diffuse subcapsular renal bleeding (Fig. 3), ovarian hemorrhage (13), and hemarthros (14). A severe secondary hyperparathyroidism may lead to spontaneous parathyroid hemorrhage with a rapidly enlarging cervical mass (15). Today, modern imaging techniques should be applied early in order to identify the bleeding site and to allow active therapeutic measures (i.e., evacuation of the hematomas).

A. Reasons for the Bleeding Tendency in the Chronic Dialysis Patient

Heparin has to be considered as a main cause of increased bleeding, besides the uremic platelet dysfunction and the platelet activation (with consecutive thrombocytopenia) induced by interaction between blood and artificial surfaces. The platelet count in the HD/HF patient is usually in the lower normal range. In some patients platelet counts decrease further during the chronic maintenance haemodialysis. A thrombocytopenia may develop as a consequence of splenomegaly (chronic hepatitis; hemolytic anemia, etc.) or of drugs (heparin itself, antibiotics, digitoxin, quinine, quinidine, carbamazepin, etc.). If the heparin dose is not adjusted to platelet counts, an imbalance between anticoagulation and hemostasis will occur, with the danger of bleeding. A significant amount of heparin is physiologically neutralized by anionic platelet constituents (platelet factor 4, beta thromboglobulin, thrombospondin); they are not available in the case of thrombocytopenia. Furthermore, UFH aggravates the platelet dysfunction by inhibiting platelet adenylate cyclase, which leads to reduction in the threshold for platelet activation (16,17).

1. Heparin-Induced Thrombocytopenia

Heparin-induced thrombopenia (HIT) is relatively common (see also contribution of Davenport this issue). It may be non-immunologically (type 1) or immunologically mediated (type 2). Type 1 usually occurs in the first few days after administration of heparin, the thrombocytopenia is moderate (rarely <100,000/μl), re-

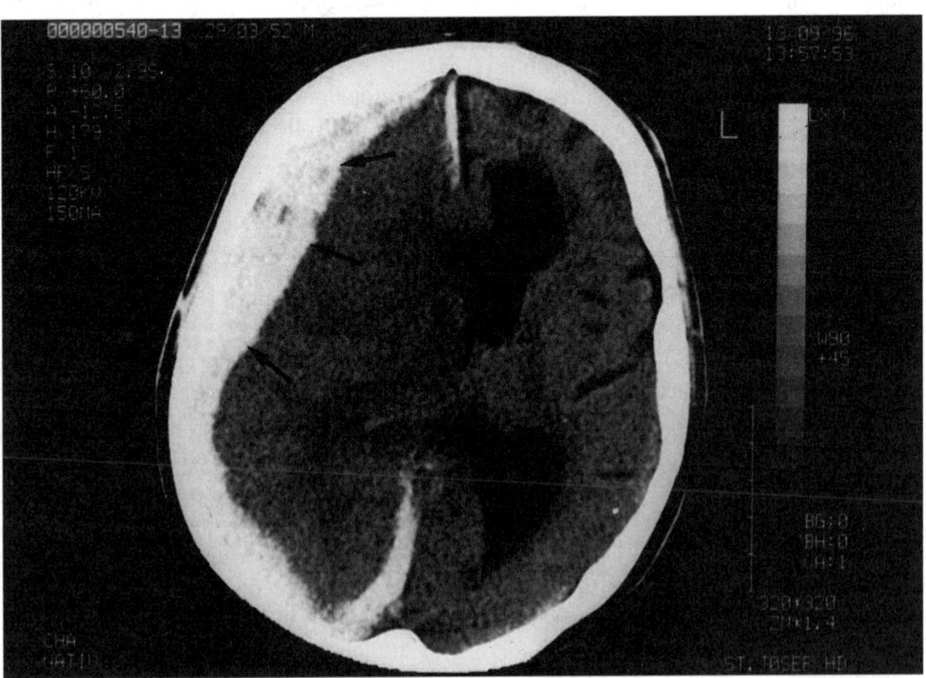

Fig. 1 Spontaneous subdural hematoma in a 45-year-old male patient after 11 months on chronic hemodialysis.

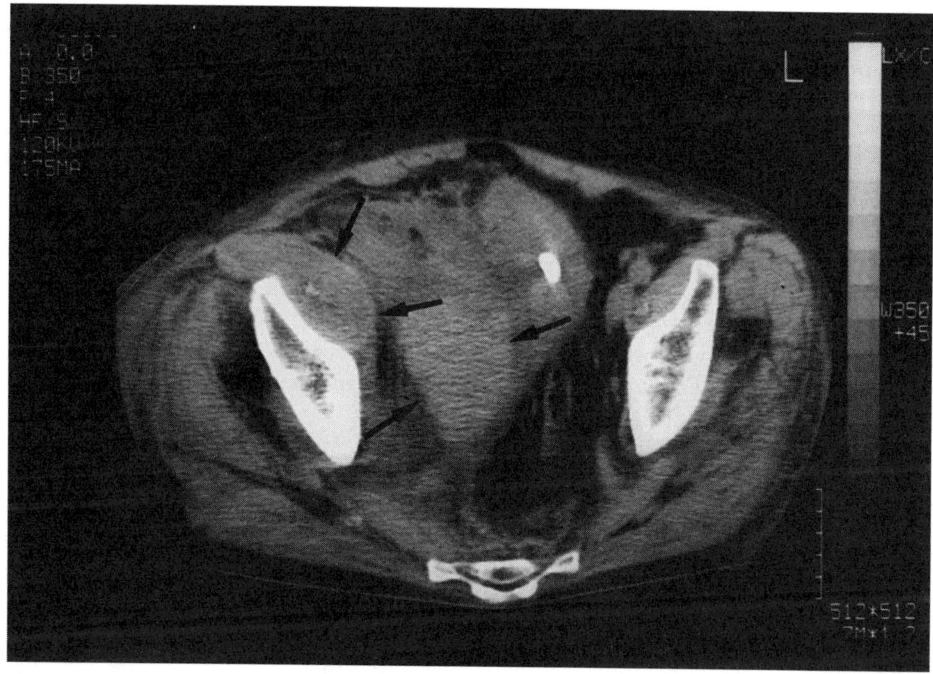

Fig. 2 Large retroperitoneal hematoma in a 55-year-old male patient 5 months after beginning of chronic hemodialysis.

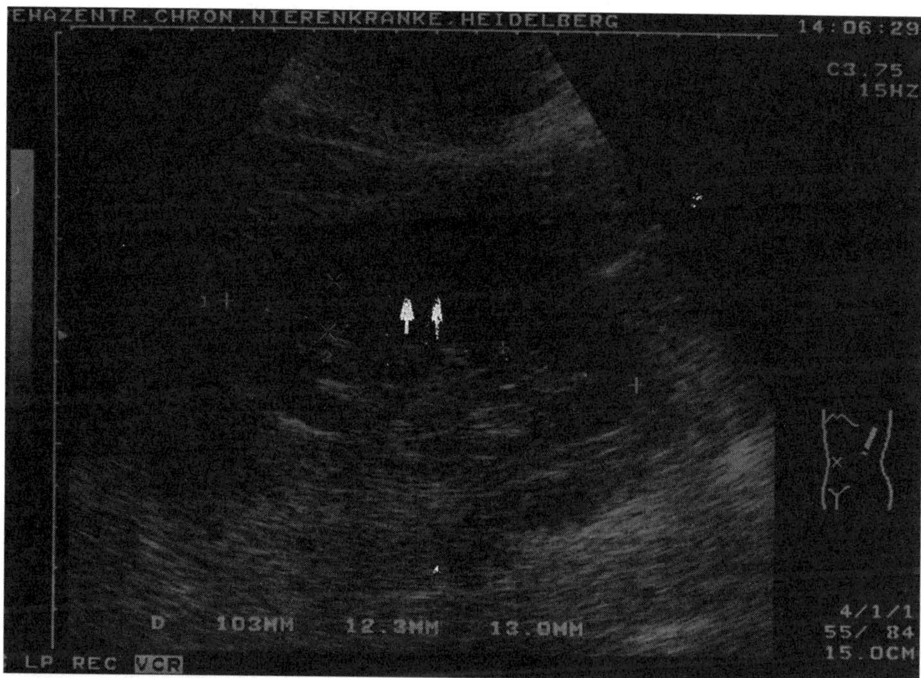

Fig. 3 Spontaneous subcapsular renal hemorrhage in a 66-year-old male patient with IgA nephropathy 6 months after beginning of chronic hemodialysis.

versible and without associated clinical complications. Type 2 usually appears between days 6 and 12 after initiation of heparin treatment but may also occur later and is accompanied by relevant hemostatic disorders (18). Type 2 is more common with UFH than with LMWH (19). A multimeric platelet factor 4 (PF 4)/heparin) complex is the target for antibodies generated by heparin (20) for type 2. Heparin dependent IgG activates platelets via their Fc receptors. Recommended tests for detection of HIT type 2 are C14-serotonin release (21) and/or a platelet aggregation test (22), both in presence of heparin. Furthermore, a microtiter based heparin-induced platelet activation assay (HIPA) (23) and an ELISA based on heparin/PF4 coating of microtiter wells (24) have been described. The most sensitive and specific tests are the C14 serotonin release, the heparin/PF4 ELISA and the HIPA test.

The clinical manifestation of HIT is variable (25). Some patients have severe bleeding, some may develop thrombotic complications (white clot syndrome). One complication of HIT type 2 is adrenal hemorrhagic infarction (26). Thrombotic complications may appear despite normal or even very low platelet counts (27). The frequency of HIT on chronic hemodialysis patients was reported to be 2–4% (28–30). Yamamoto et al. (28) attributed the presence of HIT in their patients to increased clot formation in dialyzers and extracorporeal circuits and decreases in platelet counts. In contrast to the report of Yamamoto et al., Greinacher et al. (29) found neither increased hemorrhage nor vessel occlusion. They argued that hemodialysis patients have a lower risk of developing HIT because of an impairment of the immune system. These authors advise that an alternative anticoagulation in dialysis patients is only justified if patients with HIT become clinically symptomatic. Boon et al. (30) confirmed the different long term effect of UFH and LMWH on generation of HIT in dialysis patients (mean duration of haemodialysis between 36 and 45 months). Whereas with UFH the frequency was 2.3%, HIT in LMWH treated patients was only 0.3%. In their patients only 1 had mild thrombocytopenia, and no other clinical manifestation of HIT was noted. It should, however, be realized that a HIT might occur late up to 6 years after initiation of maintenance haemodialysis (31).

2. Heparin-Induced Skin Lesions

Heparin-induced allergic skin lesions are rare. They appear usually within 1–2 weeks after heparin application and occasionally thereafter. The skin lesions are located either at or at far distance from the injection site, manifesting as itchy erythematous plaques (Fig. 4). Skin necrosis is an infrequent complication of heparin therapy, and may occur in patients with heparin antibodies from type 2 HIT, but mostly without thrombocytopenia (32,33). Heparin-induced skin necrosis usually appears in middle-age obese women between days 5 and 15 after beginning heparin treatment, but they may also occur later (31,34). This skin necrosis is characterized by the formation of one or more painful red plaques with or without necrotic skin lesions on the abdominal wall, upper and lower extremities, nose and dorsum of the hands (35) (Fig. 5). The histopathology comprises endothelial injury with hemorrhage or thrombosis and inflammatory reactions with or without pericellular infiltrates of dermal venules and capillaries; the arterioles

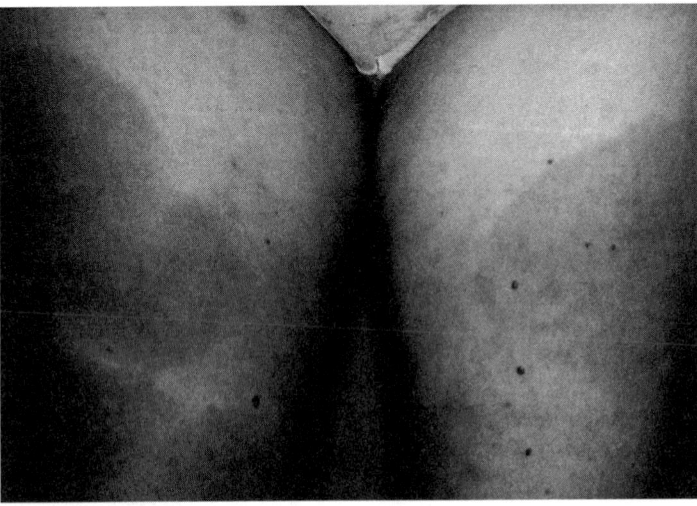

Fig. 4 Allergic skin reaction on unfractionated heparin in a 52-year-old female patient 38 days after beginning of chronic hemodialysis. The heparin allergy was proven by skin test.

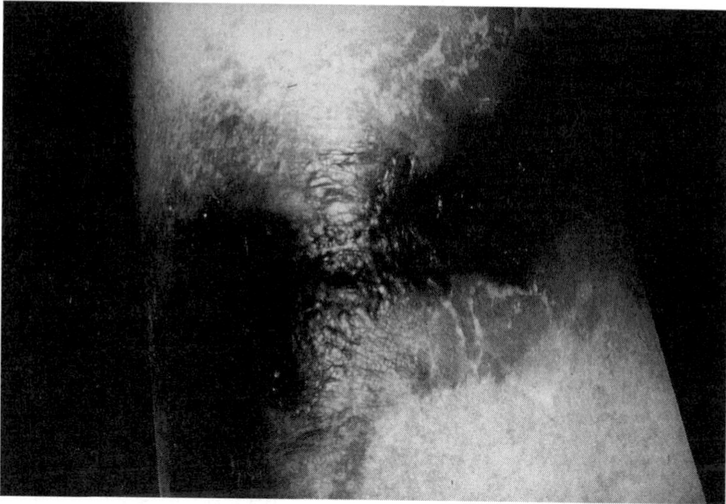

Fig. 5 Heparin-induced skin necrosis with a positive HIT test in a 66-year-old female patient 18 days after beginning of chronic hemodialysis.

are spared (36). The necrotic lesions resemble those of coumarin necrosis. Whether protein C deficiency might stimulate the formation of skin necrosis as observed in patients with end-stage renal failure and calciphylaxis (37) has not been examined in more detail. It is of note that HD/HF will transiently decrease protein C levels (38), and heparin itself accelerates the inhibition of protein C by protein C inhibitor (39). In most cases, heparin-induced skin lesions appear at the site of (subcutaneous) injection (40,41), but is has also been observed with intravenous UFH administration (42). It was claimed that bovine heparin more frequently generates such lesions than porcine mucosal heparin (43). LMWH can also induce a skin necrosis (44) distant from injection sites, and antibodies against LMWH have been detected. This observation is important because s.c. LMWH today is more often used for prevention of thrombosis in hemodialysis patients with prosthetic vascular access. Skin necrosis by s.c. heparin has been reported in a patient on peritoneal dialysis (45). Since heparin-induced skin necrosis may herald the clinical manifestation of HIT a test to exclude HIT should be performed in every case.

III. OTHER SIDE EFFECTS OF LONG-TERM ANTICOAGULATION WITH HEPARIN IN CHRONIC HEMODIALYSIS/HEMODIAFILTRATION PATIENTS

A. Hyperkalaemia

While bleeding, thrombocytopenia, and cutaneous hypersensitivity are well documented complications of UFH administration, the inhibition of aldosterone production leading to hyperkalemia is neglected (46,47). Animal experiments demonstrated that this inhibition is dependent on time and dosage. The maximum of inhibition is reached 4–5 days after UFH application. The adrenal zona glomerulosa is the target of heparin and the steroidgenesis at the step of 18-hydroxylase is suppressed (48). Given over years, heparin causes adrenal atrophy of the zona glomerulosa (49). According to a study of Siebels et al. (50), a critical UFH dosage of 15000 IU/day in subjects with normal body weight leads to hypoaldosteronism. This dosage is usually given during a hemodialysis session. Although hyperkalemia is not a problem during hemodialysis this might be relevant

1. if the patients need a high potassium content in the dialysate (in order to prevent cardiac arrhythmia)
2. if they are treated with drugs interfering with mineralocorticoid metabolism, i.e., ACE inhibitors (51) or NSAIDS, or
3. if they have diabetes mellitus.

Hyperkalemia is also observed during treatment with LMWH (50,52,53) in a dosage exceeding 3000 anti fXa U in individuals with normal body weight. This dosage is exceeded during hemodialysis with LMWH. With the advent of hirudin as alternative anticoagulant the contribution of heparin to hyperkalemia on maintenance dialysis might be better assessed (54).

B. Heparin-Related Osteoporosis

Long-term treatment with UFH can cause bone demineralization. Although infrequent this complication may gain clinical relevance in predisposed subjects (malnourished children, pregnant women and in the elderly) (55). The concomitant application of steroids might aggravate the effect of heparin on the bone. It has been suggested that the heparin-induced osteoporosis is related to dose and duration of application. In animal models this has been well documented for both UFH and LMWH (56). Since hyperparathyreoidism with its consequences on bone structure is common and predominates among chronic dialysis patients it is difficult to decide to what extent, if at all, the long-term heparin administration might contribute to renal bone disease.

IV. THERAPEUTIC CONSIDERATIONS

A. Heparinization for Hemodialysis

UFH is the agent of choice in preventing clot formation in the extracorporeal circuit. Inadequate anticoagulation leads to filter and/or extracorporeal circuit clotting, resulting in blood loss and anemia. Dialysis efficiency is reduced as evaluated by creatinine or urea clearance. Therefore optimal anticoagulation is desired. Optimal anticoagulation can be controlled by detection of thrombin generation in plasma, i.e., measurement of prothrombin fragments (F_{1+2}), thrombin/antithrombin complexes (TAT) or fibrin split products (D-dimers). The dose of heparin required to achieve this goal varies, however, and is dependent on the biocompatibility of membranes, construction of the dialyzer and roller pump segment, besides the individual patient's sensitivity. Higher heparin doses are needed if patients have higher body weight and higher hematocrit. The mean heparin half-life on hemodialysis is 0.86 ± 0.06 hours (57) and is not different from normal subjects. The heparin clearance for dialysis patients is almost wholly by nonrenal routes, since clearance by either the dialyzer or the minimal amount of residual renal function is small. After administration of UFH a major part is sequestered in the RES. In order to saturate the RES a certain amount of UFH has to be administered as a loading dose (usually 2500–5000 U). Due to the short half-life of UFH repeated doses of UFH have to be given, usually as continuous infusion (1500 U/hour) because a continuous heparin infusion is safer than intermittent injections for the prevention of thrombotic events, but also for the reduction of major bleeding (58). The effect of UFH can be monitored by prolongation of clotting times or increased antifactor Xa activity, as outlined in Table 1. The most reliable clotting test is the WBPTT; this method reflects the coagulation process more precisely than aPTT or thrombin time because it includes blood cells that are involved in blood coagulation as well (59). ACT is most widely used because it is an automated method and produces rapid results. Potential inaccuracies in the monitoring of heparin activity by ACT may occur in the presence of activated or lysed platelets as observed in intraoperative monitoring (60). The whole-blood clotting methods are not sensitive to LMWH (61). Measurement of LMWH requires a specific chromogenic substrate assay to determine the inhibition of factor Xa.

Table 1 Adjustment of Clotting Tests by UFH to Perform Adequate Hemodialysis

Clotting test	Target time/activity
aPTT	80–120 s
WBPTT	120–160 s
Thrombin time	50–70 s
ACT	150–200 s
Anti-factor Xa	>0.5 U/mL

B. Preventive Measures in Patients at Risk for Bleeding

The balance between prevention of clotting and bleeding is not easy to sustain in those patients who are at risk of bleeding. The risk of bleeding can be judged by the criteria of Swartz (62). Patients at very high risk are those with active bleeding at the time of dialysis, at high risk with active bleeding or surgical/traumatic wounds within 3 days or dialysis via femoral vessel cannula. Additional risk factors are thrombocytopenia and aspirin or coumarin, usually applied for the prevention of fistula thrombosis.

The following therapeutic measures are recommended to stop bleeding (Table 2): anticoagulation with heparin must be minimized (priming of the extracorporeal circuit with heparin, but discarding the fluid) and reduction of the loading dose to 2000 U followed by small heparin boli (500–1000 IU within 15–30 min) with frequent control of clotting time. In case of severe bleeding heparin administration should be interrupted. Heparin-free dialysis is possible if a high blood flow is guaranteed (>250 ml/min) and the patient is not overhydrated. Flushing of the dialyzer with 100–150 ml saline every 20–30 min is mandatory to remove small thrombi. The risk of clotting in the dialyzer increases if erythrocyte concentrates are given [this can be circumvented by the insertion of a three-way stop-

Table 2 Therapeutic Measures in Chronic Dialysis Patients with Bleeding

Acute bleeding	Chronic bleeding
Reduce heparin (mini-dosage) with frequent control of clotting times	Elimination of drugs interfering with hemostasis
Red blood cell concentrates (HCT > 30%)	RHu-EPO to increase hematocrit >30% with concomitant iron substitution, if required
Desmopressin	LMWH instead of UFH
Heparin-free dialysis	
Citrate as anticoagulant	
Heparinoid in case of HIT	

cock, which allows direct infusion of the blood into the venous side (63)] and if dialysis time exceeds 3 hours (64).

A further alternative as anticoagulant for UFH is the use of citrate (65–70). In a non-randomized study of Ward and Mehta (66) comparing UFH with citrate and no anticoagulation (flushing with saline) new bleeding events occurred in 26% of the patients during heparin-dialysis, even in low-risk patients, but none with citrate. Clotting occurred mainly in the saline group. The regional citrate hemodialysis may be complicated by metabolic alkalosis, particularly if high doses of citrate are required. Therefore, frequent control of the acid-base status is mandatory. Cardiac arrest may occur during bicarbonate dialysis (67). The citrate solution, if sterilized in glass bottles, contains 2–3 μg aluminum/mmol citrate, which can be prevented by sterilizing the solution in polypropylene bottles (68). Dialysis with citrate may induce a rise in total calcium concentration during and postdialysis (69). The long-term use of citrate anticoagulation may be accompanied by neurologic symptoms if the bicarbonate buffer content of the dialysate is not reduced to <30 mmol (69,70). The documented complications of regional citrate anticoagulation can be minimized by substituting hypertonic trisodium citrate for heparin, adjusting an arterial ACT of 150–200 sec and by reduction of ultrafiltration (69).

The bleeding tendency in chronic HD/HF patients may be reduced if UFH is replaced by LMWH (71). LMWH has a similar antithrombotic activity as UFH but a lower hemorrhagic tendency, although the half-life of LMWH is doubled in patients with renal failure. Therefore, in the majority of cases a bolus administration of LMWH (5000 a F Xa U) is sufficient to perform a 4-hour dialysis. Various studies with LMWH in dialysis patients clearly show that the anti-factor Xa levels in plasma must exceed 0.5 U/ml to prevent clot formation. Anti-factor Xa levels >0.5 U/ml, which are achieved with these LMWH boli, particularly during the first hour after bolus administration will, however, simultaneously increase bleeding tendency. Therefore, this mode of administration is not to be recommended in patients at risk of bleeding (72). They should receive lower LMWH boli and decreased doses of LMWH for continuous infusion as outlined by Schrader et al. (71).

If the prolongation of bleeding time indicates a platelet defect as underlying cause of acute bleeding the administration of desmopressin (DDAVP) (0.3 μg kg^{-1} iv) is helpful (73). This is particularly important in those cases where acetylsalicylic acid is given for prevention of vascular access thrombosis. Desmopression releases high molecular weight von Willebrand factor (vWF) multimers that are effective in overcoming functional platelet defects. A similar effect is obtained if desmopressin is repeated 12 hours after the first application, but it loses its efficacy the next day because of exhaustion of the vWF stores. Since erythrocytes are central to interaction between platelets and vessel wall, a low hematocrit (<30%) will support the uremic platelet defect. Therefore, red blood cell concentrates must be applied to elevate the hematocrit above 30% (2). Recombinant erythropoetin (rHu-EPO) (120–450 U/kg/week) is helpful in patients with low normal platelet counts since it increases not only the hematocrit but also platelet counts and improves platelet function (74,75; see Remuzzi this book). The effect of rHu-EPO will, however, not be obvious before the fourth to sixth week of treatment. It has definitively reduced the bleeding tendency of the chronic dialysis patient.

A heparin-induced hypersensitivity (HIT type 2; heparin-induced skin necrosis) should lead to its cessation. If the patient has a recent or new thrombosis that requires anticoagulation, a low molecular weight heparinoid (Orgaran, Org 10172) containing a mixture of heparan-, dermatan- and chrondroitin sulphate, but no heparin, is now available. It has a low cross reaction rate (about 10%) to the heparin-dependent antibody (76). For adequate dialysis, application of a bolus of 3750 U of Orgaran (after priming the dialyzer with 1500 U, but discarding the fluid) is recommended in order to maintain anti-factor Xa levels between 0.5 and 0.8 U/ml plasma in patients with a normal body weight. If dialysis is performed daily, the next Orgaran bolus should only amount to 2500 U. With a body weight of

<55 kg or >90 kg the doses should be reduced or increased by 10–20% (77,78). The criteria for judging adequacy of the Orgaran therapy are an increase of platelet counts, cessation of clotting in the extracorporeal circuit, and resolution of thrombotic events. As a further therapeutic alternative dermatan may be administered (79). Since dermatan sulphate was also used successfully as an anticoagulant in hemodialysis (80) this compound needs further evaluation. Recombinant hirudin (81) is also recommended for treatment of HIT on hemodialysis (82). Low-flux polysulfone dialyzers and an intravenous bolus of 0.14 mg/kg achieved efficient hemodialysis for 4.5 hours. Although the long plasma half-life (54) in uremia and the lack of an antidote precluded hirudin in HD/HF until now, some decisive amendments have been attained recently. Monitoring of blood hirudin concentration is now possible by means of the ecarin clotting time (83). Furthermore, it was realized that permeability of hirudin through dialyzer membranes was different (none through low-flux, partially through high-flux membranes) (82). Therefore plasma hirudin levels on dialysis may now be adjusted by applying different dialysis membranes.

As another therapeutic alternative the administration of intravenous immunoglobulins (84) and/or plasmapheresis (85) in severe HIT might be considered. The use of low molecular weight heparins in patients with HIT should be avoided since they have a high cross reactivity with UFH (79–94%); moreover unfavourable outcomes with LMWH have been reported (25).

REFERENCES

1. Riesman D. Hemorrhages in the course of Bright's disease with special reference to the occurrence of a hemorrhagic diathesis of nephrotic origin. Am J Sci 1907; 134:709–716.
2. Livio M, Gotti E, Marchesi E, Mecca G, Remuzzi G, de Gaetano G. Uremic bleeding: role of anemia and beneficial effect of red cell transfusions. Lancet 1982; II:1013–1015.
3. Andrassy K. Bleeding in acute renal failure. In: Bihari D, Neild G, eds. Acute Renal Failure in the Intensive Therapy Unit. London: Springer-Verlag, 1988:243–252.
4. Boyle JM, Johnston B. Acute upper gastrointestinal hemorrhage in patients with chronic renal disease. Am J Med 1983; 75:409–412.
5. Maher EP, Hamilton Dutoit S, Baillod RA, Sweny P, Moorhead JF. Gastrointestinal complications of dialysis-related amyloidosis. Br Med J 1988; 297:265–266.
6. Talalla A, Halbrook H, Barbour BH, Kurze T. Subdural hematoma associated with long-term hemodialysis for chronic renal disease. JAMA 1970; 212:1847–1849.
7. Alfrey AC, Goss JE, Ogden DA, Vogel JHK, Holmes JH. Uremic hemopericardium. Am J Med 1968; 391–400.
8. Galen MA, Steinberg SM, Lowrie EG, Lazarus JM, Hampers CL, Merrill JP. Hemorrhagic pleural effusion in patients undergoing chronic hemodialysis. Ann Int Med 1975; 82:359–361.
9. Milutinovich J, Follette WC, Scribner BH. Spontaneous retroperitoneal bleeding in patients on chronic hemodialysis. Ann Int Med 1977; 86:189–192.
10. Slusher MM, Hamilton RW. Spontaneous hyphema during hemodialysis (letter). N Engl J Med 1975; 293:561.
11. Ellison RT, Corrao WM, Fox MJ, Braman SS. Spontaneous mediastinal hemorrhage in patients on chronic hemodialysis. Ann Int Med 1981; 95:704–706.
12. Borra S, Kleinfeld M. Subcapsular liver hematomas in a patient on chronic hemodialysis. Ann Int Med 1980; 93:574–575.
13. Biggers JA, Remmers AR, Glassford DM, Sarles HE, Lindley JD, Fish JC. The risk of anticoagulation in hemodialysis patients. Nephron 1977; 18:109–113.
14. Marino C, Kazdin H. Spontaneous hemarthrosis in a patient treated with hemodialysis for chronic renal failure (letter). Arthr Rheumat 1982; 25:1387.
15. Roma J, Carrio J, Pascual R, Oliva JA, Mallafre JM, Montolio J. Spontaneous parathyroid hemorrhage in a hemodialysis patient. Nephron 1985; 39:66–67.
16. Fabris F, Fussi F, Casonato A, Visentin L, Randi M, Smith MR, Girolami A. Normal and low molecular weight heparins: interaction with human platelets. Eur J Clin Invest 1983; 13:135–139.
17. Amsterdam A, Reches A, Amir Y, Mintz Y, Salomon Y. Modulation of adenylate cyclase activity by sulfated glycosaminoglycans. Biochim Biophys Acta 1978; 544: 273–283.
18. King DJ, Kelton JG. Heparin-associated thrombocytopenia. Ann Int Med 1984; 100:535–540.
19. Warkentin TE, Levine MN, Hirsh J, Horsewood P, Roberts RS, Gent M, Kelton JG. Heparin-induced thrombocytopenia in patients treated with low molecular-weight heparin or unfractionated heparin. N Engl J Med 1995; 332:1330–1335.
20. Greinacher A, Pötzsch B, Amiral J, Dummel V, Eichner A, Mueller-Eckhart C. Heparin-associated thrombocytopenia: isolation of the antibody and characterization of a multimolecular PF 4-heparin complex as the major antigen. Thromb Haemost 1994; 71:247–251.
21. Sheridan D, Carter C, Kelton JG. A diagnostic test for heparin-induced thrombocytopenia. Blood 1986; 67: 27–30.
22. Chong BH, Burgess J, Ismail F. The clinical usefulness of the platelet aggregation test for the diagnosis of heparin-induced thrombocytopenia. Thromb Haemost 1993; 69:344–350.

23. Greinacher A, Michels I, Kiefel V, Mueller-Eckhardt C. A rapid and sensitive test for diagnosing heparin-associated thrombocytopenia. Thromb Haemost 1991; 66: 734–736.
24. Amiral J, Bridey F, Dreyfus M, Vissac AM, Fressinaud W, Wolf M. Platelet factor 4 complexed to heparin is the target for antibodies against generated in heparin-induced thrombocytopenia. Thromb Haemost 1992; 68: 95–96.
25. Chong BH. Heparin-induced thrombocytopenia. Austr NZ J Med 1992; 22:145–152.
26. Arthur CK, Grant SJB, Murray WK, Isbister JP, Stiel JN, Lauer CS. Heparin-associated acute adrenal insufficiency. Austr NZ J Med 1985; 15:454–455.
27. Hach-Wunderle V, Kainer K, Krug B, Müller-Berghaus G, Pötzsch B. Heparin-associated thrombosis despite normal platelet counts. Lancet 1994; 344:469–470.
28. Yamamoto S, Koide M, Matsuo M, Suzuki S, Ohtaka M, Saika S, Matsuo T. Heparin-induced thrombocytopenia in hemodialysis patient. Am J Kidney Dis 1996; 28:82–85.
29. Greinacher A, Zinn S, Wizemann U, Birk W. Heparin-induced antibodies as a risk factor for thromboembolism and hemorrhage in patients undergoing chronic hemodialysis. Lancet 1996; 348:764.
30. Boon DMS, van Vliet HHDM, Zietse R, Kappers-Klunne MC. The presence of antibodies against a P F4-heparin complex in patients on hemodialysis. Thromb Haemost 1996; 76:480.
31. Bredlich RO, Stracke S, Gall H, Proebstle TM. Heparinassoziiertes Thrombozytenaggregationssyndrom mit Hautnekrosen an der Haemodialyse. Dtsch Med Wschr 1997; 122:328–332.
32. Tuneu A, Moreno A, de Moragas JM. Cutaneous reactions secondary to heparin injections. J Am Acad Dermatol 1985; 12:1072–1077.
33. Warkentin TE. Heparin-induced skin lesions. Br J Haematol 1996; 92:494–497.
34. Humphries JE, Kaplan DM, Bolton WK. Heparin skin necrosis: delayed occurrence in a patient on hemodialysis. Am J Kidney Dis 1991; XVII:233–236.
35. O'Toole RD. Heparin. Adverse reaction (letter). Ann Int Med 1973; 79:759.
36. Sallah S, Thomas DP, Roberts HR. Warfarin and heparin-induced skin necrosis and the purple toe syndrome: infrequent complications of anticoagulant treatment. Thromb Haemost 1997; 78:785–790.
37. Mehta RL, Scott G, Sloand JA, Francis CW. Skin necrosis associated with acquired protein C deficiency in patients with renal failure. Am J Med 1990; 88:252–257.
38. Alegre A, Vicente V, Gonzalez R. Effect of hemodialysis on protein C levels. Nephron 1987; 46:386–387.
39. Heeb MJ, Espana F, Griffin JH. Activation and complexation of protein C by two major inhibitors in plasma. Blood 1989; 73:446–454.
40. Hill J, Caprini JA, Robbins J. An unusual complication of minidose heparin therapy. Clin Orthop 1976; 118: 130–132.
41. Hall JC, McConahay D, Gibson D. Heparin necrosis: an anticoagulation syndrome. JAMA 1980; 244:1831–1832.
42. Kelly RA, Gelfand JA, Pincus SH. Cutaneous necrosis caused by systemically administered heparin. JAMA 1981; 246:1582–1583.
43. Stricker H, Lämmle B, Furlan M, Sulzer I. Heparin-dependent in vitro aggregation of normal platelets by plasma of a patient with heparin-induced skin necrosis: specific diagnostic test for a rare side effect. Am J Med 1988; 85:721–724.
44. Balestra B, Quadri P, Biasiutti FD, Furlan M, Lämmle B. Low molecular weight heparin-induced thrombocytopenia and skin necrosis distant from injection sites. Eur J Haematol 1994; 53:61–63.
45. Levine LE, Bernstein JE, Soltani K, Medenica MM, Yung CW. Heparin-induced cutaneous necrosis unrelated to injection sites. A sign of potentially lethal complications. Arch Dermatol 1983; 119:400–403.
46. Phelps KR, Oh MS, Carroll J. Heparin-induced hyperkalemia: report of a case. Nephron 1980; 25:254–258.
47. Sherman RA, Ruddy MC. Suppression of aldosterone production by low-dose heparin. Am J Nephrol 1986; 6:165–168.
48. Kutyrina I, Nikishova A, Tareyeva I. Effects of heparin induced aldosterone deficiency on renal function in patients with chronic glomerulonephritis. Nephrol Dial Transpl 1987; 2:219–233.
49. Wilson E, Goetz F. Selective hypoaldosteronism after prolonged heparin administration. Am J Med 1964; 36: 635–640.
50. Siebels M, Andrassy K, Vecsei P, Seelig HP, Back T, Nawroth P, Weber E. Dose dependent suppression of mineralocorticoid metabolism by different heparin fractions. Thromb Res 1992; 66:467–473.
51. Durand D, Ader JL, Rey JP, Tran-Van T, Lloveras JJ, Bernadet P, Suc JM. Inducing hyperkalemia by converting enzyme inhibitors and heparin. Kidney Int 1988; 34(suppl 25):196–197.
52. Levesque H, Verdier S, Cailleux N, Legrand E, Gancel A, Basuyau JP, Borg JY, Moore N, Courtois H. Low molecular weight heparins and hypoaldosteronism. Br Med J 1990; 300:1437–1438.
53. Canova CR, Fischler MP, Reinhart WH. Effect of low-molecular weight heparin on serum potassium. Lancet 1997; 349:1447–1448.
54. Vanholder R, Camez A, Veys N, van Loo A, Dhondt AM, Ringoir S. Pharmacokinetics of recombinant hirudin in hemodialyzed end-stage renal failure patients. Thromb Haemost 1997; 77:650–655.
55. Bardin T, Lequesne M. The osteoporosis of heparinotherapy and systemic mastocytosis. Clin Rheumatol 1989 8(suppl 2):119–123.

56. Mätzsch T, Bergqvist D, Hedner U, Nilsson B, Ostergaard P. Effects of low molecular weight heparin and unfragmented heparin on induction of osteoporosis in rats. Thromb Haemost 1990; 63:505–509.
57. Farrell PC, Ward RA, Schindhelm K, Gotch FA. Precise anticoagulation for routine hemodialysis. J Lab Clin Med 1978; 92:164–176.
58. Salzman EW, Deykin D, Shapiro RM, Rosenberg R. Management of heparin therapy. N Engl J Med 1975; 292:1046–1050.
59. Congdon JE, Kardianl CG, Wallin JD. Monitoring heparin therapy in hemodialysis. JAMA 1973; 226:1529–1533.
60. Bode AP, Lust RM. Masking of heparin activity in the activated coagulation time (ACT) by platelet procoagulant activity. Thromb Res 1994; 73:285–300.
61. Greiber S, Weber U, Galle J, Brämer P, Schollmeyer P. Activated clotting time is not a sensitive parameter to monitor anticoagulation with low molecular weight heparin in hemodialysis. Nephron 1997; 76:15–19.
62. Swartz RD. Hemorrhage during high-risk hemodialysis using controlled heparinization. Nephron 1981; 28:65–69.
63. Sepulveda S, Davis L, Schwab SJ. Blood transfusion during heparin-free treatment. Kidney Int 1997; 51: 2015–2021.
64. Caruana RJ, Raja RM, Bush JV, Kramer MS, Goldstein SJ. Heparin free dialysis: comparative data and results in high risk patients. Kidney Int 1987; 31:1351–1355.
65. Flanigan M, von Brecht J, Freeman Rm, Lim VS. Reducing the hemorrhagic complication of hemodialysis: a controlled comparison of low-dose heparin and citrate anticoagulation. Am J Kidney Dis 1987; IX:147–153.
66. Ward DM, Mehta RL. Extracorporeal management of acute renal failure patients at high risk of bleeding. Kidney Int 1993; 43(suppl 4):237–244.
67. Charney DI, Salmond R. Cardiac arrest after hypertonic citrate anticoagulation for chronic hemodialysis. ASAIO Trans 1990; 36:M217–M219.
68. Janssen MJFM, Deegens JK, Kapinga TH, Beukhof JR, Huijgens PC, van Loenen AC, van der Meulen J. Citrate compared to low molecular weight heparin anticoagulation in chronic hemodialysis patients. Kidney Int 1996; 49:805–813.
69. Flanigan MJ, Pillsbury L, Sadewasser BSN, Lim, VS. Regional hemodialysis anticoagulation: hypertonic trisodium citrate or anticoagulant citrate dextrose-A. Am J Kidney Dis 1996; 27:519–524.
70. van der Meulen J, Janssen MJE, Langendijk PNJ, Bouman AA, Oe PL. Citrate anticoagulation and dialysate with reduced buffer content in chronic hemodialysis. Clin Nephrol 1992; 37:36–41.
71. Schrader J, Stibbe W, Armstrong VW, Kandt M, Muche R, Köstering H, Seidel D, Scheler F. Comparison of low molecular weight heparin to standard heparin in hemodialysis/hemofiltration. Kidney Int 1988; 33:890–896.
72. Andrassy K. Low molecular weight heparin and haemodialysis: neutralization by protaminchloride. Blood Coagulation Fibrinolysis 1993; 4(suppl 1):39–43.
73. Mannucci PM, Remuzzi G, Pusineri F, Lombardi R, Valsecchi D, Mecca G, Zimmerman T. Deamino-8-D-arginine vasopressin shortens bleeding time in uremia. N Engl J Med 1983; 308:8–12.
74. Moia M, Mannucci PM, Vizzotto L, Casati S, Cattaneo M, Ponticelli C. Improvement in the haemostatic defect of uremia after treatment with recombinant human erythropoetin. Lancet 1987; II:1227–1229.
75. Cases A, Escolar G, Reverter JC, Ordinas A, Lopez-Pedret J, Revert L, Castillo R. Recombinant human erythropoetin treatment improves platelet function in uremic platelets. Kidney Int 1992; 42:668–672.
76. Magnani HN. Heparin-induced thrombocytopenia (HIT): an overview of 230 patients treated with Orgaran (Org 10172). Thromb Haemost 1993; 70:554–561.
77. Chong BH, Magnani HN. Orgaran in heparin-induced thrombocytopenia. Haemostasis 1992; 22:85–91.
78. Greinacher A, Alban S. Heparinoide als eine Alternative für die parenterale Antikoagulation bei Patienten mit Heparin-induzierter Thrombozytopenie. Haemostaseologie 1996; 16:41–49.
79. Agnelli G, Iorio A, de Angelis V, Nenci GG. Dermatan sulphate in heparin-induced thrombocytopenia. Lancet 1994; 344:1295–1296.
80. Ryan KE, Lane DA, Flynn A, Ireland H, Boisclair M, Shepperd J, Curtis JR. Antithrombotic properties of dermatan sulphate (MF 701) in haemodialysis for chronic renal failure. Thromb Haemost 1992; 68:563–569.
81. Markwardt F. The development of hirudin. Thromb Res 1994; 74:1–23.
82. Nowak G, Bucha E, Brauns I, Czerwinski R. Anticoagulation with r-Hirudin in regular haemodialysis with heparin-induced thrombocytopenia. Wien Klin Wschr 1997; 109/110:354–358.
83. Nowak G, Bucha E. Quantitative determination of hirudin in blood and body fluids. Sem Thromb 1996; 22: 197–202.
84. Prall A, Nechwatal R, Riedel H, Mäurer, W. Therapie des Heparin-induzierten Thrombose-Thrombozytopeniesyndroms mit Immunglobulinen. Dtsch Med Wschr 1992; 117:1838–1842.
85. Brady J, Riccio JA, Yumen OH, Makary AZ, Greenwood SM. Plasmapheresis. A therapeutic option in the management of heparin-associated thrombocytopenia with thrombosis. Am J Clin Pathol 1991; 96:394–397.

7

Complications of Hemoperfusion

James F. Winchester
Georgetown University Medical Center, Washington, D.C.

I. INTRODUCTION

Hemoperfusion (1) is the technique of passing blood through a bed of particles contained within a device, usually cylindrical, to which blood lines and a blood pump are attached (Fig. 1A). It differs (1) from hemodialysis in that blood comes in direct contact with the membrane-coated sorbent particle and not a continuous dialysis membrane, and (2) from plasmapheresis in that no plasma is separated from blood. Hemoperfusion can be combined with any renal replacement therapy, usually hemodialysis, to increase efficiency and maintain the temperature of blood (Fig. 1B). The particles are usually inorganic (activated charcoal, neutral or ion exchange resins), but devices under development may contain cells on the dialysate side of a hemodialysis membrane [hepatosomes (2) or renal tubule cells (3)], immobilized antibiotics for removal of endotoxin [polymyxin B (4)], immobilized antibodies (5), or coated gets (6). Some similar commercially available systems use fluidized sorbents in dialysis fluid (charcoal and a cation exchanger) on one side of a cellulosic dialysis membrane (7,8) or sorbents coupled with "push-pull" plasma exchange to allow direct contact of plasma with sorbents for removal of toxins in hepatic failure (9); the main advantage over direct contact hemoperfusion is the absence of thrombocytopenia since contact of blood is restricted to the hemodialysis/pheresis membrane. This discussion will focus on inorganic hemoperfusion in light of the paucity of clinical reports of developmental devices.

II. CLINICAL INDICATIONS FOR HEMOPERFUSION

Hemoperfusion has been used in poisoning (drug and chemical exposures), hepatic failure (drug-induced, fulminant hepatic failure, etc.), and in treatment of uremia and its complications (e.g., aluminum toxicity, when hemoperfusion in patients pretreated with deferoxamine removes complexed aluminum-deferoxamine molecules). In poisoning hemoperfusion is particularly useful in removing lipid-soluble drugs, such as barbiturates, glutethimide, and theophylline. On the other hand, water-soluble drugs such as lithium and chemicals that cause an acidosis (methanol, ethylene glycol, and salicylate) are best treated with hemodialysis. Selection of a particular device from Table 1 depends on local availability, cost and shelf life, and polymer coating: all devices listed have a high capacity for lipid-soluble drugs (XAD4 resin columns have the highest capacity for lipid-soluble drugs, but they also have the most effect on removing platelets, since the particles do not have a polymer coating). It is impossible to give accurate estimations of the number of devices used per annum throughout the world, since such figures are not published: I estimate about 3000 devices a year (mostly for poisoning), are used throughout the world.

III. SORBENTS

Adsorbent charcoal is commonly used in the form of free crushed, extruded, or bead forms. Older, and aban-

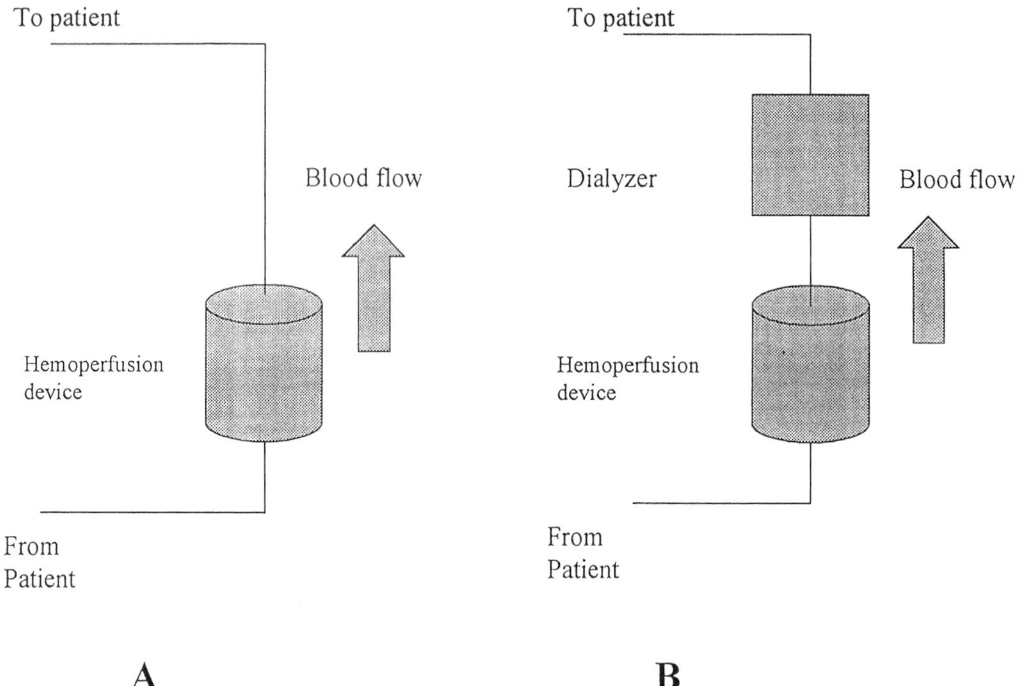

Fig. 1 Hemoperfusion (A) and hemoperfusion combined with hemodialysis (B).

doned, devices consisted of a spiral of adhesive membrane support to which particles of charcoal were fixed. Resin hemoperfusion devices had in the past contained ion-exchange resins. Today resin hemoperfusion cartridges contain neutral resins most commonly of the cross-linked polystyrene resin series (XAD-4, XAD-7, etc., Rohm and Haas, Philadelphia, PA). Table 1 lists some of the clinically available devices. The quantity of sorbent contained in, and the volume of, the device varies between manufacturers: a rule of thumb is that a large quantity/volume is used for adults and a smaller quantity/volume is used for the treatment of children. The starting material for the preparation of activated (a condition in which the sorbent is induced to have a large surface area for sorption) charcoal determines the shape of the particle. For instance, wood and other organic materials such as coconut shells are burned and crushed to yield irregular-shaped particle sizes, while more uniform particles can be made from extruded peat and petroleum droplets. The smooth round petroleum-based charcoals are more resistant to attrition and therefore small particle (''fines'') generation than other charcoals. Resins can also be pyrolized to make charcoal (carbon).

IV. ANTICOAGULANTS

For the conduct of hemoperfusion it is necessary to use anticoagulants. Most commonly heparin is the choice, but other anticoagulants have been used (prostacyclin, acid-citrate dextrose). More heparin is required than is

Table 1 Some Commercially Available Hemoperfusion Devices

Manufacturer	Device	Sorbent type	Amount of sorbent	Polymer coating
Gambro	Adsorba	Norit	100 or 300 g	Cellulose acetate
Organon-Teknika	Hemopur 260	Norit extruded charcoal	260 g	Cellulose acetate
Smith and Nephew	Hemocol or Haemocol	Sucliffe Speakman charcoal	100 or 300 g	Acrylic hydrogel
Braun	Haemoresin	XAD-4 resin	350 g	None

used in hemodialysis, and the goal is to achieve an activated clotting time (ACT) similar to that needed for hemodialysis. Optimization of anticoagulation in large measure reduces the loss of platelets and fibrinogen, as does coating of particles by synthetic ultra-thin membranes. When combined with hemodialysis, there may be a change in anticoagulant requirements: monitoring of ACT and adjustment of heparin dosing should be done.

V. COMPLICATIONS

The most common complications of hemoperfusion are shown in Table 2. Complications relate to mechanical design or use faults, incompatibility of blood-surface interaction, and the nature of substances adsorbed or released by the sorbent.

A. Mechanical

Particle embolization, a feature of the early poorly washed hemoperfusion devices, has been improved by selecting charcoal resistant to attrition (petroleum based or pyrolized resin charcoal, polystyrene resins) (10,11), by using polymer coating techniques (12), and by washing procedures applied on a commercial scale, each of which reduces particulate matter to acceptable infusion fluid limits (required by federal or other agencies). Failure to circulate blood flow in a laminar fashion through cylindrical devices (by placing the device in a vertical position) causes "channeling," where blood is forced along a path along the device perimeter or in a path in minimal contact with sorbent, which leads to significant reduction in efficiency of sorption. Air bubbles may be introduced during filling of the devices or during set-up with saline infusion containing air, resulting in air-blood interaction and blood clotting or reduced sorption surface, and should be avoided. Using sorbent particles of varying size leads to compaction of small particles against larger ones, and hence to unacceptably high hydraulic pressures within devices, and mechanical hemolysis. Selection of optimal and uniform particles sizes overcomes this problem. Most device housings are sealed with plastic glues, which occasionally can be disrupted (particularly when high pressures are developed inside the column), causing blood leaks. All devices should be closely inspected prior to use. A 1–2°C fall in blood temperature may occur across the devices, which are not heated. Rarely is this a problem, except in the hypothermic patient; combination with hemodialysis overcomes this problem. If devices containing limited quantities of sorbent are used, the device may become saturated with a particular species of chemical; this may also be seen in drug overdose patients, necessitating a change in cartridge to maintain efficient drug removal. In children it is possible to use large (adult) extracorporeal blood volume–containing devices, provided that the devices are primed with anticoagulated whole blood (13).

B. Incompatible Blood-Surface Interface

Profound platelet depletion seen with early uncoated charcoal hemoperfusion devices (14–16) has been overcome with the introduction of microencapsulation techniques; current hemoperfusion devices produce platelet losses of 30% or less (Fig. 2). In one severely poisoned patient the combination of salicylate-induced platelet sensitivity and hemoperfusion produced a profound platelet loss (Fig. 2) (17). Using collodion (cellulose nitrate), with or without albumin, improves platelet losses considerably (18–20). Other polymer

Table 2 Complications Arising During Hemoperfusion

Mechanical	Related to incompatible blood-surface interface	Substances adsorbed or released by the sorbent
Particle embolization	Thrombocytopenia	Hypocalcemia
Channeling	Platelet aggregates	Hypoglycemia
Air trapping	Leukopenia	Pyrogenic reaction
Packing of adsorbent	Complement activation	Trace metal and hormone removal
Hemolysis	Fibrinogen depletion and adsorption	Charcoal residuals
Temperature reduction		
Saturation of adsorbent by chemical species		

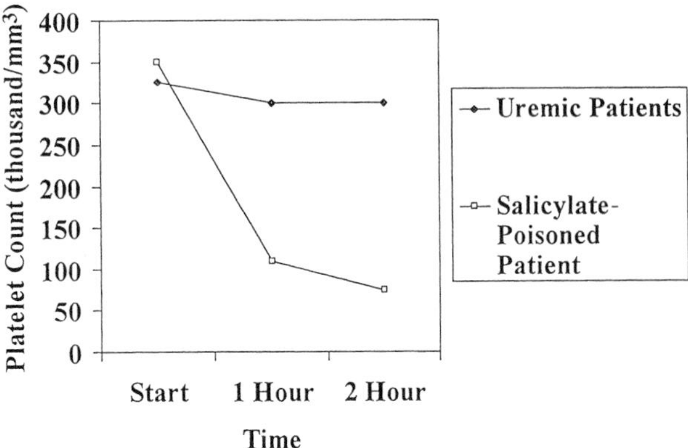

Fig. 2 Platelet counts in uremic patients (mean of five subjects), and one patient severely poisoned with salicylate, in response to coated charcoal hemoperfusion. [Personal observations]

coatings, such as hydrophilic methacrylate, also have been associated with minimal change in platelets during treatment (21). Transient leukopenia, similar to that observed during hemodialysis, occurs during hemoperfusion in humans and may be a result of complement activation by surface contact, with margination of leukocytes similar to that observed during hemodialysis (22). Adsorption or activation of coagulation factors has also been observed during clinical hemoperfusion. The most significant change is a minor reduction in the fibrinogen concentration and fibronectin (23), even with polymer-coated activated charcoal devices (24), but no appreciable changes in coagulation factors II–XII have been observed as a response to charcoal hemoperfusion in uremic patients. The side effects outlined above, although minor in nature, have stimulated the search for more biocompatible activated carbon adsorbents in the form of carbon-containing membranes and fibers (25,26).

Hemostatic changes are particularly severe in patients with hepatic failure and may be associated with the production of platelet aggregates (27), with the possibility that these produce vasoactive amines responsible for hypotension observed frequently during hemoperfusion in hepatic coma. This has not been observed in uremic patients treated with charcoal hemoperfusion. Agents to reduce platelet aggregability such as sulfinpyrazone or aspirin can reduce platelet adhesion to activated charcoal in an ex vivo hemoperfusion test system (28). Prostacyclin adjunctive to heparin, or alone, has been used in humans undergoing hemoperufsion for hepatic coma (29). Additionally, other coagulation disturbances may be prevented with prostacyclin (30).

Hemoperfusion devices may possess a large residual blood; where measured, clinically acceptable mean residual blood volumes of between 3.1 and 7 mL were observed (31,32).

C. Substances Adsorbed or Released by the Sorbent

Small quantities of calcium and glucose are removed, usually with finite saturation characteristics in the first hour of hemoperfusion; replacement with intravenous 10% calcium chloride and 5% dextrose, respectively, correct the abnormalities. Pyrogenic reactions observed with early charcoal hemoperfusion devices are not observed with modern hemoperfusion devices that have been subjected to large-scale washing techniques. The use of ion-exchange resins and nonionic resins that are not specifically prepared for medical use can be associated with pyrogenic events. The XAD series of resins are pyrogen free. Hormones and trace metals can be adsorbed by activated charcoal devices (33,34), but sine these devices are not used repetitively there is little likelihood of deficiency states being induced. A postulated complication of repetitive therapy relates to the effect of charcoal residuals, particularly hydrocarbons, on those charcoals prepared from petroleum or pitch. In addition, metallic or other contaminants within the carbon may theoretically produce cumulative toxicity, although these contaminants can be substantially reduced with special washing techniques (35).

REFERENCES

1. Samtleben W, Gurland HJ, Lysaght MJ, Winchester JF. Plasma exchange and hemoperfusion. In: Replacement of Renal Function by Dialysis. Dordrecht: Kluwer Academic Publisher; 1996:472–500.
2. Fremond B, Joly A, Desille M, Desjardins JF, Campion JP, Clement B. Cell-based therapy of acute liver failure: the extracorporeal bioartifical liver. Cell Biol Toxicol 1996; 12:325–329.
3. Humes HD, Mackay SM, Funke AJ, Buffington DA. The bioartificial renal tubule assist device to enhance CRRT in acute renal failure. Am J Kidney Dis 1997; 30(5 suppl 4):S28–S31.
4. Jaber BL, Barrett TW, Cendoroglo Neto M, Sundaram S, King AJ, Pereira BJ. Endotoxin removal by polymyxin-B immobilized polystyrene-derivative fibers during in vitro hemoperfusion of 10% human plasma. ASAIO J 1998; 44:54–61.
5. Xu Y, Lorf T, Sablinski T, Gianello P, Bailin M, Monroy R, Kozlowski T, Awwad M, Cooper DK, Sachs DH. Removal of anti-porcine natural antibodies from human

and nonhuman primate plasma in vitro and in vivo by a Galalpha1-3Galbeta1-4betaGlc-X immunoaffinity column. Transplantation 1998; 65:172–179.
6. Bosch T, Schmidt B, Kleophas W, Otto V, Samtleben W. LDL hemoperfusion—a new procedure for LDL apheresis: biocompatibility results from a first pilot study in hypercholesterolemic atherosclerosis patients. Artif Organs 1997; 21:1060–1065.
7. Ash SR. Hemodiabsorption in treatment of acute hepatic failure and chronic cirrhosis with ascites. Artif Organs 1994; 18:355–362.
8. Ash SR, Blake DE, Carr DJ, Carter C, Howard T, Makowka L. Neurologic improvement of patients with hepatic failure and coma during sorbent suspension dialysis. ASAIO Trans 1991; 37:M332–M334.
9. Ash SR, Blake DE, Carr DJ, Harker KD. Push-pull sorbent based pheresis for treatment of acute hepatic failure: the BioLogic-detoxifier/plasma filter System. ASAIO J 1998; 44:129.
10. Asher WJ. Introduction to sorbents. In: Giordano C, ed. Sorbents and Their Clinical Applications. New York: Academic Press, Inc., 1980:3.
11. Denti E, Walker JM. Activated carbon: properties, selection and evaluation. In: Giordano C, ed. Sorbents and Their Clinical Applications. New York: Academic Press, Inc., 1980:101.
12. Denti E, Luboz MP, Tessore V. Adsorption characteristics of cellulose acetate charcoals. J Biomed Mater Res 1975; 9:143.
13. Mauer S, Chavers BM, Kjellstrand CM. Treatment of an infant with severe chloramphenicol intoxication, using charcoal-column hemoperfusion. J Pediatr 1980; 96:136.
14. Yatzidis H. A convenient hemoperfusion micro-apparatus over charcoal for the treatment of endogenous and exogenous intoxications. Its used as an artificial kidney. Proc Eur Dial Transplan Assoc 1964; 1:83.
15. Dunea G, Kolff WJ. Clinical experience with the Yatzidis charcoal artificial kidney. Trans Am Soc Arhf Intern Organs 1965; 11:178.
16. Hagstam KE, Larsson LE, Thysell H. Experimental studies on charcoal hemoperfusion in phenobarbital intoxication and uremia, including histopathologic findings. Acta Med Scand 1966; 180:593.
17. Winchester JF, Forbes CD, Lang D, Courtney JM, Prentice CRM. Platelet function regulating agents—experimental data relevant to renal disease. In: Mitchell JRA, Domenet IG, eds. Thromboembolism—A New Approach to Therapy. New York: Academic Press, 1977: 83–103.
18. Chang TMS. Semipermeable aqueous microcapsules (artificial cells): with emphasis on experiments in an extracorpeal shunt system. Trans Am Soc Artif Intern Organs 1966; 12:13.
19. Odaka M, Tabata Y, Kobayashi H, Nomura Y, Soma M, Hirasawa H, Sato H, Suenaga E, Nabeta K. Three hour maintenance hemodialysis combining direct hemoperfusion and hemodialysis. Proc Eur Transplant Assoc 1976; 13:257.
20. Ota K, Ohta T, Kobayashi M, Yoshida S, Kaneko, Agishi T, Sugihara M. Petroleum based activated charcoal for direct haemoperfusion. Proc Eur Dial Transplant Assoc 1976; 13:250.
21. Stefoni S, Feliciangeli G, Coli L, Bonomini V. Evaluation of a new coated charcoal for hemoperfusion in uremia. Int J Artif Organs 1979; 2:320.
22. Craddock PR, Fehr J, Brigham KL, Kronenherg R, Jacobs HS. Complement and leukocyte-mediated pulmonary dysfunction in hemodialysis. N Engl J Med 1977; 296:769.
23. Pott G, Voss B, Lohmann J, Zundorf P. Loss of fibronectin in plasma of patients with shock and septicaemia and aher haemoperfusion in patients with severe poisoning. J Clin Chem Clin Biochem 1982; 20:333.
24. Winchester JF, Ratcliffe JG, Carlyle E, Kennedy AC. Solute, amino acid, and hormone changes with coated charcoal hemoperfusion in uremia. Kidney Int 1978; 14:74.
25. Gurland HJ, Fernandez JC, Samtleben W, Castro LA. Sorbent membranes used in a conventional dialyzer format: In vitro and clinical evaluation. Artif Organs 1978; 2:372.
26. Davis TA, Cowsar DR, Harrison SD, Tanquary AC. Artificial carbone hbers for hemoperfusion. Trans Am Soc Artif Intern Organs 1974; 20:353.
27. Weston MJ, Langley PG, Rubin MH, Hanid MA, Mellon P, Williams R. Platelet function in fulminant hepatic failure and effect of charcoal haemoperfusion. Gut 1977; 18:897.
28. Winchester JF, Forbes CD, Courtney JM, Reavey M, Prentice CRM. Effect of sulphinpyrazone and aspirin on platelet adhesion to activated charcoal and dialysis membranes in vitro. Thromb Res 1977; 11:443.
29. Gimson AE, Langley PC, Hughes RD, Canalese J, Mellon PG, Williams R, Woods HF, Weston MJ. Prostacyclin to prevent platelet activation during charcoal hemoperfusion in fulminant hepatic failure. Lancet 1980; 1:173.
30. Woods HF, Weston MJ, Bunting S, Moncada S, Vane J. Prostacyclin eliminates the thrombocyopenia associated with charcoal hemoperfusion and minimizes heparin and fibrinogen consumption. Artif Organ 1980; 4: 176.
31. Stefoni S, Coli L, Feliciangeli G, Baldrati L, Bonomini V. Regular hemoperfusion in regular dialysis treatment. A long-term study. Int J Artif Organs 1980; 3:348.
32. Chang TMS, Chirito E, Barre B, Cole C, Hewish M. Clinical performance characteristics of a new combined system for simultaneous hemoperfusion-hemodialysis-ultrafiltiation in series. Trans Am Soc Artif Inter Organs 1975; 21:502.
33. Kokot F, Pietrek J, Seredynski M. Influence of hemoperfusion on plasma levels of hormones and B-methy-

lidigoxin. Proc Eur Dial Transplant Assoc 1978; 15: 604.
34. Cornelis R, Ringoir S, Mees L, Hoste J. Behavior of trace metals during hemoperfusion. Miner Electrolyte Metab 1980; 4:113.
35. Fennimore JC, Kolthammer JC, Lang SM. Evaluation of hemoperfusion systems: in vitro methods related to performance and safety. In: Kenedi RM, Courtney JM, Gaylor JDS, Gilchrist T, eds. Artificial Organs. London: MacMillan, 1977:148–157.

8

Complications of Peritoneal Access in Acute and Chronic Peritoneal Dialysis

Madhukar Misra, Zbylut J. Twardowski, and Ramesh Khanna
University of Missouri–Columbia, Columbia, Missouri

I. INTRODUCTION

The peritoneal catheter is a lifeline for the peritoneal dialysis patient. Still the most widely used catheter for continuous ambulatory peritoneal dialysis (CAPD), the double-cuff silicone Tenckhoff catheter was developed in 1968 for treatment of patients with intermittent peritoneal dialysis (1). Catheter-related complications are increased in CAPD due to higher intra-abdominal pressure and numerous daily manipulations. Modifications of catheter design, placement techniques, meticulous postoperative care, and a standardized break in procedure have contributed to overall increased longevity, better catheter function and a reduction in catheter-related complications such as catheter-tip migration, dialysate leaks, and exit-site infections. Catheter exit-site and tunnel infections are, however, frequent in patients on CAPD and are the major causes of increased morbidity, prolonged antibiotic therapy, recurrent peritonitis, and catheter failure. A 1987 National CAPD registry report mentioned that 12.4% of catheters are removed because of exit or tunnel infection (2). This chapter will present practical aspects of complications and the management of peritoneal access in both acute and chronic peritoneal dialysis.

Peritoneal access may be required for peritoneal dialysis in both acute and chronic situations. For acute peritoneal dialysis, the access may be achieved by either rigid or soft catheters.

A. Rigid Catheters

Stylocath (Abbott Laboratories, North Chicago, IL) and the Trocath (Baxter Healthcare Corporation, Deerfield, IL) are the two most widely used rigid catheters in North America. It is important to realize that proper assessment and preparation prior to catheter insertion prevents complications and improves outcome.

B. Assessment of the Patient and Preinsertion Preparation

Nowadays, the rigid catheter is used as an access for peritoneal dialysis only under emergent situations. One of the major advantages of the rigid catheter is that it may be inserted at the bedside with very minimal preparation. Equipment required for paracentesis is all that is needed. Presence of extreme obesity or a history of previous abdominal surgery are contraindications for bedside insertion, since abdominal adhesions increase the risk of inadvertent viscus perforation. In addition, this approach should not be used in children except by an experienced pediatric nephrologist or a nephrologist with a pediatrician in attendance. The presence of a standby surgeon is mandatory in the event of a nephrologist implanting the catheter in order to deal with unexpected complications. Needless to say, all observers and persons in the immediate area, including the patient, should wear surgical masks.

A detailed description of insertion methodology of peritoneal dialysis catheters is beyond the scope of this chapter and may be found elsewhere (3). In this chapter, we will restrict the discussion to acute and chronic complications of peritoneal access.

II. COMPLICATIONS OF RIGID CATHETER INSERTION

Table 1 shows the complications of rigid catheter insertion.

A. Bloody Effluent

In approximately 30% of all cases blood will appear in the dialysate effluent after the first exchange (4,5) following catheter implantation. This bleeding (usually minor) comes from the small vessels in the abdominal wall. Bleeding usually stops after three to four exchanges unless the procedure has damaged a major vessel or the patient has a bleeding disorder. Minor bleeding can usually be controlled by pressure applied over the catheter insertion site. Occasionally, a transfusion of fresh blood will stop the bleeding. The catheter may become obstructed if the bleeding is copious; in this event, addition of 1000 units of heparin to each liter of dialysate will minimize the risk of obstruction. Though heparin (MW 15,000 daltons) prevents clot formation in the peritoneal cavity, its systemic absorption is poor and thus does not influence systemic coagulation.

B. Dialysis-Solution Leak

After rigid catheter insertion, this problem is encountered in 14–36% of patients (4–6). Factors predisposing patients to an increased risk of dialysis solution leak from the catheter exit site include frequent manipulation of the catheter to improve drainage, a catheter that is improperly secured to the skin, and being elderly or debilitated. In the latter group the risk of external leak is higher because of lax abdominal walls. The presence of a large intra-abdominal mass, such as polycystic kidneys, may cause high intra-abdominal pressure and promote an external dialysis solution leak after the standard 2-L volume has been instilled.

Table 1 Complications of Rigid Catheter Insertion

Bleeding
Dialysis-solution leak
Poor drainage
Extraperitoneal space penetration
Viscus perforation
Peritonitis
Abdominal pain
Loss of rigid catheter in the peritoneum

C. Fluid Extravasation

Dialysis fluid may extravasate into the abdominal wall, particularly in patients who have had a previous abdominal operation or multiple catheter insertions. This complication usually results from tears in the peritoneum or represents an infusion of dialysate into the potential space between the layers of abdominal wall. Dialysis fluid may enter the pleural cavity (7–9) in rare situations. Peritoneal dialysis may have to be discontinued and the patients switched to hemodialysis in such a situation. A traumatic or a congenital defect in the diaphragm may result in acute hydrothorax.

D. Inadequate Drainage

Problems with adequate drainage are not infrequent during initial dialysis. One or more of the following factors may be responsible: loss of siphon effect, one-way obstruction, and/or incorrect placement of the catheter. One-way (outflow) catheter obstruction may have multiple causes. Particularly following major hemorrhage or peritonitis, fibrin or blood clots may be trapped in the catheter and block the terminal holes. Extrinsic pressure on the catheter from adjacent organs such as a sigmoid colon full of feces or a distended bladder may also present as poor outflow. Omental wrapping is likely if the catheter is misplaced into the upper abdomen.

Accidental penetration of the extraperitoneal space by the catheter may occasionally cause poor drainage. In such cases, continued infusion may produce further dissection, thus entrapping the fluid and making the fluid unavailable for drainage. Previous intra-abdominal operations or peritonitis may lead to adhesions and loculation of fluid leading to poor drainage. Such compartmentalization of fluid not only diminishes the surface area available for dialysis, but may seriously reduce ultrafiltration capacity. The incidence of this complication is low, varying between 0.5 and 1.3% (6,10,11).

E. Perforation or Laceration

Bedside insertion of the catheter resulting in complications such as perforation or laceration of internal organs has been frequently reported. These organs include the bowel, bladder, liver, a polycystic kidney, aorta, mesenteric artery, and hernia sac (10–16). Predisposing factors comprise abdominal adhesions and distention due to paralytic ileus or bowel obstruction, and unconscious, cachectic, or heavily sedated patients. Bowel perforation may be heralded by sudden, sharp or severe abdominal pain followed by watery diarrhea and poor drainage of dialysis solution, which may be cloudy, foul-smelling, or mixed with fecal material. Such a situation requires prompt removal of the catheter, allowing the perforation to seal off completely in about 12–24 hours. Bowel perforation can be serious and may be fatal in rare cases (17). Bladder injury may be avoided by prior voiding and/or urethral catheterization before the catheter insertion (18).

F. Peritonitis

Following the use of stylet catheter, the incidence of peritonitis was 2.5% of all dialyses (19). It almost doubled when the duration of dialysis was longer than 60 hours.

G. Abdominal Pain

Approximately 56–75% of patients encounter pain in the abdomen with the first use of the catheter (4). Catheter-related pain occurs when the catheter impinges on any of the viscera. Pain may occur during inflow and outflow of dialysis solution and also when the solution is dwelling. Outflow pain is due to entrapment of omentum in the catheter during the siphoning action of fluid drainage. Constant pain during dialysis indicates pressure effects on intra-abdominal organs and often produces continuous rectal or low back pain and may require an adjustment in catheter position.

H. Loss of Part or All of the Rigid Catheter

When the catheter is manipulated with the trocar in place, part or all of the catheter may be lost (4,13,19). The distal end of the catheter may be amputated after intra-abdominal kinking of the catheter, followed by manipulation. The presence of broken catheters within the abdominal cavity, however, does not cause symptoms or ill effects. Broken catheters have been found lying freely in the peritoneal cavity without causing a peritoneal reaction; they have also been found walled off by mesentery without an inflammatory reaction. During laparoscopy, Stein (20) discovered such a catheter in a patient who had previous peritoneal dialysis on a routine postmortem examination. Exploration to retrieve the catheter is unnecessary because laparotomy is more hazardous than leaving the catheter in a severely ill patient. The incidence of catheter loss into the peritoneal cavity has been greatly reduced since the introduction of a catheter design that incorporates a metal disk with a central hole.

III. COMPLICATIONS OF SOFT-CATHETER INSERTION

Since rigid catheters are associated with a high frequency of dialysis solution leaks and poor drainage (necessitating frequent catheter manipulation and resultant peritonitis), some centers prefer to insert single or double-cuff Tenckhoff or swan-neck Tenckhoff catheters for the treatment of acute renal failure. Tenckhoff recommended using a single-cuff catheter for acute cases (1). For treatment of chronic renal failure only soft catheters are used. Several modifications in the design of soft catheters have been made over the years. A brief description of these modifications is provided here for a better understanding of these improvements in catheter design.

The Tenckhoff catheter, swan neck catheter, and Toronto Western Hospital catheter (Figs. 1 and 2) are the most commonly used catheters in chronic peritoneal dialysis. The Tenckhoff catheter is available in straight and coiled intra-abdominal configurations (single or double cuffed). Of the various types of soft catheters available for chronic peritoneal dialysis, the use of catheters with a bent intramural segment (swan-neck catheters) has increased significantly. The swan-neck design enables catheter placement in an arcuate tunnel with both external and internal segments of the tunnel directed downward without stress. Features reducing the exit/tunnel infection rates (Table 2) include downward-directed exit, two cuffs, and short sinus. The intercuff bend permanently eliminates the Silastic® resilience force or the "shape memory," which tends to extrude the external cuff. Downward peritoneal entrance tends to keep the tip in the true pelvis, reducing its migration. Pericatheter leaks are decreased due to insertion through the rectus muscle. Lower exit/tunnel infection rates curtail peritonitis episodes. Swan-neck versions of the different catheters in use include the Tenckhoff catheter, Missouri straight and coiled cath-

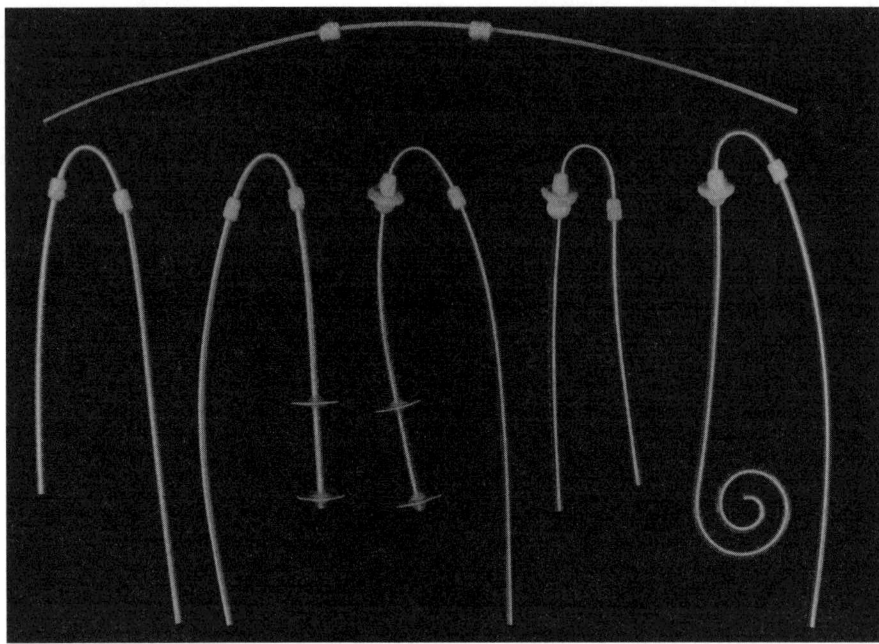

Fig. 1 (Top) Double-cuff Tenckhoff catheter with straight intraperitoneal segment. (Bottom) Five catheters, each with a bent intramural segment. Left-to-right: (1) swan-neck straight Tenckhoff, (2) swan-neck Tenckhoff with intraperitoneal disks, (3) swan-neck with bead, flange, and intraperitoneal disks for left tunnel, (4) swan-neck Missouri 2 straight for left tunnel, (5) swan-neck Missouri 2 coiled for left tunnel.

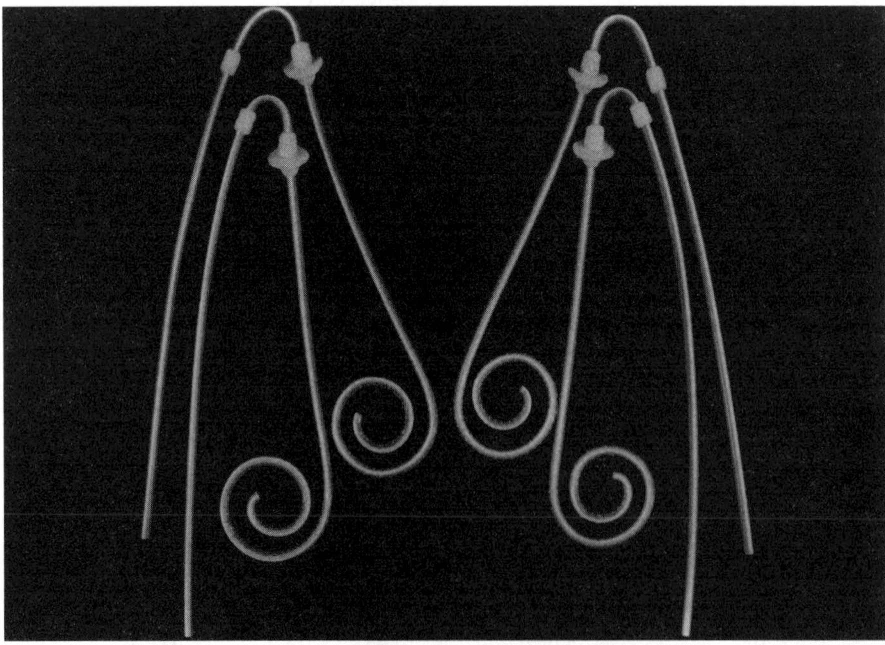

Fig. 2 Swan-neck Missouri 2 (upper) and 3 (lower) catheters with coiled intraperitoneal segments. Left-tunnel catheters to the right; right tunnel catheters to the left. The intercuff distance is 5 cm in Missouri 2 and 3 cm in Missouri 3 catheters. Stripes are to the front. The catheters for left and right tunnels are mirror images of each other.

Table 2 Features of Swan-Neck Catheter that Prevent Complications

Complication	Feature preventing complication
Exit/Tunnel infection	Downward exit, double cuff, short sinus
External cuff extrusion	Permanent bend between cuffs
Intraperitoneal tip migration	Downward intraperitoneal entrance
Pericatheter leak	Insertion through the rectus muscle
Peritonitis	Decreased tunnel infections
Infusion/Pressure pain	Coiled intraperitoneal tip

eter, Missouri presternal catheter, and Moncrief-Popovich catheter. Also, the use of catheters with a coiled intraperitoneal segment has significantly gone up in North America (21). Catheters with a coiled intraperitoneal segment minimize infusion and pressure pain.

The presternal catheter (Fig. 3) was designed primarily to decrease infectious complications in special categories of patients. The chest is a sturdy structure; when the catheter exit is located on the chest wall, the minimal wall motion decreases the chances of trauma and contamination. A chest exit also decreases the chances of contamination in patients with abdominal ostomies and in children with diapers. A loose garment usually worn on the chest may exert less pressure on the exit. Clinical surgical experience indicates the wounds heal better after thoracic surgery than after abdominal surgery; this may be because there is less mobility in the chest, or there may be other reasons. Obese patients have higher exit-site infection rates and a tendency to poor wound healing, particularly after abdominal surgery. If fat thickness per se is responsible for quality of healing and susceptibility to infection, then an exit on the chest, where there is a relatively thinner layer of subcutaneous fat, may be preferred for obese patients. All these favorable factors, together with easy exit-site care using a magnifying mirror, significantly reduce exit-site infections. The location of the catheter exit on the chest is particularly advantageous in small children owing to the greater distance from the diaper area and lesser trauma during crawling/creeping. There may be psychosocial advantages also for a chest exit. A chest exit location allows a deep tub bath without the risk of exit contamination. A long catheter tunnel combined with three cuffs may hinder pericatheter bacterial penetration into the peritoneal cavity, thus reducing the incidence of peritonitis (22–25).

The implantation of chronic dialysis catheters may be done by blind (Tenckhoff trocar) method, peritoneoscopically, Seldinger's method, or by surgical dissection. Surgical placement is mandatory for catheters with stabilizing devices at the parietal surfaces (Toronto Western, swan-neck Missouri, and swan-neck presternal). A subcutaneous tunnel of 3–7 cm is fashioned through the abdominal wall to an exit site laterally. Postoperatively, careful and meticulous catheter and exit-site care ensure excellent subsequent function.

A. Early Complications of Soft Catheters

Early complications post–soft-catheter insertion are similar to those after implantation of the rigid catheter, but their frequency is lower, particularly with surgical and peritoneoscopic insertion.

1. Bleeding

Blood-tinged dialysate is common postimplantation, but severe bleeding occurs very rarely with surgical insertion.

2. Dialysate Leak

If ambulatory peritoneal dialysis is postponed for at least 10 days after implantation (26), dialysate leaks are unlikely. With swan-neck Missouri and swan-neck presternal catheters, which utilize stabilizing devices at the peritoneal surfaces, this complication is particularly rare. Serous drainage from the exit may be confused with an early leak, which is usually external. A higher glucose concentration in the drainage than in simultaneously measured blood glucose concentration supports the diagnosis of a leak. The leak may resolve by temporarily switching to small-volume supine dialysis or short-term hemodialysis. Some authors recommend antibiotics for dialysate leaks from the exit site (27), since they are often associated with infection.

3. Obstruction

Table 3 presents the most common causes of peritoneal catheter obstruction and their treatment.

Two-way obstruction is usually due to a closed tubing clamp or kinking of the catheter or extension tubing. Major hemorrhage or peritonitis may also completely block the catheter lumen by fibrin or blood clots.

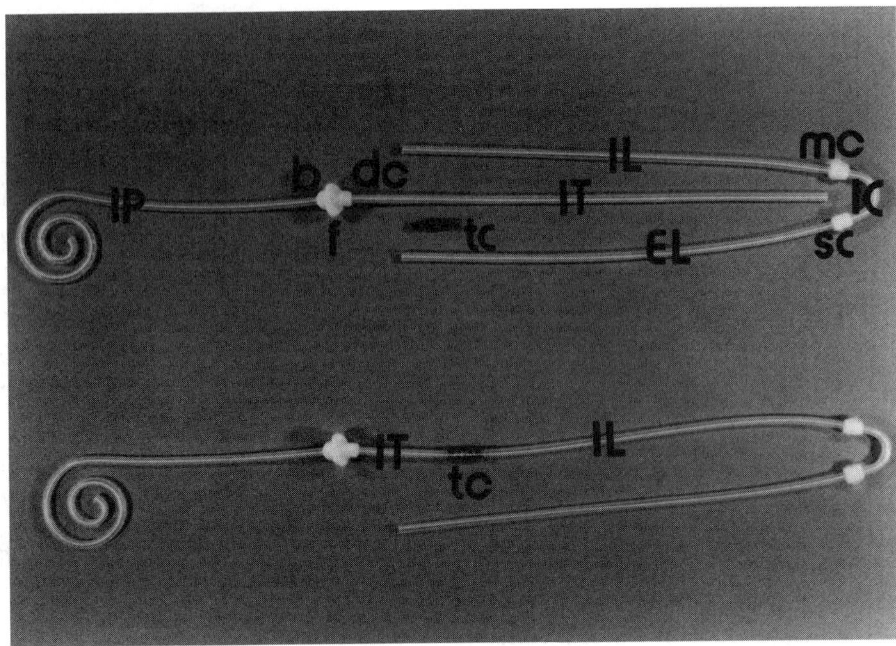

Fig. 3 Two tubes of the swan-neck presternal peritoneal catheter before (top) and after (bottom) connection. Both tubes and bead are made of silicon rubber molded in the shapes as shown. A flange and all cuffs are made of woven polyester fibers. The proximal (upper, chest) tube (PT) consists of an intratunnel limb (IL), medial (center) cuff (mc), intercuff segment (IC), superficial cuff (sc), and external limb (EL); 1–2 cm of the external limb adjacent to the superficial cuff is intended to be in the sinus tract of the tunnel (from the cuff to the exit). The distal (abdominal, lower) tube (DT) consists of an intratunnel segment (IT), deep (distal, preperitoneal) cuff (dc), flange (f), bead (b), and intraperitoneal segment (IP). After implantation (bottom), the intratunnel limb (IL) of the chest tube and the intratunnel segment (IT) of the abdominal tube are trimmed to the size of the tunnel and coupled with the titanium connector (tc).

One-way obstruction is usually equated with the failure to drain; fluid can be infused, but cannot be drained. Extrinsic pressure on the catheter tip from adjacent organs such as a sigmoid colon full of feces or a distended bladder may cause poor outflow. Among all the known causes of catheter obstruction, constipation is the most common. Fecal loading of the colon resulting in poorly functioning catheter is very often relieved by simple bowel-emptying measures like laxatives and enema. Omental wrapping is likely if the catheter is misplaced into the upper abdomen. One-way obstruction may be caused by fibrin or blood clots if only a few proximal side holes remain open, which then become easily blocked by adjacent organs. Emptying the bladder and using laxatives may restore catheter function if there is occlusion by bladder or bowel. A clot may be prevented by rinsing out blood from the peritoneal cavity and using heparin and/or dislodged by pushing into the peritoneal cavity or pulling by suction using a syringe filled with heparinized saline. Urokinase (Abbokinase) 5000 IU diluted in normal saline may be instilled into the catheter if these maneuvers are unsuccessful. Urokinase may relieve the obstruction in 10–15% of cases (28). Catheter kinking in the tunnel usually leads to two-way obstruction, recognizable on an abdominal film in two views. Surgical correction is usually required.

Table 3 Early Catheter Obstruction

Cause of obstruction	Prevention/Treatment
Occlusion by bowel	Laxatives
Occlusion by bladder	Empty bladder
Clot	Rinse out blood
	Heparin, urokinase
	Dislodge
Omental wrap	Partial omentectomy
Multiple adhesion	Adhesiolysis
Kink in the tunnel	Surgical correction

A reversed one-way obstruction occurs when the fluid can be drained but the next infusion cannot be performed. This is extremely rare. We observed such a case recently (29). The catheter tip was obstructed with a clot, which was causing inflow obstruction. Suction with a syringe removed the clot. We speculated that the clot was firmly anchored in the catheter tip and that only a few proximal side holes were opened. The outflow was not obstructed because the catheter tip must have been located in a large pocket of free space. The clot behaved like an accordion. During drainage the clot became stretched and narrowed (like an accordion bellow in extension) and fluid was able to flow through some of the side holes. During infusion the clot buckled up and widened (like a compressed accordion bellow), completely occluding the central lumen and side holes.

A catheter adhering to the peritoneum may be another reason for obstruction. This complication was found in children who have undergone partial omentectomy at the time of insertion of a single-cuff, straight Tenckhoff catheter. Repositioning of such catheters may be attempted by various methods utilizing either a steel trocar, a pliable copper thread, or a guide wire. The basic principles of this manipulation involve the following: after localization of the catheter adherence site, using a strict sterile technique, a blunted steel trocar is inserted into the catheter and gently advanced until the trocar tip is 5–7 cm proximal to the tip of the catheter. The deep cuff is used as a fulcrum and short and rapid whiplash motions are made (whiplash technique) (30) and the catheter is then freed from the adherence point. The catheter tip is then, under fluoroscopy, repositioned to a new site. Applying the same principle, a pliable copper thread (in adults) (31) or a guide wire (32,33) (in upper abdominal translocation) have been used for catheter manipulation. These methods are not without risks. There is inherent risk of wire fracture leading to catheter perforation and recurrent peritonitis. We do not use these methods in our institution.

Functioning catheters may migrate out of true pelvis for various reasons. This is documented frequently on abdominal x-rays (34). While about 20% of x-rays showed the catheter tip translocated to the upper abdomen, only 20% of these translocated catheters (4% of the total) were obstructed. The remaining functioning malpositioned catheters were either permanently translocated or repositioned spontaneously to the true pelvis. About 3% of catheters in our series were obstructed with the tip in the true pelvis (35).

While the great majority of malpositioned catheters are not obstructed, a catheter with its tip in the upper abdomen is still about six times more likely to be obstructed than a normally positioned catheter. The migration of the catheter tip may, however, be the result of the obstruction rather than its cause; omentum entangling the catheter tip may be responsible for its translocation.

If in the absence of catheter kinking, the catheter does not function for two weeks even after trying the above-described maneuvers, omental wrapping or multiple adhesions are most likely, and omentectomy or adhesiolysis through laparoscopy may be required. In our experience, if this method fails to restore catheter function, the peritoneum is not fit for peritoneal dialysis because of massive adhesions. Replacement of the catheter in such a situation is usually unhelpful. The patient almost always has to be transferred to hemodialysis.

4. Viscus Perforation and Peritonitis

With surgically inserted catheters, viscus perforation is unheard of. Early peritonitis with a soft catheter is half that reported with a rigid catheter, even in treatment of acute renal failure (36).

5. Pain in the Abdomen

Mild analgesics such as acetaminophen can usually control minimal pain after catheter insertion. It is important to avoid opiates because they cause constipation and frequently vomiting, maneuvers that may increase intra-abdominal pressure and predispose the patient to pericatheter leaks (37). Abdominal pain at the catheter tip is more likely with straight catheters due to "jet effect" and tip pressure. This pain usually subsides within a few days; however, it may become chronic and require treatment (see below).

B. Late Complications of Soft Catheters

Complications are not randomly distributed throughout the life of the catheter. Table 4 represents some of the common complications occurring late in the course of the life of a peritoneal dialysis catheter. Whereas leaks and malfunctions occur shortly after catheter implan-

Table 4 Common Catheter-Related Complications

Exit/Tunnel infection
External-cuff extrusion
Catheter obstruction
Pericatheter leak/Hernias
Peritonitis
Infusion or pressure pain

tation, infectious complications lead to catheter failure later (38).

Any discussion of exit-site infection would be incomplete without information on the healing process following catheter implantation and the meticulous postoperative care that such patients require. A detailed knowledge of the various steps involved in the healing process and the appearances of normal as well as abnormal exit sites improves management and prevents long-term complications.

We have been studying the healing process of the exit after catheter implantation since 1988. Forty-three exits in 41 patients were examined weekly for 6 weeks with a magnifying loupe and macro-photographed. Cultures were taken from sterile saline sinus washouts, peri-exit smears, and nares. A detailed report of the study with over 200 color pictures of various exit appearances has recently been published (39,40). A brief summary of the findings will be provided here.

In optimally healing exits, at one week postimplantation slight tenderness is present in about one third of exits, a scab is visible in almost all exits, and epidermis surrounding the exit orifice is pale pink or pink. A small amount of serosanguineous, bloody, or serous drainage is visible around the exit in about half of patients. There is no swelling. Drainage inside the sinus is visible in almost all sinuses and is similar in character to that seen outside. There is no epithelium visible in the sinus; the sinus is lined with a white tissue, which resembles aponeurosis.

External drainage abates by week 2 and is absent by week 3. Scabs diminish by week 3 and are not seen after week 4. Exit color remains pale pink or pink throughout the 6-week period. Drainage in the sinus diminishes and most sinuses are dry at week 6. Sinus lining remains flat but is gradually transformed into plain granulation tissue. Epithelium starts entering the sinus at week 2 or 3, progresses steadily, and covers at least half of the visible sinus tract by 5 weeks after implantation. Epithelium is fragile and pale pink or, occasionally, white.

Exits that become infected early do not show signs of healing (progression of epithelium, decrease in drainage amount). Instead, the drainage becomes purulent, the sinus lining becomes composed of granulation tissue at week 1 or 2, and the tissue becomes slightly or frankly exuberant. The presence of purulent drainage and/or slightly exuberant granulation tissue in the sinus alone, without external drainage, is sufficient for diagnosis of early infection.

Early colonization of the exit was the most significant factor in determining the healing pattern; the later the colonization, the better the healing. Positive culture from either washout or peri-exit smear 1 week after implantation was associated with early exit infection, a higher peritonitis rate, and a high probability of catheter loss due to an exit/tunnel infection. Based on these results we postulated that prophylactic antibiotics should be used for at least 2 weeks after catheter implantation and sterile exit dressing procedure for the entire healing time of approximately 6 weeks (39).

Intraperitoneal antibiotic prophylaxis for 3 weeks after catheter implantation has been recently reported to prevent early exit-site colonization and lower catheter-related infection in rats. No such human studies of antibiotic prophylaxis are yet available (40).

C. Factors Influencing Exit-Site Healing

Several factors influence the healing process: tissue perfusion, mechanical factors, bacterial colonization of sinus, epithelization, use of local cleansing agents, exit direction, and systemic factors such as obesity, diabetes mellitus, and immunosuppression.

D. Care

1. Early Care

To delay bacterial colonization of the exit site and minimize trauma, the dressing should not be changed frequently. The surgical dressing is gently removed after 1 week. Sterile nonionic surfactant or saline is used to help gauze removal if it is attached to the scab. If the scab is forcibly removed the epidermal layer is broken, a new scab has to be made, and the epidermization is prolonged. Care is taken to avoid catheter pulling or twisting.

Cleansing agents should not only decrease the number of bacteria, but also be harmless to the body defenses. Strong oxidants like povidone-iodine and hydrogen peroxide are cytotoxic to mammalian cells and should not be used (42,43). Nonionic, amphophilic, nontoxic surfactants, widely used in burn wound care, facilitate necrotic tissue removal without jeopardizing body defense mechanisms (44). In agreement with the experience of others (45), we found 20% Poloxamer 188 (Shur-Clens®; Calgon Vestal Laboratories, St. Louis, MO) to be innocuous, yet excellent in cleansing the exit from contaminants.

The exit and skin surrounding the catheter are cleansed, patted dry with sterile gauze, covered with several layers of gauze dressings, and secured with air-permeable tape. The dressing is changed after another week. The quality of healing should be evaluated until the exit is healed. Weekly dressing changes may be continued throughout the 6-week healing period if drainage is minimal or absent and epithelium progresses steadily. There are two reasons for infrequent dressing changes: first, each dressing change may introduce bacteria into the exit even though a sterile procedure is used; second, the less manipulation of the catheter, the lower the chance of exit trauma. In cases with excessive bleeding or large quantities of drainage from the incision or exit, the dressing should be changed earlier and more frequently. Recently, however, we have increased the frequency of dressing changes to every other day after 2 weeks postimplantation because most of the exits are colonized by this time and the major rationale for infrequent dressing changes (avoidance of exit colonization) no longer exists. If the amount of drainage is minimal, local antibiotics according to sensitivity may be sufficient. With large drainage and overt infection, systemic antibiotics are necessary. Antibiotics should be adjusted according to the sensitivity results. The patients may shower only before the dressing change, otherwise they must take sponge baths and avoid exit wetting.

Protecting the catheter from mechanical stress seems to be extremely important, especially during break-in. Catheters should be anchored in such a way that the patient's movements are only minimally transmitted to the exit. The method of catheter immobilization is individualized, depending on exit location and shape of the abdomen. Immobilization of catheter in the chest is easier but also has to be individualized.

2. Late Care

The care following completion of healing is simpler. Simple cleaning with soap and water provides better preventive care than either povidone-iodine painting or hydrogen peroxide cleaning and, of the three methods, is the least expensive (46). Following cleansing, a sterile gauze should be used to dry the exit and the dressing well immobilized. Most of our patients use a dressing cover for 6–12 months after implantation.

A shower should be advised instead of methods involving submersion under water (i.e., Jacuzzi, hot tub, or public pool) unless watertight exit protection can be implemented. Prolonged submersion in water containing high concentrations of bacteria breeds infection and frequently leads to severe infection with consequent loss of catheter. Following wetting, meticulous care should be exercised in obtaining a well-dried exit. The swan-neck presternal catheter allows the luxury of a hot tub bath without exit-site submersion. Because of this feature this catheter was dubbed the "bathtub" catheter (23).

E. Factors Influencing Infection of a Healed Exit Site

Factors that influence whether the healed catheter tunnel becomes infected include catheter design, catheter location in the created tunnel, bacterial colonization of the sinus, *Staphylococcus aureus* nasal carriage status of the patient, catheter exit-site direction, sinus tract length, number of cuffs, and the materials used for the external cuff and the tubing in the sinus. The importance of *S. aureus* as an etiological agent of peritoneal catheter exit-site infection has been well established. Nasal carriage of *S. aureus* is reported to be common in patients undergoing dialysis (47). A recent multicenter study found an increased incidence of exit-site infection in nasal carriers of *S. aureus*: in 85% of these infections, the strain from the nares and the strain causing the infection were similar in phage typing and antibiotic profile (48). On the other hand, these findings were not confirmed in a subsequent study by Twardowski and Prowant (49). Shorter sinus tract length (50) and double-cuffed instead of single-cuffed catheters (51) may decrease bacterial colonization and exit infection. A shorter sinus tract would, however, increase the chances of cuff extrusion. Also, a recently published national study of the U.S. Renal Data System (USRDS) revealed an increased relative risk for the first peritonitis episode with a single-cuff versus a double-cuff catheter (52). Location of the deep cuff in the muscle provides better vascularization and stronger fibrous tissue ingrowth compared to a cuff located in the subcutaneous tissue. The USRDS study (52) also revealed a reduced relative risk of first peritonitis episode for lateral catheter placement in rectus muscle belly versus midline insertion with deep cuff in subcutaneous position. The tissue ingrowth into the cuff does not seem to constitute a critical barrier for spread of infection per se (53). Additionally, the external cuff anchors the catheter, restricting piston-like movements of the catheter in the sinus.

F. Exit-Site Infection

Pierratos's definition, published in 1984 (54), was agreed upon by the vast majority of *Peritoneal Dialysis Bulletin* editorial board members and has gained wide acceptance. Exit-site infection was defined as "redness or skin induration or purulent discharge from the exit-site. Formation of the crust around the exit may not indicate infection. Positive cultures from the exit site in the absence of inflammation do not indicate infection.'' The definition stressed the presence of infection even in the instances where laboratory cultures are negative and rejected the existence of infection based on a positive culture in the absence of inflammation.

Two possible exit conditions were defined: infected and uninfected. However, unlike peritonitis, which has clear-cut diagnostic criteria, the distinction between infected and noninfected exit may not be obvious and there may be a degree of overlap. This overlap stems from the delicate balance between bacteria in the sinus and host defenses. Low-grade exit infection may abate without systemic antibiotics.

We have performed 565 evaluations of 61 healed exit sites in 56 patients between 1988 and 1994. The exit and the sinus were inspected using a Zeiss prism loupe with 4.5× magnification for the presence, absence, intensity, and/or characterisics of specific attributes such as swelling, color, crust, drainage, granulation tissue, and epithelium in the sinus. Pictures of the external exit and the visible sinus tract were then drawn and photographs of the exit site and visible sinus tract were taken. As a result of this study we introduced a new classification of exit-site appearance. A detailed description of this classification was reported elsewhere (55,56). Only a brief synopsis will be given here.

The classification is based on the cardinal signs of inflammation and additional features like drainage, regression of epidermis, and exuberance (profuse overgrowth) of granulation tissue (''proud flesh''). Exuberant granulation tissue is bulging, soft, vascularized, and bleeds easily. The presence of inflammation in almost all cases is due to infection, regardless of culture results, which do not influence exit classification. Noninflamed exits with positive cultures are not infected but colonized. Previous antibiotic therapy may render cultures from infected exits negative.

Improvement of inflammation is associated with decrease of pain, induration, drainage, exuberant granulation tissue, and/or epithelialization of the sinus. Five categories of exit appearances have been recognized: perfect, good, equivocal, acutely inflamed, and chronically inflamed. Two special categories also were established: traumatized exit and external-cuff infection with or without exit infection. Drainage is the cardinal feature of infection, but in equivocal exits this may be difficult to express outside the sinus. Traumatized exits demonstrate bleeding, scab, and deterioration of exit appearance and are painful. Prophylactic antibiotics are recommended in equivocal as well as traumatized exits.

Daily or alternate-day cleansing is required for good and perfect exits. Acute and chronic exit infections need systemic antibiotics according to culture and sensitivity results. The duration of treatment is guided by the exit appearance, the goal being to achieve a good appearance.

A 2- to 4-week course of warm 3% sodium chloride compresses applied locally to the exit site for 5–10 minutes three times daily achieves excellent results in cases that failed prolonged antibiotic therapy (57). Chronic infections may require at least one daily application indefinitely.

When the external cuff is infected without involving the exit, various combinations of intermittent or chronic purulent, bloody, or gluey drainage is usually seen outside, intermittently or chronically macerated epithelium is seen in the visible sinus, and proud flesh is visible deep inside the sinus. Drainage in the sinus may be seen only after pressure on the cuff, which may show surrounding induration.

Tunnel infection with Dacron® cuff involvement cannot be cured (58); treatment with systemic antibiotics and/or cuff shaving (55,59) may prolong the life of the catheter. Cuff shaving is usually employed on failure of prolonged antibiotic treatment. In order to avoid peritonitis associated with tunnel infection, early removal of the catheter is advisable. Apparently complete remissions and patient reluctance may make this option a difficult one. Catheter removal may be safely postponed in patients with limited life expectancies and in transplant candidates. In all other patients, once the diagnosis of cuff infection is established and cure is not achieved, the catheter should be removed.

Diagnostic evaluation of cuff involvement is difficult in cases of chronic exit infection. Ultrasound has been recommended as a valuable tool in diagnosing tunnel infections (60,61). The specificity of this method is not high; only 44–80% of cases with positive findings for tunnel infection required catheter removal. A technique with higher specificity and sensitivity is needed.

Profuse drainage washes away antibiotics when used locally in acute or chronic infection. Systemic antibiotics are excreted into the drainage and provide therapeutic concentrations locally. Local antibiotics can achieve high concentrations in the sinus in equivocal, good, or perfect exits but may be useful only in equivocal exits and/or in patients with recurrent acute infections after an acute episode subsides. Mupirocin ointment for gram-positive organisms and Neosporin® (neomycin, bacitracin, polymyxin) or gentamicin ophthalmic solution or ointment for gram-positive and gram-negative organisms usually achieve excellent results. Indiscriminate use of mupirocin (which contains polyethylene glycol as an ointment base) may damage polyurethane catheters.

G. External-Cuff Extrusion

The main reason behind cuff extrusion is resilience of the catheter material (silicon rubber), forcing the catheter to regain its natural position when placed under stress and extruding the cuff in the process. This is especially likely to occur if the cuff is too close to the exit. No treatment is needed if the cuff is not infected; if infection is present, systemic antibiotics or even surgical intervention may be needed. Topical mupirocin may markedly delay cuff infection. Shaving off the infected cuff (59) may save the catheter temporarily if there is no peritonitis or deep-cuff infection. Infection is another cause of cuff extrusion due to tissue reaction while the cuff is still in the sinus. Two such extrusions were observed with swan-neck Missouri catheters (38).

H. Catheter Obstruction

In the early postoperative period, a common cause of outflow obstruction is omental "capture" of the peritoneum. Provided peritonitis can be excluded, this complication is rare as a late event. A foreign body (e.g., Silastic®) is more prone to attract omentum very early. A proteinaceous sterile biofilm catheter coating may, with passage of time, lessen the tissue reaction to Silastic.

Other frequent causes of slow drainage include catheter translocation and occlusion by bowel or fibrin clot formation and are relieved by laxatives and/or addition of heparin 500 U/L to the dialysis solution. Permanently translocated catheters may still function, and repositioning should not be attempted in these catheters. If such a complication occurs in patients who are on nocturnal peritoneal dialysis (where fast drainage is particularly important), a tidal mode of cycler dialysis may help the situation. The constant presence of some sump volume in the peritoneal cavity allows fast dialysate flow throughout the tidal exchange (62).

I. Pericatheter Leak

Dialysis solution leaks may occur months or even years after starting CAPD. The management of early and late leaks does not differ, but most late leaks usually require surgical repair. Pericatheter leaks are more likely with midline catheter insertion than with rectus muscle insertion (63,64). This complication is rarely seen with the catheters provided with a bead and polyester flange at the deep cuff (swan-neck Missouri, swan-neck presternal, Toronto Western Hospital catheter). We have not observed a single late pericatheter leak with 181 swan-neck Missouri catheters (38).

Early leaks, which are usually external, differ from the late leaks, which infiltrate the abdominal wall at sites of least resistance (i.e., sites of hernias and previous surgeries). A sudden drop of ultrafiltration follows a sudden rise in intra-abdominal pressure (heavy lifting, coughing, or straining). Mild and intermittent leaks are difficult to localize and may be associated with minimal clinical signs in the initial stages. Later abdominal wall edema may manifest with the skin resembling that of an orange (*peau d'orange*). A chronic leak is usually a sequela of an acute leak but may occur gradually. The patient is usually fluid overloaded due to poor ultrafiltration. Scrotal or perineal edema may occur due to a patent processus vaginalis or an inguinal hernia (65). Men have a 10% reported incidence of scrotal edema on CAPD (66), whereas incidence of labial edema in women is much lower (67). This may initially resolve with supine low-volume peritoneal dialysis. In the event of associated hernia, surgical repair is usually required (69). These patients will require postoperative temporary hemodialysis for 1–2 weeks.

CT scan with intraperitoneal contrast (69,70) is the best method of leak localization. This is done as follows: the peritoneal cavity is drained completely prior to the procedure. A fresh bag of 2 L dialysis solution is prepared, 100 mL of 60% diatrizoate meglumine is injected into the dialysis solution bag through the injection port, and the solution is mixed and infused into the peritoneal cavity. To increase intra-abdominal pressure (37), the patients should stand up, walk, strain, cough, and bend over for at least 30 minutes, then assume the supine position on the CT table. The images are taken every 6 mm with a 6-mm slice thickness in the region of the suspected leak; in other regions the images are taken every 12 or 24 mm with a 12-mm slice thickness.

As mentioned before, glucose-positive vaginal discharge suggests vaginal leakage of the dialysate and may often lead to recurrent fungal peritonitis (71). This has been reported to occur following erosion of the catheter through the pouch of Douglas or through the fallopian tubes (72). The former may require catheter removal, whereas the latter may improve following fallopian tubal ligation.

J. Pericatheter Hernias

Due to a higher intra-abdominal pressure, patients on peritoneal dialysis are more prone to have hernias through the abdominal wall. They may occur at the site of a preexisting defect or along the peritoneal-lined recess leading to the deep cuff (pericatheter). A large-sized abdominal incision or long deep cuff to peritoneum distance increases the chances of occurrence of hernia.

Abdominal hernias may require surgical repair if they are large or have a tenderness indicating a risk of intestinal strangulation (73,74). Intraperitoneal injection of Tc colloid and nuclear imaging of the abdomen or chest (in cases of diaphragmatic hernias causing right or left pleural effusions) (75) may delineate the anatomy of such hernias and/or fluid collection. The pericatheter hernias result from the extrusion of the deep cuff and can leak peritoneal fluid into the subcutaneous space. They should be repaired in the event of subcutaneous extravasation or if they enlarge in size. If the deep cuff of the catheter is fixed in position (e.g., Missouri or Toronto Western ball disk catheter), the chances of developing pericatheter hernias are significantly reduced.

K. Peritonitis

The intraperitoneal segment of the catheter may be colonized by bacteria that cause peritonitis or bacteria that have migrated around the catheter. These bacteria protect themselves from host mechanisms and antibiotics by synthesizing a biofilm, which may lead to recurrent peritonitis with the same organism (76).

Microabscess formation due to deep cuff infection may also cause recurrent peritonitis (77). Trauma to the bowel by the catheter may lead to peritonitis (78).

L. Infusion or Pressure Pain

Infusion pain, as its name implies, is usually most intense at the beginning of infusion but can also occur at the end of drainage. It is usually transient and does not last for more than a few weeks. It is less common with coiled catheters. Several maneuvers may help in alleviating the pain (Table 5). Decreased infusion rate is frequently helpful. If pain occurs only at the beginning of inflow and the end of outflow, incomplete drainage and/or tidal mode for nightly peritoneal dialysis may be successful (62). Alkalinization of fluid with sodium bicarbonate or use of lidocaine are sometimes effective. One may need to change and replace the catheter with a coiled catheter if all other measures fail. Negative pressure exerted on the peritoneum generally causes outflow pain.

Table 5 Maneuvers to Alleviate Infusion Pain

Slower infusion rate
Incomplete drainage
Tidal mode for nightly peritoneal dialysis
Solution alkalization (Na bicarbonate: 2–5 mEq/L)
1% Lidocaine—2.5 mL/L (50 mg/exchange)
Catheter replacement

M. Unusual Complications

1. Organ Erosion

Straight Tenckhoff and Toronto Western Hospital catheters (78–82) may damage the viscera, causing intra-abdominal bleeding and/or peritonitis, as well as lead to genital edema due to peritoneal laceration late in the life of a catheter. These complications are generally the result of sustained pressure by the pointed tubing end of the straight Tenckhoff catheter or relatively sharp Silastic disks of the Toronto Western Hospital catheter. In the majority of such instances, there is history of catheter having not been used for some time (1–12 weeks) (80,81). Coiled (curled) catheters are reported to be free from this complication. This pressure necrosis of viscera may occur long after initial insertion (83). In patients with renal transplants, bowel perforation due to an unused peritoneal catheter has been reported (84).

2. Mechanical Accidents

Two instances of catheters being accidentally cut with scissors have been reported (82). This complication mostly occurs with the use of scissors during dressing changes, and we too have observed several such instances. The catheter may be punctured during the implantation procedure and shaving of the cuff, there being no self-sealing ability in the catheter material.

The catheter should be clamped immediately to avoid system contamination. Further management depends on the distance of the damaged site from the exit. For damage that is at least 15 mm from the exit, repair under sterile conditions may be attempted by using a peritoneal catheter repair kit available from the Quinton Instrument Co. Following wrapping with Betadine®-soaked gauze for 5 minutes, the catheter is transversely cut with a sterile blade proximal to the damaged site. The catheter clamp is released and the catheter is squeezed with fingers. The patient is asked to strain to allow dialysate flow from the peritoneal cavity. The flowing dialysate will flush eventual contaminants. While the fluid is still flowing, the Teflon tubing of the repair kit is inserted into the catheter as far as possible. Then the silicon rubber tubing of the repair kit is clamped to stop dialysate flow. The connection is dried with gauze. A mold is positioned over the connection and filled with sterile silicon glue. The extension tubing is connected to the catheter in the usual way. The glue cures for 72 hours. Using this method we have been able to save 10 catheters over a 12-year period.

3. Material Breakdown

Physical properties of the catheter material may sometimes give rise to problems. Barium sulphate incorporated into the catheter to render it radio-opaque has been reported to make the catheter brittle (85). Silicon rubber catheters have been observed to stretch, crack, or become brittle with age or after repeated exposure to Betadine (85). This necessitates either repair or replacement of the catheter. We have observed four such instances.

Polyurethane is even more likely to be damaged with aging because of so-called environmental stress cracking (ESC). Micro-cracks in the surface materials of a device are the result of corrosive forces of the living organism. Once the process begins, ultimate failure is inevitable (86). A recent report of localized softening leading to spontaneous extrusion of polyurethane catheter attributes the complication to polyethylene glycol used as an ointment base in mupirocin, commonly used for exit-site care (87).

4. Allergic Reaction

Eosinophilic peritonitis occurs most commonly during the postimplantation period. Although there are many possible causes for this condition (such as blood, air, and antibiotics), one cannot exclude a reaction to Silastic tubing. Postimplantation, the Silastic tubing is gradually covered with a proteinaceous biofilm, making the catheter less prone to allergic reaction. Allergic eosinophillic dermatitis due to silicon rubber has been reported (88,89).

5. Hemoperitoneum

This complication commonly occurs in women due to either ovulation or retroperitoneal menstruation. In one series, the incidence of hemoperitoneum was 6% of all patients on peritoneal dialysis (90). Seventy percent of these did not require any active intervention apart from addition of intraperitoneal heparin. Ten percent were minor bleeding episodes due to some intra-abdominal pathology. Only about 20% of such instances required active intervention. Hemoperitoneum may occur after many years of peritoneal dialysis in cases of sclerosing peritonitis (89). Blood transfusion may be required in cases of severe intraperitoneal bleed due to follicular or ovarian cyst rupture or thrombocytopenia.

IV. INDICATIONS FOR CATHETER REMOVAL

It may be necessary to remove the catheter under some conditions. These may be broadly categorized under two headings: catheter malfunction and complicating medical conditions with a functioning catheter.

A. Malfunction

When conservative measures fail, catheter removal becomes a necessity. This may be required in the following conditions: (a) intraluminal obstruction with blood or fibrin clot or omental tissue incarceration, (b) catheter-tip migration out of the pelvis with poor drainage, (c) a catheter kink along its course, or (d) catheter tip caught in adhesions following severe peritonitis. In these situations, there are usually both inflow and outflow draining problems. An accidental break in the continuity of the catheter that cannot be repaired will also require catheter removal.

B. Functioning Catheter with a Complication

Some clinical situations require catheter removal despite a functioning catheter. These consist of (a) recurrent peritonitis with no identifiable cause, (b) peritonitis due to exit-site and/or tunnel infection, (c) catheter with persistent exit-site infection, (d) tunnel infection and abscess, (e) late recurrent dialysate leak through the exit site or into the layers of the abdominal wall, (f) unusual peritonitis, i.e., tuberculosis, fungal, etc., (g) bowel perforation with multiple organism peritonitis, (h) refractory peritonitis of other causes, (i) severe abdominal pain either due to the catheter impinging on internal organs or during solution inflow, and (j) catheter-cuff extrusion with infection.

V. CONCLUSION

There have been considerable advances in peritoneal access technology over the years. Catheter design modifications, surgical refinement of insertion methods, improved understanding of postimplantation care, and better definition of factors impacting on healing and care of exit site have reduced complications and enhanced longevity of peritoneal access. Soft catheters are gradually replacing rigid catheters in the treatment of acute renal failure. Soft catheters are used exclusively for the treatment of chronic renal failure. Although the Tenckhoff catheter continues to be the most widely used catheter, swan-neck catheters are gaining widespread popularity. Early complications like bowel perforation or massive bleeding are rare following surgical implantation. Adopting measures like the use of swan-neck catheters and insertion through the rectus muscle instead of the midline has in recent years markedly reduced complications such as obstruction, pericatheter leaks, and superficial cuff extrusions.

The exit should be located in a place only minimally subjected to pressure and movement. Prophylactic antibiotic prior to implantation and a meticulous sterile surgical technique with perfect hemostasis prevent early infection. Healing of the exit lasts 4–8 weeks. During this time a nonocclusive (air-permeable) dressing changed weekly is recommended for 2 weeks and every other week thereafter. After the exit is healed, the simplest and best method of care is protection from trauma, cleansing with water and liquid soap containing mild disinfectant, and avoidance of gross exit contamination. Early antibiotics with mild infection prevent severe infection leading to catheter loss. Whereas supine peritoneal dialysis may be started immediately postimplantation, ambulatory peritoneal dialysis should be postponed for at least 10 days after implantation to avoid early leaks. The success of the catheter depends on the meticulous adherence to the details of catheter insertion and postimplantation care.

REFERENCES

1. Tenckhoff J, Schechter H. A bacteriologically safe peritoneal access device. Trans Am Soc Artif Intern Organs 1968; 14:181–187.
2. Lindblad AS, Novak JW, Stablein DM, et al. Report of the National CAPD Registry of the National Institutes of Health. National CAPD Registry of the National Institute of Diabetes and Digestive and Kidney Diseases, Potomac, Maryland, 1987:10.
3. Twardowski ZJ, Khanna R. Peritoneal dialysis access and exit site care. In: Gokal R, Nolph KD, eds. Textbook of Peritoneal Dilaysis. Dordrecht: Kluwer Academic Publishers, 1994:271–314.
4. Vaamonde CA, Michael VF, Metzger RA, Carrol KE. Complications of acute peritoneal dialysis. J Chron Dis 1975; 28:637–659.
5. Valk TW, Swartz RD, Hsu CH. Peritoneal dialysis in acute renal failure: analysis of outcome and complications. Dial Transpl 1980; 9:48–54.
6. Maher JF, Schreiner GE. Hazards and complications of dialysis. N Engl J Med 1965; 273:370–377.
7. Edward SR, Unger AM. Acute hydrothorax: a new complication of peritoneal dialysis. JAMA 1967; 199: 853–855.
8. Finn R, Jowett EW. Acute hydrothorax: complication of peritoneal dialysis. Br Med J 1970; 2:94.
9. Holm J, Lieden B, Lindgrist B. Unilateral effusion—a rare complication of peritoneal dialysis. Scand J Urol Nephrol 1971; 5:84–85.
10. Ribot S, Jacobs MG, Frankel HJ, Bernstein A. Complications of peritoneal dialysis. Am J Med Sci 1966; 252:505–517.
11. Mion CM, Boen ST. Analysis of factors responsible for the formation of adhesions during chronic peritoneal dialysis. Am J Med Sci 1965; 250:675–679.
12. Matalon R, Levine S, Eisinger RP. Hazards in routine use of peritoneal dialysis. NY State J Med 1971; 71: 219–224.
13. Henderson LW. Peritoneal dialysis. In: Massry SG, Sellers AL, eds. Clinical Aspects of Uraemia and Dialysis. Springfield, IL: Charles C. Thomas, 1976:574.
14. Simkin EP, Wright FK. Perforating injuries of the bowel complicating peritoneal catheter insertion. Lancet 1968; 1:61–67.
15. Krebs RA, Burtiss BB. Bowel perforation. JAMA 1966; 198:486–487.
16. Rigalosi RS, Maher JF, Schreiner GE. Intestinal perforation during peritoneal dialysis. Ann Intern Med 1964; 70:1013–1015.
17. Fleisher AG, Kimmelstiel FM, Lattes CG, Miller RE. Surgical complications of peritoneal dialysis cathters. Am J Surg 1985; 149:726.
18. Lovinggood JP. Peritoneal Catheter Implantation for CAPD. Perit Dial Bull 1984; 4(3):S106.
19. Smith E, Chamberlain MJ. Complications of peritoneal dialysis. Br Med J 1965; 1:126–127.
20. Stein MF Jr. Intraperitoneal loss of dialysis catheter. Ann Intern Med 1969; 71:869–870.
21. Twardowski ZJ, Nolph KD, Khanna R, Prowant BF. Computer interaction: catheters. In: Khanna R, ed. Advances in Peritoneal Dialysis. Selected Papers from the Fourteenth Annual Conference on Peritoneal Dialysis, Orlando, Florida, January, 1994. Toronto: Peritoneal Dialysis Publications, Inc., 1994:11–18.
22. Twardowski ZJ, Nichols WK, Khanna R, Nolph KD. Swan neck presternal peritoneal dialysis catheter: design, insertion, and break-in. Video produced by the Academic Support Center, University of Missouri, Columbia, MO, 1993. (Available through Accurate Surgical Instruments Co., 588–590 Richmond St. W., Toronto, Ontario, Canada M5V 1Y9.)
23. Twardowski ZJ, Nichols WK, Nolph KD, Khanna R. Swan neck presternal (''bath tub'') catheter for peritoneal dialysis. In: Khanna R, Nolph KD, Prowant BF, Twardowski ZJ, Oreopoulos DG, eds. Advances in Peritoneal Dialysis. Selected Papers from the Twelfth Annual Conference on Peritoneal Dialysis, Seattle,

Washington, February 1992. Toronto: Peritoneal Dialysis Bulletin, Inc., 1992:316–324.

24. Twardowski ZJ, Nichols WK, Nolph KD, Khanna R. Swan neck presternal peritoneal dialysis catheter. Perit Dial Int 1993; 13(suppl 2):S130–S132.
25. Twardowski ZJ, Khanna R, Nolph KD, Nichols WK. Peritoneal dialysis catheter: principles of design, implantation, and early care. Video produced by the Academic Support Center, University of Missouri, Columbia, MO, 1993. (Available through Accurate Surgical Instruments, Co., 588–590 Richmond St. W., Toronto, Ontario, Canada M5V 1Y9.)
26. Twardowski ZJ, Ryan LP, Kennedy JM. Catheter break-in for continuous ambulatory peritoneal dialysis—University of Missouri experience. Perit Dial Bull 1984; 4(suppl 3)S110–S111.
27. Holley JL, Bernardini J, Piraino B. Characteristics and outcomes of peritoneal dialysate leaks and associated infections. Adv Perit Dial 1993; 9:240.
28. Ash SR, Carr DJ, Diaz-Buxo JA. Peritoneal access devices: Hydraulic function and compatibility. In: Nissenson AR, Fine RN, Gentile DE, eds. Clinical Dialysis. 2d ed. Norwalk, CT: Appleton & Lange, 1990:212–239.
29. Twardowski ZJ, Pasley K. Reversed one-way obstruction of the peritoneal catheter (the accordion clot). Perit Dial Int 1994; 14:296–297.
30. O'Regan S, Garel L, Patriquin H, Yazbeck S. Outflow obstruction: whiplash technique for catheter mobilization. Perit Dial Int 1988; 8:265–268.
31. Honkanen E, Eklund B, Laasonen L, Ylinen K, Grönhagen-Riska C. Reposition of a displaced peritoneal catheter: the Helsinki whiplash method. In: Khanna R, Nolph KD, Prowant BF, Twardowski ZJ, Oreopoulos DG, eds. Perit Dialy Bull 1990; 6:159–164.
32. Schleifer CR, Ziemek H, Teehan BP, Benz RL, Sigler MH, Gilgore GS. Migration of peritoneal catheters: personal experience and a survey of 72 other units. Perit Dial Bull 1987; 7:189–193.
33. Yoshihara K, Yoshi S, Miyagi S. Alpha replacement method for the displacement of the swan neck catheter. In: Khanna R, Nolph KD, Prowant BF, Twardowski ZJ, Oreopoulos DG, eds. Perit Dial Bull 1993; 9:227–230.
34. Ersoy FF, Twardowski ZJ, Satalovich RJ, Ketchersid T. A retrospective analysis of catheter position and function in 91 CAPD patients. Perit Dial Int 1994; 14:409–410.
35. Twardowski ZJ. Malposition and poor drainage of peritoneal catheters. Semin Dial 1990; 3:57.
36. Goldsmith HJ, Edwards EC, Moorhead PJ, Wright FJ. Difficulties encountered in intermittent dialysis for chronic renal failure. Br J Urol 1966; 38:625–634.
37. Twardowski ZJ, Khanna R, Nolph KD, Scalamogna A, Metzler MH, Schneider TW, Prowant BF, Ryan LP. Intra-abdominal pressure during natural activities in patients treated with continuous ambulatory peritoneal dialysis. Nephron 1986; 44:129–135.
38. Twardowski ZJ, Prowant BF, Nichols WK, Nolph KD, Khanna R. Six year experience with swan neck catheter. Perit Dial Int 1992; 12:384–389.
39. Twardowski ZJ, Prowant BF: Exit-site healing post catheter implantation. Perit Dial Int 1996; 16(suppl 3): S51–S70.
40. Pecoits-Filho, Twardowski ZJ, Khanna R, Kim Y-L, Goel S, Moore H. The effect of antibiotic prophylaxis on the healing of exit sites of peritoneal dialysis catheters in rats. Perit Dial Int 1998; 18:60–63.
41. Twardowski ZJ, Prowant BF. Appearance and classification of healing peritoneal catheter exit sites. Perit Dial Int 1996; 16(suppl 3):S71–S93.
42. Van den Broek PJ, Buys LF, Van Furth R. Interaction of povidone-iodine compounds, phagocytic cells, and macro-organisms. Antimicrob Agents Chemother 1982; 22:593–597.
43. Iwasaki N, Kamoi K, Bae RD, Tsutsui T. Cytotoxicity of povidone-iodine on cultured mammalian cells. J Jpn Assoc Periodont 1989; 31:836–842.
44. Laufman H. Current use of skin and wound cleansers and antiseptics. Am J Surg 1989; 157:359–365.
45. Bryant CA, Rodeheaver GT, Reem EM, Nitcher LS, Kennedy JC, Edlich RF. Search for a nontoxic surgical scrub solution for periorbital lacerations. Ann Emerg Med 1984; 13:317–319.
46. Prowant BF, Schmidt LM, Twardowski ZJ, Griebel CK, Burrows L, Ryan LP, Satalowich RJ. Peritoneal dialysis catheter exit site care. Am Nephr Nurs Assoc J 1988; 15:219–222.
47. Davis SJ, Ogg CS, Cameron JS, Poston S, Nobble W. Staphylococcus nasal carriage, exit site infection and catheter loss in patients treated with continuous ambulatory peritoneal dialysis. Perit Dial Int 1989; 9:61–64.
48. Luzar MA, Coles GA, Faller B, Slingeneyer A, Dah GD, Briat C, Wone C, Knefati Y, Kessler M, Peluso F. Staphylococcal aureus nasal carriage and infection in patients on continuous ambulatory peritoneal dialysis. N Engl J Med 1990; 322:505–509.
49. Twardowski ZJ, Prowant BF. Staphylococcal aureus nasal carriage is not associated with an increased incidence of exit site infection with the same organism. Perit Dial Int 1993; 13(2):S306–S309.
50. Tenckhoff H. Home peritoneal dialysis. In: Massry SG, Sellers AL, eds. Clinical Aspects of Uremia and Dialysis. Springfield, IL: Charles C. Thomas Publ., 1976: 583–615.
51. Twardowski ZJ, Nolph KD, Khanna R, Prowant BF, Ryan LP. The need for a "swan neck" permanently bent, arcuate peritoneal dialysis catheter. Perit Dial Bull 1985; 5:219–223.
52. U.S. Renal Data System, USRDS 1992 Annual Data Report VI. Catheter-related factors and peritonitis risk in CAPD patients. Am J Kidney Dis 1992; 5(S2):48–54.
53. Twardowski ZJ, Dobbie JW, Moore HL, Nichols WK, DeSpain JD, Anderson PC, Khanna R, Nolph KD, Loy

TS. Morphology of peritoneal dialysis catheter tunnels. Macroscopy and light microscopy. Perit Dial Int 1991; 11:237–251.
54. Pierratos A: Peritoneal dialysis glossary. Perit Dial Bull 1984; 4:2–3.
55. Twardowski ZJ, Prowant BF. Exit-site study methods and results. Perit Dial Int 1996; 16(suppl 3):S6–S31.
56. Twardowski ZJ, Prowant BF. Classification of normal and diseased exit sites. Perit Dial Int 1996; 16(suppl 3): S32–S50.
57. Strauss FG, Holmes D, Nortman DF, Friedman S. Hypertonic saline compresses: therapy for complicated exit site infections. In: Khanna R, Nolph KD, Prowant BF, Twardowski ZJ, Oreopoulos DG, eds. Advances in Peritoneal Dialysis. Selected Papers from the Thirteenth Annual Conference on Peritoneal Dialysis, San Diego, California, March 1993. Toronto: Peritoneal Dialysis Bulletin, Inc., 1993:248–250.
58. Tenckhoff H. Home peritoneal dialysis. In: Massry SG, Sellers AL, eds. Clinical Aspects of Uremia and Dialysis. Springfield, IL: Charles C. Thomas Publ., 1976: 583–615.
59. Nichols WK, Nolph KD. A technique for managing exit site and cuff infection in Tenckhoff catheters. Perit Dial Bull 1983; 3(suppl 4):S4–S5.
60. Domico J, Warman M, Jaykamur S, Sorkin MI. Is ultrasonography useful in predicting catheter loss? In: Khanna R, Nolph KD, Prowant BF, Twardowski ZJ, Oreopoulos DG, eds. Advances in Peritoneal Dialysis. Selected Papers from the Thirteenth Annual Conference on Peritoneal Dialysis, San Diego, California, March 1993. Toronto: Peritoneal Dialysis Bulletin, Inc., 1993: 231–232.
61. Plum J, Sudkamp S, Grabensee G. Results of ultrasound-assisted diagnosis of tunnel infections in continuous ambulatory peritoneal dialysis. Am J Kidney Dis 1994; 23:99–104.
62. Twardowski ZJ. Tidal peritoneal dialysis. In: Nissenson AR, Fine RN, eds. Dialysis Therapy. Philadelphia: Hanley & Belfus, Inc., 1993:153–156.
63. Helfrich GB, Pechan BW, Alijani MR, Bernard WF, Rakowski TA, Winchester JF. Reduced catheter complications with lateral placement. Perit Dial Bull 1983; 3(suppl 4):S2–S4.
64. Twardowski ZJ, Nolph KD, Khanna R, Prowant BF, Ryan LP. The need for a "swan neck" permanently bent, arcuate peritoneal dialysis catheter. Perit Dial Bull 1985; 5:219–223.
65. Cooper JC, Nicholls AJ, Simms JM, Platts MM, Brown CB, Johnson AG. Genital oedema in patients treated by continuous ambulatory peritoneal dialysis: an unusual presentation of inguinal hernia. Br Med J 1983; 286: 983.
66. Tzamaloukas AH, Gibel LJ, Eisenberg B, et al. Scrotal edema in patients on CAPD: Causes, differential diagnosis and management. Dial Transplant 1992; 21:581.
67. Kopecky RT, Funk MM, Kreitzer PR. Localized genital edema in patients undergoing continuous ambulatory peritoneal dialysis. J Urol 1985; 124:880.
68. Schleifer CR, Morfesis FA, Cupit M, Chen C, Smink RD. Management of Hernias and Tenckhoff catheter complications in CAPD. Perit Dial Bull 1984; 4:146.
69. Twardowski ZJ, Tully RJ, Nichols WK, Sunderrajan S. Computerized tomography in the diagnosis of subcutaneous leak sites during continuous ambulatory peritoneal dialysis (CAPD). Perit Dial Bull 1984; 4:163–166.
70. Twardowski ZJ, Tully RJ, Ersoy FF, Dedhia NM. Computerized tomography with and without intraperitoneal contrast for determination of intra-abdominal fluid distribution and diagnosis of complications in peritoneal dialysis patients. ASAIO Transactions 1990; 36:95–103.
71. Khanna R, Oreopoulos DG, Vas S, et al. Fungal peritonitis in patients undergoing chronic intermittent or continuous peritoneal dialysis. Proc Eur Dial Transplant Assoc 1980; 17:291.
72. Caporale N, Perez D, Alegre S. Vaginal leak of peritoneal dialysis liquid. Perit Dial Int 1991; 11:284.
73. Khanna R, Nolph KD. Ultrafiltration failure and sclerosing peritonitis in peritoneal dialysis patients. In: Nissenson AR, Fine RN, eds. Dialysis Therapy. Philadelphia: Hanley and Belfus, 1986:122–125.
74. Rubin J, Raju S, Teal N, et al. Abdominal hernia in patients undergoing continuous ambulatory peritoneal dialysis. Arch Intern Med 1982; 142:1453–1455.
75. O'Connor J, Rutland M. Demonstration of pleuro-peritoneal communication with radionuclide imaging in a CAPD patient. Perit Dial Bull 1981; 1:153.
76. Dasgupta MK, Bettcher KB, Ulan RA, Burns V, Lam K, Dossetor JB, Costerton JW. Relationship of adherent bacterial biofilms to peritonitis in chronic ambulatory peritoneal dialysis. Perit Dial Bull 1987; 7:168–173.
77. Dimitriadis A, Antoniou S, Toliou T, Papadopoulos C. Tissue reaction to deep cuff of Tenckhoff catheter and peritonitis. In: Khanna R, Nolph KD, Prowant BF, Twardowski ZJ, Oreopoulos DG, eds. Advances in Peritoneal Dialysis. Selected Papers from the Tenth Annual Conference on Peritoneal Dialysis, Dallas, Texas, February 1990. Toronto: Peritoneal Dialysis Bulletin, Inc., 1990:155–158.
78. Grefberg N, Danielson BG, Nilsson P, Wahlberg J. An unusual complication of the Toronto Western Hospital catheter (letter). Perit Dial Bull 1983; 3:219.
79. della Volpe M, Iberti M, Ortensia A, Veronesi GV. Erosion of the sigmoid by a permanent peritoneal catheter (letter). Perit Dial Bull 1984; 4:108.
80. Jamison MH, Fleming SJ, Ackrill P, Schofield PF. Erosion of rectum by Tenckhoff catheter. Br J Surg 1988; 75:360.
81. Brady HR, Abraham G, Oreopoulos DG, Cardella CJ.

Bowel erosion due to a dormant peritoneal catheter in immunosuppressed renal transplant recipients. Perit Dial Int 1988; 8:163–165.
82. Golper TA, Carpenter J. Accidents with Tenckhoff catheters. Ann Intern Med 1981; 95:121–122.
83. Diaz-Buxo J. Mechanical complications of chronic peritoneal dialysis catheters. Semin Dial 1991; 4:106.
84. Brady HR, Abraham G, Oreopoulos DG, Cardella CJ. Bowel erosion due to a dormant peritoneal catheter in immunosuppressed renal transplant patients. Perit Dial Int 1988; 8:163.
85. Ward RA, Klein E, Wathen RL, eds. Peritoneal catheters. Perit Dial Bull 1983; 3(suppl 3):S9–S17.
86. Szycher M, Siciliano AA, Reed AM. Polyurethane in medical devices. Med Design Mater 1991; 18–25.
87. Rao SP, Oreopoulos DG, Unusual complications of a polyurethane PD catheter. Perit Dial Int 1997; 17(4): 410–412.
88. Kurihara S, Tani Y, Tateishi K, Yuri T, Kitada H, Sugishita N, Fukuda Y, Ishikawa I, Shinoda A, Hayakawa Y. Allergic eosinophilic dermatitis due to silicone rubber: a rare but troublesome complication of the Tenckhoff catheter. Perit Dial Bull 1985; 5:65–67.
89. Prowant BF, Schmidt LM, Twardowski ZJ, Taylor HM, Ryan LP, Satalowich RJ, Burrows L, Griebel CK, Burrows LM: Use of exudate smears for diagnosis of peritoneal catheter exit site infection. In: Avram MM, Giordano C, eds. Ambulatory Peritoneal Dialysis—Proceedings of the IVth Congress of the International Society for Peritoneal Dialysis, Venice, Italy, June 29–July 2, 1987. New York: Plenum Publishing Corporation, 1990:220–222.
90. Greenberg A, Bernardini J, Piraino B, Johnston J, Perlmutter J. Hemoperitoneum complicating peritoneal dialysis: single center experience and literature review. Am J Kidney Dis 1992; 29:252–256.

9

Problems of Peritoneal Membrane Failure

Simon J. Davies
North Staffordshire Hospital Trust, Stoke-on-Trent, United Kingdom

Gerald Anthony Coles and Nicholas Topley
University of Wales College of Medicine, Cardiff, United Kingdom

I. INTRODUCTION

Twenty years after its introduction, peritoneal dialysis (PD) is an established mode of treatment for end-stage renal failure; it provides both patient and clinician with an additional choice in therapy, with several positive advantages such as social independence and convenience, steady-state biochemistry, and gentle ultrafiltration. While in short-term studies (3–5 years) peritoneal dialysis has been shown to have a comparable outcome to hemodialysis (1–3), concerns still remain with respect to the medium and long term. There is a considerable drop-out rate within the first 3–5 years, and although a proportion of patients stop for transplantation, technical failure remains a frequent occurrence due to recurrent peritonitis, poor ultrafiltration, or inadequate solute clearance (2–5). Concerns about the ability of peritoneal dialysis to provide adequate long-term treatment have been increased by the results of the CAN-USA study, which clearly demonstrates that loss of residual renal function was an independent predictor of death (6). Thus, the principal challenge for peritoneal dialysis at the present time is to establish that it can provide adequate replacement of renal excretory function in the anuric patient.

It is, of course, in the anuric patient that the performance of the peritoneal membrane becomes critical, and in these circumstances membrane failure may be defined as any failure to replace renal function to an adequate degree. As first demonstrated by Twardowski, there turns out to be considerable differences between patients in their peritoneal membrane kinetics, which can influence both solute and water clearance (7). This phenomenon is made more complex by the ability of these kinetics to change with time on treatment (5,8). Preexisting membrane failure may, therefore, be revealed as a clinical problem as residual function is lost or alternatively be acquired later during the course of treatment due to damage associated with changes in membrane structure as a result of recurrent infection or exposure to bio-incompatible dialysate.

Renal excretory function can be subdivided into solute removal, particularly nitrogenous products of protein metabolism, and maintenance of fluid, electrolyte, and acid-base balance. Peritoneal failure may therefore be defined as an inability of peritoneal dialysis to replace adequately one or more of these functions. Adequacy in this context can be taken to be that level of replacement that gives optimum outcome. Thus, inadequate dialysis or failure means that patient outcome in terms of morbidity and mortality is significantly worse than the best currently being achieved.

The purpose of this chapter is to provide the practicing clinician with an overview of our current understanding of peritoneal membrane structure and function, the clinical assessment of this in the dialysis patient, and thus a framework for the recognition and management of peritoneal membrane failure.

II. PERITONEAL STRUCTURE AND FUNCTION

A. The Peritoneal Cavity

The peritoneum is a continuous, translucent serous membrane that consists of a monolayer of mesothelium

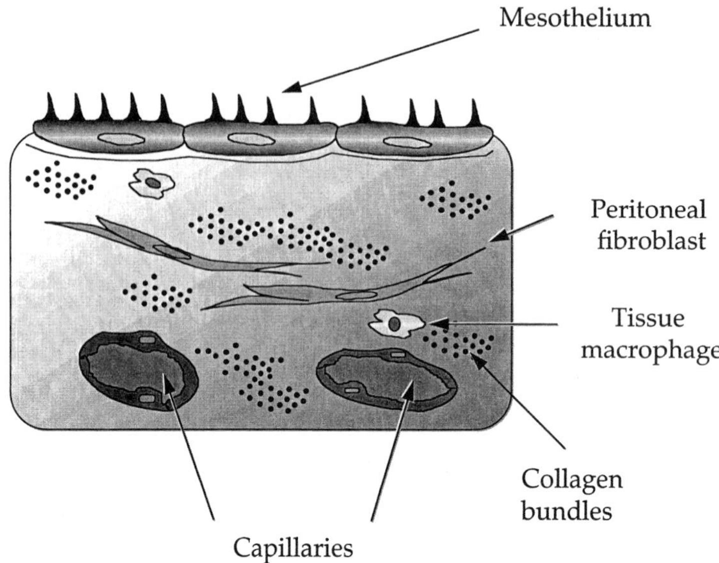

Fig. 1 Schematic representation of the structure of the peritoneal membrane.

resting on a basal lamina (Fig. 1). Below this runs a discontinuous band of elastic fibers and interwoven bundles of collagen fibers embedded in a connective tissue stroma or interstitium. The interstitium is largely composed of glycoproteins and proteoglycans (9–12). Within the submesothelial interstitium reside populations of fibroblasts and mast cells, and interspersed within it are the lymphatics and the capillary bed. The peritoneum with its mesothelial monolayer is divided into two parts: the parietal peritoneum, which bounds the outer surface of the body cavity, and the visceral peritoneum, which covers the abdominal organs. The space between these layers forms the peritoneal cavity. In addition, the greater omentum is a mesenteric apron that is continuous with the peritoneum and hangs freely into the peritoneal cavity extending from the lower border of the stomach and covering the intestines. It consists of a trabecular loose fibrous connective tissue framework covered on its surface by a continuous mesothelial monolayer and contains fibroblasts, blood, and lymphatic vessels.

B. The Mesothelium

The mesothelial layer consists of a single layer of squamous epithelial cells of mesodermal origin. In addition to the peritoneal cavity, mesothelial cell monolayers also line the pleural cavity and pericardium (13,14). The serosal surface of the mesothelium has a well-developed microvillous border. These microvilli serve to increase the peritoneal surface area, thereby facilitating absorption of materials and reducing friction and facilitating intestinal movement (Fig. 2). The mesothelial surface is also covered by a microscopic negatively charged glycocalyx composed primarily of proteoglycans (15,16). These highly glycosylated molecules are hydrophilic, and this may aid the "slippery" nature of the peritoneal surface. This is also facilitated by the ability of the mesothelial cell to secrete specific phospholipids derived from the large number of lamellar bodies easily identifiable within the cytoplasm of these cells (17–19). The mesothelial monolayer consists of a single layer of cells tightly opposed to each other with desmosomes and tight and gap junctions readily identifiable. Like endothelium, the mesothelial cell has a well-developed system of micropinocytotic vesicles and larger membrane-bound vacuoles (Fig. 3).

Over the past decade increasing interest in the role of the mesothelium in peritoneal host defence has led to the finding that these cells have considerable biosynthetic capacity and appear to contribute to peritoneal homeostasis as well as its response to infection. In this respect, the mesothelium has significant capacity to synthesize inflammatory mediators (prostaglandins, cytokines, and chemokines), mediators of fibrinolysis (tissue plasminogen activator, its inhibitor and tissue factor), growth factors, phospholipids, and proteoglycans. In addition, they express on their surface molecules important in their interaction with migrating leukocyte populations (ICAM-1 and VCAM-1) (Table 1).

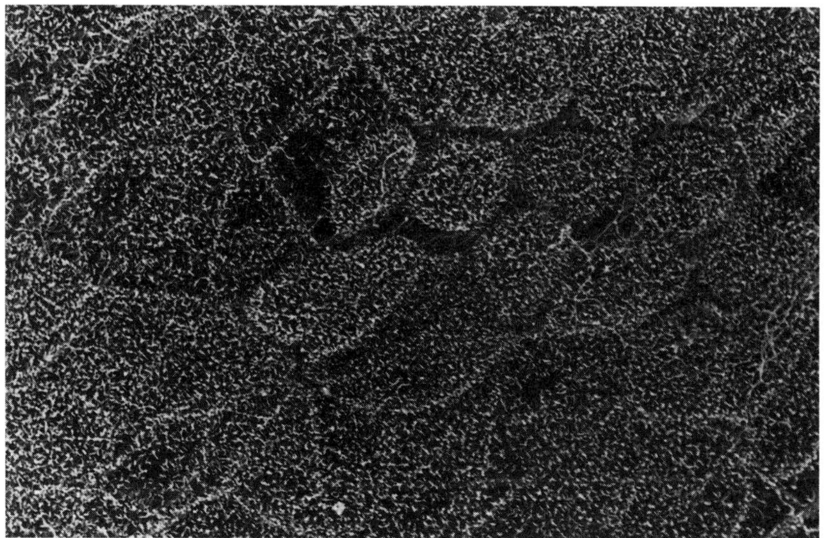

Fig. 2 Scanning electron micrograph (SEM) of the mesothelial cell surface. Note distinct cell junctions and numerous surface microvilli. (×1800).

C. The Submesothelial Interstitium

While our understanding of the contribution of the mesothelium to peritoneal homeostasis has increased significantly, our understanding of the function and changes that occur within the cellular and acellular portions of the submesothelial interstitium are still scant. This has recently increased with the isolation and characterization of peritoneal fibroblasts (that reside within the tissue) (20,21). These cells, as with mesothelial

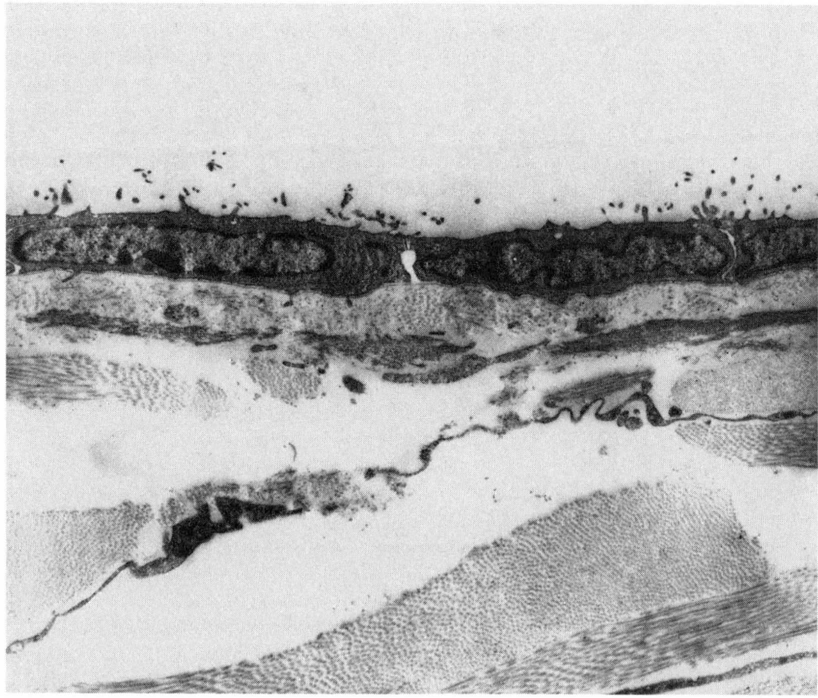

Fig. 3 Transmission electron micrograph of the mesothelial cell monolayer. Note evidence of junctional complexes between adjoining cells and numerous intracellular organelles (×10,000).

Table 1 Products of Human Mesothelium

Mediator/Molecule	Ref.
Prostaglandins (PGE_2, PGI_2)	174–176
Cytokines (IL-1, IL-6)	69,177
Chemokines (IL-8, MCP-1, RANTES)	70,77,79,178,179
Growth factors (TGF-β1, PDGF, bFGF)	180–182
Molecules important in extracellular matrix turnover (collagen I/III/IV, fibronectin, proteoglycans, metalloproteinases, hyaluronic acid)	14,183–188
Members of the fibrinolytic cascade (TPA, uPA, PAI)	189,190
Phospholipids (phosphatidyl choline, etc.)	17,18
Surface-expressed molecules (ICAM-1, VCAM-1, CD 44)	71,80,81

cells, posses significant biosynthetic capacity and thus potentially contribute to both peritoneal host defense and "fibrotic" changes in the peritoneal membrane. In the next few years further investigations will hopefully expand our understanding of the contribution of these cells to peritoneal homeostasis and to extracellular matrix turnover in the normal and dialyzed peritoneal cavity.

Within the submesothelial interstitium reside the capillaries, and while their contribution to solute and water movement is clear (see below), their function with respect to peritoneal inflammation is yet to be elucidated because these cells are difficult to isolate and culture in vitro. Significant if anecdotal evidence suggests, however, that both the structure and number of capillaries changes during peritoneal dialysis, particularly in patients with "fibrosis." These changes in capillary structure (basement membrane duplication) suggestive of diabetic-like microangiopathy and number (angiogenesis) could clearly modulate endothelial and smooth muscle cell structure and function. To date, however, there is no direct clinical or in vitro evidence of what the implication of potential alterations in capillary function might have on peritoneal function (in terms of ultrafiltration or homeostasis/inflammation).

III. MODELS DESCRIBING PERITONEAL FUNCTION

The peritoneum may be thought of most simply as a sheet or wall separating the vascular compartment from the peritoneal lumen in which there are a large number of holes (Fig. 4). These holes, usually referred to as pores, are of variable sizes, thus allowing different-sized molecules through at different rates. For small molecules, such as electrolytes, urea, creatinine, and glucose, these pores offer no effective restriction to

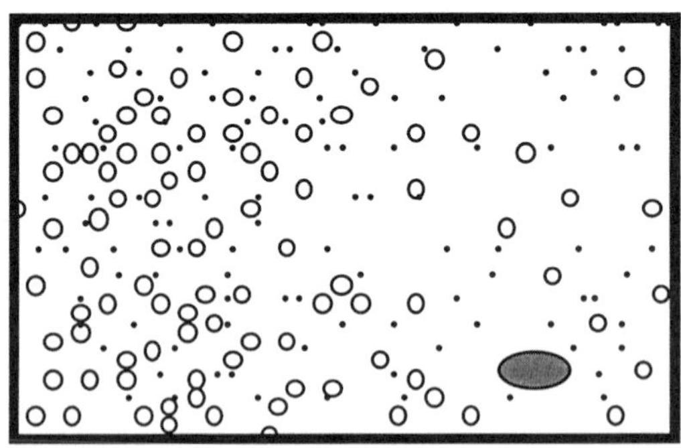

Fig. 4 Schematic diagram of the pore structure in the peritoneal membrane. The small pores (○) allow unimpeded passage of small solutes, and their total number, determined by actual membrane area × density, will determine effective peritoneal surface area. The large pores (●) allow passage of macromolecules, and their relative "size" determine intrinsic peritoneal permeability. The ultra-small pores (•) represent exclusive water channels.

movement, such that their rate of equilibration during the dialysis dwell period is determined by their total number. This in turn is determined both by the true size of the peritoneal membrane and by the density of pores within it and has led to the term effective peritoneal surface area (EPSA) (22). A good example of the influence of a change in pore density on the EPSA is one that occurs during active peritoneal inflammation, or peritonitis, when there is a rapid increase of low molecular weight solute transport, which is subsequently reversible (23).

In contrast to low molecular weight solutes, macromolecules are dependent on larger holes to pass across the peritoneum, and their rate of passage is determined both by the relative number of pores, and so the EPSA, but also by their relative size, which is a function of the intrinsic peritoneal permeability (22,24). The larger the pores, the more permeable the membrane. Thus, the loss of proteins into the dialysate in an individual patient is determined by both these factors, such that for very large molecules (e.g., IgM, 10^6daltons) the pore size (intrinsic permeability) is important, whereas for smaller proteins (e.g., albumin, 6×10^4daltons) the number of pores (EPSA) becomes the dominant factor. This is the explanation for the important inverse relationship between solute transport and plasma albumin in PD patients (25).

The passage of water across the peritoneal membrane appears to be a special case. While water is clearly small enough to pass unimpeded through holes that permit the passage of proteins and low molecular weight solutes, there is strong circumstantial evidence that specific pores exist that are exclusive for this important molecule (22,26). The existence of these pores, usually referred to as water channels, is implied both by the relative efficiency of glucose as an osmotic agent despite its relatively low molecular weight (implying that the peritoneum is acting at least in part as a truly semi-permeable membrane) and by the phenomenon of sodium (Na^+) sieving (27). Following the insertion of a hypertonic glucose solution in the peritoneum (glucose 3.86%), water passes more rapidly across than sodium, resulting in a drop in the dialysate-to-plasma ratio of this ion. In clinical terms it is likely that the existence of these pores is most relevant to the extra ultrafiltration achieved using hyper-tonic solutions, and thus the strategy for their use.

Three main properties of the peritoneum influence the passage of solutes and water across it:

1. Effective peritoneal surface area
2. Intrinsic peritoneal permeability
3. The existence of an additional water-specific pathway

This has led to the application of the "three-pore theory" (26), which has allowed estimates to be made of the relative proportion and size of these theoretical pores, confirming that it is the effective peritoneal surface area that is clinically the most important variable of peritoneal function. It has a profound effect on the osmotic gradient achieved with glucose during the dialysis dwell (thus influencing ultrafiltration) (28), it is the principal determinant of peritoneal albumin losses, and it has a considerable influence on the choice of dialysis strategy to achieve optimal solute clearances. Furthermore, it appears to be the membrane factor that varies most between individuals and is most likely to change with time on treatment (5,8,29).

However, two other factors have a significant impact on net fluid removal in the PD patient. These are the hydrostatic pressure across the peritoneal membrane (30) and the net reabsorption that occurs continually throughout the dialysis cycle (22,31). Variations in the hydrostatic gradient occur due to changes in pressure within the peritoneal lumen due to two main factors—the intraperitoneal fill volume and whether the patient is lying recumbent or standing and walking, in which case the pressures increase often above the hydrostatic pressure within the capillaries. Thus there will be a trade-off between the volume instilled, particularly during the daytime, and the net ultrafiltration achieved, which one should be aware of (30,32).

The reabsorption of water that occurs throughout the dialysis cycle, often referred to as the effective lymphatic absorption rate, has an important influence on net fluid removal (22,31). It is constant throughout the dwell period but does appear to differ substantially between individuals. The precise route of water disappearing from the peritoneum remains controversial, but clinically it is important, resulting in net positive fluid balance after longer dwell periods.

IV. CORRELATION BETWEEN ANATOMICAL STRUCTURE AND MODELS OF FUNCTION

There is a growing consensus that the effective barrier or wall between vascular compartment and peritoneal lumen is the endothelium of the peritoneal capillary circulation. Pore theory predicts that the vast majority of holes in this barrier, through which low molecular weight solutes pass, are 40–50 Å in diameter and are likely to represent the intercellular gaps between capillary endothelial cells (26). Their number or density, which reflects the effective peritoneal surface area, will, therefore, be determined by the number of perfused capillaries and not the intrinsic permeability of the membrane. The acute increase in effective peritoneal surface area during peritonitis, referred to above, results from the alterations in the peritoneal capillary bed associated with local increased concentrations in vasodilatory prostaglandins and other vascular mediators (33). This process accounts to a large degree for the acute deterioration in ultrafiltration that occurs during infections (23).

In contrast, pore theory predicts that macromolecules pass through a very much smaller number (<0.1%) of holes of larger diameter (150 Å), for which the anatomical structure is less clear (26). It is, however, likely that it is not simply a function of the size of a hole but also of the structure of the surrounding interstitium, which will restrict the rate at which macromolecules can reach the peritoneal lumen. The more interstitial fibrosis and thickening there is present, the greater the restriction there will be on macromolecular transport and the lower the measured intrinsic peritoneal permeability will be. As with effective peritoneal surface area, there is also an increase in intrinsic permeability during active peritonitis that recovers with the resolution of the infection (23).

The anatomical equivalent of the specific water channel is an ultra-small pore (<5 Å) thought to be the aquaporin-1 molecule. Its presence has been demonstrated in peritoneal capillary endothelial cells (34), and it has been proposed to be a potential important target for dialysis solution–induced peritoneal damage, such as glycosylation following continuous exposure to high glucose concentrations (22).

V. CHANGES IN PERITONEAL FUNCTION WITH TIME ON DIALYSIS

Most cross-sectional studies have suggested that the ultrafiltration capacity of the peritoneum deteriorates with time (35,36). These studies are confounded by the effect of loss of residual renal function, which results in the peritoneal problem coming to light, combined with the high drop-out rates in PD. There is, however, increasing evidence from longitudinal cohort studies that effective peritoneal surface area, as measured by the mass transfer coefficients or dialysate-to-plasma ratios of small solutes, increases with time (5,8,37,38). This effect appears to be the case despite a higher drop-out rate in patients with more rapid solute transport (39). The predominant effect of peritonitis, particularly when severe, also appears to be an increase in solute transport, although not a necessary accompaniment to these changes (8). While increased transport, and thus EPSA, appears to be a particular problem beyond 3 years of treatment, it is important to point out that there is considerable patient variability, and it is difficult to extrapolate mean values in cohort studies to the individual.

The evidence for changes in intrinsic peritoneal permeability with time on treatment is considerably less robust, partially because this is rarely measured. In one case-matched study comparing patients treated for 5 years with PD compared to those starting treatment, there appeared to be a significant reduction in peritoneal permeability with time (36) despite increased effective peritoneal surface area. This would be in keeping with an increase in peritoneal fibrosis, but longitudinal cohort studies have not confirmed this as yet, although numbers and period of follow-up are not sufficient to exclude this possibility (29). Little is known about the longitudinal changes in transcellular water channels, although the closest clinical correlate with loss of sodium sieving is the duration of dialysis treatment (27).

VI. BIOCOMPATIBILITY AND THE PERITONEAL MEMBRANE

Clinical data on changes in peritoneal membrane function with time on PD together with limited observations made in peritoneal biopsy specimens and extrapolations made from in vitro experiments present unequivocal evidence that the nature of the peritoneal membrane changes with time on dialysis (9–12,40–45). Unfortunately, despite more than 20 years of opportunity to study these presumed structural changes, there is no precise definition of what these are (except in the case of sclerosing peritonitis or sclerosing encapsulating peritonitis) and no knowledge about the factors responsible in their etiology. The limited evidence available suggests that, as in other organ systems, changes in the peritoneal membrane are "fibrotic" in character and result in eventual sclerosis or thickening of the membrane either with or without apparent mesothelial cell alterations.

A. Peritoneal Host Defense

In an attempt to understand the potential changes that might occur in the peritoneal membrane with time on

PD, a significant amount of research effort has been invested in understanding the inflammatory and humoral immune status (46–50) in the dialyzed peritoneum both during stable treatment and especially during episodes of peritonitis (51–59). Simultaneously, a large body of observations, mainly based on in vitro systems, have attempted to define the contribution of resident and infiltrating peritoneal cell populations to the activation, amplification, and resolution of peritoneal inflammation (for reviews, see Refs. 60,61). Much of this work is derived from early studies on dialysis fluid biocompatibility and initially involved the characterization of peritoneal "host defense" status (62–65). While these initial studies defined the nature of humoral and cellular host defense against infection and were seminal in defining our understanding of peritoneal inflammation, research over the succeeding 10 years has produced a more contemporary view of the contribution of various humoral and cellular components to this process (50,60,66,67). Central in this effort has been the understanding of the pivotal role played by the resident cells of the peritoneal membrane (in particular the mesothelium) in controlling peritoneal homeostasis and its response to inflammation (68–71). In addition, our increasing knowledge of the importance of the cell-cell interactions (between resident and infiltrating cells) has revealed the complexity of inflammatory reactions within the peritoneum and has identified links in basic cellular mechanisms to inflammatory processes occurring at other biological membranes in the body (gut, lung, and urinary tract) (60,72–75).

B. Inflammation in the Peritoneal Cavity

Current dogma, based on ex vivo measurements of intraperitoneal mediator levels in PD patients during peritonitis, stable dialysis, and in vitro cell culture systems, provides the following scenario. Inflammatory activation within the peritoneal cavity proceeds in a coordinate manner. The normal peritoneal cavity contains a small resident population of leukocytes, predominantly tissue macrophages (64,76). In PD patients this number is substantially increased and the dialysis procedure itself results in a constant flux of mononuclear cells as a result of their loss in drained effluent (64,76).

Inflammation in the dialyzed peritoneum thus involves an initiation phase resulting from the activation of resident phagocytes, and probably the mesothelium, by invading microorganisms (or their secreted products) (77,78) and an amplification phase, which results in mesothelial cell activation by peritoneal macrophage-derived pro-inflammatory cytokines (such as IL-1β and TNF-α). This process results in the generation of the chemotactic signals via creation of a gradient of chemotactic cytokines (specific for individual leukocyte subpopulations) in the recruitment of these inflammatory cells to the site of activation (68–70,79). This infiltration process is being facilitated by the upregulation of leukocyte specific adhesion molecules of the immunoglobulin superfamily (ICAM-1 and VCAM-1/2) on the mesothelial surface (71,80–82). Leukocyte infiltration is tightly controlled such that initially polymorphonuclear leukocytes predominate (6–24 hours) and are subsequently replaced by mononuclear cells (mononuclear phagocytes and T and B lymphocytes) (58). This switch in leukocyte phenotype appears also to be controlled by specific mesothelial cell–derived chemokines and is presumed to represent the resolution of infection/inflammation, although much less is understood about this process and the return to tissue homeostasis (83).

C. The Link Between Inflammation and Membrane Dysfunction

In understanding how structural changes can occur over time in the dialyzed peritoneal membrane, it is first important to understand which factors might contribute to this process. As will be discussed later, continuous exposure to bioincompatible dialysis solutions potentially contributes directly to cell activation and "profibrotic" events or indirectly increases the peritoneum's susceptibility to infection by downregulating host defense status (50). While there is little direct evidence to support this, there is clearly a link between peritoneal inflammation and membrane function in PD patients (8) (as noted above). In extending this argument we must make the assumption that functional changes in the peritoneal membrane (ultrafiltration, solute clearance, etc.) are linked to the changes in its structure that we know (based on biopsy evidence) to occur in long-term PD patients. Our increasing understanding of peritoneal inflammatory processes and how these events are paralleled in other organ systems also allows us (to some extent) to extrapolate from current understanding of fibrotic processes in these organs to events that might contribute to structural alterations in the peritoneal membrane (84).

It is assumed that in response to repeated episodes of inflammatory activation (although in long-term patients a single episode of peritonitis might be sufficient) in a peritoneal membrane presumably sensitized by years on dialysis changes occur in the peritoneal membrane that initiate a "fibrotic" response. At this juncture it is important to define the process of fibrotic development (hypercellularity and changes in extracellular matrix turnover and deposition over months or years that may eventually lead to irreparable deposition of a dense collagenous matrix, occlusion of blood vessels, and loss of mesothelium) to avoid confusion with sclerosing membrane syndromes (85,86). Data from many centers have clearly identified sclerosing peritonitis or, in its most severe form, sclerosing encapsulating peritonitis (SEP) both histologically and functionally. This is a rare if increasing complication in PD (0.5–0.9% of the overall PD population) and is manifested mostly in long-term patients (>8 years on therapy) where its incidence rises to 15–20% of patients on PD for more than 8 years (87). Its incidence does not appear (based on currently available data) to be related to the patients' peritonitis history, however, it is usually precipitated by an infective episode (85,86,88). The increasing numbers of patients on long-term PD (>8 years) has meant that the total numbers of episodes of SEP have increased but the overall frequency of its occurrence has not changed, strongly suggesting that time on PD is the most important factor in its initiation (87) and that a "sensitization" process occurs in the long-term dialyzed peritoneum.

In defining "fibrotic" changes within the peritoneum, however, we wish to focus on those events that potentially occur continuously over time (from initiation of the therapy) that impact on peritoneal membrane dysfunction. Although we still understand little about the time course over which these changes occur, we assume that they have a cumulative effect over years on PD.

D. Mechanisms of Fibrosis

As mentioned previously, the precise mechanisms by which peritoneal fibrosis is initiated are poorly understood. Data from studies of pulmonary, hepatic, renal, and skin fibrosis indicate that in these organs fibrosis involves a series of overlapping phases, which eventually lead to irreparable damage to the interstitium of the tissue involved (89–94). These studies show that the initiation is related to ongoing inflammation and that the presence of macrophages is important for its development. The initial activation stage appears to be followed by a period of matrix remodeling followed by increased collagen deposition and eventually tissue fibrosis. The precise signals that lead to the switching on of the fibrogenic process are unclear. It appears that in the early stages of inflammation, there is an infiltration of activated macrophages and a release of cytokines and growth factors (89,95). This process provides the cellular signals for both the attraction and activation of interstitial fibroblasts and appears to result in increased matrix deposition (89).

To date, studies of the development of peritoneal fibrosis in continuous ambulatory PD (CAPD) patients are limited to histological examination of biopsy or autopsy material (96,97). These indicate that the process described for other tissues approximates that which occurs in the peritoneal membrane. First, there appears to be little (or insufficient) evidence that the uraemic state per se is responsible for the development of fibrosis (96,98). Second, the fibrotic process is in some cases associated with ongoing mild or chronic peritoneal membrane inflammation. Third, it appears that the peritoneal fibroblast is principally responsible for the observed increases in collagen deposition.

These observations led to in vitro investigations of the potential role of peritoneal interstitial fibroblasts in contributing to fibrotic events within the peritoneal membrane. Although these studies are in their infancy, it is already clear that these cells have significant biosynthetic capacity and are clearly capable of contributing to both inflammatory and fibrotic processes within the peritoneum (20,21). These studies have shown that these cells respond to activation (by peritoneal effluents isolated during episodes of peritonitis) with increased proliferation and collagen synthesis. Interestingly, using a three-dimensional cell culture system in an attempt to mimic their in vivo environment, we have recently observed that repeated activation of peritoneal fibroblasts is required for sustained cell hyperplasia and extracellular matrix (collagen and fibronectin) synthesis. These data are of interest when taken in the context of the clinical evidence that loss of ultrafiltration appears to occur more rapidly in patients who suffer repeated or prolonged episodes of peritonitis (8) (see earlier). Furthermore, Rubin et al. reported that autopsy evidence of significant peritoneal fibrosis was only found in patients who had severe or repeated peritoneal inflammation (96).

VII. BIOINCOMPATIBILITY AND THE PERITONEAL MEMBRANE

Laboratory-based research over the past 15 years has resulted in extensive delineation of the potential effects of peritoneal dialysis fluid (PDF) components on peritoneal (and other surrogate) cell functions (65,99–104). While these studies were initially aimed at providing the rationale for the peritoneal cavity's susceptibility to infection by modulating host defense mechanisms, more recently they have provided the basis for our understanding of the potential of PDF components to modulate peritoneal membrane structure and function in long-term PD. Part of the rationale for these studies is based on clinical evidence that loss of ultrafiltration can also occur in patients without a significant history of peritoneal infection, leading to the suggestion that "other factors," such as continuous exposure to PDF components, might play an important role in the process.

A contemporary view of PDF biocompatibility therefore divides the effects of PDF components into: (a) "acute" effects, which have a predominantly inhibitory outcome and result from short-term (minutes to hours) exposure to specific PDF components, and (b)"chronic" effects, which result from prolonged or repeated exposure (hours to years) to PDF. Interestingly, various PDF components can have both acute and chronic effects, indicating their potential to modify peritoneal homeostasis by several mechanisms (see below) (Fig. 5).

A. Acute Effects of PDF: Impact on Peritoneal Host Defense

As mentioned previously, laboratory-based in vitro experiments as well as more limited animal experiments and ex vivo studies in PD patients have clearly identified that almost all components of conventional PDF levels (acidic lactate-buffered PDF containing 1.36 or 3.86% glucose) which are present at unphysiological concentrations are capable of modulating cell function (67,100,104–110). These include acidic pH (5.2–5.5), which is necessary to prevent the caramelization of glucose during its routine heat sterilization, lactate concentration (40 mM), which is used as the buffering system, and glucose concentration (75–214 mM) and associated hyperosmolality (350–500 mOsm/kg) necessary to produce an osmotically active solution. Additional studies have also identified that the heat sterilization process also gives rise to bioactive metabolites resulting from the chemical breakdown of glucose (111–114). In vitro these glucose degradation products (GDP) have been shown to modulate cell functions (115,116). In addition to their direct modulatory effects on cell function, these highly biologically active compounds are also potentially important intermediates and catalysts in the formation of advanced glycation end product (AGE) formation, the potential impact on peritoneal membrane structure and function of which will be discussed later (117).

Hand in hand with the identification of the components present in PDF that modulate cell function has been the delineation of the mechanism by which the undesirable effects are mediated. Many of the early studies using extended exposure protocols indicated significant loss of viability in all cell types. Such extended exposure periods are, however, of little clinical relevance since infused solutions are equilibrated by absorption and diffusion (64,100). While there is some

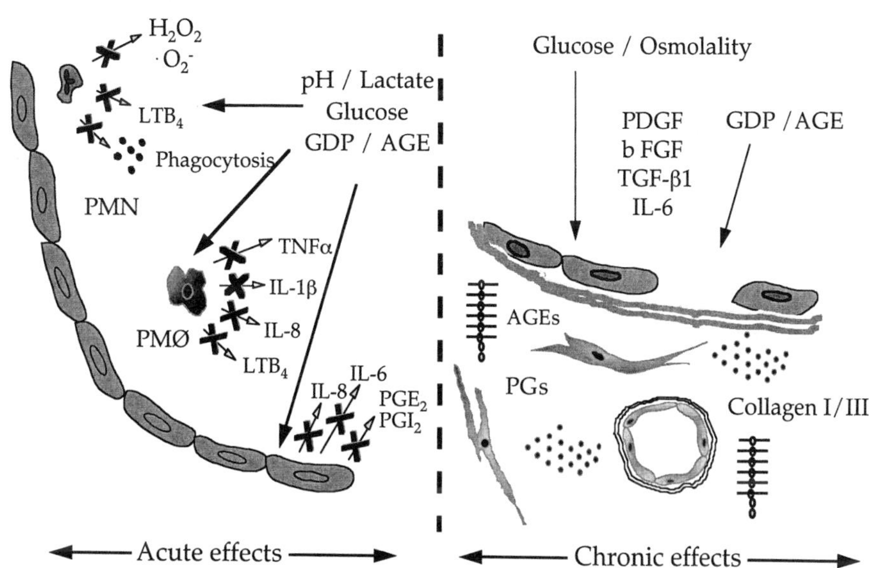

Fig. 5 Schematic representation of the acute and chronic effects of PDF components on peritoneal cell function and structure.

debate as to the time period over which this equilibration process occurs in the peritoneal cavity, ex vivo studies in which peritoneal macrophages are studied after isolation from PDF infused into patients for short time periods (usually 20–30 min) clearly show inhibition of their function. These data indicate that even for a short period the infused PDF retains its inhibitory potential in vivo. In addition, since most patients are either performing four bag exchanges per day in CAPD or infusing larger volumes of PDF in automated therapies, the cumulative effect of repeated infusion of unphysiological solutions over long periods of time must be taken into account when considering the effect of PDF in the peritoneal cavity (see later).

In more physiological experimental systems (acute exposure or simulated equilibration), the most profound effect PDF on cell function is related to the combination of low pH and lactate concentration (65,118,119). Even after very short exposure periods these components rapidly lower intracellular pH ($[pH])_i$) in all cell types studied (118). This acidification is associated with a rapid depletion of cellular ATP levels, which appears to be a central mechanism by which cell functional inhibition is mediated (120).

The extremely high glucose concentrations and associated hyperosmolality also modulate cell function following acute exposure (121). This effect is also associated with a depletion of cellular ATP levels. Although the cellular mechanisms whereby these effects are mediated is not fully delineated, recent data from our laboratory suggest that the acute effects of glucose (per se) on cell function are related to polyol pathway activation, intracellular sorbitol accumulation, and simultaneous ATP depletion (Kaur and Topley, unpublished data).

The mechanism by which GDP modulate cell function has not so far been identified, however, the pattern and degree of inhibition would suggest that similar mechanisms are operating at the subcellular level. The manifestation of these inhibitory events may be the reduction in steady-state mRNA levels for various mediators; in this respect recent data have clearly demonstrated that cytokine (IL-6 and TNF-α) as well as cyclooxygenase mRNA levels are reduced in mononuclear leukocytes and mesothelial cells following acute exposure to PDF (120,122).

B. Chronic Effects of PDF: Impact on the Structure of the Peritoneal Membrane

Over the past few years our increased awareness of the need to preserve the function of the peritoneal membrane have focused attention on the identification of those factors that modulate peritoneal membrane function with time. While the link between structural and functional alterations in the peritoneal membrane is hypothetical (see earlier), the little evidence that exists from examination of peritoneal biopsies indicates that structural changes do occur in the dialyzed membrane, and it is therefore a logical step to suggest that these "changes" are linked to functional changes such as ultrafiltration and solute clearance. This direction of thought has also been applied to PDF biocompatibility since despite the evidence that solution components are capable of modulating cell function in vitro and ex vivo, there is, to date, little evidence that this impacts on peritoneal membrane structure and function (see later).

As discussed earlier, however, PD patients are exposed to unphysiological levels of PDF components throughout their time on dialysis (approximately 3000 L/yr), although the "equilibration process" results in some PDF components reaching physiological levels at some stage during the dwell. Many, however, do not, and those that do may be at unphysiological levels for a significant period of the dwell. For example, glucose is infused at between 75 and 214 mM and at the end of a standard 4-hour dwell will have reached 20–30 and 75–90 mM (100). As the physiological glucose concentration is between 5 and 10 mM, the potential impact is clear. In addition, repeated infusion of solutions could theoretically lead to the accumulation of nonmetabolizable compounds in the tissues of the peritoneal membrane or systematically (as occurs with maltose following polyglucose infusion), the potential cumulative effects of this remains to be defined (123).

There is increasing evidence of chronic effects of PDF components on cell function, which at least provide some rationale for the argument that solution biocompatibility might have an impact on the structure/function of the peritoneal membrane. The most compelling of this relates to the effects of glucose on peritoneal cell function in vitro and in vivo and is closely related to studies in diabetes and diabetic nephropathy on the modulating influence of glucose on cell and organ function (124,125).

Initial studies in cultured mesothelial cells exposed to D-glucose for extended periods demonstrated reduced cellular proliferation; this effect appeared to be osmolality independent and paralleled observations made in phagocytic leukocytes (121,126). In both systems exposure to glucose concentrations above 75 mM resulted in significant cytotoxicity as evidenced by increased lactate dehydrogenase (LDH) release. Subsequent studies by Kumano et al. demonstrated that prolonged exposure to D-glucose was associated with increased mesothelial cell expression of fibronectin mRNA, an effect that was D-glucose specific and independent of osmolality (127). Our own studies have examined the effect of glucose on mesothelial cell transforming growth factor-β1 (TGF-β1) expression. In these experiments chronic (1–7 days) exposure of cells to glucose resulted in an increase in TGF-β1 mRNA and protein secretion (128).

Effects of chronic glucose exposure have also been observed in the peritoneal cavity of experimental animals and in PD patients. Using the ''imprint'' model, Gotloib et al. have clearly demonstrated that long-term exposure to glucose alters mesothelial cell structure and function (105–107). In vivo the stimulatory effects of glucose may occur over an even shorter time scale; Fujimori et al. recently demonstrated that intraperitoneal interleukin-6 levels correlate directly with the glucose content in the infused PDF (129). The implication of these latter findings is unclear, but continuous modulation or activation of IL-6 synthesis might have long-term consequences on the control of inflammation within the peritoneal cavity (51,54,69,130).

Our understanding of the mechanism by which glucose achieves these diverse effects is becoming increasingly more clear. Parallel experimentation in proximal tubular cells suggests that modulation of the polyol pathway plays a significant role in cell activation by glucose (131). This is clearly an area requiring further investigation.

As mentioned earlier, continuous exposure of tissues to high concentrations of glucose (such as those present in PDF) can result in the formation of AGE, a process that is facilitated in PDF by the presence of GDP, many of which catalyze or are components in the Maillard or late AGE-formation reactions (111–114,117). Examination of biopsies from the peritoneal membrane of PD patients clearly demonstrates the presence of AGE modified proteins (132,133). These could result from in situ formation due to high concentrations of glucose in the dialysate. Alternatively, they could have been deposited (trapped) by diffusion from the blood since increased levels of AGE are found in the serum of PD patients. Although their functional significance remains to be determined, data from other cell systems suggest that AGE modification of proteins modifies their metabolic fate (e.g., reduces collagen turnover) and can in some cases cause direct cell activation (134). The implication of increased cellular activation and decreased extracellular matrix turnover for the development of fibrotic changes within the peritoneal cavity is clear. Nakayama et al. (135) have reported that with increasing time on PD there is more AGE deposition in the peritoneum, particularly in vascular walls. As noted in other studies, there was also increased peritoneal permeability with longer treatment. Whether these two observations are related remains unproven, though in vitro the occupancy of endothelial cell AGE receptors is associated with increased permeability (136). In a recent study Honda et al. (137) examined peritoneal biopsies of patients with clinical ultrafiltration failure for evidence of interstitial and vascular changes. They concluded, in this small study, that there was extensive deposition of collagen IV and laminin in vessel walls and evidence of vascular smooth muscle degeneration. They attributed these changes to continuous exposure to ''certain toxic factors'' such as hyperosmolality and low pH (and presumably glucose) and suggested that these changes might be linked to changes in peritoneal membrane function.

VIII. CLINICAL ASSESSMENT OF PERITONEAL FUNCTION

A. The Peritoneal Equilibration Test

The peritoneal equilibration test (PET), following its introduction by Twardowski, has become the standard clinical tool worldwide for the assessment of peritoneal function (7,28). It measures two variables: the dialysate-to-plasma ratio of small solutes (glucose and creatinine), referred to as ''solute transport,'' and the net volume of ultrafiltration achieved after a standard 4-hour dwell using 2 L of medium-strength (2.27% glucose) dialysate.

While less precise than the measurement and calculation of mass transfer coefficients, solute transport as expressed by the dialysate-to-plasma ratio of creatinine at 4 hours represents a much simpler and perfectly adequate measure of effective peritoneal surface area. It is frequently expressed as a categorical variable (low: <0.5; low average: 0.5–0.65; high average: 0.65–0.8; high: >0.8), despite the fact that it is continuous, and it is important to recognize that these original categories were based upon the standard deviation of the distribution obtained from the first 100 patients in whom the test was performed. It does not necessarily follow, therefore, that these categories correspond to the clinical problem encountered in an individual patient, although they remain a useful guide.

An alternative way of expressing solute transport is as a continuous variable on a two-dimensional plot against the net ultrafiltration (Fig. 6) (28). This ap-

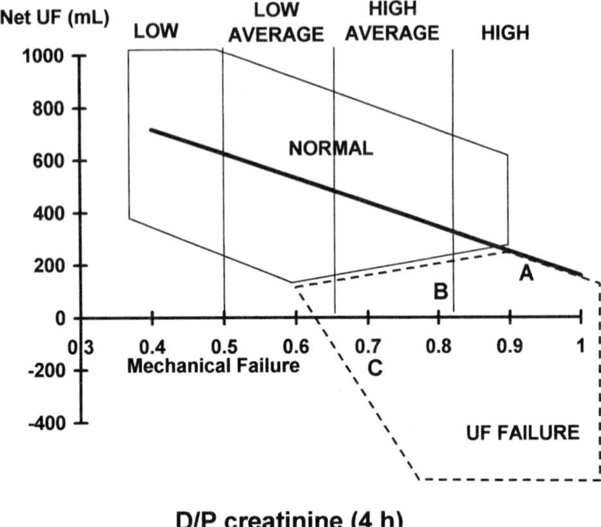

Fig. 6 Two-dimensional plot for data obtained from a standard PET. The negative regression line (y = 1090 − 931x) demonstrates the negative relationship between high solute transport and ultrafiltration. Categories for solute transport and regions associated with ultrafiltration and mechanical failure are indicated. PET results from patients with high solute (A), intermediate (B), and high absorption (C) failure are plotted.

proach has several advantages. First, it is immediately apparent whether the ultrafiltration volume obtained is appropriate for a given solute transport by comparing with the inverse relationship between these two variables previously defined for this test. Second, it allows the ready distinction between mechanical drainage problems and definition of ultrafiltration failure type. Third, it allows the plotting of serial PET results on a single chart, which facilitates the longitudinal tracking of peritoneal function. Patients tend to cluster their results in one region of the chart, allowing the relatively easy identification of a significant change in peritoneal function or equally a suspect test. Conversely, it is possible for patients to appear to switch categories (e.g., low average to high average) and yet have no clinically significant change in their peritoneal function.

The precise procedure for performing the PET has been described in detail elsewhere (7,8,28); there are, however, several points worth emphasizing that will be covered here.

1. It is important to discuss with the local chemistry laboratory the nature of the test, the dilutions of sample that will be required, and the interaction between the high glucose concentrations and the local assay for creatinine. This will allow the calculation of the appropriate correction factor to be used, allowing comparison of data with other units and the literature.
2. In preparing for the PET, patients should use their usual overnight dialysis regime (dwell length and glucose concentration) and should never be ''dry.'' This is to ensure as much as possible that the residual peritoneal volume is constant. If the patient is dry, lack of residual volume due to its reabsorption will result in underestimation of ultrafiltration.
3. In draining out both before and at the end of the test, the patient should be instructed to continue until the flow of dialysate has stopped rather than using a specific time limit. If drainage is particularly slow, this should be noted as it suggests a mechanical problem and will aid in interpretation of the test. Again, the residual peritoneal volume, if not typical, will influence the test result. Patients using disconnect systems should be careful not to allow excessive amounts of dialysate to enter the drainage bag during the flush procedure.
4. The measurement of solute transport using this method is relatively robust with a coefficient of variation in the region of 5% using the value obtained at 4 hours. No additional information is obtained from the values measured at 2 hours, which have a greater variability and are time consuming. The glucose at 4 hours must be measured to allow calculation of the creatinine concentration (see above) but provides no additional information, although it acts as a useful internal quality control if a calculation error is suspected.
5. In contrast to the solute transport, the variability in the measurement of net ultrafiltration is much greater despite the precautions mentioned above. Care should be taken not to overinterpret a result, and where possible interpretation should done in conjunction with knowledge of the volumes obtained from each exchange during the previous 24 hours. This will allow one to see if the value is consistent and so reduce sampling error.
6. The PET is not a substitute for measuring the peritoneal dialysis dose. The 4-hour D/P creatinine does not reflect the average over a 24-hour period, which will be affected by dwell lengths, and there is still a need to measure the total

dialysate volume drained from the patient over the day.

An alternative to the standard or short PET is the Standard Peritoneal Permeability Assessment (SPA) introduced by Krediet and coworkers (138). In its original form, it employed a 1.36% glucose exchange combined with instilled intraperitoneal dextran as a large molecular weight marker to calculate changes in peritoneal volumes. The glucose concentration has been revised to 3.86% to provide data for sodium sieving in the same test (see below), and a net drainage volume of 400 mL or less indicated ultrafiltration failure (139). Otherwise it is technically similar to the standard PET, provided the same precautions are observed (Table 2).

B. Measurement of Fluid Reabsorption (Relative Lymphatic Absorption)

The estimation of fluid reabsorption from the peritoneal cavity, whether by lymphatics or capillaries due to the oncotic pressure difference between blood and dialysate, remains difficult and controversial. The method involves measuring the rate of disappearance of a macromolecular marker, e.g., dextran, and at present is a research rather than a clinical tool (138). However, there are clues that will suggest that it is a significant problem, e.g., patients whose net ultrafiltration on the PET test is consistently less than would be expected from the relationship described by the regression line in Fig. 6 (28). Equally, patients in whom the net reabsorption of fluid following a long dwell is excessive are likely to have this problem. In both situations the likelihood of it contributing to peritoneal failure is increased if sodium sieving has been demonstrated to be normal.

C. Assessing Intrinsic Peritoneal Permeability

Measurement of intrinsic peritoneal permeability is complex and involves the estimation of the restriction coefficient of one or more macromolecules (24). As with estimates of lymphatic absorption, this remains a research tool, perhaps as a marker for interstitial fibrosis. At present there is no evidence that either absolute or interpatient differences in intrinsic peritoneal permeability influence clinical aspects of peritoneal function.

D. Measurement of Sodium Sieving

The purpose for measuring sodium sieving is twofold. First, it is helpful in the diagnosis of membrane failure (see below). Second, it will draw attention to the impact sodium sieving will have on the relative removal of salt and water from the patient. It is most easily measured by calculating the dialysate to plasma ratio of sodium one hour after the instillation of a hypertonic (3.86% glucose) exchange (22,139). A lower ratio (0.81–0.85) implies that sodium sieving occurs, whereas a higher ratio (0.87–0.94) indicates that this process has become much less efficient due to a clinically significant loss in the number of ultrasmall pores. Where possible, this test should include the measurement of the net ultrafiltration at 4 hours, where a value of less than 400 mL should raise concerns of ultrafiltration failure (139). It has been suggested that this test be combined with the standard PET to reduce workload by utilizing a 3.86% rather than a 2.27% glucose exchange and the taking of a sample at one hour. The disadvantage of this approach is that many nephrologists will have considerable historical data on their patients using the standard PET method or alternatively use the short version of the PET, in which only the sample obtained at 4 hours is used. Under these circumstances it is easy to proceed to a 3.86% exchange in selected patients.

E. Ex Vivo Markers of Peritoneal Structural Changes

One of the significant advantages that PD provides is access to dialysis effluent within which various parameters can be assessed. Indeed measurements (of mediator levels and the cellular components) in drained effluent have provided the basis for our understanding of the process of peritoneal inflammation in vivo (51,52,54–59,140). The ready access to this material has made it an attractive proposition within which to measure levels of markers that might be indicative of changes in the function of the membrane or its constitutive parts. In this respect, markers of mesothelial cell mass/turnover (CA125) (141–143), markers of endothelial cell function (factor VIII), and presumed fibrotic or wound-healing markers (pro-collagen I/III, hyaluronic acid, and TGF-β1) have been measured in PD patients at various points during treatment. Unfortunately, however, despite initial promise, particularly with CA125 as a mesothelial cell marker (and thus an indicator of mesothelial cell damage), the data provided so far have been cross-sectional and have produced conflicting results in different centers as to the relationship between it and time on PD (142,144). There are only limited data correlating membrane functional changes with dialysate levels in CA125, and this is

Table 2 Comparison of Peritoneal Equilibration Test (PET) with Standard Peritoneal Permeability Analysis (SPA)

Parameter	PET	SPA
Dwell length	4 hours	4 hours
Solution (glucose)	2.27%	1.36% or 3.86%*
Solute transport characteristics	D/P_{creat} ratio at 4 hours (corrected for glucose). D/P_{creat} and $MTAC_{creat}$ correlate well, although there is systematic error. For practical purposes the D/P_{creat} is independent of glucose concentration, so values obtained using PET and SPA are interchangeable. *Typical range of values:* D/P_{creat} 0.4–1.0.	Mass transfer area coefficient ($MTAC_{creat}$) or D/P ratio in simplified form of test. MTAC corrects for the convective component, and requires accurate measurement of intraperitoneal volumes before and after dwell (see below). *Typical range of values:* ($MTAC_{creat}$ 5.0–19.3 mL/min/1.73 m^2.
Ultrafiltration	Net UF volume at 4 hours. See Table 3 for values that are associated with clinical UF failure.	Uses instilled dextran 70 (1 g/L) as a volume marker to establish residual volume, effective lymphatic absorption, and transcapillary ultrafiltration. In the simplified version a net UF volume of <400 mL using 3.86% exchange suggests UF failure.
Sodium sieving	This is not part of the routine PET and requires the use of a 3.86% exchange if done as part of the SPA. It can either be expressed as the simple $D/P[Na^+]$ at 1 hour (see Table 3) or be corrected for diffusion by subtracting the gradient of $D/P[Na^+]$ at 1 hour achieved with a 1.36% exchange from that achieved with 3.86% exchange. A corrected gradient of less than 5 mmol/L may indicate impaired transcellular water transport. There is, however, a relationship between solute transport status and Na^+ sieving measured in this way, due to the more rapid loss of osmotic gradient in high transport patients.	
Intrinsic peritoneal permeability	Not applicable.	By measuring clearances of a number of proteins of varying sizes (β_2-microglobulin), a restriction coefficient is calculated that equates to the intrinsic permeability.

*Modified version of the test was a 3.86% exchange.

mostly in patients with sclerosing peritonitis, where the complete loss of mesothelium is evidenced by low or undetectable CA125 levels (145). There is clearly a need for longitudinal studies on CA125 and other markers in individual patients to define the variability and thus the usefulness of these tests. Only when such data are available can definitive links between these markers and clinical changes in peritoneal function be established or refuted.

IX. RECOGNITION OF PERITONEAL FAILURE

A. Peritoneal Function and Solute Removal

It is not the purpose of this chapter to define adequate solute removal for the PD patient, and the complications related to inadequate delivery of dialysis dose are discussed elsewhere. However, peritoneal function does have an important influence on delivered dose primarily by influencing the net ultrafiltration achieved and thus the convective component to solute clearance.

Difficulties are likely to be experienced in achieving adequate clearances in the anuric patient at either end of the solute transport spectrum. For patients with low solute transport, and thus a low effective peritoneal surface area it will be difficult to achieve targets (e.g. 60 liters creatinine clearance/week/1.73 m^2) in those with a large body surface area (146). When the PET was initially described this was considered potentially to be the principle limiting factor of peritoneal function. In practice, however, this has not turned out to be the case partially because it affects very few patients, (most large patients have D/P creatinine ratios of >0.6), but also because large patient size has not been found to be associated with adverse outcome in PD (39,147). In fact there is increasing evidence that low solute transport patients do well on peritoneal dialysis. Nevertheless, it remains an important consideration, and will have a greater impact if the chosen method of dialysis measurement is the creatinine rather than the urea clearance.

For patients with high solute transport, the principle effect on achieved dialysis dose results from the relatively poor ultrafiltration achieved in these patients, and thus the reduced convective clearance. The differences between estimates of creatinine and urea clearances will be much more, and creatinine clearance targets will be easier to achieve in these patients.

B. Peritoneal Function and Inadequate Fluid Removal—Ultrafiltration Failure

It is in the area of fluid removal from the PD patient that assessment of peritoneal function is most important. Ultrafiltration failure may be defined from two standpoints: from the assessment of peritoneal function or from a clinical approach to the patient. The former may use a definition derived from peritoneal function testing, such as the failure to achieve more than 400 mL net fluid removal following a 4-hour hypertonic dialysate exchange (139) or less than 200 mL following a PET (see Table 3) (28). The latter would define ultrafiltration failure as the inability to remove sufficient water (and salt, see below) to enable the patient to maintain their designated dry weight, while allowing an adequate fluid intake and avoiding dialysis regimes that result in excessive dialysate calorie intake and weight gain. This approach, while more clinically relevant, has the disadvantage of being less precise due to the difficulties in assessing true dry weight in PD patients and is confounded by other variables such as residual renal function and changing body composition. In practice, one will use a combination of both in the assessment of the patient.

Patients with ultrafiltration failure have been found to have peritoneal function that differs from normal in three ways: they may have high effective peritoneal surface areas as measured by solute transport, high relative lymphatic absorption rates resulting in reduced net fluid removal, or impaired transcellular water transport as evidenced by reduced sodium sieving (27,28,35,139). In the majority of such patients there is a combination of these problems, and the relative contribution of each factor is not always clear. A combination of the PET and sodium sieving test in most cases will give one sufficient information to diagnose the cause of the problem, and thus proceed to a rational approach to therapy.

The diagnostic ranges of results obtained from the standard PET and sodium sieving tests are summarised in Table 3, which should be read in conjunction with Fig. 6 where sample patients have been plotted. It should be emphasized, however, that in assessing the patient with ultrafiltration failure that it is also useful to examine the total regime that the patient is using, with the results of net ultrafiltration achieved with each individual exchange as well as the total for a 24-hour period. It is difficult to imagine how an anuric PD patient can sustain adequate nutrition on less than 1000 mL ultrafiltration per day, particularly in view of sodium balance (see below), and it is likely that this should be a minimum target for such patients. Equally, it is important to know if any of the individual exchanges result in the development of a positive balance, as this will result in a particular problem when trying to achieve target dry weights.

Table 3 Values from PET and Sodium Sieving Used to Define Ultrafiltration Failure

A. Peritoneal equilibration test	D/P_{creat} at 4 hours	Net UF volume (mL)
High solute transport UF failure (see example A, Fig. 6)	>0.85	<250
High effective lymphatic absorption (see example C, Fig. 6)	<0.75	<150
Mixed type UF failure (see example B, Fig. 6)	0.75–08.5	<220
B. Sodium sieving test	**D/P [Na+] at 1 hour using 3.86% glucose exchange**	
Impaired sodium sieving	>0.87	

C. Problems of Electrolyte Balance

Generally there are no problems associated with potassium removal in PD patients, for whom hyperkalaemia is rarely a problem. It is possible that with time and the development of malnutrition that PD patients become total body deficient in potassium, but this cannot be considered a direct result of membrane failure.

In contrast, the removal of sodium from the anuric PD patient is critically dependent on ultrafiltration and thus peritoneal membrane function (148). This is best illustrated by an example calculation of an anuric patient, with a plasma sodium concentration of 140 mmol/L, using dialysate containing 132 mmol/L, on a daily regime of 10 L. If no net ultrafiltration were achieved, then the maximum possible sodium removal per day, assuming complete equilibration with plasma, would be 80 mmol. In fact, due to the phenomenon of sodium sieving and incomplete equilibration during shorter dwells, this is likely to be an overestimate. Even allowing for gastrointestinal and sweat losses, this would not be sufficient to maintain balance. However, for every 100 mL of ultrafiltrate there is the potential to increase sodium removal by 10–14 mmol, depending on the sodium sieving. Thus, both theoretically and empirically (148) the net sodium removed is very dependent on the ultrafiltration achieved. The actual values obtained can easily be measured when assessing dialysis adequacy, and this should be done routinely in the anuric patient. It is also important to realize the impact of sodium sieving on the relative proportion of sodium to water removal in certain situations. For example, in patients having relatively high volume but short dwells with medium or high glucose concentrations, as may occur in patients on APD, ultrafiltration may appear adequate but sodium losses relatively low. This would be further exacerbated in the presence of dry days or net fluid absorption during the long daytime dwell period (149).

D. Problems of Acid-Base Correction

At present there are no firm data suggesting a trend to increasing acidosis in patients with deteriorating peritoneal function in terms of solute or fluid removal. There are no studies reporting isolated problems with acid-base balance. In general the acid-base status of the patient is determined by the concentration of potential buffer, lactate, or bicarbonate in the dialysate (150). Stein et al. reported that patients' nutrition is better if they are maintained with a dialysate containing a higher buffer concentration (40 mmol/L) as compared to a lower one (35 mmol/L) (151).

E. Other Problems Associated with High Effective Peritoneal Surface Area

In addition to the problems associated with peritoneal ultrafiltration, patients with high effective peritoneal surface areas are at additional risk for two other problems: excessive peritoneal protein losses and increased dialysis calorie load, which may contribute to obesity.

One of the undesirable systemic effects of peritoneal dialysis is the loss of plasma proteins into the dialysate, which can constitute between 5 and 15 g per day (152). The majority of the protein lost is in the form of albumin, and for reasons explained above albumin clearances are increased in high solute transport patients. This compounds the problem of hypoalbuminemia and edema in individuals who are already at risk of overhydration from poor ultrafiltration further reduces plasma refilling. While co-morbidity and nutritional state remain important determinants of the plasma albumin, it is important to recognize that this problem is often due to peritoneal function.

The absorption of glucose from the peritoneum is bimodal in the PD population (153), due to the synergistic effects of increased fractional absorption and higher dialysate glucose concentrations required by patients with greater effective peritoneal surface areas. While this does not always lead to excessive fat gain and may in some cases provide a useful energy source (154), there is no doubt that in some patients this can lead to significant and problematic obesity.

X. TREATMENT STRATEGIES FOR PERITONEAL FAILURE

A. Peritoneal Function and Dialysis Prescription

In prescribing peritoneal dialysis the principal aim is to use a regime that maximizes the total volume of dialysate drained from the patient. This is usually limited first by the maximum volume that the patient can tolerate, which should and will be greater in larger patients, and second by the patients' peritoneal function. Table 4 shows the suggested possible regimes that can be used according to patient size and effective peritoneal surface area. The actual volumes used will depend upon the target of clearance required, the amount of residual renal function, and the volumes tolerated by the patient.

Table 4 Potential PD Regimes According to Patient Size and Solute Transport

	Effective peritoneal surface area (solute transport from PET)			
Body surface area	Low (D/P_{creat} <0.5)	Low-average (D/P_{creat} 0.5–0.65)	High-average (D/P_{creat} 0.65–0.81)	High (D/P_{creat} >0.81)
Small (<1.71)	Use CAPD regimes with 21 dwells; if anuric may require extra exchanges; alter glucose according to solute transport.		Use combination of short dwells, e.g., APD overnight with glucose polymer for long dwells.	
Medium (1.71–2.0)	Use 2.5–3.1 exchanges, 5 or 6 per day, avoid short dwells and consider hemodialysis.	Use CAPD regimes with dwell volumes according to patient size; larger anuric patients may require an extra dwell period during the night (CAPD patients) or the day (APD patients). Those with higher solute transport will require higher glucose concentrations.		
Large (>2.0)			As patient size increases, use larger dwell volumes and add a further daytime dwell period.	

B. Strategies in the Management of Ultrafiltration Failure

In designing a regime for the patient with clinical evidence of ultrafiltration failure, the first step is to establish when, if at all, during the 24 hours the patient is developing positive fluid balance. Unless this is put right, the ability to achieve adequate fluid removal during the remainder of the day will be compromised. If this proves impossible using the strategies described, then it is likely that the patient will need to be switched to hemodialysis. Augmentation of residual urine volumes with diuretics may be considered, but this is unlikely to be a long-term solution.

In addition to the standard range of glucose concentrations available, there are now a variety of therapeutic procedures that can be adopted to improve ultrafiltration, and a logical approach to their use is described in the algorithm (Fig. 7). These can be broadly divided into two categories: approaches that allow manipulation of dwell length and those that exploit alternative osmotic agents, although both may be combined into the same regime.

The development of automated devices of increasing reliability has allowed one to manipulate the regime to a considerable degree. For example, a single long dwell in the daytime can be combined with four or five short dwells overnight using automated peritoneal dialysis. Alternatively, five equally spaced dwells throughout the 24-hour period may be used with an overnight assist device. In general terms, the patient with clinically relevant ultrafiltration failure will have little or no residual renal function, and thus the use of regimes that are dry either during the night or day are to be avoided in order to obtain adequate clearances.

The most important development in the field of alternative osmotic agents has been the introduction of high molecular weight glucose polymers (Icodextrin) (155). This solution is able to create an oncotic pressure across the peritoneal membrane and achieve ultrafiltration despite being iso-osmolar with plasma (156). It is ideally suited to improving ultrafiltration in patients with a high effective peritoneal surface area because it achieves most of its effects through the intercellular pores. It is important to recognize that the longer the dwell period, the better the ultrafiltration will be, at least up to 12 hours, e.g., in patients on APD (157). Original concerns regarding its safety appear to have been answered, although it is only licensed for use in one exchange per day (158). It may have particular advantages in reducing total calorie intake in patients in whom obesity is a problem or in situations where exposure of the peritoneum to glucose is being avoided. There is already evidence to suggest that its use may reverse some of the peritoneal changes associated with ultrafiltration, including reducing effective peritoneal surface area and enhancing transcellular water transport.

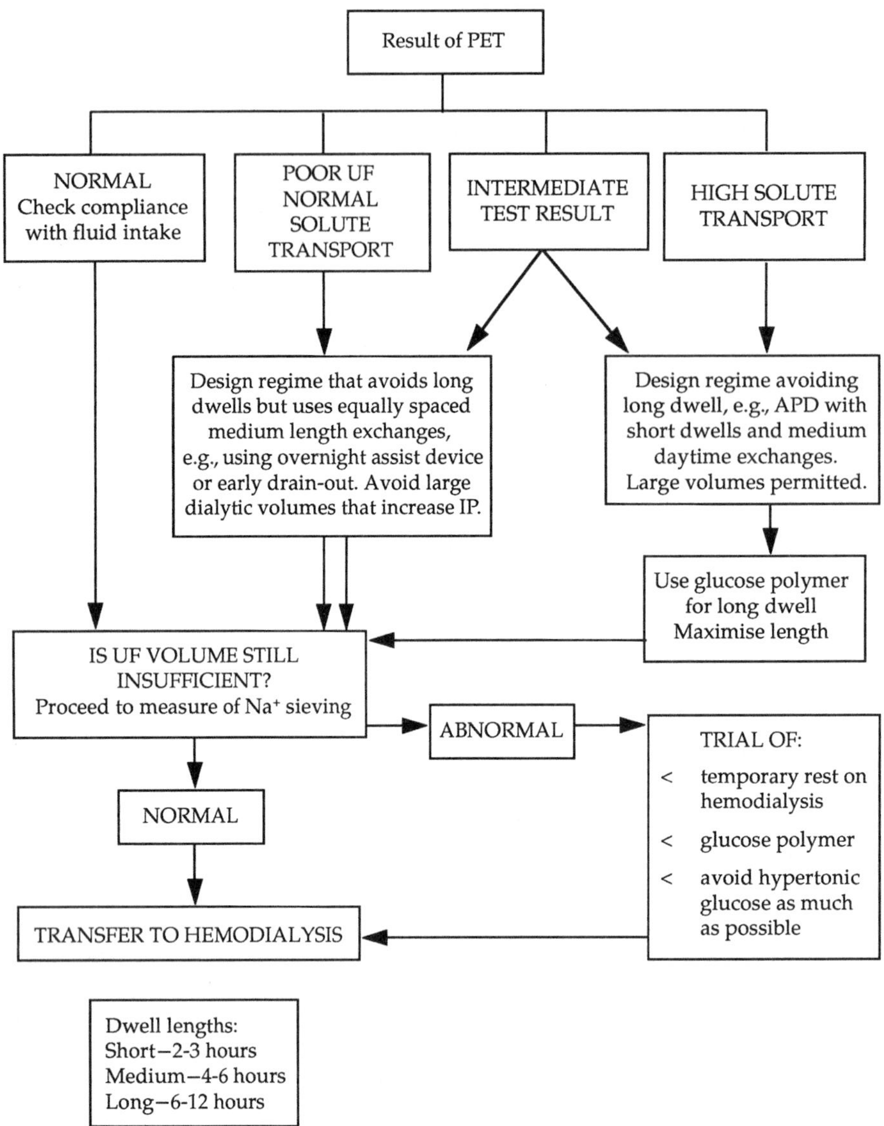

Fig. 7 Algorithm for the management options of ultrafiltration failure.

Other nonglucose solutions include amino acids and glycerol, although the latter is not generally available. These have no specific role in ultrafiltration failure except as part of a glucose-free regime, which may allow peritoneal recovery.

C. Improving Sodium Balance

As indicated above, the best way to ensure that the patient has sufficient sodium removal is to establish adequate ultrafiltration (148). It is important to recognize, however, that in reality sodium does not fully equilibrate between plasma and dialysate, particularly in shorter dwells where higher glucose concentrations will result in excessive water removal—in effect due to the sieving of sodium. It is, therefore, necessary to measure the total sodium removal, particularly in edematous anuric patients, to establish the actual amount and match where possible to the dietary intake. Other approaches to this problem are currently being developed, in particular the use of dialysate solutions with a low sodium content (159,160). Sodium concentrations ranging from 98 to 128 mmol/L have been assessed with conflicting results. Some have reported little value in the higher range but the development of concerning clinical symptoms (161), while others have found the ultra-low dialysate sodium solutions to be well tolerated and clinically efficacious (159,160,162). These differences are difficult to understand but may represent variability in dietary salt intake.

D. Improving Acid-Base Balance

As noted previously, acidosis has not been recognized as a feature of impaired peritoneal function. It is, however, important to correct any tendency to a low plasma bicarbonate, and improvement has been shown to reduce protein degradation and increase nutrition (163). Malnutrition is an important adverse risk factor for survival during PD, and any measure that will prevent the occurrence of protein calorie depletion should be implemented. At present it appears that either 40 mmol/L lactate or bicarbonate dialysate are better than lower concentrations of these ions at improving plasma bicarbonate concentrations. In addition, mmol for mmol they appear to be equipotent. In addition, patient nutrition appears to be better when using a 40 mmol/L concentration (151). The question of whether bicarbonate dialysate should be used because of enhanced biocompatibility profile will be considered later.

E. Enhancing Biocompatibility of Peritoneal Dialysis

At this point it must be reemphasised that the vast majority of evidence for PDF "bioincompatibility" is the result of in vitro experimentation. While much of this evidence is very persuasive of in vivo consequences, in many cases proof based on in vivo observation is lacking. Thus, although ex vivo studies suggest the bioincompatible nature of conventional lactate-buffered PDF containing glucose (108–110,164), data from long-term observations in PD patients are required to definitively identify which PDF components have an impact (or not) on peritoneal host defense and the structure or function of the peritoneal membrane.

Despite this lack of real in vivo evidence that PDF components directly affect peritoneal host defense or contribute to loss of membrane function, the weight of in vitro and ex vivo evidence, together with our increased understanding of the potential chronic effects of exposure to supra-physiological concentrations of PDF components, have resulted in the search for alternative solution formulations. These alternative solution formulations can be divided into (a) those that replace or reduce glucose concentration with an alternative osmotic agent, e.g., polyglucose, glycerol, amino acids, or a combination of these, and (b) those that create a neutral or near neutral pH solution either by replacing lactate as a buffer and/or preparing the solutions in dual chamber bags such that the glucose can be sterilized separately, e.g., bicarbonate, bicarbonate in combination with glycyl-glycine or lactate, or conventional lactate solution at pH 6.8 (165) (these solutions have the added advantage of reduced GDP content as a result of the sterilization of glucose at low pH). Many of these solutions have undergone phase II or phase III trials, and some have been introduced into clinical practice over the past few years. At present it is too early to assess whether any of these will impact on peritoneal membrane function. In vitro and ex vivo and animal studies, however, suggest that many of these formulations show significantly improved parameters of host defense compared to conventional acidic lactate-buffered solutions (107,110,122,166–173). It will be years, however, before the long-term effects of potentially more biocompatible PDF on peritoneal structure and function are definitively identified. Their introduction, however, allows us a unique opportunity to assess their impact compared to conventional solutions on peritoneal membrane longevity.

While there is strong theoretical, circumstantial, and in vitro evidence linking peritoneal damage to toxic or unphysiological constituents within dialysis fluid, proving direct cause and effect has been difficult. This is due in part to the relatively long period over which peritoneal damage occurs and in part to the need, in the case of glucose, to use ever-increasing concentrations to maintain adequate fluid balance, thus setting up a viscious circle. It has often been noted that a rest from PD results in some recovery of ultrafiltration capacity (38), and recent evidence from a group of patients with severe ultrafiltration failure treated with glucose-free PD (glycerol and icodextrin) for several months found an improvement in both solute transport and sodium sieving (145). In another randomized trial using icodextrin versus glucose for the long day dwell in patients treated with automated peritoneal dialysis, those patients in the icodextrin group had a significant improvement in their ultrafiltration, although the mechanism is less clear (22). It does seem likely, therefore, that strategies designed to avoid excessive glucose exposure may either reverse or prevent the development of peritoneal damage.

XI. WHAT WE DON'T UNDERSTAND ABOUT THE PROCESS OF PERITONEAL STRUCTURE/ FUNCTION CHANGES

Although our understanding of "fibrotic" processes is increasing largely as a result of in vitro experiments, many questions remain about the mechanisms by which structural alterations in the peritoneum are initiated and what factors are directly responsible or contributory to this process. In answering these questions we are severely hampered by the fact that there is no real description from PD patients of what these so-called "fibrotic" changes are or the time course over which they occur. Peritoneal biopsy data are to date very limited, and it is impossible to decide based on such a small uncontrolled sample size if the reported changes are representative for all patients. Clearly, there is the need to define the structure of the peritoneal membrane in normal, uremic, and dialyzed individuals and, where possible, to define the nature and time course of the changes that occur. Only then will we be able to define which factors contribute to membrane dysfunction and design therapeutic interventions to reduce these negative consequences and increase peritoneal membrane longevity.

XII. CONCLUSIONS

This chapter has attempted to link what is currently known about peritoneal structure and function to the clinical problems experienced in the management of PD patients. As our understanding of this membrane improves, it provides us with an increasingly rational approach to therapeutic manipulation. Hopefully, this, combined with the increasing number of treatment options available, should make it possible to enhance treatment quality and improve patient and technique survival on this modality.

REFERENCES

1. Maiorca R, Cancarini GC, Camerini C, Brunori G, Manili L, Movilli E, Feller P, Mombelloni S. Is CAPD competitive with haemodialysis for long-term treatment of uraemic patients? [review]. Nephrol Dial Transplant 1989; 4:244–253.
2. Maiorca R, Vonesh E, Cavalli PL, De Vecchi A, Giangrande A, La Greca G, Scarpione LL, Bragantini L, Cancarini GC, Cantaluppi A, Castelnova C, Castiglioni A, Poisetti P, Viglino G. A multi-centre, selection adjusted comparison of patient and technique survivals on CAPD and hemodialysis. Perit Dial Int 1990; 11:118–127.
3. Fenton SSA, Schaubel DE, Desmeules M, Morrison HI, Mayo Y, Copleston P, Jeffrey JR, Kjellstrand CM. Hemodialysis versus peritoneal dialysis: a comparison of adjusted mortality rates. Am J Kidney Dis 1997; 30:334–342.
4. Lupo A, Tarchini R, Cancarini GC, Catizone L, Cocchi R, De Vecchi A, Viglino G, Salomone M, Segoloni G, Giangrande A. Long-term outcome in continuous ambulatory peritoneal dialysis: a 10-year survey by the Italian Cooperative Peritoneal Dialysis Study Group. Am J Kidney Dis 1994; 24:826–837.
5. Davies SJ, Phillips L, Griffiths A, Russell L, Naish PF, Russell GI. What really happens to people on long-term peritoneal dialysis? Kidney Int. 54:2207–2217.
6. Churchill DN, Taylor DW, Keshaviah PR. Adequacy of dialysis and nutrition in continuous peritoneal dialysis: association with clinical outcome. J Am Soc Nephrol 1996; 7:198–207.
7. Twardowski ZJ, Nolph KD, Khanna R, Prowant BF, Ryan LP, Moore HL, Nielsen MP. Peritoneal equilibration test. Perit Dial Bull 1987; 7:138–147.
8. Davies SJ, Bryan J, Phillips L, Russell GI. Longitudinal changes in peritoneal kinetics: the effects of peritoneal dialysis and peritonitis. Nephrol Dial Transplant 1996; 11:498–506.
9. Gotloib L, Shostack A. Ultrastructural morphology of the peritoneum: new findings and speculations on transfer of solutes and water during peritoneal dialysis. Perit Dial Bull 1987; 7:119–129.
10. Gotloib L, Shostak A. The functional anatomy of the peritoneum as a dialysing membrane. In: Twardowski ZJ, Nolph KD, Khanna R, eds. Peritoneal Dialysis. New York: Churchill Livingstone, 1990:1–27.
11. Di Paolo N, Sacchi G, De Mia M, Gaggiotti E, Capotondo L, Rossi P, Bernini M, Pucci A, Sabatelli P, Alessandrini C. Morphology of the peritoneal membrane during continuous ambulatory peritoneal peritoneal dialysis. Nephron 1986; 44:204–211.
12. Di Paolo N, Sacchi G, Buoncristiani V. The morphology of the human peritoneum in CAPD patients. In: Maher J, ed. Frontiers in Peritoneal Dialysis. New York: Field Rich, 1985:11–19.
13. Satoh K, Prescott SM. Culture of mesothelial cells from bovine pericardium and characterisation of their arachidonate metabolism. Biochim Biophys Acta 1987; 930:283–296.
14. Rennard SI, Jaurand M-C, Bignon J, Kawanami O, Ferrans VJ, Davidson J, Crystal RG. Role of pleural mesothelial cells in the production of the submesothelial connective tissue matrix of lung. Am Rev Respir Dis 1984; 130:267–274.
15. Gotloib L, Shostack A, Jaichenko J. Ruthenium-red-stained anionic charges of rat and mice mesothelial

cell and basal lamina: the peritoneum is a negatively charged dialyzing membrane. Nephron 1988; 48:65–70.

16. Gotloib L, Shustak A, Jaichenko J. Loss of mesothelial electronegative fixed charges during murine septic peritonitis. Nephron 1989; 51:77–83.
17. Beavis J, Harwood JL, Coles GA, Williams JD. Intraperitoneal phosphatidyl choline levels in patients on continuous ambulatory peritoneal dialysis do not correlate with adequacy of ultrafiltration. J Am Soc Nephrol 1993; 3:1954–1960.
18. Beavis J, Harwood JL, Coles GA, Williams JD. Synthesis of phospholipids by human peritoneal mesothelial cells. Perit Dial Int 1994; 14:348–355.
19. Dobbie JW, Pavlina T, Lloyd J, Johnson RC. Phosphatidylcholine synthesis by peritoneal mesothelium: its implication for peritoneal dialysis. Am J Kid Dis 1988; 12:31–36.
20. Jörres A, Ludat K, Lang J, Sander K, Gahl GM, Frei U, DeJonge K, Williams JD, Topley N. Establishment and functional characterization of human peritoneal fibroblasts in culture: regulation of interleukin-6 production by pro-inflammatory cytokines. J Am Soc Nephrol 1996; 72:2192–2201.
21. Beavis MJ, Williams JD, Hoppe J, Topley N. Human peritoneal fibroblast proliferation in 3-dimensional culture: modulation by cytokines, growth factors and peritoneal dialysis effluent. Kidney Int 1997; 51:205–215.
22. Krediet RT, Ho-Dac-Pannekeet M, Struijk DG. Preservation of peritoneal membrane function. Kidney Int 1996; 50:S62–S68.
23. Krediet RT, Zuyderhoudt FM, Boeschoten EW, Arisz L. Alterations in the peritoneal transport of water and solutes during peritonitis in continuous ambulatory peritoneal dialysis patients. Eur J Clin Invest 1987; 17: 43–52.
24. Krediet RT, Struijk DG, Koomen GC, Zemel D, Boeschoten EW, Hoek FJ, Arisz L. Peritoneal transport of macromolecules in patients on CAPD. Contrib Nephrol 1991; 89:161–174.
25. Blake PG, Flowerdew G, Blake RM, Oreopoulos DG. Serum albumin in patients on continuous ambulatory peritoneal dialysis—predictors and correlations with outcomes. J Am Soc Nephrol 1993; 3:1501–1507.
26. Rippe B, Stelin G, Haraldson B. Computer simulations of peritoneal fluid transport in CAPD. Kidney Int 1991; 40:315–325.
27. Monquil M, Imholz AL, Struijk DG, Krediet RT. Does impaired transcellular water transport contribute to net ultrafiltration failure during CAPD. Perit Dial Int 1995; 15:42–48.
28. Davies SJ, Brown B, Bryan J, Russell GI. Clinical evaluation of the peritoneal equilibration test. A population based study. Nephrol Dial Transplant 1993; 8: 64–70.
29. Struijk DG, Krediet RT, Koomen GCM, Boeschoten EW, Hoek FJ, Arisz L. A prospective study of peritoneal transport in CAPD patients. Kidney Int 1994; 45:1739–1744.
30. Durand P-Y, Chanliau J, Gamberoni J, Hestin D, Kessler M. Intraperitoneal hydrostatic pressure and ultrafiltration volume in CAPD. Adv Perit Dial 1993; 9: 46–48.
31. Struijk DG, Imholz AL, Krediet RT, Koomen GC, Arisz L. Use of the disappearance rate for the estimation of lymphatic absorption during CAPD [review]. Blood Purif 1992; 10:182–188.
32. Imholz AL, Koomen GC, Struijk DG, Arisz L, Krediet RT. Effect of an increased intraperitoneal pressure on fluid and solute transport during CAPD. Kidney Int 1993; 44:1078–1085.
33. Steinhauer HB, Schollmeyer P. Prostaglandin mediated loss of proteins during peritonitis in continuous ambulatory peritoneal dialysis. Kidney Int 1986; 29: 584–590.
34. Pannekeet MM, Mulder JB, Weening JJ, Struijk DG, Zweers MM, Krediet RT. Demonstration of aquaporin-CHIP in peritoneal tissue of uremic and CAPD patients. Perit Dial Int 1996; 16(suppl 1):S54–7.
35. Heimburger O, Waniewski J, Werynski A, Tranaeus A, Lindholm B. Peritoneal transport in CAPD patients with permanent loss of ultrafiltration capacity. Kidney Int 1990; 38:495–506.
36. Struijk DG, Krediet RT, Koomen GC, Hoek FJ, Boeschoten EW, Reijden HJ, Arisz L. Functional characteristics of the peritoneal membrane in long-term continuous ambulatory peritoneal dialysis. Nephron 1991; 59:213–220.
37. Blake PG, Abraham G, Sombolos K, Izatt S, Weissgarten J, Ayiomamitis A, Oreopoulos DG. Changes in peritoneal membrane transport rates in patients on long term CAPD. Adv Perit Dial 1989; 5:3–7.
38. Selgas R, Fernandez-Reyes MJ, Bosque E, Bajo MA, Borrego F, Jimenez C, Del Peso G, de Alvaro F. Functional longevity of the human peritoneum: how long is continuous peritoneal dialysis possible? Results of a prospective medium long-term study. Am J Kidney Dis 1994; 23:64–73.
39. Davies SJ, Phillips L, Russell GI. Peritoneal solute transport predicts survival on CAPD independently of residual renal function. Nephrol Dial Transplant 1998; 13:962–968.
40. Gotloib L, Shostack A, Bar-Sella P, Cohen R. Continuous mesothelial injury and regeneration during long term peritoneal dialysis. Perit Dial Bull 1987; 7:148–155.
41. Di Paolo N, Sacchi G. Peritoneal vascular changes in continuous ambulatory peritoneal dialysis (CAPD): an in vivo model for the study of diabetic microangiopathy. Perit Dial Int 1989; 9:41–45.
42. Dobbie J, Zaki M, Wilson L. Ultrastructural studies on the peritoneum with special reference to chronic

ambulatory peritoneal dialysis. Scott Med J 1981; 26: 213–223.

43. Dobbie J, Lloyd J, Gall C. Categorization of ultrastructural changes in peritoneal mesothelium, stroma and blood vessels in uremia and CAPD patients. In: Khanna R, Nolph K, Prowant B, Twardowski Z, Oreopoulos D, eds. Toronto: Perit Dial Int Inc., 1990:3–12.
44. Dobbie JW. Pathogenesis of peritoneal fibrosing syndromes (sclerosing peritonitis) in peritoneal dialysis. Perit Dial Int 1992; 12:14–27.
45. Dobbie JW. Ultrastructure and pathology of the peritoneum in peritoneal dialysis. In: Gokal R, Nolph KD, eds. The Textbook of Peritoneal Dialysis. Dordrecht: Kluwer Academic Publishers, 1994:17–44.
46. Coles GA. Immunoglobulin and complement. Contrib Nephrol 1990; 85:24–29.
47. Coles GA, Minors SJ, Horton JK, Fifield R, Davies M. Can the risk of peritonitis be predicted for new continuous ambulatory peritoneal dialysis (CAPD) patients? Perit Dial Int 1989; 9:69–72.
48. Coles GA, Alobaidi HMM, Topley N, Davies M. Opsonic activity of dialysis effluent predicts those at risk of *Staphylococcus epidermidis* peritonitis. Nephrol Dial Transplant 1987; 2:359–365.
49. Holmes C, Lewis S. Host defense mechanisms in the peritoneal cavity of continuous ambulatory peritoneal dialysis patients. 2. Humoral defenses. Perit Dial Int 1991; 11:112–117.
50. Holmes CJ. Peritoneal host defense mechanism in peritoneal dialysis. Kidney Int 1994; 46:S58–S70.
51. Zemel D, ten Berge RJM, G. SD, Bloemena E, Koomen GCM, Krediet RT. Interleukin-6 in CAPD patients without peritonitis: relationship to the intrinsic permeability of the peritoneal membrane. Clin Nephrol 1992; 37:97–103.
52. Zemel D, ten Berge RJM, Koomen GCM, Struijk DG, Krediet RT. Serum interleukin-6 in continuous ambulatory peritoneal dialysis patients. Nephron 1993; 64:320–321.
53. Zemel D, Krediet RT, Koomen GCM, Kortekaas WMR, Geertzen HGM, ten Berge RJM. Interleukin-8 during peritonitis in patients treated with CAPD; an in vivo model of acute inflammation. Nephrol Dial Transplant 1994; 9:169–174.
54. Zemel D, Koomen GCM, Hart AAM, ten Berge RJM, Struijk DG, Krediet RT. Relationship of TNFα, interleukin-6, and prostaglandins to peritoneal permeability for macromolecules during longitudinal follow-up of peritonitis in continuous ambulatory peritoneal dialysis. J Lab Clin Med 1994; 122:686–696.
55. Zemel D, Imholz ALT, de Wart DR, Dinkla C, Struijk DG, Krediet RT. The appearance of tumor necrosis factor-α and soluble TNF-receptors I and II in peritoneal effluent during stable and infectious CAPD. Kidney Int 1994; 46:1422–1430.
56. Zemel D, Betjes MGH, Dinkla C, Struijk DG, Krediet RT. Analysis of inflammatory mediators and peritoneal permeability to macromolecules shortly before the onset of overt peritonitis in patients treated with CAPD. Perit Dial Int 1994; 15:134–141.
57. Moutabarrik A, Nakanishi I, Namiki M, Tsubakihara Y. Interleukin-1 and its naturally occurring inhibitor in peritoneal dialysis patients. Clin Nephrol 1995; 43: 243–248.
58. Brauner A, Hylander B, Wretlind B. Interleukin-6 and interleukin-8 in dialysate and serum from patients on continuous ambulatory peritoneal dialysis. Am J Kid Dis 1993; 22:430–435.
59. Brauner A, Hylander B, Wretlind B. Tumor necrosis factor-α, interleukin-1β, and interleukin-1 receptor antagonist in dialysate and serum from patients on continuous ambulatory peritoneal dialysis. Am J Kid Dis 1996; 27:402–408.
60. Topley N, Jörres A, Mackenzie R, Coles GA, Williams JD. Interactions of macrophages and mesothelial cells in peritoneal host defence. Nieren Hochdruckkr 1994; 23:S88–S91.
61. Topley N, Davenport A, Li F-K, Fear H, Williams JD. Activation of inflammation and leukocyte recruitment into the peritoneal cavity. Kidney Int 1996; 50:S17–S21.
52. Duwe AK, Vas SI, Weatherhead JW. Effects of the composition of peritoneal dialysis fluid on chemiluminescence, phagocytosis and bactericidal activity in vitro. Infect Immun 1981; 33:130–135.
63. Alobaidi HM, Coles GA, Davies M, Lloyd D. Host defence in continuous ambulatory peritoneal dialysis: the effect of the dialysate on phagocyte function. Nephrol Dial Transplant 1986; 1:16–21.
64. Alobaidi H. Host Defence in CAPD: A Laboratory and Clinical Investigation. University of Wales, 1986.
65. Topley N, Alobaidi HM, Davies M, Coles GA, Williams JD, Lloyd D. The effect of dialysate on peritoneal phagocyte oxidative metabolism. Kidney Int 1988; 34:404–411.
66. Topley N, Mackenzie R, Jörres A, Coles GA, Williams JD. Cytokine networks in CAPD: interactions of resident cells during inflammation in the peritoneal cavity. Perit Dial Int 1993; 13:S282–S285.
67. Topley N, Williams JD. Effect of peritoneal dialysis on cytokine production by peritoneal cells. Blood Purif 1996; 14:188–197.
68. Topley N, Petersen MM, Mackenzie R, Kaever V, Neubauer A, Stylianou E, Coles GA, Davies M, Jörres A, Williams JD. Human peritoneal mesothelial cell prostaglandin synthesis: induction of cyclooxygenase mRNA by peritoneal macrophage derived cytokines. Kidney Int 1994; 46:900–909.
69. Topley N, Jörres A, Luttmann W, Petersen M, Lang M, Thierausch K-H, Müller C, Coles G, Davies M, Williams J. Human peritoneal mesothelial cells syn-

thesize IL-6: induction by IL-1β and TNFα. Kidney Int 1993; 43:226–233.

70. Topley N, Brown Z, Jörres A, Westwick J, Coles GA, Davies M, Williams JD. Human peritoneal mesothelial cells synthesize IL-8: synergistic induction by interleukin-1β and tumor necrosis factor α. Am J Pathol 1993; 142:1876–1886.
71. Liberek T, Topley N, Luttmann W, Williams JD. Adherence of neutrophils to human peritoneal mesothelial cells: role of intercellular adhesion molecule-1. J Am Soc Nephrol 1996; 7:208–217.
72. Madara JL. Pathobiology of the intestinal epithelial barrier. Am J Pathol 1990; 137:1273–1281.
73. Agace WW, Hedges SR, Ceska M, Svanborg C. Interleukin-8 and the neutrophil response to mucosal gram negative infection. J Clin Invest 1993; 92:780–785.
74. Hedges S, Svensson M, Svanborg C. Interleukin-6 response of epithelial cell lines to bacterial stimulation in vitro. Infect Immun 1992; 60:1295–1301.
75. Simon RH, Paine III R. Participation of alveolar epithelial cells in lung inflammation. J Lab Clin Med 1995; 126:108–118.
76. Cichocki T, Hanicki Z, Sulowicz W, Smolenski O, Kopec J, Zembala M. Output of peritoneal cells into peritoneal dialysate. Nephron 1983; 35:175–182.
77. Visser CE, Steenbergen JJE, Betjes MGH, Meijer S, Arisz L, Hoefsmit ECM, Krediet RT, Beelen RHJ. Interleukin-8 production by human mesothelial cells after direct stimulation with staphylococci. Infect Immun 1995; 10:4206–4209.
78. Visser CE, Brouer-Steenbergen JJE, Schadee-Eestermans IL, Meijer S, Krediet RT, Beelen RHJ. Ingestion of *Staphylococcus aureus*, *Staphylococcus epidermidis* and *Escherichia coli* by human peritoneal mesothelial cells. Infect Immun 1996; 64:3425–3428.
79. Zeillemaker AM, Mul FPJ, Hoynck van Papendrecht AAGM, Kuijpers TW, Roos D, Leguit P, Verbrugh HA. Polarized secretion of interleukin-8 by human mesothelial cells: a role in neutrophil migration. Immunol 1995; 84:227–232.
80. Andreoli SP, Mallett C, Williams K, McAteer JA, Rothlein R, Doerschuk CM. Mechanisms of polymorphonuclear leukocyte mediated peritoneal mesothelial cell injury. Kidney Int 1994; 46:1100–1109.
81. Cannistra SA, Ottensmeier C, Tidy J, DeFranzo B. Vascular cell adhesion molecule-1 expressed by peritoneal mesothelium partly mediates the binding of activated human T lymphocytes. Exp Haem 1994; 22: 996–1002.
82. Suassuna JHR, Das Neves FC, Hartley RB, Ogg CS, Cameron JS. Immunohistochemical studies of the peritoneal membrane and infiltrating cells in normal subjects and in patients on CAPD. Kidney Int 1994; 46:443–454.
83. Robson RL, Witowski J, Loetscher P, Topley N. Differential regulation of C-C and C-x-C chemokine synthesis in cytokine-activated human peritoneal mesothelial cells by IFN-γ. Kidney Int 1997; 52:1123.
84. Topley N. Membrane longevity in peritoneal dialysis: impact of infection and biocompatible solutions. Adv Ren Rep Ther. In press.
85. Campbell S, Clarke P, Hawley C, Wigan M, Kerlin P, Butler J, Wall D. Sclerosing peritonitis: identification of diagnostic, clinical, and radiological features. Am J Kidney Dis 1994; 24:819–825.
86. Nomoto Y, Kawaguchi Y, Kubo H, Hirano H, Sakai S, Kurokawa K. Sclerosing encapsulating peritonitis in patients undergoing continuous ambulatory peritoneal dialysis: a report on the Japanese sclerosing encapsulating peritonitis study group. Am J Kidney Dis 1996; 28:420–427.
87. Rigby RJ, Hawley CM. Sclerosing peritonitis: the experience in Australia. Nephrol Dial Transplant 1998; 13:154–159.
88. Holland P. Sclerosing encapsulating peritonitis in chronic ambulatory peritoneal dialysis. Clin Radiol 1990; 41:19–23.
89. Peltonen J, Kähäri L, Jaakkola S, Kähäri VM, Varga J, Uitto J, Jiminez SA. Evaluation of transforming growth factor-β and type I procollagen gene expression in fibrotic skin diseases by in situ hybridisation. J Invest Dermatol 1990; 94:365–371.
90. Wahl SM. Fibrosis: bacterial cell wall induced hepatic granulomas. In: Gallin JI, Goldstein IM, Snyderman R, eds. Basic Principles and Clinical Correlates. New York: Raven Press, 1988:841–859.
91. Elias JA, Freundlich B, Kern JA, Rosenbloom J. Cytokine networks in the regulation of inflammation and fibrosis in the lung. Chest 1990; 97:1439–1445.
92. Mauch C, Krieg T. Fibroblast-matrix interactions and their role in the pathogenesis of fibrosis. Rheum Dis Clin North Am 1990; 16:93–107.
93. Mauch C, Hatamachi A, Scharffetter K, Kreig T. Regulation of collagen synthesis in fibroblasts within a three-dimensional collagen gel. Exp Cell Res 1988; 178:493–503.
94. Kunico GS, Neilson EG, Haverty T. Mechanisms of tubulointerstitial fibrosis. Kidney Int 1991; 39:550–556.
95. Freundlich B, Bomalaski JS, Neilson E, Jiminez SA. Regulation of fibroblast proliferation and collagen synthesis by cytokines. Immunol Today 1986; 7:303–307.
96. Rubin J, Herrara GA, Collins D. An autopsy study of the peritoneal cavity from patients on continuous ambulatory peritoneal dialysis. Am J Kid Dis 1991; 17: 97–102.
97. Verger C, Luger A, Moore HL, Nolph KD. Acute changes in peritoneal morphology and transport properties with infectious peritonitis and mechanical injury. Kidney Int 1983; 23:823–831.
98. Pollock CA, Ibels LS, Eckstein RP, Graham JC, Caterson RJ, Mahoney JF, Sheil AGR. Peritoneal mor-

phology on maintenance dialysis. Am J Nephrol 1989; 9:198–204.
99. Topley N, Coles GA, Williams JD. Biocompatibility studies on peritoneal cells. Perit Dial Int 1994; 14: S21–S28.
100. Topley N. What is the ideal technique for testing the biocompatibility of peritoneal dialysis solutions. Perit Dial Int 1995; 15:205–209.
101. Topley N. Biocompatibility of peritoneal dialysis solutions and host defence. Adv Ren Rep Ther 1996; 3: 1–3.
102. Topley N, Davenport A, Li F-K, Fear H, Williams JD. Peritoneal defence in peritoneal dialysis. Nephrology 1996; 2:S167–S172.
103. Jörres A, Williams JD, Topley N. Peritoneal dialysis solution biocompatibility: inhibitory mechanisms and recent studies with bicarbonate-buffered peritoneal dialysis solutions. Perit Dial Int 1997; 17:S42–S46.
104. Jörres A, Gahl GM, Frei U. Peritoneal dialysis fluid biocompatibility: Does it really matter? Kidney Int 1994; 46:S79–S86.
105. Gotloib L, Waisbrut V, Shostak A, Kushnier R. Biocompatibility of dialysis solutions evaluated by histochemical techniques applied to mesothelial cell imprints. Perit Dial Int 1993; 13:201–207.
106. Gotloib L, Waisbrut V, Shostak A, Kusnier R. Acute and long-term changes observed in imprints of mouse mesothelium exposed to glucose-enriched, lactated, buffered dialysis solutions. Nephron 1995; 70:466–477.
107. Gotloib L, Wajsbrot V, Shostak A, Kushnier R. Population analysis of mesothelium in situ and in vivo exposed to bicarbonate-buffered peritoneal dialysis fluid. Nephron 1996; 73:219–227.
108. de Fijter CWH, Oe LP, Heezius ECJM, Donker AJM, Verbrugh HA. Low-calcium peritoneal dialysis fluid should not impact peritonitis rates in continuous ambulatory peritoneal dialysis. Am J Kid Dis 1996; 27: 409–415.
109. de Fijter CWH, Verbrugh HA, Peters EDJ, Oe PL, van der Meulen J, Verhoef J, Donker AJM. In vivo exposure to the currently available peritoneal dialysis fluids decreases the function of peritoneal macrophages in CAPD. Clin Nephrol 1993; 39:75–80.
110. de Fijter CWH, Verbrugh HA, Oe LP, Heezius E, Donker AJM, Verhoef J, Gokal R. Biocompatibility of a glucose polymer-containing peritoneal dialysis fluid. Am J Kid Dis 1993; 4:411–418.
111. Griffin JC, Marie SC. Glucose degradation in the presence of sodium lactate during autoclaving at 121°C. Am J Hosp Pharm 1958; 15:893–895.
112. Taylor RB, Jappy BM, Neil JM. Kinetics of dextrose degradation under autoclaving conditions. J Pharm Pharmacol 1971; 23:121–129.
113. Heimlich KR, Martin AN. A kinetic study of glucose degradation in acid solution. J Am Pharmacol Assoc 1960; 49:592–597.
114. Webb NE, Sperandio GJ, Martin AN. A study of the composition of glucose solutions. J Am Pharm Assoc 1958; 47:101–103.
115. Wieslander AP, Nordin MK, Kjellstrand PTT, Boberg UC. Toxicity of peritoneal dialysis fluids on cultured fibroblasts, L-929. Kidney Int 1991; 40:77–79.
116. Wieslander AP, Nordin MK, Martinson E, Kjellstrand PTT, Boberg UC. Heat sterilised PD-fluids impair growth and inflammatory responses of cultured cell lines and human leukocytes. Clin Nephrol 1993; 39: 343–348.
117. Lamb EJ, Cattell WR, Dawnay ABSJ. In vitro formation of advanced glycation end products in peritoneal dialysis fluid. Kidney Int 1995; 47:1768–1774.
118. Liberek T, Topley N, Jörres A, Petersen MM, Coles GA, Gahl GM, Williams JD. Peritoneal dialysis fluid inhibition of polymorphonuclear leukocyte respiratory burst activation is related to the lowering of intracellular pH. Nephron 1993; 65:260–265.
119. Douvdevani A, Rapoport J, Konforty A, Yulzari R, Moran A, Chaimovitz C. Intracellular acidification mediates the inhibitory effect of peritoneal dialysate on peritoneal macrophages. J Am Soc Nephrol 1995; 6:207–213.
120. Witowski J, Topley N, Jörres A, Liberek T, Coles GA, Williams JD. Effect of lactate buffered peritoneal dialysis fluids on human peritoneal mesothelial cell interleukin-6 and prostaglandin synthesis. Kidney Int 1995; 47:282–293.
121. Liberek T, Topley N, Jörres A, Coles GA, Gahl GM, Williams JD. Peritoneal dialysis fluid inhibition of phagocyte function: effects of osmolality and glucose concentration. J Am Soc Nephrol 1993; 3:1508–1515.
122. Jörres A, Gahl GM, Topley N, Neubauer A, Ludat K, Müller C, Passlick-Deetjen J. In vitro biocompatibility of alternative CAPD fluids; comparison of bicarbonate buffered and glucose polymer based solutions. Nephrol Dial Transplant 1994; 9:785–790.
123. Mistry CD, Gokal R, Peers E, et al. A randomised multicentre clinical trial comparing isoosmolar Icodextrin with hyperosmolar glucose solutions in CAPD. Kidney Int 1994; 46:496–503.
124. Ruderman NB, Williamson JR, Brownlee M. Glucose and diabetic vascular disease. FASEB J 1992; 6:2905–2914.
125. Tilton RG, Baier LD, Harlow JE, Smith SR, Ostrow E, Williamson JR. Diabetes-induced glomerular dysfunction: links to a more reduced cytosolic ratio of NADH/NAD+. Kidney Int 1992; 41:778–788.
126. Breborowicz A, Rodela H, Oreopoulos DG. Toxicity of osmotic solutes on human mesothelial cells in vitro. Kidney Int 1992; 41:1280–1285.
127. Kumano K, Schiller B, Hjelle JT, Moran J. Effect of osmotic solutes on fibronectin mRNA expression in rat peritoneal mesothelial cells. Blood Purif 1996; 14: 165–169.

128. Witowski J, Williams JD, Topley N. D-Glucose induces transforming growth factor-b1 (TGF-b1) mRNA expression and secretion in human peritoneal mesothelial cells (HPMC): effect of hyperosmolality. Peritoneal Dialysis International. In press.
129. Fujimori A, Naito H, Miyazaki T, Azuma M, Hashimoto S, Horikawa S, Tokukoda Y. Elevation of interleukin-6 in the dialysate reflects peritoneal stimuli and deterioration of peritoneal function. Nephron 1996; 74:471–472.
130. Witowski J, Jörres A, Williams JD, Topley N. Superinduction of IL-6 synthesis in human peritoneal mesothelial cells is related to induction and stabilization of IL-6 mRNA. Kidney Int 1996; 50:1212–1223.
131. Phillips AO, Steadman R, Topley N, Williams JD. Elevated D-glucose concentrations modulate TGF-β1 synthesis by human cultured renal proximal tubular cells. Am J Pathol 1995; 147:362–374.
132. Yamada K, Miyahara Y, Hamaguchi K, Nakayama M, Nakano H, Nozaki O, Miura Y, Suzuki S, Tuchida H, Mimura N, Araki N, Horiuchi S. Immunohistochemical study of human advanced glycosylation end-products (AGE) in chronic renal failure. Clin Nephrol 1994; 42:354–361.
133. Friedlander MA, Wu YC, Elgawish A, Monnier VM. Early and advanced glycosylation end products: kinetics of formation and clearance in peritoneal dialysis. J Clin Invest 1996; 97:728–735.
134. Vlassara H. Recent progress on the biologic and clinical significance of advanced glycosylation end products. J Lab Clin Med 1994; 124:19–30.
135. Nakayama M, Kawaguchi M, Yamada K, Masegawa T, Takazoe K, Katoh N, Mayakawa H, Osaka N, Yamamoto H, Ogawa H, Kubo H, Shigematsu T, Sakai O, Horiuchi S. Immunological detection of advanced glycosylation end products in the peritoneum and its possible pathophysiological role in CAPD. Kidney Int 1997; 51:182–188.
136. Esposito C, Gerlach H, Brett J, Stern D, Vlassara H. Endothelial receptor-mediated binding of glucose-modified albumin is associated with increased monolayer permeability and modulation of cell surface coagulant properties. J Exp Med 1989; 170:1387–1407.
137. Honda K, Nitta K, Horita H, Yumura W, Nihei H. Morphological changes in the peritoneal vasculature of patients on CAPD with ultrafiltration failure. Nephron 1996; 72:171–176.
138. Pannekeet MM, Imholz AL, Struijk DG, Koomen GC, Langedijk MJ, Schouten N, de Waart R, Hiralall J, Krediet RT. The standard peritoneal permeability analysis: a tool for the assessment of peritoneal permeability characteristics in CAPD patients. Kidney Int 1995; 48:866–875.
139. Ho-dac-Pannekeet MM, Atasever B, Struijk DG, Krediet RT. Analysis of ultrafiltration failure in peritoneal dialysis patients by means of standard peritoneal permeability analysis. Perit Dial Int 1997; 17:144–150.
140. Goldman M, Vandenabeele P, Moulart J, Amraoui Z, Abramowicz D, Nortier J, Vanherweghem JL, Fiers E. Intraperitoneal secretion of interleukin-6 during continuous ambulatory peritoneal dialysis. Nephron 1990; 56:277–280.
141. Visser CE, Brouwer-Steenbergen JJE, Betjes MGH, Koomen GCM, Beelen RJH, Krediet RT. Cancer antigen 125: a bulk marker for mesothelial cell mass in stable peritoneal dialysis patients. Nephrol Dial Transplant 1995; 10:64–69.
142. Ho-dac-Pannekeet MM, Hiralall JK, Struijk DG, Krediet RT. Longitudinal follow-up of CA125 in peritoneal effluent. Kidney Int 1997; 51:888–893.
143. Pannekeet MM, Koomen GCM, Struijk DG, Krediet RT. Dialysate CA125 in stable CAPD patients: no relation to transport parameters. Clin Nephrol 1995; 44: 248–254.
144. Lai KN, Lai KB, Szeto CC, Ho KKL, Poon P, Lam CWK, Leung JCK. Dialysate cell population and cancer antigen 125 in stable continuous ambulatory peritoneal dialysis patients: their relationship with transport parameters. Am J Kidney Dis 1997; 29:699–705.
145. Ho-dac-Panekeet MM. Assessment of peritoneal permeability and mesothelial cell mass in peritoneal dialysis patients: effects of non-glucose solutions. Amsterdam: 1998:271.
146. Harty J, Gokal R. The impact of peritoneal permeability and residual renal function on PD prescription. Perit Dial Int 1996; 16(suppl 1):S147–52.
147. Wang T, Heimburger O, Waniewski J, Bergstrom J, Lindholm B. Increased peritoneal permeability in CAPD results in decreased fluid and small solute removal, and lower survival. J Am Soc Nephrol 1996; 7:1468.
148. Wang T, Waniewski J, Heimburger O, Werynski A, Lindholm B. A quantitative analysis of sodium transport and removal during peritoneal dialysis. Kidney Int 1997; 52:1609–1616.
149. Freida P, Issad B, Allouache M. Relationships between fill volume, small solutes clearances, and net ultrafiltration during a standardised APD program. Perit Dial Int 1998; 18:124.
150. Feriani M, Carobi C, La Greca G, Buoncristiani U, Passlick-Deetjen J. Clinical experience with a 39 mmol/l bicarbonate-buffered peritoneal dialysis solution. Perit Dial Int 1997; 17:17–21.
151. Stein A, Moorhouse J, Iles-Smith H, Baker F, Johnstone J, James G, Troughton J, Bircher G, Walls J. Role of an improvement in acid/base status and nutrition in CAPD patients. Kidney Int 1997; 52:1089–1095.
152. Young GA, Taylor A, Kendall S, Brownjohn AM. Longitudinal study of proteins in plasma and dialysate during continuous ambulatory peritoneal dialysis (CAPD). Perit Dial Int 1990; 10:257–261.
153. Davies SJ, Russell L, Bryan J, Phillips L, Russell GI. Impact of peritoneal absorption of glucose on appetite,

protein catabolism and survival in CAPD patients. Clin Nephrol 1996; 45:194–198.

154. Bergstrom J, Furst P, Alvestrand A, Lindholm B. Protein and energy intake, nitrogen balance and nitrogen losses in patients treated continuous ambulatory peritoneal dialysis. Kidney Int 1993; 44:1048–1057.

155. Mistry CD, Gokal R. Icodextrin in peritoneal dialysis: early development and clinical use. Perit Dial Int 1994; 14:S13–S21.

156. Ho-dac-Pannekeet MM, Schouten N, Langendijk MJ, Hiralall JK, de Waart DR, Struijk DG, Krediet RT. Peritoneal transport characteristics with glucose polymer based dialysate. Kidney Int 1996; 50:979–986.

157. Posthuma N, ter Wee PM, Verbrugh HA, Oe PL, Peers E, Sayers J, Donker AJ. Icodextrin instead of glucose during the daytime dwell in CCPD increases ultrafiltration and 24-h dialysate creatinine clearance. Nephrol Dial Transplant 1997; 12:550–553.

158. Gokal R, Mistry CD, Peers E, Group. MS. A United Kingdom multicenter study of icodextrin in continuous ambulatory peritoneal dialysis. Perit Dial Int 1994; 14:S22–S27.

159. Imholz AL, Koomen GCM, Struijk DG, Arisz L, Krediet RT. Fluid and solute transport in CAPD patients using ultralow sodium dialysate. Kidney Int 1994; 46: 333–340.

160. Nakayama M, Yokoyama K, Kubo H, Matsumoto H, Hasegawa T, Shigematsu T, Kawaguchi Y, Sakai O. The effect of ultra-low sodium dialysate in CAPD. A kinetic and clinical analysis. Clin Nephrol 1996; 45: 188–193.

161. Amici G, Virga G, Da Rin G, Teodori T, Calzavara P, Bocci C. Low sodium concentration solution in normohydrated CAPD patients. Adv Perit Dial 1995; 11: 78–82.

162. Freida P, Issad B, Allouache M. Impact of a low sodium dialysate on usual parameters of cardiovascular outcome of anuric patients during APD. Perit Dial Int 1998; 18:124.

163. Graham KA, Reaich D, Channon SM, Downie S, Gilmour E, Passlick-Deetjen J, Goodship TH. Correction of acidosis in CAPD decreases whole body protein degradation. Kidney Int 1996; 49:1396–1400.

164. de Fijter CWH, Verbrugh HA, Oe LP, Peters EDJ, Van der Meulen J, Donker AJM, Verhoef J. Peritoneal defence in continuous ambulatory versus continuous cyclic peritoneal dialysis. Kidney Int 1992; 42:947–950.

165. Rippe B, Simonsen O, Wieslander A, Landgren C. Clinical and physiological effects of a new, less toxic and less acidic fluid for peritoneal dialysis. Perit Dial Int 1997; 17:27–34.

166. Topley N, Kaur D, Petersen MM, Jörres A, Williams JD, Faict D, Holmes CJ. In vitro effects of bicarbonate and bicarbonate-lactate buffered peritoneal dialysis solutions on mesothelial cell and neutrophil function. J Am Soc Nephrol 1996; 7:218–224.

167. Topley N, Kaur D, Petersen MM, Jörres A, Passlick-Deetjen J, Coles GA, Williams JD. Bio-compatibility of bicarbonate-buffered peritoneal dialysis fluids: influence on mesothelial cell and neutrophil function. Kidney Int 1996; 49:1447–1456.

168. Fischer H-P, Schenk U, Kiefer T, Hübel E, Thomas S, Yatzidis H, Mettang T, Kuhlmann U. In vitro effects of bicarbonate- versus lactate-buffered continuous ambulatory peritoneal dialysis fluids on peritoneal macrophage function. Am J Kidney Dis 1995; 26:924–933.

169. Dobos GJ, Böhler J, Kuhlmann J, Elsner J, Andre M, Passlick-Deetjen J, Schollmeyer PJ. Bicarbonate-based dialysis solutions preserves granulocyte functions. Perit Dial Int 1994; 14:366–370.

170. Manahan FJ, Ing BL, Chan JC, Gupta DK, Zhou FQ, Pal I, Rahman MA. Effects of bicarbonate-containing versus lactate-containing peritoneal dialysis solutions on superoxide production by human neutrophils. Artif Organs 1989; 13:495–497.

171. Plum J, Fusshöller A, Schoenicke G, Busch T, Erren C, Fieseler C, Kirchgessner J, Passlick-Deetjen J, Grabensee B. In vivo and in vitro effects of amino-acid-based and bicarbonate-buffered peritoneal dialysis solutions with regard to peritoneal transport and cytokines/prostanoids dialysate concentrations. Nephrol Dial Transplant 1997; 12:1652–1660.

172. Schambye HT, Flesner P, Pedersen RB, Hardt-Madsen M, Chemnitz J, Christensen HK, Detmer A, Pedersen FB. Bicarbonate- versus lactate-based CAPD fluids: a biocompatibility study in Rabbits. Perit Dial Int 1992; 12:281–286.

173. Yatzidis H. Enhanced ultrafiltration in rabbits with bicarbonate glycylglycine peritoneal dialysis solution. Perit Dial int 1993; 13:302–306.

174. Topley N, Jörres A, Petersen MM, Mackenzie R, Kaever V, Coles GA, Davies M, Williams JD. Human peritoneal mesothelial cell prostaglandin (PG) metabolism: induction by cytokines and peritoneal macrophage conditioned medium. J Am Soc Nephrol 1991; 2:432.

175. Coene MC, C. vH, Claeys M, Herman AG. Arachidonic acid metabolism by cultured mesothelial cells. Biochim Biophys Acta 1982; 710:437–445.

176. Coene MC, Solheid C, Claeys M, Herman AG. Prostaglandin production by cultured mesothelial cells. Arch Int Pharmacodyn 1981; 249:316–318.

177. Douvdevani A, Rapoport J, Konforty A, Argov S, Ovnat A, Chaimowitz C. Human peritoneal mesothelial cells synthesize IL-1α and β. Kidney Int 1994; 46: 993–1001.

178. Betjes MGH, Tuk CW, Struijk DG, Krediet RT, Arisz L, Hart M, Beelen RH. Interleukin-8 production by human peritoneal mesothelial cells in response to tumor necrosis factor α, interleukin-1, and medium conditioned by macrophages co-cultured with *Staphylococcus epidermidis*. J Inf Dis 1993; 168:1202–1210.

179. Li FK, Loetscher P, Williams JD, Topley N. Human peritoneal mesothelial cells (HPMC) synthesise the C-C chemokines MCP-1 and RANTES: induction by macrophage-derived cytokines. Proceedings of the International Society of Nephrology, 1995:445.
180. Gerwin BI, Lechner JF, Reddel RR, Young AA. Comparison of production of transforming growth factor-β and latelet derived growth factor by normal human mesothelial cells and mesothelioma cell lines. Cancer Res 1987; 89:1257–1262.
181. Bermudez E, Everitt J, Walker C. Expression of growth factor and growth factor receptor RNA in rat pleural mesothelial cells in culture. Exp Cell Res 1990; 190:91–98.
182. Offner A, Feichtinger H, Stadlmann S, Obrist P, Marth C, Klingler P, Grage B, Schmahl M, Knabbe C. Transforming growth factor-β synthesis by human peritoneal mesothelial cells. Am J Pathol 1996; 148:1679–1688.
183. Yung S, Coles GA, Williams JD, Davies M. The source and possible significance of hyaluronan in the peritoneal cavity. Kidney Int 1994; 46:527–533.
184. Yung S, Thomas GJ, Stylianou E, Williams JD, Coles GA, Davies M. Source of peritoneal proteoglycans: human peritoneal mesothelial cells synthesize and secrete mainly small dermatan sulphate proteoglycans. Am J Pathol 1995; 146:520–529.
185. Yung S, Coles GA, Davies M. IL-1β, a major stimulator of hyaluronan synthesis in vitro of human peritoneal mesothelial cells: relevance to peritonitis in CAPD. Kidney Int 1996; 50:1337–1343.
186. Marshall BC, Santana A, Xu Q-P, Petersen MJ, Campbell EJ, Hoidal JR, Welgus HG. Metalloproteinases and tissue inhibitor of metalloproteinases in mesothelial cells: cellular differentiation influences expression. J Clin Invest 1993; 91:1792–1799.
187. Harvey W, Amlot PL. Collagen production by human mesothelial cells in vitro. J Pathol 1983; 139:337–347.
188. Davilla RM, Crouch EC. Role of mesothelial and submesothelial stromal cells in matrix remodeling following pleural injury. Am J Pathol 1993; 142:547–556.
189. Thompson JN, Paterson-Brown S, Harbourne T, Whawell SA, Kalodiki E, Dudley HAF. Reduced human peritoneal plasminogen activating activity: possible mechanism of adhesion formation. Br J Surg 1989; 76:382–384.
190. van Hinsbergh CWM, van den Berg EA, Fiers W, Dooijewaard G. Tumor necrosis factor induces the production of urokinase-type plasminogen activator by human endothelial cells. Blood 1990; 75:1991–1998.

10

Complications Related to Inadequate Delivered Dose of Peritoneal Dialysis

Antonios H. Tzamaloukas
University of New Mexico School of Medicine, and Veterans Affairs Medical Center, Albuquerque, New Mexico

Thomas A. Golper
University of Arkansas for Medical Sciences, Little Rock, Arkansas, and Renal Disease Management, Inc., Youngstown, Ohio

The definition of adequacy of a dialytic treatment has a broad scope including control of biochemical and outcome parameters such as azotemia, acid-base indices, serum electrolytes, body fluid balance, nutrition, rehabilitation, and quality and length of life (1–3). Unlike hemodialysis (HD) or intermittent forms of peritoneal dialysis (PD), the pattern of serum electrolyte concentration is usually within the normal limits in most patients on continuous forms of PD. Electrolyte abnormalities (e.g., hypokalemia) in continuous PD are often the result of conditions extrinsic to the process of dialysis (e.g., gastrointestinal losses), although they can occasionally reflect nutritional status. Quality and length of life issues are primarily determined by comorbidities. For example, diabetic patients have the poorest quality of life and the shortest survival of all dialysis patients. For these reasons, adequacy of PD has been limited in many discussions to adequacy of salt and water control, adequacy of control of azotemia, and prevention of worsening uremia (4). The NKF-DOQI PD Adequacy Work Group, which both authors served on, struggled with these limitations because guideline development requires firm data. Therefore, this chapter will focus on complications of PD that relate to inadequate delivered dose of dialysis, focusing on the consequences of poor azotemic control, its recognition, and management. Fluid balance and its ramifications in PD patients will be discussed in the context of their interface with the control of azotemia and as they relate to cardiovascular comorbidities.

I. SMALL SOLUTE CLEARANCE AS AN INDEX OF AZOTEMIC CONTROL

It is now clear that the blood levels of azotemic indices are poor indicators of control of uremia by PD or HD. Patients with very low rates of removal of urea and creatinine may develop frank uremia resulting in poor protein intake, low urea-generation rate, and muscle wasting with a low creatinine-generation rate. Essentially, urea and creatinine generation shrink to accommodate the low clearances of each solute. Thus, low plasma levels of urea and creatinine do not by themselves reflect adequate dialysis and, in fact, have been shown to be predictors of short survival in both HD and PD patients.

Most clinicians believe that prevention of uremia is linked to adequate clearance of urea and creatinine (5–8). Consequently, these clearances are measured and target levels (more accurately, lowest acceptable levels) have been established for both clearances (see below).

Many investigations define adequacy of dialysis in general with respect to small solute clearance. This chapter will discuss the consequences, causes, and prevention of inadequate small solute clearance in the PD population. To set the stage for this discussion, we must mention the concerns inherent to dialytic clearances starting with the problem caused by the process of clearance normalization.

II. NORMALIZED SMALL SOLUTE CLEARANCES

In the early years of continuous ambulatory peritoneal dialysis (CAPD), the prescription of the dose of dialysis was uniform with four daily 2-L exchanges. Although this regimen is convenient, it does not take into account that the size of the individual patient affects the delivered PD dose. If the rate of production of an azotemic solute and its rate of removal (total clearance) are fixed, the size of the individual will determine the amount of the solute in the body and, in the absence of a steady state, also the blood concentration of this solute. In the original kinetic calculations showing the feasibility of CAPD, Popovich et al. introduced urea volume (equal to total body water, V) as the size indicator (9). However, the first effort to normalize urea clearance by V took place 10 years later (10). In the same year, Gotch and Sargent introduced the notion of the fractional urea clearance (Kt/V_{urea}) in their pivotal analysis of the National Cooperative Dialysis Study (NCDS) (11). From then on, urea clearance has been normalized by V.

Creatinine clearance (C_{Cr}) has traditionally been normalized by body surface area (BSA) rather than total body water (V). While one would expect that the same PD prescription should result in adequate levels for both clearances, this is often not the case. Therefore, the relationship between the two clearances generates clinical concern. Whether normalization by two different size indicators changes the relationship between the two normalized clearances is a critical confounding issue affecting virtually all the aspects of this chapter.

The relationship between V estimated by the use of height, weight, and age (12,13) and BSA estimated by the use of height and weight (14) was found to be apparently linear in normal subjects (12) and PD patients (15). However, subsequent investigations showed that this relationship is not mathematically linear. Thus, the relationship between the normalized clearances may be different from that of clearances that are not normalized. Gender and degree of obesity affect the relationship between V and BSA. Among subjects with the same height and weight (the same BSA), females have substantially lower V values than males. Also, in subjects developing obesity, V increases out of proportion to the increase in BSA (16). Clinical studies confirmed that the effect of the degree of obesity is one of the causes of discrepancy between the normalized clearances (17).

It is recognized that mathematical (artificial) distortion of the relationship between clearances can cause falsely low or high levels for one clearance (18,19), but the best way to correct this artifact is unsettled (20,21). The obvious solution is to normalize both clearances using the same size indicator (16).

III. CLINICAL CONSEQUENCES OF INADEQUATE SMALL SOLUTE CLEARANCE

Table 1 shows potential consequences of inadequate small solute clearance. We will detail the arguments regarding the linkage of the clinical manifestations of uremia to inadequate small solute clearances.

A. Uremic Manifestations as Indicators of Inadequate Clearance

The syndrome of uremia is thought to result, at least in part, from the retention of toxic metabolites that can be removed by dialysis. The NCDS showed in HD patients that inadequate urea clearance appeared to be associated with some uremic manifestations (22). The inference is that dialytic urea clearance is related to the clearance of some uremic toxins, i.e., the "urea as a surrogate marker" concept. Numerous studies suggest that a larger delivered PD dose improves patient well-being. Lameire et al. demonstrated a positive correlation between Kt/V_{urea} and protein catabolic rate and between Kt/V_{urea} and nerve conductivity and an inverse correlation between Kt/V_{urea} and hospitalization days (23). In addition, a lower peritonitis rate was observed in those CAPD patients with a higher Kt/V_{urea}. Tattersall et al. found that hospital admission rates were lower when weekly Kt/V_{urea} was >1.75, as opposed to if Kt/V_{urea} were <1.75 (24). Maiorca et al. and CAN-USA both demonstrated that an increased total delivered PD dose was associated with fewer hospitalized days (7,8). Using symptoms, nursing assessment, and clinical laboratory data, Brandes et al. reported superior outcomes with weekly PD Kt/V_{urea} of 2.3 compared to 1.5 (25). Arkouche et al. reported similar findings when

Table 1 Clinical Consequences of Inadequate Small Solute Clearance in Peritoneal Dialysis

Uremic symptoms and signs–morbidity
Supportive evidence of link with small solute clearances
Inference from hemodialysis findings (22)
Correlation of Kt/V_{urea} with nerve conduction velocity (23)
Inverse correlation of clearances with hospitalization rate (7,8,24)
Inverse correlation of clearances with symptom score (23–29)
Problems
Lack of correlation between clearances and symptoms (30–34)
Lack of specificity and sensitivity of uremic symptoms (35,36)
Malnutrition
Supportive evidence of link with small solute clearances
Frequency of anorexia in renal failure (37)
Association between inadequate small solute clearance and anorexia and wasting in peritoneal dialysis (38)
Correlation between nPNA and Kt/V_{urea} (39)
Correlation between small solute clearance and subjective global assessment (49)
Problems
nPNA does not correlate with other nutritional parameters (40)
Small solute clearances are not predictors of serum albumin (42–44)
Rising small solute clearances to adequate levels does not improve serum albumin (44)
Mortality
Supportive evidence of a link with small solute clearance
Inverse relationship between small solute clearance and mortality (6,7,23,30,50,51)
Association between low clearance and increased cardiac mortality (53)
Problems
Lack of association between low clearances and mortality (54)
Lack of a prospective interventional study

comparing patients with a weekly Kt/V_{urea} of 2.3 to those with 1.6 (26). Heaf noted superior symptom indices when total solute clearance was higher (27). Thus, it is reasonable to conclude that small solute removal is to some extent related to signs and symptoms of uremia and that lower delivered doses of PD are associated with worse or more frequent symptoms.

However, the association between low Kt/V_{urea} or normalized creatinine clearance (C_{Cr}) and the appearance of uremic manifestations in PD patients has not been as strong as we would prefer. While certain studies have reported an association between the appearance of uremic manifestations and low solute clearances (23–29), others failed to find such an association (30–33). The studies showing an association between low clearances and uremic manifestations were based on small numbers of subjects and could have been influenced because the investigators were familiar with both the clinical course of the patients *and* their clearance values. Investigators blinded to the clearance values cannot necessarily predict by clinical examination (34) whether these values are low or high. One of the problems arising from the use of uremic manifestations as indices of inadequate clearance is that the most common of the "uremic" manifestations are nonspecific and can be secondary to other comorbid conditions (35,36). An even more serious problem is the appreciation that uremic manifestations have a low sensitivity as indices of underdialysis (see below). This failure of objectivity for symptom grading supports the utilization of mortality as the prime outcome marker.

B. Malnutrition as an Indicator of Inadequate Small Solute Clearance

The association between malnutrition and low small solute clearances in PD patients is also disputed (reviewed in Ref. 3). Anorexia with low protein intake is an early manifestation of renal failure (37). Inadequate dialysis could also lead to anorexia and malnutrition with hypoalbuminemia and muscle wasting (38). In stable (noncatabolic) dialysis patients, urea-formation rate is coupled to dietary protein intake. Therefore, the easy calculation of the rate of nitrogen appearance in urea (the protein equivalent of nitrogen appearance, PNA) provides a measure of dietary protein intake (39). However, the usefulness of PNA as a nutrition indicator has been questioned (reviewed in Ref. 3). PNA normalized to body size indicators does not agree with other indices of nutrition (40), and its positive correlation with Kt/V_{urea} is largely due to mathematical coupling, at least in cross-sectional analyses (41).

Another problem with the association between low small solute clearance and malnutrition is the lack of convincing evidence that nutrition improves after an increase in dialysis clearance. This has only rarely been noted even in HD patients (42). The implications of this include that long-standing, undertreated uremia results in irreversible malnutrition and/or that there is no dialyzable anorexia-inducing solute. Small solute clearances were not identified as predictors of serum albumin concentration in PD patients by multivariate analysis (43,44). As will be discussed below, PD patients lose albumin and other proteins into effluent dialysate. On the other hand, dialytic protein losses in HD patients are generally much less, even with leaky high flux dialyzers. Furthermore, an increase in the dose of PD resulting in "adequate" clearance levels failed to raise serum albumin concentration (44). It should be noted, however, that serum albumin concentration is influenced by multiple factors, the most important of which are the type of peritoneal transport and comorbidities present. Patients characterized by high solute transport lose large amounts of albumin into the effluent dialysate and tend to have low serum albumin levels (43–45). If inflammatory co-morbid conditions are present, high levels of cytokines cause inhibition of hepatic albumin synthesis and an increase in the synthesis of acute phase reactants (46). Consequently, high levels of acute phase reactants are associated with hypoalbuminemia in PD patients (47).

Despite the difficulties in demonstrating a clear association between nutritional indices and small solute clearances in PD, this association cannot be overlooked. The association between uremia and anorexia in predialysis patients has been demonstrated (48). In addition, a CANUSA follow-up study found an association between subjective global assessment (SGA), a clinical index of nutrition, and small solute clearances (49). PD patients developing malnutrition should be evaluated for other co-morbid conditions that may be contributory. Those who have low clearances should also have their dialysis dose increased. After adequate clearances have been obtained, the progress of their nutrition should be monitored.

C. Mortality as an Index of Low Solute Clearance

The evidence linking small solute clearances to mortality in PD patients is stronger. Patient survival and delivered PD dose measured by Kt/V_{urea} were related in five cohort studies (6,7,23,30,50). De Alvaro et al. showed that patients with a weekly Kt/V_{urea} of 2.0 have a better survival than those with a Kt/V_{urea} of 1.7 per week (30). Blake et al. found that weekly Kt/V_{urea} of $\leq$1.5 was associated with an increased risk of death (50). Belgian long-term PD survivors had a Kt/V_{urea} exceeding 2.0 per week (23). Genestier et al. suggested that a weekly Kt/V_{urea} of $\geq$1.7 improved survival (6). Maiorca et al. found that weekly Kt/V_{urea} of >1.96 was associated with a better survival (7). Teehan et al. showed that a mean weekly Kt/V_{urea} of >1.89 was associated with a decreased risk of death (51). All of these studies utilized a univariate analysis that did not include confounding comorbidities. Univariate analyses may not be appropriate to evaluate the complexity of relating dose of dialysis to mortality (52). However, the CANUSA study did include analyses of confounding comorbidities (8). This multicenter prospective cohort study of 680 incident CAPD patients showed that a decrease of 0.1 in weekly Kt/V_{urea} was associated with a 5% increase in the relative risk of death, and a decrease of 5 L/week/1.73 m^2 of total creatinine clearance was associated with a 7% increase in the risk of death. The CANUSA study predicts a 75% survival at 2 years with a sustained Kt/V_{urea} of 2.0 per week. Thus, many studies have implied that survival may be enhanced by a larger delivered PD dose. These studies show that various targets ranging from a weekly Kt/V_{urea} of 1.5 to 2.0 impact survival. Figure 1 shows the calculated probability of patient survival by different levels of C_{Cr} in the CANUSA study (8).

High mortality in underdialyzed patients is not necessarily caused by uremia. In HD patients, low Kt/V_{urea} is associated with increased risk of death from coronary artery disease, other cardiac diseases, cerebrovascular accident, and other conditions except malignant neoplasms (52). Low Kt/V_{urea} has been associated with excessive cardiac mortality in PD patients with ischemic heart disease or left ventricular dysfunction (53). The low Kt/V_{urea} may reflect all the consequences of underdialysis, which may include volume overload and hypertension, both well-recognized cardiovascular risk factors, discussed further below.

One study, reported so far in abstract form, found that advanced age, wasting, and elevated blood pressure, but not small solute clearances, were predictors

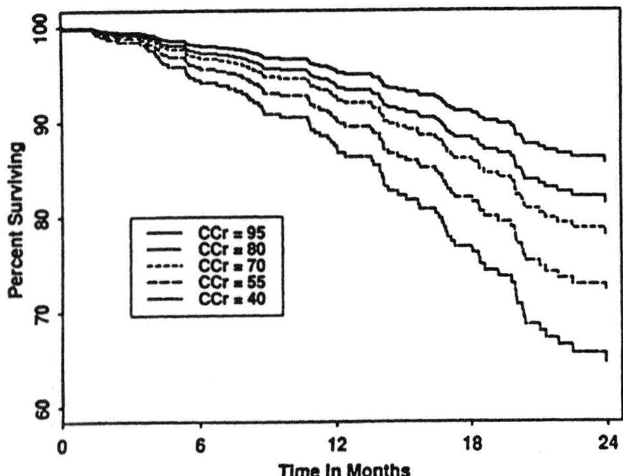

Fig. 1 Estimated probability of patient survival in the CANUSA study. Patients were stratified by Ccr. (From Ref. 8.)

of patient survival in peritoneal dialysis (54). The findings of this study appear to contrast with those of previous studies, which found an association between low clearances and high mortality (5–8). Details of the analysis performed in this last study (54) were not available at the time of writing of this chapter.

A recent report from the CANUSA study illuminates the difficulties in defining the predictors of mortality in peritoneal dialysis. Churchill et al. reported that the peritoneal transport type characterized by a peritoneal equilibration test has major effects on patient and technique survival in CAPD (55): 2-year patient survival probability was 91% in low transporters, 80% in low-average transporters, 72% in high-average transporters, and 71% in high transporters. The differences in survival were associated with differences in serum albumin (higher levels in low transporters) and in albumin losses in the dialysate (higher losses in high transporters). However, peritoneal (and total) creatinine clearance was progressively higher in higher transport groups. In the same study, low total creatinine clearance had been found by multivariate analysis to be a major predictor of high mortality (8). This effect of low creatinine clearance was found despite the adverse effect of high transport on mortality. The weight of the evidence at this point favors a linkage between small solute clearance and patient survival in peritoneal dialysis.

D. What Is Wrong With Clinical Manifestations of Uremia as Indicators of Underdialysis?

From the discussion above, it is clear that there is an effect of low solute clearance on the outcomes of PD. Yet clinical findings fail to discriminate between inadequate and adequate clearances, suggesting that the sensitivity of uremic manifestations may be low in detecting inadequate dialysis. An analogy may be helpful to explain the apparent paradox. Patients with partially treated life-threatening infections may not present with high fever, leukocytosis, and positive cultures but may still succumb to infection. In this analogy, low small solute clearances represent partial ("inadequate") treatment of advanced renal failure. Another way to view the role of dialysis is to prevent uremic symptoms in the first place. This will be a function of the timing of initiation of dialysis as well as the intensity of dialysis. Consequently, the current targets for small solute clearance in PD are at levels higher than those at which uremic manifestations may appear (35). The NKF-DOQI targets are consistent with improved survival and low morbidity (7,8).

IV. PRESCRIBING THE TYPE AND DOSE OF PD REQUIRED FOR A TARGET CLEARANCE

Recent independent recommendations agree about the target clearances (56,57). The following total (peritoneal and renal) weekly normalized clearances were recommended by the National Kidney Foundation's Dialysis Outcomes Quality Initiative (NKF-DOQI) Work Group: for CAPD, 2.0 for Kt/V_{urea} and 60 L/1.73 m^2 for C_{Cr}; for continuous cycling peritoneal dialysis (CCPD), 2.1 for Kt/V_{urea} and 63 L/1.73 m^2 for C_{Cr}; and for nightly intermittent peritoneal dialysis (NIPD), 2.2 for Kt/V_{urear} and 66 L/1.73 m^2 for C_{Cr} (57).

The prescription of the dialysis dose should take into account the patient's lifestyle choice, size, peritoneal transport characteristics, and residual renal function (RRF). Using these parameters several highly accurate computer models calculating the type and dose of PD have been developed (58–62).

Empiric approaches to the prescription of PD can also be applied. Table 2 reproduces the empiric approach to ensure that the small solute clearance targets will be achieved as suggested by the NKF-DOQI guidelines (57). This approach stratifies PD patients by lifestyle choice (CAPD vs. CCPD), residual renal function (GFR < 2 mL/min vs. GFR ≤ 2 mL/min), and size using BSA as the size indicator (BSA < 1.7 m^2 vs. BSA = 1.7–2.0 m^2 vs. BSA > 2.0 m^2). This stratification is appropriate for Kt/V_{urea}. To achieve the target C_{Cr}, patients should be stratified by peritoneal transport type in addition to lifestyle choice, size, and RRF (63).

The principle underlying the prescription of the PD schedule and dose using either a computer model or an empiric approach is that the dose of PD must be individualized. Patient size, RRF, and peritoneal transport characteristics play major roles in defining normalized clearances and must be accounted for in the technicalities of the prescription. Failure to apply this principle has been a major cause of inadequate dialysis.

V. CAUSES OF INADEQUATE SMALL SOLUTE CLEARANCE IN PD

Causes of inadequate small solute clearance can be classified as errors by the providers (PD nurses and nephrologists) and errors directly attributed to patients. Patients can make several types of errors, intentional

Table 2 An Empiric Model of Peritoneal Dialysis Prescription

1. Underlying GFR >2 mL/min	
a. Lifestyle choice: CAPD	
BSA <1.7 m^2	4 × 2.0 L exchanges/d
BSA 1.7–2.0 m^2	4 × 2.5 L exchanges/d
BSA >2.0 m^2	4 × 3.0 L exchanges/d
b. Lifestyle choice: CCPD	
BSA <1.7 m^2	4 × 2.0 L (9 h/night) + 2.0 L/d
BSA 1.7–2.0 m^2	4 × 2.5 L (9 h/night) + 2.5 L/d
BSA >2.0 m^2	4 × 3.0 L (9 h/night) + 3.0 L/d
c. Lifestyle choice: NIPD	
Usually reserved for high transporters and some patients with substantial residual renal function. See also 2c.	
2. Underlying GFR ≤2 mL/min	
a. Lifestyle choice: CAPD	
BSA <1.7 m^2	4 × 2.5 L/d
BSA 1.7–2.0 m^2	4 × 3.0 L/d
BSA >2.0 m^2	4 × 3.0 L/d (may need added nocturnal APD if clearances are not adequate)
b. Lifestyle choice: CCPD	
BSA <1.7 m^2	4 × 2.5 L (9 h/night) + 2.0 L/d
BSA 1.7–2.0 m^2	4 × 3.0 (9 h/night) + 2.5 L/d
BSA >2.0 m^2	4 × 3.0 (10 h/night) + 2 × 3.0 L/d (may need combined hemodialysis/PD or transfer to hemodialysis)
c. Lifestyle choice: NIPD	
See also 1c. If patients are high transporters, NIPD may be prescribed using kinetic modeling.	

Source: Modified from Ref. 57.

or accidental, but the list of provider errors is longer (Table 3).

A. Provider Errors

1. Selection Errors

The proper selection of patients for PD contributes to the success of the therapy. The NKF-DOQI Guidelines have identified contraindications to either initiation or continuation of PD (57). These have been categorized into absolute and relative (Table 4) contraindications. Indications for switching from PD to HD are divided into temporary or permanent reasons for the modality conversion. These include consistent failure to achieve the target clearances, failure to control fluid overload, recurrent and/or frequent peritonitis, unmanageable hypertriglyceridemia, difficult-to-overcome technical/mechanical problems, and malnutrition resistant to aggressive management (Table 5) (3,57). These conditions as reasons to terminate PD assume that HD will solve these problems. If there is not a reasonable likelihood that HD will correct these conditions, then switching from PD to HD may not be indicated. If one or more of the conditions listed is present at the time of the initiation of dialysis, HD should be considered as the first-choice dialysis method. There will be patients who insist on PD or for technical reasons cannot be placed on HD. Such high-risk patients should be monitored frequently and cautiously.

Table 3 Causes of Inadequate Small Solute Clearance in Peritoneal Dialysis

Provider-dependent
Errors in patient selection for peritoneal dialysis
Not accounting for the effects of decreasing residual renal function
Not accounting for patient size
Not accounting for peritoneal transport type
Not accounting for changes in dwell time
Not accounting for discrepancies between C_{Cr} and Kt/V_{urea}
Patient-dependent
Errors in sampling
Noncompliance

Table 4 Contraindications for Peritoneal Dialysis

Absolute contraindications
Documented loss of peritoneal membrane function, which has many potential adverse effects including inadequate clearance (62)
Psycho-neurological problems interfering with decision making and ability to perform the tasks related to PD
Abdominal mechanical problems, such as large hernias
Relative contraindications
Fresh intraabdominal foreign bodies
Dialysate leaks
Large body size
Intolerance to the required volume of dialysate
Inflammatory or ischemic bowel disease
Abdominal wall or skin infection
Morbid obesity
Severe malnutrition
Frequent attacks of diverticulitis

Table 5 Indications for Switching from Peritoneal Dialysis to Hemodialysis

Indications for temporary switching
Failure to achieve adequate solute removal (example—recent abdominal or genital surgery mandating small volume exchanges)
Failure to adequately remove salt and water by ultrafiltration (example—peritonitis causing a high transport state in setting of pre-existing volume overload)
Acute pancreatitis unresolving with conservative therapy
Catheter-related soft tissue infections requiring a short interval without a PD catheter
Minute bowel-leak associated peritonitis requiring peritoneal rest
Hydrothorax
Severe malnutrition resistant to aggressive management
Indications for permanent switching
Consistent failure to achieve solute removal targets when there are no medical, technical, or psycho-social contraindications to hemodialysis
Inadequate fluid removal by PD when there are no medical, technical, or psycho-social contraindications to hemodialysis
Unmanageably severe hypertriglyceridemia
Unacceptably frequent peritonitis or severe debilitating peritonitis
Intractable mechanical problems (examples: recurrent hydrothorax, certain major hernia conditions)
Technical inabilities
Severe malnutrition resistant to aggressive management

2. Loss of Residual Renal Function as a Cause of Underdialysis

RRF decreases in the course of PD (8). Consequently, total clearance also decreases unless the dose of PD is increased. If RRF deteriorates without commensurate increase in delivered PD dose, patients who previously had adequate clearance levels will then have inadequate clearances. The need for frequent measurement of RRF and proper increase of the PD dose has been stressed in recent guidelines (56,57).

3. Body Size as a Cause of Underdialysis

This was presented in the first section. With the recognition of the importance of size came also the recognition that there may be size limitations to any PD regimen. In addition to eliminating very large patients from consideration as PD candidates, size also influences the choice of the PD regimen. Very large patients require daily dialysate volumes exceeding the volumes delivered by traditional CAPD (65,66). Such patients can be dialyzed with a combination of several daytime CAPD exchanges and nighttime automated peritoneal dialysis (APD) (67). HD once or twice weekly can be combined with PD (57). This is described by NKF-DOQI and shown in Fig. 2. The development of anuria in large individuals may be the precipitating factor for switching to hemodialysis.

The underweight, malnourished patient presents an interesting size-related problem. The underweight patient may have adequate clearance because of small size (low V and BSA). However, if the therapeutic efforts to correct malnutrition are successful and the patient gains weight, the same dialysis dose (clearances) may result in low normalized clearances as V and BSA increase. Furthermore, if the malnutrition and small size are secondary to underdialysis, there will never be a correction of the primary problem of underdialysis. For this reason the NKF-DOQI guidelines proposed to increase the target Kt/V_{urea} and C_{Cr} in these subjects in proportion to their degree of size loss. Thus, the desired Kt/V_{urea} target is calculated by multiplying the normal size target Kt/V_{urea} (2.0 in CAPD) by the fraction $V_{desired}/V_{actual}$ and the desired target C_{Cr} is calculated by multiplying the normal size target C_{Cr} (60 L/1.73 m^2 for CAPD) by the fraction $BSA_{desired}/BSA_{actual}$ (57).

Another size-related issue is fluid overload. Fluid overload creates an even more subtle problem, because it affects the accuracy of the estimates of the normalized clearances. The anthropometric methods estimating V and BSA do not distinguish between weight gain secondary to obesity and gain from edema. In the case

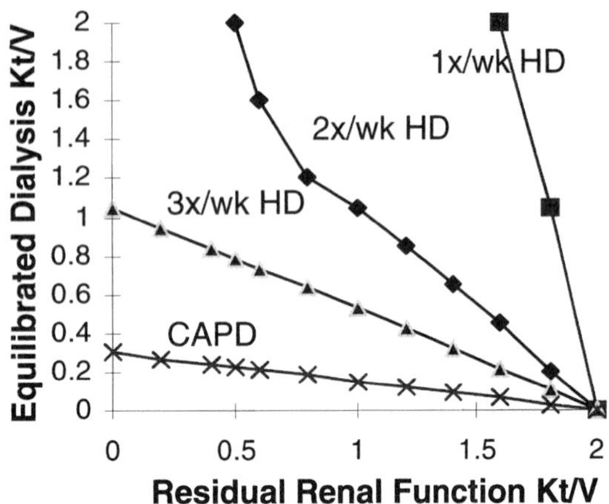

Fig. 2 This figure from the NKF-DOQI Adequacy of Peritoneal Dialysis Guidelines (57) can be used to add PD and/or HD to residual renal function or to each other. For example, PD plus residual renal function could be added on the horizontal axis and HD dose requirements determined on the vertical axis. Equivalent total dialysis doses calculated with the assumptions that K_r, K_p, and K_d are clinically equivalent clearance terms and the intermittent dialysis dose-schedule is equivalent to continuous dialysis when average predialysis BUN equals steady-state BUN of continuous therapy at equal nPCR. eK_dt/V_{urea} = the equilibrated (double-pool), delivered, and normalized hemodialysis doses. N = 1,2,3 corresponds to once, twice, and thrice weekly hemodialysis, respectively.

of edema, these methods are inaccurate in a predictable manner. The formulas estimating V may be several liters in error, even in nonedematous individuals (68–70). However, this type of error represents individual deviations and is not, for the most part (70), systematic. The formulas were derived from populations that excluded edematous subjects. If the anthropometric formula provides an accurate estimate of body water at dry weight, it will mathematically and predictably underestimate body water in edematous subjects (71). Comparison of anthropometric V to D_2O space measurements in overhydrated PD patients confirmed the mathematical prediction (72). In edematous PD patients this type of error will cause systematic underappreciation of true V and, as a consequence, overestimation of the delivered urea clearance. Whereas <40% of the weight gained during development of obesity adds to urea volume of distribution, 100% of edema weight gain adds to urea volume of distribution. The anthropometric formulas can be corrected to accurately account for the amount of excess body water if dry weight is known (71). Calculation of Kt/V_{urea} using the corrected V results in values much lower than the Kt/V_{urea} values obtained with the use of the uncorrected anthropometric formulas in PD subjects with substantial fluid overload (73). Unfortunately, the error created by fluid retention on BSA has not been estimated yet. This presents another argument favoring utilization of Kt/V_{urea}. A practical method, albeit untested in clinical trials, is to estimate fluid excess in liters (or kg) and add this directly to the calculated edema-free V. This fluid overload corrected V should then be used in the Kt/V_{urea} calculations.

Some other adverse effects of fluid retention in PD patients will be discussed here since they also relate to inadequate dialysis. Volume mediated rise in blood pressure is a common feature of renal failure. Hypertension (HT) is a well-described risk factor for the development of cardiovascular disease in all types of populations, including ESRD. Eighty percent of ESRD patients are hypertensive when they initiate dialysis, but in CAPD patients the prevalence falls to 40% by the end of the first year (74) probably secondary to salt and water removal by dialysis. Many PD patients can discontinue antihypertensive medications, particularly early in the course of PD. However, RRF may play a significant role in the maintenance of normal volume in PD patients. Faller and Lameire (75) showed that blood pressure is readily controlled in the first 3 years of PD. Later blood pressure control became problematic and more intense antihypertensive drug management was required. This may have reflected loss of RRF and its role in normalization of volume. Thus, a possible consequence of decline in RRF is overhydration. Rottembourg (76) monitored pulmonary capillary wedge pressures in CAPD patients and interpreted his findings to conclude that these patients were constantly overhydrated. The dry weight in dialysis patients is difficult to determine in general. Overt clinical features of overhydration are evident in about one fourth of patients on CAPD (77) and latent overhydration may be quite prevalent. Thus, the failure of adequate PD (plus RRF) to control volume may contribute to HT and its adverse cardiovascular sequelae.

It is possible that CAPD patients with inadequate small solute clearance could have secondary worsening of their anemia, which is usually compensated by an increased dose of erythropoietin. Erythropoietin therapy may be contributory to hypertension in dialysis patients. Eschbach et al. (78) reported that 31% of dialysis patients receiving erythropoietin had an increase in blood pressure requiring additional antihypertensive medication. Balaskas and colleagues (79) have shown that erythropoietin can be contributory to hypertension in CAPD patients. Thus, inadequate delivered dose of

PD can induce several mechanisms for exacerbating HT.

Rigorous control of blood pressure and salt and water homeostasis can favorably influence patient outcome and should be part of the definition of PD adequacy. Experience from Tassin, France (80,81), has demonstrated improved outcomes with aggressive blood pressure control and normalization of extracellular volume with long, slow HD. This approach should hold true for CAPD patients. The pathophysiology of hypertension in CAPD patients is multifactorial, resulting from the interplay of volume, cardiac, vascular, and other factors.

4. Peritoneal Membrane Function as a Cause of Underdialysis

Peritoneal membrane function can be analyzed by a standardized function test. Twardowski's peritoneal equilibration test (PET) is the most commonly used (82). This test allows the classification of peritoneal solute transport as low, low-average, high-average, and high. In CAPD patients peritoneal solute transport type has a profound effect on peritoneal creatinine clearance and an essentially negligible effect on peritoneal urea clearance (55,63,83). The consequences of this are that peritoneal transport type can be ignored in the prescription of PD for the target Kt/V_{urea} (84) but must be highly considered in the prescription of PD for the target C_{Cr} (63,85). In addition, anuric CAPD patients with low, low-average, or even high-average transport who achieve a Kt/V_{urea} of 2.0 cannot achieve a C_{Cr} of 60 L/1.73 m^2 (83). Figure 3 shows the idealized relationship between peritoneal creatinine and urea clearances (86). Both clearances were normalized by the same size indicator (V) to eliminate the distortion caused by the use of two size indicators and to show the clear effects of the transport type. The effect of the transport type is isolated by the use of the same normalized clearance (Kt/V). The clearance formula is weekly $Kt/V = 7 \times (D/P) \times Dv/V$, where D/P is the dialysate-to-plasma concentration ratio for the urea or creatinine in the clearance study data and Dv is the 24-hour drain volume. The slope $(Kt/V_{creatinnie})/(Kt/V_{urea})$ is equal to the slope $(D/P_{creatinine})/(D/P_{urea})$ because Dv and V are the same for both clearances. Figure 3 was drawn using the mean slopes $(D/P_{creatinine})/(D/P_{urea})$ in 476 clearance studies in CAPD patients with known peritoneal transport type (83). These slopes were 0.65 for low peritoneal solute transport type, 0.76 for low-average transport, 0.84 for high-average transport, and 0.92 for high transport.

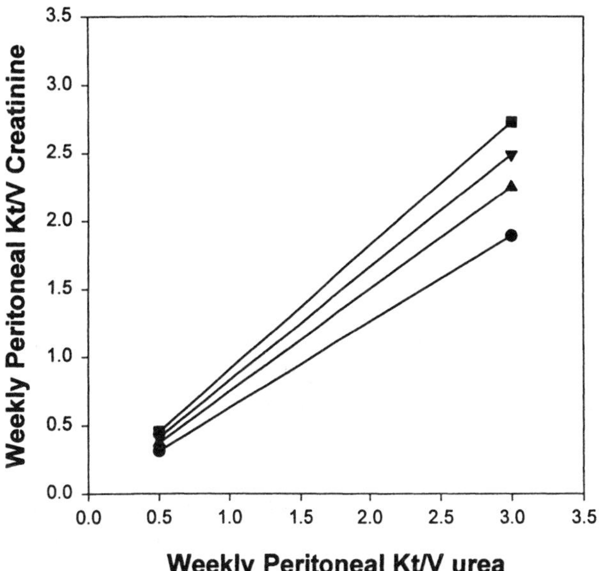

Fig. 3 Idealized relationship between peritoneal urea and creatinine clearance in patients on CAPD with different types of peritoneal solute transport. To avoid the distortion caused by the use of two different size indicators, both clearances were normalized by V. (•), Low peritoneal transport type; (▲), low-average transport; (▼), high-average transport; (■), high transport. (From Ref. 86.)

5. Problems Caused by Shortening of the Dwell Time

Shortening of the dwell time (CCPD, APD, NIPD) has more pronounced effects on C_{Cr}, particularly in low transporters, because creatinine equilibration across the peritoneal membrane is slower than that of urea (86). Thus, short dwells remove urea more quickly than creatinine in all transport types. This becomes more evident and clinically relevant with low transport characteristics. The consequence is that when the dose of PD is increased by adding APD exchanges, patients may achieve the target Kt/V_{urea}, but not the target C_{Cr} (87).

6. Problems Caused by Discrepancies Between Kt/V_{urea} and C_{Cr}

In the context of this discussion a discrepancy is present when one clearance is above and the other below the current target recommendations. One artificial source of discrepancy, the use of two different size indicators for Kt/V_{urea} and C_{Cr}, was discussed earlier. As a consequence of this phenomenon, women with adequate Kt/V_{urea} may be at risk of low C_{Cr}, while men with adequate C_{Cr} may be at risk of low Kt/V_{urea}. Underweight individuals with adequate Kt/V_{urea} may be at risk of inadequate C_{Cr}, while obese subjects with adequate C_{Cr} may be at risk of low Kt/V_{urea} (17). These types of discrepancies would be eliminated if both clearances are normalized by the same size parameter (16).

In addition to the artificial discrepancies, differences between Kt/V_{urea} and C_{Cr} are also caused by the behavior of the peritoneal membrane and residual renal function. These "physiological" discrepancies are real and require comprehension. They are found in approximately 20% of the clearance studies (85,88). The physiological discrepancies include different peritoneal transport types and shortening of the dwell time plus substantial residual renal function. Residual renal creatinine clearance, even when calculated as the average of urinary urea and creatinine clearances (57,89), is higher than urinary urea clearance (86). Therefore, subjects with substantial residual renal function and adequate C_{Cr} may be at risk of low Kt/V_{urea} (85,87). An example using average values from recent studies will illustrate this last statement: assuming that an individual on CAPD has a total creatinine clearance of 60 L/1.73 m^2 weekly, which corresponds to a $Kt/V_{creatinine}$ of 1.8 weekly (83), with 50% of his total creatinine clearance derived from residual renal function, he will have both peritoneal and urinary $Kt/V_{creatinine}$ equal to 0.90 weekly. In CAPD patients, urinary $Kt/V_{creatinine}$, corrected by averaging urea and creatinine urinary clearances, exceeds urinary Kt/V_{urea}, on the average, by 38% (90). Therefore, urinary Kt/V_{urea} will be 0.65 (0.90/1.38). Peritoneal Kt/V_{urea} exceeds peritoneal $Kt/V_{creatinine}$, on the average, by 25% (83). Therefore, peritoneal Kt/V_{urea} will be 1.13 (0.90 x 1.25), and total Kt/V_{urea} will be 1.78 (0.65 + 1.13), which is less than the target of 2.0 weekly. Thus, the greater the RRF, the more likely that C_{Cr} will exceed urea clearance, and a major discrepancy between these solute clearances will complicate defining adequacy by these measures.

The measurement of residual renal function is subjected to a relative large daily variation, mainly as a result of urine-collection errors (91). These errors will have a greater effect on C_{Cr} than on Kt/V_{urea}. In subjects with low urine flow rates and infrequent voiding, urine collection accuracy may be enhanced by using 48-hour instead of 24-hour collections (57).

The course of patients with a physiological discrepancy between Kt/V_{urea} and C_{Cr} should be monitored carefully. If the patient remains clinically stable, without uremic manifestations and with adequate nutrition, the dose of dialysis is presumably adequate, although outcomes such as survival and hospitalization rate should be tabulated in such patients. A worsening clinical or nutritional status that persists despite maximization of the PD dose, particularly when not explained by comorbidity, in a patient with a discrepancy between the two clearances should be considered as a potential indication for switching to HD (57).

7. Problems Caused by Faulty Technique

Errors in urine collection were discussed above. Errors in the measurement of clearances may be secondary to improper mixing of samples from long and short dwell time bags or errors in the sampling of blood in CCPD or NIPD. Sampling blood at the middle of the off cycler period (usually mid-day) is recommended. Analytical errors usually are secondary to interference of glucose with certain creatinine assays. The clinical laboratory should be aware whether its creatinine assay is receiving interference from glucose or not and provide its own correction factor if its assay is affected by glucose (57).

B. Patient Errors

1. Sampling Errors

Errors in urine sampling were discussed above. In addition, patients may bring for the clearance study a greater or smaller number of bags than the number of bags drained over the clearance period. Careful and detailed education of the patients and their families about the importance and the detailed procedure of obtaining an accurate clearance measurement may be the only practical way to avoid these errors. Aliquot techniques may be helpful here, but they generate their own set of potential problems.

2. Noncompliance

Noncompliance with the prescribed PD dose may take several forms including omission of one or more exchanges, poor timing, so that dwell times are too short in some exchanges and too long in others, leaving the abdomen dry for excessive time periods, inordinate long infusion or drain times, and "dumping" of part of a dialysate bag prior before filling the abdomen (92).

Estimates of the frequency of noncompliance in CAPD vary greatly (93) and are affected by the biochemical or clinical methods utilized. One method proposed comparing the measured creatinine excretion in the dialysate and urine to predicted creatinine production (94): a ratio of measured to predicted creatinine excretion exceeding 1.3 was considered an indication that the patient was noncompliant in the days before the clearance study and increased the number of exchanges on the day of the clearance study. This behavior increases the total C_{Cr} because of the unloading of the excess accumulated creatinine during the study day (94).

Using the creatinine excretion ratio, several authors reported an incidence of noncompliance between 11 and 26% (95,96). However, the measured-to-predicted creatinine ratio was theoretically shown to be neither sensitive nor specific as an index of noncompliance (97,98). Clinical studies confirmed this theoretical prediction (99,100). A deviation (increase) in total creatinine excretion exceeding 15% of a carefully determined (by several measurements) baseline excretion was proposed by NKF-DOQI as a simple screening method for noncompliance (57,101). Although this last method has not been tested, the measurements for a routine clearance study provide the means to follow creatinine excretion. Large increases in creatinine excretion have no other interpretation but that of noncompliance (57).

Using an inventory of home supplies by visiting the patients homes and counting unused bags versus prescriptions, Bernardini and Piraino found noncompliance in 40% of their Pittsburgh CAPD patients. On the average, these patients performed 75% of their prescribed exchanges (102). Using a comparable method, Fine reported only 12% noncompliance in Winnipeg CAPD patients (103). A similar difference in noncompliance between Canada and the United States was also reported in a multicenter study involving 656 CAPD patients who completed a compliance questionnaire (104).

Sevick et al. compared logs kept by the patients to counts kept by a computer chip–containing bottle cap, which recorded every opening of the bottle and the time of the opening. The patients were instructed to place all used pull tabs in the bottle (105). The number of pull tabs in the bottle was also counted. These authors reported that patient noncompliance estimated from the number of bottle openings was substantially greater than that estimated from the patient logs, that noncompliance increased with increased number of prescribed exchanges, and that dwell times were often erratic (105).

The preceding discussion summarizes hard evidence that noncompliance occurs and may be a major cause of underdialysis in PD. Patient noncompliance cannot be measured accurately by patient questionnaires. The causes of noncompliance have not been studied adequately in PD patients. By inference from studies in drug compliance, the NKF-DOQI Guidelines suggest that lack of understanding of the importance of adherence to the prescription as well as certain psychological and medical conditions, such as hostility towards authority, depression, memory impairment, financial problems, impaired mobility, language and ethnic barriers, male gender, and young age, may cause poor compliance (57).

The recommended method to prevent and treat noncompliance is education of dialysis staff, patient, and family members. The dialysis staff should have a clear understanding of the importance of small solute clearance and of the exact steps of a dialysate exchange. In addition, the dialysis staff should have developed proper teaching techniques, including visual aids that can be understood by a patient with even low educational level. Periodic retraining of both dialysis staff and patient (every 6 months or so) and psychological profiling of the patients are proposed (57). The success of these measures will require outcomes analysis.

VI. PATIENTS WITH INADEQUATE CLEARANCE STAYING ON PD

After all the factors causing low clearances have been adequately addressed, inability to achieve the target clearances should be considered a reason to switch to HD. However, as mentioned earlier, this assumes that target HD doses can be achieved. Factors contributing to inadequate delivered doses of PD could be applicable to the HD setting. A patient missing PD exchanges may also miss HD treatments or terminate the session prematurely. The two dialysis modalities should be considered as complementary methods used to obtain optimal outcomes (106). However, small subsets of PD patients who either cannot perform HD or are at excessive risk of cardiovascular mortality from HD may be maintained on PD. The first category includes patients with failures of multiple vascular accesses. Prolonged survival was reported in a small number of such patients who had suboptimal clearances (107). The second category is exemplified by patients with severe congestive heart failure. Successful PD with reasonable survival has been reported in such patients (108–113).

REFERENCES

1. Burkart JM. Adequacy of peritoneal dialysis. In: Henrich WL, ed. Principles and Practice of Dialysis. Baltimore: Williams and Wilkins 1994:111–129.
2. Ronco C. Adequacy of peritoneal dialysis is more than Kt/V. Nephrol Dial Transplant 1997; 12(suppl 1):68–73.

3. Chatoth DK, Golper TA, Gokal R. In-depth review: morbidity and mortality in defining adequacy of peritoneal dialysis: a step beyond NKF-DOQI. Am J Kidney Dis 1999; 33:617–632.
4. Tzamaloukas AH. Inadequacy of dialysis and infectious complications of continuous ambulatory peritoneal dialysis. Diagnosis, management and prevention. Am Kidney Fund Nephrol Lett 1991; 8:29–36.
5. Teehan BP, Schleifer CR, Brown J. Adequacy of continuous ambulatory peritoneal dialysis: morbidity and mortality in chronic peritoneal dialysis. Am J Kidney Dis 1994; 23:990–1001.
6. Genestier S, Hedelin G, Schaffer P, Faller B. Prognostic factors in CAPD patients: a retrospective study of a 10 year period. Nephrol Dial Transplant 1995; 10:1905–1911.
7. Maiorca R, Brunori G, Zubani R, et al. Predictive value of dialysis adequacy and nutritional indices for mortality and morbidity in CAPD and HD patients. Nephrol Dial Transplant 1995; 10:2295–2305.
8. Churchill DN, Taylor DW, Keshaviah PR. Adequacy of dialysis and nutrition in continuous peritoneal dialysis: association with clinical outcomes. J Am Soc Nephrol 1996; 7:198–207.
9. Popovich RP, Hlavinka DJ, Bormar JP, Moncrief RW, Dechard JF. The consequences of physiological resistances on metabolite removal from the patient-artificial kidney system. ASAIO Transactions 1975; 21: 108–115.
10. Teehan BP, Schleifer CR, Sigler CR, Gilgore GS. A quantitative approach to the CAPD prescription. Perit Dial Bull 1985; 5:152–256.
11. Gotch F, Sargent JA. A mechanistic analysis of the National Cooperative Dialysis Study (NCDS). Kidney Int 1985; 28:526–534.
12. Hume R,Weyers E. Relationship between total body water and body surface area in normal and obese subjects. J Clin Pathol 1971; 24:234–238.
13. Watson PE, Watson ET, Batt RP. Total body water for adult males and females estimated from simple anthropometric measurements. Am J Clin Nutr 1980; 33: 27–39.
14. Dubois D, Dubois EP. A formula to estimate the approximate body surface area if height and weight be known. Arch Intern Med 1916; 16:863–871.
15. Tzamaloukas AH, Murata GH. Body surface area and anthropometric body water in patients on continuous peritoneal dialysis. Perit Dial Int 1995; 15:284–285.
16. Tzamaloukas AH, Malhotra D, Murata GH. Gender, degree of obesity and discrepancy between urea and creatinine clearance in peritoneal dialysis. J Am Soc Nephrol 1998; 9:497–499.
17. Satko SG, Burkart JM. Frequency and causes of discrepancy between KT/V and creatinine Cl (abstr). Perit Dial Int 1997; 17(suppl. 1):S23.
18. Tzamaloukas AH. In search of the ideal V. Perit Dial Int 1996; 16:345–346.
19. Vonesh EF, Moran J. Discrepancy between urea KT/V versus normalized creatinine clearance. Perit Dial Int 1997; 17:13–16.
20. Vonesh EF. Consequences of normalizing peritoneal dialysis dose. Semin Dial 1997; 10:293–294.
21. Tzamaloukas AH, Vonesh EF. Urea clearance, creatinine clearance and size indicators in peritoneal dialysis. Semin Dial 1998; 11:192–194.
22. Lowrie EG, Laird NM, Parker TF, et al. Effect of hemodialysis prescription on patient morbidity. Report of the National Cooperative Dialysis Study. N Engl J Med 1981; 305:1176–1181.
23. Lameire NH, Vanholder R, Veyt D, Lambert M, Ringoir S. A longitudinal, five year survey of urea kinetic parameters in CAPD patients. Kidney Int 1992; 42: 426–432.
24. Tattersall JE, Doyle S, Greenwood RN, Farrington K. Kinetic modeling and underdialysis CAPD patients. Nephrol Dial Transplant 1993; 8:535–538.
25. Brandes JC, Piering WF, Peres JA, Blumenthal JS, Fritsche C. Clinical outcome of continuous ambulatory peritoneal dialysis predicts urea and creatinine kinetics. J Am Soc Nephrol 1992; 2:1430–1435.
26. Arkouche W, Delawari E, My H, Laville M, Abdullah E, Traeger J. Quantification of adequacy of peritoneal dialysis. Perit Dial Int 1993; 13(suppl. 2):S215–S218.
27. Heaf J. CAPD adequacy and dialysis morbidity: detrimental effect of a high peritoneal equilibration rate. Renal Failure 1995; 17(5):575–587.
28. Holley JL. Patient-reported symptoms and adequacy of dialysis as measured by creatinine clearance. Perit Dial Int 1993; 13(suppl. 2):S219–S220.
29. Tzamaloukas AH, Murata GH, Sena P. Assessing the adequacy of peritoneal dialysis. Perit Dial Int 1993; 13:236–238.
30. DeAlvaro F, Bajo MA, Alvarez-Ude F, et al. Adequacy of peritoneal dialysis: Does KT/V have the same predictive value as HD? A multicenter study. Adv Perit Dial 1992; 8:93–97.
31. Mooraki A, Kliger AS, Gorban-Brenan NL, Juergensen P, Brown E, Finkelstein FO. Weekly KT/V urea and selected outcomes in 56 randomly selected patients. Adv Perit Dial 1993; 9:92–96.
32. Spinowitz BS, Gupta BK, Kulpgowski J, et al. Dialysis adequacy versus metabolic factors in the clinical assessment of CAPD. Adv Perit Dial 1993; 9:295–298.
33. Goodship THJ, Passlick-Deetjen J, Ward MK, Wilkinson R. Adequacy of dialysis and nutritional status in CAPD. Nephrol Dial Transplant 1993; 8:1366–1371.
34. Tzamaloukas AH, Balaskas EV, Voudiklari S, et al. Double-blinded comparison between clinical and laboratory evaluation of CAPD adequacy (abstr). Perit Dial Int 1995; 15(suppl. 2):S61.
35. Tzamaloukas AH, Murata GH. Adequacy of continuous ambulatory peritoneal dialysis. Int J Artif Organs 1993; 16:557–562.

36. Bergstrom J. Appetite in CAPD patients. Perit Dial Int 1995; 15(suppl. 3):S181-S184.
37. Ikizler TA, Greene JH, Wingard RL, Parker DA, Hakim RM. Spontaneous dietary protein intake during progression of chronic renal failure. J Am Soc Nephrol 1995; 6:1386–1391.
38. Jones MR. Etiology of severe malnutrition: results of an international cross-sectional study in continuous ambulatory peritoneal dialysis patients. Am J Kidney Dis 1994; 23:412–420.
39. Bergstrom J, Furst P, Alverstrand A, Linholm B. Protein and energy intake, nitrogen balance and nitrogen losses in patients treated with continuous ambulatory peritoneal dialysis. Kidney Int 1993; 44:1048–1057.
40. Harty JC, Boulton H, Curwell J, et al. The normalized protein catabolic rate is a flawed marker of nutrition in CAPD patients. Kidney Int 1994; 45:103–109.
41. Harty JC, Farragher B, Boulton H, et al. Is the correlation between the normalized protein catabolic rate (NPCR) and KT/V the result of mathematical coupling? (abstract) J Am Soc Nephrol 1993; 4:407.
42. Hertel J, Lightfoot BO, Fincher ME, McConnell KR, Caruana RJ. Correlation between urea reduction rates and serum albumin levels in patients on hemodialysis. ASAIO J 41(3) 1995; M801–M804.
43. Blake PG, Flowerdew G, Blake RM, Oreopoulos DG. Serum albumin in patients on continuous ambulatory peritoneal dialysis: predictors and correlations with outcomes. J Am Soc Nephrol 1993; 3:1501–1507.
44. Malhotra D, Tzamaloukas AH, Murata GH, Fox L, Goldman RS, Avasthi PS. Serum albumin in continuous peritoneal dialysis: its predictors and relationship to urea clearance. Kidney Int 1996; 50:243–249.
45. Nolph KD, Moore HL, Prowant B, et al. Continuous ambulatory peritoneal dialysis with a high flux membrane. ASAIO J 1993; 39:904–909.
46. Malhotra D, Murata GH, Tzamaloukas AH. Serum albumin in peritoneal dialysis: clinical significance and important influences on its levels. Int J Artif Organs 1997; 20:251–254.
47. Yeun JY, Kaysen GA. Acute phase reactants and peritoneal dialysate albumin losses are the main determinants of serum albumin in peritoneal dialysis patients. Am J Kidney Dis 1997; 30:923–927.
48. Ikizler TA, Wingard RL, Hakim RM. Malnutrition in peritoneal dialysis patients: etiologic factors and treatment options. Perit Dial Int 1995; 15(5, suppl.):S63–S66.
49. McCusker FM, Teehan BP, Thorpe K, Keshaviah P, Churchill D. How much peritoneal dialysis is required for the maintenance of a good nutritional state? Kidney Int 1996; 50:S56–S61.
50. Blake PG, Balaskas E, Blake R, Oreopoulos DG. Urea kinetics has limited relevance in assessing adequacy of dialysis in CAPD. Adv Perit Dial 1992; 8:65–70.
51. Teehan BP, Schleifer CR, Brown J. Urea kinetic modeling is an appropriate assessment of adequacy. Semin Dial 1992; 5:189–192.
52. Bloembergen WE, Stannard DC, Port F, et al. Relationship of dose of hemodialysis and cause-specific mortality. Kidney Int 1996; 50:557–565.
53. Davies SJ, Bryan J, Phillips L, Russell GI. The predictive value of KT/V and peritoneal solute transport in CAPD patients is dependent on the type of comorbidity present. Perit Dial Int 1996; 16(suppl 2): S15–S162.
54. Jager KJ, Merkus MP, Dekker FW, Boeschoten EW, Krediet RT. Patient characteristics at baseline are predictors for patient survival: contribution of dialysis adequacy remains uncertain (abstr). Perit Dial Int 1998; 18(suppl. 1):S17.
55. Churchill DN, Thorpe KE, Nolph KD, Keshaviah PR, Oreopoulos DG, Page D. Increased peritoneal membrane transport is associated with decreased patient and technique survival for continuous peritoneal dialysis patients. J Am Soc Nephrol 1998; 9:1285–1292.
56. Blake P, Burkart J, Churchill D, et al. Recommended clinical practices for maximizing peritoneal dialysis clearances. Perit Dial Int 1996; 16:448–456.
57. Golper T, Churchill D, Burkart J, et al. National Kidney Foundation, DOQI—Dialysis Outcomes Quality Initiative. Clinical practice guidelines for peritoneal dialysis adequacy. Am J Kidney Dis 1997; 30(suppl. 2):S67–S136.
58. Vonesh EF, Lysacht MJ, Moran J, Farrell P. Kinetic modeling as a prescription aid in peritoneal dialysis. Blood Purif 1991; 9:247–270.
59. Gotch F, Keen M. Kinetic modeling in peritoneal dialysis. In: Nissenson AR, Fine RN, Gentile DE, eds. Clinical Dialysis. 3rd ed. East Norwalk, CT: Appleton, 1995: 343–376.
60. Roberston BC, Juacz NM, Walker PJ, Raymond KH, Taber TE, Adcock AI. A prescription model for peritoneal dialysis. ASAIO J 1995; 41:116–126.
61. Rippe B. Peritoneal dialysis capacity. Perit Dial Int 1997; 17(suppl. 2):S131–S134.
62. Vonesh EF, Burkart J, McMurray SD, Williams RF. Peritoneal dialysis kinetic modeling: validation in a multicenter clinical study. Perit Dial Int 1996; 16:471–481.
63. Rao P, Tzamaloukas AH, Murata GH, et al. Estimating the daily dialysate drain volume required for a target peritoneal creatinine clearance from body water and peritoneal transport characteristics. Adv Perit Dial 1997; 13:38–41.
64. Korbet SM, Rodby ST. Peritoneal membrane failure: differential diagnosis, evaluation and treatment. Semin Dial 1994; 7:128–137.
65. Nolph KD, Jensen RA, Khanna R, Twardowski ZJ. Weight limitations for weekly urea clearances using various exchange volumes in CAPD. Perit Dial Int 1994; 14:261–264.

66. Rocco M. Body surface area limitations in achieving adequate therapy in peritoneal dialysis patients. Perit Dial Int 1996; 16:617–622.
67. Tzamaloukas AH, Dimitriadis A, Murata GH, et al. Continuous peritoneal dialysis in overweight individuals: urea and creatinine clearances. Perit Dial Int 1996; 16:302–306.
68. Sherman RA. Quantitating peritoneal dialysis: the problem with V. Semin Dial 1996; 9:381–383.
69. Woodrow G, Oldroyd B, Turney JH, Davies PSW, Day JME, Smith MA. Measurement of total body water and urea kinetic modeling in peritoneal dialysis. Clin Nephrol 1997; 47:52–57.
70. Arkouche W, Fouque D, Pachiandi C, et al. Total body water and body composition in chronic peritoneal dialysis patients. J Am Soc Nephrol 1997; 8:1906–1914.
71. Tzamaloukas AH. Effect of edema on urea kinetic studies in peritoneal dialysis patients. Perit Dial Int 1994; 14(4):398–401.
72. Wong KC, Xiong DW, Kerr DG, et al. Kt/V in CAPD by different estimations of V. Kidney Int 1995; 48: 563–569.
73. Tzamaloukas AH, Murata GH, Dimitriadis A, et al. Fractional urea clearance in continuous peritoneal dialysis: effects of volume disturbances. Nephron 1996; 74:567–571.
74. Lameire N. Cardiovascular risk factors and blood pressure control in continuous ambulatory peritoneal dialysis. Perit Dial Int 1993; 13(suppl 2): S394–395.
75. Faller B, Lameire N. Evolution of clinical parameters and peritoneal function in a cohort of CAPD patients followed over 7 years. Nephrol Dial Transplant 1994; 9:280–286.
76. Rottembourg J. Residual renal function and recovery of renal function in patients treated by CAPD. Kidney Int 1993; 43(suppl 40):S106–S110.
77. Tzamaloukas AH, Saddler MC, Murata GH, Malhotra D, Sena P, Simon D, Hawkins KL, Morgan K, Nevarez M, Wood B, Elledge L, Gibel LJ. Symptomatic fluid retention in patients on continuous peritoneal dialysis. J Am Soc Nephrol 1995; 6:198–206.
78. Eschbach JW, Egrie JC, Downing MR, et al. The safety of epoetin alpha: results of clinical trials in the United States. In: Garland HJ, Moran J, Samtleben W, Scigalla P, Wieczorek L, eds. Erythropoietin in Renal and Nonrenal Anemias. Contrib Nephrol 1991; 88:72–80.
79. Balaskas EV, Melamed IR, Gupta A, Bargman J, Oreopoulos DG. Influence of erythropoietin on blood pressure in continuous ambulatory peritoneal dialysis patients. Perit Dial Int 1993; 13(suppl 2):S553–S557.
80. Charra B, Calemard E, Ruffet M, Chazot C, Terrat JC, Vanel T, Laurent G. Survival as an index of adequacy of dialysis. Kidney Int 1992; 41:1286–1291.
81. Charra B, Calemard E, Laurent G. Importance of treatment time and blood pressure control in achieving long term survival on dialysis. Am J Nephrol 1996; 16:35–44.
82. Twardowski ZJ, Nolph KD, Khanna R, et al. Peritoneal equilibration test. Perit Dial Bull 1987;7:138–147.
83. Tzamaloukas AH, Murata GH, Piraino B, et al. Peritoneal urea and creatinine clearances in continuous peritoneal dialysis patients with different types of peritoneal solute transport. Kidney Int 1998; 53:1405–1411.
84. Tzamaloukas AH, Murata GH, Malhotra D, Fox L, Goldman RS, Avasthi PS. The minimal dose of dialysis required for a target KT/V in continuous peritoneal dialysis. Clin Nephrol 1995; 44:316–321.
85. Tzamaloukas AH, Murata GH, Malhotra D, Fox L, Goldman RS, Avasthi PS. Creatinine clearance in continuous peritoneal dialysis: dialysis dose required for a minimal acceptable level. Perit Dial Int 1996; 16: 41–47.
86. Tzamaloukas AH, Murata GH, Malhotra D. The relationship between the clearances of urea and creatinine in peritoneal dialysis. Int J Artif Organs 1998; 21:255–258.
87. Tebeau JL, Moran JE, Vonesh EF, Pu K, Harter MC, Improvements in delivered dose utilizing a prescription management process. Perit Dial Int 1998; 18(suppl. 1):S23.
88. Chen HH, Shetty A, Afthentopoulos I, Oreopoulos DG. Discrepancy between weekly KT/V and weekly creatinine clearance in patients on CAPD. Adv Perit Dial 1995; 11:83–87.
89. Bhatla P, Moore HL, Nolph KD. Modification of creatinine clearance by estimation of residual creatinine and urea clearance in CAPD patients. Adv Perit Dial 1995; 11:101–105.
90. Tzamaloukas AH, Murata GH. The relationship between the normalized renal clearances of urea and creatinine in continuous peritoneal dialysis. Perit Dial Int 1998; 18:447–448.
91. Rodby RA, Firanek C, Cheng YG, Korbet SM. Reproducibility of studies of peritoneal dialysis adequacy. Kidney Int 1996; 50:267–271.
92. Caruana RJ, Smith KL, Hess CP, Perez JC, Cheek PL. Dialysate dumping: a novel cause of inadequate dialysis in continuous ambulatory peritoneal dialysis (CAPD) patients. Perit Dial Int 1989; 9:73–75.
93. Amici G, Viglino G, Virga G, et al. Compliance study in peritoneal dialysis using PD Adequest software. Perit Dial Int 1996; 16(suppl. 2):S176-S178.
94. Keen M, Lipps B, Gotch F. The measure of creatinine generation rate in CAPD suggests only 78% of prescribed dialysis is delivered. Adv Perit Dial 1993; 9: 73–75.
95. Warren PJ, Brandes JC. Compliance with the prescribed dialysis prescription is poor. J Am Soc Nephrol 1994; 4:1627–1629.

96. Nolph KD, Twardowski ZJ, Khanna R, et al. Predicted and measured daily creatinine production in CAPD: identifying noncompliance. Perit Dial Int 1995; 15: 22–25.
97. Tzamaloukas AH. Can excess of estimated over predicted creatinine generation be a discriminating test for non-compliance in continuous ambulatory peritoneal dialysis? J Am Soc Nephrol 1995; 6:1519–1520.
98. Tzamaloukas AH. Pharmacokinetic analysis of creatinine generation discrepancy as an index of noncompliance in CAPD. Adv Perit Dial 1996; 12:61–65.
99. Blake PG, Spanner E, McMurray S, Lindsay RM, Ferguson E. Comparison of measured and predicted creatinine excretion is an unreliable index of compliance in PD patients. Perit Dial Int 1996; 16:147–153.
100. Burkart JM, Bleyer AJ, Jordan JR, Zeigler NC. An elevated ratio of measured to predicted creatinine production in CAPD patients is not a sensitive predictor of noncompliance with the dialysis prescription. Perit Dial Int 1996; 16:142–146.
101. Johansson A-C, Attman P, Haraldsson B. Creatinine generation rate and lean body mass: a critical analysis in peritoneal dialysis patients. Kidney Int 1997; 51: 855–859.
102. Bernardini J, Piraino B. Measuring noncompliance with prescribed exchanges in CAPD and CCPD patients. Perit Dial Int 1997; 17:338–342.
103. Fine A. Compliance with CAPD prescription is good. Peri Dial Int 1997; 17:323–346.
104. Blake P, Korbet S, Blake R, et al. Admitted noncompliance [nc] with CAPD exchanges is more common in U.S. than Canadian patients (abstr). Perit Dial Int 1998; 18(suppl. 1):S12.
105. Sevick MA, Burkart J, Rocco MV, Levine D. Measurement of CAPD adherence using a novel approach (abstr). Perit Dial Int 1998; 18(suppl. 1):S27.
106. Van Biesen WA, Vigt PE, Vanholder R, Lameire NH. Integrated care can improve long-term survival (abstr). Perit Dial Int 1998; 18(suppl. 1):S56.
107. Makil D, Gibel LJ, Tzamaloukas AH. CAPD in patients with hemodialysis access failure. (abstr). Perit Dial Int 1998; 18(suppl. 1):S55.
108. Robson MD, Biro A, Knobel B, Schai C, Mordchia R. Peritoneal dialysis in refractory congestive heart failure: Part II. Continuous ambulatory peritoneal dialysis (CAPD). Perit Dial Bull 1983; 3:133–134.
109. Kim D, Khanna R, Wu G, Fountas P, Druck N, Oreopoulos DG. Successful use of continuous ambulatory peritoneal dialysis in refractory heart failure. Perit Dial Bull 1985; 5:127–130.
110. McKinnie JJ, Bourgeois RJ, Husserl FE. Long-term therapy for heart failure with continuous ambulatory peritoneal dialysis. Arch Intern Med 1985; 145:1128–1129.
111. Rubin J, Bell R. Continuous ambulatory peritoneal dialysis as a treatment of severe congestive heart failure in the face of chronic renal failure. Report of eight cases. Arch Intern Med 1986; 146:1533–1535.
112. Konig PS, Llotta K, Kronenberg F, Ioannidis M, Herld M. CAPD: a successful treatment in patients suffering with therapy-resistant congestive heart failure. Adv Perit Dial 1991; 7:97–101.
113. Stegmayr B, Banga L, Lundberg L, Wikdahl AM, Plum-Wirell M. PD treatment for severe congestive heart failure. Perit Dial Int 1996; 16(suppl. 1):S231-S235.

11

Infectious Complications and Peritonitis and Their Management

Ram Gokal
Manchester Royal Infirmary, Manchester, United Kingdom

I. INTRODUCTION

Ever since the introduction of peritoneal dialysis in the management of renal failure, complications related to the technique, in particular peritonitis and access-related problems, have bedeviled its wider use and acceptance. Even after the introduction of continuous ambulatory peritoneal dialysis (CAPD) in 1976 (1) and the subsequent technical and other advances, these problems still remain the Achilles heel of peritoneal dialysis therapy. The frequent occurrence of peritonitis remains the major complication of peritoneal dialysis (PD) and together with access-related infections accounts for considerable morbidity, hospitalization, and therapy change to hemodialysis. These aspects remain preeminent areas of research to try and minimize such complications. This chapter discusses peritonitis and catheter-related infections and their management.

II. PERITONITIS

Over the last two decades since the introduction of CAPD there have been some dramatic changes in the incidence of peritonitis related to several technological improvements, including the transfer sets to catheter connector (titaneum) and long-life tubing, which requires less frequent transfer set changes. The most important change has been the introduction of the so-called Y-set or disconnect systems (2,3). The latter was first introduced in Italy with reported rates of peritonitis of an episode every 24–36 patient-months. A multicenter study in Canada confirmed the results (4). This "flush before fill" method has now become widely accepted in its many variations, making it possible for the average unit to report an episode of peritonitis every 2 to 3 years. The U.S. Renal Data System (USRDS) reports that the time to first peritonitis of patients on a Y set was 20.6 months compared to the standard connection system, where it was 11.4 months (5).

A. Definition

The constant presence of fluid in the peritoneal cavity has certainly modified the definition and clinical features of peritonitis in CAPD. A practical definition (6) of peritonitis requires the presence of two of the following criteria in any combination:

1. Presence of organisms on gram stain or subsequent culture of PD fluid.
2. Cloudy fluid (WBC >100 cells, with greater than 50% neutrophils).
3. Symptoms of peritoneal inflammation.

In episodes of peritonitis, cloudiness of the dialysate effluent is almost invariably present (7). For practical purposes it should be seen as the earliest detector of peritoneal infection, which can be readily identified by the patient even in the absence of abdominal pain. Turbidity can be seen with cell counts greater than 100.

B. Relapse or Reinfection

These concepts are reasonably well defined, are arbitrary, and may have prognostic significance (8). Relapse is defined as occurrence of another episode of peritonitis caused by the same genus/species that caused the immediately preceding episode occurring within 4 weeks of completion of the antibiotic course. This is sometimes referred to as a recurrent episode. It indicates either inadequate treatment or possibly the opening of an abscess cavity that was previously inaccessible to treatment.

Reinfection is a new peritonitis episode beyond the 4-week period with the same organism. If reinfection occurs an internal focus or catheter source should be suspected. The debate about what constitutes reinfection or relapse continues even after clinical criteria and typing methods are used (9).

C. Signs and Symptoms

The frequency of presenting signs and symptoms of peritonitis has been well defined (7,10,11). Cloudy dialysate effluent is almost invariably present (99% of patients), while abdominal pain was present in 80–95% of cases. Gastrointestinal symptoms (nausea, vomiting, diarrhea) range from 7 to 36%, while chills were present in 12–23% of cases. Fever was often lacking and was recorded in only about one third of the cases, while abdominal tenderness was present in 80% of cases, together with rebound tenderness in 60% of the patients. Other signs and symptoms include anorexia, malaise, the occurrence of drainage problems (about 15% of cases), increased protein catabolic rate, and dialysate protein losses (12,13).

1. Cloudy Bag

Among the various manifestations of peritonitis, a cloudy peritoneal effluent is almost a constant finding. This modification of the appearance of a drained dialysate is usually sudden; it is observed without gradation from one exchange draining clear fluid to the next showing a cloudy effluent. The turbidity of the peritoneal effluent may not be easy to recognize at a glance. The patient should learn how to identify even the slight opalescence of the drain bag by bringing it before a light. The observation of a cloudy dialysate is not synonymous with peritonitis. The differential diagnosis should be made with peritoneal eosinophilia, neutrophilia, intraperitoneal bleeding, and the presence of fibrin in the peritoneal effluent.

2. Peritoneal Eosinophilia Syndrome

The syndrome of peritoneal eosinophilia is not frequent, is observed in the early stages of CAPD, and by definition cloudy fluid is always present. In contrast with infectious peritonitis, peritoneal eosinophilia is not associated with abdominal pain and is relatively asymptomatic (14). Dialysate white cell count gives values ranging from 10% reaching values of 95%. Repeated cultures of the peritoneal fluid dialysis are persistently negative. The clinical course is characterized by the rapid clearing of the dialysis effluent after a few days. There appears to be a close association of eosinophils with hypersensitivity reactions, which suggests a role for some allergenic substances or air brought into the peritoneal cavity by CAPD procedures. Specific therapy is not indicated, although at times intraperitoneal hydrocortisone is necessary (15).

D. Pathogenesis of Peritonitis

Contamination at the time of the peritoneal dialysis exchange was and still is a major cause of peritonitis (16,17). Touching the connection, dropping the tubing on the floor or table, and performing the exchange in an atmosphere filled with dust or animal hair all may lead to peritonitis. Holes in the catheter, tubing, or bags and accidental disconnections also can cause peritonitis.

Approximately 15–20% of peritonitis episodes are secondary to catheter infections (18,19). Exit site infections, especially those due to *Staphylococcus aureus* or *Pseudomonas aeruginosa*, can spread to involve the catheter tunnel and the peritoneum (20,21), which is often refractory or relapsing. In the absence of known contamination or a catheter infection, peritonitis due to gram-negative organisms are generally considered to be enteric in origin, probably due to transmural migration of bacteria across the bowel wall (22–24). Bowel perforation leads to polymicrobial peritonitis but is an unusual cause of peritonitis (25). Peritonitis has been reported following colonoscopy with polypectomy (26,27), endoscopy with sclerotherapy, and dental procedures (28). Vaginal leak of dialysate (29) and the use of intrauterine devices (30) are other unusual causes of peritonitis.

E. Microorganisms Causing Peritonitis and Portals of Entry

The most common microorganisms to cause peritonitis are listed in Table 1, which also shows the changing pattern of organisms related to the use of disconnect systems (31). The culture has no growth in up to 20% of episodes that meet the criteria for peritonitis based on cell count (31,32). Most of these episodes are due

Table 1 Microorganisms Causing Peritonitis and Change in Peritonitis Rates for Organisms with Introduction of Y-Set Systems

		Peritonitis rates (episodes/patient-year)	
Microorganisms	%	Straight line	Y-set
Gram-positive			
S. epidermidis	30–40	0.34	0.17
S. aureus	15–20	0.15	0.13
Streptococcus	10–15		
Other Gram +	2–5		
Gram-negative		0.12	0.10
Pseudomonas	5–10		
Enterobacter	5–20		
Other gram −	5–7		
Fungi	2–10	0.02	0.01
Other organisms	2–5		
Culture negative	10–30		

Source: Ref. 137.

to inadequate culture techniques or prior antibiotic therapy (7,33). Placing the effluent in blood culture bottles (16,34), the Bac-tec method (35), or concentration by filtering (36) decreases the incidence of negative cultures.

There exists a delicate balance between the invaders that gain access into the peritoneal cavity and the host defense mechanism that is present to counteract such invasions. In the intact abdomen the occasional penetrations of organisms are appropriately dealt with by such mechanisms; this is probably a frequent event, but only rarely does it lead to major infections. The situation is different for peritoneal dialysis patients. It is well known that penetration of infectious organisms into the peritoneal cavity occurs more frequently than episodes of peritonitis (37). The host defense mechanisms are thought to be impaired in peritoneal dialysis, and hence peritonitis rates will be much higher in patients undergoing peritoneal dialysis. Since the conditions that lead to peritonitis are not known, all portals of entry have to be considered seriously in order to reduce peritonitis incidence.

Surveillance cultures from abdominal skin site, throat, and hands done on peritoneal dialysis patients before they enter a dialysis program have been undertaken (7). These are the areas from which incidental contaminations of peritoneal dialysis patients can occur. It is therefore possible to generate a listing that estimates the probable route of entry from the type of organisms isolated (Table 2).

Table 2 Routes of Infections and Related Microorganisms in CAPD Peritonitis

Route	Organisms	%
Transluminal	*S. epidermidis* *Acinetobacter*	30–40
Periluminal	*S. epidermidis* *S. aureus* *Pseudomonas* Yeasts	20–30
Transmural	Gram-negatives Anaerobes	20–30
Hematogenous	Streptococci Tuberculosis	5–10
Ascending	Yeasts Lactobacilli	2–5

F. Clinical Course of Peritonitis

The incubation period of peritonitis is not well known, but it is estimated from touch contamination incidents as well as prospective studies to be usually 24–48 hours. During this period, bacteria, aligned to the peritoneal wall, multiply and are shed into the PD fluid at a time when the peritoneal network is activated, resulting in white cells emigrating out of the circulation to the area of injury. This pathogenetic mechanism of the time schedule has been cleverly studied by Zemel et al. (38), where CAPD patients stored the overnight PD effluent at 4°C for 2 days. If an episode of peritonitis occurred, two overnight bags were brought in. In this way nine episodes of peritonitis were assessed. The study found that at least 24 hours prior to clinical peritonitis (and at times up to 48 hours previously), positive bacterial cultures were present in most of the PD effluents. There was also an increase in the number of peritoneal macrophages, a moderate increase in neutrophils, and a relative phagocytic malfunction of the macrophages. It seems, therefore, that in any bacterial invasion, the host defense mechanisms need to be overwhelmed before clinical peritonitis ensues—this battle is a constantly ongoing one.

The appearance of the symptoms may be very rapid (36). In most cases of peritonitis the symptoms decrease rapidly after the initiation of therapy and disappear within 2–3 days. During this period the cell counts decrease and the bacterial cultures become negative. In the majority of the cases, positive peritoneal cultures are present only for 3–4 days. Persistence of symptoms is indicative of a complicated cause or a possible resistant organism that is not responding well to antibiotics used; these require further investigation and possible catheter removal.

G. Treatment of Peritonitis

When peritonitis occurs in patients on peritoneal dialysis, treatment should be started immediately after completion of the appropriate microbiological work-up; however, treatment has to be initiated in the absence of appropriate diagnostic information, and therefore certain arbitrary decisions have to be taken on the appropriateness of the antibiotic treatment based on the considerations presented above on causative organisms. Several protocols for antibiotic treatments have been proposed (16,17,39,40), and there is an increasing consensus towards a standardized approach combining the continuation of CAPD with intraperitoneal administration of antibiotics. Such an approach has been further emphasized in the recent update of the Advisory Committee on Peritoneal Dialysis (a subcommittee of the International Society For Peritoneal Dialysis) (41).

In their 1993 recommendations (40), the ad hoc committee advocated the use of vancomycin as the mainstay against gram-positive infections with ceftazidine or aminoglycoside covering the gram-negative organism as first-line, blind therapy in the absence of an organism being identified on gram stain at presentation. However, since publication of that report in 1993 there has been a dramatic increase in the prevalence of vancomycin-resistant microorganisms, especially enterococci (VRE), from approximately 0.5% to nearly 14%; this has been particularly evident in larger hospitals. Vancomycin resistance has been associated with resistance to other penicillins and aminoglycosides, thus presenting a treatment dilemma since many of the second-line antimicrobial agents that could be used have not been proven in therapeutic trials. This has prompted a number of worldwide agencies (42–44) to discourage routine use of vancomycin for prophylaxis and for oral use against *Clostridium difficile* enterocolitis. The major concern is that the vancomycin resistance is transmitted to staphyloccocal strains, creating an issue of major epidemiological importance. The focus, therefore, has moved away from the use of vancomycin as a first-line therapy, and the peritonitis subcommittee has reverted back to using first-generation cephalosporins in large doses.

1. Initial Empiric Antibiotic Selection

Figure 1 outlines assessment and antibiotic therapy (41). The empiric treatment is further subdivided into continuous or intermittent use in relation to residual urine output. It advocates a first-generation cephalosporin antibiotic for gram-positive and an aminoglycoside for gram-negative cover. This would prevent unnecessary exposure to vancomycin and thus prevent emergence of resistant organisms. This strategy is consistent with the desire to preserve vancomycin for use in resistant organisms. The rationale for using the recommended large dose of first-generation cephalosporin is that the organisms are in fact sensitive to the drug because of the levels achieved at the site of the infection (peritoneal cavity). It is now recognized that the antibiotic can be given as a single dose overnight with good efficacy (45). Such dosing regime is also applicable to the aminoglycosides; a single daily dose of these agents has been shown to be efficacious and may be less toxic. It is also felt that the increased bacterial killing rate associated with prolonged postantibiotic effect are obtained using once daily dosage and the oto- and nephrotoxicity can be minimized. Continuous therapy results in sustained but low serum levels, which are bactericidal but may favor toxic accumulation of these agents.

2. Modification of Treatment Regimen Once Culture and Sensitivity Results Are Known

a. Gram-Positive Microorganisms

The management of patients with gram-positive organisms on culture is shown in Fig. 2 (41). If the organism is an enterococcus, the cephalosporin is replaced with ampicillin (125 mg/L) and the aminoglycoside may be continued with one exchange per day based on sensitivity. If the organism is *S. aureus*, its sensitivity to methicillin will dictate further therapy changes. If it is sensitive to methicillin, the aminoglycoside should be discontinued, and if the clinical response is less than desired, rifampicin (600 mg/d) should be added orally to the IP cephalosporin. The use of rifampicin in areas with a high prevalence of tuberculosis cannot be advocated and other antibiotics, according to sensitivities, need to be used. If the *S. aureus* is methicillin resistant (MRSA), rifampicin should be added and the cephalosporin should be changed to clindamycin or vancomycin. The vancomycin regime is then as previously (2 g IP every 7 days). For other gram-positive organisms, such as *Staphylococcus epidermidis*, which is the most frequently identified organism in this situation, the first-generation cephalosporins are usually sufficient. However, if the organism is again methicillin resistant (MRSE), then one needs to consider use of clindamycin or vancomycin. If there is no clear

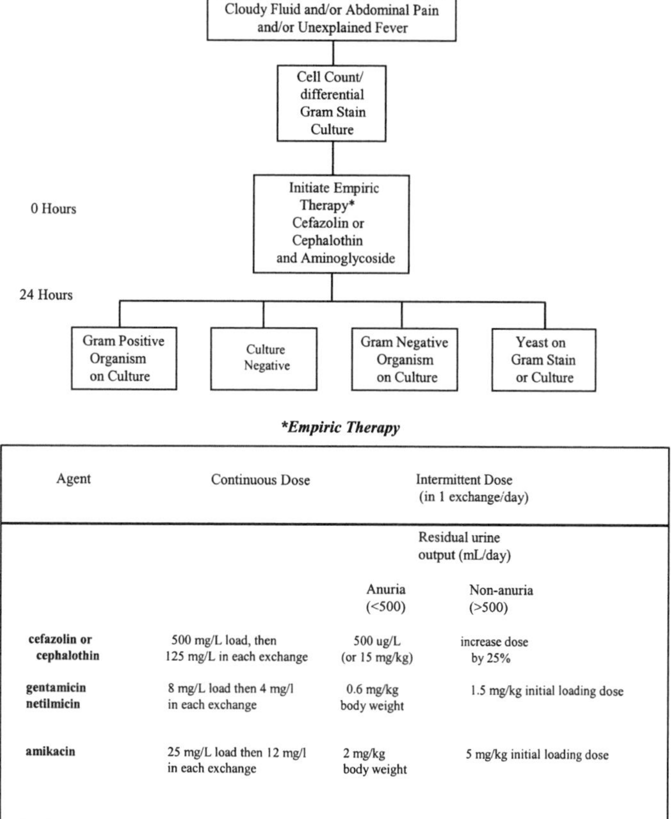

Empiric Therapy

Agent	Continuous Dose	Intermittent Dose (in 1 exchange/day)	
		Residual urine output (mL/day)	
		Anuria (<500)	Non-anuria (>500)
cefazolin or cephalothin	500 mg/L load, then 125 mg/L in each exchange	500 ug/L (or 15 mg/kg)	increase dose by 25%
gentamicin netilmicin	8 mg/L load then 4 mg/l in each exchange	0.6 mg/kg body weight	1.5 mg/kg initial loading dose
amikacin	25 mg/L load then 12 mg/l in each exchange	2 mg/kg body weight	5 mg/kg initial loading dose

Fig. 1 Assessment and therapy of patients presenting with a cloudy bag and symptoms of peritonitis. Patients with residual urine output may require 0.6 mg/kg body weight doses with increased frequency based on serum and/or dialysate levels. (From Ref. 41.)

improvement within 48 hours or if the current peritonitis episode is a recurrence or relapse, switching to an alternative agent such a clindamycin or vancomycin is warranted.

b. Limits on Vancomycin Use

Vancomycin for initial therapy is cost effective, convenient, and, in combination with a second drug for gram-negative bacilli, provides good initial coverage. However, because of the emergence of resistant strains, vancomycin use has been limited to those indications above. However, if the patient has a history of frequent methicillin-resistant staphylococcal infections or looks seriously ill, vancomycin with a second drug for gram-negative coverage is still a good choice. In addition, in the penicillin/cephalosprorin allergic patient, vancomycin could still be used, as it might in areas of the world where VRE is not a problem.

c. Once-Daily Aminoglycoside and Cephalosporin

There are limited data on treating peritonitis with once-daily aminoglycoside dosing. Low (46) performed pharmacokinetic studies of 0.6 mg/kg gentamicin in one exchange IP with a 6-hour dwell. IP levels were high throughout the 6-hour dwell but negligible thereafter. Serum levels remained low. Lai et al. (45) examined the efficacy of once-daily IP cefazolin and gentamicin (minimum dwell of 6 hours) for treatment of peritonitis. All 19 gram-positive peritonitis episodes resolved with only one infection due to *S. aureus* requiring modification of the initial therapy. Three episodes of *S. epidermidis* were resistant to both gentamicin and cephalosporin, yet responded to therapy with these agents. There were 14 gram-negative episodes; all episodes due to *P. aeroginosa* required alteration in therapy, and in spite of this three required catheter removal. These preliminary results suggest that

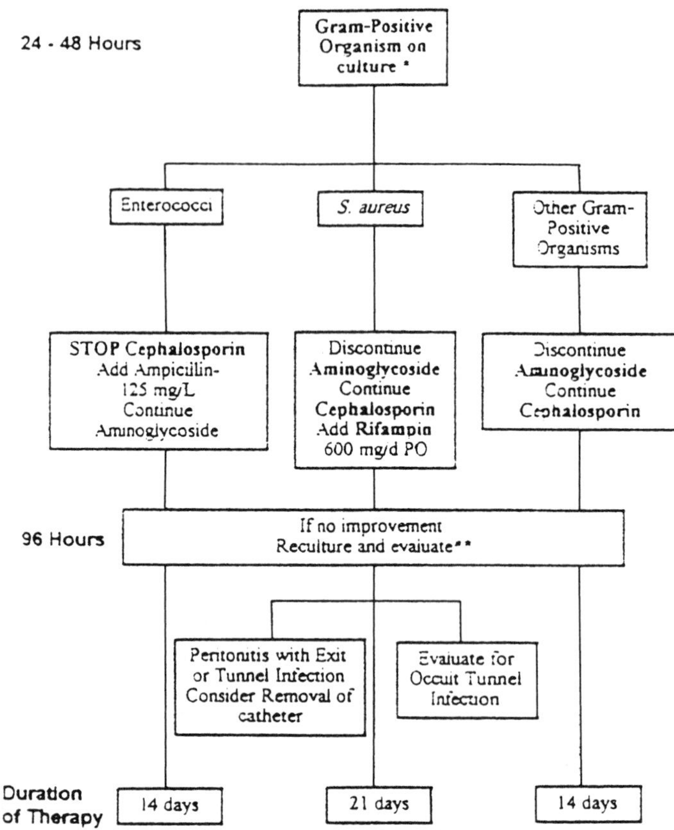

Fig. 2 Management of patients with gram-positive organisms on culture. *Choice of therapy should always be guided by sensitivity patterns. **If methicillin-resistant *S. aureus* is cultured and the patient is not responding clinically, clindamycin or vancomycin should be used. (From Ref. 41.)

the combination of a first-generation cephalosporin and gentamicin, each given in one exchange per day, is a reasonable approach to treating many peritonitis episodes. Vas et al. (47) reported on their experience of treating peritonitis with the previous protocol using vancomycin (over a time period January 1995–September 1995) and the new regime (October 1995–June 1996). Overall, there was no difference in the percentage cure rate in treating coagulase-negative staphylococci that were methicillin sensitive (92% vancomycin vs. 100% cefazolin). However, for the coagulase-negative staphylococci that were methicillin-resistant (MRSE), the cure rate was 73% for vancomycin and only 45% for cefazolin. For *S. aureus* the vancomycin treatment resulted in 58% cure as opposed to 67% for cefazolin. This was a disappointing result with both treatment protocols and is out of line with other studies, which show a higher cure rate.

Further light was thrown on this subject in a short report (48). In the setting of increasing clinical isolates of VRE in the hospital, antibiotic sensitivities to all staphylococci causing CAPD peritonitis between January and June 1996 were reviewed to see if the protocol could be changed to avoid the use of vancomycin. Fifty-eight isolates of staphylococci were reviewed; of these 17 were *S. aureus* and 39 were coagulase-negative staphylococci (CNS), comprising 15% and 35% of all positive isolates from CAPD fluid during this period. All *S. aureus* isolates were sensitive to vancomycin and rifampicin. All the CNS were sensitive to vancomycin, but only 23% were sensitive to methicillin and 44% to gentamicin. The findings suggested that at least 50% of CNS peritonitis cases would not be adequately treated if a cephalosporin was used as empiric therapy for peritonitis in CAPD. It is important, therefore, to assess the local sensitivity patterns and methicillin resistance before discarding the use of vancomycin. In addition the catheter should be carefully examined for evidence of infection (exit site and/or tunnel). If present (and cultures confirm *S. aureus* at this site also) then strong consideration should be given to rapid removal of the catheter even if the peritonitis appears to be resolving.

d. Culture-Negative Peritonitis

Occasionally (<20%) cultures may be negative for a variety of technical or clinical reasons. Care and management of such patients are shown in Fig. 3. Experience would indicate that if the patient is clinically improving after 4–5 days and there is no suggestion of gram-negative organisms on Gram stains, only the cephalosporin should be continued. Duration of therapy is 2 weeks.

e. Gram-Negative Microorganisms

The outline of care of such gram-negative peritonitis is shown in Fig. 4. The decision to discontinue the aminoglycoside and continue with the first-generation cephalosporin will be guided by in vitro sensitivity testing. If the culture report reveals multiple gram-negative organisms, it is imperative to consider the possibility of intraabdominal pathology necessitating surgical exploration. Should the culture reveal a *Pseudomonas* infection, especially *P. aeroginosa*, the aminoglycoside is continued on an increased dose and a second pseudomonal agent added to the regime as shown in Fig. 4. One needs to look carefully for evidence of catheter infection with *Pseudomonas* (which sometimes is subtle), and, if present, removal of catheter is almost mandatory.

f. Fungal Organisms

Fungal peritonitis occurs in peritoneal dialysis patients (Bayer, Johnson) at rates of 0.01–0.11/y (17,49,50). The patient appears acutely ill with severe abdominal pain and may rapidly progress to death particularly if catheter removal is delayed (51). Few reports suggest that cure can be obtained with prolonged courses of antifungal agents (52,53). Prior antibiotic therapy is a predisposing cause (54) for most cases of *Candida* peritonitis, which accounts for 75% of episodes.

Many clinicians still feel that catheter removal is indicated immediately after fungal identification by Gram stain or culture. However, if this is not the policy,

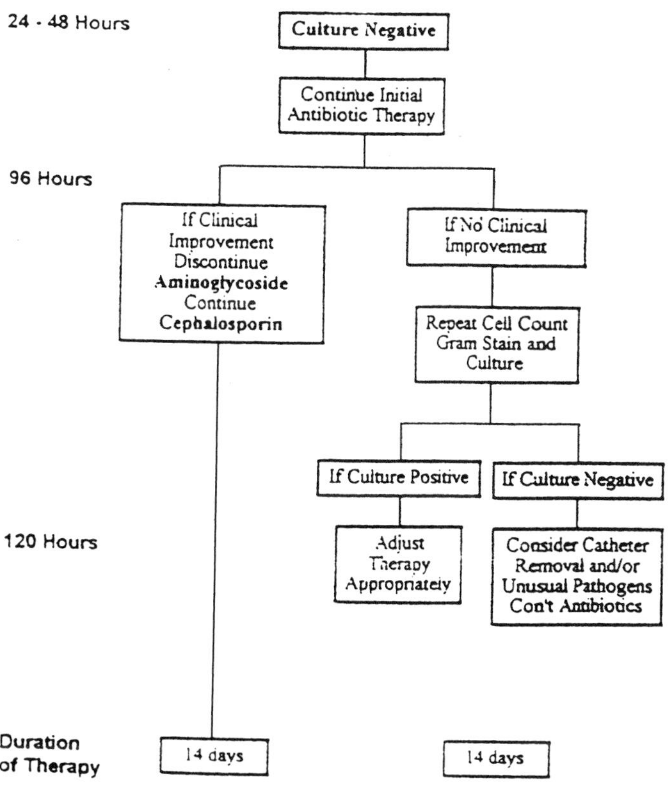

Fig. 3 Management of culture negative episodes of peritonitis. (From Ref. 41.)

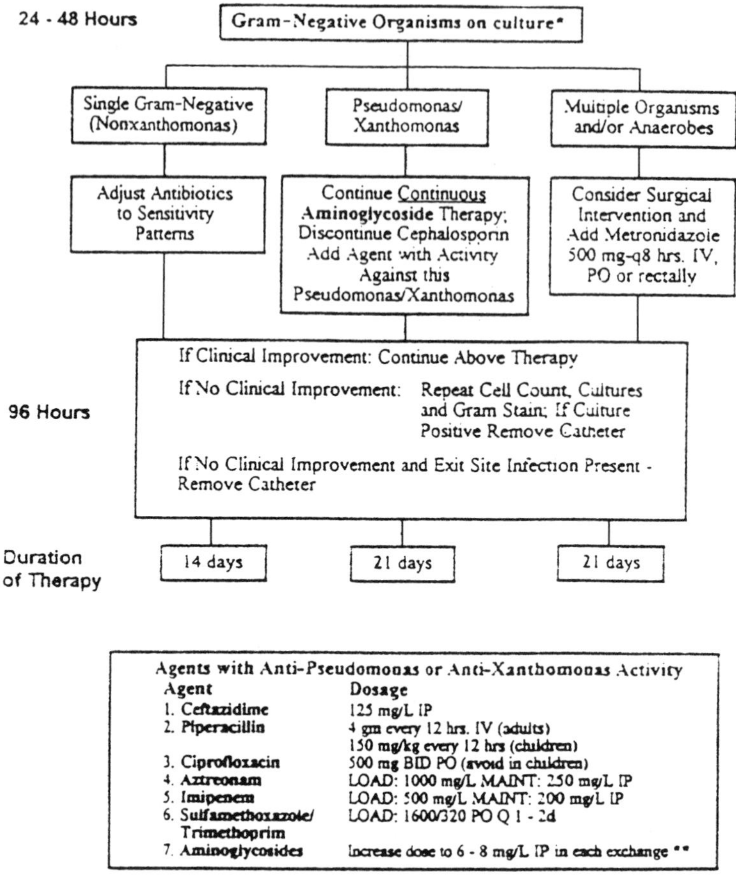

Agents with Anti-Pseudomonas or Anti-Xanthomonas Activity

Agent	Dosage
1. Ceftazidime	125 mg/L IP
2. Piperacillin	4 gm every 12 hrs. IV (adults) 150 mg/kg every 12 hrs (children)
3. Ciprofloxacin	500 mg BID PO (avoid in children)
4. Aztreonam	LOAD: 1000 mg/L MAINT: 250 mg/L IP
5. Imipenem	LOAD: 500 mg/L MAINT: 200 mg/L IP
6. Sulfamethoxazole/ Trimethoprim	LOAD: 1600/320 PO Q 1 - 2d
7. Aminoglycosides	Increase dose to 6 - 8 mg/L IP in each exchange **

Fig. 4 Management of patients with gram-negative organisms on culture. *Choice of therapy should always be guided by sensitivity patterns. **See text for discussion on intermittent dosing. (From Ref. 41.)

then a proposed regime is outlined in Fig. 5 (41). Immediate catheter removal, however, is probably still the best choice. It is imperative, if a course of treatment with antifungal agents is pursued, that the catheter be removed should there be no improvement after 4–5 days of adequate therapy. Therapy with these agents should be continued after catheter removal for at least an additional 10 days.

Prophylaxis with oral nystatin during antibiotic therapy is effective in preventing fungal peritonitis in both children and adults (55,56). Patients requiring frequent or prolonged antibiotic therapy will benefit from prophylaxis.

3. Assessment of Patients Who Fail to Demonstrate Clinical Improvement Within 48 Hours of Initiating Therapy

Most patients with peritoneal dialysis–related peritonitis will show considerable clinical improvement within 2 days of starting antibiotics. Occasionally symptoms persist beyond 48–96 hours. At 96 hours, if the patient has not shown definitive clinical improvement, a reevaluation of the clinical status is essential. One should be cognizant of potential intraabdominal or gynecological pathologies, which may require surgical intervention, or the presence of unusual pathogens such as mycobacteria, fungi, or fastidious organisms. For *S. aureus* and *P. aeroginosa* peritonitis related to catheter or tunnel infection, it is almost mandatory to remove the catheter. If anaerobic bacteria have been identified, the catheter should be removed and surgical exploration considered. Similarly if more than one gram-negative organism other than *P. aeroginosa* has been identified, catheter removal is warranted and intravenous antibiotics should be continued to 5–7 days; surgical exploration should be considered especially if there is presence of anaerobic bacteria.

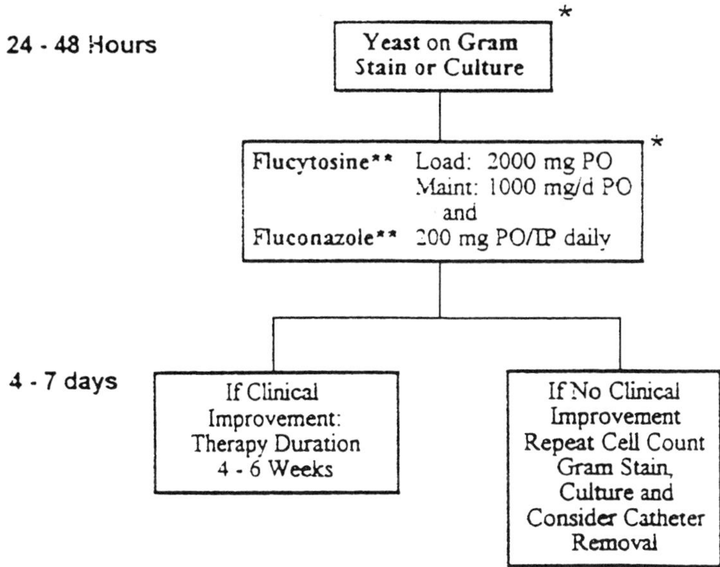

Fig. 5 Management of patients with yeasts on Gram stain or culture. *See text. **Pediatric dose: 1. Flucytosine loading dose of 50–100 mg/kg body weight po daily and maintenance dose of 25–50 mg/kg po daily; 2. Fluconazole 1–3 mg/kg body weight IP every 2 days. (From Ref. 41.)

4. Treatment of Peritonitis in APD Patients

The guidelines (41) suggest that the regimen be adjusted to around-the-clock exchanges of 3–4 hours until the fluid clears, which occurs in most cases in 24–72 hours. During this time the patient must remain connected to the cycler or may disconnect for one dwell of 24 hours as long as the full exchange is maintained. This may not be possible at home, and therefore a regime of this sort may require hospitalization. An alternative is to place the antibiotics in the long day dwell (i.e., giving the antibiotic once daily); alternatively, the patient may be switched to CAPD, with the addition of antibiotics to all exchanges. Few data have been published on this and a lot of the experience of treatment of APD peritonitis is from the pediatric literature. In all other respects the guidelines for diagnosis and treatment of peritonitis in CAPD patients can be used in APD situations.

H. Peritoneal Infections in Relation to Specific Organisms

1. Polymicrobial Peritonitis

Polymicrobial peritonitis (two or more microorganisms) occurs in about 3–6% of peritonitis episodes (25,57), and diabetes, HIV, or underlying gastrointestinal disease are not more prevalent in these patients. Only 22% required catheter removal to effect cure; most patients continue CAPD at 30 and 180 days after the episode. In the presence of two gram-negative bacilli, anaerobes, or gram-negative bacillus in combination with a fungus (58), bowel perforation may have occurred, but this is relatively uncommon. Fecal peritonitis is associated with severe symptoms, may be associated with bacteremia (59), commonly results in transfer of the patient to hemodialysis, and more often leads to death compared to other forms of peritonitis (58,60), especially if surgery is delayed. Laparotomy is required for perforation. Features helpful in determining if perforation is present include fecal matter in drained dialysate, diarrhea containing dialysate, and large volume of free air in the abdominal cavity (61). Multiple organisms should not be assumed to be due to bowel pathology but may be due to touch contamination or catheter infection (25).

Intraabdominal abscesses are rare complications of peritonitis in CAPD patients, occurring in 0.7% of peritonitis episodes (62). These are more common with peritonitis episodes due to *P. aeroginosa*, *Candida albicans*, *S. aureus*, and polymicrobial peritonitis (62). Fever, abdominal pain and tenderness, and a peripheral leukocytosis are all consistent with this diagnosis, which can then be confirmed by CT scan or ultrasound. The abscesses require drainage.

2. Acinetobacter Peritonitis

Peritonitis due to *Acinetobacter* frequently occurs within a few months of a previous episode of peritonitis due to another organism and is infrequently associated with catheter infection (63). Galvao et al. (64) suggest that this ubiquitous bacteria causes peritonitis when peritoneal host defenses are suppressed from previous peritonitis episodes. Aminoglycosides alone may result in relapse (63,64); ampicillin-sublactam or imipenem-cilastatin may be required (63). Patient drop-out from *Acinetobacter* peritonitis is 17%, which is comparable to *P. aeruginosa* peritonitis (63).

3. Mycobacterium Peritonitis

Tuberculous peritonitis is a rare occurrence in peritoneal dialysis patients. It is due to a reactivation of a latent peritoneal focus rather than a primary infection. Most patients present with fever, abdominal pain, and sometimes a cloudy effluent. The effluent white blood cells are predominately polymorphonuclear cells. This plus the absence of disease elsewhere make this a difficult diagnostic problem (25,65,66). Earlier diagnosis can be made with laparotomy and biopsy and detection of microbacterial DNA amplified by polymerase chain reaction (67). No data exist for optimal therapy or for duration of treatment—most reported cases have been treated for 9–12 months with triple therapy. Catheter removal appears not to be mandatory (66). If peritoneal dialysis is continued, ultrafiltration failure may occur but is not inevitable (65,66). In addition to *Mycobacterium tuberculosis*, peritonitis due to other mycobacteria (*M. fortuitum*, *M. kasasii*, *M. gordonae*, *M. avium-intracellulare*, *M. chelonei*, *M. gastri*) has been reported (68,69).

I. Possible Courses and Outcome of Peritonitis

It should be possible in up to 80% of cases to achieve complete cure without recourse to catheter removal. Persistent symptoms beyond 96 hours can occur in about 13–39% of episodes. Relapsing peritonitis is a feature in 8–16% of episodes, while catheter removal to effect a cure is necessary in up to 15% of cases. Death is reported in 1–3% of cases (70).

Peritonitis and peritoneal catheter infections are the cause of significant morbidity, including catheter loss (18,71,72), transfer to hemodialysis, either permanently or temporarily (19,50,73,74), and hospitalization (50,71,75). Peritonitis can lead to the patient's death, from sepsis or related complications, especially when the microorganism is gram-negative bacillus or fungus (70,71,74–76).

Peritonitis results in a marked increase in effluent protein losses, which contributes to the protein malnutrition so prevalent in PD patients (77). Ultrafiltration decreases transiently (78). The pH of the effluent falls especially in the presence of gram-negative peritonitis and contributes to impaired neutrophil activity (79). Over time, long-term PD can lead to increase in solute transport and loss of ultrafiltration (hyperpermeable membrane); this process has been shown to be exacerbated and accelerated by peritonitis proportional to the degree of inflammation and number of infections in close proximity (80). These physiological changes correspond to striking pathological changes in the peritoneal membrane (81,82). Although the changes are usually transient, peritoneal fibrosis (often referred to as sclerosing peritonitis) may result from severe episodes, a cumulative effect of multiple episodes, or episodes later in the course of peritoneal dialysis (82–84). In a recent Japanese study sclerosing peritonitis was found in 62 of 6923 patients; in these patients the peritonitis rate was 3.3 times that of the rest (85). Sclerosing peritonitis is a severe complication of peritoneal dialysis in which the patient becomes progressively more malnourished due to bowel obstruction from encasement of the bowel. Peritoneal dialysis cannot be continued once this often lethal complication occurs.

J. Peritoneal Lavage

The evidence of detrimental effect of fresh dialysis solutions on local host defense mechanism (86) has convinced most nephrologists not to undertake rapid exchange peritoneal lavage in the management of peritoneal infection. However, after a few in-and-out exchanges that remove inflammatory products and lessen abdominal pain, CAPD is resumed with long dwell exchanges. In a study by Ejlersen et al. (87) the findings of poor outcome in patients treated with 24 hours of initial lavage vindicate this policy. The dwell time may have to be shortened in cases of poor ultrafiltration as there is recognized increased permeability during an episode of peritonitis (88). The use of Icodextrin in this situation has shown improved ultrafiltration (89). Peritoneal lavage, however, remains indicated in cases of fecal peritonitis prior to surgical exploration.

K. Relapsing Peritonitis

Relapsing peritonitis is defined as occurrence of an episode of peritonitis caused by the same genus/species that caused the immediately preceding episode and occurring within 4 weeks of completion of the antibiotic course. Management strategies are similar to those used for the initial episode. Consideration here should be given to catheter-related infection as well as intraabdominal pathology. In some instances short-term interruption of peritoneal dialysis may be of value (90), as may be the use of a cytology brush (91).

L. Catheter Removal

Infections are the cause of approximately 85% of catheter removals. *S. aureus* is the organism resulting in the most catheter loss (92). Infective causes leading to catheter removal include persistent peritonitis, peritonitis associated with catheter infections, relapsing and recurrent peritonitis, polymicrobial peritonitis, and peritoneal abscess.

M. Catheter Insertion/Removal (One-Step Procedure) for CAPD Peritonitis

The optimum time between the removal of a catheter and reinsertion of a new one is not known. Usually a period of 3–4 weeks is allowed. However, recent experiences suggest that short intervals may be acceptable; indeed one could perform the removal of the old catheter and the insertion of a new one during the same operation, and this has been successfully done in a number of reports (93–96). Data would suggest that this is quite a feasible procedure which lessens hospitalization, and minimizes the use of back-up hemodialysis.

N. Use of Adjuvent Therapy and Treatment of CAPD Peritonitis

Thrombolytic therapy has been used for the treatment of recurrent peritonitis. Success is variable and Williams et al. (97) showed in a randomized study that catheter replacement was superior (14 of 17 peritonitis-free after catheter replacement as opposed to 5 of 17 with urokinase). Thrombolytic therapy should be reserved for infections for which no other cause or complication is evident and probably should be limited to coagulase-negative staphylococcus or culture-negative infection.

O. Prevention of Peritonitis in Peritoneal Dialysis

Peritonitis due to *S. epidermidis*, most often due to touch contamination at the time of the exchange, has decreased with improvements in connection technology (98). Careful selection of patients and an emphasis on training also diminish this form of peritonitis (99). *S. aureus* infections may be reduced with prophylactic antibiotics and eradication of nasal carriage (see later). The risk of *Candida* peritonitis can be reduced with oral nystatin during antibiotic therapy. Methods to diminish enteric peritonitis have not been identified. Neither daily cephalexin nor trimethoprim 160 mg/sulfamethoxazole 800 mg was effective in reducing peritonitis risk (100), although the effect of the prophylaxis on the rates of individual organisms was not reported. Constipation should be avoided, and prophylactic antibiotic therapy prior to colonoscopy is recommended (101).

III. PERITONEAL CATHETER–RELATED INFECTIONS

Colonization of the exit site with microorganisms may lead to infection of the exit site, which may spread along the subcutaneous pathway of the catheter to the inner cuff and subsequently to the peritoneum. Catheter infections, a term that includes both exit site and tunnel infections, occur at a rate of 0.6 per year, although reported figures vary dependent on the definitions used. *S. aureus* and *P. aeruginosa* are the most common and serious catheter infections, since they are difficult to resolve and frequently result in peritonitis, leading to catheter loss.

The site of the infection can be the sinus (exit-site infection) or the subcutaneous or external cuff and tunnel (tunnel infection). The preperitoneal cuff can also be infected, but this is difficult to diagnose. Infections can be acute or chronic. Acute infections last for less than 4 weeks, while chronic ones are of greater duration.

A. Exit Site Infection

This is present if there is purulent drainage at the peritoneal catheter exit site, with or without erythema (6,102). The presence of induration and tenderness worsens the prognosis (102). Twardowski and Prowant (103) have further classified the catheter-related infections into various categories (Table 3), which forms the basis of management—a regime adopted by the recent

Table 3 Exit Site Infection

	Equivocal infection	Acute infection	Chronic infection	Cuff infection
Evaluation	Culture and sensitivities on peri-exit smear. Gram stain.	Culture and sensitivities on exudate. Gram stain.	Culture and sensitivities on exudate. Gram stain.	Palpation of cuff and tunnel. Culture and sensitivities and Gram stain of exudate (spontaneous or after pressure on cuff). Ultrasound of cuff/ tunnel.
Initial therapy	Cauterize slightly exuberant granulation tissue. Topical mupirocin.	Cauterize slightly exuberant and exuberant granulation tissue. First-generation cephalosporin for gram-pos. organisms, quinolone for gram-neg. organisms, vancomycin for MRSA.	Cauterize slightly exuberant and exuberant granulation tissue. If initial therapy: first-generation cephalosporin for gram-pos. organisms; quinolone for gram-neg. organisms; vancomycin for MRSA. If previously treated: add synergistic drug or change antibiotic according to culture and sensitivities.	Cauterize slightly exuberant and exuberant granulation tissue. Initial antibiotic therapy based on Gram stain results.
48 Hours	Change to neosporin or gentamycin ointment if gram-neg. organisms on culture.	Adjust therapy according to culture and sensitivities.	Adjust therapy according to culture and sensitivities.	Adjust antibiotic according to culture and sensitivities.
Follow-up	If no improvement in 2 weeks, change to systemic antibiotic based on initial culture and sensitivities. Continue therapy 7 days past achieving a good appearance. Response to systemic antibiotic therapy is excellent with cure occurring in almost all instances.	Evaluate weekly; reculture if no improvement. Substitute another appropriate antibiotic or add a second, synergistic antibiotic. Use rifampicin as a second antibiotic for staphylococcal infections. Most acute infections respond favorably to therapy. Continue to treat for 7 days after achieving a good appearance. If accompanying peritonitis, consider catheter removal.	Evaluate every 2 weeks; reculture every 2 weeks if no improvement on appropriate therapy. If infection recurs repeatedly after achieving a good appearance: 1. consider chronic antibiotic suppression, 2. if no improvement after a month of treatment, suspect cuff infection and treat as such. If accompanying peritonitis, remove catheter.	Reevaluate every 2 weeks; reculture monthly. If no remission: 1. consider cuff shaving, 2. consider catheter replacement. If accompanying peritonitis, remove catheter.

MRSA = Methicillin-resistant *Staphylococcus aureus*.
Source: Ref. 41.

report of the ISPD committee on catheter and exit-site practices (104).

1. An Acute Exit-Site Infection

This is defined as purulent and/or bloody drainage from the exit site, which may be associated with erythema, tenderness, exuberant granulation tissue, and edema (6,103). The erythema needs to be more than twice the catheter diameter; there is regression of the epithelium in the sinus. An acute catheter infection may be accompanied by pain and the presence of a scab, but crusting alone is not indicative of infection. Purulent drainage should always be cultured. Positive cultures of normal-appearing exit sites indicate the presence of colonization, not infection.

2. Chronic Exit-Site Infection

This may be the result of an untreated or inadequately treated acute infection. It may also be a sequela of a resolved, acute infection, which recurs after withdrawal of antibiotic therapy. Symptoms of chronic infection are similar to those of acute infections; however, exuberant granulation tissue is more common both externally and in the sinus. Granulation tissue at the external exit is sometimes covered by a large, stubborn crust or scab. Pain, erythema, and swelling are frequently absent in chronic infection.

3. An Equivocal Exit Site

This is defined as purulent and/or bloody drainage only in the sinus that cannot be expressed outside, accompanied by the regression of the epithelium and occurrence of slightly exuberant granulation tissue in the sinus. Erythema may be present but with a diameter less than twice the width of the catheter. Pain, swelling, and external drainage are absent (103). The equivocal infected exit site represents low-grade infection. Although some equivocal exits improve spontaneously, most progress to overt infection if untreated.

B. Pathogens

S. aureus is responsible for the majority of exit-site and tunnel infections. *P. aeruginosa* is much less common but, like *S. aureus*, is difficult to eradicate and frequently leads to peritonitis if catheter removal is delayed. *S. epidermidis* is a relatively infrequent cause of tunnel infection in contrast to peritonitis. Other gram-positive organisms, other gram-negative bacilli, and rarely fungi account for the remaining infections.

S. aureus peritonitis occurs predominately in patients who either have or have had a history of *S. aureus* catheter infections and in patients with *S. aureus* colonization either in the nares (105–108), the skin (109), or at the peritoneal catheter exit site (109–111). Nasal carriage of *S. aureus* has been shown to be of particular importance in diabetics and immunosuppressed patients—these authors advocate prophylaxis for these patients; in nondiabetics this should be done only if two or more swabs are positive (112). Almost one half of patients carry *S. aureus* in their nares at the initiation of peritoneal dialysis, and these are the patients most likely to develop *S. aureus* exit-site and tunnel infections (113,114).

C. Tunnel Infection

Tunnel infection is present when there is pain, tenderness, erythema, induration, or any combination of these over the subcutaneous pathway of the catheter. However, many tunnel infections are occult, detected only by sonography of the subcutaneous catheter pathway (21,115). Tunnel infections are present in approximately one half of all exit-site infections, but they occasionally occur in the absence of an exit-site infection (20,21). The infection can involve the outer cuff, intercuff segment, and/or inner cuff of the catheter, and as the infection spreads along the tunnel toward the peritoneum, the risk of peritonitis greatly increases (21).

D. Treatment of Peritoneal Dialysis Catheter Infections

Therapy of exit-site infections includes local care, systemic antibiotics, and revision of the tunnel surgically and, as a last resort, replacement of the catheter. Antibiotic therapy for exit-site infection is tailored to the specific organism identified.

Exit-site, tunnel, and cuff infections require antibiotic therapy. Table 3 outlines the evaluation and treatment of exit-site and tunnel infections (7,41,104,116). Antibiotic therapy should be started immediately for tunnel and exit-site infections, pending culture results.

1. Gram-Positive Organisms

The initial antibiotic chosen should cover, at a minimum, gram-positive organisms. Oral penicillinase-resistant penicillins, oral trimethoprim/sulfamethoxazole, or cephalexin are reasonable, convenient, and cost-effective options (41,104). Vancomycin should be avoided in view of the emergence of VRE (117). Once culture results are available, the antibiotic can be adjusted. In slowly resolving or particularly severe-appearing *S. aureus* exit-site infections, rifampin 300 mg bid in adults (5–10 mg/kg bid in children) may be added.

2. Gram-Negative Organisms

Quinolones are generally used for *P. aeruginosa* catheter infections; ceftazidime may be added if necessary (118,119). Chelation interactions may occur between fluoroquinolones and concomitantly administered multivalent cations. Calcium salts, oral iron supplements, zinc, sucralfate, magnesium-aluminum antacids, and milk may reduce ciprofloxacin absorption by 75–90%; staggering of administration is advised.

3. Chronic Exit-Site Infections

Here a combination of synergistic antibiotics is preferred to a single agent to avoid emergence of resistant organisms, since the therapy is continued over a prolonged period. The response to therapy is slow, and the features of chronic infection change very slowly to an equivocal exit and then eventually to a good exit site.

4. Length of Therapy

Unfortunately, there are few data on the optimal choice and length of antibiotic therapy or the route of administration (oral, intraperitoneal, intravenous). Data on usefulness of local therapy for exit-site and tunnel infections are limited. Therapy should be continued until the exit site appears completely normal. Prolonged antibiotics may be necessary. If 3–4 weeks of antibiotics fail to resolve the infection, the catheter should be replaced. Alternatively, deroofing of the tunnel or exteriorization of the cuff may be performed while maintaining antibiotic therapy. In chronic exit-site infection, antibiotic and local care are continued until the desired features of a good exit site are achieved. Some cases of chronic infection may require long-term (6 months or more) suppressive doses of antibiotics.

5. Cuff Shaving

The superficial cuff can be completely removed (exteriorized and shaved) when antibiotics do not resolve an infection (102,120). The variety of described techniques includes debridement of the area of cellulitis and revision of the tunnel. Subsequent peritonitis with the same organism occurs in approximately half of the patients who undergo cuff shaving for *S. aureus* and may result in the eventual removal of the catheter.

6. Topical Treatment

Topical treatment may be used as an adjunct to systemic antibiotics in treatment of exit infections or as initial therapy for low-grade infection (equivocally infected exit). Topical antibiotic therapy is not appropriate for acute and chronic exit infections.

Hypertonic saline (3% NaCl solution) dressings may be beneficial in otherwise refractory episodes (121). Other topical treatments include application of soaks to the exit two to four times a day as well as the application of dry heat (121–123). Soaking solutions include 0.9% saline, sodium hypochlorite, dilute hydrogen peroxide, and povidone-iodine (123). There are no controlled studies assessing the effectiveness of these topical treatments.

Equivocally infected exit sites can be treated with either local or oral antibiotics. The topical antibiotics that have been successfully used include mupirocin, gentamicin, and neosporin. Cauterization of the slightly exuberant granulation tissue in the sinus may be necessary. Systemic antibiotics may be used in cases unresponsive to topical therapy (103).

E. Prevention of Exit-Site and Tunnel Infections

Antibiotics given at the time of catheter insertion have been identified as a way to decrease catheter-related peritonitis in animal studies (124), but definitive evidence in patients is lacking (125,126). Catheter immobilization, proper location of the exit site, sterile wound care immediately after placement of the catheter, and avoidance of trauma are all recommended and used by most centers (127,128).

A downward-directed exit site was associated with lower peritonitis rates in a report from pediatric centers in North America (129). In addition, the Network 9 study found that directing the subcutaneous portion of the catheter downward decreased the risk of peritonitis associated with exit-site and/or tunnel infection by 38%, while an upward-directed catheter had a 50% increased risk of catheter-related peritonitis, compared to horizontally directed tunnels (130). USRDS (131) reported that the relative risk of peritonitis was essentially identical for straight and bent catheters; however, when the analysis was repeated with adjustment for possible center effect, the peritonitis rate was significantly lower with permanent bent catheters.

Swan-neck catheters were designed to diminish cuff extrusions and catheter tip migration associated with straight catheter implanted in arcuate tunnels. Randomized studies comparing a swan-neck catheter to the straight Tenckhoff catheter without a preformed bend showed a lower probability for the first exit infection with the swan-neck catheter, but the survival was not different (132,133). Cuff extrusions and catheter migration were seen only in the Tenckhoff catheters. In another randomized study, there was a significantly lower rate of exit-site infections with swan-neck catheters (134).

New catheter designs or modifications have been proposed as a means of reducing peritonitis from catheter infections, but definitive studies have not yet been done (135,136).

F. Nasal Carriage of *Staphylococcus aureus* and Prevention of Catheter Infections

S. aureus nasal carriage, as defined by one positive culture from the nares, is a risk factor for *S. aureus* infection. Without prophylaxis the rates of *S. aureus* exit-site infections are about 0.34–0.41 per year (137). Prophylaxis reduces the rate to less than 50% of this. Four protocols have been demonstrated to be effective in preventing *S. aureus* catheter infections. Treatment of *S. aureus* nasal carriage with intranasal mupirocin twice daily for 5 days is effective in lowering *S. aureus* catheter infections in nasal carriers (138,139). The therapy must be either repeated monthly or repeated when the nose culture again becomes positive for *S. aureus*. The disadvantages of the intranasal approach are expense and the need for repeated nose cultures (if therapy is based on positive cultures only). Alternative approaches to decreasing *S. aureus* infections that are not dependent on obtaining nose cultures include cyclical rifampin 600 mg per day for 5 days given every 12 weeks or mupirocin to the exit site as part of routine daily care (140,141). Prophylactic use of rifampin leads to significant side effects in 12% of patients, as well as rifampin resistance, obviating the use of this drug for therapy. Therefore the use of rifampin for prophylaxis is not recommended. All approaches reduced *S. aureus* exit-site infections to one third of the previous rate.

G. Trauma to Catheter Tract

Twardowski and Prowant (142) found that documented trauma preceded exit-site deterioration in all exit sites previously classified as perfect and half of these previously classified as good. The proposed definition of trauma is anything that breaks the integrity of the skin at the exit site or the epithelium or granulation tissue in the sinus.

H. Recommendations for Prophylaxis

Patients who are nasal carriers of *S. aureus* may receive prophylaxis; no one regimen of eradication is superior. As a maneuver to prevent exit-site infections, application of mupirocin to the exit site as part of the daily routine is advocated. Trauma to the catheter tract should be avoided by proper immobilization and should be reported to the dialysis unit if it causes severe pain or bleeding or if there is subsequent deterioration of the exit-site appearance with redness, exudate, persistent pain, or tenderness.

REFERENCES

1. Popovich RP, Moncrief JW, Dechard JB, Bomer JB, Pyle WK. The definition of a normal portable/wearable equilibrium peritoneal dialysis technique. Abst Am Soc Artif Intern Organs 1976; 5:64.
2. Buoncrustiani C, Bianca P, Cozzani M. A new safe simple connection system for CAPD. Int J Urol Nephrol 1980; 1:50–53.
3. Majorca R, Cantaluppi A, Cancarini GC, Scalamogna A, Broccoli R, Graziani G, Brasa S, Ponticelli C. Prospective controlled trial of a Y connector and disinfectant to prevent peritonitis in CAPD. Lancet 1983; ii:642–644.
4. Canadian CAPD Clinical Trials Group. Peritonitis in CAPD: a multicentre, randomised clinical trial comparing the Y connector disinfectant system to standard system. Perit Dial Int 1989; 9:159–163.
5. VI Catheter related factors and peritonitis risk in CAPD patients. USRDS 1992 Annual Report. Am J Kidney Dis 1993; 20(suppl 2):48–54.
6. Pierratos A. Peritoneal dialysis glossary. Perit Dial Bull 1984; 4:2–3.
7. Keane WF, Vas SI. Peritonitis. In: Gokal R, Nolph KD, eds. The Textbook of Peritoneal Dialysis. Dordrecht: Kluwer Academic Publishers, 1994:473–502.
8. Al Wali W, Baillod R, Brumfitt W, Hamilto-Miller JM. Differing prognostic significance of re-infection and relapse in CAPD peritonitis. Nephrol Dial Transplant 1992; 7:133–136.
9. Brown AL, Stephenson JR, Baker LR, Tabaqchali S. Recurrent CAPD peritonitis caused by coagulase-negative staphylococci: reinfection or relapse determined by clinical criteria and typing methods. J Hosp Inf 1991; 18:109–115.

10. Tzamaloukas AH. Peritonitis in peritoneal dialysis patients: an overview. Adv Renal Replac Ther 1996; 3: 232–236.
11. Peterson DK, Matzke GR, Keane WF. Current concepts in the management of peritonitis in CAPD patients. Rev Infect Dis 1987; 9:604–612.
12. Lindholm B, Bergstrom J. Nutritional requirement of peritoneal dialysis. In: Gokal R, Nolph KD, eds. The Textbook of Peritoneal Dialysis. Dordrecht: Kluwer Academic Publications, 1994:443–472.
13. Rubin J, Flynn MA, Nolph KD. Total body potassium —a guide to nutritional health in patients undergoing CAPD. Am J Clin Nutr 1981; 34:94–98.
14. Gokal R, Ramos JM, Ward MK, Kerr DNS. "Eosinophilic peritonitis" in CAPD. Clin Nephrol 1981; 15: 328–330.
15. Salgia P, Manos J, Gokal R. Cutaneous manifestations heralding eosinophilic peritonitis. Perit Dial Bull 1984; 4:265.
16. Report of the Working Party BASC. Diagnosis and Management of Peritonitis in CAPD. Lancet 1987; 1: 845–849.
17. Tranaeus A, Heimburger O, Lindholm B. Peritonitis in CAPD: diagnostic findings, therapeutic outcomes and complications. Perit Dial Int 1989; 13:179–190.
18. Golper TA, Hartstein A. Analysis of the causative pathogens on uncomplicated CAPD associated peritonitis: duration of therapy, relapses and prognosis. Am J Kidney Dis 1986; 7:141–145.
19. Piraino B, Bernadini J, Sorkin M. The influence of peritoneal catheter exit site infections on peritonitis tunnel infections and catheter loss on CAPD. Am J Kidney Dis 1986; 8:436–440.
20. Piraino B, Bernadini J, Sorkin M. Five year study of the microbiological results of exit site infections and peritonitis in CAPD. Am J Kidney Dis 1987; 4:281–286.
21. Plum J, Sudkamp S, Grabansee B. Results of ultrasound assisted diagnosis of tunnel infections in CAPD. Am J Kidney Dis 1994; 23:99–104.
22. Scheinburg FB, Seligman AM, Fine J. Transmural migration of intestinal bacteria. N Engl J Med 1950; 242: 747–751.
23. Steiner RW, Halasz NA. Abdominal catastrophes and other unusual events in CAPD. Am J Kidney Dis 1990: 15:1–7.
24. Wood CJ, Fleming V, Turnridge J, Thompson N, Atkins RC. Campylobacter peritonitis in CAPD: Report of eight cases and a review of the literature. Am J Kidney Dis 1992; 19:162–166.
25. Holley JL, Bernadini J, Piraino B. Polymicrobial peritonitis in patients on CAPD. Am J Kidney Dis 1992; 19:162–166.
26. Ray SM, Piraino B, Holley J. Peritonitis following colonoscopy in a peritoneal dialysis patient. Perit Dial Int 1990; 10:97–98.
27. Holley J, Seibert D, Mos A. Peritonitis following colonoscopy and polypectomy: A need for prophylaxis? Perit Dial Bull 1987; 7:105.
28. Kiddy K, Brown P, Michael J, Adu J. Peritonitis due to *Streptococcus viridans* in patients receiving CAPD. Brit Med J 1985; 290:969–970.
29. Coward RA, Gokal R, Wise M. Peritonitis associated with vaginal leakage of dialysis fluid in CAPD. Br Med J 1982; 284:1529.
30. Korzets A, Chagnac A, Ori Y, Zerin D, Levi J. Pneumococcal peritonitis complicating CAPD: Was the indwelling intrauterine device to blame? Clin Nephrol 1991; 35:24–25.
31. Holley JL, Bernadini J, Piraino B. Infecting organisms in CAPD patients on the Y set. Am J Kidney Dis 1994; 23:569–573.
32. Bunke M, Brier ME, Golper TA. Culture negative CAPD peritonitis: The Network 9 Study. Adv Perit Dial 1994; 10:174–178.
33. Eisele G, Adewunni C, Bailie CR, Yocum D, Venezia R. Surreptitious use of antimicrobial agents by CAPD patients. Perit Dial Int 1993; 13:315–317.
34. Ryan S, Fessia S. Improved method for recovering of peritonitis causing micro-organisms from peritoneal dialysis. J Clin Microbiol 1987; 25:383–384.
35. Lye W, Wong PL, Leong SO, Lee EJC. Isolation of organisms in CAPD peritonitis: a comparison of two techniques. Adv Perit Dial 1994; 10:166–168.
36. Vas S. Microbiological aspects of CAPD. Kidney Int 1983; 23:83–92.
37. Williams PS, Hendy MS, Ackrill P. Routine daily surveillance cultures in management of CAPD patients. Perit Dial Bull 1987; 7:183–186.
38. Zemel D, Betjes M, Dinkla C, Struijk DG, Krediet RT. Analysis of inflammatory mediators and peritoneal permeability to macromolecules shortly before the onset of overt peritonitis in patients treated with CAPD. Perit Dial Int 1995; 15:134–141.
39. The Ad-Hoc Advisory Committee on Peritonitis Management. CAPD peritonitis treatment recommendations: 1989 update. Perit Dial Int 1989; 9:247–256.
40. Keane W, Everett ED, Golper TA et al. Peritoneal dialysis related peritonitis treatment recommendations: 1993 update. Perit Dial Int 1993; 13:14–28.
41. Keane W, Alexander SR, Bailie GR, Boeschoten E, Gokal R, Golper T, Holmes C, Huang C-C, Kawaguchi Y, Piraino B, Riella M, Schaefer F, Vas S. Peritoneal dialysis-related peritonitis treatment recommendations: 1996 update. Perit Dial Int 1996; 16:557–573.
42. Nosocomial enterococci resistant to Vancomycin. United States 1989-1993. MMWR CDC Surveill Summ 1993; 42:597–599.
43. Commentary. Vancomycin-resistant *Staphylococcus aureus*: Apocalypse now? Lancet 1997; 350:1670–1673.

44. CDC. *Staphylococcus aureus* with reduced susceptibility to vancomycin. United States, MMWR 1997; 46:765–766.
45. Lai MN, Kao MT, Chen CC, Cheung SY, Chung WK. Intraperitoneal once-daily dose of cefazolin and gentamicin for treating CAPD peritonitis. Perit Dial Int 1997; 17:87–89.
46. Low CL. Pharmacokinetics of once daily IP gentamicin in CAPD patients. Perit Dial Int 1996; 16:379–384.
47. Vas SI, Bargman J, Oreopoulos DG. Treatment of PD patients of peritonitis caused by gram positive organisms with a single daily dose of antibiotics. Perit Dial Int 1997; 17:91–93.
48. Sandoe JAT, Gokal R, Struthers K. Vancomycin-resistant enterococci and emperical vancomycin for CAPD peritonitis. Perit Dial Int 1997; 17:617–618.
49. Rotillar C, Black J, Winchester J, Rakowski TA, Mosher WF, Mazzori MJ, Amcranzavi M, Garaguzi V, Alijani MR, Angy WP. Ten years experience with CAPD. Am J Kidney Dis 1991; 17:156–164.
50. Pollock CA, Ibels LS, Caterson RJ, Mahony JF, Waugh BA, Cocksedge B. CAPD—eight years of experience at a single centre. Medicine 1989; 68:293–308.
51. Kerr CM, Perfect JR, Craven PC, Juvgeusin JH, Drutz DJ, Shelburne JD, Gallis HA, Gutman RA. Fungal peritonitis in patients on CAPD. Ann Intern Med 1983; 99:334–337.
52. Lee Sh, Chiang SH, Hseih SJ, Shen HM. Successful treatment of fungal peritonitis with intracatheter antifungal retention. Adv Perit Dial 1995; 11:172–175.
53. Benevent D, Peyronnet P, Lagarde C, Leroux-Robert C. Fungal peritonitis in patients on continuous ambulatory peritoneal dialysis. Three recoveries in 5 cases without catheter removal. Nephron 1985; 41: 203–206.
54. Johnson RJ, Ramsey PG, Gallagher N, Ahmed S. Fungal peritonitis in patients on peritoneal dialysis. Am J Nephrol 1985; 5:169–175.
55. Robitaille P, Meerouani, A, Clermont MJ, Ebert E. Successful antifungal prophylaxis in chronic peritoneal dialysis: a pediatric experience. Perit Dial Int 1995; 15:77–78.
56. Zaruba K, Peters J, Jungbluth H. Successful prophylaxis for fungal peritonitis in patients on CAPD: six years' experience. Am J Kidney Dis 1991; 17:43–46.
57. Kiernan L, Finkelstein FO, Kliger FS, Gorban-Brennan N, Juergensen P, Mooraki A, Brown E. Outcome of polymicrobial peritonitis in continuous ambulatory peritoneal dialysis patients. Am J Kidney Dis 1995; 25:461–464.
58. van der Reijden HJ, Struijk DG, van Ketel RJ, Kox C, Krediet RT, Arisz L. Fecal peritonitis in patients on continuous ambulatory peritoneal dialysis, an endpoint in CAPD? Adv Perit Dial 1988; 4:198–203.
59. Morduchowicz G, van Dyk FJ, Wittenberg C, Winler J, Boner G. Bacteremia complicating peritonitis in peritoneal dialysis patients. Am J Nephrol 1993; 13: 278–280.
60. Tzamaloukas AH, Murata GH, Fox L. Death associated with Pseudomonas peritonitis in malnourished elderly diabetics on CAPD. Perit Dial Int 1993; 13:241–242.
61. Tzamaloukas AH, Obermiller LE, Gibel LJ, Murata GH, Wood B, Simon D, Erickson DG, Kanig SP. Peritonitis associated with intra-abdominal pathology in continuous ambulatory peritoneal dialysis patients. Perit Dial Int 1992; 13(suppl 2):S335–S337.
62. Boroujerdi-Rad H, Juergensen P, Mansourian V, Kliger AS, Finkelstein FO. Abdominal abscesses complicating peritonitis in continuous ambulatory peritoneal dialysis patients. Am J Kidney Dis 1994; 23:717–721.
63. Lye WC, Lee EJC, Ang KK. Acinetobacter peritonitis in patients on CAPD: characteristics and outcome. Adv Perit Dial 1991; 7:176–179.
64. Galvao C, Swartz R, Rocher L, Reynolds J, Starmann B, Wilson D. Acinetobacter peritonitis during chronic peritoneal dialysis. Am J Kidney Dis 1989; 14:101–104.
65. Cheng IKP, Chan PCK, Chan MK. Tuberculous peritonitis complicating long-term peritoneal dialysis. Am J Nephrol 1989; 9:155–161.
66. Mallat SG, Brensilver JM. Tuberculous peritonitis in a CAPD patient cured without catheter removal: Case report, review of the literature, and guidelines for treatment and diagnosis. Am J Kidney Dis 1989; 13: 154–157.
67. Vas SI. Renaissance of tuberculosis in the 1990's: lesson for the nephrologist. Perit Dial Int 1994; 14:209–214.
68. Dunmire RB, Breyer JA. Nontuberculous mycobacterial peritonitis during continuous ambulatory peritoneal dialysis: case report and review of diagnostic and therapeutic strategies. Am J Kidney Dis 1991; 18: 126–130.
69. White R, Abreo K, Flanagan R, Gadallah M, Krane K, El-Shahawy M, Shakamuri S, McCoy R. Nontuberculous mycobacterial infections in continuous ambulatory peritoneal dialysis patients. Am J Kidney Dis 1993; 22:581–587.
70. Tzamaloukas AH. Peritonitis in peritoneal dialysis patients: An overview. Adv Ren Replac Therap 1996; 3: 232–236.
71. Gokal R, Francis DMA, Goodship THJ, Bint AJ, Ramos JM, Ferner RE, Proud G, Ward MK, Kerr DNS. Peritonitis in continuous ambulatory peritoneal dialysis. Lancet 1982; 2:1388–1391.
72. Gokal R, King J, Bogle S, Marsh F, Oliver D, Jakubowski C, Hunt L, Baillod R, Ogg C, Ward M, Wilkinson R. Outcome in patients on continuous ambulatory peritoneal dialysis and haemodialysis: 4 year

analysis of a prospective multicentre study. Lancet 1987; x:1105–1109.
73. Gokal R, Bogle S, Hunt L, Marsh F, Oliver D, Jakubowski C, Baillod R, Ogg C, Ward M, Wilkinson R. CAPD peritonitis still a major problem in CAPD: result of a multicentre study. J Nephrol 1989; 2:95–99.
74. Woodrow G, Turney JH, Brownjohn AM. Technique failure in peritoneal dialysis and its impact on patient survival. Perit Dial Int 1997; 17:360–364.
75. Ataman R, Burton PR, Gokal R, Brown CB, Marsh FP, Walls J. Long-term CAPD-some UK experience. Clinical Nephrol 1988; 30(suppl 1):S71–S75.
76. Fried LF, Bernardini J, Johnston JR, Piraino B. Peritonitis influences mortality in peritoneal dialysis patients. J Am Soc Nephrol 1996; 7:2176–2182.
77. Rubin J, McFarland S, Hellems EW, Bower JD. Peritoneal dialysis during peritonitis. Kidney Int 1981; 19: 460–464.
78. Raja RM, Kramer SM, Barber K. Solute transport and ultrafiltration during peritonitis in CAPD patients. ASAIO J 1984; 7:8–11.
79. Sennesael JJ, De Smedt GC, Van der Niepen P, Verbeelen DL. The impact of peritonitis on peritoneal and systemic acid-base status of patients on continuous ambulatory peritoneal dialysis. Perit Dial Int 1994; 14: 61–65.
80. Davies SJ, Bryan J, Phillips L, Russell GI. Longitudinal changes in peritoneal kinetics: the effects of peritoneal dialysis and peritonitis. Nephrol Dial Transplant 1996; 11:498–506.
81. Dobbie JW, Henderson I, Wilson LS. New evidence on the pathogenesis of sclerosing encapsulating peritonitis (SEP) obtained from serial biopsies. Adv Perit Dial 1987; 3:138–149.
82. Dobbie JW. Pathogenesis of peritoneal fibrosing syndromes (sclerosing peritonitis) in peritoneal dialysis. Perit Dial Int 1992; 12:14–27.
83. Selgas R, Fernandez-Reyes MJ, Bosque E, Bajo MA, Borrego F, Jimenez C, Del Peso G, De Alvaro F. Functional longevity of the human peritoneum: How long is continuous peritoneal dialysis possible? Results of a prospective medium long-term study. Am J Kidney Dis 1994; 23:64–73.
84. Slingeneyer A. Preliminary report on a cooperative international study on sclerosing encapsulating peritonitis. Contrib Nephrol 1987; 57:239–247.
85. Nomoto Y, Kawaguchi Y, Kubo H, Hirano H, Sakai H, Kurokawa K. Sclerosing encapsulating peritonitis in patients undergoing CAPD: a report of the Japanese Sclerosing Encapsulating Peritonitis Study Group. Am J Kidney Dis 1996; 28:420–427.
86. Liberek T, Topley N, Jorres A, Coles GA, Gahl GM, Williams J. Peritoneal dialysis fluid inhibition of phagocytic function: effects of osmolality and glucose concentration. J Am Soc Nephrol 1993; 3:1508–1515.
87. Ejlersen E, Brandi L, Lokkegaard H, Ladefoged J, Kopp R, Haarh P. Is initial (24 hours) lavage necessary in treatment of CAPD peritonitis? Perit Dial Int 1991; 11:38–42.
88. Pannekeet MM, Zemel D, Koomen GC, Struijk DG, Krediet RT. Dialysate markers of peritoneal tissue during peritonitis and in stable CAPD. Perit Dial Int 1995; 15:217–225.
89. Gokal R, Mistry CD, Peers EM, and the MIDAS Study Group. Peritonitis occurrence in a multicentre study of Icodextrin and Glucose in CAPD. Perit Dial Int 1995; 15:226–230.
90. Locatelli A, Quiroga MA, De Benedetti L, Gomez M, Barone R, Baron MC. Treatment of recurrent and resistant CAPD peritonitis by temporary withdrawal of PD without removal of catheter. Adv Perit Dial 1995; 11:176–178.
91. Ha SK, Seo JK, Lee SY, Lee CK, Lee JI, Kim SJ, Park CJ, Kim DH. Successful use of cytology brush in the treatment of relapsing CAPD peritonitis. Nephrol Dial Transplant 1997; 12:1997–1999.
92. Weber J, Mettang T, Hubel E, Kiefer T, Kuhlmann U. Survival of 138 surgically placed straight double-cuff Tenckhoff catheters in patients on continuous ambulatory peritoneal dialysis. Perit Dial Int 1993; 13:224–227.
93. Paterson AD, Bishop MC, Morgan AG, Burden RP. Removal and replacement of Tenckhoff catheter at a single operation. Successful treatment of resistant peritonitis in continuous ambulatory peritoneal dialysis. Lancet 1986; 2:1245–1247.
94. Swartz R, Messana J, Reynolds J, Ranjit U. Simultaneous catheter replacement and removal in refractory peritoneal dialysis infection. Kidney Int 1991; 40: 1160–1165.
95. Posthuma N, Borgstein BJ, Eijsbouts Q, Wee PM. Simultaneous peritoneal dialysis catheter insertion and removal in catheter related infections without interruption of peritoneal dialysis. Nephrol Dial Transplant 1998; 13:700–703.
96. Mayo RR, Messana JM, Boyer CJ, Swartz RD. Pseudomonas peritonitis treated with simultaneous catheter replacement and removal. Perit Dial Int 1995; 15:389–390.
97. Williams AJ, Boeltis I, Johnson BF, Raftrey AT, Cohen GL, Moorhead PJ, El Nahas AM, Brown C. Tenckhoff catheter replacement or intraperitoneal urokinase: a randomised trial in the management of recurrent CAPD peritonitis. Perit Dial Int 1989; 9:65–67.
98. Churchill DN. CAPD peritonitis: a critical appraisal of prophylactic strategies. Semin Dial 1991; 4:94–100.
99. Fellin G, Gentile MG, Cancarini G, Lupo A, Salomone M, Tarchini R, Segoloni GP, Fursaroli M, Maiorca S, Piccoli G. Peritonitis in CAPD: role of patients and staff. A report from the Italian CAPD study group. Adv Perit Dial 1988; 4:165–168.
100. Churchill DN, Taylor W, Vas SI, Singer J, Beecroft ML, Wu G, Manuel A, Paton T, Walker S, Smith EFM,

Oreopoulos DG. Peritonitis in CAPD patients: a randomized clinical trial of cotrimoxazole prophylaxis. Perit Dial Int 1988; 8:125–128.

101. Oreopoulos DG. Prevention of peritonitis in patients undergoing CAPD. Perit Dial Bull 1986; 6:2–4.

102. Abraham G, Savin E, Ayiomamitis A, Izatt S, Vas SI, Mathews RE, Oreopoulos DG. Natural history of exit-site infection in patients on continuous ambulatory peritoneal dialysis. Perit Dial Int 1988; 8:211–216.

103. Twardowski ZJ, Prowant BF. Classification of normal and diseased exit sites. Perit Dial Int 1996; 16(suppl 3):S32–50.

104. Gokal R, Alexander S, Ash S, Chen TW, Danielson A, Holmes C, Joffe P, Moncrief J, Nichols K, Piraino B, Prowant B, Slingeneyer A, Stegmayr B, Twardowski Z, Vas S. Peritoneal Catheters and exit site practices toward optimum peritoneal access: 1998 update. Perit Dial Int 1998; 18:11–33.

105. Oxton LL, Zimmerman SW, Roecker EB, Wakeen M. Risk factors for peritoneal dialysis related infections. Perit Dial Int 1994; 14:137–144.

106. Piraino B, Perlmutter JA, Holley JL, Bernardini J. *Staphylococcus aureus* peritonitis is associated with *Staphylococcus aureus* nasal carriage in peritoneal dialysis patients. Perit Dial Int 1993; 13(suppl 2):S332–S334.

107. Sesso R, Draibe S, Castelo A, Sato I, Leme I, Barbosa D, Ramos O. *Staphylococcus aureus* skin carriage and development of peritonitis in patients on continuous ambulatory peritoneal dialysis. Clin Nephrol 1989; 31: 264–268.

108. Sewell CM, Clarridge J, Lacke C, Weinman EJ, Young EJ. Staphylococcal nasal carriage and subsequent infection in peritoneal dialysis patients. JAMA 1982; 248:1493–1495.

109. Pignatari A, Pfaller M, Hollis R, Sesso R, Leme I, Herwaldt L. *Staphylococcus aureus* colonization and infection in patients on continuous ambulatory peritoneal dialysis. J Clin Microbiol 1990; 28:1898–1902.

110. Swartz R, Messana J, Starmann B, Weber M, Reynolds J. Preventing *Staphylococcus aureus* infection during chronic peritoneal dialysis. J Am Soc Nephrol 1991; 2:1085–1091.

111. Davies SJ, Ogg CS, Cameron JS, Ponton S, Noble WC. *Staphylococcus aureus* nasal carriage, exit-site infection and catheter loss in patients treated with continuous ambulatory peritoneal dialysis (CAPD). Perit Dial Int 1989; 9:61–64.

112. Vychytil A, Lorenz M, Schneider B, Horl W, Haag-Weber M. New strategies to prevent *Staphylococcus aureus* infections in peritoneal dialysis patients. J Am Soc Nephrol 1998; 9:669–676.

113. Luzar MA, Brown CB, Balf D, Hill L, Issad B, Monnier B, Moulart J, Sabatier JC, Wauquier JP, Peluso F. Exit site care and exit site infection in continuous ambulatory peritoneal dialysis: results of a randomized multicenter trial. Perit Dial Int 1990; 10:25–29.

114. Luzar MA. Exit site infection in continuous ambulatory peritoneal dialysis: a review. Perit Dial Int 1991; 11:333–340.

115. Korzets Z, Erdberg A, Golan E, Ben-Chitrit S, Verner M, Rathaus V, Bernheim J. Frequent involvement of the internal cuff segment in CAPD peritonitis and exit-site infection—an ultrasound study. Nephrol Dial Transplant 1996; 11:336–339.

116. Twardowski ZJ, Prowant BF. Current approaches to exit site infections in patients on peritoneal dialysis. Nephrol Dial Transplant 1997; 12:1284–1295.

117. Golper TA, Tranaeus A. Vancomycin revisited. Perit Dial Int 1996; 16:116–117.

118. Taber TE, Hegeman TF, York SM, Kinney RA, Webb DH. Treatment of pseudomonas infections in peritoneal dialysis patients. Perit Dial Int 1991; 11:213–216.

119. Kazmi HR, Raffone FD, Kliger AS, Fenkelstein FO. Pseudomonas exit site infections in CAPD patients. J Am Soc Nephrol 1992; 2:1498–1501.

120. Scalmogna A, Castelnovo C, De Vecchi A, Ponticelli C. Exit site and tunnel infection in CAPD patients. Am J Kidney Dis 1991; 18:674–677.

121. Strauss FG, Holmes D, Nortman DF, Friedman F. Hypertonic saline compresses: therapy for complicated exit site infections. Adv Perit Dial 1993; 9:248–250.

122. Gokal R, Ash SR, Helfrich BG, et al. Peritoneal catheters and exit site practices: Toward optimum peritoneal access. Perit Dial Int 1993; 13:29–39.

123. Prowant BF, Warady BA, Nolph KD. Peritoneal dialysis catheter exit site care: Results of an international study. Perit Dial Int 1993; 13:149–154.

124. Pecoits-Filho R, Twardowski ZJ, Khanna R, Kim Y-L, Goel S, Moore H. The effect of antibiotic prophylaxis on the healing of exit sites of peritoneal dialysis catheters in rats. Perit Dial Int 1998; 18:60–63.

125. Bennett-Jones DN, Martin J, Barratt AJ, Duffy TJ, Naish PF, Aber GM. Prophylactic gentamicin in the prevention of early exit site infections and peritonitis in CAPD. Adv Perit Dial 1988; 4:147–150.

126. Newman LN, Tessman M, Hanslik T, Schulak J, Mayes J, Friedlander M. A retrospective view of factors that affect catheter healing: Four years of experience. Adv Perit Dial 1993; 9:217–222.

127. Copley JB, Smith BJ, Koger DM, Rodgers DJ, Fowler M. Prevention of postoperative peritoneal dialysis catheter related infections. Perit Dial Int 1988; 8:195–197.

128. Turner K, Edgar D, Hair M, Uttley L, Sternland R, Hunt L, Gokal R. Does catheter immobilization reduce exit-site infections in CAPD patients? Adv Perit Dial 1992; 8:265–268.

129. Warady BA, Sullivan EK, Alexander SR. Lessons from the peritoneal dialysis patient database: a report of the North American Paediatric Renal Transplant Co-operative Study. Kidney Int 1996; 49(suppl 53): S68–S71.

130. Golper TA, Brier ME, Bunke M, Schreiber M, Bartlett DK, Hamilton RW, Strife F, Hamburger RF. Risk factors for peritonitis in long term peritoneal dialysis: the Network 9 Peritonitis and Catheter survival studies. Am J Kidney Dis 1996; 38:428–436.
131. U.S. Renal Data System. USRDS 1996 Annual Data Report. Bethesda, MD: National Institutes of Health, National Institute of Diabetes and Digestive and Kidney Disease, 1996:C.5.
132. Eklund BH, Honkanen EO, Kalan AR, Kyllonen LE. Catheter configuration and outcome in CAPD: a prospective comparison of two catheters. Perit Dial Int 1994; 14:70–74.
133. Eklund BH, Honkanen EO, Kalan AR, Kyllonen LE. Peritoneal Dialysis Access: Prospective randomised comparison of the Swan Neck and Tenckhoff catheters. Perit Dial Int 1995; 15:353–356.
134. Lye WC, Kour N-W, van der Straaten J, Leong S-O, Lee E. A prospective randomised comparison of the Swan neck, coiled and straight Tenckhoff catheters in patients on CAPD. Perit Dial Int 1996; 16(supp 1): S333–335.
135. Moncrief J, Popovich RP, Broadrick LJ, He A, Simmons E, Tate RA. The Moncrief-Popovich catheter: a new peritoneal access technique for patients on peritoneal dialysis. ASAIO J 1993; 39:62–65.
136. Catizone L, Cantaluppi A, Peluso F, Zucchelli P. A new catheter to prevent exit site infections in peritoneal dialysis. Adv Perit Dial 1992; 8:283–287.
137. Holley JL, Bernadini J, Piraino B. Infecting organisms in CAPD patients on the Y-set. Am J Kidney Dis 1994; 23:569–573.
138. Mupirocin Study group. Nasal mupirocin prevents S. aureus exit site infection during peritoneal dialysis. J Am Soc Nephrol 1996; 7:2403–2408.
139. Perez-Fontan M, Garcia-Falcon T, Rosalie M, Rodrigues-Carmona A, Adeva M, Rodrigues-Lozana I, Moncalion J. Treatment of Staph. aureus nasal carriages in CAPD with Mupirocin: long term results. Am J Kidney Dis 1993; 22:708–712.
140. Zimmerman SW, Ahrens E, Johnson CA, Craig W, Leggatt J, O'Brien M, Oxton M, Rocker EP, Engeseth S. Randomised controlled trial of prophylactic rifampin for PD related infections. Am J Kidney Dis 1991; 18:225–231.
141. Bernardini J, Piraino B, Holley JL, Johnstone JR, Lukes R. Randomised trial of Staph. aureus prophylaxis in PD patients: mupirocin calcium ointment 2% applied to the exit site versus oral rifampin. Am J Kidney Dis 1996; 26:695–700.
142. Twardowski ZJ, Prowant BF. Exit-site study methods and results. Perit Dial Int 1996; 16(suppl 3):S6–31.

12

Problems with Anticoagulation for Continuous Renal Replacement Therapies

Andrew Davenport
The Royal Free Hospital, London, United Kingdom

I. INTRODUCTION

Continuous renal replacement therapies (CRRTs) are increasingly being advocated to treat acute renal failure in the intensive care and high-dependency setting. The gradual removal of plasma water and azotemic toxins during CRRT provides a major advantage over intermittent dialysis techniques. However, to achieve control of azotemia comparable to daily intermittent hemodialysis/hemofiltration, the CRRT extracorporeal circuit must function continuously, 24 hours a day, day after day (1). Anticoagulants are therefore routinely used to help maintain and maximize the life of the CRRT circuit by attempting to prevent coagulation within the hemofilter/hemodialysis circuit. Inadequate anticoagulation leads initially to reduced efficiency of the CRRT circuit in terms of both solute and water clearance, followed by premature clotting of the circuit, resulting in blood loss, treatment "downtime," and the additional financial costs and nursing time involved in setting up a new CRRT circuit. Excessive anticoagulation, on the other hand, may result in bleeding complications (usually minor), with a reported incidence ranging from <5% up to 26% of treatments (2,3) and, on occasion, proving fatal (4).

This chapter will review the complications of anticoagulants currently used for extracorporeal CRRT circuits in terms of both the patient and the anticoagulant.

II. PATIENT-DRIVEN COMPLICATIONS OF ANTICOAGULATION IN CRRT

The majority of patients treated by CRRT are critically ill patients admitted to an intensive care unit setting with multiple organ failure. These patients may be at increased risk of hemorrhage due to loss of clotting factors, increased fibrinolysis due to disseminated intravascular coagulopathy, and/or thrombocytopenia. Some patients will have a prothrombotic tendency due to a reduction in the natural inhibitors of the coagulation cascades.

III. SPECIFIC CONDITIONS

A. Trauma and Immediately Postsurgery

Many patients who develop acute renal failure (ARF) following multiple trauma have been multiply transfused with plasma expanders and blood. High doses of gelatin-based colloid expanders have been reported to interfere with the interaction between circulating platelets and endothelial-derived von Willebrand factor (vWF), resulting in decreased platelet activation (5). The combination of high-volume resuscitation with gelatin-based expanders and blood may lead to a reduction in coagulation serine proteases, fibrinogen, and platelets in patients who may have undergone recent surgery or have occult intra- or retroperitoneal hemorrhage and therefore may lead to an increased risk of hemorrhage during CRRT if an extracorporeal anticoagulant is used.

B. Intracranial Surgery

Patients who develop ARF following neurosurgery usually do so in the setting of multiple trauma with hypotension or secondary to sepsis and/or aminoglycoside-induced renal failure. Monitoring of intracranial pressure (ICP) currently requires invasive monitoring using epidural, subdural, intraparenchymal, or intraventricular pressure transducers. Intraventricular catheters are associated with the greatest risk of hemorrhage, whereas epidural monitors have the lowest risk (6). Although hemorrhage may be fatal, small bleeds around the catheter/transducer lead to damping of the signal and thereby inaccurate pressure recording. Because CRRT is preferable to intermittent therapy due to the greater stability of cerebral blood flow and perfusion, it is equally important that any anticoagulant used does not provoke intracerebral or extradural hemorrhage. In the past, anticoagulation with standard unfractionated heparin has been reported to be associated with fatal hemorrhage, with hemorrhage around the intracranial pressure-monitoring device (4). Although prostacyclin, citrate, and nafamostat have been reported to have caused fewer or no hemorrhages at the site of ICP monitors, we currently use anticoagulant-free CRRT circuits in all patients in whom the ICP is measured. Even so, in our experience, computer tomography (CT) brain scans do show a small incidence of subdural/extradural hemorrhage.

C. Liver Disease

Because many of the serine protease coagulation factors are hepatically synthesized, many patients with liver disease will have abnormal prothrombin ratios (PTR) and activated partial thromboplastin times (APPT). In chronic liver disease, patients may have a degree of thrombocytopenia due to splenomegaly and splenic sequestration. Thus many patients with chronic liver disease may require little or no anticoagulation for CRRT. However, because the liver also synthesises anticoagulants, some patients will have a tendency to thrombus. In addition to those presenting with the Budd-Chiari syndrome, patients with acute hepatic failure often require extracorporeal anticoagulants (7). Indeed, the introduction of artificial hepatic assist devices has shown the difficulty in maintaining the integrity of these extracorporeal circuits, with doses of up to 10,000 IU/h of heparin required at times (8).

D. Multiorgan Failure Due to Sepsis

Several studies have shown that critically ill patients are a heterogeneous group with abnormalities in both the clotting cascades and also platelet function reported. In the majority of patients the clotting cascades are activated, as evidenced by a reduction in circulating factor XII, prekallikrein, and factor VII with an increase in fibrinogen (Fig. 1) (9). In addition, the natural anticoagulants antithrombin III, protein C, and protein S are often reduced (Fig. 2) (10), tipping the balance towards a coagulopathy. Thus, many patients with the sepsis syndrome have evidence of increased thrombotic activity with both detectable circulating thrombin-antithrombin III complexes (TATs) and prothrombin breakdown products (PF1 and PF2). Fibrinolysis is often enhanced, as shown by increased D dimer concentrations. However, many other studies have reported an increase in plasminogen activator inhibitor (PAI), which would tend to reduce plasminogen activation and so reduce fibrinolysis (Fig. 3) (9).

Platelets can be activated by the release of vWF, thromboxane A_2, thrombin, arachidonic acid, and prostaglandins G_2 and H_2, which are synthesized by activated endothelium, as found in critically ill patients with the sepsis syndrome (11). In addition, cathepsin G and platelet activation factor, released from activated polymorphonuclear cells, can also cause platelet activation and aggregation. The majority of patients with the sepsis syndrome have a reduced peripheral platelet count and evidence of in vitro platelet activation (11). Many of these patients will also have evidence of increased nitric oxide production, which will tend to prevent local endothelial platelet activation and aggregation but will not prevent platelet contact activation and aggregation in the extracorporeal circuit.

Patients in the intensive care unit are a heterogeneous group, some with active oozing from vascular access sites yet apparently normal laboratory coagulation studies and thromboelastogram, others with marked thrombocytopenia coupled with abnormal coagulation studies and thromboelastogram with no evidence of hemorrhage. This may reflect that in vivo the major determinant in platelet–vessel wall interaction is blood flow, and therefore laboratory tests of platelet function may not necessarily reflect the in vivo situation (12).

While in the intensive care unit, patients may be given drugs that interfere with platelet function. Many currently used antibiotics can result in reduced platelet

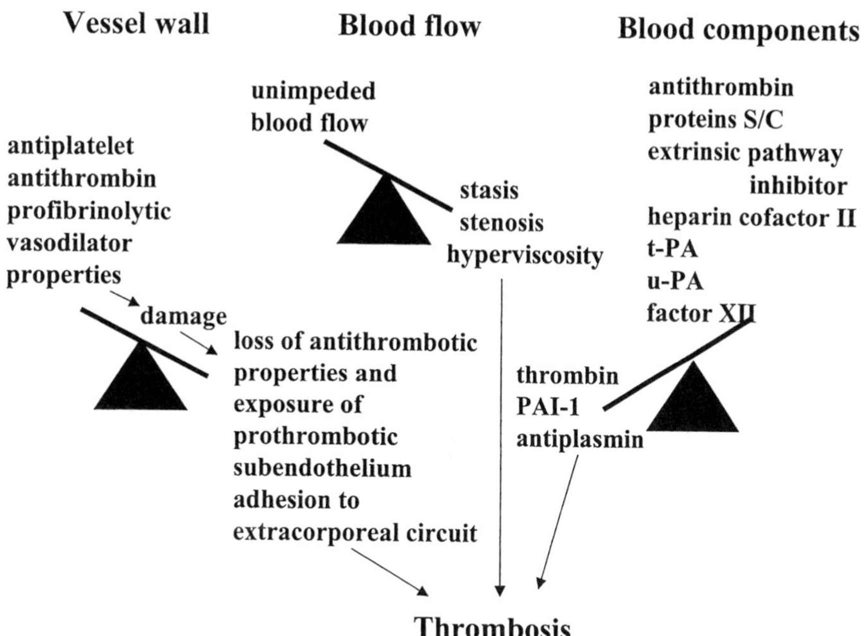

Fig. 1 Virchow's classic triad of thrombosis developing in areas of vessel wall damage coupled with blood flow abnormality and prothrombotic coagulation factors.

function and/or thrombocytopenia. Such antibiotics include penicillins, cephalosporins, aztreonam, aminoglycosides, tetracyclines, rifampicin, and sulfonamides. Nitroprusside and glyceryl trinitrate may act as nitric oxide donors and increase endothelial nitric oxide production; similarly prostacyclin, used to reduce pulmonary vascular resistance or improve tissue blood supply, will reduce platelet adhesion.

E. Post–Cardiac Surgery

ARF is more common in patients who have had a reduced cardiac output during surgery and in those with a prolonged cardiac bypass circuit time. There are differences between the CRRT circuit and that of the cardiac bypass in terms of blood pump speeds and the extracorporeal temperature. Patients undergoing major cardiac surgery often return from cardiac bypass with a marked thrombocytopenia. This is due to events occurring in the extracorporeal circuit, resulting in both platelet fragmentation and functional changes (13). Platelets show a reduced in vitro aggregation response to ADP and collagen and were shown to have a reduction in surface membrane receptors, both surface glycoproteins [GpIb (vWF receptor) and GpIIb/IIIa (mainly fibrinogen receptor)] and loss of the α-granules (13). Electron microscopy showed that these platelets had undergone a conformational change from the normal resting discoid shape to the active form—elongated, thin, with many pseudopodia. These changes reflect the hypothermia of cardiac surgery coupled with mechanical stress of the pumped circuit and adhesion to the extracorporeal circuit. This latter is due to the deposition of fibrinogen on both the plastic of the extracorporeal lines and the hemofilter, which then leads to platelet adhesion through the GpIIb/IIIa receptor.

In addition, contact activation of the extrinsic clotting cascade by the extracorporeal circuit leads to utilization of the natural anticoagulants, such as antithrombin III (ATIII). Thus, subsequent anticoagulation with heparin may not be as effective as anticipated due to the reduction in ATIII (Table 1).

The changes that occur during cardiac extracorporeal bypass are much greater than those during a standard intermittent hemodialysis treatment (14) and reflect the longer duration of circuit time during cardiac bypass, the higher blood flows achieved with an occlusive pump, and hypothermia.

F. Postpartum Acute Renal Failure

Several of the naturally occurring anticoagulants, antithrombin III, protein S, and protein C are lower during normal pregnancy and lower still in twin pregnancies (Table 1) (13). Postpartum acute renal failure is usually due to a small vessel coagulopathy, as found in

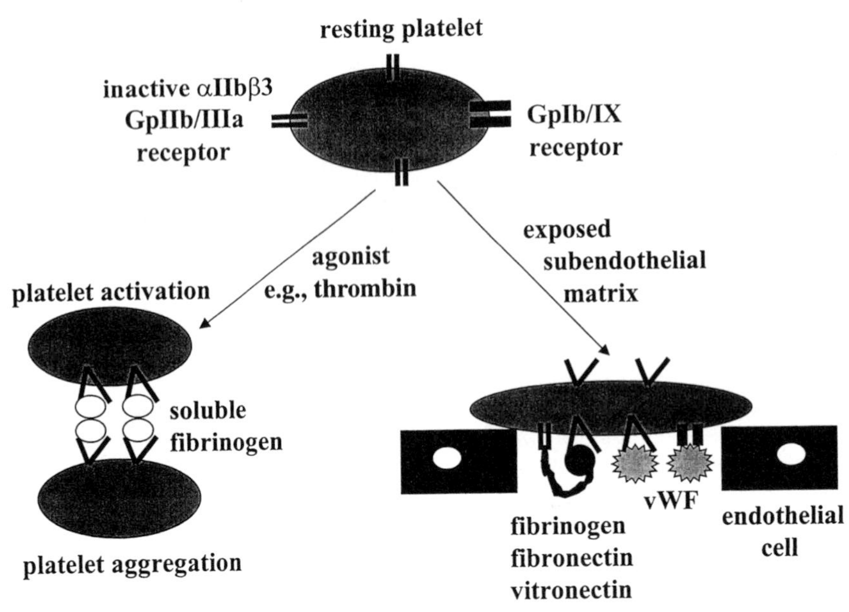

Fig. 2 Platelet activation following exposure to circulating agonist or subendothelial matrix.

hemolytic uremic syndrome (HUS), lupus anticoagulant (antiphospholipid) syndrome, or disseminated intravascular coagulation. The combination of the natural loss of anticoagulants coupled with excess intravascular coagulation and thrombocytopenia in cases of HUS can lead to shortened CRRT circuit life. Anticoagulation is then a balance between the risks of uterine hemorrhage and the need for anticoagulation in those patients at risk of thrombosis and effective CRRT circuit duration. Prostacyclin has been advocated as the anticoagulation of choice in HUS-associated renal failure due to the reduction in endothelial prostacyclin pro-

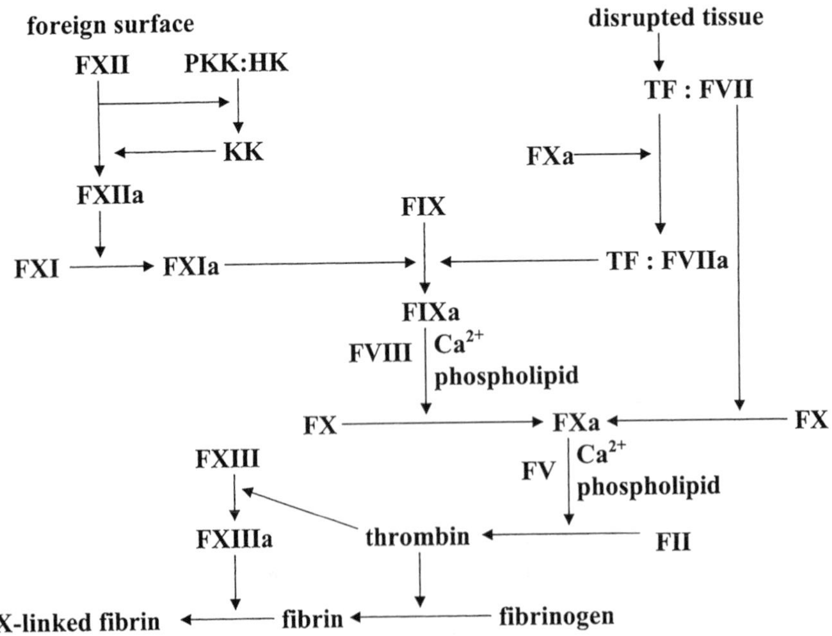

Fig. 3 Extrinsic and intrinsic (contact) coagulation pathways. PKK = Prekallikrein; HK = high molecular weight kallikrein; KK = kallikrein; TF = tissue factor.

Table 1 Acquired Causes of Deficiency in the Natural Anticoagulants

Antithrombin III	Protein C[a]	Protein S
Liver disease	Liver disease	Liver disease
	Liver transplantation	
DIC	DIC	DIC
Cardiac bypass surgery	Cardiac bypass surgery	Cardiac bypass surgery
Twin pregnancy	Twin pregnancy	Pregnancy
Nephrotic syndrome	Hemodialysis	SLE
Protein-losing enteropathy		Anti-cardiolipin Ab
Major surgery		
Acute thrombosis		
Drugs	Drugs	Drugs
Heparin	Warfarin	Warfarin
Asparaginase	Asparaginase	
	Cancer chemotherapy	Cancer chemotherapy
Estrogens		Estrogens

[a]Patients with factor V Leiden have reduced binding of protein C to factor V and therefore have a functional protein C deficiency.

duction (15). In those patients with lupus anticoagulant–associated central venous thrombosis or other thrombotic disease, large doses of heparin may be required due to the low levels of ATIII, and this may lead to increased uterine hemorrhage.

G. Pediatrics

To minimize the extracorporeal blood volume, pediatric CRRT circuits utilize smaller-diameter tubing and a dialyzer. These modifications increase the relative surface area of the circuit and thus increase contact activation and hemoconcentration within the dialyzer. This, coupled with the smaller-caliber, high-resistance, vascular access required, means that clotting within the pediatric CRRT circuit is more problematic than in the adult.

IV. EFFECT OF EXTRACORPOREAL CRRT CIRCUIT ON BLOOD COAGULATION

Compared to intermittent hemodialysis and/or hemofiltration, patients treated by CRRT have their blood exposed to the extracorporeal circuit on a continuous basis, potentially for a prolonged period. Previous work has shown that platelets are activated during conventional intermittent hemodialysis by flow through the dialyzer membrane and the coagulation cascades activated by exposure to plastic surfaces (16). This raises the question as to whether continued exposure to the extracorporeal circuit produces changes in platelet function or coagulation cascades resulting in increased extracorporeal clotting or increased risk of hemorrhage to the patient.

A. Platelet Function

Peripheral platelet counts have been reported either not to change or to decrease during prolonged treatment with CRRT (17,18). This reduction in platelet count appears to be greatest in patients anticoagulated with standard unfractionated heparin and less in those given prostacyclin or no anticoagulation at all (19). In vitro studies of platelet function during CRRT revealed a marked decrease in maximum platelet aggregation in response to collagen (from 28% to 5%), adrenaline (from 39% to 10%), and ADP (from 44% to 16%). These changes in laboratory assessment of platelet function occurred within 24 hours of starting CRRT, at a time when there was no change in the peripheral platelet count (20). Although there were major changes in these in vitro tests of platelet function, there were no clinical sequelae, such as major hemorrhage. As hematocrit and blood flow are critical in initiating platelet aggregation, it may be that these in vitro tests do not accurately reflect in vivo activity. Our own experience is that there is no systematic change in platelet function during CRRT as assessed by serial thromboelastography. Indeed, some proinflammatory cytokines, such as platelet-activating factor, are removed during hemofiltration, and these losses may counterbalance other changes (21). This is supported by a study from the

University of Vienna, which showed that with heparin anticoagulation there was no change in the bleeding time during the first 24 hours of CRRT using an in vitro model of a damaged blood vessel to assess platelet function (18). Interestingly, bleeding times have been reported to increase following a routine 4-hour hemodialysis. This was associated with a reduction in platelet surface glycoprotein receptors (GpIb) (from 38% to 24%) and in vitro reduction of platelet aggregation with thrombin (from 55% to 20%) (22). Thus, although platelets are activated during intermittent hemodialysis, prolonged exposure to the extracorporeal circuit during CRRT does not result in any adverse clinical effect.

B. Coagulation Factors

The exposure of blood to an extracorporeal circuit results in plasma protein adsorption. The interaction between these proteins with the artificial surface can initiate the activators of both the intrinsic and extrinsic clotting cascades. Factor XII can be directly activated by negatively charged membranes, such as polyacrylonitrile and polymethylmethacrylate (23), thus facilitating the conversion of high molecular weight kallikrein and prekallikrein through to kallikrein (24), thus potentially initiating the intrinsic cascade (Fig. 3). Not only can the coagulation cascade be activated, but some of the natural inhibitors also decrease (25). Some studies have demonstrated an increase in intravascular thrombosis during hemodialysis, with increased circulating TATs detected (26,27). Kallikrein activation will result in complement activation and also lead to increased conversion of plasminogen to plasmin and therefore potentially increase fibrinolysis.

Granulocyte activation occurs during passage through the hemodialysis circuit, with release of elastase and cathepsin G (23). These enzymes tip the balance towards fibrinolysis by modifying plasminogen to a more active form and inactivating the inhibitors of plasmin and plasminogen activation (C1-inhibitor, α_2-antiplasmin, and PAI-1). In addition, these neutrophil enzymes can degrade fibrin and also inhibit coagulation by degrading several of the coagulation proteins, including factors V, VII, VIII, IX, XII, and XIII. Monocyte and other mononuclear cell activation during dialysis results in the upregulation of cell adhesion molecules and integrins; these latter include the vitronectin receptor, allowing binding to vWF, fibrinogen, and thrombospondin (26). Activation then results in the release of "tissue factor," which can initiate activation of the extrinsic clotting cascade.

Despite these changes during intermittent hemodialysis, CRRT has not been reported to result in changes in the clotting cascade. Standard anticoagulation tests are either normal or not changed by CRRT (unless patients were treated with heparin) (18). More sophisticated studies measuring prekallikrein and factor XII have similarly reported that CRRT does not lead to activation of the intrinsic coagulation pathway (28). Treatment with CRRT has not been observed to result in increased intravascular thrombosis, as most studies have failed to document significant changes in TATs (29). However, TATs have been reported to increase immediately prior to dialyzer/hemofilter clotting (28). Similarly, the natural anticoagulants like ATIII have not been shown to be affected by CRRT (21). In keeping with stable TATs, CRRT has been observed not to result in increased fibrinolysis, as shown by stable fibrinopeptide A concentrations (29).

Thus, despite the procoagulant effects of intermittent hemodialysis, CRRT has been shown by several groups not to directly affect the coagulation cascades.

V. EFFECT OF CRRT CIRCUIT DESIGN ON CIRCUIT LIFE

Several centers have observed longer CRRT circuit duration with spontaneous CAVHF/CAVHD when compared to pumped CVVHF/CVVHD (4,30). Pumped and spontaneous circuits differ in the length of extracorporeal tubing, and therefore pumped circuits are associated with greater extracorporeal cooling. In addition, pumped circuits have a mechanical occlusive roller pump and a venous air detector, both of which may cause platelet activation (31). This suggests that the design of the extracorporeal circuit may have an effect on circuit life, which is supported by Kramer's original observation that the development of a femoral arterial access catheter for CAVHF resulted in both a longer duration of the CAVHF circuit and a marked reduction in the incidence of hemorrhage, because less heparin was required to maintain the circuit (2). Observations on which part of the extracorporeal circuit initiates clotting have suggested that the most common site is the hemofilter/dialyzer, followed by the vascular access site and then the venous air detector (32–34).

A. Vascular Access

Spontaneous CRRT circuits have traditionally employed femoral arterial and venous vascular access catheters or arterio-venous shunts. The main resistance, and therefore the greatest fall in perfusion pressure in the spontaneous circuit, is the arterial access site (35). This led to the development of specially designed femoral arterial access catheters, with a diameter ≥2 mm and a shortened length (8–10 cm), to provide reduced resistance to flow (35) and to maximize laminar flow within the access device (31). Using these catheters over a mean arterial blood pressure range of 60–120 mmHg, blood flow is greater with the femoral arterial catheter than with a radial arterio-venous shunt (36).

Arterio-venous fistulae and shunts result in a change in blood flow from laminar to turbulent flow. This has been shown to result in activation of the coagulation pathways due to endothelial activation by the turbulent blood. Reports have shown evidence of intravascular thrombosis with increased TATs, PF-1, and PF-2 and plasmin-α_2 antiplasmin complexes (37), coupled with endothelial activation, with the release of t-PA and u-PA (37). In clinical practice CAVHF circuits lasted longer and required less heparin with femoral arterial access when compared to A-V shunts (30,35,38). Despite using shunts, the average life of the hemofilter/hemodialyzer was reported to be in excess 48 hours (39,40).

Spontaneous CRRT requires arterial access, and in the elderly patient with atheromatous vessels, large-bore femoral catheter insertion and A-V shunt formation may be problematical. In the earlier reports of CAVHF, femoral arterial damage was noted, ranging from local hemorrhage through to arteriovenous fistula formation, mycotic aneurysm formation, and arterial occlusion (2,3,35,38). In addition spontaneous CRRT circuits depend upon the patient's mean arterial blood pressure, which in critically ill patients may be labile, and a sudden decline in blood pressure can result in filter clotting. Thus, most centers now treat patients with pumped CRRT circuits, which only require venous access. Interestingly, the reported circuit duration was less with pumped systems, ranging from less than 24 to 48 hours (4,19,30,34). Similarly, although circuit duration is less in the pediatric CRRT experience, arteriovenous circuits survived longer than the corresponding pumped circuit (41).

Work studying vascular access in chronic dialysis patients has shown that the site of the tip of the double lumen venous catheter is an important factor in determining the risk of fibrin deposition at the tip and in the side holes of the catheter, reducing effective flow and leading to catheter malfunction. Thus, for internal jugular catheters, left-sided placement and, more importantly, the position of the catheter tip high in the superior vena cava were most likely to lead to catheter occlusion (42,43). This is thought to be due to local turbulence in blood flow in the superior vena cava, especially when the central venous pressure is low. To prevent premature clotting of subclavian or jugular central venous catheters, these should be positioned at the caval-atrial junction or within the right atrium. Because of this difficulty in positioning, some groups have reported improved circuit life using femoral venous access (44). However, if the femoral catheter is short and lies in the iliac veins, then clotting is more problematic than if the catheter is longer and lies within the inferior vena cava.

Most venous access catheters are silastic dual lumen catheters designed to be inserted via a Seldinger technique. Care with insertion is required to prevent damage to the tip during insertion, which can lead to increased blood flow turbulence and premature clotting. Unlike the single lumen catheter, most dual lumen catheters do not have two circular lumena. Invariably one lumen is compressed into a D shape. This results in increased resistance to blood flow and a reduction in flow, with an increase in nonlaminar blood flow and therefore increases the likelihood of platelet activation and contact cascade activation (Fig. 4). This has been shown to have clinical consequences in hemodialysis patients, with better flows and greater solute removal obtained with dual circular lumen catheters (45). This accords with our own clinical experience of using two single circular lumen lines compared to those with a D-shaped lumen. Similarly, in the pediatric field it can be technically difficult to insert dual lumen vascular access catheters due to the size of the veins, and some centers recommend the insertion of two single lumen catheters (46). Typically the internal diameter of the two single lines is greater than that of the circular/D-shaped line, thus reducing the resistance to blood flow (45). More recently heparin-bonded access lines have been introduced and reported to reduce the incidence of fibrin deposition on the catheter tip with greater patency times in children.

No CRRT circuit can function without good access, whatever anticoagulant is used. In one recent study reduced blood pump speed, a surrogate for access malfunction, was a strong predictor for premature circuit failure (32). Further progress needs to be made in developing vascular access catheters made of nonthrombogenic material that do not lead to the activation of platelets and coagulation pathway proteins which can be inserted atraumatically and optimally positioned. It may well be that two single lumen lines allowing greater laminar blood flow (as used in CAVHF) provide better access than one double lumen catheter.

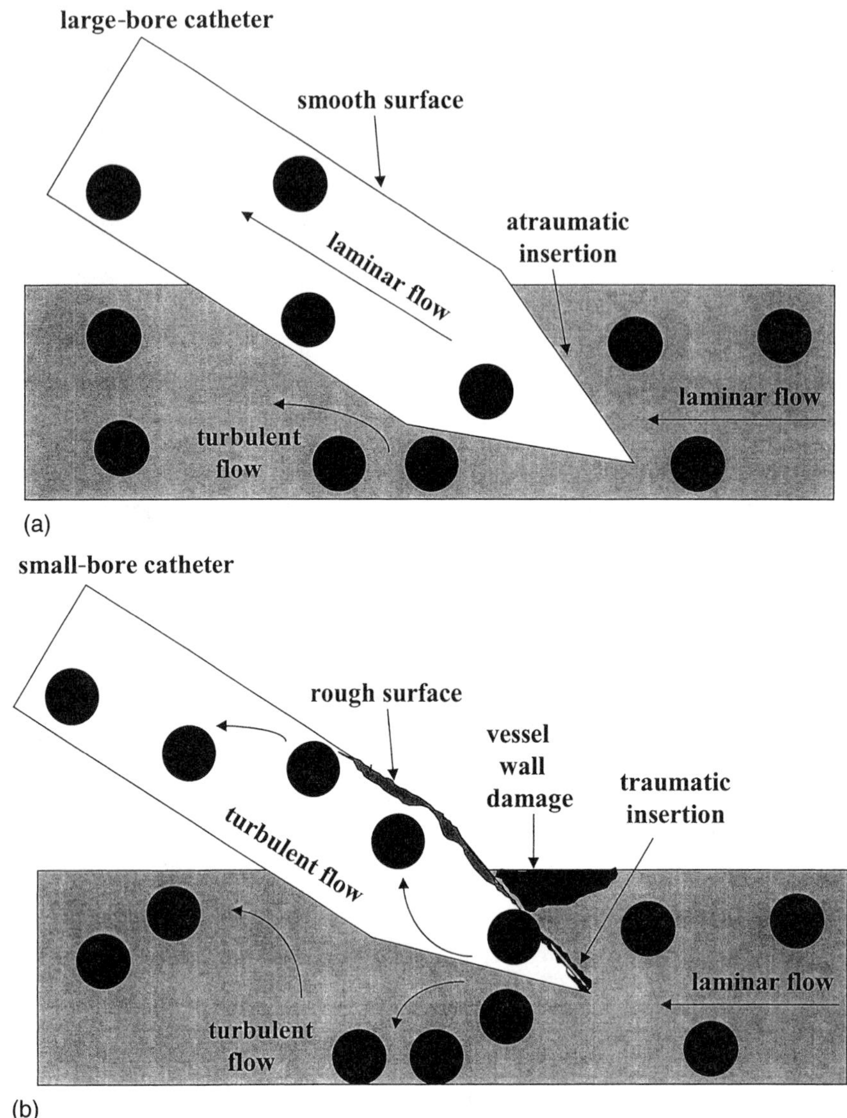

Fig. 4 (a) Good vascular access. (b) Vascular access problems resulting in turbulent blood flow following insertion of high-resistance small-diameter catheter, with vessel wall and catheter damage following traumatic insertion, resulting in platelet and contact cascade activation.

B. Extracorporeal Lines

All CRRT circuits rely on blood lines, and these should be made with a smooth internal biocompatible surface that minimizes platelet adhesion and activation and the adsorption of coagulation pathway and prothrombogenic (e.g., vWF) proteins. Complement activation has been reported to be increased using silicon lines compared to polyvinylchloride (Polaschegg, unpublished data), but there is a paucity of data as yet on the effect of different polymer blood lines and the risk of circuit failure due to clotting (47).

Spontaneous CRRT lines are usually much shorter than those used with pumped circuits. This results in reduced thermal losses, which may play a role in the accelerated intrinsic coagulation system activation and platelet aggregation observed in cardiac bypass extracorporeal circuits (13). Similarly, shorter lines result in less protein adsorption and contact activation.

Pediatric patients require narrow-diameter tubing, because the extracorporeal volume can be critical in neonates and critically ill infants (41,46). The initial greater flow achieved with pumped circuits often resulting in hemodynamic instability (46). The use of narrow-diameter tubing increases the relative surface area and therefore increases contact activation. This may account for the shortened circuit life in the pediatric experience of CRRT and the persistent longer duration of spontaneous circuits, with their shorter lines, than pumped circuits (41,46,48).

C. Extracorporeal Blood Pump

Currently most blood pumps in pumped CRRT circuits are roller pumps, which are designed to be occlusive or at least partially occlusive, depending upon the thickness of the blood tubing and the elasticity of the spring clips in the pump head. Thus blood is drawn out of the access device and delivered in a sawtooth flow profile to the hemofilter/hemodialyzer membrane. The actual pulsatile pressure profile will depend upon both the blood pump speed and the physical characteristics of the tubing. In one study, the mean maximum pressure between the blood pump and the dialyzer inlet was 202 mmHg with an average blood pump speed of 200 mL/min, but in one third of CRRT circuits studied peak pressures of >300 mmHg were recorded (32). This is in keeping with an earlier study (49), which reported similar high prefilter pressures when a blood pump was used in the circuit (31). The variability in the sawtooth profile is greatest for the occlusive pump head. This pattern of blood flow is obviously nonlaminar, and any turbulence is likely to increase the risk of premature clotting by the mechanical activation of platelets, circulating monocytes, and leukocytes (13).

More recently a different blood pump has been developed (Fresenius Accumen, Fresenius, Walnut Creek, CA), which utilizes a bellows design to propel the blood. This system is designed to reduce the sawtooth blood flow, and may be able to reduce clotting in the CRRT circuit, by reducing contact activation. As yet, this system is only in the clinical trial stage.

D. Hemofilter/Hemodialyzer

Clotting within the hemofilter/dialyzer membrane is the most common cause of premature clotting within the CRRT circuit, with studies reporting membrane clotting accounting for 40–63% of all circuit losses (32,33). This is due to platelet and clotting cascade activation within the dialyzer predominantly due to contact activation. When exposed to a foreign surface, such as the extracorporeal circuit, platelet adherence is rapid (25). Although the number of platelets available for hemostasis depends upon the peripheral platelet count, it is more dependent upon the hematocrit (50), because the transport of circulating platelets towards the dialyzer membrane surface is mediated by red blood cells. This transport process is increased with both increasing hematocrit and blood flow and also by both larger and less deformable red blood cells (51).

Spontaneous circuits require low-pressure, high–hydraulic permeability hemofilters/hemodialyzers for optimal function, because at increased resistance due to the filter/dialyzer geometry blood flow no longer is laminar and increased clotting ensues (52). Parallel plate hemofilters/dialyzers generally have the lowest resistance to flow and provide better convective and diffusive clearances (53) with longer filter/dialyzer patency and lower anticoagulant requirement (35). If hollow fiber designs are used, these should be of a relatively short fiber length coupled with a larger cross-sectional area (35). However, in pumped CRRT circuits, high pressures can be generated (32), resulting in nonlaminar blood flow with increased turbulence recorded with flat plate designs (49) and increased premature clotting (54). Thus, for pumped CRRT circuits hollow fiber membrane design is superior.

Ideally all membranes should have a smooth inert biocompatible and nonthrombogenic surface. The membrane composition and surface charge will determine the deposition of circulating plasma proteins, including albumin, complement, fibrinogen, and vWF, onto the membrane surface. Polyacrylonitrile membranes are highly negatively charged and are known to adsorb plasma proteins and various proinflammatory cytokines and growth factors onto their surface. In one single-center study the use of this highly negatively charged membrane was reported to result in reduced CRRT circuit patency compared to a polyamide membrane (44). However, a long hollow fiber membrane design was used in this study with a spontaneous circuit. It was most likely that the increased flow resistance within the polyacrylonitrile membrane led to the reduced performance. This is supported by another group, who reported marked differences between membranes when used as hemofilters but found no differences when using the same membranes as dialyzers (44). When the effect of CRRT on the contact coagulation cascade using a polyacrylonitrile membrane was critically assessed, polyacrylonitrile membranes were not shown to cause any activation of the intrinsic pathway, nor was there any evidence of increased intravascular clotting (28). This latter finding is supported by clinical studies comparing the same two membranes, which did not show any membrane effect on filter/dialyzer patency rates (4). Similarly, a further multicenter trial did not show any difference between polyacrylonitrile and polysulfone membranes in terms of the duration of CRRT (55). Most studies have reported that synthetic membranes require less anticoagulation than corresponding cellulosic membranes, suggesting that platelet aggregation and activation of the clotting system is yet another marker of membrane bioincompatibility (56). Whereas activation of the extrinsic clotting cascade was thought to be mainly due to contact activation with the extracorporeal circuit, data from cardiopulmonary bypass has shown that monocyte activation is the key event in activation of clotting cascades, which may explain why continued clotting cascade activation does not appear to occur during CRRT.

Membrane biocompatibility varies from membrane to membrane. In general the passage of blood across a cellulosic-based membrane results in greater activation of plasma complement proteins, more severe peripheral leukopenia and thrombocytopenia, and the generation of proinflammatory cytokines and polymorphonuclear leukocyte activation, as evidenced by elastase release, than the synthetic membranes (57). Although polysulfone and polyacrylonitrile membranes appear to be the least bioincompatible, other factors including membrane geometry, sterilization method, and dialysate composition can all affect the blood-dialyzer membrane interaction (57). Similarly, membrane bioincompatibility is greater with higher blood pump speeds due to nonlaminar turbulent blood flow through the membrane.

E. Predilution or Postdilution Fluid Replacement

The design of the CRRT circuit can also predispose to increased clotting within the fibers of the hemofilter/dialyzer membrane. If a postdilutional hemofiltration circuit is used with large ultrafiltrate volumes, this will lead to increased hemoconcentration and oncotic pressure due to plasma water losses during the passage of blood through the membrane (36). Because platelet interactions with the membrane are dependent upon red blood cell transport, increasing the hematocrit during transit along the membrane can increase platelet transport to the membrane surface (50,51). Similarly, increased protein concentration can lead to increased protein deposition on the membrane, which could then increase activity of the contact coagulation cascade due to deposition of factor XII. In the development of CAVHF techniques, one group advocated the use of negative pressure applied to the ultrafiltrate channel to increase the ultrafiltrate (58). Although this may temporarily increase the ultrafiltrate rate, it also increases hematocrit and protein deposition on the membrane leading to premature clotting and reduced membrane patency.

Predilution, on the other hand, reduces the hematocrit and protein concentration entering the hemofilter/hemodialyzer. This has been clinically reported to both increase membrane patency rates (25,59) and reduce anticoagulant requirements (58,60).

F. Venous Air Detection Chamber

Gretz and colleagues (34) demonstrated that the venous air detection chamber in the pumped CRRT circuit is another vulnerable site for clotting to develop. They showed that not only was there a combination of stagnant blood with a turbulent inflow, predisposing to clotting, but also that the air/blood interface at the top of the chamber was important in determining premature clotting of the circuit (34). In one other study clotting starting in the venous bubble trap was the cause of premature circuit in 7.5% of circuits (32). Thus, by deliberately infusing the postdilutional replacement fluid into the venous air detection chamber to prevent an air/blood interface, they showed an increased filter patency and duration of the CRRT circuit. Venous air detection chambers are a safety feature of the pumped CRRT circuits. More recently, an alternative circuit has been designed that uses an air porous plastic diaphragm as the blood pump, which extrudes air so no separate venous air trap is required. This system, by removing the venous air detector chamber, may prove of benefit in considering future designs to achieve anticoagulant-free CRRT.

G. Dialysate/Substitution Fluid

Pre- and postdilution fluid replacement with normal saline, 5% dextrose, commercially available lactate-based substitution fluid with and without glucose, lactate-free and bicarbonate fluids have not been reported to affect filter/dialyzer clotting (61). Similarly the same fluids and peritoneal dialysis fluid, when used as dialysate, have not been observed to have any discernable affect on membrane patency (41,62,63). In theory the use of a high glucose concentration in the dialysate/substitution fluid could lead to changes in red blood cell rheology (51), with increased risk of clotting within the extracorporeal circuit (50).

H. Priming the Circuit

Most centers rinse the hemofilter/dialyzer and extracorporeal lines with normal saline containing 5000 IU unfractionated heparin (28,32), although the amount varies from 2,500 to 20,000 IU (34,62,63). Similarly, the priming volumes also vary, ranging from 1.0 to 4.5 L (28,32,64). Because heparin can be adsorbed to the plastic blood tubing and membrane, these differences in priming may have a clinical effect on membrane patency. The average circuit life reported was 30 hours for the group using a 1 L rinsing cycle (32), 48 hours when 2 L were used (64), and 44 hours when larger volumes were employed (28). This would suggest that a 2 L priming volume with 5000 IU of heparin maximizes membrane patency.

I. Albumin Precoating

In vitro studies showed that precoating a polyacrylonitrile dialyzer membrane with albumin (1.5 $\mu g/cm^2$) resulted in the deposition of 80 platelets/mm^2, compared to 35,800/cm^2 when fibrinogen (2.0 $\mu g/cm^2$) was coated onto the membrane (14). In clinical practice, albumin precoating of plasma exchange circuits was observed to reduce platelet accumulation and thrombus formation from 44% to 5% (66). One study in patients with hepatic and renal failure reported that precoating the CRRT circuit with 4.5% albumin and heparin resulted in a median reduction in the peripheral platelet count of 13%, compared to 23% in those anticoagulated with prostacyclin and 32% with heparin alone (67). Following albumin-heparin priming, anticoagulation free CRRT circuits significantly outlasted those with standard heparin priming followed by either heparin or prostacyclin anticoagulation (67). This finding has not been universal, however, and may reflect differences in the albumin priming procedure and patient populations (68).

J. The Effect of CRRT on Anticoagulants

Some anticoagulants are removed during hemofiltration and/or dialysis. Heparin, both standard unfractionated heparin (5–35 kDa, mean 13 kDa) and the smaller forms (2–8 kDa, mean 5 kDa), are charged molecules with minimal loss during CRRT (69). The proteoglycans dermatan and heparan sulfate are similarly too charged to be significantly removed during CRRT (70). Although recombinant hirudin is too large to be removed by low flux membranes (<5 kDa), it is cleared by higher-flux membranes, with greater losses during dialysis than hemofiltration (71). On the other hand, the serine protease inhibitors nafamostat and gabexate mesilate are rapidly cleared by dialysis, with less removed during hemofiltration (72). Similarly, some 20% of prostacyclin is removed during hemofiltration, with an estimated 25–30% cleared with continuous dialysis (73). Citrate has the greatest clearance of all anticoagulants during CRRT, losses again being greater with dialysis (33). Removal of calcium and citrate within the hemofilter/dialyzer may have a beneficial effect in preventing platelet aggregation and activation and activation of the final common coagulation pathway, because these are calcium-dependent reactions.

VI. ANTICOAGULATION FOR CRRT

A. Standard Unfractionated Heparin

Structure: Unfractionated heparin is a mixture of glycosaminoglycan composed of alternating residues of D-glycosamine and uronic acid (5–100 kDa).

Action: All heparin molecules contain a unique pentasaccharide structure, which has high-affinity binding to antithrombin. After its reaction with heparin, antithrombin undergoes conformational change, which increases its ability to inactivate the serine proteases thrombin, factor Xa, and factor IXa. Thrombin is most sensitive to this interaction, with heparin binding to both thrombin and antithrombin. Heparin cofactor II is also catalyzed by heparin, but the anticoagulant effect is only achieved at high levels of heparin and is specific for thrombin (74). In addition, heparin reduces the adhesion of platelets to injured arterial walls and to collagen, probably by maintaining vessel wall electronegativity (25).

Clinical use: Standard heparins are the most commonly used anticoagulants for CRRT.

Half-life: Half-life time is 40–120 minutes.

Dosage schedule: The CCRT circuit is primed with 2 L normal saline with 2,500–10,000 IU standard heparin. A loading dose of heparin (5–10 IU/kg) at the start of CRRT is followed by a maintenance dose of 3–12 IU/kg/h (33,44,75).

Monitoring: The whole blood clotting time (WBCT) and the activated coagulation time (ACT) are the most common bedside tests of heparin anticoagulation. Fresh unanticoagulated whole blood samples should be rapidly delivered into a glass tube at 37°C. The procedure with ACT is similar, but uses an activator of the intrinsic coagulation system. Both are prone to error depending on sampling errors, volumes tested, and test tube sizes, and both require regular quality control. In addition, the results are dependent upon the level of coagulation factors, platelets, and hematocrit.

The activated partial thromboplastin time (APTT) is a laboratory test on plasma separated from citrated blood. APTT should be measured in conjunction with a prothrombin time, which, although little affected by heparin, provides valuable information about coagulation factor levels (Fig. 5).

Centers differ not only in the monitoring tests performed and their frequency, but also the site at which samples are taken (44,59,62). As discussed above, bedside tests are affected by hemoconcentration and platelet count. Thus, results of WBCT and ACT taken from the same patient will differ, during hemofiltration with postdilutional fluid replacement, if taken prior to and postfilter, simply due to ultrafiltration increasing hematocrit and platelet concentration causing shorter times postfilter. To overcome these technical problems, most units check coagulation times immediately prior to the filter/dialyzer; if anticoagulation is required, it must be maximum during flow through the dialyzer membrane, as this is the primary site for clotting to develop (4,59).

Thus, whereas the expected WBCT for hemodialysis would be 15–20 minutes, the corresponding time for CRRT would be 10–15 minutes prior to and 6–10 minutes after the dialyzer/hemofilter. For ACT, hemodialysis would be 200–240 seconds, CRRT 180–240 seconds pre- and 160–200 seconds postfilter/dialyzer, and for the APTT, hemodialysis would be 120–160 seconds and for CRRT 45–80 seconds prefilter and 35–45 seconds postfilter/dialyzer.

Filter patency rates: Filter patency has not been proven to be determined either by the total heparin dose or by APPT or other clotting studies (19,28,30,44). Very few studies have reported either that increased heparin administration resulted in increased filter patency (36) or that increased APTT was associated with prolonged circuit life (44). Van der Wetering and colleagues reported a reduced filter patency rate with systemic APTT times less than 35 seconds (54). However, several groups have observed that lower doses of heparin can be used in patients with thrombocytopenia without any reduction in filter patency or circuit life (19,21,59).

Advantages: The one advantage of heparin, apart from cost, is that the dose can be adjusted according to bedside monitoring tests. Most centers have experience with heparin and have developed their own protocols. Compared to the low molecular weight and synthetic heparins, the half-life is shorter and therefore overanticoagulation can be corrected more quickly by reduction in dosage or with protamine, depending upon the clinical situation.

Minor complications: Because heparin is a charged molecule it may adsorb to the plastic tubing, especially when infused in a high concentration (e.g., 1 mL/h of a 1000 IU/L solution). Thus, to achieve thorough mixing, heparin should be infused at a low concentration but high volume (e.g., 2.5–10 IU/mL at 100–200 mL/h) (21). Others have devised a Venturi mixing chamber to achieve thorough mixing (59).

Heparin may induce a state of thrombocytopenia, usually in a time- and dose-dependent manner, which

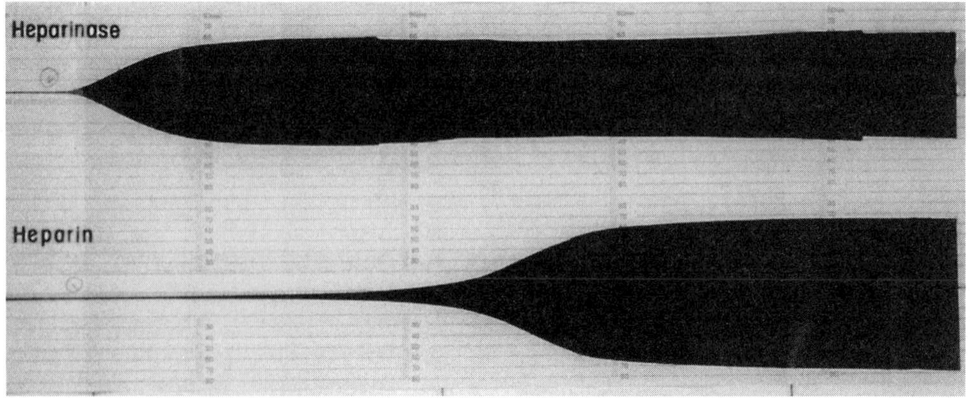

Fig. 5 Thromboelastograph recording from a patient treated by CRRT with a heparin infusion of 1000 IU/h with a systemic APPT of 50 s. The sample was divided into two, one treated with heparinase. The delayed clot formation due to the action of heparin is shown.

may occur in patients treated by CRRT for protracted periods. This responds to a reduction in dosage and is termed heparin-induced thrombocytopenia type I.

Major complications: Hemorrhage is the major complication of heparin anticoagulation. One group reported an incidence of major hemorrhage of >100% (54). Most studies have reported an incidence of around 25%, with some 3.5–10% of deaths being directly attributable to problems with anticoagulation during CRRT (4,54). Although the absolute amount of heparin has not been shown to be related to the incidence of hemorrhage (19), this may be due to the heterogeneity of the patient populations in terms of the levels and balance of coagulation and anticoagulant factors but also the variability in heparin half-live (ranging from 0.66 to 4.5 hours) (59). However, monitoring of systemic blood samples has shown that at a APTT of 15–35 seconds the incidence of de novo patient hemorrhage was 2.9 per 1000 hours of CRRT, which increased to 7.4 at an APTT of 45–55 seconds (54).

Less commonly severe thrombocytopenia may develop, with agglutination of platelets and paradoxical thrombosis, either arterial and/or venous. This syndrome occurs more commonly with bovine (up to 5%) than with porcine heparin (1% or less) and is usually due to the presence of an antibody, IgG isotype, directed against a multimolecular complex of heparin and platelet factor 4 (75). This heparin-induced thrombocytopenia type II, or heparin-associated antibody (HAT), has a peak time of onset after 5–12 days of heparin exposure. The HAT syndrome can cause both bleeding and thrombotic complications and can promote clotting in extracorporeal circuits. In most cases this is associated with a precipitous fall in the peripheral platelet count, although rarely the platelet count can be maintained. Recovery requires the avoidance of heparin. In cases of HAT associated with major thrombosis, prostacyclin or synthetic heparinoids have been used to both maintain CRRT circuit and systemic anticoagulation and to prevent extension of the thrombosis (64). Although citrate is an effective extracorporeal anticoagulant, it does not provide systemic anticoagulation in cases complicated by major arterial or venous thrombosis.

The routine laboratory method for detecting heparin-dependent antibodies uses a platelet aggregation assay, utilizing platelets from normal healthy donors, the patient's plasma, and the same heparin preparation as that administered to the patient. This screening test may be negative in up to 50% of cases (64), and if HAT is clinically suspected, a more sensitive ELISA test using PF4 complexed with heparin should be performed.

B. Regional Heparinization

Regional heparinization was developed to achieve maximum anticoagulation during passage through the hemofilter/dialyzer but with minimum systemic effects, thereby reducing the risk of patient hemorrhage yet achieving prolonged membrane patency and extracorporeal life.

Structure: This small basic protein is derived from sperm or mature testes of fish (genera *Oncorhynchus*, *Salmo*, or *Trutta*).

Action: Cationic groups of protamine bind to anionic heparin, preventing heparin binding to ATIII and heparin cofactor II, thus neutralizing any free heparin and reducing the systemic effects of extracorporeal anticoagulation.

Clinical use: This procedure is suited to patients who are at increased risk of hemorrhage.

Half-life: Protamine binds rapidly to free heparin, but the complex is then taken up by the reticuloendothelial system, broken down, and the protamine released. This results in an increase in protamine half-life with dose and duration of therapy.

Dosage schedule: The CCRT circuit is primed with 2 L normal saline with 2,500–10,000 IU standard heparin. A loading dose of heparin (5–10 IU/kg) is administered at the start of CRRT, followed by a maintenance dose of 3–12 IU/kg/h (33,44,75). Protamine infusion postfilter is started at a rate calculated on the basis of 1 mg of protamine neutralizing 100 IU of standard heparin (13).

Monitoring: Regular monitoring of the APTT both pre– and post–heparin infusion and postprotamine is required, followed by adjusting either the dose of heparin or protamine and/or both and then reassessment (59). Too little protamine puts the patient at risk of hemorrhage; conversely, too much protamine may cause the CRRT circuit to clot or the patient to react adversely to protamine.

Filter patency: Comparison of regional heparinization during spontaneous CRRT using a dialyzer with standard low-dose heparin (500 IU/h) was reported to result in a mean 33% increase in filter life (30). When the same center compared data for a corresponding pumped CRRT circuit, again the mean circuit life was 29% longer with regional heparinization (30). These data favor the use of regional heparinization in increasing circuit patency.

Advantages: Centers that advocate regional heparinization have reported both improved filter patency rates and fewer hemorrhagic complications despite similar APTTs (30,59).

Complications: Unfortunately in clinical practice the half-life of heparin is dose dependent and increases with prolonged administration. The heparin-protamine complex is taken up by the reticuloendothelial system and broken down, with the release of heparin back into the circulation (13). Thus the protamine infusion has to be adjusted to the needs of the individual patient. In clinical practice, the amount of protamine required to neutralize 100 IU heparin varies more than threefold, making it difficult to successfully establish regional heparinization with simple standardized protocols (59).

Protamine has a number of potentially adverse clinical effects, including hypotension due to the combination of reduced cardiac output and decreased systemic vascular resistance, increased pulmonary vascular resistance, bronchospasm, and decreased platelet function (25). When given in large boluses to reverse heparin-associated hemorrhage, protamine can also cause severe anaphylactic reactions, but these are unlikely when infused during CRRT at the low doses used in clinical practice (0.6–2 mg/100 IU heparin) (59).

Regional heparinization cannot be used with heparin-coated hemofilters/dialyzers because the protamine binds to the heparin coating, neutralizing its effect. Protamine has less effect on neutralizing low molecular weight heparins (LMWHs) than standard heparin, due to the smaller size of the molecule and the reduced charge. In view of the increased half-life of the LMWHs, regional heparinization with protamine is not recommended.

Because patients are given standard heparin, they can still develop the side effects of heparin (see above). Indeed, in some series there has been no proven reduction in the incidence of hemorrhagic events during regional heparinization compared to standard heparin anticoagulation during CRRT (30).

C. Antithrombin III Supplementation and Heparin

Antithrombin III (ATIII) levels are often reduced in critically ill patients with renal failure. Studies have shown that conventional heparin anticoagulation is much less likely to prevent circuit thrombosis during CRRT in patients with acquired antithrombin III deficiency (76).

Structure: The natural serpin protein is synthesized in the liver and vascular endothelium.

Action: As with most serpins, it forms a 1:1 irreversible complex with target protease. By binding thrombin, it inhibits the action of thrombin. ATIII is also an important physiological inhibitor of factor Xa and kallikrein. It can also bind most of the other serine protease coagulation factors (13,74).

Clinical use: Use has been evaluated in clinical conditions of ATIII deficiency—liver disease, cardiac bypass surgery, and septic shock.

Half-life: Following bolus dose, there is large interpatient variation between 2 and 12 hours.

Dosage schedule: For intermittent dialysis, a loading dose of 3000 IU provides normal ATIII levels for at least hours (27). In CRRT, a lower loading dose of 1000 IU, with a continuous infusion of 250–500 IU/hr, has been suggested. Standard heparin is then given as a loading dose (5–10 IU/kg) at the start of CRRT, followed by a reduced maintenance dose of 3–5 IU/kg/h, adjusted to WBCT or ACTT (75).

Monitoring: As for standard heparin (see above).

Filter patency rates: Studies have failed to show any significant duration of extracorporeal circuit life and/or small molecular weight solute clearance, suggesting no difference in membrane patency (27).

Advantages: Reduction in the total amount of standard heparin is required to maintain a target whole blood clotting time (27). However, the reduction in heparin dose has not been shown to significantly reduce the incidence of hemorrhage.

Complications: This procedure involves increased complexity and greatly increased cost with no major clinical advantage. Studies have shown that the infusion of ATIII does not reduce extracorporeal clotting, as shown by the failure to decrease the generation of TATs. In addition, patients are treated with heparin and are at risk for all the complications of heparin therapy.

D. Low Molecular Weight Heparins

LMWHs are obtained by the chemical or enzymatic depolymerization of various chains of standard heparin.

Structure: LMWH is a glycosaminoglycan with a molecular weight of 5 kDa.

Action: LMWH, by comprising fewer than 18 saccharides, cannot bind to both ATIII and thrombin simultaneously, thus losing antithrombin activity compared to standard heparin. Because inactivation of factor Xa does not require direct heparin binding, LMWH by activating AT-III retains anti-Xa activity.

Clinical use: LMWHs have been shown superior to standard heparin for the prevention of deep venous thrombosis and the treatment of venous embolic events, due to the lower complication rate. Thus, LMWHs were advocated to be the anticoagulant of choice for CRRT circuits in patients at high risk of hemorrhage.

Half-life: The currently available LMHs—dalteparin, enoxaparin, and nadroparin—differ in size, half-life, and biological activity (77). The terminal half-life is much greater for the LMWHs than for unfractionated heparin, with enoxaparin having the longest at 27.7 hours (77). Half-lives are increased in renal failure because in healthy subject LMWHs are degraded in the proximal tubules (59).

Dosage schedule: Initially most centers either used a loading dose followed by a continuous infusion (78) or gave further bolus doses every 6 hours (79). More recently LMWHs have been shown to be effective when started as a continuous infusion without a loading dose (e.g., dalteparin 600 IU/h), achieving a mean anti-factor Xa activity of 0.49 IU/mL (therapeutic range for systemic anticoagulation 0.3–0.8 IU/mL) within one hour of starting CRRT (69).

Monitoring: LMWH by activating AT-III retains anti-Xa activity. Thus, when monitoring the affect of anticoagulation with LMWH, there is only a modest affect on the APTT, and special assays are required to determine the inhibition of factor Xa. Some commercial kits for testing factor Xa activity include purified ATIII. Thus, although they are an assay of heparin or LMWHs, these kits are a poor indicator of heparin anticoagulation, especially in critically ill patients who are usually ATIII deficient. Hence it is most important when LMWHs are used to seek an assay that omits exogenous ATIII so that the LMWH dose can be titrated against anticoagulant activity, otherwise anti-factor Xa activity and the effect of LMWH on anticoagulation may not correlate.

The recommended anti-factor Xa activity range for standard intermittent hemodialysis is 0.2–0.4 U/mL. Whereas anti-factor Xa activity of ≥0.25 IU/mL using enoxaprin prevented clotting (79), dalteparin has been reported to require higher levels (0.47–0.79 IU/mL) (78). Thromboelastography can also be used to monitor anticoagulation, as the reaction time is correlated with anti-factor Xa activity (78).

Filter patency rates: Studies using LMWH have shown that filter patency depends upon the degree of anticoagulation. For dalteparin, lower doses (antifactor Xa activity 0.27–0.53 IU/mL) resulted in reduced dialyzer patency and premature circuit clotting compared to higher doses (0.47–0.79 IU/kg), as assessed by urea filtration ratios (78).

Advantages: LMWHs have been reported to reduce bleeding from needle puncture sites at the end of intermittent dialysis, and one study reported a reduced incidence of bleeding compared to standard heparin in patients with a moderate risk of hemorrhage (80).

Monitoring can be done at the bedside, using a thromboelastograph, and adjusting the infusion rate according to the reaction time.

Complications: LMWHs are more expensive than standard heparin and require more complicated monitoring, which may not be readily available, especially out of normal service hours. Several groups have reported increased hemorrhage in patients treated with LMWHs (44,81), which may be due to the combination of difficulty in titrating the initial bolus dose and the continuous infusion rate to achieve target anti-factor Xa activity, coupled with a laboratory test which included purified ATIII. If overanticoagulated, unlike standard heparin, protamine has only a partial effect, and fresh frozen plasma may therefore be required to control hemorrhage because of the prolonged half-life of the LMWHs.

When first introduced, LMWHs were tried in patients with HAT syndrome. However, it is now recognized that immune-mediated thrombocytopenia may also rarely occur with the LWMHs. Thus, in patients with HAT, in vitro testing for cross-reactivity should be determined prior to using LMWH, because in the great majority of patients with HAT cross-reactivity is the rule; dalteparin 89%, nadroparin 86%, and enoxaparin 83%, and, therefore, LMWHs should be avoided (82).

E. Dermatan Sulfate

Dermatan and chondroitin sulfate are natural anticoagulants synthesized by endothelial cells and present in the extracellular matrix.

Structure: Dermatan sulfate is a charged sulfated glycosaminoglycan, but with a lower charge density than heparin.

Action: Dermatan sulfate primarily works through the binding and activation of heparin cofactor II to inhibit thrombin formation.

Clinical use: Dermatan sulfate is currently only used for intermittent hemodialysis.

Half-life: The half-life of dermatan sulfate ranges from 2 to 6 hours.

Dosage schedule: A single loading dose of 6 mg/kg has been recommended for a standard 4-hour intermittent dialysis treatment. Standard schedules for CRRT have not been established.

Monitoring: Extracorporeal circuits can be maintained at lower APTT times than during standard heparin (i.e., for hemodialysis 80–120 s and for CRRT 35–45 s postfilter/dialyzer).

Filter patency: Studies from hemodialysis suggest that dermatan sulfate increases filter patency, which may be due to reduced platelet activation compared to heparin (83).

Advantages: This procedure requires simple laboratory monitoring tests of anticoagulation, coupled with reduced systemic anticoagulation and platelet activation. There are few clinical data, but as yet bleeding episodes and thrombocytopenia have not been reported.

Disadvantages: These include high cost and limited experience in CRRT.

F. Synthetic Heparins/Heparinoids

These agents are known as heparinoids because of the pentasaccharide group. Danaparoid (orgaran) was the first to become commercially available, although others are entering clinical trials.

Structure: Heparinoids are glycosaminoglycurons that contain five or fewer polysaccharide residues with a pentasaccharide group.

Action: The action of these agents is similar to that of the LWMHs. Synthetic heparinoids may have an additional advantage over standard and LMWHs in that heparin can paradoxically increase intrinsic coagulation cascade activity due to the activation of factor XI by fibrin-bound thrombin. For example, standard heparin increases this reaction 68-fold, compared to LMWH (dalteparin), which increased it 12-fold, whereas danapranoid only caused a 3-fold increase and another experimental synthetic pentasaccharide had no affect on the intrinsic clotting cascade following the addition of fibrin-bound thrombin (84).

Clinical use: Heparinoids can usually be used in patients who have developed the HAT syndrome with standard and LMWHs, as there is very little cross-reactivity (<10%) (82). We recently used danaparoid in such a case complicated by iliac vein thrombosis, with no hemorrhagic problems during CRRT, and coupled with dialyzer patency and circuit life in excess of 24 hours.

Half-life: Half-life activity against both factor Xa and IIa is greater for danaparoid (18–25 h) compared to the LMWHs, yet following bolus administration the initial effect on anti-IIa activity is least with danaparoid (77).

Dosage schedule: We currently start with a bolus dose of 2500 IU of danaparoid followed by an infusion of 400 IU/h, then adjust the rate (usually between 200 and 400 IU/h) to the desired APTT.

Monitoring: Unlike LMWHs, danaparoid can be monitored by not only anti-factor Xa activity but also APTT, as there is a correlation between anti-Xa activity and APTT (88).

Filter patency: In cases of HAT, it is our clinical experience that danaparoid results in prolonged circuit duration compared to LMWHs, prostacyclin, and anticoagulation free circuits. However, there are too few data on the use of heparinoids in uncomplicated cases to know whether there is any benefit.

Advantages: Heparinoids can be used in cases of HAT, when not only an extracorporeal anticoagulant but also systemic anticoagulation is required to prevent extension of venous or arterial thrombosis. Monitoring can be with standard laboratory tests rather than requiring anti-factor Xa activity, as with the LMWHs.

Synthetic heparinoids have not been widely used, and therefore their safety profile in terms of bleeding risk is unknown. However, our limited clinical experience and that of others (85) suggests that the risk of hemorrhage is substantially less than that with standard heparin and that filter patency and CRRT circuit life are similar to those of other anticoagulants.

Complications: These agents are much more expensive than standard heparin. The longer half-life of plasma anti-Xa activity could cause problems with overanticoagulation during CRRT if too great an infusion dose is used. If overanticoagulated, unlike standard heparin, protamine has only a partial effect, and fresh frozen plasma may therefore be required to control hemorrhage because of the prolonged half-life of the heparinoids. In ≤10% of cases of HAT there may be cross-reactivity with the synthetic heparinoids (85).

G. Heparin-Coated Extracorporeal Circuits

Heparin bonding of cardiopulmonary and extracorporeal oxygenation circuits has been shown to result in a reduction in heparin requirement and risk of hemorrhage. Heparin bonding of CRRT circuits has been attempted by various groups, who circulated high concentrations of either heparin (34) or heparin-albumin solutions prior to commencing treatment (67). Phase III clinical trials with a heparin-bonded membrane (Duraflo, Baxter, Deerborne, IL) are currently underway.

Action: Heparin binds to extracorporeal lines and/or dialyzer and is designed to reduce extracorporeal platelet, leukocyte activation, and thrombogenesis (86). The amount of heparin released from the membrane is very small (<1%), and we and others have not noted any change in APTT during treatment.

Filter patency: In our experience, anticoagulant free circuits utilizing heparin-bonded dialyzers can operate in excess of 48 hours. Other groups using heparin-coated CRRT circuits in patients with liver disease have also reported circuit lives in excess of 40 hours (67). Initial results in ICU patients again suggest less platelet activation and both prolonged filter patency and circuit life (87).

Advantages: Heparin-bonded CRRT circuits allow the possibility of using no additional anticoagulation. Provided filter patency and circuit life exceeds 48 hours, after which the use of heparin-bonded CRRT circuits will increase. Similarly, the frequency of hemorrhage is much lower than during standard heparin CRRT, and in our own experience it is not significantly different from CRRT circuits with no anticoagulation.

Complications: Heparin-bonded membranes and lines increase costs. Despite heparin bonding of the membrane, we have found that the most common site of CRRT circuit clotting remains the hemofilter/dialyzer (32). As yet, no patient treated with a heparin-bonded circuit has developed either type of heparin-associated thrombocytopenia.

H. Regional Citrate Anticoagulation

Sodium citrate has been used as an anticoagulant for many years.

Structure: Citrate is a six-carbon molecule with a molecular weight of 160 daltons. It is an intermediate of the tricarboxylic acid cycle.

Action: Citrate chelates ionized calcium, which is necessary for the coagulation cascade, and prevents clotting when the ionized calcium is $\leq$0.25 mmol/L (normal 1.1–1.3).

Clinical use: Citrate is used in several centers as the extracorporeal anticoagulant of choice for all patients, whereas in other centers it is reserved for those at high risk of hemorrhage.

Half-life: The half-life of citrate is very short because it is readily removed by dialysis, reducing systemic anticoagulation, and neutralized when returned to the central venous blood.

Dosage schedule: Regional citrate CRRT circuits do not require priming with heparinized saline. Most centers have used 0.14 molar trisodium citrate (4% solution), infused prior to the dialyzer at a ratio of citrate flow to blood flow of 3–4%. It is recommended that when the citrate infusion is set up, citrate be infused as close to the arterial/venous access catheter as possible to both maximize mixing and allow anticoagulation of the entire extracorporeal circuit. In clinical practice, the initial citrate infusion is usually set at 170 mL/h for a blood flow rate of 100 mL/min. Thereafter, the infusion rate is adjusted according to postfilter WBACT times, aiming for a WBACT of 180–220 seconds with a citrate infusion rate of 100–200 mL/h (62,75).

When regional citrate anticoagulation is used, the predilutional fluid must not contain calcium or bicarbonate; therefore 0.9% saline is often used (62). A special hyponatremic dialysate (117 mmol/L) is required containing no calcium or alkali (33), with a relatively high chloride content of 122.5 mmol/L (75). The hyponatremic dialysate is required because of the high sodium load prefilter due to the combination of trisodium citrate and normal saline predilution. Dextrose is added to the dialysate to maintain osmolality. Infusion of calcium or bicarbonate prior to or as dialysate would affect ionized calcium concentrations and therefore interfere with citrate anticoagulation.

As calcium is complexed with citrate and lost into the dialysate, calcium is infused as calcium chloride centrally to maintain a normal ionized calcium returning to the patient (33). Most patients requiring 40–45 mL/h of a 0.735% calcium chloride solution (1 mEq/10 mL) to maintain a normal systemic ionized calcium (75).

Monitoring: Bedside monitoring with estimation of whole blood activated clotting times can be performed, aiming for a WBACT of 190–275 seconds, and the citrate infusion adjusted accordingly. Initially the WBACT should be measured every 2 hours until a stable infusion rate has been achieved. In addition to monitoring the anticoagulation, it is recommended that regular biochemical monitoring also be required, with measurement of the ionized calcium, electrolytes, and bicarbonate every 12 hours and adjustment of the calcium infusion as needed (75).

Filter patency: Several centers have found regional citrate anticoagulation to be very effective, in terms of both dialyzer membrane patency and circuit life, with filter patency and circuit life prolonged for 4–6 days. These results are substantially better than those reported with other anticoagulants.

Advantages: Regional citrate anticoagulation is inexpensive and can be readily monitored at the bedside. For extracorporeal use it has advantages over heparin with a marked reduction in the incidence of hemorrhagic complications reported (73); one center reported no hemorrhagic complications during more than 10,000 hours of CRRT (75). Citrate anticoagulation does not lead to platelet activation, which may be why circuit life and filter patency are so prolonged compared to heparin. The alkalinization associated with citrate may be an advantage when managing patients with lactic acidosis.

Complications: A drawback of citrate anticoagulation is the complexity of the CRRT circuit and the requirement for a specialized dialysate/substitution fluid. Currently these fluids are not commercially available, and therefore for successful regional citrate anticoagulation a center must have access to a sterile fluids manufacturer to produce the volumes of fluid required. However, those centers that have been able to manufacture their own fluids continue to use citrate, showing that the benefits outweigh the inconvenience.

Because each citrate molecule is eventually metabolised, mainly in the liver, to three bicarbonate molecules, alkalosis may occur. To help prevent alkalosis, normal saline is given as a predilution fluid and calcium is given as calcium chloride. By giving a high chloride load the risk of developing metabolic alkalosis is reduced (88). These biochemical disturbances most commonly occur with pumped hemofiltration circuits, because the clearance of citrate is less than during dialysis which leads to excessive alkalosis (75). Up to 26% of patients will develop a mild metabolic alkalosis, more commonly in those with hepatic dysfunction and patients requiring support with large amounts of blood products (containing acid citrate dextrose anticoagulant). Alkalosis can be simply managed by either reducing the citrate infusion rate if the WBACT is high or increasing bicarbonate losses and chloride gain. This can be done most effectively by increasing the dialysate flow or less effectively by increasing the predilution normal saline infusion, because both fluids will result in greater bicarbonate losses in the filter/dialyzer and provide additional chloride. In extreme cases the alkalosis can be controlled by titrating the infusion rate of a 0.2 M HCl through a major vein (75).

Hypercitratemia has been reported in 10–15% of patients—usually those with some degree of hepatic dysfunction. This can usually be readily corrected by reducing the rate of the citrate infusion to 1.5–2.5% of the blood flow. In most cases this occurs in the setting of alkalosis, but it may also develop in cases of severe tissue acidosis. Hypernatremia has also been reported in less than 10% of patients (44), more commonly during hemofiltration, because the prefilter sodium load cannot be removed as well as during dialysis.

Occasionally, despite titrating the citrate dose according to ACT and calcium infusion according to ionized calcium concentration, patients may develop hypercitratemia, hypercalcemia, and metabolic acidosis (89). This usually occurs in the setting of acute renal failure with muscle damage and initial hypocalcemia. Despite a normal ionized plasma calcium, total plasma calciums in excess of 4.0 mmol/L have been observed in association with hypercitratemia (plasma citrate > 20 mmol/L, normal range 0.07–0.14 mmol/L) (89). Such hypercitratemia suggests hepatic dysfunction, and if the citrate cannot be metabolized through to bicarbonate, then the patient will become acidotic due to the loss of plasma bicarbonate through the dialyzer.

More recently, anticoagulation with isotonic acid citrate dextrose has been introduced, rather than trisodium citrate. This may reduce the incidence of biochemical abnormalities observed with citrate anticoagulation.

I. Prostacyclin

Prostacyclin is a natural anticoagulant produced by endothelial cells via the breakdown of arachidonic acid.

Structure: Prostacyclin is one of the prostaglandins, a group of polyunsaturated fatty acids, containing a cyclopentane ring with two side chains.

Action: Prostacyclin (PGI_2) blocks platelet activation and aggregation and promotes vasodilatation through the suppression of platelet cyclic AMP. Although other prostanoids (PGE_1 and PGE_2) have similar antiplatelet activities, they are not as potent as PGI_2 (28).

Clinical use: PGI_2 was first used to maintain charcoal hemoperfusion extracorporeal circuits in patients with liver disease to prevent platelet activation. Subsequently, PGI_2 has been shown to be effective in maintaining extracorporeal circuits in patients at risk of hemorrhage, initially in hemodialysis patients and more recently during CRRT (4,31). In addition, PGI_2 may also offer a benefit in improving tissue oxygen delivery, especially in patients with liver failure (90).

Half-life: The half-life of PGI_2 can be measured in minutes. Once infused, some PGI_2 is lost in the filtrate/dialysate, some is bound to albumin, and free PGI_2 is metabolized in the lungs (21).

Dosage schedule: Most centers use a standard infusion of 5 ng/kg/min, with a range of 2.5–10. The CCRT circuit is rinsed with heparinized saline prior to starting treatment. Prior to commencing CRRT, PGI_2 should be infused systematically, starting initially at 0.5 ng/kg/min, after which the dose is slowly increased to 5 ng/kg/min. Once this dose has been achieved, CRRT is commenced and the infusion site switched to the CRRT circuit (4).

Monitoring: PGI_2 does not affect standard anticoagulation tests, apart from the bleeding time (18), and it is therefore difficult to titrate the dose to any individual patient. Thromboelastography shows the effect of PGI_2 by reducing the maximum amplitude of the trace. However, as PGI_2 is rapidly bound to platelets, changes in dosage have no discernible effect on the thromboelastograph tracing once the platelets are saturated with PGI_2 (91).

Filter patency: PGI_2 has been successfully used as an anticoagulant in both pediatric (73) and adult acute renal failure (4) because platelet activation appears to be the key to clotting developing within the CRRT circuit (28). However, the effect of PGI_2 on filter patency and circuit life varies from center to center. In spontaneous circuits, PGI_2 has been reported to improve filter patency and circuit life in both children and adults when compared to standard heparin (4,73). In pumped CRRT circuits, some studies have observed an improvement in filter patency (18,55) and circuit life compared to heparin, whereas others did not (4,28).

Advantages: Anticoagulation with PGI_2 has been reported by many groups to significantly reduce the incidence of hemorrhage when compared to standard heparin, and it is used in many centers for patients at serious risk of hemorrhage (18,21,55). By reducing platelet activation, PGI_2 also reduces leukocyte activation and cytokine generation, leading to improved circuit biocompatibility compared to standard heparin. PGI_2 may also help improve tissue oxygen delivery, which may be important in patients with sepsis syndrome and those with liver failure where there is evidence of tissue hypoxia (90).

Disadvantages: The systemic vasodilatory effects of PGI_2 include hypotension due to reduced systemic and pulmonary vasodilatation. Because the half-life of PGI_2 is some 2 minutes, these side effects can be readily reversed by reducing or stopping the infusion. These vasodilatory changes can lead to an imbalance between tissue oxygen delivery and oxygen requirement, for example, in the lung increased shunting, in the heart reduced coronary perfusion, and in the brain cerebral hypoxia and increased intracranial pressure (91). These adverse effects can be reduced by optimizing cardiac filing pressures prior to the administration of PGI_2 and by giving albumin solutions that bind free PGI_2 (4). In addition, infusing PGI_2 prior to the filter reduces the systemic effects, because up to 40% is removed during passage through the dialyzer (73).

The other prostanoids, PGE_1 and PGE_2, have similar antiplatelet activities, but they are not as potent as PGI_2 and their systemic vasodilatatory effects should be minimal (28).

Although PGI_2 is an effective anticoagulant, its cost has reduced its widespread use. Occasionally PGI_2 is used in patients with other complications, such as pulmonary hypertension and acute liver failure, where its effects on tissue blood flow are thought to have a beneficial effect (81,90).

J. Heparin and Prostacyclin

Clinical use: Some groups have added PGI_2 to patients anticoagulated with standard heparin, who had repeated clotting of the CRRT circuit, to good effect (38,40).

Dosage schedule: Several centers have used a combination of PGI_2 (2–6.5 ng/kg/min) and standard heparin (200–350 IU/h) (18,39,40).

Monitoring: (See under heparin and PGI_2.) Most centers monitor as for standard heparin.

Filter patency: The combination of heparin and PGI_2 has been reported to achieve CRRT circuit lives of >48 hours (40). Other studies observed that the combination increased hemofilter/dialyzer patency when compared to heparin and PGI_2 alone, with filter patency maintained for up to 80 hours (44).

Advantages: The combination of heparin and PGI_2 results in greater filter patency (55) and circuit duration (38,40).

Complications: Apart from the additional cost and complexity of the circuit, careful comparison of the combination of heparin and PGI_2 showed no increase in the incidence of hemorrhage in one study (18), whereas in another, although the frequency was less than that for heparin, it was greater than that for PGI_2 alone (44).

K. Serine Protease Inhibitors

Aprotinin, gabexate, and nafamostat mesylate are serine protease inhibitors and were initially introduced to reduce hemorrhage.

1. Aprotinin

Structure: Aprotinin is a member of the bovine serpin superfamily and is a serine protease inhibitor.

Action: Bleeding is reduced due to inhibition of activation of kallikrein, trypsin, and plasmin. At the higher doses used during CRRT or cardiopulmonary bypass, aprotinin also inhibits antiplasmin (13). The effects of aprotinin on the coagulation system depend upon the circulating plasma concentration, because its affinity for plasmin is much greater than that for kallikrein (74). Thus, at a plasma concentration of 125 kIU/mL (kallikrein inactivation units), aprotinin inhibitis fibrinolysis and complement activation. At higher concentrations (200 kIU/mL) kallikrein activation will be reduced (13), which may have additional benefits in the critically ill patient by improving cardiovascular stability. Reduced kallikrein activation will decrease blood coagulation activated by contact with anionic surfaces and the plastic of the extracorporeal circuit (16). In addition, by reducing neutrophil activation, and therefore cathepsin G release, aprotinin will also reduce secondary platelet activation by neutrophils.

Clinical use: We have used aprotinin in cases of postoperative hemorrhage following liver transplantation, when conservative management is appropriate and the patient must be anticoagulated due to an underlying prothrombotic condition (e.g., Budd-Chiari syndrome secondary to paroxysmal nocturnal hemoglobinuria or another prothrombotic state).

Half-life: Aprotinin has an elimination half-life of 2 hours.

Dosage schedule: Cardiopulmonary bypass circuits and extracorporeal oxygenators use an initial loading dose of 2×10^6 kIU followed by a maintenance infusion of 500,000 kIU/h. However, for CRRT we have used aprotinin at an infusion rate of 50,000 kIU/h. The CRRT circuit was initially primed with heparinized saline and predilution fluid replacement.

Monitoring: Aprotinin reduces activation of the intrinsic coagulation cascade, resulting in prolongation of the WBCT, ACT and KCCT. We have aimed for a predialyzer KCCT of 40–70 seconds.

Filter patency: In combination with predialyzer fluid replacement, we have experienced membrane patency in excess of 48 hours.

Advantages: Aprotinin allows anticoagulation and the maintenance of extracorporeal circuits in cases of patients with active hemorrhage who require anticoagulation to protect from an underlying prothrombotic tendency. Monitoring can be done at the bedside or by simple standard laboratory tests.

Complications: Unfortunately, the current costs of aprotinin preclude its general use.

2. Nafamostat Mesylate

Gabexate maleate, a short-acting serine protease (half-life = 80 s), which acts at the same sites as ATIII (16), has been replaced by nafamostat mesylate (MW = 540 daltons) in clinical practice.

Structure: 6-Amido-2-naphthyl *p*-guanidinobenzoate dimethanesulfonate.

Action: This agent inhibits the action of thrombin, factor Xa and XIIa.

Clinical use: Used extensively in Japan, nafamostat has been reported to reduce the incidence of hemorrhage compared to heparin and LMWH in high-risk patients (92,93).

Dose schedule: Because nafamostat is removed during its passage through the extracorporeal circuit, the recommended infusion rate is greater for hemodiafiltration circuits (0.3 mg/kg/h) than for hemofiltration (0.1 mg/kg/h).

Half-life: Nafamostat has a half-life of 5–8 minutes (92).

Monitoring: By inhibiting thrombin, factor Xa, and XIIa, nafamostat prolongs the WBCT, ACT, and APTT, thus allowing bedside monitoring (72). A strong positive correlation has been reported between plasma nafamostat concentration and the ACT (92). Thus, with a short half-life the infusion rate can be adjusted according to the bedside ACT (target 150 s) to achieve adequate anticoagulation.

Filter patency: Treatment with nafamostat has been shown to result in an increase in thrombin–antithrombin III complexes and prothrombin fragments during CRRT (44,93). Thus, nafamostat does not prevent the development of intravascular/extracorporeal clotting and may not result in prolonged hemofilter/dialyzer patency and circuit life (58).

Advantages: Because nafamostat is readily removed during hemofiltration and dialysis (40%) (72), anticoagulation is maximum at entry to the hemofilter/dialyzer and the concentration returning to the patient is reduced, with systemic concentrations being <4% of the prehemofilter concentration (92). Not surprisingly, the incidence of reported hemorrhage (4%) was much less than that with standard heparin (67%) and LMWH (29%) (92,93).

Complications: Treatment with nafamostat is currently estimated at $300 per day. Nafamostat is readily adsorbed to the negatively charged polyacrylonitrile membrane, making initial dosing schedules problematical. In hemodialysis, some patients developed a syndrome of myalgia and arthralgia.

Rarely, nafamostat has been reported to cause eosinophilia and bone marrow suppression in hemodialysis patients. As yet, bone marrow suppression has not been reported during CRRT.

L. Hirudin

Hirudin, which comes from leeches, and its recombinant forms are direct inhibitors of thrombin.

Structure: Hirudologue is a synthetic recombinant form of hirudin.

Action: Hirudin is the most potent inhibitor of thrombin known. It also inhibits the action of factor IXa.

Clinical use: Experience with hirudin has mainly been following cardiac angioplasty, and for intermittent hemodialysis, although some centers are now reporting their experience using hirudin for CRRT (71).

Dosage schedule: Most centers have reported using intermittent boluses followed by an infusion. This has led in many cases to over anticoagulation, and therefore a continuous infusion is now the preferred option, although the dose infused varies from 0.003 to 0.013 mg/kg/h, depending upon the individual patient and also the membrane used. Hirudin appears to be adsorbed to polyacrylonitrile and some other high flux membranes, but it is not affected when low flux polysulphone and/or cellulose based membranes are used. This membrane effect may account for the wide discrepancy in dosage schedules.

Monitoring: Although in theory the effect of hirudin can be monitored at the bedside by both the ACT and APTT, in practice these measurements have not provided an accurate assessment of anticoagulation. This may be due to differences in membrane adsorption, as ideally the ACT and APTT are measured pre-dialyzer/hemofilter. Hirudin activity can also be assessed by functional assays of the hirudin-thrombin complex.

Filter patency: Preliminary data suggests that anticoagulation with hirudin is equally effective as heparin, but not as good as citrate.

Complications: Difficulties in obtaining a standard dosage schedule have resulted in either an excess of hemorrhage, due to over anticoagulation coupled with the relatively long half life, or circuit clotting due to inadequate anticoagulation. Hopefully, with greater clinical usage these initial problems will be overcome. Hemorrhage requires prompt treatment with fresh frozen plasma.

M. Platelet Antibodies

Trials are currently in progress assessing the benefits of using recombinant monoclonal antibodies to platelet glycoprotein surface receptors (GpIIb/IIIa) in patients undergoing coronary artery angioplasty and stenting. Platelets are the major factor in determining clot formation in the extracorporeal circuit (19,44); the effectiveness of platelet antibodies given as a bolus at the start of CRRT on membrane patency and circuit life remains to be determined.

N. Low Molecular Weight Dextrans

Low molecular weight dextrans (LMWDs) were introduced as an artificial blood substitute and then used in vascular surgery to prevent graft thrombosis.

Structure: LMWDs are produced by the digestive action of strains of *L. mesenteroides* on sucrose.

Action: LMWDs, when infused in large volumes, inhibit the action of vWF, and also have a fibrinoplastic effect, weakening fibrin formation and polymerization. They accelerate the action of thrombin in converting fibrinogen to fibrin, which then makes the clot more amenable to fibrinolysis by plasmin (74). In addition, LMWDs are also adsorbed onto platelet membranes, reducing platelet function by preventing platelet aggregation (13).

Clinical use: Limited clinical data are available.

Dosage schedule: One controlled trial used a 10% LMWD solution–infused prefilter at a rate of 25 mL/h.

Monitoring: In doses of up to 1.5 g/kg LMWDs do not affect standard laboratory clotting tests, but do increase the bleeding time. Thus, the only bedside test able to monitor the effects of LMWDs is the thromboelastograph.

Filter patency rates: In one small study the CRRT mean circuit duration was reported in excess of 30 hours (94) but did not differ from that of predilution alone.

Advantages: By reducing platelet activation and in combination with their effects on fibrin formation, LMWDs in theory should be effective extracorporeal anticoagulants.

Complications: Unless a thromboelastograph is used, the anticoagulant effects of LMWDs are difficult to assess. Thus, patients may be either under- or over-anticoagulated.

LMWDs have been reported to increase the incidence of acute renal failure in patients following cardiac bypass surgery. It is unknown whether the daily administration of 500–1000 mL of LMWD leads to additional renal damage and delay in the recovery from acute renal failure.

Due to the effect of LMWDs on clot stability, it is advised that they not be used in neurosurgical cases requiring CRRT and other clinical conditions in which a secondary hemorrhage could have major adverse consequences.

O. No Anticoagulation

Ideally, all CRRT circuits would be anticoagulant free to reduce the risk of potential hemorrhage.

Action: To achieve successful anticoagulation-free CRRT, thought is required in the design of the circuit (Fig. 6). The two most effective mechanical methods of maintaining the extracorporeal circuit involve preventing stagnation and reducing blood viscosity

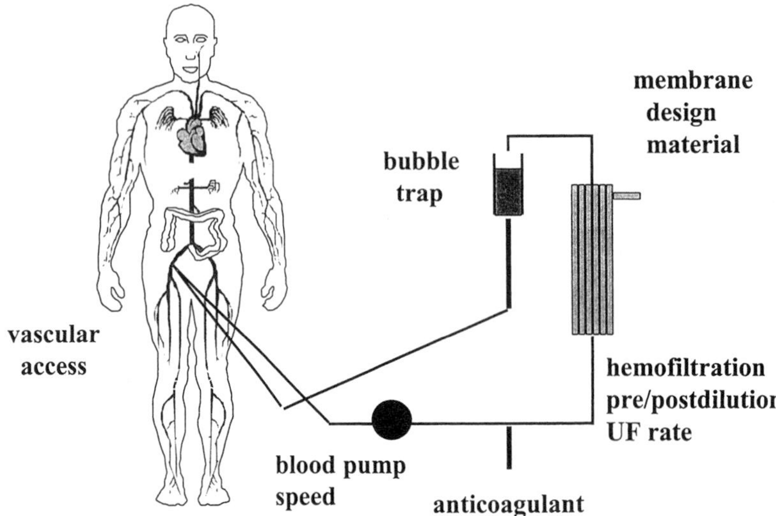

Fig. 6 CRRT circuit: the key sites of contact activation are membrane, vascular access, blood pump, and venous air detector. The sites of thrombus formation are membrane, venous air detector, and vascular access.

(50,51). The slowest flow in the circuit is through the hemofilter/dialyzer, leading to red blood cell aggregation (21). Activation of platelets and leukocytes accelerates this cellular aggregation. Thus, the anticoagulation-free CRRT circuit starts with a low-resistance vascular access designed to produce laminar flow with minimal contact activation. Then there should be a minimum of blood lines to reduce the length of the extracorporeal circuit and to reduce contact activation and thermal losses, with a minimum of joints or connectors to reduce unnecessary turbulent flow (31). Stasis in the venous air detector chamber should be minimized; we routinely return postfilter fluid into the air detector chamber to reduce the air/blood interface and reduce stasis (21). A biocompatible membrane is required to reduce contact activation (24,26). Paradoxically, high blood pump speeds are to be avoided, as they can increase contact activation (31). Blood viscosity can be reduced during passage through the hemofilter/dialyzer by giving prefilter fluid (60) and by avoiding excessive blood transfusion.

Clinical use: Anticoagulation-free CRRT is traditionally used in patients at high risk of hemorrhage or actively bleeding. Most groups have observed that patients with thrombocytopenia can be successfully treated without anticoagulation (19,54). Depending upon the balance between coagulation cascade activation and fibrinolysis, patients with coagulopathies and liver disease may also be managed without anticoagulants.

Dosage schedule: Most centers prime the CRRT with heparinized saline and then rinse with saline. Thereafter the key is effective predilution (1.0–2.0 L/h) to minimize hemoconcentration within the hemofilter/dialyzer. Dialysis is preferable to hemofiltration to minimize ultrafiltration losses and hemoconcentration within the dialyzer.

Monitoring: We use the urea dialysate-to-plasma ratio to assess whether a hemofilter/dialyzer is developing clotting within the membrane and should be exchanged.

Filter patency: Several groups, including pediatric centers, have tried anticoagulant-free CRRT circuits, both spontaneous and pumped, in patients adjudged to be at risk of hemorrhage and have found that circuit life was similar to that achieved with their standard anticoagulant regimen (30,41).

Advantages: No anticoagulation obviates the need for special monitoring of extracorporeal anticoagulation. In cases of patients at risk of hemorrhage, if hemorrhage does continue or develops during CRRT, then extracorporeal anticoagulants cannot be implicated.

Disadvantages: Without careful thought as to the design of the CRRT circuit, especially with inadequate vascular access, anticoagulant-free CRRT circuit life and filter patency may be reduced, preventing successful treatment.

VII. SUMMARY

To reduce the incidence of iatrogenic hemorrhage, ideally all CRRT circuits should be anticoagulant free. This can be accomplished by careful design of the circuit and choice of patient—thrombocytopenic or at risk of hemorrhage. The advent of heparin-bonded membranes, lines, and vascular access catheters may help achieve the goal of no additional anticoagulant. In addition, the development of new blood pump technology will help reduce contact activation and do away with a separate venous air detector chamber.

Some patients, however, will develop premature clotting of the CRRT circuit; provided this is not due to inadequate vascular access, anticoagulation is required. Of the currently available regimens, citrate and the synthetic heparinoids appear to have the greatest safety profile in terms of reducing the risk of hemorrhage.

Systemic anticoagulation may be required as part of the general management of patients in acute renal failure treated by CRRT (e.g., postcardiac surgery, major venous thrombosis). Under these circumstances, anticoagulation with heparin or LMWHs appears appropriate, and if heparin-associated antibodies develop, a heparinoid can be substituted if systemic anticoagulation is required.

ACKNOWLEDGMENTS

I wish to acknowledge the help and support of my colleagues Paul Sweny, Doreen Browne, and George Collee and the nursing staff of the intensive care unit at the Royal Free Hospital.

REFERENCES

1. Macias WL, Clark WR. Azotemia control by extracorporeal therapy in patients with acute renal failure. New Horizons 1995; 3:688–698.
2. Kramer P, Böhler J, Kehr A, Gröne HJ, Schrader J, Matthaei D, Scheler F. Trans Am Soc Atif Intern Organs 1982; 28:28–32.
3. Olbricht C, Mueller C, Schurek HJ, Stolte H. Treatment of acute renal failure in patients with multiple organ failure by continuous spontaneous hemofiltration. Trans Am Soc Artif Intern Organs 1982; 28:33–37.
4. Davenport A, Will EJ, Davison AM. Comparison of the use of standard heparin and prostacyclin anticoagulation in spontaneous circuits in patients with combined acute renal and hepatic failure. Nephron 1994; 66:431–437.
5. Tabuchi N, de Haan J, Gallandat Huet RC, Boonstra PW, van Oeveren W. Gelatin use impairs platelet adhesion during cardiothoracic surgery. Thromb Haemostasis 1995; 74:1447–1151.
6. Blei A, Olafsson S, Webster S, Levy R. Complications of intracranial pressure monitoring in fulminant hepatic failure. Lancet 1993; 341:157–158.
7. Atillasoy E, Berk PD. Extracorporeal liver support: historical background and critical analysis. In: Lee WM, Williams R, eds. Acute Liver Failure. Cambridge University Press, 1997:223–244.
8. Ellis AJ, Sussman NL, Kelly JH, Williams R. Clinical experience with an extracorporeal liver assist device. In: Lee WM, Williams R, eds. Acute Liver Failure. Cambridge University Press, 1997:255–266.
9. Hesselvik F, Blomback M, Brodin B, Maller R. Coagulation fibrinolysis and kallikrein systems in sepsis: relation to outcome. Crit Care Med 1989; 17:724–733.
10. Hesselvik JF, Malm J, Dahlback B, Blomback M. Protein C, protein S and C4b binding protein in severe infection and septic shock. Thromb Hemostat 1991; 65:126–129.
11. Bone RC, Balk RA, Cerra FB, Dellinger RP, Fein AM, Knaus WA, Schein RM, Sibbald WJ. Definitions for sepsis and organ failure and guidelines for the use of innovative therapies in sepsis. The ACCP/SCCM Consensus Conference Committee. American College of Chest Physicians/Society of Critical Care Medicine. Chest 1992; 101:1644–1655.
12. Rabelink TJ, Zwaginga JJ, Koomans HA, Sixma JJ. Thrombosis and hemostasis in renal disease. Kid Int 1994; 46:287–296.
13. Hunt BJ. Acquired coagulation disorders. In: Weatherall DJ, Ledingham DJJ, Warrell DA, eds. Oxford Texbook of Medicine. 3d ed. Oxford Medical Publishers, 1996:3653–3661.
14. Cazenave JP, Mulvihill. Interactions of blood with surfaces: hemocompatibility and thromboresistance of biomaterials. Contrib Nephrol 1988; 62:118–127.
15. Neild GH, Barratt TM. Acute renal failure associated with microangiopathy. In: Davison AM, Cameron JS, Grünfeld J-P, Kerr DNS, Ritz E, Winearls CG, eds. Oxford Textbook of Renal Medicine. 2nd ed. Oxford Medical Publications, 1649–1666.
16. Schmidt B, Mujais SK. Evaluation of dialysis membrane-blood compatibility: experimental methods. Contrib Nephrol 1995; 113:32–44.
17. Barraud F, Ferrand E, Hira M, Chagneau C, Pourrat O, Robert R. Variation of platelet count during continuous

venovenous hemofiltration. Proceedings Continuous Hemofiltration Therapies in the ICU, Paris, 1996, p. 12.
18. Langenecker SA, Felfernig M, Werba A, Mueller CM, Chiari A, Zimpfer M. Anticoagulation with prostacyclin and heparin during continuous venovenous hemofiltration. Crit Care Med 1994; 22:1774–1781.
19. Martin PY, Chevrolet JC, Suter P, Favre H. Anticoagulation in patients treated by continuous veno-venous hemofiltration: a retrospective study. Am J Kidney Dis 1994; 24:806–812.
20. Boldt J, Menges T, Wollbruck M, Sonneborn S, Hempelmann G. Continuous hemofiltration and platelet function in critically ill patients. Crit Care Med 1994; 22:1150–1160.
21. Davenport A, Kirby SA. Hemofiltration/dialysis treatment in patients with acute renal failure. Care Crit Ill 1996; 12:54–58.
22. Sloand JA, Sloand EM. Studies on platelet membrane glycoproteins and platelet function during hemodialysis. J Am Soc Nephrol 1997; 8:799–803.
23. Churchill DN. Efficiency and biocompatibility of membranes. Contrib Nephrol 1995; 113:60–71.
24. Hakim RM. Clinical implications of hemodialysis membrane biocompatibility. Kidney Int 1993; 44:484–494.
25. Webb AR, Mythen MG, Jacobson D, Mackie IJ. Maintaining blood flow in the extracorporeal circuit: hemostasis and anticoagulation. Intensiv Care Med 1995; 21: 84–93.
26. Schmidt B, Mujais SK. Evaluation of dialysis membrane-blood compatibility: experimental methods. Contrib Nephrol 1995; 113:32–44.
27. Langley PG, Keays R, Hughes RD, Forbes A, Delvos U, Williams R. Antithrombin III supplementation reduces heparin requirement and platelet loss during hemodialysis of patients with fulminant hepatic failure. Hepatol 1991; 14:251–256.
28. Salmon J, Cardigan R, Mackie I, Cohen SL, Machin S, Singer M. Continuous venovenous hemofiltration using polyacrylonitrile filters does not activate contact system and inrinsic system coagulation pathways. Intensiv Care Med 1997; 23:38–43.
29. Stefanidis I, Hägel J, Kierdorf H, Maurin N. Influencing hemostasis during continuous venovenous hemofiltration after acute renal failure: comparison with hemodialysis. Contrib Nephrol 1995; 116:140–144.
30. Bellomo R, Teede H, Boyce N. Anticoagulant regimens in acute continuous hemodiafiltration: a comparative study. Intensiv Care Med 1993; 19:329–332.
31. Davenport A. The coagulation system in the critically ill patient with acute renal failure and the effect of an extracorporeal circuit. Am J Kidney Dis 1997; 30(suppl 4):S20–27.
32. Holt AW, Bierer P, Berstein AD, Bury LJ, Vedig AE. Continuous renal replacement therapy in critically ill patients: monitoring circuit function. Anaesth Intens Care 1996; 24:423–429.
33. Mehta RL. Anticoagulation strategies or continuous renal replacement therapies: what works? Am J Kidney Dis 1996; 28(suppl 3):S8–S14.
34. Gretz N, Quintel M, Ragaller M, Odenwälder W, Bender HJ, Rohmeiss P, Strauch M. Low-dose heparinization for anticoagulation in intensive care patients on continuous hemofiltration. Contrib Nephrol 1995; 116:130–135.
35. Ronco C. Continuous renal replacement therapies for the treatment of acute renal failure in intensive care patients. Clin Nephrol 1993; 40:187–198.
36. Golper TA. Continuous arteriovenous hemofiltration in acute renal failure. Am J Kidney Dis 1985; 6:373–386.
37. Erdenm Y, Haznedaroglu IC, Celik I, Yalcin AU, Turgan C, Caglar S. Coagulation, fibrinolysis and fibrinolysis inhibitors in hemodialysis patients: contribution of arteriovenous fistula. Nephrol Dial Transplant 1996; 11: 1299–1305.
38. Olbricht CJ, Schurek HJ, Tytul S, Muller C, Stolte H. Comparison between Scribner shunt and femoral catheters as vascular access for continuous arteriovenous hemofiltration. In: Kramer P, ed. Arteriovenous Hemofiltration. Berlin: Springer-Verlag, 1985:57–66.
39. Weiss L, Danielson BG, Wikström B, Hedstrand U, Wahlberg J. Continuous arteriovenous hemofiltration in the treatment of 100 critically ill patients with acute renal failure: report on clinical outcome and nutritional aspects. Clin Nephrol 1989; 31:184–189.
40. Stevens PE, Davies SP, Brown EA, Riley B, Gower PE, Kox W. Continuous arteriovenous hemodialysis in critically ill patients. Lancet 1988; ii:150–152.
41. Smoyer WE, McAdams C, Kaplan BS, Sherbottle JR. Determinants of survival in pediatric continuous hemofiltration. J Am Soc Nephrol 1995; 6:1401–1409.
42. McLaughlin K, Jones B, Mactier R, Porteus C. Long-term vascular access for hemodialysis using silicon dual lumen catheters with guidewire replacement of catheters for technique salvage. Am J Kidney Dis 1997; 29: 553–559.
43. Jean G, Chazot C, Vanel T, Charra B, Terrat JC, Calemard E, Laurent G. Central venous catheters for hemodialysis: looking for optimal blood flow. Nephrol Dial Transplant 1997; 12:1689–1691.
44. Favre H, Martin Y, Stoermann C. Anticoagulation in continuous extracorporeal renal replacement therapy. Semin Dial 1996; 9:112–118.
45. Athirakul K, Conlon P, Schwab S. Cuffed central venous hemodialysis catheters and adequacy of dialysis. J Am Soc Nephrol 1996; 7:1402.
46. Zobel G, Ring E, Kuttnig M, Grubbauer HM. Continuous arteriovenous hemofiltration versus continuous venovenous hemofiltration in critically ill pediatric patients. Contrib Nephrol 1991; 93:257–260.
47. Cicchetti T, Senatore RP, Fransima F, Ferrari S, Striano U, Milei M, Cosentino S. Dialysis treatment using an

ethylene vinyl alcohol membrane and no anticoagulation for chronic uremic patients. Artif Organs 1993; 17: 816–819.
48. Zobel G, Ring E, Rödel S. Prognosis in pediatric patients with multiple organ system failure and continuous extracorporeal renal support. Contrib Nephrol 1995; 116:163–168.
49. Davenport A, Will EJ, Davison AM. The effect of the direction of dialysate flow on the efficiency of continuous arteriovenous hemodialysis. Blood Purif 1990; 8: 329–336.
50. Turitto VT, Weiss HJ, Baumgartner HR. Rheological factors influencing platelet interaction with vessel wall surfaces. J Rheol 1979; 23:735–749.
51. Aarts PAMM, Heethaar RM, Sixma JJ. Red blood cell deformibility influences platelet vessel wall interaction in flowing blood. Blood 1983; 62:214–217.
52. Olbricht CJ, Haubitz M, Häbel U, Frei U, Koch K-M. Continuous arteriovenous hemofiltration: in vivo functional characteristics and its dependence on vascular access and filter design. Nephron 1990; 55:49–57.
53. Yohay DA, Butterly DW, Schwab SJ, Quarles LD. Continuous arteriovenous hemodialysis: effect of dialyzer geometry. Kidney Int 1992; 42:448–451.
54. Van der Wetering J, Westendorp RGJ, van der Hoeven JG, Stolk B, Feuth JDM, Chang PC. Heparin use in continuous renal renal replacement therapies: the struggle between filter coagulation and patient hemorrhage. J Am Soc Nephrol 1996; 7:145–150.
55. Silvester W, Honoré P, Sieffert E, Valentine J, Wagle S, Smithies M, Bihari D. Effect of heparin, prostacyclin or combination, and effect of polyacrylonitrile or polysulphone membranes on filter survival in critically ill patients on continuous venovenous hemofiltration. Proceedings Continuous Hemofiltration Therapies in the ICU, Paris, 1996, p. 16.
56. Lang S, Küchle C, Fricke H, Schiffl H. Biocompatible intermittent hemodialysis. New Horizons 1995; 3:680–687.
57. Lane DA, Bowry SK. The scientific basis for selection of measures of thrombogenicity. Nephrol Dial Transplant 1994; 9(suppl 2):18–28.
58. Kaplan AA, Longnecker RE, Folkert VW. Suction assisted continuous arteriovenous hemofiltration. Trans Am Soc Artif Intern Organs 1983; 29:408–413.
59. Kaplan AA. Continuous arteriovenous hemofiltration-and related therapies. In: Jacobs C, Kjellstrand KE, Koch KM, Winchester JF, eds. Replacement of Renal Function by Dialysis. 4th ed. Boston: Kluwer Academic Publishers, 19xx:390–417.
60. David S, Cambi V. Hemofiltration: predilution versus post dilution. Contrib Nephrol 1992; 96:77–85.
61. MacLean AG, Goddard J, Harber M, Niadoo R, Davenport A, Sweny P. Lactate free dialysate for continuous hemodiafiltration. Effects on control of acidosis, blood pressure and inotrope requirement. Am Soc Nephrol 1996; 7:1413.
62. Mehta RL, McDonald BR, Aguilar MM, Ward DM. Regional citrate anticoagulation for continuous arteriovenous hemodialysis in critically ill patients. Kidney Int 1990; 38:976–981.
63. Ward DM, Mehta RL. Extracorporeal management of acute renal failure patients at risk of high bleeding. Kidney Int 1993; (suppl 41):S237–S244.
64. Samuelsson O, Amiral J, Attman P-O, Bennegård K, Biörck S, Larsson G, Tengborn L. Heparin-induced thrombocytopenia during continuous hemofiltration. Nephrol Dial Transplant 1995; 10:1768–1771.
65. Ronco C, Brendolan A, Bragantini L, Chiaramonte S, Feriani M, Fabris A, Dell'Aquila R, LaGreca G, Milan M. Continuous arteriovenous hemofiltration with AN69S membrane; procedures and experience. Kidney Int 1988; 33(suppl 24):S150–S153.
66. Mulvihill JN, Cazenave JP, Faradji A, Oberling F. Reduction de l'adhesion des plaquettes et de la formation d'un thrombus dans les circuits extracorporels de plasmapherese apres passivation des surfaces par l'albumine. 8eme Congr int CEC, Paris, 1983, p. 134.
67. Ellis A, Wendon JA, Williams R. Effect of albumin priming on hemofiltration circuits. 13th European Crit Care Meeting, Athens, 1996, p. 362.
68. Reeves JH, Seal PF, Voss AL, O'Connor C. Albumin priming does not prolong hemofilter life. ASAIO J 1997; 43:193–196.
69. Singer M, McNally T, Screaton G, Mackie I, Machin S, Cohen SL. Heparin clearance during continuous venovenous hemofiltration. Intensive Care Med 1994; 20: 212–215.
70. Nurmohamed MT, Knipscheer HC, Stevens P, Krediet RT, Roggekamp MC, Berckmans, ten Cate JW. Clinical experience with a new antithrombotic (dermatan sulfate) in chronic dialysis patients. Clin Nephrol 1993; 39:166–171.
71. Vanholder RC, Camez AA, Veys NM, Soria J, Mirshahi M, Sorai C, Ringoir R. Recombinant hirudin: a specific thrombin inhibiting anticoagulant for hemodialysis. Kidney Int 1994; 1754–1759.
72. Morikawa K, Akizawa T, Koshikawa S. Application for FUT-175, protease inhibitor, for an anticoagulant to hemodialysis. Jpn J Artif Organs 1983; 12:75.
73. Zobel G, Trop M, Muntean W, Ring E, Gleispach TA. Anticoagulation for continuous arteriovenous hemofiltration in children. Blood Purif 1988; 6:90–95.
74. Mackie IJ, Bull HA. Normal hemostasis and its regulation. Blood Rev 1989; 3:237–250.
75. Ward DM. The approach to anticoagulation in patients treated with extracorporeal therapy in the ICU. Adv Renal Replacement Ther 1997; 4:160–173.
76. Bastien O, French P, Paulus S, Filley S, Berruyer M, Dechavanne M. Antithrombin III deficiency during continuous veno-venous hemofiltration. Contrib Nephrol 1995; 116:154–158.
77. Stiekema JC, Van Griensen JM, Van Dinther TG, Cohen AF. A cross over comparison of the anti-clotting effects

of three low molecular weight heparins and glycosaminoglycuron. Br J Clin Pharmacol 1993; 36:51–56.

78. Jeffrey RF, Khan AA, Douglas JT, Will EJ, Davison AM. Anticoagulation with low molecular weight heparin (fragmin) during continuous hemodialysis in the intensive care unit. Artif Organs 1993; 17:717–720.
79. Wynckel A, Bernieh B, Toupance O, N'Guyen PH, Wong T, Lavaud S, Chanard J. Guidelines to the use of enoxparin in slow continuous dialysis. Contrib Nephrol 1991; 93:221–224.
80. Hory B. Hemodialysis with low molecular weight heparin versus standard heparin to standard heparin in hemodialysis/hemofiltration. Am J Med 1988; 84:566–567.
81. Davenport A. CRRT in the management of patients with liver disease. Seminar Dial 1996; 9:78–84.
82. Vun CM, Evans S, Chong BH. Cross reactivity study of low molecular weight heparins and heparinoid in heparin-induced thrombocytopenia. Thromb Res 1996; 81:525–532.
83. Nurmohamed MT, Knipscheer HC, Stevens P, Krediet RT, Roggekamp MC, Berckmans RJ, Ten Cate JW. Clinical experience with a new antithrombotic (dermatan sulfate) in chronic hemodialysis patients. Clin Nephrol 1993; 39:166–171.
84. von dem Borne PA, Meijers JC, Bouma BN. Effect of heparin on the activation of factor XI by fibrin bound thrombin. Thromb Haemostasis 1996; 76:347–353.
85. Mahul P, Raynaud J, Favre JP, Jospe R, Decousus H, Auboyer C. Heparin-induced thrombopenia during hemodialysis in intensive care: use of a low molecular weight heparinoid, ORG 10172 (Orgaran). Ann Fr Anesth Reanim 1995; 14:29–32.
86. Bannan S, Danby A, Cowan D, Ashraf S, Martin PG. Low heparinization with heparin-bonded bypass circuits: is it a safe strategy? Ann Thorac Surg 1997; 63: 663–668.
87. Sieffert E, Matéo J, Deligeon N, Payen D. Continuous venovenous hemofiltration using heparin coated or non heparin coated membranes in critically ill patients. Proceedings Continuous Hemofiltration Therapies, Paris, 1996, pp. 14–15.
88. Davenport A, Worth DP, Will EJ. Hypochloraemic alkalosis after high flux continuous hemofiltration and continuous arteriovenous hemofiltration with dialysis. Lancet 1988; i:658.
89. Nowak MA, Campbell TE. Profound hypercalcaemia in continuous venovenous hemofiltration dialysis with trisodium citrate anticoagulation and hepatic failure. Clin Chem 1997; 43:412–413.
90. Ellis A, Wendon J. Circulatory, respiratory, cerebral and renal derangements in acute liver failure: pathophysiology and management. Semin Liver Dis 1996; 16:379–388.
91. Davenport A, Will EJ, Davison EM. The effect of prostacyclin on intracranial pressure in patients with acute hepatic and renal failure. Clin Nephrol 1991; 25:151–157.
92. Ohtake Y, Hirasawa H, Sugai T, Oda S, Shiga H, Matsuda K, Kitamurs. Nafamostat mesylate as anticoagulant in continuous hemofiltration and continuous hemodialysis. Contrib Nephrol 1991; 93:215–217.
93. Shigemoto T, Shimaoka H, Atagi K, Satani M. Optimal anticoagulation during continuous hemofiltration and continuous hemodialysis for patients with multiple organ failure. Jpn J Artif Organs 1994; 23:380–384.
94. Palevsky PM, Burr R, Moreland L, Tokiwa Y, Greenberg A. Failure low molecular weight dextran to prevent clotting during continuous renal replacement therapy. ASAIO J 1995; 41:847–849.

13

Complications of Fluid Management in Continuous Renal Replacement Therapies

Ravindra L. Mehta
University of California, San Diego, San Diego, California

Fluid management is an integral component in the management of patients with acute renal failure (ARF) in the intensive care unit (ICU) setting. In the presence of a failing kidney, fluid removal is often a challenge and requires the use of high-dose diuretics with a variable response. It is often necessary in this setting to institute dialysis for volume control rather than metabolic control. Continuous renal replacement therapy (CRRT) techniques offer a significant advantage over intermittent dialysis for fluid control, however, if not carried out appropriately they can result in major complications. In order to utilize these therapies for their maximum potential, it is necessary to recognize the factors that influence fluid balance and have an understanding of the principles of fluid management with these techniques (1–4).

Over the last decade there has been a general trend to use aggressive fluid resuscitation for patients with multiorgan failure to achieve supranormal levels of oxygen delivery. This has been largely based on the findings of several studies that have shown that survival in critically ill surgical patients is associated with supranormal levels of cardiac output, oxygen delivery, and oxygen utilization (5,6). Although this concept has now been questioned (7,8), it is still an important factor in the management of the ICU patient. The end result is often a markedly edematous patient with fluid sequestration in all organs. Third spacing of fluids is common and fluid removal by glomerular filtration is limited by plasma refilling from the interstitial compartment. Most surgeons and intensivists who believe in the value of supranormal oxygen delivery are willing to accept edema as a side effect of fluid resuscitation, however, there is evidence to suggest that fluid overload by itself may be an important factor contributing to an adverse outcome. Lowell et al. (9) have shown that in a group of surgical patients mortality was related to the extent of fluid overload, with a 100% mortality in patients with more than 20% increase in fluid from baseline. This can be explained if one recognizes that the consequences of fluid excess are not limited to superficial edema but result in myocardial and gut edema, thereby compromising vital organ functions and promoting local ischemia. It is therefore essential that the strategy of fluid management be viewed in the context of permitting support without compromising vital organ function. The goals of fluid management in this setting are to remove fluid without compromising cardiac output, compensate for the increased fluid given to achieve hemodynamic stability, and maintain urine output. To achieve these goals it would be ideal to have the capability of unlimited fluid removal so that any amount of fluid intake can be easily accommodated without fluid retention and to have the ability to alter the rate of fluid removal at will. While glomerular filtration can easily achieve the first goal, it is extremely difficult to alter the rate of urine formation. CRRT techniques offer the flexibility required to achieve these goals.

I. PRINCIPLES OF FLUID MANAGEMENT WITH CRRT

CRRT techniques have two inherent characteristics that allow their use as highly effective methods of fluid control: utilization of highly permeable membranes and the continuous nature of the technique (10). Both of these factors permit unlimited fluid removal, which is limited only by the primary driving force (mean arterial pressure for nonpumped systems and pump speed for pumped systems) and the efficacy of the filter over time. The ability to remove large volumes of fluid can be manipulated in several different ways for fluid balance. As shown in Table 1, there are three levels of intervention. In Level 1 the ultrafiltrate volume obtained is limited to match the anticipated needs for fluid balance. This calls for an estimate of the amount of fluid to be removed over 8–24 hours and subsequent calculation of the ultrafiltration rate. This strategy is similar to that commonly used for intermittent hemodialysis and differs only in that the time to remove fluid is 24 hours instead of 3–4 hours. For example, if it is estimated that 4 L of fluid need to be removed over a 24-hour period, the ultrafiltration rate is set at approximately 170 mL/h. With this method the CRRT technique is used essentially as a means of achieving a fixed output per hour, but no attempt is made to manipulate the ultrafiltration rate or accommodate changes in fluid intake. As a consequence, replacement fluid may not be used and net fluid balance achieved may vary significantly from desired balance at the end of the time period. In some instances no attempt is made to set a particular ultrafiltrate rate, and fluid removed at the end of each time period (8–24 hours) is simply tabulated and listed as an output. Thus there is minimal control for fluid management.

In Level 2 the ultrafiltrate volume every hour is deliberately set to be greater than the hourly intake, and net fluid balance is achieved by hourly replacement fluid administration. In this method a greater degree of control is possible and fluid balance can be set to achieve any desired outcome. The success of this method depends on the ability to achieve ultrafiltration rates, which always exceed the anticipated intake. This allows flexibility in manipulation of the fluid balance so that for any given hour the fluid status could be net negative, positive, or even. A key advantage of this technique is that the net fluid balance achieved at the end of every hour is truly a reflection of the desired outcome. For instance, as described in the example previously, if 4 L of fluid are to be removed over 24 hours, the desired outcome every hour is −170 mL/h. This implies that the ultrafiltration rate should be ≥170 mL/h + intake every hour. The net fluid balance desired may or may not be achievable, however, this method permits control of overall fluid management using the CRRT technique. The amount of replacement fluid needed to achieve fluid balance is easily calculated using a flow sheet.

Level 3 extends the concept of Level 2 intervention to target the desired net balance every hour to achieve a specific hemodynamic parameter, e.g., central venous pressure (CVP), pulmonary artery wedge pressure (PAWP), or mean arterial pressure (MAP). Once a desired value for the hemodynamic parameter is determined, fluid balance can be linked to that value. For example, if it is desirable to keep a patients PAWP

Table 1 Approaches to Fluid Management

	Level 1	Level 2	Level 3
Component			
UF volume	Limited	>Intake	>Intake
Replacement	Minimal	Adjusted to achieve fluid balance	Adjusted to achieve fluid balance
Fluid balance	8-hourly	Hourly	Hourly, targeted
UF Pump	Yes	Yes	No
Advantages			
Simplicity	+++	++	+
Fluid balance	+	+++	+++
Regulate volume	+	++	+++
CRRT as support	+	++	+++
Disadvantages			
Nursing effort	+	++	+++
Errors in fluid balance	+	++	+++
Hemodynamic instability	+++	++	+
Fluid overload	+++	+	+

Table 2 Sliding Scale for Volume Adjustment

Target parameter[a] (mmHg)	
Desired volume change (mL/h)	
PAWP <6	+175 mL and notify nephrologist on call
PAWP 6–8	+125 mL
PAWP 9–11	+75 mL
PAWP 12–14	Zero balance
PAWP 15–17	−50 mL

[a]Pulmonary artery wedge pressure.

between 14 and 16 mmHg, a sliding scale for hourly fluid management can be formulated so that for PAWP values of 12–14 mmHg net fluid balance is maintained at zero, for values >14 mmHg fluid is removed, and for values <12 mmHg fluid is replaced (Table 2). In essence this method maximally utilizes the capacity of CRRT techniques to control fluids. A key issue to recognize here is that by incorporating this level, CRRT techniques have tremendous flexibility and are not simply devices for fluid removal but allow overall control of fluid management as fluid regulatory devices. This external control is a key advantage over intermittent hemodialysis. Additionally it can be viewed as an advantage over the normal kidney wherein there is limited control possible. In general, greater control calls for more effort and consequently results in improved outcomes.

II. PRACTICAL ISSUES IN FLUID MANAGEMENT

A. Prescription

This is a key issue in the proper use of these techniques and one that is often misunderstood. When CRRT techniques are utilized, a prescription for fluid management requires consideration not only of the type and quantity of different fluids used for replacement or dialysate but also the desired goals for the patient in the short term (24–48 h) and over a longer period of time. This calls for a team approach with consultation between the intensivist, nephrologist, pharmacist, nutritionist, and ICU and dialysis nursing staff. For instance, a patient with a hypercatabolic state and metabolic acidosis may require custom compositions of the replacement fluids and dialysate and an ongoing evaluation of the nutritional effects. Definition of fluid goals for each time period should be multidisciplinary and reflect a thorough understanding of the patient's condition and the CRRT technique. We have found that targeted intervention (Level 3) is easier to achieve, quantitate, and monitor and generally facilitates understanding between different care providers. For example, it is usually easier to agree on a target hemodynamic parameter (PAWP) that can be optimized than it is to decide on a patient's overall volume status. The fluid-management prescription is therefore somewhat dynamic and subject to frequent modifications depending upon the clinical condition. It has been our experience that frequent consultations between intensivists and nephrologists on establishing target parameters are extremely useful in this regard.

B. Establishing a Sliding Scale

In order to use Level 3 fluid management effectively the following are required:

1. The hourly UF volume should be in excess of all intakes every hour.
2. Hemodynamic targets should be selected for ease of measurement and to reflect overall parameter desired for stability (usual choices are CVP, PAWP, MAP, systolic BP)
3. Accurate record of all intakes and outputs should be kept and used for hourly calculations.

The parameter can be adjusted based on patient status and the scale adjusted as needed to achieve a goal. The main aim is to target fluid management to a hemodynamic parameter, thereby using CRRT as a fluid regulatory device. Table 2 shows an example of a sliding scale. In the example shown, the sliding scale is weighed more heavily for giving fluid back when the parameter is low. This can be adjusted depending on the circumstance, but we have found that it is safer to be slow in fluid removal and more aggressive in fluid repletion to maintain stability.

C. Fluid Balance

Most current CRRT techniques require an hourly or more frequent assessment of fluid balance. The process, although labor intensive, is fairly simple, provided a separate flowsheet is used for the calculations. Table 3 shows examples of a net balance of −100, +200, and 0 mL/h. The third column depicts a situation in which the desired balance of −100 mL for the hour could not be achieved because the ultrafiltration rate was lower than the intake. As shown, the 8-hour totals reflect the net balance, having accounted for all intakes and outputs. A stepwise approach in the flowsheet captures all

Table 3 Flow Sheet Calculations for Fluid Management in CRRT

		Hours										
		06	07	08	09	10	11	12	13	14	8	Total
1A	UF output	1600		1600		1200		1600				
1B	Dialysate infused	1000		1000		1000		1000				
1C	Actual UF out	600		600		200		600				
2	Additional out	100		100		50		0				
3	Total out	700		700		250		600				
4	All intake except replacement	400		400		400		750				
5	Hourly fluid balance	−300		−300		150		150				
6	Desired outcome	−100		200		−100		0				
7	Calc replacement	200		500		0		0				
8	Actual net balance	−100		200		150		150				400

the relevant data and translates it into an action plan to achieve a predetermined fluid goal. It is important to reiterate that using this approach, fluid replacement always follows fluid removal and is usually an hour behind. From a nursing perspective the hourly measurement of ultrafiltrate and calculation of replacement fluids necessary is tedious, but this can be minimized by some of the newer devices now available. The newer generation of pumped systems use meticulous balancing devices (e.g., Hospal Prisma, Braun Diapact, Baxter BM25) or volumetric control (e.g., Kimal Hygeia Plus, Fresenius ADM08) to achieve an ongoing fluid balance (11). While these systems provide the ability to maintain a set fluid balance and eliminate the hourly measurements, unfortunately all of these devices in their current configurations permit the use of the pumps for fluid removal only, thereby limiting their application as Level 2 and 3 methods. As newer integrated systems become available, targeted fluid balance will be more automated and less prone to errors. In the interim, a standardized approach to fluid balance is crucial to the success of these techniques.

D. Monitoring

Ongoing monitoring should involve checks on the composition of the fluids prescribed and determination that they are infusing in the right site. For instance, marked changes in the composition of blood can occur if a calcium solution intended for intravenous infusion is inadvertently infused as a dialysate fluid. The nursing staff, pharmacists, and physicians should independently verify the accuracy of the fluids. Rapid changes in fluid status are easily achieved with CRRT techniques. However, controlled fluid management necessitates periodic assessment of nursing interventions. In our center the hemodialysis nurses check the flowsheets maintained by the ICU nurses every 12 hours. These are additionally checked by the nephrologist for accuracy. Monitoring also involves evaluation for leaks from the ultrafiltrate bag and changes in fluid infusion rates and composition.

III. COMPLICATIONS RELATED TO FLUID MANAGEMENT

Table 4 shows the main complications associated with fluid management in CRRT. As discussed above, problems can arise in any of the major components. These are described further.

A. Prescription

Complications related to the prescription of fluid regulation can occur secondary to inappropriate goals, the volume of fluid removed or replaced, and the composition of fluid. As discussed above, setting targets for fluid removal or replacement is a crucial element in the control of fluids in CRRT. In practice this is achieved by an overall assessment of the patient's volume status. Often this task is difficult because it is dependent on a knowledge of the hydration state (total body water), the capacity of the circulatory system (resistance and compartmental distribution), and the content of osmotically active solutes. In critically ill patients it is difficult to assess the hydration state, particularly if large volumes of fluid have been used for resuscitation in short periods of time. Records of weights are often erroneous given the difficulty in weighing patients with multiple tubes on ventilators, and estimates of fluid losses can

Table 4 Complications Secondary to Fluid Management in CRRT

Variable	Parameter	Complication
Prescription	Inappropriate goal	Volume depletion
	Amount of fluid removed	Fluid overload
	Rate of fluid removal	Hypotension
		Hemodynamic instability
Fluid balance	Measurement	
	Manual	Inaccurate measurement
	Automated	Pump errors
	Recording	
	charting	
	calculations	Inaccurate fluid balance
	Timing of replacement	
	Delayed	
	Immediate	Hemodynamic instability
Fluid composition	Replacement fluid	Electrolytes, acid base problems
	Dialysate	Catabolic rate
	Drug delivery	Infection risk
	Nutrition	Inappropriate dosing
		Over- and underfeeding
Equipment	Nonintegrated pumps	Increased filter clotting
	Inaccurate balancing	Backfiltration
		Fluid overload or depletion
	Temperature control	Hypothermia
Management	Interference	Inappropriate goal
	Changed orders, boluses	Inadequate fluid balance

be wrong in patients with large insensible losses (e.g., patients with burns and open wounds). Assessment of circulatory capacitance is helped by measurement of central filling pressures, cardiac output, and systemic vascular resistance, however, these are also prone to measurement errors. While it is possible to assess the solute content by sequential measurement of blood chemistries, dilution of solutes by large volumes of fluid and compartment redistribution can significantly affect solute concentrations.

It is thus fairly common to find that a patient with marked edema and several liters of fluid excess may have a limited intravascular volume. In this situation, although fluid removal is required, it may be initially necessary to maintain an adequate intravascular volume by a combination of altering the composition of fluids infused (colloids and blood products) and influencing the systemic resistance. If CRRT is used to remove fluid without recognition of these factors, the rate of fluid removal may greatly exceed the capacity of the patient to mobilize fluid from the interstitial and intracellular compartments to the intravascular compartment, which will result in hemodynamic instability, evidenced by a decrease in blood pressure and organ perfusion. Similarly, an underestimation of the patients volume requirements could result in an inadequate rate of fluid removal resulting in worsened fluid overload. Both of these events are more likely with Level 1 fluid management because the fluid removal with CRRT is not directly linked to patient-driven parameters and is dependent on physician assessment of a fluid goal. In our experience over the last 5 years, it is evident that use of Level 2 and 3 fluid-management strategies minimize these problems. Which parameters should be used to regulate fluid management is often dependent on the availability of information (e.g., Swan-Ganz catheter). We have found that commonly monitored parameters (e.g., CVP or mean arterial pressure) can be easily used for this purpose.

Although several publications have suggested that CRRT provides improved hemodynamic stability, particularly in comparison to intermittent hemodialysis (12–17), it is difficult to establish a clear relationship with fluid removal or replacement and hypotension in most patients. The inherent complexity of the underlying illness in multiorgan failure is as likely to influence blood pressure in the ICU patients as is CRRT. Manns et al. compared the effects of IHD and CVVHD on residual kidney function in critically ill patients with ARF (12) and found that patients treated with IHD had a 25% decline in creatinine and urea clearance during and following IHD in comparison to a 7% decline in those on CVVHD. One explanation offered for this finding was the 7% reduction in mean arterial pressure (MAP) during IHD and maintained hemodynamic stability in CVVHD despite lower starting MAP. While these findings are relevant to demonstrate the operational differences in CRRT and IHD, it is important to recognize that the period of observation for CRRT was limited to the initial 6 hours of the procedure. In actual practice fluctuations in arterial pressure and other hemodynamic parameters are common in CRRT, and it is often difficult to ascertain the relationship between these changes and fluid removal. Problems are more likely if fluid management incorporates a Level 1 approach because there is often no compensation for hemodynamic changes. Recognition of these issues is important for prevention of these complications.

B. Fluid Balance

As described earlier different strategies are used for achieving fluid balance in CRRT. Accurate fluid balance requires three steps: a method to accurately measure fluid changes (intakes and outputs) over a period of time, a technique to record these changes and perform calculations for establishing interval fluid balance, and a mechanism for making changes in the fluid removal or replacement rates to correct any discrepancy in the desired fluid balance. Complications can arise related to each of these steps. Measurement of fluid intake and output related to CRRT can be done manually using a graduated cylinder to measure the ultrafiltrate and dialysate (if dialysate is used) and recording of the volume delivered through infusion pumps (dialysate and replacement fluid). Inaccuracies in manual measurement can result in errors in fluid balance, and the process is also somewhat tedious and prone to accidental spills with potential exposure of personnel to infectious material. An alternative method is to control the rate of the ultrafiltrate (and dialysate out) using an infusion pump. Several problems can result from this approach:

1. Most infusion pumps commonly available in the ICU have flow rates of up to 1 L per hour and may limit fluid rates. In such situations two pumps or special infusion pumps (e.g., Baxter Gemini with flow rates of 2–4 L/h) may need to be used.
2. Infusion pumps have inaccuracies of 5–15% and may lead to substantial errors in fluid balances if they are not assessed with manual measurement of fluids (19,20). Baldwin et al. (20) compared the volume delivered based on the readout from an infusion pump to actual measured volume over a 24-hour period and found discrepancies ranging from 1100 to 1800 mL.
3. Because the infusion pumps are not integrated and linked to the blood pump, an alarm condition on the blood pump side resulting in stoppage of the blood pump will cause continued fluid removal from the ultrafiltrate side resulting in an increased tendency for the filter to clot. Similarly, an alarm condition in the infusion pump will result in a reduced removal of fluid as the blood pump will continue to operate. If an infusion pump is used to control the volume of ultrafiltrate it is important to measure the volume removed periodically to ensure accuracy of collection and that alarm conditions are corrected immediately. Newer CRRT systems address this problem by integrating the pumps and providing a method of measuring fluid balance on a scale (Hospal Prisma, Braun Diapact, Baxter BM25) or volumetrically (Kimal Hygeia Plus) (11).

While these methods are accurate, it is important to emphasize that the machine records only fluids within the system and does not include any fluids given outside the system. Accidental bumping of the equipment may require a recalibration of the scales.

A second step in fluid balance is recording the fluids in and out of the CRRT system and incorporating this information in the overall fluid balance for the patient. Several individual methods are used, and no standard approach is currently followed. Some users record the information as part of the routine ICU flowsheet, while others use a separate CRRT flowsheet. We favor the use of a separate sheet, as described earlier, because it permits calculations easily and can be used to guide therapy. Regardless of what tool is used for charting the frequency of recording, data should be consistent (usually every hour). Inaccuracies in recording on paper flow sheets can result in calculation errors. We have found that the extent of error is also influenced by the familiarity of the nursing personnel with CRRT. Because these procedures typically go over several days, different nursing personnel will likely care for the same patient. A standardized flowsheet and a defined protocol for charting is a necessary step to reduce errors (22,23).

A key step for fluid balance is to perform calculations for fluid balance to allow for any discrepancies to be corrected. There is considerable variation in this area because some users will not include fluid boluses in the calculations under the assumption that these are being given to restore intravascular fluid. Inconsistencies in data recording and inclusion in the calculations will result in significant deviations in fluid balance from day to day. Similarly, computation errors in the calculations lead to inaccurate fluid balance and contribute to under- or overhydration. As described earlier, our approach is to include all intakes and outputs in the fluid balance calculations and to use the concept of a desired hourly fluid balance. Appropriate instruction and ongoing in-servicing of personnel performing CRRT is essential to eliminate these errors. Periodic audits of the charting should also be done. In our center this is the responsibility of a dialysis nurse and is done every 12 hours (10).

A final step in fluid balance is the designated action taken in response to the calculations. Depending upon the approach and frequency of calculations, adjustments to the ultrafiltration rate, blood flow rate, dialysate flow rate, or replacement fluid rate may be required. Some CRRT systems are designed to permit manipulation only of the blood flow rate (BFR) and dialysate and replacement flow rates, and the UFR is defined by the machine (PRISMA), whereas other systems allow the UFR also to be adjusted. Understanding the conditions imposed by the CRRT system is key for proper fluid balance. Nonintegrated CRRT systems (Hospal BSM22, Baxter BM11) that do not have fluid-balancing capability rely on the hourly adjustments made in replacement fluid rate or ultrafiltration rate to achieve fluid balance. In each of these systems fluid removal usually precedes fluid replacement and can result in large imbalances contributing to hemodynamic instability. In general there is always some lag time from the time fluid is removed to when it is replaced. In order to minimize this lag time, it is advisable to initiate the replacement fluid as close to the time that fluid is first removed; e.g., when a new CRRT procedure is started, it is helpful to keep the net fluid balance zero or positive for the first 2–3 hours, and fluid replacement should commence at the time CRRT is initiated or within a short period of time (5–15 min). If a Level 2 or 3 fluid-management strategy is utilized, replacement fluid will lag approximately an hour behind. If an integrated CRRT system with fluid-balancing capability (e.g., Hospal Prisma) is used, a zero or negative fluid balance can be achieved in real time, however, because the fluids infused or removed outside the CRRT system are not counted for real time, fluid balance does not occur. Thus, it is important to have a standardized protocol for making changes in the rates of various fluids at the end of every hour based on the system in place.

C. Fluid Composition

One of the major advantages of CRRT is that the composition of replacement fluid and dialysate can be modified to achieve any specific change in plasma composition (23). For instance, the concentration of sodium bicarbonate can be varied to correct metabolic acidosis and concentration of potassium, and other ions can similarly be adjusted. Several centers use standard hemofiltration solutions (e.g., Hospal Hemosol, Baxter hemofiltration solution), which have predetermined concentrations of base (usually lactate) and ions; however, in many instances customized solutions with varying composition need to be made (23–32). When customized solutions are utilized, it is important to ensure that the concentration of various ions is as prescribed. This is particularly important for potassium and calcium concentrations, which can result in significant toxicity. Although not well reported in the literature, there have been reports of patient deaths related to an inadvertent mixing of a high concentration of potassium in the dialysate. Another issue is to safeguard against the inadvertent use of a solution as a dialysate when it is intended for intravenous infusion. For instance, when citrate anticoagulation is used, a 0.1 mEq/mL calcium chloride solution is infused through a central line to maintain the ionized calcium levels in the normal range. We have had two occasions when the calcium chloride solution was inadvertently infused as dialysate, resulting in marked hypercalcemia. As a consequence a protocol is needed that clearly identifies each bag of solution with a color code to identify its purpose, route of infusion, and contents. The pharmacist who prepares the solutions cross-checks the content, and the ICU nurse stores the solutions in separate areas for dialysate and replacement fluid (22). This has prevented any further problems. In the last 2 years there have been several publications commenting on the beneficial role of bicarbonate as buffer instead of lactate (24–31). Use of lactate ions as base has been associated with an increase in urea generation (24). Additionally, the capacity to convert lactate to bicarbonate may be impaired in the setting of hypotension and MOF, resulting in lactate accumulation (25). Hilton et al. (24,29) have shown that use of bicarbonate-based solutions is associated with improved hemodynamic stability, although no difference was found by Thomas et al. (25) comparing lactate- and bicarbonate-based solutions. A recently completed multicenter study in Germany has further shown that use of lactate-based substitution fluids is associated with reduced hemodynamic stability in comparison to bicarbonate-based solutions (A. Riegel, personal communication). Similarly Kierdorf et al. (31) have demonstrated an increase in nitrogen generation possibly related to increased catabolism in patients given lactate-based solutions. These findings are similar to those of Olbricht et al. (32), suggesting that lactate-based solutions may have some deleterious effects.

A practical issue with use of bicarbonate-based solutions is that it is difficult to store premixed bicarbonate solutions (33–35). Paganini et al. (33) advocated preparing a nonsterile bicarbonate solution using a standard hemodialysis machine. This method has been used successfully at the Cleveland clinic and at other centers (34), but it is unclear what is the risk for infection, particularly if the solutions are stored for several hours or days prior to use. This is particularly important if there is any backfiltration, as may occur in a nonintegrated CRRT system using a infusion pump to control the ultrafiltrate. Another factor to consider is that premixed solutions containing calcium and bicarbonate show evidence of microprecipitation of calcium carbonate crystals, which should be avoided (35).

D. Equipment

Currently several new integrated systems are available for CRRT (11), but many centers use older systems with one to two pumps (Baxter BM11, Hospal BSM 22) or have configured home-made systems using blood pumps from hemodialysis machines. More recently the Fresenius 2008H machine has been modified to reduce the dialysate flow to 100 mL/min, and this system is being utilized to provide variations of CRRT, e.g., extended daily dialysis or slow, low-efficiency dialysis (36,37). The choice of equipment can result in errors in fluid balance and management as pointed out earlier and needs to be considered. A key area is the cooling effect of the replacement fluid and dialysate. It is now well recognized that there is a significant drop in core temperature if the solutions are not heated (38–40). Studies comparing the effect of cold versus warm substitution fluids in intermittent hemofiltration have shown that there is improved hemodynamic stability in cold hemofiltration related to an increase in peripheral vascular resistance (39). Effects of cooling in CRRT are not clearly defined. Matamis et al. (40) found a decrease in energy requirements (38,40) and that hemodynamic stability may be impaired. It is recommended that replacement solutions and dialysate should be heated prior to infusion. This is easily achieved with the newer CRRT systems, which have a heater in line, but requires an external heater to be placed in line for the nonintegrated systems. The effect on temperature is particularly important for techniques using high-volume hemofiltration (41). The site of delivery of replacement fluid, i.e., prefilter or postfilter, may also have an effect on circuit clotting by influencing the filtration fraction (see Chapter 12).

E. Management

CRRT systems are prone to interference from outside. Because the system runs continuously and several personnel are typically involved in the delivery of care, there is increased opportunity for error. For instance, it is fairly common for a hypotensive episode to be treated with aggressive fluid resuscitation outside of the CRRT system, which can lead to major changes in fluid balance. It is imperative that changes in orders for fluid management be relegated to the physicians managing the CRRT system (42,43). If emergent changes are required for CRRT, it is important that the fluid calculations be included in the CRRT system. We have found that use of Level III management reduces the interference and subsequent fluid balance problems.

IV. SUMMARY

Fluid management is an integral component of CRRT systems, but it is the least standardized area. As a consequence, several complications can occur. Recognition of the areas where complications may occur is an important step in prevention. Fluid management continues to be a major area in CRRT, which requires close attention.

REFERENCES

1. Forni LG, Hilton PJ. Continuous hemofiltration in the treatment of acute renal failure. N Engl J Med 1997; 336(18):1303–1309.
2. Golper TA. Indications, technical considerations, and strategies for renal replacement therapy in the intensive care unit. J Intensiv Care Med 1992; 7:310–317.
3. Davenport A, Will EJ, Davidson AM. Improved cardiovascular stability during continuous modes of renal

replacement therapy in critically ill patients with acute hepatic and renal failure. Crit Care Med 1993; 21: 328–338.

4. van Bommel EFH. Are continuous therapies superior to intermittent hemodialysis for acute renal failure on the intensive care unit? Nephrol Dial Transplant 1995; 311–314.
5. Bland RD, Shoemaker WC, Abraham E, Cobo JC. Hemodynamic and oxygen transport patterns in surviving and non-surviving postoperative patients. Crit Care Med 1985; 13:85–90.
6. Tuschmidt J, Fried J, Astiz M, Rackow E. Elevation of cardiac output and oxygen delivery improves outcome in septic shock. Chest 1992; 102:216–220.
7. Hayes MA, Timmins AC, Yau EHS, Palazzo M, Hinds CJ, Watson D. Elevation of systemic oxygen delivery in the treatment of critically ill patients. N Engl J Med 1994; 330:1717–1722.
8. Gattinoni L, Brazzi L, Pezosi P, Latini R, Togeni A, Resentia A, Fumagali A. For the SVO_2 Collaborative Group: a trial of goal oriented hemodynamic therapy in critically ill patients. N Engl J Med 1995; 333:1025–1032.
9. Lowell JA, Schifferdecker C, Driscoll DF, Benotti PN, Bistrian BR. Postoperative fluid overload: not a benign problem. Crit Care Med 1990; 18:728–733.
10. Mehta RL. Fluid management in continuous renal replacement therapy. Sem Dial 1996; 9:140–144.
11. Ronco C, Brendolan A, Bellomo R. Current technology for continuous renal replacement therapies. In: Ronco C, Bellamo R, eds. Critical Care Nephrology. Dordrecht: Kluwer Academic Publishers, 1998: 1269–1308.
12. Manns M, Sigler MH, Teehan BP. Intradialytic renal haemodynamics—potential consequences for the management of the patient with acute renal failure [editorial]. Nephrol Dial Transplant 1997; 12(5):870–872.
13. van Bommel EF, Ponssen HH. Intermittent versus continuous treatment for acute renal failure: Where do we stand? Am J Kidney Dis 1997; 30(5 suppl 4):S72–79.
14. Manns M, Sigler MH, Teehan BP. Continuous renal replacement therapies: an update. Am J Kidney Dis 1998; 32(2):185–207.
15. Lameire N, Van Biesen W, Vanholder R, Colardijn F. The place of intermittent hemodialysis in the treatment of acute renal failure in the ICU patient. Kidney Int 1998; 66(suppl):S110–119.
16. Bellomo R, Ronco C. Continuous versus intermittent renal replacement therapy in the intensive care unit. Kidney Int 1998; 66(suppl):S125–128.
17. Misset B, Timsit JF, Chevret S, Renaud B, Tamion F, Carlet J. A randomized crossover comparison of the hemodynamic response to intermittent hemodialysis and continuous hemofiltration in ICU patients with acute renal failure. Intensiv Care Med 1996; 22(8):742–746.
18. van Bommel EF. Are continuous therapies superior to intermittent haemodialysis for acute renal failure on the intensive care unit? Nephrol Dial Transplant 1995; 10(3):311–314.
19. Roberts M, Winney RJ. Errors in fluid balance with pump control of continuous hemodialysis. Int J Artif Organs 1992; 15:99–102.
20. Baldwin IC, Elderkin TD. Continuous hemofiltration: nursing perspectives in critical care. New Horizons 1995; 3(4):738–747.
21. Baldwin IC. Training, management, and credentialing for CRRT in the ICU. American J Kidney Dis 1997; 30(5 suppl 4):S112–116.
22. Martin RK, Jurschak J. Nursing management of continuous renal replacement therapy. Sem Dial 1996; 9: 192–199.
23. Marcias WL. Choice of replacement fluid/dialysate anion in continuous renal replacement therapy. Am J Kidney Dis 1996; 28(suppl 3):S15–S20.
24. Hilton PJ, Taylor J, Forni LG, Treacher DF. Bicarbonate-based haemofiltration in the management of acute renal failure with lactic acidosis. QJM 1998; 91(4):279–283.
25. Thomas AN, Guy JM, Kishen R, Geraghty IF, Bowles BJ, Vadgama P. Comparison of lactate and bicarbonate buffered haemofiltration fluids: use in critically ill patients. Nephrol Dial Transplant 1997; 12(6):1212–1217.
26. Benjamin E. Continuous venovenous hemofiltration with dialysis and lactate clearance in critically ill patients. Crit Care Med 1997; 25(1):4–5.
27. Levraut J, Ciebiera JP, Jambou P, Ichai C, Labib Y, Grimaud D. Effect of continuous venovenous hemofiltration with dialysis on lactate clearance in critically ill patients. Crit Care Med 1997; 25(1):58–62.
28. Morgera S, Heering P, Szentandrasi T, Manassa E, Heintzen M, Willers R, Passlick-Deetjen J, Grabensee B. Comparison of a lactate-versus acetate-based hemofiltration replacement fluid in patients with acute renal failure. Renal Failure 1997; 19(1):155–164.
29. Wright DA, Forni LG, Carr P, Treacher DF, Hilton PJ. Use of continuous haemofiltration to assess the rate of lactate metabolism in acute renal failure. Clin Sci 1996; 90(6):507–510.
30. Marangoni R, Civardi F, Masi F, Savino R, Cimino R, Colombo R, Maltagliati L. Lactate versus bicarbonate on-line hemofiltration: a comparative study. Artif Organs 1995; 19(6):490–495.
31. Kierdorf H, Leue C, Heintz B, Riehl J, Melzer H, Sieberth HG. Continuous venovenous hemofiltration in acute renal failure: Is a bicarbonate- or lactate-buffered substitution better? Contrib Nephrol 1995; 116:38–47.
32. Olbricht CJ, Huxmann-Näägeli D, Bischoff H. Bicarbonate instead of lactate buffered substitution solution for continuous hemofiltration in intensive care. Anasth Intensivther Notfallmed 1990; 25(2):164–167.

33. Leblanc M, Moreno L, Robinson OP, Tapolyai M, Paganini EP. Bicarbonate dialysate for continuous renal replacement therapy in intensive care unit patients with acute renal failure. Am J Kidney Dis 1995; 26(6): 910–917.
34. Schwab G, Gregory MJ. Rapid production of bicarbonate-based dialysate for continuous veno-venous hemodiafiltration. Blood Purif 1999; 17:27.
35. Maccariello ER, Boechat L, Pagani JR, Ruffier C, Ruffier J, Rocha E. Single bag bicarbonate solutions in CRRT: Is that safe? Blood Purif 1999; 17:27.
36. Hu KT, Yeun JY, Craig M, Tarne P, Depner TA. Extended daily dialysis: an alternative to continuous venovenous hemofiltration in the intensive care unit. Blood Purif 1999; 17:28.
37. Chatoth DK, Shaver MR, Golper TA. Daily 12 hour sustained low efficiency dialysis (SLED) for the treatment of critically ill patients with acute renal failure: initial experience. Blood Purif 1999; 17:29.
38. Yagi N, Leblanc M, Sakai K, Wright EJ, Paganini EP. Cooling effect of continuous renal replacement therapy in critically ill patients. Am J Kidney Dis 1998; 32(6): 1023–1030.
39. van Kuijk WH, Hillion D, Savoiu C, Leunissen KM. Critical role of the extracorporeal blood temperature in the hemodynamic response during hemofiltration. J Am Soc Nephrol 1997; 8(6):949–955.
40. Matamis D, Tsagourias M, Koletsos K, Riggos D, Mavromatidis K, Sombolos K, Bursztein S. Influence of continuous haemofiltration-related hypothermia on haemodynamic variables and gas exchange in septic patients. Intensiv Care Med 1994; 20(6):431–436.
41. Bellomo R, Baldwin I, Cole L, Ronco C. Preliminary experience with high-volume hemofiltration in human septic shock. Kidney Int 1998; 66(suppl):S182–185.
42. Bellomo R, Cole L, Reeves J, Silvester W. Who should manage CRRT in the ICU? The intensivist's viewpoint. Am J Kidney Dis 1997; 30(5 suppl 4):S109–111.
43. Mehta RL, Martin R. Initiating and implementing a continuous renal replacement therapy program: requirements and guidelines. Sem Dialysis 1996; 9:80–87.

14

Problems of Solute Removal in Continuous Renal Replacement Therapies

William R. Clark
Baxter Healthcare Corp., and Indiana University School of Medicine, Indianapolis, Indiana

Michael A. Kraus
Indiana University School of Medicine, Indianapolis, Indiana

Bruce A. Mueller
Purdue University, West Lafayette, Indiana

I. INTRODUCTION

Renal replacement therapy (RRT) is required in a significant percentage of patients with acute renal failure (ARF), particularly those in an intensive care unit (ICU) setting (1). Whether intermittent hemodialysis (IHD) or continuous renal replacement therapy (CRRT) is employed, one of the foremost objectives is the removal of blood solutes that are retained as a consequence of decreased or absent glomerular filtration. With regard to solute removal, the above RRT options differ substantially in several respects. The primary mechanism of removal, the solute molecular weight (MW) removal spectrum, the rate of solute removal, and the overall (cumulative) removal all may differ significantly between the above therapies. Based on these differences, the complications related to solute removal vary according to the specific RRT being employed.

Prior to gaining insight into the solute removal–related complications in ARF, a thorough understanding of the mechanisms by which solute removal is achieved by RRT is necessary. Therefore, this chapter first provides a comprehensive overview of solute mass transfer for hemodialyzers and hemofilters used in ARF. This overview sets the stage for a discussion of the possible ways in which solute removal may be impaired in RRT used in ARF. For the purposes of this chapter, complications related to solute removal and impairment in solute removal, relative to that which is expected (i.e., prescribed), are considered synonymous.

II. FUNDAMENTAL MECHANISMS OF EXTRACORPOREAL SOLUTE AND WATER REMOVAL

A. Membrane Flux

The water permeability (flux) characteristics of an extracorporeal membrane are primarily determined by mean pore size. For analytical purposes, a common practice is to model the pores of a hollow fiber membrane as a series of parallel cylinders (2). (Of note, the path that pores take within an extracorporeal membrane is actually tortuous. However, the cylindrical model has been found to be a reasonable representation of the actual clinical situation.) In this model, fluid flow through the pore is quantified by use of the Hagen-Poisseuile law (2). According to this equation, the volumetric rate of fluid flow is proportional to the fourth power of the pore radius for a given transmembrane pressure. Therefore, a relatively small increase in mean pore size has a relatively large impact on the ultrafiltration capabilities of the membrane.

B. Solute Removal by Diffusion

Diffusion involves the mass transfer of a solute in response to a concentration gradient. For the extracorporeal removal of a retained solute in an ARF patient, this concentration gradient exists across a semipermeable membrane in a hemodialyzer or hemofilter. The inherent rate of diffusion of a solute is termed its diffusivity (3), whether this is in solution (such as dialysate and blood) or within an extracorporeal membrane. Diffusivity in solution is inversely proportional to solute molecular weight and directly proportional to solution temperature. Solute diffusion within a membrane is influenced by both membrane thickness (diffusion path length) and membrane diffusivity (4), which is a function of both pore size and number (density).

In conventional IHD, the overall mass transfer coefficient–area product (KoA) is used to quantify the diffusion characteristics of a particular solute-membrane combination (5). The overall mass transfer coefficient is the inverse of the overall resistance to diffusive mass transfer, the latter being a more applicable quantitative parameter from an engineering perspective:

$$\mathrm{Ko} = \frac{1}{\mathrm{Ro}}$$

The overall mass transfer resistance can be viewed as the sum of resistances in series (3):

$$\mathrm{Ro} = \mathrm{Rb} + \mathrm{Rm} + \mathrm{Rd}$$

where Rb, Rm, and Rd are the mass transfer resistances associated with the blood, membrane, and dialysate, respectively. In turn, each resistance component is a function of both diffusion path length (x) and diffusivity (D):

$$R_O = (x/D)_B + (x/D)_M + (x/D)_D$$

The diffusive mass transfer resistance of both the blood and dialysate compartments for a hemodialyzer is primarily due to the unstirred (boundary) layer just adjacent to the membrane (6). Minimizing the thickness of these unstirred layers is primarily dependent on achieving relatively high shear rates, particularly in the blood compartment (7). For similar blood flow rates, higher blood compartment shear rates are achieved with a hollow fiber dialyzer than with a flat plate dialyzer. Indeed, based on the blood and dialysate flow rates (generally at least 250 and 500 mL/min, respectively) achieved in contemporary IHD with hollow fiber dialyzers, the controlling diffusive resistance is that due to the membrane itself.

Another approach to quantifying diffusive mass transfer specifically through an extracorporeal membrane is use of Fick's law of diffusion:

$$N = D(dC/dx)$$

where N is mass flux (mass removal rate normalized to membrane surface area), D is membrane diffusivity, an intrinsic membrane property for the particular solute being assessed, and dC/dx is the change in solute concentration with respect to distance. This equation also can be expressed in a more applicable, integrated form:

$$N = D(\Delta C/\Delta x)$$

Thus, for a given concentration gradient across a membrane, the rate of diffusive solute removal is directly proportional to the membrane diffusivity and indirectly proportional to the effective thickness of the membrane.

As described above, membrane diffusivity is determined both by the pore size distribution and the number of pores per unit membrane area (pore density). Diffusive mass transfer rates within a membrane decrease as solute molecular weight increases due not only to effect of molecular size itself, but also to the resistance provided by the membrane pores (8). The difference in mean pore sizes between low-permeability dialysis membranes (e.g., regenerated cellulose) and high-permeability membranes (e.g., polysulfone, polyacrylonitrile, cellulose triacetate) has a relatively small impact on small solute (urea, creatinine) diffusivities. This is related to the fact that even low-permeability membranes have pores sizes that are significantly larger than the molecular sizes of these solutes. However, as solute molecular weight increases, the tight pore structure of the low-permeability membranes plays an increasingly constraining role such that diffusive removal of solutes larger than 1000 daltons is minimal by these membranes. On the other hand, the larger pore sizes that characterize high-flux membranes account for their higher diffusive permeabilities. In fact, based on the flow rates typically used in high-flux IHD, diffusion is the primary removal mechanism for solutes as large as inulin (5200 daltons) for all high-permeability membranes (9) and even β_2-microglobulin (11,000 daltons) for certain high-permeability membranes (10,11).

C. Solute Removal by Convection

Convective solute removal is primarily determined by the sieving properties of the membrane used and the ultrafiltration rate. The mechanism by which convection occurs is termed solvent drag. If the molecular dimensions of a solute are such that sieving does not occur, the solute is swept ("dragged") across the membrane in association with ultrafiltered plasma water. Thus, the rate of convective solute removal can be modified either by changes in the rate of solvent (plasma water) flow or in the mean effective pore size of the membrane.

Both the water and solute permeability of an ultrafiltration membrane are influenced by the phenomena of secondary membrane formation (12) and concentration polarization (13). The exposure of an artificial surface to plasma results in the nonspecific, instantaneous adsorption of a layer of proteins, the composition of which generally reflects that of the plasma itself. Therefore, plasma proteins such as albumin, fibrinogen, and immunoglobulins form the bulk of this secondary membrane. This layer of proteins, by serving as an additional resistance to mass transfer, effectively reduces both the water and solute permeability of an extracorporeal membrane. Evidence of this is found in comparisons of solute sieving coefficients determined before and after exposure of a membrane to plasma or other protein-containing solution (8). In general, the extent of secondary membrane development and its effect on membrane permeability is directly proportional to the membranes adsorptive tendencies (i.e., hydrophobicity). Therefore, this process tends to be most evident for high-flux synthetic membranes, such as polyacrylonitrile, polysulfone, and polymethylmethacrylate.

Although concentration polarization (13) primarily pertains to plasma proteins, it is distinct from secondary membrane formation. Concentration polarization specifically relates to ultrafiltration-based processes and applies to the kinetic behavior of an individual protein. Accumulation of a plasma protein that is predominantly or completely sieved (rejected) by a membrane used for ultrafiltration of plasma occurs at the blood compartment membrane surface. This surface accumulation causes the protein concentration just adjacent to the membrane surface (i.e., the submembranous concentration) to be higher than the bulk (plasma) concentration. In this manner, a submembranous (high) to bulk (low) concentration gradient is established, resulting in "back-diffusion" from the membrane surface out into the plasma. At steady state, the rate of convective transport to the membrane surface is equal to the rate of backdiffusion. The polarized layer of protein is the distance defined by the gradient between the submembranous and bulk concentrations. This distance (or thickness) of the polarized layer, which can be estimated by mass balance techniques, reflects the extent of the concentration polarization process.

By definition, concentration polarization is applicable in clinical situations in which relatively high ultrafiltration rates are used. Therefore, in ARF, concentration polarization may play a significant role in CVVH and CVVHDF, and the specific operating conditions used in these therapies influence the polarization process. Conditions that promote the process are high ultrafiltration rate (high rate of convective transport), low blood flow rate (low shear rate), and the use of postdilution (rather than predilution) replacement fluids (increased local protein concentrations) (14).

The extent of the concentration polarization determines its effect on actual solute (protein) removal. In general, the degree to which the removal of a protein is influenced is directly related to that protein's extent of rejection by an individual membrane. In fact, concentration polarization actually enhances the removal of a molecular weight class of proteins (30,000–70,000 daltons) that otherwise would have minimal convective removal. This is explained by the fact that the pertinent blood compartment concentration subjected to the ultrafiltrate flux is the high submembranous concentration primarily rather than the much lower bulk concentration. Therefore, the potentially desirable removal of certain proteins in this size range in ARF patients has to be weighed against the undesirable increase in convective albumin losses. This concern is particularly relevant in light of the growing interest in the use of high-volume hemofiltration ($\geq$6 L/h) for the treatment of septic conditions (with or without ARF) (15,16).

On the other hand, the use of very high ultrafiltration rates in conjunction with other conditions favorable to protein polarization may significantly impair overall membrane performance. The relationship between ultrafiltration rate and transmembrane pressure (TMP) is linear for relatively low ultrafiltration rates, and the positive slope of this line defines the ultrafiltration coefficient of the membrane. However, as ultrafiltration rate further increases, this curve eventually plateaus (13). At this point, maintenance of a certain ultrafiltration rate is only maintained by a concomitant increase in TMP. At sufficiently high TMP, fouling of the membrane with denatured proteins may occur and an irreversible decline in solute and water permeability of the membrane ensues. Therefore, the ultrafiltration rate (and associated TMP) used for a convective therapy with a specific membrane needs to fall on the initial (linear) portion of the UFR versus TMP relationship with avoidance of the plateau region.

Convective solute removal can be quantified in the following manner (17):

$$N = (1 - \sigma)Jv\ Cm$$

where N is the convective flux (mass removal rate per unit membrane area), Jv is the ultrafiltrate flux (ultrafiltration rate normalized to membrane area), Cm is the mean intramembrane solute concentration, and σ is the reflection coefficient, a measure of solute rejection. As Werynski and Waniewski have explained (17), the parameter $(1 - \sigma)$ can be viewed as the membrane resistance to convective solute flow. If σ equals 1, no convective transport occurs, while a value of 0 implies no resistance to convective flow. Of note, the appropriate blood compartment concentration used to determine Cm is the submembranous concentration rather than the bulk phase concentration. Therefore, this parameter is significantly influenced by the effects of concentration polarization.

It is useful to individually assess the parameters on the right-hand side of the above equation and the manner in which changes in these parameters may affect the rate of convective solute transport. During a RRT, changes in the permeability properties of the hemofilter membrane or in the operating conditions may alter these parameters. However, a complex interplay exists between these parameters, and the net effect of changes in hemofilter membrane permeability or RRT operating conditions may be difficult to predict. To illustrate this point, the effect of a progressive decrease in membrane permeability as a membrane becomes fouled with proteins can be assessed. As a membrane becomes fouled with plasma proteins, the resistance to convective solute flow (σ) increases such that the parameter $(1 - \sigma)$ decreases. In addition, fouling may result in a decrease in ultrafiltrate flux (Jv) despite attempted increases in TMP. This phenomenon is most relevant for CRRT systems operated without a blood pump, such as CAVH and CAVHD. However, when the membranes become irreversibly fouled (i.e., gel formation occurs), even a hemofilter used in a venovenous system loses ultrafiltration capabilities. Finally, polarization of solute at the membrane surface due to the fouling causes an increase in the submembranous blood compartment concentration but a decrease in the filtrate concentration. The net effect on Cm, which essentially is a mean of the submembranous and filtrate concentrations, is difficult to predict and depends on the specific solute in question. In general, however, except for relatively large proteins capable of only minimal convective transport (e.g., albumin), fouling results in a decrease in Cm because the decrease in filtrate concentration is predicted to be greater than the increase in the submembranous concentration.

D. Interaction Between Diffusion and Convection

In IHD and some continuous therapies, diffusive and convective solute removal occur simultaneously. However, the effect of this combination on the total removal of a specific solute differs between intermittent and slow continuous therapies. In IHD, diffusion and convection interact in such a manner that total solute removal is significantly less than what would be expected if the individual components are simply added together. This phenomenon is explained in the following way. Diffusive removal results in a decrease in solute concentration in the blood compartment along the axial length (i.e., from blood inlet to blood outlet) of the hemodialyzer/hemofilter. As convective solute removal is directly proportional to the blood compartment concentration, convective solute removal decreases as a function of this axial concentration gradient. On the other hand, hemoconcentration resulting from ultrafiltration of plasma water causes a progressive increase in plasma protein concentration and hematocrit along the axial length of the filter. This hemoconcentration and resultant hyperviscosity causes an increase in diffusive mass transfer resistance and a decrease in solute transport by this mechanism. The effect of this interaction on overall solute removal in IHD has been analyzed rigorously by numerous investigators (17,18). The most useful quantification has been developed by Jaffrin (18):

$$Kt = Kd + Qf \times Tr$$

where Kt is total solute clearance, Kd is diffusive clearance under conditions of no ultrafiltration, and the final term is the convective component of clearance. The latter term is a function of the ultrafiltration rate (Qf) and an experimentally derived transmittance coefficient (Tr), such that:

$$Tr = S(1 - Kd/Qb)$$

where S is solute sieving coefficient. Thus, Tr for a particular solute is dependent on the efficiency of diffusive removal. At very low values of Kd/Qb, diffusion has a very small impact on blood compartment concentrations and the convective component of clearance closely approximates the quantity $S \times Qf$. However, with increasing efficiency of diffusive removal (i.e., increasing Kd/Qb), blood compartment concentrations are significantly influenced. The result is a decrease in Tr and, consequently, in the convective contribution to total clearance.

Due to the markedly lower flow rates used in CRRT, the effect of simultaneous diffusion and convection on overall solute removal is quite different. Based on a comparison of clearances, the rate of diffusive removal of small solutes in CAVHD, CVVHD, or CVVHDF (17–34 mL/min) (19–23) is only approximately 5–15% of the rate achieved in IHD. Therefore, the small solute concentration gradient along the axial length of the filter (i.e., extraction) is minimal compared to that which is seen in an IHD setting, in which extraction ratios of 50% or more are the norm. This difference is demonstrated in the following comparison of CVVHD and IHD, both operated in the pure dialysis (diffusive) mode. For typical blood and dialysate flow rates of 300 and 500 mL/min, respectively, an expected diffusive urea clearance is approximately 200 mL/min for a high-efficiency dialyzer used in an ARF IHD application. Based on this clearance and an assumed arterial line BUN of 60 mg/dL, the resultant venous line BUN is 20 mg/dL. This significant decrease in the BUN occurring along the axial length of the dialyzer reduces potential convective solute removal, as explained above. On the other hand, typical blood and dialysate flow rates in a strictly diffusive CVVHD procedure are 200 and 17 mL/min, respectively (21,22), which result in a urea clearance of 17 mL/min due to saturation of the effluent dialysate stream (dialysis equilibrium) (20–22). Based on this clearance and the same arterial line BUN of 60 mg/dL, the resultant venous line BUN is 55 mg/dL. Thus, the minimal diffusion-related change in small solute concentrations along the filter allows any additional clearance related to convection to be simply additive to the diffusive component. Indeed, in a classic paper (20), Sigler and Teehan demonstrated this lack of interaction between diffusion and convection in a series of patients treated with CAVHD operating at a dialysate flow rate of 1 L/h and an ultrafiltration rate range of 4 to 10 mL/min.

III. SOLUTE REMOVAL MECHANISMS: INTERMITTENT HEMODIALYSIS VERSUS CRRT

Application of the above principles allows a comparison of solute-removal mechanisms for extracorporeal RRT used in ARF (Table 1). Solutes are divided into four categories: small solutes (<300 daltons), middle molecules (500–5,000 daltons), low molecular weight (LMW) proteins (5,000–50,000 daltons), and large proteins (>50,000 daltons). Except for the LMW protein category, the prototypical molecules (surrogates) in each category are similar for both ESRD and ARF. These common prototypical solutes are (a) urea, creatinine, phosphate, and amino acids (small solutes), (b) vitamin B_{12}, vancomycin (24,25), and inulin (middle molecules), and (c) albumin (large molecules). For the LMW protein category, β_2-microglobulin is the focus in ESRD therapies (26), while inflammatory mediators, such as complement pathway products (MW 9–23 kDa) and cytokines (MW 15–50 kDa), are more of interest in the ARF setting (27–30).

Table 1 Determinants of Solute Removal in IHD and CRRT

	IHD	CRRT
Small solutes (mw < 300)	Diffusion: Q_B Q_D Membrane thickness	Diffusion: Q_D Convection: Q_F
Middle molecules (mw = 500–5,000)	Diffusion Convection: Q_F SC	Convection: Q_F Diffusion
LMW proteins (mw = 5,000–50,000)	Convection Diffusion Adsorption: site availability	Convection Adsorption: site availability
Large proteins (mw > 50,000)	Convection	Convection

Q_B, blood flow rate; Q_D, dialysate flow rate; Q_F, ultrafiltration rate; SC, sieving coefficient.
Source: Ref. 62.

As is the case in ESRD, optimized removal of solutes in the small solute, middle molecule, and LMW protein categories and minimal removal of albumin are therapy goals in ARF. However, as Table 1 indicates, the mechanisms by which solute removal within a particular category occurs may differ significantly between the two types of therapies. For patients receiving IHD, small solute removal occurs almost exclusively by diffusion (24). As such, optimized small solute removal is achieved by employing dialysis conditions that minimize diffusive mass transfer resistances, such as high flow rates and thin membranes (2). Likewise, for solutes in the middle molecule category, removal by high-flux IHD occurs predominantly by diffusion (31). Although LMW protein removal by high-flux dialyzers occurs primarily by convection or adsorption, diffusion can even play a significant role in the removal of solutes in the class (e.g., β_2-microglobulin) for some membranes (32). Only for a solute whose molecular weight is similar to or larger than that of albumin is convection essentially the sole removal mechanism during high-flux IHD. Recent ESRD data (33) demonstrate total protein losses during high-flux dialysis may be significant (up to 15–20 g per treatment), at least for certain membrane-reuse combinations. Protein losses for IHD have not been quantified in ARF.

The predominant mass transfer mechanism for each class of solutes may be significantly different for the slow continuous therapies. Small solute removal can occur exclusively by convection in CVVH (34,35), predominantly by diffusion in CVVHD (21,22), or by approximately equal contributions of both diffusion and convection in CVVHD (23). For a properly functioning filter, small solute sieving coefficients during CVVH are close to unity (36,37) such that clearances for these solutes are primarily determined by the ultrafiltration rate and the mode of replacement fluid administration (predilution vs. postdilution) (38). For the diffusion-based continuous therapies employing dialysate flow rates of 2 L/h or less, urea and creatinine clearances approximate the effluent dialysate flow rate because of the existence of dialysis equilibrium (20–22). For middle molecule removal, Jeffrey et al. (25) have recently shown that convection is more important than diffusion for a surrogate solute (vancomycin: MW, 1448) when the same ultrafiltration rate (CVVH) and effluent dialysate flow rate (CVVHD) of 25 mL/min (1.5 L/h) is used. As the relative importance of convection increases with solute molecular weight, transmembrane removal of LMW proteins in ARF patients occurs almost exclusively by this mechanism. However, adsorptive removal of inflammatory mediators in this class has also been demonstrated, and considerable controversy currently exists as to whether convection or adsorption optimizes mediator removal. Finally, in contrast to the above IHD data for ESRD patients, Mokrzycki and Kaplan (39) have recently reported a relatively modest mean total protein loss of 1.6 g/day in seven CRRT patients.

IV. REMOVAL OF SMALL NITROGENOUS WASTE PRODUCTS IN ARF

A. Factors Influencing Small Solute Removal in ARF

Factors that influence and impair small solute removal in ARF can be either patient related or therapy related. In the latter category, some of these factors are directly related to filter performance, while others relate to other aspects of the RRT.

Protein hypercatabolism, total body water, and body size are all patient-related factors that significantly impact the degree to which small solute removal provides azotemia control in ARF. Acute renal failure in the ICU epitomizes a non–steady-state condition, as urea generation rates and protein catabolic rates (PCRs) have been reported to vary on a daily basis (40,41). Protein hypercatabolism is nearly always present in this setting, with net normalized PCR (nPCR) values of 1.5 g/kg/day or greater and net nitrogen deficits of 6 g/day or greater routinely reported (40,42–44).

The nPCR values in ARF are reflective of the metabolic perturbations associated with ARF. The manner in which nPCR changes with time in critically ill patients treated with a CRRT has been reported to be quite variable. Clark et al. (40) found a linear relationship between nPCR and time, ranging from 1.5 to 1.9 g/kg/day over the first several days of therapy in patients treated with CVVH. On the other hand, Chima et al. (41) described an essentially random variation of nPCR with time in patients receiving CAVH.

Body size and the extent of volume overload in ARF patients are also critical considerations in RRT prescription. For both nonuremics and patients with ESRD, numerous previous investigations have documented that total body water closely approximates urea distribution volume, with values reported to be 0.55–0.60 L/kg of lean body mass (45–48). However, the relationship between V and lean body mass in ARF patients is not nearly as well defined. Several factors in ARF make determination of this relationship quite difficult. These factors include severe volume overload and ongoing catabolism of lean body mass.

Clark et al. (49) recently reported a mean V of 65% of body weight in a group of 11 hypercatabolic ARF patients whose mean IHD characteristics included 13 dialyses over a 24-day period. In concert with catabolism-induced loss of lean body mass, volume overload most likely accounts for the markedly higher fractional urea distribution volumes in ARF than those in ESRD patients and normal individuals. On the other hand, Clark et al. (50) found the mean value of V to be 0.55 L/kg of body weight in a group of 11 critically ill patients receiving CVVH at steady state.

As shown recently by Evanson et al. (51), failure to account for these volume disturbances may result in large discrepancies between prescribed and delivered HD doses. In a group of 45 patients who received a total of 136 HD treatments, these investigators used dialyzer KoA, prescribed blood flow rate and time, and a value of V equal to 0.60 × pre-HD body weight to estimate prescribed Kt/V. Delivered Kt/V was estimated by an equation employing pre-HD and post-HD BUN values, a technique that may be problematic in ARF (see below). Nonetheless, a significant difference was observed between prescribed and delivered Kt/V per treatment (1.26 ± 0.45 vs. 1.04 ± 0.49, respectively; mean ± SD). This difference appeared to be related primarily to the use of an estimated V, for prescription purposes, that was significantly less than the actual (kinetically derived) V. Our group has also highlighted the detrimental effect on expected small solute removal if volume overload is neglected (52). In addition, the large discrepancy between prescribed and delivered ARF dialysis doses observed in the Evanson et al. study has been corroborated by others (53).

Severe volume overload may also adversely influence small solute removal in relation to the large ultrafiltration requirements during IHD. During the relatively short duration of IHD (compared to CRRT), rapid osmolarity changes occur as large solute loads are removed from hypercatabolic patients. Especially in the early phase of a dialysis treatment, these osmolar changes may create a gradient for water movement from the intravascular space to the interstitial space. This water movement, in combination with the intravascular volume depletion occurring by extracorporeal ultrafiltration, may cause significant hypotension. A potential solution to this problem is the use of sequential ultrafiltration/dialysis (54), which involves an increase in overall treatment time if total urea removal is to be maintained. On the other hand, total urea removal is sacrificed if treatment time is kept constant. Dialytic sodium modeling is an alternative solution to this problem, but formal reports describing its use in ARF are presently lacking.

A number of RRT-related factors also influence small solute removal. Access recirculation may adversely affect the small solute clearances of any RRT. Although extensively investigated in ESRD patients with permanent (nonpercutaneous) vascular accesses (55,56), the determinants of percutaneous access recirculation in ARF patients are not as well characterized. Percutaneous catheters designed for long-term use in chronic hemodialysis have been shown by Twardowski et al. (57) to have very low (≈2%) degrees of recirculation. At a blood flow rate of 250 mL/min, Kelber et al. (58) reported comparably low values for subclavian and internal jugular catheters used for IHD in ARF. However, mean recirculation was 10% for 24 cm femoral catheters while shorter (15 cm) femoral catheters exhibited an even greater value of 18%. At a blood flow rate of 400 mL/min, the value of this latter measurement increased to 38%. These data have recently been corroborated by Leblanc et al. (59).

For small solutes, diffusive mass transfer resistances are an important consideration, and failure to apply the general principles discussed above may result in impaired removal. A widespread misconception is that because of the relatively open pore structure of highly permeable dialyzers (Kuf > 20 mL/h/mmHg), their urea removal capabilities are necessarily superior to those of low-permeability dialyzers (Kuf < 10 mL/h/mmHg). However, the thicknesses of highly permeable synthetic membranes (≥25 μm) are substantially larger than those of low-flux cellulosic membranes, most of which have thicknesses of <10 μm (2). At blood flow rates (<300 mL/min) typically employed in ARF, the urea clearances for the two types of dialyzers are actually very similar. Thus, the enhanced diffusivity of urea in highly permeable synthetic membranes is negated by the large diffusive resistance associated with their relatively thick structures.

To illustrate this point, in vitro urea clearances for a low-flux modified cellulosic dialyzer (Hemophan membrane: thickness ≈8 μm) and a high-flux polyacrylonitrile dialyzer (AN69 membrane: thickness ≈25 μm) can be compared. At an in vitro blood flow rate of 200 mL/min, the urea clearance of a 0.9 m^2 Hemophan dialyzer (117 mL/min) is actually about 6% greater than that (166 mL/min) of a AN69 dialyzer with comparable surface area (1.0 m^2) (60). Although increasing blood flow rate would have a relatively greater impact on urea clearance for the high-flux dialyzer, this comparison still attests to the importance of membrane thickness in determining small solute clearances. In addition, this comparison confirms the importance of using fundamental mass transfer principles in choosing an extracorporeal device for ARF patients.

Once an extracorporeal device and a specific RRT is chosen, adequate therapy prescription and delivery is imperative so that a selected target for metabolic control can be achieved. Two issues are pertinent in this regard. First, as previously discussed and as is the case in chronic hemodialysis, the amount of prescribed therapy is nearly always greater than the amount delivered (51,53). Second, at present, exactly what should be the targets for metabolic control in both IHD and CRRT remain to be defined (see below). Nonetheless, the clinician needs to have a specific target in mind when a RRT is prescribed.

B. Avoidance of Underdialysis: Use of Urea Kinetic Methods to Guide Therapy Prescription

The recognition that both morbidity and mortality are inversely related to delivered HD dose in ESRD patients has substantially changed clinical practices in the United States (60a,60b). A number of urea-based quantification methods that differ greatly in complexity and usefulness now are used in this setting. Investigators have recently begun to extrapolate some of these ESRD quantification techniques to the ARF setting. Examples of this are discussed below.

We have recently developed a computer-based model designed to permit individualized RRT prescription for ARF patients (61). The critical input parameter is the desired level of metabolic control, which is the time-averaged BUN (BUN_a) or steady-state BUN (BUN_s) for IHD or CRRT, respectively. The basis for the model was a group of 20 patients who received uninterrupted CRRT for at least 5 days. In these patients, the nPCR increased linearly ($r = 0.97$) from 1.55 ± 0.14 g/kg/day (mean ± SEM) on day 1 to 1.95 ± 0.15 g/kg/day on day 6. The daily value of G, determined from the above linear relationship, was employed to produce BUN versus time curves by the direct quantification method for simulated patients of varying dry weights (50–100 kg) who received variable CRRT clearances (500–2000 mL/h). Steady-state BUN versus time profiles for the same simulated patient population treated with IHD regimens ($K = 180$ mL/min; $t = 4$ hr per treatment) of variable frequency were generated by use of the variable-volume single pool kinetic model. From these profiles, regression lines of required IHD frequency (per week) versus patient weight for desired BUN_a values of 60, 80, and 100 mg/dL were obtained. Regression lines of required CRRT urea clearance (mL/h) versus patient weight for desired BUN_s values of 60, 80, and 100 mg/dL were also generated. The required amounts of IHD (treatment frequency) and CRRT (urea clearance) at these three levels of azotemic control were compared.

The results of these analyses appear in Table 2 and Figs. 1 and 2. For the attainment of intensive metabolic control (BUN_a = 60 mg/dL) at steady state, a required treatment frequency of 4.4 dialyses per week is predicted for a 50-kg patient. However, the model predicts that the same degree of metabolic control cannot be achieved even with daily IHD therapy in hypercatabolic ARF patients weighing more than 90 kg. Conversely, for the attainment of intensive CRRT metabolic control (BUN_s = 60 mg/dL), required urea clearances of approximately 900 and 1900 mL/h are predicted for 50-kg and 100-kg patients, respectively. Therefore, this model suggests that for many patients, rigorous azotemia control equivalent to that readily attainable with most CRRTs can only be achieved with intensive IHD regimens. Therefore, these modeled data suggest that the complication of inadequate azotemic control is less likely to occur in hypercatabolic ARF patients if a CRRT is used.

We also assessed the effect of variable IHD intermittence by plotting both IHD BUN_a and CRRT BUN_s versus the ratio $nPCR/(Kt/V)_d$, where the denominator in the latter term represents the normalized daily therapy dose. As previously predicted and shown for patients with nESRD (45) and ARF (40), a linear relationship was observed when these regression analyses

Table 2 Continuous Renal Replacement Therapy Clearance Rate (mL/h)/Intermittent Hemodialysis Frequency (per week) Requirements for Varying Levels of Azotemia Control[a]

Weight (kg)	BUN = 60 mg/dL	BUN = 80 mg/dL	BUN = 100 mg/dL
50	886/4.4	668/3.2	535/<3.0
60	1097/5.2	823/3.8	649/3.0
70	1300/6.0	977/4.4	763/3.5
80	1500/6.9	1123/5.0	886/4.0
90	1686/NA	1279/5.6	1018/4.5
100	1911/NA	1432/6.2	1133/5.0

[a]BUN value is either continuous renal replacement therapy steady-state BUN or intermittent hemodialysis time-averaged BUN.
NA, not achievable with daily dialysis.
Source: Ref. 61.

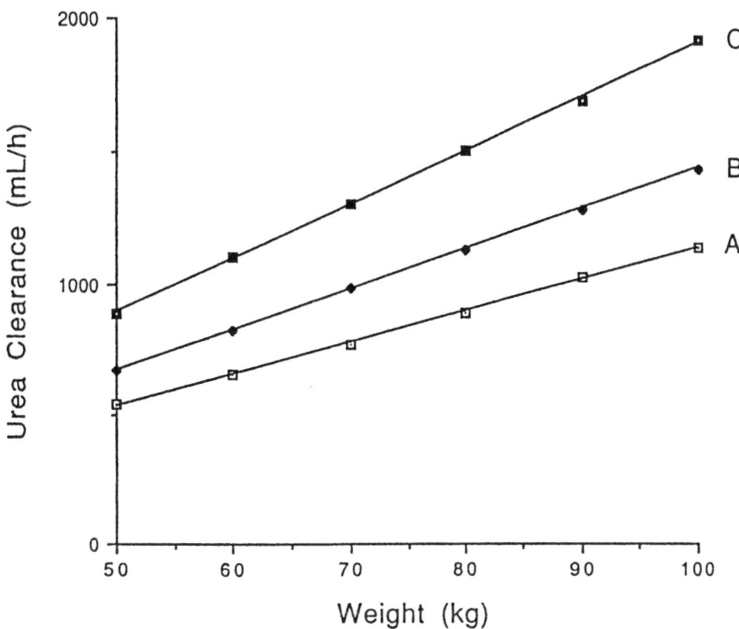

Fig. 1 Predicted CRRT urea clearance required for the attainment of varying desired levels of steady-state azotemia control (BUNs). The clearances shown are for patients ranging in size from 50 to 100 kg. The target BUNs values for curves A, B, and C are 100, 80, and 60 mg/dL, respectively. (From Ref. 61.)

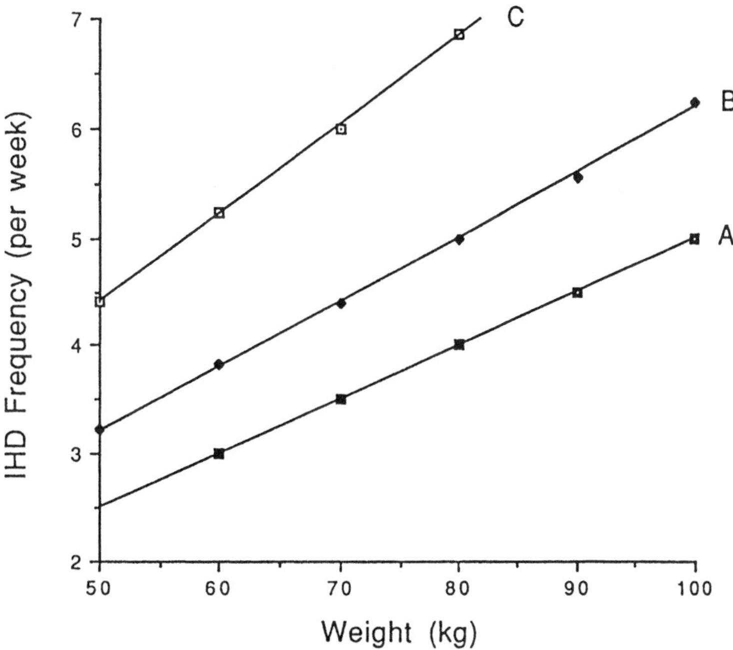

Fig. 2 Predicted IHD frequencies required for the attainment of varying desired levels of time-averaged azotemia control (BUNa). The frequencies are shown for patients ranging in size from 50 to 100 kg. The target BUNa values for curves A, B, and C are 100, 80, and 60 mg/dL, respectively. (From Ref. 61.)

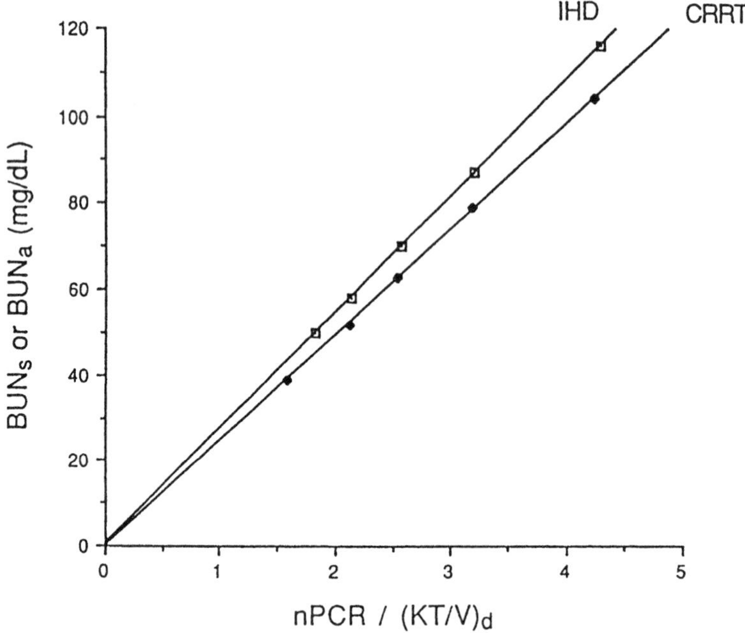

Fig. 3 Steady-state RRT azotemia control versus the ratio nPCR/(Kt/V)d. The curves are shown for a patient of 70 kg dry weight. The CRRT line represents BUNs values, whereas the IHD line represents BUNa values. (From Ref. 61.)

were performed (Fig. 3). The two regression lines shown are for simulated patient of dry weight 70 kg. Because nPCR was constant in these steady state simulations (1.95 g/kg/day), variations in the abscissa were attributable entirely to changes in $(Kt/V)_d$. In turn, changes in therapy dose were related to changes in K for CRRT and in treatment frequency for IHD. Therefore, the points determining the CRRT line represent K values ranging from 750 mL/h [highest $nPCR/(Kt/V)_d$ value] to 2000 mL/h [lowest $nPCR/(Kt/V)_d$ value]. Conversely, the points on the IHD line represent treatment frequencies ranging from three per week [highest $nPCR/(Kt/V)_d$ value] to seven per week [lowest $nPCR/(Kt/V)_d$ value]. This figure shows that the degree of divergence between the CRRT BUN_s and IHD BUN_a lines decrease with increasing IHD frequency [i.e., decreasing $nPCR/(Kt/V)_d$]. This convergence shows that the inherent inefficiency associated with an intermittent therapy, relative to that of a continuous therapy, decreases with increasing frequency. Therefore, if IHD is the chosen therapy and the complication of inadequate metabolic control is to be avoided, high therapy frequency has specific benefits (62). In addition to the benefits specifically pertaining to the kinetics of solute removal, increased IHD frequency may result in decreased ultrafiltration requirements per treatment. The avoidance of hypotensive episodes related to rapid ultrafiltration rates may also indirectly improve solute removal by decreasing the risk of therapy interruptions.

C. Small Solute Control in ARF: Effect of Amount of Delivered Therapy on Outcome

Based on presently available data, precise targets for optimal metabolic control are not able to be provided for ARF patients treated with either IHD or CRRT. However, at least for IHD, rough guidelines exist. Kjellstrand has suggested that IHD should be initiated before the BUN reaches 100 mg/dL and that therapy should be delivered at a level to maintain the pre-dialysis BUN below 100 mg/dL (63). Support for these recommendations is found in early comparative studies in which groups of patients received substantially different levels of IHD therapy (64–66). In these investigations, survival was directly correlated with IHD intensity as measured by predialysis BUN, which ranged from approximately 90 to 150 mg/dL.

In a more contemporary study, Gillum et al. (67) reported results from a multicenter, prospective study in which the effect of dialysis intensity on survival in patients with ARF was investigated. In this trial, a total of 34 patients with diverse ARF etiologies received either "intensive" or "nonintensive" dialysis. Daily dialysis of 5–6 hours per treatment was generally prescribed in the intensive group, while the regimen in the nonintensive group consisted of 5-hour treatments administered daily to every third day. Mean predialysis azotemia control achieved in the two groups was very close to the target BUN and serum creatinine values of 60 and 5 mg/dL, respectively (intensive group), and 100 and 9 mg/dL, respectively (nonintensive group). However, prescribed blood and dialysate flow rates were not provided. In addition, data permitting an estimation of the rate of interdialytic urea generation were not reported. Therefore, neither dialysis dose nor PCR could be estimated. Nevertheless, survival in the intensively treated group (41%) did not differ significantly from that in the nonintensive group (52%).

Although serum creatinine was used as an efficacy parameter in the above study, recent data suggest that this parameter should not be used in this manner. Our group recently quantified steady-state creatinine kinetic parameters in a group of 11 critically ill ARF patients who received CVVH (68). In these patients, of whom four were women, the mean pretreatment serum creatinine was 5.6 ± 2.6 mg/dL, while the value was 3.4 ± 1.7 mg/dL at steady state, which occurred after a mean treatment period of approximately one week. A significant linear relationship was observed between steady-state serum creatinine and both creatinine generation rate and lean body mass. Normalized to body weight, mean lean body mass was found to be 0.51 ± 0.09 kg/kg, a value significantly lower than previously reported for both normal and ESRD patients. These data suggest that the steady-state serum creatinine is best viewed as a nutritional parameter rather than a therapy efficacy parameter in this patient population. Indirect support for this contention comes from recent data of Paganini et al. (53), who report that death is associated with a low rate of rise of serum creatinine in the ICU ARF population (see below).

In a recent study of 58 consecutive ICU ARF patients receiving IHD at the Cleveland Clinic, Tapolyai et al. (69) correlated patient outcome (survival vs. death) with a variety of patient-related and dialysis-related parameters. Patient demographics, hemodynamic status, and illness severity scores were similar in surviving and nonsurviving patients. Dialysis dose for each treatment was estimated by calculation of single-pool Kt/V. The prescribed Kt/V was not significantly different between the two groups. However, the mean delivered Kt/V per treatment was significantly higher among survivors (survivors: 1.09; nonsurvivors: 0.89). Although the actual Kt/V determination method was not specified in this preliminary report, these data suggest that survival in critically ill patients is correlated directly with delivered IHD dose.

In a more recent publication (53), the Cleveland Clinic group has extended this analysis. These investigators assessed outcome in 842 ICU ARF patients who received RRT between 1988 and 1994 at their institution. The Cleveland Clinic Foundation (CCF) ARF scoring system (70) was employed to estimate illness severity. In this system, 23 different demographic, clinical, and laboratory parameters are used to produce a score ranging from 0 (low mortality) to 20 (high mortality). Eight factors were found to be associated strongly with poor patient outcome, including need for mechanical ventilation, leukopenia, thrombocytopenia, number of nonrenal organ system failure, and a low rate of increase in the serum creatinine. When patient outcome was adjusted for the CCF outcome score, survival was correlated with delivered IHD ($Kt/V > 1.0$ per treatment).

In a prospective study, Schiffl et al. (71) randomized 72 ICU ARF patients to either daily IHD or every other day IHD. Overall mortality in this study was 35% but was significantly lower in the daily IHD group (21%) than in the alternate day group (47%). Using weekly Kt/V as the discriminating parameter, these investigators observed a significantly lower mortality in the high-dose group ($Kt/V > 6.0$ per week; 16%) than in the low-dose group ($Kt/V < 3.0$ per week; 57%).

Both of the above studies have employed a single-pool quantification technique developed specifically for the ESRD population (72). The equation used in these studies contains constants accounting for the effects of intradialytic urea generation and ultrafiltration on delivered dose. However, these constants were generated from ESRD patients. Therefore, extrapolation of this or any other equation developed specifically for ESRD patients to ARF patients may be problematic, as recently demonstrated by Lo et al. (73).

Recent studies also suggest that the intensity of CRRT influences outcome. Data from Storck et al. (74) suggest that greater intensity of CRRT produces is associated with better patient outcomes. In this study, patients were treated with either CAVH or CVVH such that a wide range of ultrafiltration rates was obtained. Survival was found to be significantly higher in the CVVH group than in the CAVH group, in which the mean ultrafiltration rates were 15.5 and 7.5 L/day, respectively. Whether the superior survival in the patients treated with CVVH rather than CAVH was related to the former's greater convective removal of small solutes or larger substances could not be determined from the data provided. In addition, data from Paganini et al. suggest that a steady-state BUN of ≤45 mg/dL is associated with a favorable outcome in CRRT patients (53).

D. Small Solute Removal Capabilities of Renal Replacement Therapies Used in Acute Renal Failure

The first extensive description of the use of CAVH in patients with ARF was published by Lauer et al. in 1983 (75). An average ultrafiltrate production rate of 10 L/day obtained in these patients allowed BUN values to be maintained below 90 mg/dL. Urea nitrogen removal was reported to range between 4 and 12 g/day. Notably, a blood pump resulting in blood flow rates as high as 200 mL/min was used in some patients. Kaplan et al. (76) treated a series of 15 patients with postdilution CAVH, which was associated with a mean daily ultrafiltrate production rate of 13.7 L/day. In all but three patients, BUN values were kept below 100 mg/dL. For treatments in which ultrafiltrate production fell below 400 mL/h, wall vacuum suction (200 mmHg) was applied to the filtrate line. In neither of these reports were estimates of protein catabolic rate provided.

Following its initial description by Geronemus and Schneider (19), Sigler and Teehan (20) assessed azotemia control by CAVHD in a series of 15 critically ill patients who received this therapy over a mean duration of 159 hours. Blood flow rates ranging from 40 to 180 mL/min resulted in a mean ultrafiltration rate of 6.9 L/day while the dialysate flow rate was consistently 1 L/h. From this combination of operating parameters, a mean whole blood urea clearance of 23.8 mL/min (34.3 L/day) was obtained. In turn, pretreatment and posttreatment BUN values were 76 and 50 mg/dL, respectively. As in the above CAVH studies, the degree of protein catabolism for these patients was not reported.

With an increasing awareness of the complications and limitations of continuous arteriovenous therapies, the use of continuous venvenous therapies (21–23,34,35) has steadily increased over the past several years. Macias et al. (34) described their experience with blood pump–assisted hemofiltration (CVVH) in a series of 25 patients who were treated for a mean duration of 7.7 days. The mean blood flow and ultrafiltration production rates were 147 mL/min and 879 mL/h (21.1 L/day), respectively. Azotemia control was characterized by a decrease in the BUN from 89 mg/dL pre-CVVH to 79 mg/dL at the cessation of treatment.

More recent reports have described the use of CVVHD (21,22) and CVVHDF (23) in ARF patients. Ifedoria et al. (22) employed CVVHD in a series of patients with the following operating parameters: blood flow rate, 100 mL/min; inlet dialysate flow rate, 5–30 mL/min; and ultrafiltration rate, up to 300 mL/h. The latter two parameters were varied to meet solute and volume removal requirements, respectively. The achieved blood urea clearances of 10–40 mL/min resulted in a fall in the BUN from a mean pretreatment value of 82 mg/dL to a mean value of 54 mg/dL after 48–72 hours of therapy. Although the dialysate flow rates typically used in CVVHDF are similar to those used in CVVHD, ultrafiltration rates in the former are significantly greater. In a CVVHDF system described by Mehta (23), the dialysate flow rate was 1 L/h and the ultrafiltration rate approximately 0.7 L/h. The resultant urea clearances, which had approximately equal diffusive and convective components, approached 45 L/day. This investigator has reported the routine attainment of steady-state BUN values in the 40–50 mg/dL range, even in hypercatabolic patients.

V. DIALYTIC REMOVAL OF OTHER SMALL SOLUTES IN ACUTE RENAL FAILURE

Because derangements in phosphate balance (77) and amino acid profiles (78) are commonly found in ARF, the extracorporeal removal of these compounds is an important consideration. Although the apparent molecular weight of inorganic phosphate is relatively low, hydration of this charged molecule renders its effective molecular weight much larger. In addition, the kinetics of phosphate removal during IHD is controlled by compartmentalization related to relatively slow internal mass transfer (79). Therefore, phosphate is relatively inefficiently removed during IHD, especially when a low-flux dialyzer is employed.

Phosphate removal is much more effective in CRRT due to the greater use of large-pore membranes and the combination of long treatment time and relatively low rate of extracorporeal removal, the latter of which renders intercompartment mass transfer of much less importance. The difference between IHD and CRRT with respect to phosphate removal is clearly demonstrated by the need for phosphate supplementation in the two therapies. Phosphate supplementation is required to prevent the development of hypophosphatemia in a large percentage of patients treated with CRRT employing both diffusion and convection (80). On the other hand, the need for phosphate supplementation is relatively rare in patients treated with IHD, except possibly in malnourished patients who have an anabolic response to nutritional supplementation.

Unlike urea, creatinine, and phosphate, amino acids are not waste products and the concentrations of these solutes do not rise predictably in ARF. However, they are small solutes that can be appreciably removed by extracorporeal therapies used in ARF. This dialytic removal of amino acids is important in the critically ill ARF patient for two reasons. First, ARF commonly results in perturbations in both plasma muscle amino acid profiles, such that individual amino acid concentrations may be abnormally elevated or depleted. Therefore, the dialytic removal of those amino acids whose plasma concentrations are already low due to ARF itself is particularly undesirable. Second, extracorporeal removal renders a certain fraction of amino acids infused as part of a parenteral nutrition formulation to be not available for systemic incorporation. Recent data suggest that the extent of this fractional amino acid removal is RRT dependent. Hynote et al. (81) measured amino acid clearances in a group of five ICU ARF patients treated with IHD. These investigators used total dialysate collections to measure clearance and total removal during both low-flux and high-flux treatments using unsubstituted cellulosic and polysulfone dialyzers, respectively. Treatments were performed for an average duration of 3 hours per session with a blood flow rate of 200–300 mL/min and a dialysate flow rate of 500 mL/min. For all treatments, the mean amino acid clearances were 107 and 150 mL/min in the low-flux and high-flux arms, respectively ($p = 0.01$), while the mean amino acid removal amounts were 5.2 and 7.3 g/treatment, respectively ($p = 0.05$). Based on total dialytic removal, extracorporeal losses represented 7.2% of the infused amino acids in the low-flux arm and 10.1% in the high-flux arm.

Frankenfeld et al. (82) quantified amino acid removal in ARF patients treated with CRRT. These investigators measured amino acid clearance and total extracorporeal removal by CAVHD for 17 patients in whom varying dialysate flow rates were employed. In addition, the effluent filtrate to blood urea nitrogen concentration ratio (FUN:BUN) was also measured to provide an estimate of filter efficacy. The dialysate flow rate was set at either 15 or 30 mL/min. Both effluent dialysate volume and FUN:BUN were found to be significant predictors of amino acid losses such that:

$$\text{Total amino acid losses (g/12 h)} = -2.0 + \text{effluent volume} \times 0.273 + \text{FUN:BUN} \times 2.97$$

In aggregate, these two studies demonstrate that for ARF patients receiving both parenteral nutrition and RRT, dialytic amino acid removal causes the amount of delivered therapy to be less than that prescribed. This effective reduction in the delivered dose must be considered when parenteral nutrition is provided in the ARF setting.

VI. DIALYTIC REMOVAL OF MIDDLE MOLECULES IN ACUTE RENAL FAILURE

For the characterization of dialyzer performance, vitamin B_{12} (molecular weight, 1355 daltons) is widely used as an in vitro middle molecule surrogate. However, this solute has little relevance in in vivo dialyzer evaluations due to its extensive plasma protein binding. A more relevant middle molecule is vancomycin (molecular weight, 1448 daltons) for several reasons. First, the drug is commonly used in patients with acute renal failure and assays for serum concentration determinations are widely available. Second, vancomycin is minimally protein bound in patients with renal failure (83) and available to be removed by extracorporeal techniques. Finally, the drug's volume of distribution is well characterized (84) and, although it has a slightly larger range, it approximates that of urea.

Numerous studies have assessed the dialytic removal of vancomycin both in ESRD and ARF patients. Contrary to the negligible removal of vancomycin during IHD with low-flux unsubstituted cellulosic dialyzers (85), substantial diffusive removal of this drug is achieved with high-flux IHD (85–90). However, initial reports of this latter phenomenon overestimated the actual extent of removal by failing to account for the significant rebound that occurs after high-flux IHD (86). This post-IHD rebound is explained by the slower rate of vancomycin mass transfer between well-perfused compartments of the body (i.e., extracellular space) and poorly perfused compartments (i.e., intracellular space), relative to the rate of dialytic transmembrane mass transfer (68). As is the case for urea, the extent of vancomycin rebound is directly related to dialyzer clearance of the drug. Due to the difficulty in predicting post-IHD vancomycin rebound and its effect on drug dosing in high-flux IHD, many clinicians favor the use of low-flux dialyzers for patients receiving vancomycin.

Due to the much slower rate of extracorporeal removal of vancomycin during CRRT, the disequilibrium between body compartments described above for high-flux IHD is not a major consideration. As described previously (25), recent data suggest convection is a more efficient removal mechanism than diffusion when typical blood and dialysate flow rates are used in CRRT. For convection-based CRRT, in vivo sieving coefficients of vancomycin have been reported in the 0.8–0.9 range (91). Therefore, total (daily) drug removal tends to be somewhat higher in CVVH than in CVVHD when ultrafiltrate and effluent dialysate volumes, respectively, are the same. Vancomycin dosing needs to account for the variable extent of extracorporeal drug removal by the different therapies used in ARF.

VII. DIALYTIC REMOVAL OF PLASMA PROTEINS IN ACUTE RENAL FAILURE

The identification of β_2-microglobulin as a precursor molecule in the development of dialysis-related amyloidosis established low-molecular weight proteins as a new class of uremic toxins (92). In response to this discovery, significant effort has been directed toward developing membranes and treatment strategies that optimize β_2-microglobulin removal. However, efforts to enhance β_2-microglobulin removal by increasing membrane permeability have been limited by the concomitant need to minimize the removal of other proteins, such as albumin (93).

In some critically ill patients with ARF, LMW proteins also represent a class of molecules considered "toxic." However, specifically in the case of patients with sepsis or multisystem organ failure, the specific toxins are inflammatory mediators, such as cytokines and complement pathway products. The topic of mediator removal is not discussed further here, as this subject in the context of high-volume hemofiltration is addressed in detail elsewhere in this book. However, it is worth noting that the same general constraint of minimizing albumin removal while maximizing LMW protein removal, described above for ESRD therapies, applies to the use of CRRT in sepsis-related conditions. In this regard, Mokrzycki and Kaplan (39) have recently measured total protein losses in a series of ARF patients treated with CRRT. Both CVVH and CVVHDF were employed in this study, such that daily filter output volumes ranged from approximately 1000 to 2000 mL/h. High-flux polysulfone dialyzers and polysulfone hemofilters were used. A direct relationship between dialysate/ultrafiltrate total protein concentration and serum total protein concentration was observed. When the CVVH and CVVHDF data were combined, the mean daily total protein loss was found to be 1.6 g. However, when relatively high-volume CVVH (approximately 2000 mL/h ultrafiltration rate) was used, the daily loss was found to be as high as 7.5 g.

Although the study suggests that albumin removal by the continuous therapies is clinically acceptable, it must be borne in mind that the ultrafiltration rates and membrane used were typical for conventional CRRT. However, some investigators have recently proposed the use of both high ultrafiltration rates (up to 6 L/h) and hemofilters of increased permeability (15,16) specifically to enhance the removal of inflammatory mediators. Although both of these therapy modifications may enhance mediator elimination, the undesirable convective removal of albumin may also be expected to increase substantially. In light of the pervasive extent of both somatic and visceral malnutrition in this patient population, quantification of albumin losses will have to be performed as the use of high-volume hemofiltration increases.

Table 3 Complications Related to Solute Removal in CRRT

Solute	CRRT role	Root cause	Clinical consequence
Nitrogenous wastes	Inadequate removal	Filter dysfunction Inadequate Rx	Poor metabolic control
Water-soluble vitamins	Excessive removal	Inadequate supplementation	Metabolic disorders
Amino acids	Excessive removal	Inadequate supplementation	Malnutrition; negative nitrogen balance
Phosphate	Excessive removal	Inadequate supplementation	Hypophosphatemia
Drugs (vancomycin, aminoglycosides)	Excessive removal	Inadequate supplementation	Antimicrobial therapy failure
Large proteins	High ultrafiltration rate or filter porosity	—	Hypoproteinemia

VIII. SUMMARY AND CONCLUSIONS

Table 3 attempts to summarize the complications of CRRT potentially related to solute removal. Certain complications are related to inadequate solute removal, such as inadequate metabolic control related to insufficient small solute removal, which in turn may be due to filter dysfunction or an inadequate prescription. However, most of the complications are iatrogenic in origin, typically being related to inadequate supplementation of solutes that are relatively efficiently removed by CRRT.

There is a growing interest in defining the adequacy of solute removal by ARF dialytic therapies. At present, for neither IHD nor CRRT is adequate therapy defined, although some recent preliminary data exist for IHD. In addition, techniques specifically designed to measure the delivered dialysis dose in ARF have not been developed and validated. As is the case for chronic hemodialysis, the future of therapy quantification may rest in on-line quantification (94).

REFERENCES

1. Douma C, Redekop W, Van Der Meulen J, Van Olden R, Haeck J, Struijk D, Krediet R. Predicting mortality in intensive care patients with acute renal failure treated with dialysis. J Am Soc Nephrol 1997; 8:111–117.
2. Lysaght M. Evolution of hemodialysis membranes. Contrib Nephrol 1995; 113:1–10.
3. Colton C, Lowrie E. Hemodialysis: physical principles and technical considerations. In: Brenner B, Rector F, eds. The Kidney. 2d ed. Philadelphia: W.B. Saunders Co., 1981:2425–2489.
4. Colton C. Analysis of membrane processes for blood purification. Blood Purif 1987; 5:202–251.
5. Sargent J, Gotch F. Principles and biophysics of dialysis. In: Maher J, ed. Replacement of Renal Function by Dialysis. 3rd ed. Dordrecht: Kluwer Academic Publishers, 1989:89–91.
6. Colton CK, Lysaght M. Membranes for hemodialysis. In: Jacobs C, ed. Replacement of Renal Function by Dialysis. 4th ed. Dordrecht: Kluwer Academic Publishers, 1995:107–108.
7. Henderson LW. Biophysics of ultrafiltration and hemofiltration. In: Jacobs C, ed. Replacement of Renal Function by Dialysis. 4th ed. Dordrecht: Kluwer Academic Publishers, 1995:114–118.
8. Ofsthun NJ, Zydney AL. Importance of convection in artificial kidney treatment. Contrib Nephrol 1994; 108: 53–70.
9. Scott MK, Mueller BA, Clark WR. Effect of membrane type on the performance of bleach-reprocessed high-flux dialyzers (abstr). J Am Soc Nephrol 1997; 8:172A.
10. Naitoh A, Tatsuguchi T, Okada M, Ohmura T, Sakai K. Removal of beta-2-microglobulin by diffusion alone is feasible using highly permeable dialysis membranes. Trans Am Soc Artif Intern Organs 1988; 34:630–634.
11. Mineshama M, Hoshino T, Era K, Kitano Y, Suzuki T, Sanaka T, Teraoka S, Ahishi T, Ota K. Difference in β_2-microglobulin removal between cellulosic and synthetic polymer membrane dialyzers. Trans Am Soc Artif Intern Organs 1990; 36:M643–M646.
12. Rockel A, Hertel J, Fiegel P, Abdelhamid S, Panitz N, Walb D. Permeability and secondary membrane formation of a high flux polysulfone hemofilter. Kidney Int 1986; 30:429–432.
13. Kim S. Characteristics of protein removal in hemodiafiltration. Contr Nephrol 1994; 108:23–37.
14. Henderson LW. Pre vs post dilution hemofiltration. Clin Nephrol 1979; 11:120–124.
15. Grootendorst AF, Van Bommel EFH, Van Der Hoven B. High-volume hemofiltration improves hemodynamics of endotoxin-induced shock in the pig. Intensive Care Med 1992; 18:235–240.
16. Grootendorst AF, Van Bommel EFH, Van Leengoed LAMG, Van Der Hoven B. Infusion of ultrafiltrate from endotoxemic pigs depresses myocardial performance in normal pigs. J Crit Care 1993; 8:161–169.
17. Werynski A, Waniewski J. Theoretical description of mass transport in medical membrane devices. Artif Organs 1995; 19:420–427.
18. Jaffrin M. Convective mass transfer in hemodialysis. Artif Organs 1995; 19:1162–1171.
19. Geronemus R, Schneider N. Continuous arteriovenous hemodialysis: a new modality for treatment of acute renal failure. Trans Am Soc Artif Intern Organs 1984; 30:610–612.
20. Sigler MH, Teehan BP. Solute transport in continuous hemodialysis: a new treatment for renal failure. Kidney Int 1987; 32:562–571.
21. Relton S, Greenberg A, Palevsky P. Dialysate and blood flow dependence of diffusive solute clearance during CVVHD. ASAIO J 1992; 38:691–696.
22. Ifedoria O, Teehan B, Sigler M. Solute clearance in continuous venovenous hemodialysis. ASAIO J 1992; 38:697–701.
23. Mehta RL. Therapeutic alternatives to renal replacement for critically ill patients in acute renal failure. Semin Nephrol 1994; 14:64–82.
24. Scott MK, Mueller BA, Clark WR. Vancomycin mass transfer characteristics of high flux cellulosic dialyzers. Nephrol Dial Transplant 1997; 12:2647–2653.
25. Jeffrey RF, Khan AA, Prabhu P, Todd N, Goutcher E, Will EJ, Davison AM. A comparison of molecular clearance rates during continuous hemofiltration and hemodialysis with a novel volumetric continuous renal replacement system. Artif Organs 1994; 18:425–428.
26. Clark WR, Macias WL, Molitoris BA, Wang NHL. Membrane adsorption of β_2-microglobulin: equilibrium

and kinetic characterization. Kidney Int 1994; 46:1140–1146.

27. Pascual M, Schifferli JA. Adsorption of complement factor D by polyacrylonitrile dialysis membranes. Kidney Int 1993; 43:903–911.
28. Goldfarb S, Golper TA. Proinflammatory cytokines and hemofiltration membranes. J Am Soc Nephrol 1994; 5: 228–232.
29. Bellomo R, Tipping P, Boyce N. Tumor necrosis factor clearances during veno-venous hemodiafiltration in the critically ill. Trans Am Soc Artif Intern Organs 1991; 37:M322–M323.
30. Riera JA, Vela JL, Quintana MJ, Lopez E, de Solo B, Checa A. Cytokines clearance during venovenous hemofiltration in the trauma patient. Am J Kidney Dis 1997; 30:483–488.
31. Scott MK, Mueller BA, Clark WR. Dialyzer-dependent changes in solute and water permeability with bleach reprocessing. Am J Kidney Dis. In press.
32. Clark WR, Macias WL, Molitoris BA, Wang NHL. Plasma protein adsorption to highly permeable hemodialysis membranes. Kidney Int 1995; 48:481–488.
33. Kaplan AA, Halley SE, Lapkin RA, Graeber CW. Dialysate protein losses with bleach processed polysulphone dialyzers. Kidney Int 1995; 47:573–578.
34. Macias WL, Mueller BA, Scarim SK, Robinson M, Rudy D. Continuous venovenous hemofiltration: an alternative to continuous arteriovenous hemofiltration and hemodiafiltration in acute renal failure. Am J Kidney Dis 1991; 18:451–458.
35. Canaud B, Garred L, Christol J, Anbas S, Beraud J, Mion C. Pump-assisted continuous venovenous hemofiltration for treating acute uremia. Kidney Int 1988; 33: S154–S156.
36. Golper T, Erbeck K, Roberts P, Price J. Small solute sieving coefficients using hemodialyzers as filters in continuous venovenous hemofiltration (abstr). J Am Soc Nephrol 1992; 3:367.
37. Schaeffer J, Olbricht CJ, Koch KM. Long-term performance of hemofilters in continuous hemofiltration. Nephron 1996; 72:155–158.
38. Ofsthun NJ, Colton CK, Lysaght MJ. Determinants of fluid and solute removal rates during hemofiltration. In: Henderson L, Quellhorst E, Baldamus C, Lysaght M, eds. Hemofiltration. Berlin: Springer-Verlag, 1986:17–39.
39. Mokrzycki M, Kaplan AA. Protein losses in continuous renal replacement therapies. J Am Soc Nephrol 1996; 7:2259–2263.
40. Clark WR, Alaka KJ, Mueller BA, Macias WL. A comparison of metabolic control by continuous and intermittent therapies in acute renal failure. J Am Soc Nephrol 1994; 4:1413–1420.
41. Chima CS, Meyer L, Hummell AC, Bosworth C, Heyka R, Paganini E, Werynski A. Protein catabolic rate in patients with acute renal failure on continuous arteriovenous hemofiltration and total parenteral nutrition. JASN 1993; 3:1516–1521.
42. Feinstein EI, Blumenkrantz MJ, Healy M, Koffler A, Silberman H, Massry S, Kopple J. Clinical and metabolic responses to parenteral nutrition in acute renal failure. Medicine 1981; 60:124–137.
43. Feinstein EI, Kopple JD, Silberman H, Massry SG. Total parenteral nutrition with high or low nitrogen intakes in patients with acute renal failure. Kidney Int 1983; 26:S319–S323.
44. Ikizler TA, Greene JH, Wingard RL, Hakim RM. Nitrogen balance in acute renal failure (ARF) patients (abstr). JASN 1995; 6:466.
45. Gotch F. Kinetic modeling in hemodialysis. In: Nissenson A, Fine R, Gentile D, eds. Clinical Dialysis. 2nd ed. Norwalk: Appleton and Lange, 1990:118–146.
46. Watson P, Watson I, Batt R. Total body water volumes for adult males and females estimated from simple anthropometric measurements. Am J Clin Nutr 1980; 33: 27–39.
47. Hume R, Weyers E: Relationship between total body water and surface area in normal and obese subjects. J Clin Pathol 1974; 24:234–238.
48. Malina R. Quantification of fat, muscle, and bone in man. Clin Orthop Relat Res 1969; 65:9–38.
49. Clark WR, Alaka KJ, Mueller BA, Macias WL. Comparison of metabolic control by intermittent versus continuous renal replacement therapy in patients with acute renal failure (abstr). Trans Am Soc Artif Intern Organs 1993; 39:95.
50. Clark WR, Murphy MH, Alaka K, Mueller BA, Pastan SO, Macias WL. Urea kinetics in continuous hemofiltration. ASAIO J 1992; 38:M664–M667.
51. Evanson J, Hakim R, Wingard R, Knights S, Schulman G, Ikizler T, Himmelfarb J. Assessment of dialysis dose in acute renal failure patients (abstr). J Am Soc Nephrol 1996; 7:1512.
52. Clark WR, Mueller BA, Kraus MA, Macias WL. Solute control by extracorporeal therapies in acute renal failure. Am J Kidney Dis 1996; 28(suppl 3):S21–S27.
53. Paganini EP, Tapolyai M, Goormastic M, Halstenberg W, Kozlowski L, Leblanc M, Lee JC, Moreno L, Sakai K. Establishing a dialysis therapy/patient outcome link in intensive care unit acute dialysis for patients with acute renal failure. Am J Kidney Dis 1996; 28(suppl 3):S81–S89.
54. Wehle B, Asaba H, Castenfors J. Hemodynamic changes during sequential ultrafiltration and dialysis. Kidney Int 1979; 15:411–418.
55. Sherman R. The measurement of dialysis access recirculation. Am J Kidney Dis 1993; 22:616–621.
56. Windus D. Permanent vascular access: A nephrologist's view. Am J Kidney Dis 1993; 21:457–471.
57. Twardowski Z, Van Stone J, Jones M, Klusmeyer M, Haynie J. Blood recirculation in intravenous catheters for hemodialysis. J Am Soc Nephrol 1993; 3:1978–1981.

58. Kelber J, Delmez J, Windus D. Factors affecting delivery of high-efficiency dialysis using temporary vascular access. Am J Kidney Dis 1993; 22:24–29.
59. Leblanc M, Fedak S, Mokris G, Paganini E. Blood recirculation in central temporary catheters for acute hemodialysis. Clin Nephrol 1996; 45:315–319.
60. Van Stone J: Hemodialysis apparatus. In: Daugirdas J, Ing T, eds. Handbook of Dialysis. 2d ed. Boston: Little, Brown and Company, 1994:32–38.
60a. Clark WR, Rocco MV, Collins AJ. Quantification of hemodialysis: analysis of methods and the relevance to patient outcome. Blood Purif 1997; 15:92–111.
60b. NKF-DOQI Hemodialysis Adequacy Work Group. Clinical practice guidelines for hemodialysis adequacy. Am J Kidney Dis 1997; 30(suppl 2):S15–S66.
61. Clark WR, Mueller BA, Kraus MA, Macias WL. Extracorporeal therapy requirements for patients with acute renal failure. J Am Soc Nephrol 1997; 8:804–812.
62. Clark WR, Ronco C. Renal replacement therapy quantification in acute renal failure: solute removal mechanisms and dose quantification. Kidney Int 1998; 53(suppl 66):S133–S137.
63. Kjellstrand C, Jacobson S, Lins L. Acute renal failure. In: Maher J, ed. Replacement of Renal Function by Dialysis. 3rd ed. Dordrecht: Kluwer Academic Publishers, 1989:616–649.
64. Gornick C, Kjellstrand C. Acute renal failure complicating aortic aneurysm surgery. Nephron 1983; 35:145–157.
65. Matas M, Payne W, Simmons R, Buselmeier T, Kjellstrand C. Acute renal failure following blunt civilian trauma. Ann Surg 1977; 185:301–306.
66. Kleinknecht D, Jungers P, Chanard J, Barbanel C, Ganeval D. Uremic and non-uremic complications in acute renal failure: evaluation of early and frequent dialysis on prognosis. Kidney Int 1972; 1:190–196.
67. Gillum DM, Dixon BS, Yanover MJ, Kelleher S, Shapiro M, Benedetti R, Dillingham M, Paller M, Goldberg J, Tomford R, Gordon J, Conger JD. The role of intensive dialysis in acute renal failure. Clin Nephrol 1986; 25:249–255.
68. Clark WR, Mueller BA, Kraus MA, Macias WL. Quantification of creatinine kinetic parameters in patients with acute renal failure. Kidney Int 1998; 54:554–560.
69. Tapolyai M, Fedak S, Chaff C, Paganini E. Delivered dialysis dose may influence ARF outcome in ICU patients (abstr). JASN 1994; 5:530.
70. Paganini EP, Halstenberg W, Goormastic M. Risk modeling in acute renal failure requiring dialysis: the introduction of a new model. Clin Nephrol 1996; 44:206–211.
71. Schiffl H, Lang S, Konig A, Held E. Dose of intermittent hemodialysis and outcome of acute renal failure: a prospective randomized study (abstr). J Am Soc Nephrol 1997; 8:290A.
72. Daugirdas JT. Second generation logarithmic estimates of single-pool variable volume Kt/V: an analysis of error. J Am Soc Nephrol 1993; 4:1205–1213.
73. Lo AJ, Depner TA, Chin ES, Craig MA. Urea disequilibrium contributes to underdialysis in the intensive care unit (abstr). J Am Soc Nephrol 1997; 8:287A.
74. Storck M, Hartl W, Zimmerer E, Inthorn D. Comparison of pump-driven and spontaneous hemofiltration in postoperative acute renal failure. Lancet 1991; 337:452–455.
75. Lauer A, Saccaggi A, Ronco C, Belledonne M, Glabman S, Bosch J. Continuous arteriovenous hemofiltration in the critically ill patient. Ann Intern Med 1983; 99:455–460.
76. Kaplan A, Longnecker R, Folkert V. Suction-assisted continuous arteriovenous hemofiltration. Trans Am Soc Artif Intern Organs 1983; 29:408–413.
77. Locatelli F, Pontoreiero G, DiFilippo S. Electrolyte disorders and substitution fluid in continuous renal replacement therapy. Kidney Int 1998; 53(suppl 66):S151–S155.
78. Ikizler TA, Himmelfarb J. Nutrition in acute renal failure patients. Adv Renal Replace Ther 1997; 4(suppl 1):54–63.
79. Clark WR, Leypoldt JK, Henderson LW, Scott MK, Mueller BA, Vonesh EF. Quantifying the effect of changes in the hemodialysis prescription on effective solute removal with a mathematical model. J Am Soc Nephrol 1999; 10:601–610.
80. Cottrell A, Mehta RL. Phosphate kinetics in continuous renal replacement therapy (abstr). J Am Soc Nephrol 1992; 3:360.
81. Hynote E, McCamish M, Depner T, Davis P. Amino acid losses during hemodialysis: Effects of high-solute flux and parenteral nutrition in acute renal failure. JPEN 1995; 19:15–21.
82. Frankenfeld D, Badellino M, Reynolds N, Wiles C, Siegel J, Goodzari S. Amino acid losses and plasma concentration during continuous hemofiltration. JPEN 1993; 17:551–561.
83. Tan CC, Lee HS, Ti TY, Lee EJC. Pharmacokinetics of intravenous vancomycin in patients with end-stage renal disease. Ther Drug Monitor 1990; 12:29–34.
84. Rodvold K, Blum R, Fischer J. Vancomycin pharmacokinetics in patients with various degrees of renal function. Antimicrob Agents Chemother 1988; 32:848–852.
85. Bastani B, Spyker D, Minocha A, Cummings R, Westervelt F. In vivo comparison of three different hemodialysis membranes for vancomycin clearance: cuprophan, cellulose acetate, and polyacrylonitrile. Dial Transplant 1988; 17:527–528.
86. Lanese D, Alfrey A, Molitoris B. Markedly increased clearance of vancomycin during hemodialysis using polysulfone membranes. Kidney Int 1989; 35:1409–1412.

87. Quale J, O'Halloran J, DeVincenzo N, Barth R. Removal of vancomycin by high-flux hemodialysis membranes. Antimicrob Agents Chemother 1992; 36:1424–1426.
88. Bohler J, Reetze-Bonorden R, Keller E, Kramer A, Schollmeyer P. Rebound of plasma vancomycin levels after hemodialysis with highly permeable membranes. Eur J Clin Pharmacol 1992; 42:635–640.
89. DeSoi C, Sahm D, Umans J. Vancomycin elimination during high-flux hemodialysis: Kinetic model and comparison of four membranes. Am J Kidney Dis 1992; 20: 354–360.
90. Pollard T, Lamposona V, Akkerman S. Vancomycin redistribution: dosing recommendations following high-flux hemodialysis. Kidney Int 1994; 45:232–237.
91. Golper T, Marx M. Drug dosing adjustments during continuous renal replacement therapy. Kidney Int 1998; 53(suppl 66):S165–S168.
92. Geyjo F, Odani S, Yamada T. β_2-Microglobulin: a new form of amyloid protein associated with chronic hemodialysis. Kidney Int 1986; 30:385–390.
93. Kaplan AA, Halley S, Lapkin R, Graeber C. Dialysate protein losses with bleach processed polysulphone dialyzers. Kidney Int 1995; 47:573–578.
94. Canaud B, Bosc JY, Leblanc M, Vaussenat F, Leray-Moragues H, Garred LJ, Mathieu-Daude JC, Mion C. On-line dialysis quantification in acutely ill patients: preliminary clinical experience with a multipurpose urea sensor monitoring device. ASAIO J 1998; 44:184–190.

15

Cardiac Disease in Hemodialysis and Peritoneal Dialysis Patients

Patrick S. Parfrey
Health Sciences Centre, Memorial University, St. John's, Newfoundland, Canada

Norbert Lameire
University Hospital of Gent and University of Gent, Gent, Belgium

I. INTRODUCTION

Cardiac disease exerts a major influence on the morbidity and mortality of dialysis patients, as demonstrated by the frequent occurrence of heart failure and ischemic heart disease (1), very high mortality rates (2), and high proportion of cardiac deaths (2). These adverse events can usually be attributed to disorders of cardiac muscle structure and function and/or disorders of perfusions (3). Hemodynamic, metabolic, and other risk factors are prevalent in dialysis patients, which predispose to various cardiac disorders, some of which may be amenable to intervention (4–6).

II. EPIDEMIOLOGY

A. Mortality

Relative to the general population, death rates are extremely high among end-stage renal disease (ESRD) patients, and the major cause of death is cardiac (7) (Fig. 1). Of deaths classified as cardiac, cardiac arrest was the attributed cause of death in 39% of cases, followed by acute myocardial infarction (24%) (7) (Fig. 2).

B. Impact of Geography

Data on cardiovascular mortality in ESRD patients should be interpreted with the differences in geographical distribution of cardiovascular mortality in the general population in mind. This is well illustrated in Europe, where there is a well-known north/south gradient in prevalence of cardiovascular disease, mainly coronary heart disease, in the general population: a lower prevalence in most Mediterranean countries and a higher prevalence in northern Europe (8,9). However, over the last decade a remarkable shift in this gradient from a north/south towards a more east/west direction has occurred (9).

Despite a decline in cardiovascular mortality in the general population, the distribution of causes of death in ESRD patients had not changed substantially in the past decade. Moreover, there were no significant differences in the proportion of these causes between patients older and younger than 65 years of age, nor were there differences between diabetic patients and patients with other renal diseases. The 1991 report of the EDTA Registry (10) pointed out great differences in both the total and cardiovascular mortality in ESRD patients between northern and southern Europe. The death rate from myocardial ischemia and infarction was four times greater in northern than in southern European males and five times more common in northern European females than in southern European females.

An age- and sex-specific analysis of mortality from ischemic heart disease in diabetic and nondiabetic patients with ESRD in Italy and the United Kingdom revealed that the death rate was three to four times higher

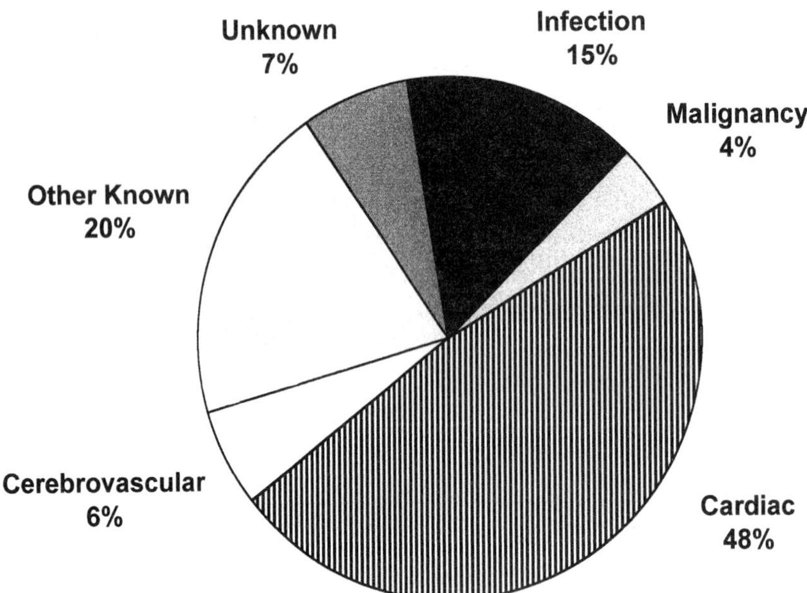

Fig. 1 Percent distribution of causes of death for all ESRD patients over the age of 20 years, 1991–1993. (From Ref. 7.)

in the United Kingdom than in Italy in all age groups and both sexes (10). It would thus appear that the mortality differences between these representative northern and southern European countries are not purely due to differences in age, sex, or the proportion of patients with diabetic ESRD.

There was a relatively constant 16- to 19-fold higher death rate in patients with ESRD as compared with the general population in both countries. Thus, the increased mortality from ischemic heart disease appears to relate to the presence of ESRD and additional factors such as diabetes superimposed on underlying funda-

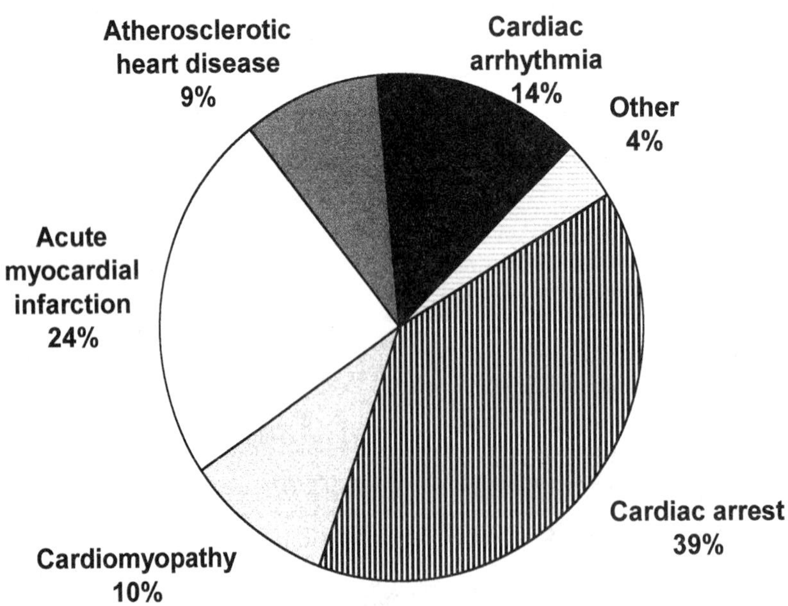

Fig. 2 Percent distribution of specific cardiac causes of death among all cardiac causes for all ESRD patients, 1991–1993. (From Ref. 7.)

mental genetic and/or environmental differences in susceptibility to cardiovascular disease in different populations (9).

C. Hemodialysis versus Peritoneal Dialysis

Most reports have similar survival in chronic ambulatory peritoneal dialysis (CAPD) and in-center hemodialysis (HD) patients (11–20). However, differences in outcomes have recently been reported from national registries. The Canadian Organ Replacement Register (21) reveals that among patients who spent at least 90% of their time on either CAPD or HD, those who received CAPD seem to have better survival than patients receiving only HD. There is a higher probability of patient survival with CAPD in Canada compared with the United States (22). In the latter country patients treated with CAPD had a 19% higher mortality rate than those receiving any form of HD (23). This increase in risk was greatest in diabetics of any age and in nondiabetics above age 55. The excess all-cause mortality observed in peritoneal dialysis (PD)–treated patients was accounted for, in decreasing order, by infection (35%), acute myocardial infarction (24%), other cardiac causes (16%), cerebrovascular disease (8%), withdrawal (8%), and malignancy (6%) (24). Also, a recent Italian analysis has shown that patients treated by PD had a relative risk of death of 1.4 compared with patients on HD (25), and decreased survival in peritoneal dialysis patients was reported from Australia and New Zealand (26).

In three Canadian centers the outcomes of hemo- and peritoneal dialysis patients were compared using intention-to-treat analysis (based on the mode of therapy at 3 months) and efficacy analysis (patients treated exclusively by either modality of treatment) (27). After adjustment was made for PD patients being less likely to have chronic hypertension and more likely to have diabetes, ischemic heart disease, and cardiac failure at baseline, a biphasic mortality pattern was observed (Fig. 3). For the first 2 years after starting dialysis therapy, there was no statistically significant difference in mortality. After 2 years, mortality was 57% greater among PD patients in the intention-to-treat analysis and 127% greater in the efficacy analysis. The Canadian Organ Replacement Register study found significantly higher mortality rates on hemodialysis compared with CAPD/CCPD (chronic cycling peritoneal dialysis) in the first 2 years of follow-up, after adjustments for age, primary renal diagnosis, comorbid conditions, and center size (28).

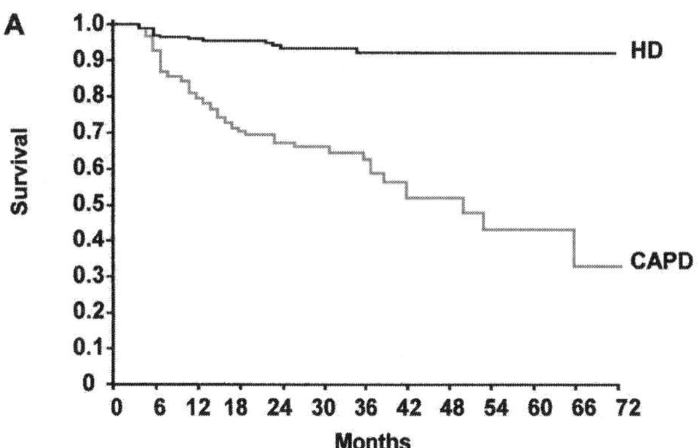

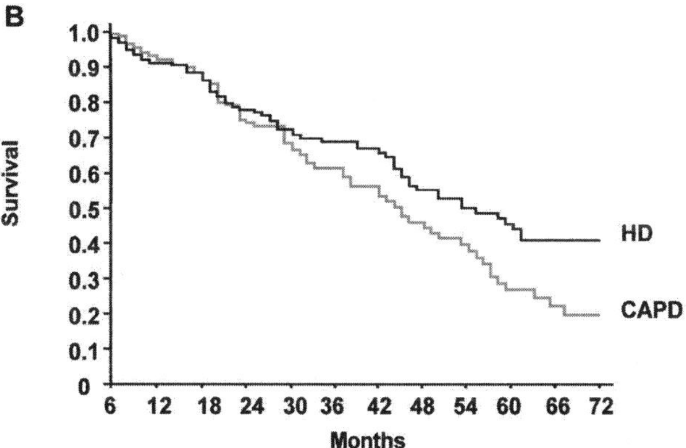

Fig. 3 Survival in a cohort of patients treated with hemo- (■) or peritoneal dialysis (---). (A) The survival according to mode of dialysis therapy at 3 months. (B) The survival in patients treated exclusively with one mode of dialysis therapy. (From Ref. 27.)

Most of the above-mentioned data were obtained at a time when the delivery of peritoneal dialysis was inadequate, the importance of residual renal function was poorly understood, and the contribution of comorbid conditions was often not taken into account. Also one must be aware of selection bias (29). Selecting younger and healthier kidney transplant candidates with sufficient residual renal function, fewer cardiovascular risk factors, and for whom CAPD was the first renal replacement therapy significantly improved the overall and cardiovascular survival at 3 and 5 years of follow-up.

Mortality data in earlier individual center reports (reviewed in Ref 30) and more recent reports (16,25, 31–34), with one exception (35), suggest that, like in hemodialysis, cardiovascular disease was by far the most common cause of death in PD patients. Also, in the recent CANUSA study on adequacy and nutrition in CAPD patients (32), 75% of the deaths during the 2-year study period were cardiovascular in nature.

D. Morbidity

In a prospective study of new dialysis patients, followed for a mean of 41 months, 133 patient had heart failure at baseline and 56% (N = 75) had recurrent heart failure during follow-up. Two hundred and ninety-nine were free of heart failure on initiation of dialysis and 25% (N = 76) developed de novo heart failure (5). In patients treated only with peritoneal dialysis, 16.5% developed de novo heart failure versus 28.1% of those treated only with hemodialysis (p = 0.02) (27). In the same cohort 22% (N = 95) had ischemic heart disease at baseline and 78% did not. Twelve percent (N = 41) of the latter group subsequently developed de novo ischemic heart disease (6).

A large cohort (N = 496) of new Canadian hemodialysis patients were followed for a mean of 218 days (1). During this period there were 30 ischemic events (myocardial infarction or angina) requiring hospitalization, giving a probability of 8% per year, and there were 40 episodes of pulmonary edema requiring hospitalization or additional ultrafiltration, giving a probability of 10% per year. In a group of 31 PD patients only 15 had no evidence of ischemic heart disease (36). De novo appearance of ischemic heart disease in CAPD patients has been reported to be 8.8% after one year and 15% after 2 years (37).

On average, hospital admission rates per patients year were 14% higher for PD patients than for HD patients after adjustment for race, age, gender, and cause of ESRD. However, the causes of this higher hospital admission rates in PD patients were not studied (38). Table 1 shows the number of hospital admission days per year at risk over the years 1979–84, 1985–89 and 1990–95 for the main causes (i.e., cardiovascular problems, infections, and other problems) in PD patients in the Gent unit. It appears that the hospitalization rate is decreasing with time, both for cardiovascular morbidity and infectious problems. These results must, however, be interpreted with caution in view of the change in selection policy that occurred in the Gent unit, with the preferential acceptance in the PD program of younger kidney transplant candidates who had fewer cardiovascular handicaps.

III. PATHOGENESIS

A. Myocardial Disease

Maintenance of normal left ventricular (LV) wall stress necessitates the development of LV hypertrophy (Fig. 4) if LV pressure rises or LV diameter increases. This is initially a beneficial adaptive response (3). However, continuing LV overload leads to maladaptive myocyte changes and myocyte death, which may be further exacerbated by diminished perfusion, malnutrition, uremia, and hyperparathyroidism (3,4). This loss of myocytes will predispose to LV dilatation and ultimately systolic dysfunction. In addition, myocardial fibrosis occurs, which will not only diminish cardiac compliance but also attenuate the hypertrophic response to pressure overload (3).

Disorders of LV structure include concentric LV hypertrophy, a response to LV pressure overload, and LV dilatation with hypertrophy, a response to LV volume overload (3). These structural abnormalities predispose to diastolic dysfunction, in which diminished compliance results in a higher-than-normal change in LV pressure for a given change in LV volume. Ultimately failure of the pump function of the heart (systolic dysfunction) occurs. Both diastolic and systolic dysfunction predispose to symptomatic left ventricular failure, a frequent occurrence in dialysis patients and a harbinger for early death (4,5). In the presence of LV hypertrophy (LVH), impairment of coronary perfusion may be catastrophic, resulting not only in regional impairment of LV contraction, but also in LV dilatation and systolic dysfunction (6).

Hemodialysis patients provide the quintessential model for overload cardiomyopathy, because LV pressure overload occurs frequently from hypertension and occasionally from aortic stenosis, and LV volume over-

Table 1 Number of Hospitalization Days (Training Excluded) per Year and Causes of Hospitalization in Peritoneal Dialysis Patients at the University Hospital Gent

Years	Cardiovascular	Infections	Other	Total
1979–1984	10.7	13.2	2.5	26.4
1985–1989	8.5	11.0	3.4	22.9
1990–1995	6.3	7.8	2.6	16.7

Source: Ref. 29.

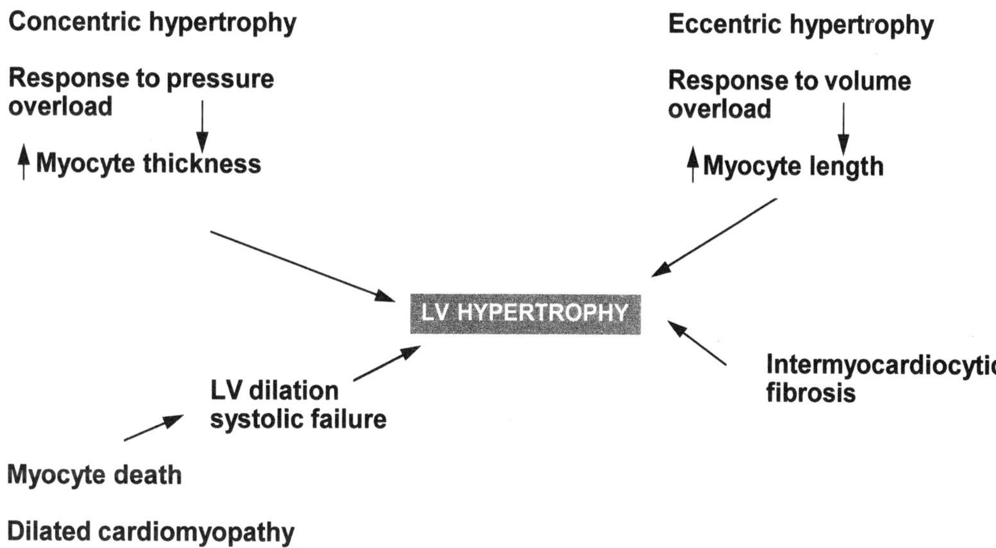

Fig. 4 Causes of left ventricular hypertrophy.

load is ubiquitous due to the presence of an arteriovenous fistula, anemia, and hypervolemia (3).

The ill effects of hypertension have been attributed to a reduction in the caliber or the number of arterioles, resulting in increased peripheral resistance. This definition does not take into account the fact that blood pressure fluctuates during the cardiac cycle and that systolic and diastolic blood pressures are merely the limits of this oscillation. By using Fourier analysis, the blood pressure curve can be decomposed into its steady and oscillatory components (39). The steady component, that is, mean blood pressure, is determined exclusively by cardiac output and total peripheral resistance (pressure and flow are considered constant over the time). The oscillatory component (oscillation around this mean) is pulse pressure that is determined by the pattern of LV ejection, the viscoelastic properties of large conduit arteries (arterial distensibility), and intensity and timing of arterial wave reflections (39). Therefore, pressure overload may be primarily related to increased peripheral resistance (with increased diastolic and mean pressure) or to decreased arterial distensibility and early return of arterial wave reflections (with increased systolic pressure and wide pulse pressure) (39).

Flow overload also leads to vascular remodeling and parallel development of arteriosclerosis in the peripheral arteries (40). Several determinants of systolic and pulse pressure are altered in ESRD patients, including decreased arterial compliance and an early return of arterial wave reflections, which are independent factors associated with the extent of LVH (40–43). Decreased arterial compliance and functional alterations observed in ESRD are associated with remodeling of conduit arteries, characterized by arterial dilatation (40,44) and intima-media hypertrophy (40,45). These arterial changes resemble those that occur with aging, such as arteriosclerosis, which is primarily medial, characterized by diffuse dilatation and stiffening of major arteries (39,46). These changes must be distinguished from atherosclerosis, which is focal, nonuniformly distributed, primarily intimal, inducing occlusive lesions and compensatory focal enlargement of arterial diameters (39,46).

Arterial walls are exposed to the influence of mechanical factors, such as flow and pressure stresses, which act as mechanical stimuli for remodeling. Experimental and clinical studies have shown that chronically increased arterial flow led to increased internal arterial dimensions and arterial wall remodeling with a compensatory increase in arterial wall thickness (47,48). The consequence of structural and functional changes of the arterial system in uremic patients is increased pulsatile work of the heart, which accounts in part for the development of parallel LV and vascular adaptation in chronic uremia (Fig. 5) (3).

B. Disorders of Perfusion

Coronary artery disease is the usual cause of symptoms of ischemic heart disease in dialysis patients (49). However, nonatherosclerotic disease, resulting from

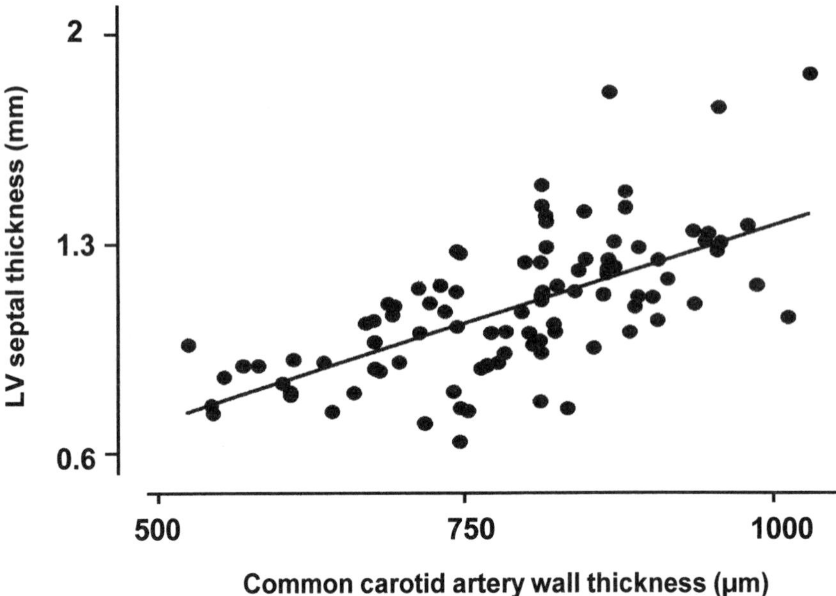

Fig. 5 The correlation between common carotid artery wall thickness and LV septal thickness in dialysis patients. (From Ref. 3.)

small vessel disease and/or from the underlying cardiomyopathy, may account for a substantial minority of cases of symptomatic ischemic heart disease (6,49). Multiple factors contribute to the vascular pathology of chronic uremia (Fig. 6), including chronic injury to the vessel wall, prothrombotic factors, lipoprotein interactions, proliferation of smooth muscle, increased oxidant stress, diminished antioxidant stress, hyperhomocysteinemia, hypertension, diabetes, and smoking (3).

IV. CARDIAC STRUCTURE AND FUNCTION

A. Prevalence

Figure 7 shows the patterns of LV hypertrophy seen on echocardiography. In the Canadian cohort of 432 dialysis patients, followed from the initiation of end-stage renal disease therapy, only 16 % had a normal echocardiogram on starting dialysis (50). Forty-one percent had concentric LV hypertrophy, 28% LV dilatation, and 16% systolic dysfunction. This implies that causes of LV dysfunction occur in the predialysis phase of chronic renal failure. Two hundred and seventy-five patients had a follow-up echocardiogram 17 months after starting dialysis therapy (4). The proportion of those who had a normal echocardiogram was 13%, with concentric LV hypertrophy 40%, with LV dilatation 26%, and with systolic dysfunction 20% (4).

B. Echocardiographic Outcome

In a subgroup of dialysis patients with normal echocardiogram on starting dialysis (N = 30), 32% had developed concentric LV hypertrophy, 16% LV dilatation, and 3% systolic dysfunction in the second year after starting dialysis (4). In 229 patients maintained exclusively on hemodialysis, LV cavity volume increased by 7 mL/m^2 during 1-year follow-up, and LV mass increased by 36 g/m^2 (27). One might expect that blood flow would not increase as much in peritoneal dialysis patients as in hemodialysis patients, because there is no vascular access and less variable fluctuations in salt and water status. In 70 patients treated exclusively with peritoneal dialysis, LV cavity volume decreased by 5 mL/m^2 during 1-year follow-up (27). When compared to hemodialysis patients, the differences in the changes in LV volume approached statistical significance (p = 0.06).

In 55 normotensive CAPD patients who were on treatment for a mean of 28.8 ± 24.9 months, a high prevalence of left atrial dilatation and left ventricular hypertrophy was found (51). The latter was mainly the result of septal thickening. The degree of ventricular hypertrophy in these patients was related to the amount of hypercirculation and to the quality of the blood purification. In this study the majority of patients with left ventricular hypertrophy had the asymmetrical, septal form of left ventricular hypertrophy. The direct cor-

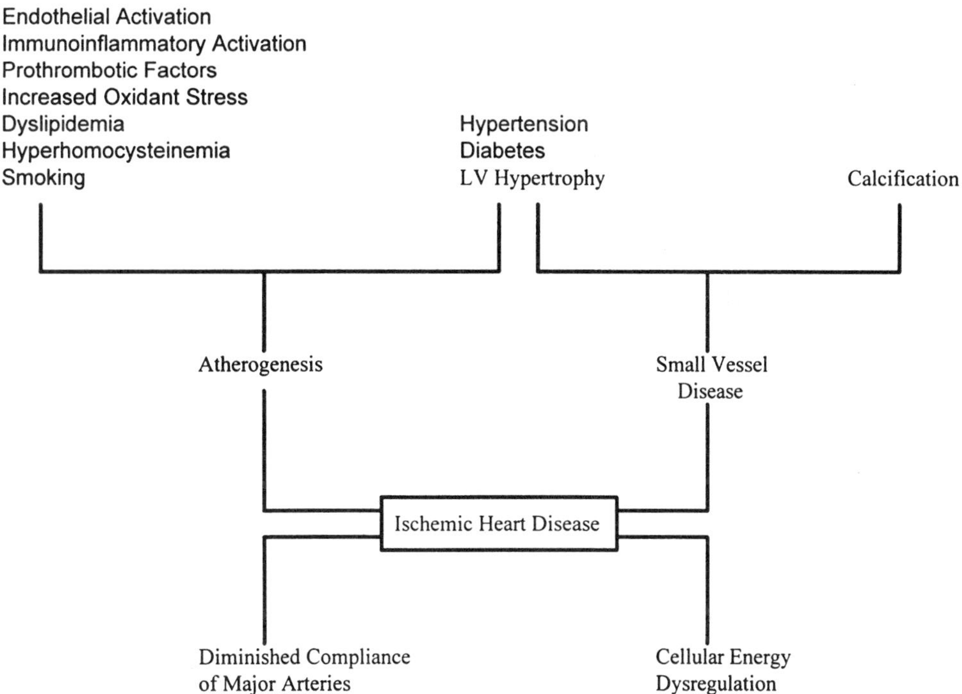

Fig. 6 Causes of ischemic heart disease in chronic uremia.

relation between left atrial diameter and left ventricular muscle mass suggests impaired left ventricle diastolic filling. Abnormal diastolic left ventricular filling in CAPD patients has been found (52,53) in patients both with and without left ventricular hypertrophy, in whom a disturbed ratio between the ventricular rapid filling in protodiastole and the filling due to atrial contraction exists, with a greater than normal atrial contribution.

After initiation of CAPD therapy, regression as well as progression in left ventricular hypertrophy has been described. Prospective studies did not show a deterioration in left ventricular function up to 2 years after CAPD (54). Others did not observe changes in left ventricular mass, ejection fraction, or left ventricular telediastolic dimension, despite a fall in blood pressure (54,55). On the other hand, a regression of left ventricular hypertrophy and consequently of the impaired diastolic compliance responsible for the hypertrophic hyperkinetic or ischemic myocardiopathy has been found in many CAPD patients (52,55–57). CAPD, started in patients with severe left ventricular systolic dysfunction and renal failure, led to a substantial improvement in isotopic left ventricular ejection fraction, functional status, and blood pressure control (58). However, many of these beneficial effects have been observed only in the first years after start of PD therapy. As has been pointed out, the prevalence of left ventricular hypertrophy significantly decreased during the first 2–3 years but rose later again in a cohort of 24 CAPD patients who were continuously treated for at least 5 years (30).

C. Clinical Outcome

Echocardiographic disorders of the left ventricle predispose to cardiac failure and to earlier death (Fig. 8) (4). One- and 2-year survival rates of 90 and 64%, respectively, have been reported in systolic dysfunction patients treated with CAPD (58). A group of 21 CAPD patients who were followed for 18 months had an initial prevalence of left ventricular hypertrophy of 52%. The mortality was 25% and 56% in the group with moderate and severe left ventricular hypertrophy, respectively. All deaths were due to cardiovascular events (59).

D. Impact of Intraperitoneal Infusion Volume

A significant decrease in left ventricular internal dimensions in diastole from the infusion of 3 L or more of dialysate has been observed (60). This was correlated with the rise in intra-abdominal pressure. These

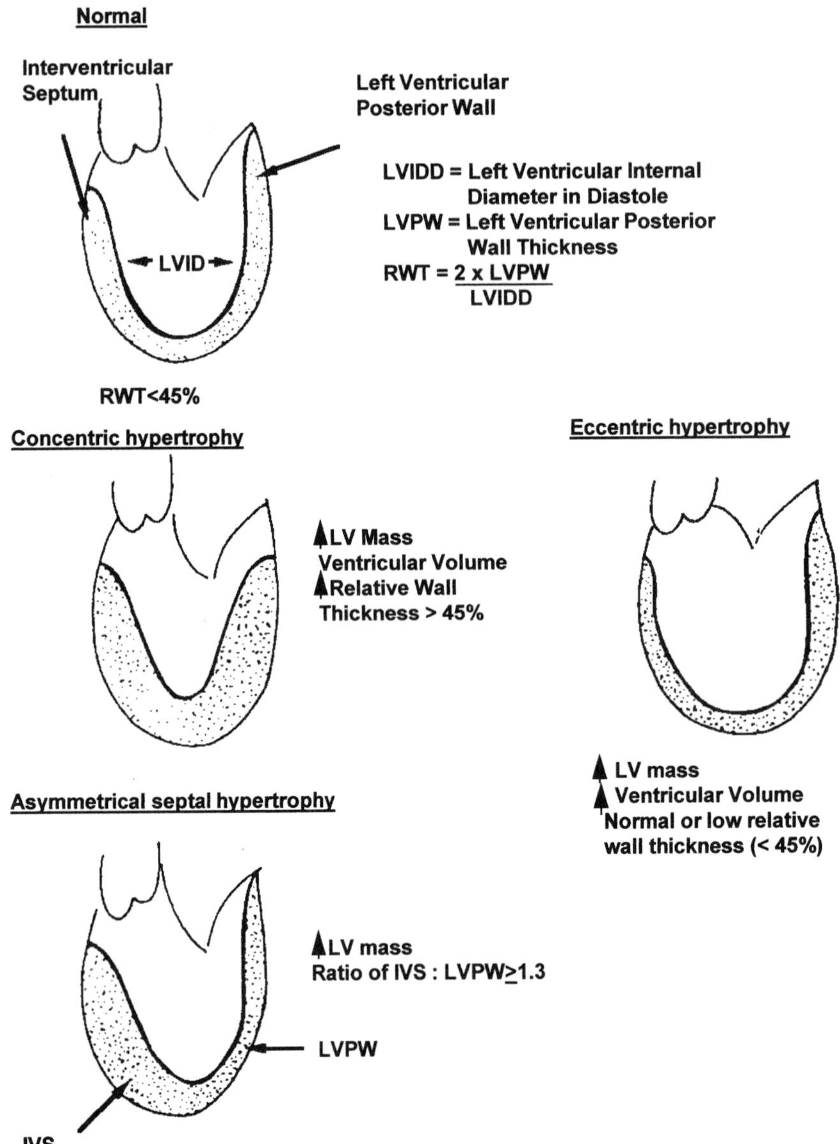

Fig. 7 Patterns of left ventricular hypertrophy observed on echocardiography. LVID = Left ventricular end diastolic internal decimeter; RWT = relative wall thickness; IVS = interventricular septal wall thickness in diastole; LVPW = left ventricular posterior wall thickness in diastole. (From Ref. 28.)

effects were confined to the subgroup of patients with an increased left ventricular wall thickness. Infusion of 1 or 2 L did not affect systolic function (60). Although some studies (61,62) have found a fall in cardiac output (using dye dilatation method) after infusion of similar exchange, most studies did not find any difference, whether impedance cardiography (63), Doppler echocardiography (64), or thermodilution (65,66) methods were used.

V. CARDIAC ARRHYTHMIAS

A. Hemodialysis

In patients without renal failure, left ventricular hypertrophy and coronary heart disease appear to be associated with an increased risk of arrhythmias. As outlined above, these cardiac diseases are among the most prevalent in ESRD patients. In addition, serum electro-

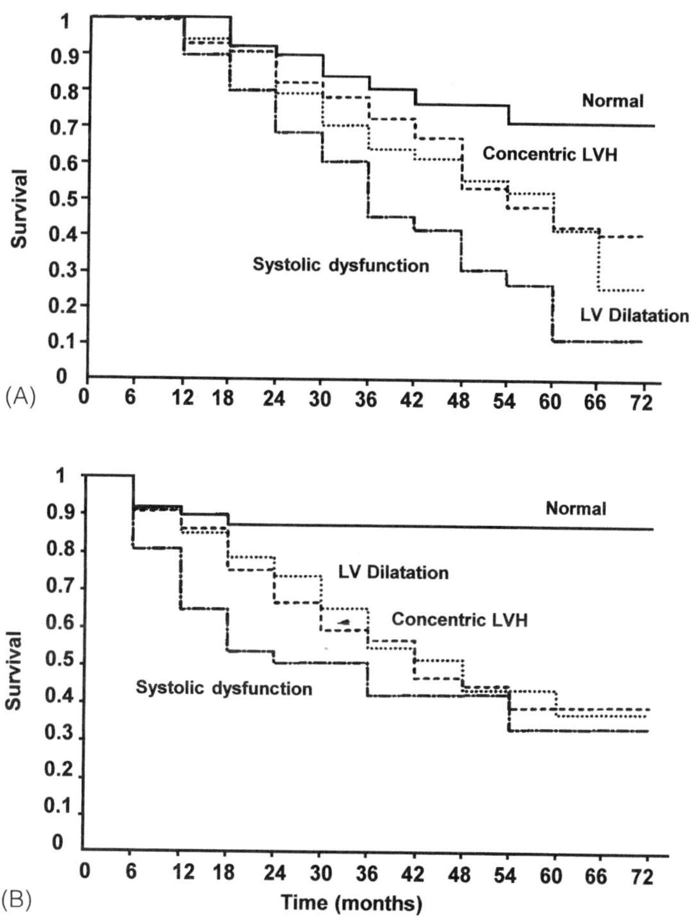

Fig. 8 Time to onset of heart failure (A) and to death (B) in patients starting dialysis therapy who have systolic dysfunction, concentric LV hypertrophy, LV dilatation, or normal echocardiogram. (From Ref. 4.)

lyte levels that can affect cardiac conduction, including potassium, calcium, magnesium, and hydrogen, are often abnormal or undergo rapid fluctuations during hemodialysis. For all these reasons, cardiac arrhythmias should be common in these patients. The presence of all of these confounding factors explains why the assessment and interpretation of arrhythmias in hemodialysis patients is difficult.

In cross-sectional studies of patients with end-stage renal disease, the prevalence of atrial arrhythmias was between 68 and 88%, ventricular arrhythmias were present in 56–76% of patients, and premature ventricular complexes were found in 14–21% (67–69). Older age, preexisting heart disease, left ventricular hypertrophy, and use of digitalis therapy were associated with higher prevalence and greater severity of cardiac arrhythmias (70). There is a considerable variation in the frequency and severity of arrhythmias during hemodialysis, as well as in the interdialytic period. Because of these factors, there is no consensus on the frequency of arrhythmias in end-stage renal disease patients or their clinical significance.

Coronary artery disease has been associated with a higher frequency of arrhythmias in some (71,72), but not all studies on hemodialysis (68,69). Also, the association with left ventricular hypertrophy has not been well documented in ESRD, and whether or not left ventricular hypertrophy is a cause of fatal arrhythmias (sudden death) in dialysis patients has not been clarified. There are also conflicting data about the effect of dialysis, and various dialysis compositions and dialysis protocols on the occurrence of rhythm disturbances. Some studies show higher incidence of premature ventricular contractions during dialysis or in the immediate postdialysis period (67,69), whereas in others no differences could be observed (68). Most of the atrial arrhythmias are of low clinical and hemodynamic significance, except the bradyarrhythmias and atrial tachyarrhythmias.

The majority of the premature ventricular contractions are unifocal and below 30 per hour, but high-grade ventricular arrhythmias like multiple premature ventricular contractions, ventricular couplets, and ventricular tachycardia were found in 27% of 92 patients with 24-hour Holter monitoring (73). The finding of high-grade ventricular arrhythmias in the presence of coronary artery disease was associated with increased risk of cardiac mortality and sudden death (72,74). Whereas the dialysis method, membrane, and buffer used do not seem to have a direct effect on the incidence of arrhythmias (75), dialysis-associated hypotension seems to be an important factor in precipitating high-grade ventricular arrhythmias, irrespective of the type of dialysis (75,76).

Use of digoxin in hemodialysis patients has raised concern regarding precipitation of arrhythmias, especially in the immediate postdialysis period, when both hypokalemia and relative hypercalemia may occur (71,72,77). Keller et al. (78) studied 55 patients in a crossover study of "on-and-off" digoxin and found no increase in incidence of arrhythmias when patients were on the drug.

B. Peritoneal Dialysis

Holter monitoring of cardiac rhythm of 21 CAPD patients revealed a high frequency of atrial and/or ventricular premature beats (79). There were no differences in the type and freqency of the extrasystoles between the day on CAPD and the day on which dialysis was deliberately withheld. It seems that, in contrast with hemodialysis, CAPD is by itself not responsible for provoking or aggravating arrhythmias. The arrhythmias are more a reflection of the patient's age, underlying ischemic heart disease, or an association with left ventricular hyperthrophy (80,81).

A recent study (82) in which 27 CAPD patients were compared with 27 hemodialysis patients revealed that severe cardiac arrhythmias occurred in only 4% of CAPD and in 33% of the hemodialysis group. Patients in both groups were matched for age, sex, duration of treatment, and etiology of chronic renal failure The lower frequency of left ventricular hypertrophy, the maintenance of a relatively stable blood pressure, the absence of sudden hypotensive events, and the significantly lower incidence of severe hyperkalemia in patients on peritoneal dialysis (83) may explain the lower incidence of severe arrhythmias in CAPD patients.

VI. RISK FACTORS FOR CARDIAC DISEASE

The risk factors can be categorized as hemodynamic, metabolic, or other. Circumstantial evidence and longitudinal studies support several risk factors as important for the development of cardiac disease (Fig. 9), but no clinical trials have demonstrated that any risk factor intervention leads to clinical benefit in dialysis patients.

A. Cardiovascular Risk at Onset of Dialysis

It is remarkable that the high rate of cardiovascular morbidity and mortality in ESRD patients is occurring at a time when the prevalence of coronary artery disease is declining in the general population. This discrepancy is in part due to the demographics of patients about to be started on dialysis: about one third are diabetic, the average age is now over 60 years, approximately 16% are over 74 years of age, and many patients have underlying cardiac disease (84). Among new patients starting dialysis in the United States, 41% had coronary artery disease and 41% had heart failure (7).

Because heart disease, or at least several of its risk factors, often antedate dialysis or even precede renal failure, the high mortality due to cardiovascular causes in both the HD and PD populations could be explained by the acceptance of these high-risk patients who are given a dialysis opportunity despite adverse odds. This may be particularly relevant in PD because, in the past and probably still today, many dialysis programs preferentially reserve PD for the patient handicapped by cardiac disease on the premise that this continuous dialysis technique offers some advantages over the intermittent HD mode of treatment This may not now happen in the United States. The USRDS 1992 Annual Data Report (85) showed a 6–17% reduction in the relative count of risk factors in PD compared to HD patients within all age and diabetes subgroups.

In all of above-mentioned studies except one (86), where the morbidity and mortality of PD and HD patients have been compared, cardiovascular, cerebrovascular, and peripheral vascular comorbidity at the start of dialysis was associated with increased relative risk of death in both dialysis modalities. The impact of the presence of heart failure when starting dialysis on subsequent survival is shown in Fig. 10A and the impact of ischemic heart disease in Fig. 10B (5,6).

Table 2 shows the prevalence of several cardiovascular risk factors at the initiation of chronic PD in two recently published series (16,29). Between 1979 and

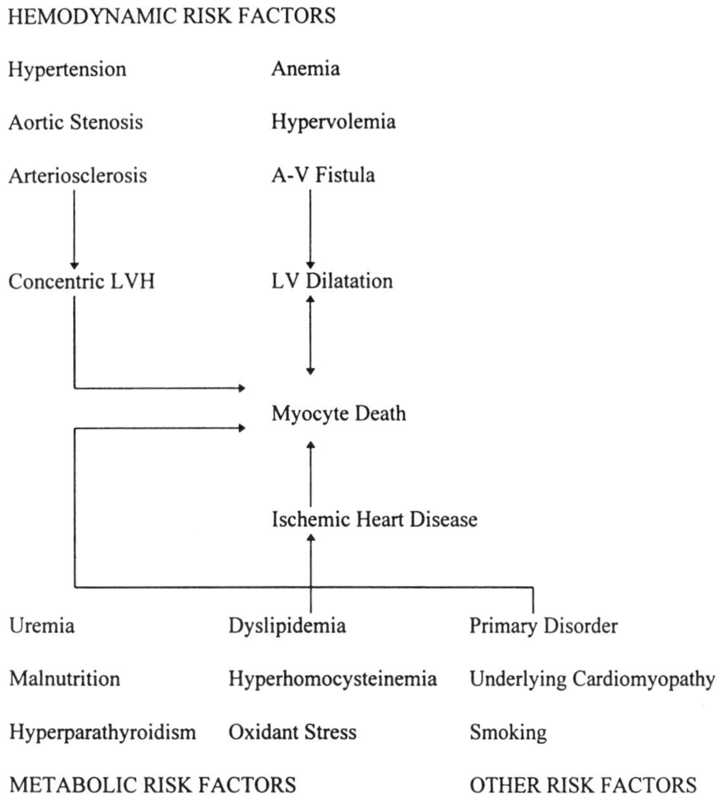

HEMODYNAMIC RISK FACTORS

Hypertension	Anemia
Aortic Stenosis	Hypervolemia
Arteriosclerosis	A-V Fistula
↓	↓
Concentric LVH	LV Dilatation

Concentric LVH → Myocyte Death; LV Dilatation ↔ Myocyte Death; Ischemic Heart Disease → Myocyte Death; Metabolic and other risk factors → Myocyte Death / Ischemic Heart Disease

Uremia	Dyslipidemia	Primary Disorder
Malnutrition	Hyperhomocysteinemia	Underlying Cardiomyopathy
Hyperparathyroidism	Oxidant Stress	Smoking
METABOLIC RISK FACTORS		OTHER RISK FACTORS

Fig. 9 Risk factors for cardiac disease in chronic uremia.

the end of 1995, 300 end-stage renal failure patients (mean age 57.7 ± 2.8 years) were trained on CAPD in Gent and survived at least one month on this therapy. A total of 59 patients were suffering from diabetic nephropathy (29). In Brescia, 297 patients (38 patients suffering from diabetic nephropathy) started PD between 1981 and 1993 (16). It is remarkable that the distribution of the several cardiovascular risk factors is very similar between both centers. Whereas the survival at 1 year was not influenced by the number of risk factors, patients with seven to eight risk factors already showed a statistically lower survival in the second year compared to the other groups. When patients with five or more risk factors are considered, their survival is significantly lower from the fourth year on of treatment with CAPD.

B. Mode of Dialysis Therapy

The hemodialysis state constitutes a condition of hemodynamic overload and metabolic perturbation lethal in its impact on the heart. Renal transplantation is the best model of what happens to the heart when uremia is treated properly. Although hypertension usually persists, as does the fistula and perhaps hypervolemia, anemia is corrected, as is the metabolic perturbation. Following renal transplantation, concentric LV hypertrophy and LV dilatation improves, but the most striking observation is the improvement in systolic dysfunction (87). It is not known which adverse risk factors characteristic of the uremic state have been corrected to produce the improvement in LV contractility. Dialysis provides inadequate treatment of the uremic state, but the target quantity of dialysis, which may limit the contribution of "uremic toxins" to cardiac dysfunction, is unknown. A current trial ongoing in the United States comparing two quantities of hemodialysis may be helpful in this regard.

In the Canadian studies, the hemodynamic benefit of peritoneal dialysis described earlier did not translate into increased survival. In fact, hemodialysis had a late survival advantage over peritoneal dialysis (Fig. 3) because of the adverse impact of hypoalbuminemia in the latter group. Mean serum albumin in peritoneal dialysis patients in the first 2 years of therapy accounted for 65% of the increase in subsequent mortality (27). It

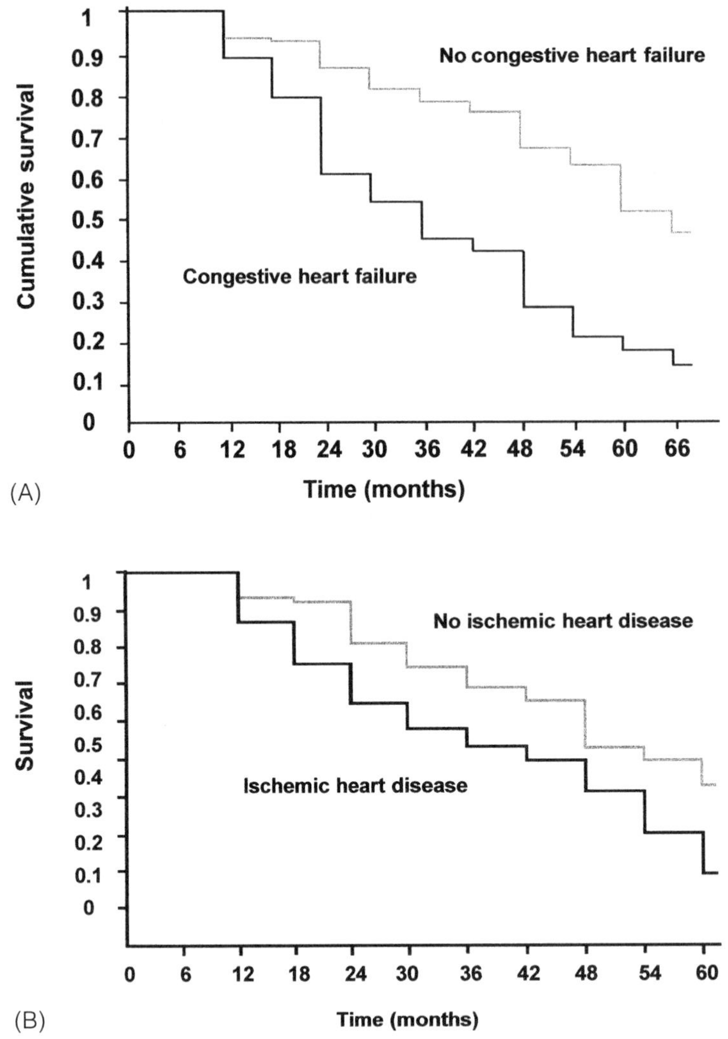

Fig. 10 Unadjusted mortality in dialysis patients (A) with and without heart failure at the start of dialysis therapy (from Ref. 5) and (B) with and without ischemic heart disease at start (from Ref. 6).

appears that the path to cardiac death is different for hemodialysis and peritoneal dialysis patients. Thus, in hemodialysis patients a higher proportion developed cardiac failure, which was associated with hypertension and anemia and predisposed to cardiac death. In peritoneal dialysis patients mortality was associated predominantly with hypoalbuminemia, which predisposed to death in unknown fashion.

VII. HEMODYNAMIC RISK FACTORS

A. Volume Overload

In comparison with age-, sex-, and blood pressure–matched nonuremic controls, the LV diastolic diameter (50,88–92) is increased in ESRD patients. The changes are moderate, with values usually lying around the normal upper limits, but true LV dilatation is observed in 32–38% of patients (50,90). The ventricular enlargement is probably attributable to chronic volume/flow overload and high-output state associated with three factors: salt and water retention (93–96), arteriovenous shunts (90,95,97), and anemia (3,41,51,96,98,99). It also may occur in response to myocyte death.

B. Salt and Water Retention

It is believed that peritoneal dialysis, because it is a continuous process, is better at controlling salt and water overload than hemodialysis. However, many CAPD

Table 2 Presence of Cardiovascular Risk Factors at Start of PD

Risk factors	Gent N = 300 (%)	Brescia N = 297 (%)
Peripheral vascular disease	115 (38)	65 (22)
Cardiomegaly	183 (61)	—
Hypertension	173 (58)	231 (78)
Anemia	220 (73)	—
Heart failure	69 (23)	—
Dyslipidemia	66 (22)	90 (30)
Cerebrovascular disease	10 (3)	54 (18)
Ischemic cardiopathy	56 (19)	74 (25)
Arrhythmia	—	39 (13)
Diabetes (all)	59 (20)	63 (21)

Source: Ref. 29.

patients are actually fluid overloaded (100). Some hemodynamic studies performed at the moment of renal transplantation of CAPD patients show that they are constantly overhydrated (100). The overhydration is further demonstrable when CAPD patients are transferred to HD. Table 3 shows the evolution of body weight and blood pressure in a series of 35 CAPD patients 3 months after transfer to HD. A remarkable reduction of 4.2 kg in "dry" weight from CAPD to the prehemodialysis body weight and a significant decrease in diastolic blood pressure was observed.

Clinical features of symptomatic fluid gain may occur in 25% of CAPD patients (101). Peripheral edema (100%), pulmonary congestion (80%), pleural effusions (76%), and systolic and diastolic hypertension were the most common manifestations of the symptomatic fluid gain. A hyperpermeable membrane with high peritoneal solute transport is a risk factor for this complication. Latent overhydration is particularly frequent in patients with diabetic nephropathy (102).

The disappearance of the residual renal function not only has a negative impact on the adequacy of peritoneal dialysis but may contribute to the volume overload of the patient in case of poor peritoneal ultrafiltration (103–106).

Faller and Lameire (107) found that peritoneal ultrafiltration declined as a result of previous use of a dialysate containing acetate rather than lactate. However, a gradual increase in the daily use of more hypertonic bags was also noted in the patients who were never exposed to acetate. Selgas et al. (108) followed the long-term peritoneal function of 56 patients with at least 3 years on CAPD. They concluded that after 5–11 years, the human peritoneum showed functional stability in patients with a low peritoneal inflammation rate. However, patients with frequent and/or prolonged peritonitis showed a significant decrease in ultrafiltration capacity and an increase in peritoneal creatinine diffusion capacity.

In a most recent analysis (109), including 38 patients with at least 5 years on CAPD, similar results were obtained, i.e., a decrease in ultrafiltration and an increase in the mass transport rate of creatinine with time. Nine patients who reached 8 years on CAPD had lost half of their ultrafiltration capacity compared with the baseline value. The fluid volume status in these patients remained adequate since they used more hypertonic dialysate.

Importantly, the loss of ultrafiltration in association with peritoneal hyperpermeability (ultrafiltration loss type I) may recover by introducing 4-week peritoneal "rest periods."

C. Anemia

In ESRD patients, an association between LV dilatation and anemia has been observed. After adjusting for age,

Table 3 Evolution of Body Weight and Blood Pressure in Patients Transferred from CAPD to Hemodialysis (N = 28)

	Before transfer	After transfer
Body weight (kg)	66.6 ± 2.3	62.4 ± 2.4[a]
Systolic blood pressure (mmHg)	145 ± 4.8	144 ± 3.8
Diastolic blood pressure (mmHg)	82 ± 2.3	76 ± 1.3[a]
Antihypertensive medication (number of patients)	13/28	10/28

[a] $p < 0.05$.
Source: Adapted from Refs. 16, 29.

Table 4 Association Between Anemia (Effect of a Fall in Mean Hemoglobin Level of 1 g/dL) and Clinical Outcomes in the Combined Group of Hemodialysis and Peritoneal Dialysis Patients

Outcome	Risk ratio (*p*)
De novo ischemic heart disease	No association
De novo cardiac failure	1.28 (0.017)
Death	1.14 (0.024)

Note: The covariates entered in each multivariate analysis were age, diabetes mellitus, ischemic heart disease (excluded for the outcomes de novo and recurrent ischemic heart disease), and the average monthly mean arterial blood pressure, serum albumin, and hemoglobin level before the index event.
Source: Adapted from Ref. 99.

diabetes, ischemic heart disease, blood pressure, and serum albumin levels, each 10 g/L decrease in mean hemoglobin level was independently associated with the presence of LV dilatation (odds ratio: 1.46 for each 10 g/L decrease) (99). Anemia was independently associated with the development of de novo cardiac failure, as well as overall mortality (Table 4). The time to onset of heart failure according to level of hemoglobin up to development of heart failure or final follow-up is shown in Fig. 11. This effect was more readily apparent in hemodialysis patients than peritoneal dialysis patients, possibly because the latter group had higher mean hemoglobin levels while on dialysis therapy (9.6 ± 1.5 vs 8.4 ± 1.4 g/dL; $p < 0.0001$) (99). A number of other investigators have noted an independent association between anemia and mortality (110,111).

There have been several studies examining the effect of partial correction of anemia with rHuEpo on echocardiographic abnormalities. Most of these have had small numbers of patients and have been before-after surveys without a control group. In spite of these limitations, the studies have consistently shown that treating anemia leads to a decrease in hypoxic vasodilatation, an increased peripheral resistance, reduced cardiac output, and partial reversal of LV dilatation and hypertrophy (89,112–123). None of the published literature has had adequate power to test the hypothesis that improvement of echocardiographic parameters will reduce cardiac morbidity or mortality.

D. Hypertension

The relationship between systemic blood pressure and LV mass has been examined in experimental uremia (124) and in cross-sectional studies of ESRD patients (41,91,96,125–127). However, in a preferable design (a longitudinal study), the importance of raised systolic blood pressure in the development of LV hypertrophy was shown (128). The independent association of hypertension with concentric hypertrophy has been reported in dialysis patients (129).

Hypertension is a common finding in dialysis pa-

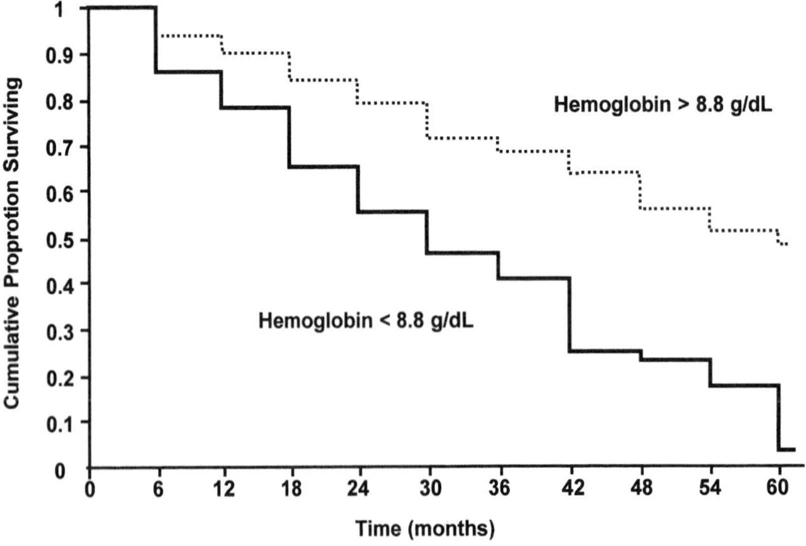

Fig. 11 Time to onset of heart failure by level of hemoglobin measured up to development of heart failure or final follow-up, adjusted for age, diabetes, ischemic heart disease, mean blood pressure, and serum albumin level. (From Ref. 99.)

tients. Approximately 80% of patients are hypertensive at the initiation of dialysis. However, in hemodialysis the prevalence falls to 25–30% by the end of the first year, due largely to volume control (130).

Early reports documented improved blood pressure control and impressive regression of left ventricular hypertrophy in CAPD patients (57). Saldanha and colleagues (131) recently followed the time sequence of changes in blood pressure, body weight, and hematocrit in two groups of CAPD patients. The first group of patients was transferred from HD to CAPD, while the second group was treated with CAPD without previous other dialysis treatment. The patients coming from HD manifested a progressive fall in blood pressure in the first months after they were treated with CAPD. An approximately similar but less important fall in blood pressure was observed in the new CAPD patients during the first 2 years of their dialysis treatment. Whereas approximately 60% of the HD patients did not need antihypertensive therapy, this decreased to 40% after the transfer to CAPD. This effect was transient as the number of patients who needed more antihypertensive drug treatment subsequently increased with time. In the new CAPD patients, there was an initial increase in patients who did not need antihypertensive drug therapy, but as in the first group, the patients who needed more drug therapy became larger with time. Also, in the long-term study of 23 CAPD patients followed for at least 7 years, no significant changes in blood pressure were found, but an increased requirement for antihypertensive medication was noted (132). This has recently been confirmed by Amann et al. (13). It thus seems that the blood pressure can be readily controlled in CAPD patients during the first 2–3 years of dialysis, but that once the residual renal function is very low or absent, the control becomes more difficult and the patients need a higher number of antihypertensive drugs.

Hypertension is a well-established risk factor for LV hypertrophy, coronary artery disease, stroke, and death in the general population (133). It has been widely held that hypertension is a major cause of mortality in dialysis patients (134–138). The evidence to support this notion is conflicting. In the widely quoted study of Charra et al. (134), patients received very large amounts of dialysis, with a mean achieved KT/V of 1.67; 5-year survival was an unheard-of 87%. In this study, 98% of patients achieved normotension without the need for antihypertensive agents. The authors speculate that lack of hypertension or toxic antihypertensive drugs accounted for much of the excellent survival achieved in their study. Although the survival statistics are highly impressive, this study is an inadequate vehicle to assess the impact of hypertension in the study population. Conversely, two very large epidemiological studies have suggested that low (139,140), not high, blood pressure is independently associated with mortality in ESRD.

In the Canadian cohort, mean arterial blood pressure levels were 101 ± 11 mm Hg (129). An inverse relationship between blood pressure levels and mortality was observed, with an (adjusted) increase in mortality of 22% for each 10 mmHg decrease in the mean arterial blood pressure distribution curve. Conversely, even within this range, rising blood pressure was independently associated with an increase in LV mass index and cavity volume on follow-up echocardiography, de novo ischemic heart disease, and de novo cardiac failure (Table 5). These effects were evident even within a range of blood pressure considered to be "normotensive." It was apparent in this data set that the inverse association between blood pressure and mortality was a statistical epiphenomenon. High blood pressure predisposed to the development of cardiac disease, but low blood pressure was a marker for the pressure of cardiac disease. Thus the inverse correlation was attributable to the large burden of cardiac failure, a very lethal occurrence, for which low blood pressure was the single greatest predictor of subsequent death. The bottom line from this study was that lower blood pressure was highly desirable in dialysis patients, at least before the onset of cardiac failure (129).

The time to onset of heart failure by level of mean arterial pressure (measured up to development of heart failure or final follow-up) is shown in Fig. 12. The group with mean blood pressure greater than 108

Table 5 Association Between Blood Pressure (Effect of a Rise in Mean Arterial Blood Pressure Level of 10 mmHg) and Clinical Outcomes in the Combined Group of Hemodialysis and Peritoneal Dialysis Patients

Outcome	Risk ratio (p)
De novo ischemic heart disease	1.39 (0.051)
De novo cardiac failure	1.44 (0.007)
Death	0.82 (0.009)

Note: The covariates entered in each multivariate analysis were age, diabetes mellitus, ischemic heart disease (excluded for the outcomes de novo and recurrent ischemic heart disease), and the average monthly mean arterial blood pressure, serum albumin, and hemoglobin level before the index event.
Source: Ref. 129.

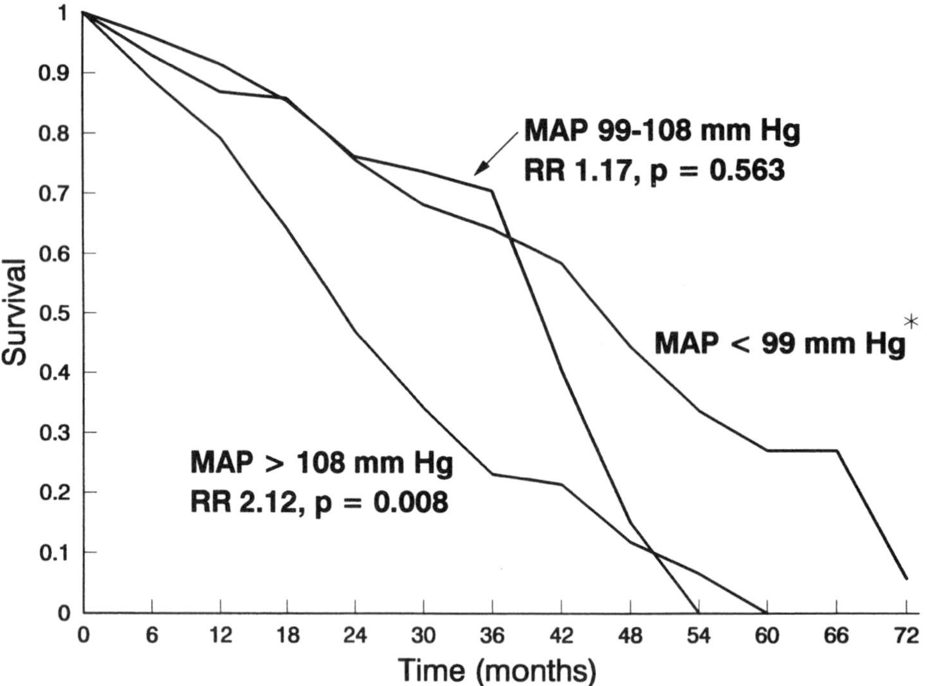

Fig. 12 Time to onset of heart failure by mean arterial blood pressure, measured up to development of heart failure, or final follow-up, adjusted for age, diabetes, ischemic heart disease, hemoglobin, and serum albumin level. (From Ref. 129.)

mmHg was at much higher risk than those with pressure below 99 mmHg. The intermediate group did not have an increased rate of heart failure until after 3 years (129).

E. Aortic Stenosis

Aortic sclerosis occurs frequently in hemodialysis patients. Eventually acquired aortic stenosis may occur in a minority of patients (141), and this will induce further concentric LV hypertrophy. Progression of calcific aortic stenosis may be very rapid, especially in association with autonomous hyperparathyroidism (142).

VIII. METABOLIC RISK FACTORS

A. Hypoalbuminemia

Hypoalbuminemia and dialysis intensity have been shown repeatedly to be perhaps the most critical predictors of outcome in ESRD patients (32,51,110,143–151). In these studies the relationship between hypoalbuminemia and mortality was especially strong; this observation, coupled with the fact that cardiovascular disease far overshadows any other cause of death in ESRD, suggests that the adverse impact of hypoalbuminemia might be mediated via cardiac disease. In the Canadian study, mean serum albumin levels were 3.9 ± 0.4 g/dL in hemodialysis patients, compared with 3.5 ± 0.5 g/dL in peritoneal patients ($p < 0.0001$) (152). Among hemodialysis patients, each 1 g/dL fall in mean serum albumin was independently associated with the development of de novo and recurrent cardiac failure, de novo and recurrent ischemic heart disease, cardiac mortality, and overall mortality. Among peritoneal dialysis patients, hypoalbuminemia was independently associated with progressive LV dilatation on serial echocardiograms, de novo cardiac failure, and overall mortality (Table 6) (152). Hemodialysis was associated with a survival advantage compared with peritoneal dialysis, which was apparent after 2 years. The lower serum albumin level of peritoneal dialysis patients in the first 2 years of therapy explained 65% of this excess mortality (27). How hypoalbuminemia might lead to coronary artery disease and cardiomyopathy in dialysis patients is a matter of pure speculation given our current knowledge.

There is indirect evidence that uremia is cardiotoxic in human ESRD. In the National Cooperative Dialysis Study, there were more cardiac events in patients who were randomized to receive less intensive dialysis (153). Churchill et al. found that more intensive dial-

Table 6 Association Between Mean Serum Albumin and Clinical Outcomes (Effect of a 10 g/L Fall), Analyzed Separately in Hemodialysis (N = 261) and Peritoneal Dialysis (N = 171) Patients

	Hemodialysis		Peritoneal dialysis	
Outcome	Relative risk	*p*	Relative risk	*p*
Ischemic heart disease				
De novo	5.29	0.001	No association	No association
Recurrrent	4.24	0.005	No association	No association
Cardiac failure				
De novo	2.22	0.001	4.16	0.003
Recurrent	3.84	0.003	No association	No association
Mortality				
All-cause	4.33	<0.001	2.06	<0.001
Cardiac	5.60	0.001	No association	No association
Noncardiac	3.58	<0.001	3.52	<0.001

Note: The covariates entered in each multivariate analysis were age, diabetes mellitus, ischemic heart disease (excluded for the outcomes de novo and recurrent ischemic heart disease), and the average monthly mean arterial blood pressure, serum albumin, and hemoglobin level before the index event.
Source: Adapted from Ref. 152.

ysis ameliorated cardiac abnormalities in a randomized crossover trial (154).

B. Abnormal Calcium-Phosphate Homeostasis

In the Canadian study, hypocalcemia was strongly associated with ischemic heart disease, even after adjustment with covariates (155). Another group has shown that low calcium levels are independently associated with mortality in a very large cross-section of dialysis patients (156). Hypocalcemia-induced hyperparathyroidism may lead to profound disturbances of myocardial bioenergetics and myocardial ischemia (157). Hyperparathyroidism has also been associated with dyslipidemia (158) and LV hypertrophy (159). Death of myocytes may be caused by hyperparathyroidism (160). Interstitial myocardial fibrosis is a prominent finding in uremia, and parathyroid hormone is a permissive factor in the genesis of this fibrosis (161). Extensive fibrosis may be responsible for attenuation of the hypertrophic response to pressure overload and may contribute to the development of dilated cardiomyopathy and heart failure in subjects with secondary hyperparathyroidism (162).

C. Dyslipidemia

ESRD is associated with both quantitative and qualitative lipid disturbances. Peritoneal dialysis patients have more adverse lipid profiles than hemodialysis patients: high cholesterol, high triglyceride, decreased HDL, and high LDL levels (163). Several studies have shown that ESRD patients tend to have higher lipoprotein Lp(a) levels than the general population (164–166). Qualitative abnormalities are also common in ESRD. The abnormalities seen in ESRD patients include (a) a defect in postprandial lipid disposal, exposing the vasculature to high chylomicron remnant concentrations, (b) elevated intermediate-density lipoprotein levels, (c) increased heterogeneity of LDL and HDL apoproteins, (d) abnormalities of size and composition of LDL and HDL particles, (e) increased LDL susceptibility to oxidation, and (f) altered cell surface LDL epitope recognition (167–170).

In general, the design of studies relating outcome to lipid status in ESRD has been suboptimal. The situation is confounded by the observation that low serum cholesterol levels, probably indicative of malnutrition, may be independently associated with mortality in ESRD (156). Recent reports, however, have associated dyslipidemia with cardiac death in diabetic ESRD patients (171,172), lipoprotein(a) levels with cardiovascular disease (173), and vascular access loss (174) in ESRD patients.

D. Hyperhomocysteinemia

This abnormality is common in patients with end-stage renal disease and may contribute to the development of atherosclerosis and thromboembolic vascular disease in these patients (175–181).

E. Oxidant Stress

The oxidative modification of LDL in the vascular wall may be an important step in atherogenesis (182–184). Increased oxidant stress occurs in end-stage renal failure (185–188). It may result from reduced concentrations of endogenous antioxidants (189,190) and increased oxidant production from acidosis and abnormal metabolism (187) and from ongoing low-grade inflammatory processes (191,192). Dysregulation in the balance between proinflammatory cytokines and their inhibitors has been shown, which may contribute to the uremia-related chronic immunoinflammatory disorder (191,192). The evidence to support the presence of oxidized LDL in dialysis patients is contradictory (193–195), although increased titers of autoantibodies against oxidized LDL, compared with normal controls, have been reported (196).

IX. OTHER RISK FACTORS

A. Smoking

Smoking is a powerful risk factor for coronary artery disease in the general population (197), in hemodialysis patients (139), and especially in diabetics with ESRD (198).

B. Diabetes Mellitus

Diabetic nephropathy is the most common cause of ESRD. It is widely recognized that this patient group is at a very high risk of cardiovascular disease. In the Canadian study, diabetes was independently associated with concentric LV hypertrophy on baseline echocardiography (odds ratio 2.4) (21), the development of de novo ischemic heart disease (relative risk 4.0) (19), overall mortality (relative risk 2.0), and mortality after 2 years (relative risk 1.9) (199).

There is considerable evidence for a specific diabetic cardiomyopathy in patients without ESRD, manifested by LV diastolic dysfunction, which is believed to be associated with microvascular coronary disease (200–203). LV hypertrophy is found more frequently in hypertensive diabetics than hypertensive nondiabetics (204). In a postmortem study hypertensive-diabetic hearts were heavier and had more fibrosis than diabetic nonhypertensive and hypertensive nondiabetic hearts (205).

Diabetes mellitus is an independent risk factor for the development of coronary artery disease in the general population, quite apart from the excessive burden of other risk factors, such as hypertension and dyslipoproteinemia (206,207). Defining ischemic heart disease on the basis of clinical symptoms almost certainly underestimates the degree of coronary artery disease in diabetic patients, in whom there is a very marked prevalence of silent ischemic heart disease. It has been estimated that about a third of asymptomatic diabetic patients on renal replacement therapy have 50% or more stenosis of at least one coronary artery (208–210). This prevalence rises markedly with age. Manske et al. (208) found that 88% of asymptomatic diabetics undergoing pretransplantation screening coronary angiography had significant arterial stenosis. In patients younger than 45 years of age, only those with each of certain characteristics—diabetes less than 5 years, normal ST segments on electrocardiography, and a smoking history less than 5 pack-years—could be predicted not to have angiographic coronary artery disease with any degree of confidence (sensitivity 97%; negative predictive accuracy 96%) (208). These latter studies are likely subject to selection bias; it is probable that the true prevalence of asymptomatic coronary artery disease is much higher when the diabetic-ESRD population is considered in its entirety.

C. Valvular Calcifications in PD Patients

Chronic renal failure has been suggested as a risk factor for mitral annular calcification (211–213), a degenerative process of the mitral annulus. This abnormality derives its clinical significance from related consequences such as mitral insufficiency or stenosis, cardiac arrhythmias such as atrial fibrillation, infectious endocarditis, arterial emboli, heart failure, and stroke (211).

A nonselected CAPD population was studied by echocardiography at the start of therapy and every 1–1.5 years thereafter. Seventeen patients of the 135 studied showed mitral annular calcification at the start of dialysis. In these patients, high systolic blood pressure and left ventricular hypertrophy were related to this abnormality. Of 76 patients included in the follow-up study, another 17 patients developed mitral annual calcification de novo after a mean time of 49.7 ± 26.9 months of CAPD. The most remarkable and almost constant association found at echocardiography was the presence of left atrial dilatation. In the patients who developed mitral annular calcification, only duration of CAPD seemed to favor its appearance. Other risk factors such as severe hyperparathyroidism and/or hypertension with left ventricular hypertrophy could not be found as independent risk factors.

X. SCREENING FOR CARDIOVASCULAR DISEASE

A. Clinical Assessment of Cardiac Status

Obviously the least costly and least invasive step in assessing cardiac status is an initial and periodic history and physical examination. There is good evidence, however, that this alone is not sufficiently sensitive. As in the general population, a significant proportion of cardiac events are asymptomatic in ESRD patients. Diabetics, in particular, have a very high incidence of silent ischemia (214). In a series of 100 diabetics with ESRD, 75% of the patients with angiographically demonstrated CAD had no typical angina symptoms (210).

B. Noninvasive Testing for Cardiomyopathy

Echocardiographic assessment of patients with ESRD is useful in the evaluation of left ventricular structure and function, as well as in the detection of pericardial effusion and coexisting valvular lesions. Its usefulness might be reduced in dialysis patients by failure to standardize the time at which echocardiography is performed. The test should therefore be undertaken when the patient is euvolemic (94).

Echocardiography is indicated in dialysis patients with heart failure because the identification of diastolic dysfunction might preclude treatment with digoxin or vasodilators that induce increased cardiac contractility. It should probably be recommended as a screening tool for asymptomatic manifestations of cardiomyopathy if targeted treatment of potential risk factors might result. It is our practice to obtain echocardiograms on starting dialysis therapy and to repeat them if clinical problems develop or at 2-year intervals. Doppler echocardiography provides information about the blood flow velocity within the cardiac chambers, across valves, and in great vessels, from which hemodynamic assessment of the heart and measurements of diastolic function can be made.

M-mode echocardiography is most useful for estimating left ventricular wall thickness and left ventricular size. Quantification of the degree of change in left ventricular size in systole compared with diastole allows the calculation of fractional shortening, a measure of systolic function. Calculation of the left ventricular mass index provides a measure of LVH.

C. Noninvasive Testing for Coronary Artery Disease

Exercise-based stress tests for coronary artery disease (CAD) are not useful in patients on dialysis. Very few patients achieve adequate exercise levels, lowering the sensitivity of the test substantially. Thallium-201 myocardial imaging used with pharmacological stressors has a moderate degree of sensitivity for detecting CAD, but the results are variable and the accuracy is reduced in dialysis patients (215). This test is no more predictive of future cardiac events than a history of CAD or an abnormal baseline electrocardiogram (216)

Echocardiography has proved to be useful in the detection of CAD. Besides demonstrating the presence of CAD, it can provide information concerning the location and extent of ischemia. It also has the advantage of being independent of the electrocardiogram and is therefore useful in patients with an abnormal baseline electrocardiogram, which would preclude stress electrocardiography. Both regular treadmill exercise and pharmacological stressors have been employed.

Dobutamine stress echocardiography is promising, with perhaps the highest degree of sensitivity in detecting CAD in ESRD patients (217). It is not, however, available in all centers.

Table 7 summarizes the most useful noninvasive screening tests for coronary artery disease in dialysis patients compared to nonuremic patients.

D. Coronary Angiography

Cardiac catheterization and coronary angiography remains the "gold standard" for the diagnosis of CAD. It is also essential for the performance of PTCA and before revascularization surgery. The major disadvantages of this mode of investigation are its relatively high cost and relatively high side-effect profile (232) and the fact that patients are frequently hospitalized to have it done. From a renal perspective the major disadvantage is the significant incidence of radiocontrast nephropathy. This might not be a concern in anuric hemodialysis patients, but it is a major problem in patients with peritoneal dialysis who strongly depend on the residual renal function for adequacy of dialysis. Patients with symptomatic ischemic heart disease should be investigated with coronary angiography if revascularization is considered a reasonable option.

E. Screening for Cardiac Arrhythmias

The predictive value of Holter monitoring in the primary treatment of arrhythmias is not proven, and the criteria for prediction of efficacy of a specific antiarrhythmic drug are not clear. Although the test has several limitations, the major advantage is ease of technique and noninvasiveness (233).

Table 7 Approximate Sensitivities and Specificities of Noninvasive Testing for Coronary Artery Disease

	Patients without renal disease		Patients with renal disease		
Test	Sensitivity (%)	Specificity (%)	Sensitivity (%)	Specificity (%)	Ref.
Exercise electrocardiogram	50–85	85	[a]	[a]	218
Exercise thallium-201	82	91	67	62	219–221
Dipyridamole thallium-201	79	76	37–86	73–79	222–225
Adenosine thallium-201	83	75			226
Exercise echocardiography	76–84	95	[a]	[a]	227,228
Dobutamine echocardiography	72–89	85–95	69–95	95	227, 229–231
Dipyridamole echocardiography	52–60	95			227

[a]The sensitivity and specificity of exercise-based tests is adversely affected by the limited exercise capacity of uremic patients. Insufficient data available.

Electrophysiological testing has been shown to be more accurate in predicting response and prognosis with specific antiarrhythmic agents (234) but has the disadvantage of being invasive and carries the risk of provoking dangerous arrhythmias. Signal-averaged electrocardiogram is being used to identify patients with the substrate for ventricular arrhythmias and a high risk of sudden death (235). The use of this technique in dialysis patients has not yet been fully studied.

XI. MANAGEMENT

A. Volume Overload

From a pathogenetic perspective it is highly likely that the continuing LV volume overload in dialysis patients is detrimental to the heart. Little attention has been given to obsessive maintenance of euvolemia, probably because there is no easily used method to assess blood volume. Similarly, little attention has been given to limiting blood flow rates in fistulas and grafts. An analogy could be made between our failure to limit LV volume overload in dialysis patients and lack of interest in tight blood sugar control in diabetes mellitus, in that it was highly likely that poor blood sugar control was related to long-term complications of diabetes but it took many years to convince patients and doctors that obsessive control of blood sugar levels was beneficial (236).

B. Anemia

Evidence-based recommendations for the clinical use of erythropoietin have been published recently (237). The target hemoglobin for erythropoietin is under review. Currently there are several ongoing clinical trials to assess the risks and benefits of complete normalization of hematocrit in ESRD patients compared to current practice of partial correction of anemia. Whether complete correction of anemia leads to regression of LV abnormalities, prevention of heart failure and improved survival, and whether the cost of such an approach in terms of finances, hypertension (238,239), and vascular access loss (238,240–244) is worth the effort are areas of practical concern to patients, health care personnel, and health finance agencies.

Recently, a randomized controlled trial in the United States comparing mortality after correction of anemia with erythropoietin to partial correction of anemia in hemodialysis patients with symptomatic cardiac disease was terminated because of increased mortality and vascular access loss in the intervention group targeted to a normal hematocrit (287). Clearly, in patients with symptomatic heart disease, particularly ischemic heart disease, the target hemoglobin should be no higher than 100–110 g/L. The target hemoglobin in those with asymptomatic cardiac disease is unknown.

C. Hypertension

Numerous trials in the 1970s and 1980s confirmed that treating blood pressure levels greater than 160/95 was beneficial. The reduction in the incidence of stroke, on average by 41%, was more dramatic than the reduction seen in coronary heart disease, which averaged 14% (245). More recently, it has been shown that treating hypertension is at least as beneficial in elderly subjects (246). It has also been demonstrated that isolated systolic blood pressure should be treated in this group of patients (246). Several points regarding these trials are worth noting. β-Blockers and diuretics formed the cornerstone of therapy in these studies. The use of combinations of agents was the rule rather than the exception. None of these trials was designed to determine how much blood pressure should be reduced, and to date there are no published studies that determine the efficacy of angiotensin-converting enzyme (ACE) inhibitors and calcium channel blockers in reducing hard cardiovascular endpoints compared with longer established agents, principally β-blockers and diuretics. Several ongoing trials, which should be completed between 1997 and 2003, address these key issues (reviewed in Ref. 247). Calcium channel blockers and ACE inhibitors are commonly prescribed antihypertensive agents in ESRD patients. The use of calcium channel blockers, especially the use of short-acting dihydropyridines, has come under scrutiny on the basis of retrospective epidemiological studies showing an association with increased mortality (248). Such a study design is obviously less than ideal because it cannot control for all biases that lead a physician to pick one agent over another. Several ongoing randomized controlled trials are assessing whether long-acting calcium channel blockers are safe.

Aggressive control of blood pressure reduces the rate of nephron loss in progressive renal impairment in the predialysis phase. This has been shown in diabetic (249) and nondiabetic nephropathy (250). This effect has been most clearly shown with ACE inhibitors but also with calcium channel blockers. Even in patients who become dependent on dialysis, an intervention that slows the rate of loss of residual renal function would be highly desirable. Whether ACE inhibitors or calcium channel blockers still have this effect after the onset of dialysis therapy is unknown.

The regression of LV hypertrophy lacks a therapeutic trial to demonstrate its benefits in terms of morbidity and mortality. In essential hypertension with blood pressure lowering the decrease in LV hypertrophy is determined by pretreatment LV mass index, magnitude of blood pressure lowering, duration of therapy, and antihypertensive drug class (251). Rank order for regression of LV hypertrophy was ACE inhibition, calcium channel blockers, and β-blockers. In hemodialysis patients an ACE inhibitor perindopril did induce regression of LV hypertrophy (252).

D. Hyperlipidemia

In nonrenal patients aggressive lowering of LDL cholesterol delayed progression of atherosclerosis in saphenous vein coronary artery bypass grafts (253) and antidyslipidemic therapy prevented myocardial infarction and death (254). Five years of treatment of dyslipidemia in patients with and without known atherosclerosis prevented myocardial infarction or cardiovascular death. The number needed to treat to prevent one event was 16 patients in those with known atherosclerosis and 53 in those without known atherosclerosis. The evidence for the economic attractiveness of secondary prevention in patients with coronary artery disease and serum cholesterol levels between 5.5 and 8 mmol/L is good (255). It remains to be determined whether aggressive therapy of dyslipidemia has an impact on patient outcome in ESRD. Depending on the patient's life expectancy, we recommend treatment of hyperlipidemia in those with known coronary artery disease. The primary prevention of hyperlipidemia is a more difficult issue, but we recommend treatment of severe hyperlipidemia (serum cholesterol ≥8 mmol/L). If the patient is likely to survive long enough (e.g., 2 years) to obtain benefit from treatment of mild hyperlipidemia, then perhaps this should be undertaken.

E. Hyperhomocysteinemia

Administration of folic acid reduced plasma homocysteine levels in patients with chronic renal failure. This response may be seen in the presence of high circulating folate levels before the administration of additional vitamin. In a placebo-controlled, 8-week trial (256) in 27 PD and HD patients, the plasma homocysteine concentration could be lowered from 29.5 to 21.9 μmol/L with supraphysiological doses of vitamins that are cofactors in homocysteine metabolism: folic acid (15 mg/day), vitamin B_6 (100 mg/day), and vitamin B_{12} (1 mg/day). The normal homocysteine level is <15 μmol/L, so this regimen was only partially effective. A 26% decline in mean levels with a normalization of homocysteine levels occurred in 5 of 15 patients versus 0 of 12 placebo-treated patients. The efficacy of this approach in preventing atherosclerosis in both HD and PD patients remains to be determined.

Another approach, a 3-month treatment with fish oil, did not improve serum levels of homocysteine or the lipid profile of CAPD patients (257).

F. Management of Heart Failure

ACE inhibitors have been clearly shown to improve symptoms, morbidity, and survival in nonuremic individuals with heart failure (258–260). ACE inhibitors are efficacious in the prevention of heart failure in asymptomatic patients whose left ventricular ejection fraction is less than 35% (259) and in patients after myocardial infarction with an ejection fraction of 40% or less (261). It seems reasonable to extrapolate these results to the dialysis population and to recommend their use in patients with diastolic and systolic dysfunction. A word of caution on the use of ACE inhibitors in heart failure is needed. By reducing both the systemic and intra-adrenal formation of angiotensin II, thereby removing the stimulatory effect of this hormone on adrenal aldosterone release, ACE inhibitors can induce or aggravate hyperkalemia in dialysis patients (262). Effective therapy of the hyperkalemia in this setting includes limiting potassium intake, discontinuing the ACE inhibitor, or the concomitant use of low doses (such as 5 mL with meals) of the potassium-binding resin sodium polystyrene sulfonate (Kayexalate™).

The use of digoxin and vasodilators is probably different for those with systolic and diastolic dysfunction. Digoxin should probably be prescribed in those dialysis patients with heart failure who have systolic dysfunction (with or without atrial fibrillation) (263). On the other hand, it should be avoided in dialysis patients with normal systolic function and heart failure, because the increased contractility induced by digoxin could worsen diastolic function. Nitrates and hydralazine have been shown to improve symptoms and survival in the nonuremic population with heart failure (264). However, they increase myocardial contractility and may induce a deterioration of diastolic function.

Low-dose β-blocking agents improve New York Heart Association functional class and left ventricular ejection fraction in patients with idiopathic and ischemic dilated cardiomyopathy (265). The effect of β-blockers on survival is not resolved. A new agent, Carvedilol, has unique characteristics that distinguish it from other β-blockers including α blockade and antioxidant properties. Two recent studies (266,267) suggest a reduced mortality and hospitalization in nonrenal patients with heart failure, but the evidence is incomplete to recommend its routine use.

No data exist concerning the efficacy of drug therapy in heart failure in dialysis patients despite the fact that the etiology of heart failure is different from that in nonrenal patients. The use of hemofiltration in chronic heart failure has been essentially developed by Canaud et al. (268). In this setting, ultrafiltration may be implemented by different modalities (269, 270). Isolated ultrafiltration is a plasma water filtration without any fluid replacement. This technique is intended to restore the sodium balance in patients suffering from large extracellular fluid overload. The simple SCUF circuit can be used. Hemofiltration may also be performed with a certain amount of volume compensation. In this case, the CAVH or CVVH can be applied where both water-sodium balance is restored and biological or metabolic disorders are corrected.

G. Impact of CAPD in Heart Failure

Several papers report on the treatment with peritoneal dialysis of patients suffering from heart failure (54,271–273). Subjective clinical improvement is in general noted with a decrease in dyspnea, recovery of autonomy, and even occasionally a recovery of the professional activities of the patients. This functional improvement is due to the progressive and smooth ultrafiltration, resulting in sometimes impressive losses of body weight and improvement in cardiac performance. The objective data on patient survival in these series can be summarized as follows: of a total of 40 adult patients, 23 (75%) died after a mean survival period of 7 months in patients with organic renal failure and 14 months in patients with functional renal failure. The majority of the patients die relatively early and mostly because of cardiac reasons. During the treatment with CAPD a fall in the elevated ANP, renin and aldosterone levels have been observed (274).

H. Coronary Artery Revascularization

Dialysis patients fulfilling the anatomical criteria used in the general population are likely to benefit from coronary revascularization. Generally accepted criteria are (a) one-, two-, or three-vessel disease with angina refractory to medical management, when the intent is to relieve symptoms, (b) left main coronary artery disease, and (c) triple-vessel disease associated with ventricular dysfunction or easily inducible ischemia, when the intent is to improve survival. Coronary artery bypass surgery appears to be an effective means of relieving chest pain in patients with ESRD. The surgical mortality in 296 patients reported up to 1993 was 9% (275), which is higher than the 3% mortality observed in nonrenal patients. This may relate more to the level of LV function than to other factors associated with ESRD (275).

Although the data on outcome of coronary artery bypass surgery in ESRD are limited, there is even less information on angioplasty outcomes. If surgery is chosen in symptomatic patients, it is associated with greater initial morbidity than angioplasty but is more effective in the relief of angina and prevents the need for repeated procedures in the following 2–3 years (276–278).

In view of the limited life expectancy of many dialysis patients with coronary artery disease, angioplasty may be preferred in some patients because of the lower rate of initial morbidity and the possibility that the patient may be dead before subsequent revascularization procedures are required. The decision to opt for surgery in dialysis patients is more difficult because their survival is influenced by multiple factors other than coronary artery disease. Although angioplasty may be an attractive option in dialysis patients for relief of symptoms, many patients would not be optimal candidates because of recent myocardial infarction, previous revascularization, occluded coronary arteries, complex coronary stenosis, or some degree of narrowing of the left main coronary artery. It is clear that data on the outcome of medical therapy compared with angioplasty and bypass grafting in ESRD patients is necessary to enhance decision making.

Rinehart et al. (279) reported the outcomes of angina, myocardial infarction, cardiac death, and all-cause death following percutaneous transluminal coronary angioplasty (PTCA) or coronary artery bypass grafting (CABG) in a total of 84 chronic dialysis patients with symptomatic coronary artery disease. Only 4 patients were treated with peritoneal dialysis. It appeared that the postoperative risk of angina and the combined endpoints of angina, myocardial infarction, and cardiovascular death were significantly greater following PTCA than CABG. One needs to be aware of selection bias in the choice of revascularization procedures in interpreting this study. However, it appears that a high restenosis rate after RTCA is a problem in ESRD.

Reports on the efficacy of elective coronary stenting undertaken during cardiac catheterization compared with balloon angioplasty indicate that stenting decreases the need for repeated revascularization (280,281). In patients with isolated stenosis, stenting reduced the recurrence of angina when compared to angioplasty (282). Initially, stenting required intensive antithrombin and antiplatelet therapy and, consequently, a prolonged hospital stay (282). Recent studies show that vascular complications are far less problematic and lengths of stay are shorter in the era of aspirin and ticlopidine, rather than warfarin, after stenting (283). If the impressive early data are associated with long-term benefits, this procedure may be useful in a subset of dialysis patients with coronary artery disease.

I. Cardiac Arrhythmias

The following factors should be taken into consideration in the management of arrhythmias in dialysis patients

1. Asymptomatic, nonsustained supraventricular arrhythmias and unifocal premature ventricular contractions that are not associated with symptoms and/or hemodynamic compromise usually do not require therapy. If however, the same rhythm disturbances are present in a setting of coronary heart disease, pericarditis, or severe cardiomyopathy, treatment may be indicated.

Some patients will require only short-term treatment during or immediately after dialysis, and the approach is very similar to that used for nonuremic patients.

2. Drug therapy of arrhythmias in dialysis patients is more complicated compared with nonuremic patients because of possible alterations in pharmacokinetics, protein binding, as well as additional drug clearance during dialysis. Also, drug interactions should be kept in mind because dialysis patients are often on multiple medications. Many of the drugs used to treat arrhythmias may themselves become arrhythmogenic under certain conditions. The decision to treat arrhythmias with a specific drug should therefore be taken after carefully considering the risk-benefit ratio and after consulting an experienced cardiologist. Recently published pharmacokinetic data on antiarrhythmic drugs in renal failure are available and should be consulted (233).

3. Emergency treatment of symptomatic supraventricular tachyarrhythmias include cardioversion and/or digoxin and verapamil for younger patients with good left ventricular function, followed by quinidine. Systemic anticoagulation is indicated in patients with chronic atrial fibrillation to decrease the risk of thromboembolic events.

Sustained ventricular tachycardia should be treated urgently with lidocaine followed by quinidine or mexiletine. Ventricular fibrillation should be managed with defibrillation followed by lidocaine.

Bradyarrhythmias may require permanent placement of a pacemaker in patients with syncope caused by sinus node dysfunction, sick sinus syndrome, high degree atrial ventricular block, and carotid sinus hypersensitivity.

4. Treatment of underlying cardiac disorders and correction of precipitable factors are of primary importance in the prevention of cardiac arrhythmias. These treatments include correction of anemia, adjustments of potassium in the dialysate solution, especially in patients treated with digoxin, to prevent hypokale-

mia, and prevention of severe hyperkalemia before dialysis, as well as prevention of hypomagnesemia and hypercalcemia. Recently an interesting new model of hemodialysis potassium removal on the control of ventricular arrhythmias has been described (284). By decreasing the intrahemodialysis dialysate potassium concentration and maintaining a constant plasma-dialysate potassium gradient, it was possible to reduce the arrhythmogenic effect compared to standard hemodialysis with a constant dialysate potassium concentration and decreasing plasma-dialysate potassium gradient.

J. Pericarditis

Pericarditis occurred 161 times in 136 of 1058 patients undergoing chronic dialysis during a period of 13.7 years (285). Cardiac tamponade occurred during 27 episodes, while pretamponade occurred in 30. Tamponade was less frequent and resolution of pericarditis without invasive intervention more frequent when pericarditis occurred within 2 weeks of initiation of chronic dialysis. Similarly, resolution with conservative therapy was more frequent with first episodes than with recurrences, and when pericarditis occurred within 3 months of initiation of chronic dialysis. The overall survival was 89.7% and was the same irrespective of the duration of dialysis or whether the pericarditis was a first episode or a recurrence. It is recommended that patients with pericarditis and no hemodynamic alterations receive intensive hemodialysis, with careful hemodynamic and echocardiographic monitoring, as primary treatment. Invasive intervention is indicated if cardiac tamponade or pretamponade develops, if a pericardial effusion increases progressively in size, or if a large effusion persists after 10–14 days of intensive dialysis. The invasive intervention of choice is either formal pericardiectomy or subxiphoid pericardiotomy with intrapericardial steroid instillation. Since pericardiocentesis has proven to be a high-risk procedure, it is reserved for emergency circumstances and is then preferably performed in the operating room just prior to induction of anesthesia for definitive surgical drainage.

REFERENCES

1. Churchill DN, Taylor DW, Cook RJ, La Plante P, Barre P, Cartier P, Fay W, Goldstein M, Jindal K, Mandin H, McKenzie JK, Muirhead N, Parfrey PS, Posen GA, Slaughter D, Ulan RA, Werb R. Canadian Hemodialysis Morbidity Study. Am J Kidney Dis 1992; 19:214–234.
2. US Renal Data System: USRDA 1991 Annual Report. Bethesda, MD: The National Institute of Diabetes and Digestive and Kidney Diseases, 1991.
3. London G, Parfrey PS. Cardiac disease in chronic uremia: pathogenesis. Adv Renal Replac Ther 1997; 4: 194–211.
4. Parfrey PS, Foley RN, Harnett JD, Kent GM, Murray DC, Barre PE. The outcome and risk factors for left ventricular disorders in chronic uremia. Nephrol Dial Transpl 1996; 11:1277–1285.
5. Harnett JD, Foley RN, Kent GM, et al. Congestive heart failure in dialysis patients: prevalence, incidence, prognosis, and risk factors. Kidney Int 1996; 49: 1428–1434.
6. Parfrey PS, Foley RN, Harnett JD, Kent GM, Murray D, Barre PE. Outcome and risk factors of ischemic heart disease in chronic uremia. Kidney Int 1996; 49: 1428–1434.
7. Bloembergen WE. Cardiac disease in chronic uremia: epidemiology. Adv Renal Replac Ther 1997; 4:185–193.
8. World Health Organisation: World Health Statistics Annual for 1993. Geneva: WHO, 1995.
9. WHO Monica Project: Geographical variation in the major risk factors for coronary heart disease in men and women aged 35–64 years. World Health Stat Q 1988; 41:115–136.
10. Raine AEG, Margreiter R, Brunner FP, Ehrich JHH, Geerlings W, Landais P, Loirat C, Mallick NP, Selwood NH, Tufveson G, Valderrabano F. Report on management of renal failure in Europe, XXII, 1991. Nephrol Dial Transplant 1992; 7(suppl 2):7–35.
11. Nelson CB, Port FK, Wolfe RA, Guire KE. Comparison of continuous ambulatory peritoneal dialysis and hemodialysis patient survival with evaluation of trends during the 1980s. J Am Soc Nephrol 1992; 3:1147–1155.
12. Held PJ, Port FK, Turenne MN, Gaylin DS, Hamburger RJ, Wolfe RA. Continuous ambulatory peritoneal dialysis and hemodialysis: comparison of patient mortality with adjustment for comorbid conditions. Kidney Int 1994; 45:1163–1169.
13. Tzamaloukas AH, Yuan ZY, Balaskas E, Oreopoulos DG. CAPD in end-stage patients with renal disease due to diabetes mellitus—an update. Adv Perit Dial 1992; 8:185–191.
14. O'Donoghue D, Manos J, Pearson R, Scott P, Bakran A, Johnson R, Dyer P, Martin S, Gokal R. Continuous peritoneal dialysis and renal transplantation: a ten-year experience in a single center. Perit Dial Int 1992; 12: 242, 245–249.
15. Nissensen AR, Gentile DE, Soderblom RE, Oliver DF, Brax C. Morbidity and mortality of continuous ambulatory peritoneal dialysis: regional experience and long-term prospects. Am J Kidney Dis 1986; 7:229–234.

16. Maiorca R, Cancarini GC, Zubani R, Camerini C, Manili L, Brunori G, Movili E. CAPD viability: a long-term comparison with hemodialysis. Perit Dial Int 1996; 16:276–287.
17. Gentil MA, Carrazio A, Pavon MI, Rosado M, Castillo D, Ramos B, Algarra GR, Tejuca F, Banasco VP, Milan JA. Comparison of survival in continuous ambulatory peritoneal dialysis and hospital hemodialysis: a multicentric study. Nephrol Dial Transplant 1991; 6: 444–451.
18. Serkes KD, Blagg CR, Nolph KD, Vonesh EF, Shapiro F. Comparison of patient and technique survival in continuous ambulatory peritoneal dialysis (CAPD) and hemodialysis: a multicenter study. Perit Dial Int 1990; 10:15–19.
19. Wolfe RA, Port FK, Hawthorne VM, Guire KE. A comparison of survival among dialytic therapies of choice: in-center hemodialysis versus continuous ambulatory peritoneal dialysis at home. Am J Kidney Dis 1990; 15:133–140.
20. Maiorca R, Cancarini GC, Brunori G, Camerini C, Manili L. Morbidity and mortality of CAPD and hemodialysis. Kidney Int 1993; 43(suppl 40):S4–S15.
21. Fenton SD. Renal replacement therapy in Canada 1981-1992. In: Jacobs C, Kjellstrand CM, Koch KM, Winchester JF, eds. Replacement of Renal Function by Dialysis. 4th ed. Dordrecht: Kluwer Academic, 1996: 1406–1422.
22. Churchill DA, Thorpe KE, Vonesh EF, et al. Lower probability of patient survival with continuous peritoneal dialysis in the United States compared with Canada. J Am Soc Nephrol 1997; 8:965–971.
23. Bloembergen WE, Port FK, Mauger EA, Wolfe RA. A comparison of mortality between patients treated with hemodialysis and peritoneal dialysis. J Am Soc Nephrol 1995; 6:177–183.
24. Bloembergen WE, Port FK, Mauger EA, Wolfe RA. A comparison of causes of death between patients treated with hemodialysis and peritoneal dialysis. J Am Soc Nephrol 1995; 6:184–191.
25. Locatelli F, Marcelli D, Conte F,Limido A, Lonati F, Malberti F, Spotti D. 1983 to 1992: Report on regular dialysis and transplantation in Lombardy. Am J Kidney Dis 1995; 25:196–205.
26. Disney APS. Demography and survival of patients receiving treatment for chronic renal failure in Australia and New Zealand: report on dialysis and renal transplantation treatment from the Australia and New Zealand Dialysis and Transplant Registry. Am J Kidney Dis 1995; 25:165–175.
27. Foley RN, Parfrey PS, Harnett JD, et al. Mode of dialysis therapy and mortality in end-stage renal disease. J Am Soc Nephrol 1998; 9:267–276.
28. Fenton SSA, Schaubel DE, Desmeules M, Morrison HI, Mao Y, Copleston P, Jeffery JR, Kjellstrand CM. Hemodialysis versus peritoneal dialysis: a comparison of adjusted mortality rates. Am J Kidney Dis 1997; 30:334–342.
29. Lameire N, Vanholder RC, Van Loo A, Lambert MC, Vijt D, Van Bockstaele L, Vogeleere P, Ringoir SM. Cardiovascular diseases in peritoneal dialysis patients: the size of the problem. Kidney Int 1996; 50(suppl 56):S28–S36.
30. Lameire N, Bernaert P, Lambert MC, Vijt D. Cardiovascular risk factors and their management in patients on continuous ambulatory peritoneal dialysis. Kidney Int 1994; 46(suppl 48):S31–S38.
31. Viglino G, Cancarini GC, Catizone L, Cocchi R, De Vecchi A, Lupo A, Salomone M, Segoloni GP, Giangrande A. Ten years experience of CAPD in diabetics: comparison of results with non-diabetics. Nephrol Dial Transplant 1994; 9:1443–1448.
32. Canada-USA (CANUSA) Peritoneal Dialysis Study Group. Adequacy of dialysis and nutrition in continuous peritoneal dialysis. Association with clinical outcomes. J Am Soc Nephrol 1996; 7:198–207.
33. Genestier S, Hedelin G, Schaffer P, Faller B. Prognostic factors in CAPD patients: a retrospective study of a 10-year period. Nephrol Dial Transplant 1995; 10: 1905–1911.
34. United States Renal Data System. USRDS 1995 Annual Data Report. U.S. Department of Health and Human Services. Bethesda, MD: The National Institutes of Health, National Institute of Diabetes and Digestive and Kidney Diseases, August 1995.
35. Burton PR, Walls J. Selection-adjusted comparison of life-expectancy of patients on continuous ambulatory peritoneal dialysis, hemodialysis, and renal transplantation. Lancet 1987; 1:1115–1118.
36. Gault MH, Longerich L, Prabshakaran V, Purchase L. Ischemic heart disease, serum cholesterol and apolipoproteins in CAPD. Trans Am Soc Artif Intern Organs 1991; 37:M513–M514.
37. Wu G and the University of Toronto Collaborative Dialysis Group. Cardiovascular deaths among CAPD patients. Perit Dial Bull 1983; 3(suppl 3):S23–S26.
38. Habach G, Bloembergen WE, Mauger EA, Wolfe RA, Port FK. Hospitalization among United States dialysis patients: hemodialysis versus peritoneal dialysis. J Am Soc Nephrol 1995; 5:1940–1948.
39. Nichols WW, O'Rourke MF. Vascular impedance. In McDonald's Blood Flow in Arteries: Theoretic, Experimental and Clinical Principles. London: Edward Arnold Publisher, 1991.
40. London GM, Guerin AP, Marchais SJ, et al. Cardiac and arterial interactions in end-stage renal disease. Kidney Int 1996; 50:600–608.
41. Greaves SC, Gamble GD, Collins JF, et al. Determinants of left ventricular hypertrophy and systolic dysfunction in chronic renal failure. Am J Kidney Dis 1994; 24:768–776.

42. London GM, Guerin AP, Pannier B, et al. Increased systolic pressure in chronic uremia: role of arterial wave reflections. Hypertension 1992; 20:10–19.
43. Marchais SJ, Guerin AP, Pannier B, et al. Wave reflections and cardiac hypertrophy in chronic uremia: influence of body size. Hypertension 1993; 22:876–883.
44. Barenbrock M, Spieker C, Laske V, et al. Studies of the vessel wall properties in hemodialysis patients. Kidney Int 1994; 45:1397–1400.
45. Kawagishi T, Nishizawa Y, Konishi T, et al. High-resolution B-mode ultrasonography in evaluation of atherosclerosis in uremia. Kidney Int 1995; 48:820–826.
46. O'Rourke M. Mechanical principles in arterial disease. Hypertension 1995; 26:2–9.
47. Kamiya A, Togawa T. Adaptive regulation of wall shear stress to flow change in the canine carotid artery. Am J Physiol 1980; 239:H14-H21.
48. Langille BL, O'Donnell F. Reductions in arterial diameters produced by chronic decrease in blood flow are endothelium-dependent. Science 1986; 231:405–407.
49. Rostand RG, Kirk KA, Rutsky EA. Dialysis ischemic heart disease: insights from coronary angiography. Kidney Int 1984; 25:653–659.
50. Foley RN, Parfrey PS, Harnett JD, et al. Clinical and echocardiographic disease in patients starting end-stage renal disease therapy. Kidney Int 1995; 47:186–192.
51. Hüting J, Kramer W, Reitinger J, Kuhn K, Wizemann V, Schutterle G. Cardiac structure and function in continuous ambulatory peritoneal dialysis: influence of blood purification and hypercirculation. Am Heart J 1990; 119:334–352.
52. Hüting J, Kramer W, Reittinger J, Kuhn K, Schutterle G, Wizemann V. Abnormal diastolic left ventricular filling by pulsed Doppler echocardiography in patients on continuous ambulatory peritoneal dialysis. Clin Nephrol 1991; 36:21–28.
53. Buonchristiani U, Gamberi G, Misuri S, Carobi C, Giombini L, Di Paolo N. Diastolic left ventricular malfunction in CAPD patients. In: Ota K, Maher J, Winchester J, Hirszel P, eds. Current Concepts in Peritoneal Dialysis. Excerpta Medica, 1992:681–686.
54. Tabacchi GC, Castiglioni A, Lola P, Giangrande A. Echocardiographic evaluation of left ventricular function in patients on CAPD. Perit Dial Bull 1987; 2(suppl 7):S75.
55. Mousson C, Tanter Y, Chalopin JM, Rebibou JM, Dentan G, Morelon P, Rifle G. Traitement de l'insuffisance cardiaque congestive au stade terminal par dialyse péritonéale continue. Evolution à long terme. Presse Med 1988; 17:1617–1620.
56. Deligiannis A, Paschalidou E, Sakellariou G, Vargemezis V, Geleris P, Kontopoulos A, Papadimitriou M. Changes in left ventricular anatomy during haemodialysis, continuous ambulatory peritoneal dialysis and after renal transplantation. Proc EDTA-ERA 1984; 21: 185–189.
57. Leenen FHH, Smith DL, Khanna R, Oreopoulos DG. Changes in left ventricular hypertrophy and function in hypertensive patients started on continuous ambulatory peritoneal dialysis. Am Heart J 1985; 110:102–106.
58. Hébert JJ, Falardeau M, Pichette V, et al. Continuous ambulatory peritoneal dialysis for patients with severe left ventricular systolic dysfunction and end stage renal disease. Am J Kidney Dis 1995; 25:761–768.
59. Eisenberg M, Prichard S, Barre P, Patton R, Hutchinson T, Sniderman A. Left ventricular hypertrophy in end-stage renal disease on peritoneal dialysis. Am J Cardiol 1987; 60:418–419.
60. Franklin JO, Alpert MA, Twardowski ZJ, Khanna R, Nolph KD, Morgan RJ, Kelly Dl. Effect of increasing intra-abdominal pressure on left ventricular function in continuous ambulatory peritoneal dialysis. Am J Kidney Dis 1988; 12:291–298.
61. Swartz C, Onesti G, Mailloux L, et al. The acute hemodynamic and pulmonary perfusion effects of peritoneal dialysis. Trans Am Soc Artif Intern Organs 1969; 15:367–372.
62. Pacifico AD, Lasker N, Frank MJ, Levinson GE. Cardiovascular function in peritoneal dialysis. Tran Am Soc Artif Intern Organs 1966; 11:86–90.
63. Kong CH, Raval U, Thompson FD. Effect of two liters of intraperitoneal dialysate on the cardiovascular system. Clin Nephrol 1986; 26:134–139.
64. Vandenbogaerde J, Matthys E, Everaert J, Colardyn F, Lameire N. The influence of dialysate exchange on cardiac output in CAPD patients. Perit Dial Bull 1987; 7:242–244.
65. Acquatella H, Perez-Rojas M, Burger B, Guinand-Baldo. Left ventricular function in terminal uremia. Nephron 1978; 22:160–174.
66. Schurig R, Gahl G, Schartl M, Becker H, Kessel M. Central and peripheral haemodynamics in longterm peritoneal dialysis patients. Proc EDTA 1979; 16:165–170.
67. Kimura, K, Tabei, K, Asano, J, Hosoda, S. Cardiac arrhythmias in hemodialysis patients. A study of incidence and contributory factors. Nephron 1989; 53: 201–207.
68. Wizemann, V, Kramer, W, Thormann, J, Kindler M, Schütterle G. Cardiac arrhythmias in patients on maintenance hemodialysis: causes and management. Contrib Nephrol 1986; 52:42–53.
69. Gruppo Emodialisi e Pathologia Cardiovasculari. Multicentre cross-sectional study of ventricular arrhythmias in chronically hemodialysed patients. Lancet 1988; 6:305–309.
70. Wizemann V, Kramer W. Cardiac arrhythmias in end-stage renal disease: prevalence, risk factors, and man-

agement. In: Parfrey PS, Harnett JD, eds. Cardiac Dysfunction in Chronic Uremia. Boston: Kluwer Academic Publishers, 1992:67.

71. Blumberg A, Hausermann M, Strub B, et al. Cardiac arrhythmias in patients on maintenance hemodialysis. Nephron 1983; 33:91–95.
72. D'Elia JA, Weinrauch LA, Gleason RE, Hampton LA, Smith-Ossman S, Yoburn DC, Kaldany A, Healy RW, Stevens Leland O. Application of the ambulatory 24-hour electrocardiogram in the prediction of cardiac death in dialysis patients. Arch Int Med 1988; 148: 2381–2385.
73. Niwa A, Taniguchi K, Ito H, Nakagawa S, Takeuchi J, Sasaoka T, Kanayama M. Echocardiographic and Holter findings in 321 uremic patients on maintenance hemodialysis. Jpn Heart J 1985; 26:403–411.
74. Sforzini S, Latini R, Mingadi G, Vincent A, Redaelli B. Ventricular arrhythmias and four-year mortality in hemodialysis patients. Lancet 1992; 339:212–213.
75. Wizemann V, Kramer W, Funke T, Schütterle G. Dialysis-induced cardiac arrhythmias: fact or fiction? Nephron 1985; 39:356–360.
76. Qellhorst E, Scheunemann B, Hildebrand U. Hemofiltration: an improved method of treatment for chronic renal failure. Contrib Nephrol 1985; 4:194–211.
77. Morrison G, Michelson EL, Brown S, Morganroth J. Mechanism and prevention of cardiac arrhythmias in chronic hemodialysis patients. Kidney Int 1980; 17: 811–819.
78. Keller F, Weinmann J, Schwarz A, et al. Effect of digitoxin on cardiac arrhythmia in hemodialysis patients. Klin Wschr 1987; 65:1081–1086.
79. Peer G, Korzets A, Hochhauzer E, Eschcar Y, Blum M, Avram A. Cardiac arrhythmia during chronic ambulatory peritoneal dialysis. Nephron 1987; 45:192–195.
80. McLenachan JM, Dargie HJ. Ventricular arrhythmias in hypertensive left ventricular hypertrophy. Am J Hypert 1990; 3:735–740.
81. Canziani ME, Saragosa MA, Draibe SA, Barbieri A Ajzen H. Risk factors for the occurrence of cardiac arrhythmias in patients on continuous ambulatory peritoneal dialysis. Perit Dial Int 1993; 13(suppl 2): S409–S411.
82. Canziani ME, Cendoroglo Neto M, Saragoça MA, Cassiolato MA, Ramos OL, Ajzen H, Draibe SA. Hemodialysis versus continuous ambulatory peritoneal dialysis: effects on the heart. Artif Organs 1995; 19: 241–244.
83. Tzamaloukas A, Avasthi P. Temporal profile of serum potassium concentration in nondiabetic and diabetic outpatients on chronic dialysis. Am J Nephrol 1987; 7:101–109.
84. Rostand SG, Rutsky EA. Coronary artery disease in end-stage renal disease. In: Henrich W, ed. Principles and Practices of Dialysis. Baltimore: Williams & Wilkins, 1994, pp. 181–195.
85. USRDS 1992 Annual Data Report. Am J Kidney Dis 1992; 20(suppl 2):20–26.
86. Schrander-van de Meer AM , Van Saase JLCM, Roodvoets AP, et al. Mortality in patients receiving renal replacement therapy, a single center study. Clin Nephrol 1995; 43:174–179.
87. Parfrey PS, Harnett JD, Foley RN, Kent GM, Murray DC, Barre PE, Guttmann RD. Impact of renal transplantation on uremic cardiomyopathy. Transplantation 1995; 60:908–914.
88. Lai KN, Ng J, Whitford J, et al. Left ventricular function in uremia: echocardiographic and radionuclide assessment in patients on maintenance hemodialysis. Clin Nephrol 1985; 23:125–133.
89. Low I, Grutzmacher P, Bergmann M, et al. Echocardiographic findings in patients on maintenance hemodialysis substituted with recombinant human erythropoietin. Clin Nephrol 1989; 31:26–30.
90. London GM, Fabiani F. Left ventricular dysfunction in end-stage renal disease. Echocardiographic insights. In: Parfrey PS, Harnett JD, eds. Cardiac Dysfunction in Chronic Uremia. Boston: Kluwer Academic Publishers, 1992, pp. 117–138.
91. London GM, Marchais SJ, Guerin AP, et al. Cardiovascular function in hemodialysis patients. In: Grunfeld JP, Bach JF, Funck-Brentano JL, et al., eds. Advances in Nephrology. Vol. 20. St. Louis: Mosby Year Book, 1991, pp. 249–274.
92. Hutting J, Kramer W, Schutterle G, et al. Analysis of left ventricular changes associated with chronic hemodialysis: a non-invasive follow up study. Nephron 1988; 49:284–290.
93. Chaignon M, Chen WT, Tarazi RC, et al. Effect of hemodialysis on blood volume distribution and cardiac output. Hypertension 1981; 3:327–332.
94. Harnett JD, Murphy B, Collingwood P, et al. The reliability and validity of echocardiographic measurement of left ventricular mass in hemodialysis patients. Nephron 1993; 65:212–214.
95. London GM, Marchais SJ, Guerin AP, et al. Cardiac hypertrophy and arterial alterations in end-stage renal disease: hemodynamic factors. Kidney Int 1993; 43(suppl 41):S42–S49.
96. Hutting J, Kramer W, Schutterle G, et al. Analysis of left ventricular changes associated with chronic hemodialysis: a non-invasive follow up study. Nephron 1988; 49:284–290.
97. Ahearn DJ, Maher JF. Heart failure as a complication of hemodialysis fistula. Ann Intern Med 1972; 70: 201–204.
98. Gerry JL, Baird MG, Fortuin NJ. Evaluation of left ventricular function in patients with sickle cells anemia. Am J Med 1976; 60:968–972.
99. Foley RN, Parfrey PS, Harnett JD, et al. The impact of anemia on cardiomyopathy, morbidity and mortality

in end-stage renal disease. Am J Kidney Dis 1996; 28: 53–61.

100. Rottembourg, J. Residual renal function and recovery of renal function in patients treated by CAPD. Kidney Int 1993; 43(suppl 40):S106–S110.

101. Tzamaloukas AH, Saddler MC, Murata GH, et al. Symptomatic fluid retention in patients on continuous peritoneal dialysis. J Am Soc Nephrol 1995; 6:198–206.

102. Mulec H, Blohmé G, Kullenberg K, Nyberg G, Björck S. Latent overhydration and nocturnal hypertension in diabetic nephropathy. Diabetologia 1995; 38:216–220.

103. Lameire N. The impact of residual renal function on the adequacy of peritoneal dialysis. Nephron 1997; 77: 13–28.

104. Lameire N. Cardiovascular risk factors and blood pressure control in continuous ambulatory peritoneal dialysis. Perit Dial Int 1993; 13(suppl 2):S394–S395.

105. Davies SJ, Bryan J, Phillips L, Russel GI. The predictive value of KT/V and peritoneal solute transport in CAPD patients is dependent on the type of comorbidity present. Perit Dial Int 1996; 16(suppl I): S158–S162.

106. Heimburger O, Waniewski J, Werynski A, Tranaeus A, Lindholm, B. Peritoneal transport in CAPD patients with permanent loss of ultrafiltration capacity. Kidney Int 1990; 38:495–506.

107. Faller B, Lameire N. Evolution of clinical parameters and peritoneal function in a cohort of CAPD patients followed over 7 years. Nephrol Dial Transplant 1994; 9:280–286.

108. Selgas R, Fernandez-Reyes MJ, Bosque E, et al. Functional longevity of the human peritoneum: how long is continuous peritoneal dialysis possible? Results of a prospective medium long-term study. Am J Kidney Dis 1994; 23:64–73.

109. Selgas R, Bajo MA, Del Peso G, Jimenez C. Preserving the peritoneal membrane in long-term peritoneal dialysis patients. Sem Dial 1995; 8:326–332.

110. Yang CS, Chen SW, Chiang CH, et al. Effects of increasing dialysis dose on serum albumin and mortality in hemodialysis patients. Am J Kidney Dis 1996; 27: 380–386.

111. Lowrie EG, Huang NL, Lew NL, et al. The relative contribution of measured variables to death risk among hemodialysis patients. In: Friedman EA, ed. Death on Hemodialysis: Preventable or Inevitable? Dordrecht: Kluwer Academic Publishers, 1994:121–141.

112. London GM, Zins B, Pannier B, et al. Vascular changes in hemodialysis patients in response to recombinant human erythropoietin. Clin Nephrol 1989; 31:26–30.

113. Macdougall IC, Lewis NP, Saunders MJ, et al. Long-term cardiorespiratory effect of amelioration of renal anemia by erythropoietin. Lancet 1990; 335:489–493.

114. Canella G, LaCanna G, Sandrini M, et al. Renormalization of high cardiac output and left ventricular size following long-term recombinant human erythropoietin treatment of anemia dialyzed uremic patients. Clin Nephrol 1990; 34:272–278.

115. Silberberg J, Racine N, Barre PE, et al. Regression of left ventricular hypertrophy in dialysis patients following correction of anemia with recombinant human erythropoietin. Can J Cardiol 1990; 6:1–4.

116. Low-Friedrich I, Grutzmacher P, Marz W, et al. Therapy with recombinant human erythropoietin reduces cardiac size and improves cardiac size in chronic hemodialysis patients. Am J Nephrol 1991; 11:54–60.

117. Pascual J, Teruel JL, Moya JL, et al. Regression of left ventricular hypertrophy after partial correction of anemia with erythropoietin in patients on hemodialysis: a prospective study. Clin Nephrol 1991; 35:280–287.

118. Tagawa H, Nagano M, Saito H, et al. Echocardiographic findings in hemodialysis patients treated with recombinant human erythropoietin: proposal for a hematocrit most beneficial to hemodynamics. Clin Nephrol 1991; 35:35–38.

119. Goldberg N, Lundin AP, Delano B, et al. Changes in left ventricular size, wall thickness, and function in anemic patients treated with recombinant human erythropoietin. Am Heart J 1992; 124:424–427.

120. Martinez-Vea A, Bardaji A, Garcia C, et al. Long-term myocardial effects of correction of anemia with recombinant human erythropoietin in aged patients on hemodialysis. Am J Kidney Dis 1992; 19:353–357.

121. Fellner SK, Lang RM, Neumann A, et al. Cardiovascular consequences of the correction of the anemia of renal failure with erythropoietin. Kidney Int 1993; 44: 1309–1315.

122. Morris KP, Skinner JR, Hunter S, et al. Short term correction of anemia with recombinant human erythropoietin and reduction of cardiac output in end-stage renal failure. Arch Dis Child 1993; 68:644–648.

123. Rogerson ME, Kong CH, Leaker B, et al. The effect of recombinant human erythropoietin on cardiovascular responses to postural stress in dialysis patients. Clin Autonom Res 1993; 3:271–274.

124. Mall G, Rambausek M, Neumeister A, et al. Myocardial interstitial fibrosis in experimental uremia: implications for cardiac compliance. Kidney Int 1988; 33: 804–811.

125. Himelman RB, Landzberg JS, Simonson JS, et al. Cardiac consequences of renal transplantation: changes in left ventricular morphology and function. J Am Coll Cardiol 1988; 12:915–923.

126. London GM, Marchais SJ, Safar ME, et al. Aortic and large artery compliance in end-stage renal failure. Kidney Int 1990; 37:137–142.

127. Conlon PJ, Walshe JJ, Heinle SK, Minda S, Krucoff M, Schwab SJ. Predialysis systolic blood pressure cor-

relates strongly with mean 24-hour systolic blood pressure and left ventricular mass in stable hemodialysis patients. J Am Soc Nephrol 1996; 7:2658–2663.
128. Harnett JD, Kent GM, Barre PE, et al. Risk factors for the development of left ventricular hypertrophy in a prospectively followed cohort of dialysis patients. J Am Soc Nephrol 1994; 4:1486–1490.
129. Foley RN, Parfrey PS, Harnett JD, et al. Impact of hypertension on cardiomyopathy, morbidity and mortality in end stage renal disease. Kidney Int 1996; 49: 1379–1385.
130. Zucchelli P, Santoro A, Zuccala A. Genesis and control of hypertension in hemodialysis patients. Semin Nephrol 1988; 8:163.
131. Saldanha LF, Weiler E, Gonick HC. Effect of continuous ambulatory peritoneal dialysis on blood pressure control. Am J Kidney Dis 1993; 21:184–188.
132. Faller B, Lameire N. Evolution of clinical parameters and peritoneal function in a cohort of CAPD patients followed over 7 years. Nephrol Dial Transplant 1994; 9:280–286.
133. Kannel WB. Role of blood pressure in cardiovascular disease: The Framingham Study. Angiology 1975; 26: 1–14.
134. Charra B, Calemard E, Ruffet M, et al. Survival as an index of adequacy of dialysis. Kidney Int 1992; 41: 1286–1291.
135. Degoulet P, Legrain M, Reach I, et al. Mortality factors in patients treated by chronic hemodialysis. Nephron 1982; 31:103–110.
136. Neff MS, Eiser AR, Slifkin RF, et al. Patients surviving 10 years of dialysis. Am J Med 1983; 74:996–1004.
137. Fernandez JM, Carbonell ME, Mazzuchi N, et al. Simultaneous analysis of mortality and morbidity factors in chronic hemodialysis patient. Kidney Int 1992; 41: 1029–1034.
138. Tomita J, Kimura G, Inove T, et al. Role of systolic blood pressure in determining prognosis of hemodialyzed patients. Am J Kid Dis 1995; 25:405–412.
139. U.S. Renal Data System 1992 Annual Report, IV. Comorbid conditions and correlations with mortality risk among 3,399 incident hemodialysis patients. Am J Kidney Dis 1992; 20(Suppl 2):32–38.
140. Iseki K, Miyasato F, Tokuyama K, et al. Low diastolic blood pressure, hypoalbuminemia, and risk of death in a cohort of hemodialysis patients. Kidney Int 1997; 51:1212–1217.
141. Raine AEG. Acquired aortic stenosis in dialysis patients. Nephron 1994; 68:159–168.
142. McFalls EO, Archer SL. Rapid progression of aortic stenosis and secondary hyperparathyroidism. Am Heart J 1990; 120:206–208.
143. Owen SR, Lew NL, Yan Liu SM, et al. The urea reduction ratio and serum albumin concentrations as predictors of mortality in patients undergoing hemodialysis. N Engl J Med 1993; 329:1001–1006.
144. Held PJ, Levin NW, Bovbjerg RR, et al. Mortality and duration of hemodialysis treatment. JAMA 1991; 265: 871–875.
145. Collins AJ, Ma JZ, Umen A, et al. Urea index and other predictors of hemodialysis patient survival. Am J Kidney Dis 1994; 23:272–282.
146. Gotch F, Sargent J. A mechanistic analysis of the National Cooperative Dialysis Study. Kidney Int 1985; 28:526–534.
147. Parker TF, Husni L, Huang W, et al. Survival of hemodilaysis in the U.S. is improved with a greater quantity of dialysis. Am J Kidney Dis 1994; 23:670–680.
148. Iseki K, Kawazoe N, Fukiyama K. Serum albumin is a strong predictor of death in chronic dialysis patients. Kidney Int 1993; 44:115–119.
149. Spiegel DM, Breyer JA. Serum albumin: a predictor of long-term outcome in peritoneal dialysis patients. Am J Kidney Dis 1994; 23:283–285.
150. Acchiardo SR, Moore LW, La Tour PA. Malnutrition as the main factor in the morbidity and mortality of hemodialysis patients. Kidney Int 1983; 24(suppl 16): 199–203.
151. Kopple JD. Effect of malnutrition on morbidity and mortality in maintenance dialysis patients. Am J Kidney Dis 1994; 24:1002–1009.
152. Foley RN, Parfrey PS, Harnett JD, et al. Hypoalbuminemia, cardiac morbidity and mortality in end-stage renal disease. J Am Soc Nephrol 1996; 7:728–736.
153. Lowrie EG, Laird NM, Parker TF, et al. Effect of the hemodialysis prescription on patient morbidity. Report from the National Co-operative Dialysis Study. N Engl J Med 1981; 305:1176–1181.
154. Churchill DN, Taylor DW, Tomlinson DW, et al. Effects of high flux hemodialysis on cardiac structure and function among patients with end-stage renal failure. Nephron 1993; 65:573–577.
155. Foley RN, Parfrey PS, Harnett JD, et al. Hypocalcemia, morbidity, and mortality in end-stage renal disease. Am J Nephrol 1996; 16:386–393.
156. Lowrie EG, Lew NL. Death risk in hemodialysis patients: the predictive value of commonly measured variables and an evaluation of death rate differences between facilities. Am J Kidney Dis 1990; 15:458–482.
157. Massry SG, Smorgorzewski M. Mechanisms through which parathyroid hormone mediates its deleterious effects on organ function in uremia. Semin Nephrol 1994; 14:219–231.
158. Lacour B, Basile C, Drueke T, et al. Parathyroid function and lipid metabolism in the rat. Miner Elect Metab 1982; 7:157–165.
159. Stefenelli T, Mayr H, Bergler-Klein J, et al. Primary hyperparathyroidism: Incidence of cardiac abnormalities and partial parathyroidectomy. Am J Med 1993; 95:197–202.

160. Bogin E, Massry SG, Harary I. Effect of parathyroid hormone on rat heart cells. J Clin Invest 1981; 67: 1215–1227.
161. Amann K, Wiest G, Klaus G, et al. The role of parathyroid hormone in the genesis of interstitial cell activation in uremia. J Am Soc Nephrol 1994; 4:1814–1819.
162. London GM, Fabiani F, Marchais SJ, et al. Uremic cardiomyopathy: an inadequate left ventricular hypertrophy. Kidney Int 1987; 31:973–980.
163. Totao RD, Lena Vega GL, Grundy SM. Mechanisms and treatment of dyslipidemia of renal diseases. Curr Opin Nephrol Hypertension 1993; 2:784–790.
164. Auguet T, Senti M, Rubies-Prat J, et al. Serum lipoprotein(a) concentrations in patients with chronic renal failure receiving hemodialysis: influence of apolipoprotein(a) genetic polymorphism. Nephrol Dial Transplant 1993; 8:1099–1103.
165. Webb AT, Reaveley DA, O'Donnell M, et al. Lipoprotein(a) in patients on maintenance hemodialysis and continuous ambulatory peritoneal dialysis. Nephrol Dial Transplant 1993; 8:609–613.
166. Thillet J, Faucher C, Issad B, et al. Lipoprotein(a) in patients treated by continuous ambulatory peritoneal dialysis. Am J Kidney Dis 1993; 22:226–232.
167. Weintraub M, Burstein A, Rassin T, et al. Severe defect in clearing postprandial chylomicron remnants in dialysis patients. Kidney Int 1992; 42:1247–1252.
168.. Joven J, Vilella E, Ahmed S, et al. Lipoprotein heterogeneity in end stage renal disease. Kidney Int 1992; 42:1247–1252.
169. Maggi E, Bellazzi R, Falaschi F, et al. Enhanced LDL oxidation in uremic patients: an additional mechanism for accelerated atherosclerosis? Kidney Int 1994; 45: 876–883.
170. Reade V, Tailleaux A, Reade R, et al. Expression of apolipoprotein B epitopes in low density lipoproteins of hemodialyzed patients. Kidney Int 1993; 44:1360–1365.
171. Tschope W, Koch M, Thomas B, et al. Serum lipids predict cardiac death in diabetic patients on maintenance hemodialysis. Results of a prospective study. The German Study Group Diabetes and Uremia. Nephron 1993; 64:354–358.
172. Tschope W, Koch M, Thomas B, et al. Survival and predictors of death in dialyzed diabetic patients. Diabetologia 1993; 36:1113–1117.
173. Cressman MD, Heyka RJ, Paganini EP, et al. Lipoprotein(a) is an independent risk factor for cardiovascular disease in hemodialysis patients. Circulation 1992; 86:475–482.
174. Goldwasser P, Michel MA, Collier J, et al. Prealbumin and lipoprotein(a) in hemodialysis: Relationship with patients and vascular access survival. Am J Kidney Dis 1993; 22:215–225.
175. Bostom AG, Lathrop L. Hyperhomocysteinemia in end-stage renal disease: prevalence, etiology, and potential relationship to arteriosclerotic outcomes. Kidney Int 1997; 52:10–20.
176. Gupta A, Robinson K. Hyperhomocysteinemia and end stage renal disease. J Nephrol 1997; 10:77–84.
177. Bachmann J, Tepel M, Raidt H, Riezler R, Graefe U, Zappia V. Hyperhomocysteinemia and the risk of vascular disease in hemodialysis patients. J Am Soc Nephrol 1995; 6:121–125.
178. Dennis VW, Robinson K. Homocysteinemia and vascular disease in end-stage renal disease. Kidney Int 1996; 57(suppl):S11.
179. Robinson K, Gupta A, Dennis V, Arheart K, Chaudhary D, Green R, Vigo P, Mayer EL, Selhub J, Kutner M, Jacobson DW. Hyperhomocysteinemia confers an independent increased risk of atherosclerosis in end-stage renal disease and is closely linked to plasma folate and pyridoxine concentrations. Circulation 1996; 94:2743–2748.
180. Hultberg B, Andersson A, Sterner G. Plasma homocysteine in renal failure. Clin Nephrol 1993; 40:230–234.
181. Kim S, Hirose S, Tamura H, Nagasawa R, Tokushima H, Mitarai T, Isoda K. Hyperhomocysteinemia as a possible role for atherosclerosis in CAPD patients. Adv Perit Dial 1994; 10:282–285.
182. Witzum JL, Steinberg D. Role of oxidized low density lipoprotein in atherogenesis. J Clin Invest 1991; 88: 1785–1792.
183. Morel DW, DiCorleto PE, Chisholm GM. Endothelial and smooth muscle cells alter low density lipoprotein in vitro by free radical oxidation. Arteriosclerosis 1984; 4:357–364.
184. Stiko-Rahm A, Hultgardh-Nilsson A, Regnstrom J, et al. Native and oxidized LDL enhances production of PDGF AA and the surface expression of PDGF receptors in cultured human smooth muscle cells. Arterioscler Thromb 1992; 12:1089–1099.
185. Roselaar SE, Nazhat NB, Winyard PG, et al. Detection of oxidants in uremic plasma by electron spin resonance spectroscopy. Kidney Int 1995; 48:199–206.
186. Witko-Sursat V, Friedlauder M, Capeillere-Blandin C, et al. Advanced oxidation protein products as a novel marker of oxidative stress in uremia. Kidney Int 1996; 49:1304–1313.
187. Price SR, Mitch WE. Metabolic acidosis and uremic toxicity: protein and amino acid metabolism. Semin Nephrol 1994; 12:232–237.
188. Miyata T, Wada Y, Cai Z, et al. Implications of an increased oxidative stress in the formation of advanced glycation end products in patients with end stage renal failure. Kidney Int 1997; 51:1170–1181.
189. Ono K. The effect of vitamin C supplementation and withdrawal on the mortality and morbidity of regular hemodialysis patients. Clin Nephrol 1989; 31:31–34.
190. Cohen JD, Viljoen M, Clifford D, et al. Plasma vitamin E levels in a chronically hemolyzing group of dialysis patients. Clin Nephrol 1986; 25:42–47.

191. Pereira BJG, Shapiro L, King AJ, et al. Plasma levels of IL1-Beta, TNF-alpha and their specific inhibitors in underdialyzed chronic renal failure, CAPD and hemodialysis patients. Kidney Int 1994; 45:890–896.
192. Descamps-Latscha B, Herbelin A, Nguyen AT, et al. Balance between IL1-Beta, TNF-alpha, and their specific inhibitors in chronic renal failure and maintenance dialysis: relationships with activation markers of T cells, B cells, and monocytes. J Immunol 1995; 154:882–892.
193. Maggi E, Bellazzi R, Falaschi F, et al. Enhanced LDL oxidation in uremic patients: an additional mechanism for accelerated atherosclerosis? Kidney Int 1994; 45: 876–883.
194. Sutherland WHF, Walker RJ, Ball MJ, et al. Oxidation of low density lipoproteins from patients with renal failure or renal transplants. Kidney Int 1995; 48:227–236.
195. Schultz T, Schiffl H, Scheithe R, et al. Preserved antioxidative defense of lipoproteins in renal failure and during hemodialysis. Am J Kidney Dis 1995; 25:564–571.
196. Maggi E, Bellazi R, Gazo A, et al. Autoantibodies against oxidatively-modified LDL in uremic patients undergoing dialysis. Kidney Int 1994; 46:869–876.
197. Kannel WB. Update on the role of cigarette smoking in coronary artery disease. Am Heart J 1981; 101: 319–328.
198. McMillan MA, Briggs JD, Junor BJ. Outcome of renal replacement therapy in patients with diabetes mellitus. BMJ 1990; 301:540–544.
199. Foley RN, Calleton BF, Parfrey PS, Harnett JD, Kent GM, Murray D, Barre PE. Cardiac disease in diabetic end-stage renal disease. Diabetologia 1997; 40:1307–1312.
200. Shapiro LM, Howatt AP, Calter MM. Left ventricular function in diabetes mellitus I. Methodology and prevalence and spectrum of abnormalities. Br Heart J 1981; 45:122–128.
201. Shapiro LM, Leatherdale BA, MacKinnon J, et al. Left ventricular function in diabetes mellitus II. Relation between clinical features and left ventricular function. Br Heart J 1981; 45:129–132.
202. Thuesen L, Christiansen JS, Mogensen CE, et al. Echocardiographic-determined left ventricular wall characteristics in insulin dependent diabetic patients. Acta Med Scand 1988; 224:343–348.
203. Galderisi M, Anderson KM, Wilson PWF, et al. Echocardiographic evidence for a distinct diabetic cardiomyopathy (The Framingham Heart Study). Am J Cardiol 1991; 68:85–89.
204. Grossmann E, Shemesh J, Shamiss A, et al. Left ventricular mass in diabetes-hypertension. Arch Intern Med 1992; 152:1001–1004.
205. van Hoeven KH, Factor SM. A comparison of the pathological spectrum of hypertensive diabetic and hypertensive-diabetic heart disease. Circulation 1990; 82:848–885.
206. Kannel WB, McGee DL. Diabetes and cardiovascular disease: The Framingham Study. JAMA 1979; 241: 2035–2038.
207. Valsania P, Zarich SW, Kowalchuk GJ, et al. Severity of coronary artery disease in young patients with insulin-dependent diabetes mellitus. Am Heart J 1991; 122:695–700.
208. Manske CL, Thomas W, Wang Y, et al. Screening diabetic transplant candidates for coronary artery disease: identification of a low risk subgroup. Kidney Int 1993; 44:617–621.
209. Weinrauch L, D'Elia EA, Healy RW, et al. Asymptomatic coronary artery disease: an assessment of diabetics evaluated for renal transplantation. Circulation 1978; 58:1184–1190.
210. Braun WE, Phillips DF, Vidt DG. Coronary artery disease in 100 diabetics with end stage renal disease. Transplant Proc 1984; 16:603–607.
211. Fernandez-Reyes MJ, Bajo MA, Robles P, et al. Mitral annular calcification in CAPD patients with a low degree of hyperparathyroidism. An analysis of other possible risk factors. Nephrol Dial Transpl 1995; 10: 2090–2095.
212. Hüting J. Progression of valvular sclerosis in end-stage renal disease treated by long-term peritoneal dialysis. Clin Cardiol 1992; 15:745–750.
213. Hüting J. Predictive value of mitral and aortic valve sclerosis for survival in end-stage renal disease on continuous ambulatory peritoneal dialysis. Nephron 1993; 64:63–68.
214. Chiariello M, Indolfi C, Cotecchia MR, Sifola C, Romano M, Condererlli M. Asymptomatic transients ST changes during ambulatory ECG monitoring in diabetic patients. Am Heart J 1985; 110:529–534.
215. Murphy SW, Parfrey PS. Screening for cardiovascular disease in dialysis patients. Curr Opin Nephrol Hypertension 1996; 5:532–540.
216. Morrow CE, Schwartz ES, Sutherland DE, Simmons RL, Ferguson RM, Kjellstrand CM, Najarian JS. Predictive value of thallium stress testing for coronary and cardiovascular events in uremic diabetic patients before renal transplantation. Am J Surg 1983; 146: 331–335.
217. Bates JR, Sawada SG, Segar DS, et al. Evaluation using dobutamine stress echocardiography in patients with insulin dependent diabetes mellitus before kidney and/or pancreas transplantation. Am J Cardiol 1996; 77:175–179.
218. Coley CM, Eagle KA. Preoperative assessment and perioperative management of cardiac ischemic risk in noncardiac surgery. Curr Probl Cardiol 1996; 5:290–382.
219. Okada RD, Boucher CA, Straus HW, Pahost GM. Exercise radionucleotide imaging approaches to coronary artery disease. Am J Cardiol 1980; 46:1188–1204.

220. Kotler TS, Diamond GA. Exercise thallium 201 scintiography in the diagnosis and prognosis of coronary artery disease. Ann Intern Med 1990; 113:684–702.
221. Holley JL, Fenton RA, Arthur RS. Thallium stress testing does not predict cardiovascular risk in diabetic patients with end stage renal disease undergoing cadaveric renal transplantation. Am J Med 1991; 90: 563–570.
222. Go RT, Marwick TH, MacIntyre WJ, Saha JB, Neumann DR, Underwood PA, Simplendorfer CC. A prospective comparison of rubidium 82 PET and thallium 201 SPECT myocardial perfusion imaging utilizing a single dipyridamole stress in the diagnosis of coronary artery disease. J Nucl Med, 1990; 31:1899–1905.
223. Dahan M, Lagallicier B, Himbert D, Faraggi M, Aubrey N, Siohan N, Siohan P, Viron B, Gourgon R, Mignon F. Diagnostic value of myocardial thallium stress scintiography in the detection of coronary artery disease in patients undergoing chronic hemodialysis. Arch Mal Coeur 1995; 88:1121–1123.
224. Boudreau RJ, Strony JT, du Cret RP, Kuni CC, Wang Y, Wilson RF, Schwartz JS, Castaneda-Zuniga WR. Perfusion thallium imaging of type I diabetes patients with end stage renal disease: comparison of oral and intravenous dipyridamole administration. Radiology 1990; 175:103–105.
225. Marwick TH, Steinmuller DR, Underwood DA, Hobbs RT, Raymundo TG, Swift C, Braun WE. Ineffectiveness of dipyridamole SPECT thallium imaging as a screening technique for coronary artery disease in patients with end stage renal failure. Transplantation 1990; 49:100–103.
226. Coyne EP, Belvedere DA, Van de Streek PR, Weiland FL, Evans RB, Spaccavento LJ. Thallium-201 scintiography after intravenous infusion of adenosine compared with exercise thallium testing in the diagnosis of coronary artery disease. J Am Coll Cardiol 1991; 17:1289–1294.
227. Dagianti A, Penco M, Agati L, Sciomer S, Dagianti A, Rosanio S, Fedele F. Stress echocardiography: comparison of exercise, dipyridamole and dobutamine in detecting and predicting the extent of coronary artery disease. J Am Coll Cardiol 1995; 26:18–25.
228. Marwick TH, Nemec JJ, Pashkow FI, Stewart WJ, Salcedo EE. Accuracy and limitations of exercise echocardiography in routine clinical settings. J Am Coll Cardiol 1992; 19:74–81.
229. Sawada SG, Segar DS, Ryan T, Brown SE, Dohan AM, Williams R, Fineberg NS, Armstrong WF, Feigenbaum H. Echocardiographic detection of coronary artery disease during dobutamine infusion. Circulation 1991; 83:1605–1614.
230. Reis G, Marcovitz PA, Leichtman AB, Merion RM, Fay WP, Werns SW, Armstrong WF. Usefulness of dobutamine stress echocardiography in detecting coronary artery disease in end-stage renal disease. Am J Cardiol 1995; 75:707–710.
231. Albanese J, Nally J, Marwick T, D'Hondt AM, Wijins W, Van Ypersele C. Dobutamine echocardiography is effective in the non-invasive detection of prognostically important coronary artery disease in patients with end-stage renal diseast (abstr). J Am Soc Nephrol 1994; 5:322.
232. Barett BJ, Parfrey PS, Vavasour HV, O'Dea F, Kent GM, Stone E. A comparison of non-ionic, low osmolality radio-contrast agents with ionic, high-osmolality agents during cardiac catheterization. N Engl J Med 1992; 326:431–436.
233. Venkatesan J, Henrich WL. Cardiac disease in chronic uremia: management. Adv Ren Repl Ther 1997; 4: 249–266.
234. Wilber DJ, Garan H, Finkelstein D, et al. Out-of-hospital cardiac arrest: use of electrophysiologic testing in the prediction of long-term outcome. N Engl J Med 1988; 318:19–24.
235. Cripps T, Bennett ED, Carom AJ, et al. High gain signal averaged electrocardiogram combined with 24-hour monitoring in patients early after myocardial infarction for bedside prediction of arrhythmic events. Br Heart J 1988; 60:181–187.
236. Diabetes Control and Complications Trial (DCCT) Research Group. Effect of intensive diabetes management on macrovascular events and risk factors in the Diabetes Control and Complications Trial. Am J Cardiol 1995; 75:894–903.
237. Muirhead N, Bergman J, Burgess E, Jindal KK, Levin A, Nolin L, Parfrey P. Evidence based recommendations for the clinical use of recombinant human erythropoietin. Am J Kidney Dis 1995; 26:S1–S24.
238. Winearls CG, Oliver DO, Pippard MJ, et al. Effect of human erythropoietin derived from recombinant DNA on the anemia of patients maintained by chronic hemodialysis. Lancet 1986; ii:1175–1177.
239. Eschbach JW, Egrie JC, Downing MR, et al. Correction of the anemia of end-stage renal disease with recombinant human erythropoietin. N Engl J Med 1987; 316:73–78.
240. Casati S, Passerini P, Campise MR, et al. Benefits and risks of protracted treatment with human recombinant erythropoietin in patients having hemodialysis. BMJ 1987; 295:1017–1020.
241. Paganini EP, Latham D, Abdulhadi M. Practical considerations of recombinant human erythropoietin therapy. Am J Kidney Dis 1989; 14:19–25.
242. Sundal E, Kaeser U. Correction of anemia of chronic renal failure with recombinant human erythropoietin: safety and efficacy of one year's treatment in a European Multicentre Study of 150 hemodialysis-dependent patients. Nephrol Dial Transpl 1989; 4:979–987.
243. Canadian Erythropoietin Study Group. Association between recombinant human erythropoietin and quality of life and exercise capacity of patients receiving hemodialysis. BMJ 1990; 300:573–578.

244. Churchill DN, Muirhead N, Goldstein M, et al. Probability of thrombosis of vascular access among hemodialysis patients treated with recombinant human erythropoietin. J Am Soc Nephrol 1994; 4:1809–1813.
245. Collins R, Peto R, MacMahon S, et al. Blood pressure, stroke and coronary heart disease. Part 2, short-term reductions in blood pressure: over-view of randomized drug trials in their epidemiological context. Lancet 1990; 225:827–838.
246. Lever AF, Ramsay LE. Treatment of hypertension in the elderly. J Hypertens 1995; 13:571–579.
247. Hanssen L. The benefits of lowering elevated blood pressure: a critical review of studies of cardiovascular morbidity and mortality in hypertension. J Hypertens 1996; 14:537–544.
248. Furberg CD, Psaty BM, Meyer JV. Nifedipine: dose-related increase in mortality in patients with coronary heart disease. Circulation 1995; 92:1326–1331.
249. Lewis EJ, Hunsicker LG, Bain RD, Rohde RD. The effect of angiotensin-converting-enzyme inhibition on diabetic nephropathy. N Engl J Med 1993; 329:1456–1462.
250. Maschio G, Alberti D, Janin G, et al. Effect of the angiotensin-converting-enzyme inhibitor benazepril on the progression of chronic renal insufficiency. N Engl J Med 1996; 334:939–945.
251. Schneider RE, Martas P, Klingbeil A. Reversal of left ventricular hypertrophy in essential hypertension. A meta-analysis of randomized double-blind studies. J Am Med Assn 1996; 275:1507–1513.
252. London GM, Pannier B, Guerin AP, et al. Cardiac hypertrophy, aortic compliance, peripheral resistance, and wave reflection in end-stage renal disease: comparative effects of ACE inhibition and calcium channel blockade. Circulation 1994; 90:2786–2796.
253. The Post Coronary Artery Bypass Graft Trial Investigators: The effect of aggressive lowering of low density lipoprotein cholesterol levels and low dose anticoagulation on obstructive changes in saphenom vein coronary artery bypass grafts. N Engl J Med 1997; 336:153–162.
254. Rembold CM. Number needed to treat analysis of the prevention of myocardial infarction and death by antidyslipidemic therapy. J Fam Pract 1996; 42:577–586.
255. Johannesson M, Jonsson B, Kjekshus J, et al for Scandinavian Simvastatin Survival Study Group. Cost effectiveness of simvastatin treatment to lower cholesterol levels in patients with coronary artery disease. N Engl J Med 1997; 336:332–336.
256. Bostom AG, Shemin D, Lapane KL, Hume AL, Yoburn D, Nadeau MR, Bendich A, Selhub J, Rosenberg IH. High dose B-vitamin treatment of hyperhomocysteinemia in dialysis patients. Kidney Int 1996; 49: 147–152.
257. Holdt B, Korten G, Knippel M, Lehman JK, Claus R, Holtz M, Hausmann S. Increased serum level of total homocysteine in CAPD patients despite fish oil therapy. Perit Dial Int 1996; 16(suppl 1):S246–S249.
258. The CONSENSUS Trial Study Group. Effects of enalapril on mortality in severe congestive heart failure: results of the Cooperative North Scandinavian Enalapril Survival Study (CONSENSUS). N Engl J Med 1987; 316:1429–1435.
259. The SOLVD Investigators. Effect of enalapril on survival in patients with reduced left ventricular ejection fractions and congestive heart failure. N Engl J Med 1991; 325:293–302.
260. Yusuf B, Pepine CJ, Gares C, Pouleur H, Salem D, Kostis J, Benedict C, Rousseau M, Bourassa M, Pitt B. Effect of enalapril on myocardial infarction and unstable angina in patients with low ejection fractions. Lancet 1992; 340:1173–1178.
261. Pfeffer MA, Braunwald E, Moyé LA, Basta L, Brown EJ, Cuddy TE, Davis BR, Geltman EM, Goldman S, Flaker GC, et al. Effect of captopril on mortality and morbidity in patients with left ventricular dysfunction after myocardial infarction. N Engl J Med 1992; 327: 669–677.
262. Oster JR, Materson BJ. Renal and electrolyte complications of congestive heart failure and effects of treatment with angiotensin-converting enzyme inhibitors. Arch Intern Med 1992; 152:704–710.
263. The Digitalis Investigation Group. The effect of digoxin on mortality and morbidity in patients with heart failure. N Engl J Med 1997; 336:525–533.
264. Cohn JH, Archibald DG, Ziesche S, Franciosa JA, Hartson WE, Tristani FE, Dunkman WB, Jacobs W, Francis GS, Flohr KH, et al. Effect of vasodilator therapy on mortality in chronic congestive heart failure: results of a Veterans Administration Cooperative Study. N Engl J Med 1986; 314:1547–1552.
265. Zaremski DG, Nolan PE, Srack MK, Lui CY. Meta-analysis of the use of low dose beta blockers in idiopathic or ischemic dilated cardiomyopathy. Am J Cardiol 1996; 77:1247–1250.
266. Parker M, Briston MR, Cohn JN, et al. for the U.S. Carvedilol Heart Failure Study Group. The effect of carvedilol on morbidity and mortality in patients with chronic heart failure. N Engl J Med 1996; 334:1349–1355.
267. Australia/New Zealand Heart Failure Research Collaborative Group. Randomized placebo controlled trial of Carvedilol in patients with congestive heart failure due to ischemic heart disease. Lancet 1997; 349:375–380.
268. Canaud B, Christol JP, Klouche K, Beraud JJ, Ferriere M, Grolleau R, Mion C. Slow continuous ultrafiltration: a means of unmasking myocardial functional reserve in end stage cardiac disease. In: Sieberth HG, Mann H, Stummvoll HK, eds. Third International Conference on Continuous Hemofiltration. Basel: Karger, 1990:79–83.

269. Simpson IA, Rae AP, Simpson K, Gribben J, Boulton Jones JM, Allison ME, Hutton I. Ultrafiltration in the management of refractory congestive heart failure. Br Heart J 1986; 55:344–347.
270. Rimondini A, Cipolla CM, Della Bella P, Grazi S, Sisillo E, Susini G, Guazzi MD. Hemofiltration as short-term treatment for refractory congestive heart failure. Am J Med 1987; 83:43–48.
271. Mckinnie JJ, Bourgeois RJ, Husserl FE. Longterm therapy for heart failure with continuous ambulatory peritoneal dialysis. Arch Int Med 1985; 145:1128–1129.
272. Rubin J, Ball R. Continuous ambulatory peritoneal dialysis as treatment of severe congestive heart failure in the face of chronic renal failure. Report of eight cases. Arch Int Med 1986; 146:1533–1535.
273. Konig PS, Lhotta K, Kronenberg F, Joannidis M, Herold M. CAPD: a successful treatment in patients suffering from therapy-resistant congestive heart failure. Adv Perit Dial 1991; 7:97–101.
274. Lai KN, Li PKT, Woo KS, Lui SF, Leueng JCK, Law E, Nicchols MG. Vasoactive hormones in uremic patients on continuous ambulatory peritoneal dialysis. Clin Nephrol 1991; 35:218–223.
275. Ko W, Kreiger KH, Isom OW. Cardiopulmonary bypass procedures in dialysis patients. Ann Thorac Surg 1993; 55:677–684.
276. Hillis LD, Rutherford JD. Coronary angioplasty compared with bypass grafting. N Engl J Med 1994; 331: 1086–1087.
277. Hamm CW, Reimers J, Ischinger T, Rupprecht H-J, Berger J, Bleifeld W, for the German Angioplasty Bypass Surgery Investigation. A randomized study of coronary angioplasty compared with bypass surgery in patients with symptometic multivessel coronary disease. N Engl J Med 1994; 331:1037–1043.
278. King SB, Lembo NJ, Weintraub WS, Kosinski AS, Barnhart HX, Kutner MH, Alazraki NP, Guyton RA, Zhao X-Q for the Emory Angioplasty Versus Surgery Trial (EAST). A randomized trial comparing coronary angioplasty with coronary bypass surgery. N Engl J Med 1994; 331:1044–1050.
279. Rinehart AL, Herzog CA, Collins AJ, Flack JM, Ma JZ, Opsahl JA. A comparison of coronary angioplasty and coronary artery bypass grafting in chronic dialysis patients. Am J Kidney Dis 1995; 25:281–290.
280. Fischman DL, Leon MB, Baim DS, Schatz RA, Savage MP, Penn I, Detre K, Vehtri L, Ricci D, Nobuyoshi M, et al. for the Sent Restenosis Study Investigators. A randomized comparison of coronary-stent placement and balloon angioplasty in the treatment of coronary artery disease. N Engl J Med 1994; 331: 496–501.
281. Serruys PW, De Jaegere P, Kiemeneij F, Macaya C, Rutsch W, Heyndrickx G, Emanuelsson H, Marco J, Legrand V, Materne P, et al. for the Benestent Study Group: A comparison of balloon-expandable-stent implantation with balloon angioplasty in patients with coronary artery disease. N Engl J Med 1994; 331: 489–495.
282. Versaci F, Gaspardone A, Tomai E, et al. A comparison of coronary artery stenting with angioplasty for isolated stenosis of the proximal left anterior descending coronary artery. N Engl J Med 1997; 336:817–822.
283. Schomig A, Neumann FJ, Kastrati A, et al. A randomized comparison of anti-platelet and anti-coagulant therapy after coronary artery stents. N Engl J Med 1996; 334:1084–1089.
284. Redaelli B, Locatelli F, Limido D, Andrulli S, Signorini MG, Sforzini S, Bonoldi L, Vincenti A, Cerutti S, Orlandini G. Effect of a new model of hemodialysis potassium removal on the control of ventricular arrhythmias. Kidney Int 1996; 50:609–617.
285. Rutsky EA, Rostand SG. Treatment of uremic pericarditis and pericardial effusion. Am J Kidney Dis 1987; 10:2–8.
286. Foley RN, Parfrey PS, Harnett JD. Left ventricular hypertrophy in dialysis patients. Sem Dial 1992; 5:34, 1992.
287. Besarab A, Bolton K, Egrie JC et al. The effects of normal as compares with low hematocrit values in patients with cardiac disease who are receiving hemodialysis and Epotin. N Eng J Med 1998; 339:584–590.

16

Hematological Problems and Their Management in Hemodialysis and Peritoneal Dialysis Patients

Iain C. Macdougall
King's College Hospital, London, United Kingdom

I. INTRODUCTION

It has been recognized for over 150 years that the major hematological complication of chronic renal failure is a progressive and often severe chronic anemia (1). Although this is multifactorial, by far the main cause of this is inadequate production of the hormone erythropoietin by the diseased kidneys (2), resulting in a normochromic normocytic hypoproliferative anemia. Untreated, this not only causes the debilitating symptoms of extreme tiredness and lethargy, muscle fatigue, cold intolerance, and exertional dyspnea associated with anemia, but it has also been shown to be a major contributory factor to the high prevalence of cardiovascular disease in dialysis patients, with consequent increased morbidity and mortality (3).

In the 1970s and early 1980s, the management of renal anemia consisted of androgen therapy, iron supplementation, vitamin supplements, and repeated blood transfusions. None of these measures was adequate in achieving satisfactory or sustained correction of the anemia, which has only been possible since the introduction of recombinant human erythropoietin (epoetin) therapy in the late 1980s. This latter treatment has transformed the management of renal anemia as well as the lives of the numerous patients worldwide who have received this therapy. Many studies have confirmed the improvements in quality of life, exercise capacity, and cardiac function associated with epoetin treatment, and there is now preliminary evidence that there is a reduction in long-term cardiovascular morbidity and mortality (4,5). The advent of epoetin therapy has, however, brought its own problems such as functional iron deficiency and epoetin resistance, and much attention has been focused on ways of optimizing the response by means of intravenous iron supplementation and other adjuvant therapies.

Disorders of white cell and platelet function have also been described in renal failure, but these are of secondary importance compared with those related to the red cell. The majority of this chapter is therefore devoted to the anemia of renal failure and its management, with lesser prominence given to the leukocyte and platelet disorders.

II. ANEMIA OF CHRONIC RENAL FAILURE

As renal function declines, there is a progressive worsening of anemia, which becomes particularly evident once the serum creatinine rises above 300 μmol/L or the GFR falls below 30 mL/min (6). The severity of the anemia parallels fairly closely the degree of renal impairment, and its major cause is loss of the cells in the kidney responsible for the synthesis and secretion of erythropoietin. This results in an inappropriately low level of erythropoietin circulating in the blood for the degree of anemia (Fig. 1) (2). Other factors have, however, been implicated in the pathogenesis of renal anemia, including iron deficiency, blood loss, folate deficiency, hyperparathyroidism with marrow fibrosis,

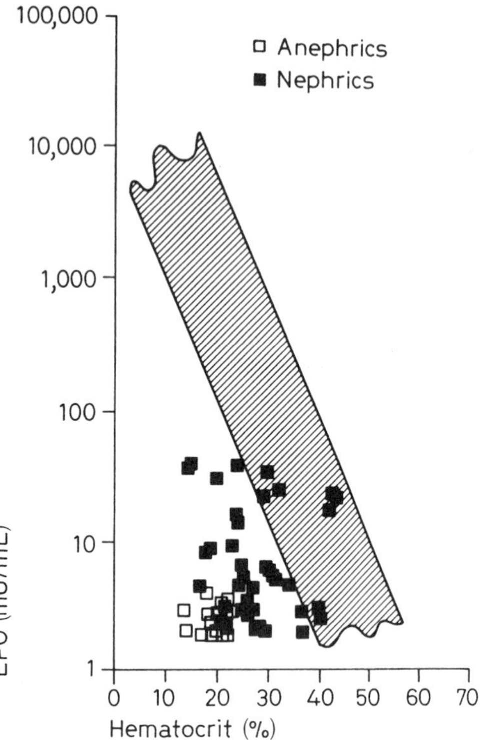

Fig. 1 Relationship between serum erythropoietin levels and hematocrit in patients with chronic renal failure. The hatched area shows the normal relationship in healthy control subjects and patients with non-renal anemias. (Taken from Ref. 2, used with permission.)

aluminum toxicity, and suppression of erythropoiesis by "uremic inhibitors" (7).

The peripheral blood film from a patient with uncomplicated renal anemia usually reveals normochromic normocytic red cells, occasionally with fragmented red cells or "burr" cells. The reticulocyte count is inappropriately low for the degree of anemia, and ferrokinetic studies confirm the reduced erythropoietic activity. Cellularity of the bone marrow may be decreased, normal, or increased, and blood volume studies show a reduced red cell mass but normal total blood volume (8).

III. PREVALENCE OF ANEMIA IN DIALYSIS PATIENTS

By the time the patient with chronic renal failure reaches the need for dialysis, the hemoglobin is often around 6–8 g/dL, and only about 3% of such patients have a normal hematocrit (9). There may, however, be some improvement after institution of dialysis, particularly peritoneal dialysis. Before the introduction of erythropoietin therapy in the late 1980s, around 10% of dialysis patients were regularly transfusion-dependent, and many more required an occasional top-up transfusion.

Generally, hemodialysis patients tend to have a higher prevalence and greater severity of anemia than peritoneal dialysis patients. Various factors have been suggested to explain this, including a greater degree of blood loss or hemolysis in hemodialysis patients and better removal of "middle molecules" inhibitory to erythropoiesis in peritoneal dialysis patients. Sequential comparative studies of changes in hemoglobin concentration after starting dialysis have shown a greater initial increase in continuous ambulatory peritoneal dialysis (CAPD) patients compared with those on hemodialysis, but after 5 years there is no longer any difference. Likewise, studies of red cell mass in hemodialysis and CAPD patients suggest that there is little difference between the two modalities of treatment (10).

The severity of the anemia in dialysis patients is independent of the etiology of end-stage renal failure, with the exception of patients with adult polycystic kidney disease, who tend to have higher hemoglobin concentrations (11). This is thought to be due to increased production of erythropoietin by the cells lining the cysts, resulting in enhanced serum erythropoietin levels (12). Indeed, it has been shown that interstitial cells in the cyst walls of patients with autosomal dominant polycystic kidney disease express erythropoietin mRNA, and cysts derived from proximal tubules, but not those derived from distal tubules, have been found to contain increased concentrations of bioactive erythropoietin (13). Serum erythropoietin levels in patients with polycystic kidneys are, on average, twice as high as in patients with end-stage renal disease of noncystic origin (12). Similarly, a marked increase in hemoglobin concentration and even polycythemia can also occur in dialysis patients who develop acquired cystic disease of the kidneys (14).

IV. PATHOGENESIS OF RENAL ANEMIA

A. Erythropoietin Production

It is generally accepted that insufficient erythropoietin production is the major reason for the anemia associated with end-stage renal disease (7). Plasma erythropoietin concentrations are usually inappropriately low for the severity of anemia (2). This is particularly true for anephric patients, who tend to have more severe anemia, but even in these individuals erythropoietin levels are still measurable (15). In this situation, erythropoietin is probably produced by the liver (16).

Interestingly, the inability of erythropoietin production to respond to the degree of anemia appears to be independent of the cause of end-stage renal disease. It is still uncertain whether the reduced erythropoietin levels are a consequence of destruction of the cells producing the hormone, or a transformation of the cells that results in a loss of their ability to produce the hormone, or a lack of the appropriate signals that normally stimulate erythropoietin production. It is known that severely damaged kidneys can sometimes produce supranormal amounts of erythropoietin (17) and that a reversible inhibition of erythropoietin production occurs in acute renal failure (18), and hence disturbance of the normal control mechanisms may also be playing a part. Furthermore, even in uremia, erythropoietin production can be increased in response to stimuli such as hypoxic hypoxia (19) and also suppressed in response to blood transfusions or immunomodulatory cytokines.

B. "Uremic Inhibitors" of Erythropoiesis

Studies dating from the 1970s have shown that serum from uremic individuals potently inhibits growth of erythroid progenitor cells in culture (20). Further experiments to define which factor or factors in uremic serum cause this effect have been fruitless. Addition of urea, creatinine, or guanidinosuccinic acid added separately to the culture medium failed to have any effect (21). Other candidate "uremic inhibitors" have included polar lipids, arsenic, spermine, spermidine, vitamin A, and parathyroid hormone, but none has survived rigorous scientific testing. The fact that renal anemia often improves to some extent after starting regular dialysis also supports the theory that a "uremic substance" removed by dialysis is toxic to the bone marrow.

C. Hyperparathyroidism

There are two possible mechanisms by which hyperparathyroidism might exacerbate renal anemia. The first is by direct suppression of erythroid progenitor cell growth by parathyroid hormone, as mentioned above (22), and the second is via its effect in inducing marrow fibrosis and thereby reducing the pool of erythroid progenitor cells in the bone marrow (23). An improvement in anemia has been found following parathyroidectomy (24), and a reduction in PTH levels induced by high-dose vitamin D supplementation has also been shown to result in an improved response to epoetin therapy (25,26).

D. Aluminum Toxicity

Aluminum overload is now much less common with the introduction of water deionizers and the reduced usage of aluminum-containing phosphate binders. In the past, however, aluminum toxicity was associated with a microcytic anemia (27), which improved after desferrioxamine chelation therapy (28). The mechanism by which aluminum toxicity exacerbates anemia is poorly understood, but may be due to interference with iron transport and/or its utilization, inhibition of heme synthesis, or increased hemolysis due to an increase in red cell fragility.

E. Iron and Folate Deficiency

Hemodialysis patients have up to five times the amount of iron loss as nonuremic individuals (4–5 mg per day compared with 1–2 mg), which is partly due to losses in the dialyzer (10), occult gastrointestinal bleeding (29), and repeated phlebotomy. Folate is readily removed by hemodialysis so excessive losses of this hematinic substance are also present in such patients (30). Many patients on dialysis suffer from poor appetite, and hence dietary insufficiency may exacerbate these deficiencies.

F. Hemolysis

Many patients with uremia have a shortened red cell life span due to low-grade hemolysis or hypersplenism. This appears to be related to the degree of uremia (31) and can improve after initiation of regular dialysis. However, hemodialysis may also exacerbate a more severe hemolysis, which has been attributed to several toxins including formaldehyde (32), copper, chloramine, and nitrates.

V. CLINICAL CONSEQUENCES OF RENAL ANEMIA

As with other causes of chronic anemia, there are various consequences of longstanding renal anemia in terms of both symptoms and organ function. Patients complain of tiredness, lethargy, muscle fatigue, reduced exercise capacity, poor concentration, impaired memory and intellectual ability, breathlessness at rest and on exercise, angina, palpitations, loss of appetite, reduced libido, and a sensation of feeling cold. Tests of exercise physiology using a treadmill or bicycle ergometry confirm the decrease in exercise capacity and indicate a reduced maximum oxygen consumption (VO_2 max) and anaerobic threshold (33). Cardiac output increases to compensate for the lowered oxygen-carrying capacity of the blood, and this is achieved by an increase in both stroke volume and heart rate (34). There is a compensatory hypoxia-induced vasodilatation, which lowers the systemic vascular resistance, and severe cases can result in high-output cardiac failure. Changes in muscle metabolism occur with increased lactate production on exercise, and there is a shift in the hemoglobin-oxygen dissociation curve. Electrophysiological tests of the brain, including measurement of P3 latencies, indicate impaired cognitive function (35), and various abnormalities of endocrine function have been attributed to chronic renal anemia.

Severe renal failure is often associated with a bleeding tendency, characterized by a prolonged skin bleeding time (36). This is due to abnormalities of platelet function, and anemia is a major factor. Correction of the anemia by either blood transfusion (37) or erythropoietin therapy (38) usually results in a return of the bleeding time to normal. Several mechanisms are involved in this process, including greater interaction of platelets with the vessel wall, enhanced ADP production, and an improvement in platelet function.

VI. OTHER HEMATOLOGICAL EFFECTS ASSOCIATED WITH CHRONIC RENAL FAILURE

A. Leukocyte Abnormalities

The major hematological abnormality in chronic renal failure relates to the erythroid lineage, with inadequate red cell production due to a relative erythropoietin deficiency. However, abnormalities of white cell and platelet function have also been reported (39).

In the myeloid lineage, a reduction in the capacity of the bone marrow to generate granulocytes has been documented in renal failure, and there is enhanced peripheral consumption of neutrophils by the dialyzer in hemodialysis patients (40). Thus, some dialysis patients may show a borderline neutropenia. The oxidative metabolism of granulocytes is altered in chronic renal failure (41), and there is increased production of free oxygen radicals by polymorphonuclear cells in patients on regular dialysis (42). The phagocytic activity of granulocytes is impaired in chronic renal failure once the glomerular filtration rate decreases to less than 10 mL/min (42).

Altered monocyte function has also been reported in dialysis patients; various studies have documented defective antigen presentation (43), a decrease in chemotactic response (44), and a reduction in phagocytic activity (45). In vitro production of several cytokines (interleukin-1, interleukin-6, and tumor necrosis factor) from monocytes in uremic patients is altered, partly affected by the nature of the dialysis membrane (46). Oxidative damage of the monocyte membrane has also been observed in patients with uremia; this is reversible by administering an antioxidant such as vitamin E (47).

The immune response in chronic renal failure is altered largely due to changes in both T- and B-lymphocyte function (48). Thus, there is a reduced capacity of T cells to form colonies (49), a reduced production of IL-2 by T cells (50), altered T-lymphocyte function in hemodialysis patients, which is improved by high-flux dialysis with polysulfone membrane (51), and a suboptimal antibody response to hepatitis B and influenza vaccines in hemodialysis patients (52).

The clinical implications of these impaired granulocyte, monocyte, and lymphocyte functions contribute to the chronic immunodeficiency state that is characteristic of uremia. This causes cutaneous anergy, prolonged allograft survival, and an increased incidence of infection due to gram-negative organisms and mycobacteria. In spite of continuing improvements in hemodialysis techniques, the immune response of uremic patients remains poor.

B. Platelet Abnormalities

The main defect in the megakaryocytic lineage in uremia relates to abnormalities of platelet function, causing hemostatic problems characterized by a prolonged bleeding time (36). This is only partly corrected by regular dialysis and seems to be due to a defect in activation of the glycoprotein adhesion receptors causing both impaired platelet aggregation and adhesion to endothelium (53). Platelet volume and the circulating platelet mass are reduced in chronic renal failure, possibly due to a reduction in thrombopoietin concentrations or activity (54). The mean platelet life span is reduced in uremic patients with a GFR of 15–30 mL/min; this is corrected to normal after no less than 12 months of treatment with regular hemodialysis (55). The platelet membrane is affected by increased activity of free oxygen radicals in chronic renal failure; this is reversed by vitamin E (56). Platelets in uremia also release diminished quantities of ATP, show a selective defect in the pool of deposited serotonin, and have an increased ability to synthesize thromboxane A_2 (57).

The functional platelet defect of uremia is reversed transiently by the administration of DDAVP (desmopressin) (58) or conjugated estrogens (59) intravenously. The mechanism by which DDAVP causes this effect is possibly the release of von Willebrand factor multimers from storage sites into the plasma. Estrogens may act by inhibiting vascular prostacyclin. Correction of anemia by blood transfusion or recombinant human erythropoietin also reverses the prolonged bleeding time of uremia.

VII. MANAGEMENT OF RENAL ANEMIA

The management of anemia in renal failure has been transformed over the last decade by the introduction of recombinant human erythropoietin into clinical practice. Several other factors, however, have also been shown to play a part, and these too deserve a mention.

A. Hematinic Supplements

Patients with chronic renal failure are prone to develop deficiencies of vitamins and minerals necessary for red cell production (particularly iron, vitamin B_{12}, and folate) as a result of dietary restrictions, poor appetite, and increased dialyzer and gastrointestinal blood losses. Patients on hemodialysis have on average iron losses of 4–5 mg per day compared with the normal loss of 1 mg daily. Likewise, there are increased folate losses through the process of dialysis (30). Since it is easy to measure blood levels of these hematinics and to treat any deficiencies that develop, it is important that dialysis patients are screened for vitamin B_{12}, folate, and iron deficiency on a regular basis, and supplements given as required.

B. Dialysis

A spontaneous improvement in anemia is seen in some patients during the first few months after starting dialysis, which may be related to the intensity of dialysis treatment and to an enhanced red cell survival (60). The improvement in hemoglobin concentration is initially greater with CAPD than with hemodialysis (61), but after 5 years there is little difference between the two modalities (62). Serum erythropoietin levels are decreased or unchanged after dialysis is instituted (61), suggesting that other mechanisms are involved. It has also been shown that underdialysis may confer some resistance to erythropoietin therapy (63), and increasing the dialysis prescription may itself cause an improvement in hemoglobin concentration in hemodialysis patients receiving erythropoietin.

C. Androgen Therapy

Androgens were shown more than 20 years ago to improve the anemia in dialysis patients. These agents increase erythropoiesis by stimulating endogenous erythropoietin production, either from residual renal tissue or from the liver (60,64). They may also increase the sensitivity of erythroid precursor cells to erythropoietin. In some renal patients, androgens allowed partial correction of anemia with a reduction in transfusion requirements (65), but they tend to be beneficial in mild cases only and are limited by a high incidence of side effects such as virilization, muscle and liver damage, and cholestasis (66). In developed countries they have little role to play nowadays, but in countries with a poorer economic status they have been advocated as a cheaper alternative to erythropoietin.

D. Blood Transfusions

Before the advent of erythropoietin therapy, many patients with renal failure required repeated blood transfusions in order to avoid the symptoms and complications of severe anemia. This had several disadvantages and drawbacks:

1. Frequent blood transfusion results in suppression of residual endogenous erythropoietin production and hence erythroid activity.
2. Repeated blood transfusions cause iron overload and tissue iron accumulation, with possible long-term deleterious effects on the heart, liver, pancreas, and endocrine glands.
3. Blood transfusion exposes the dialysis patient to the risk of infection from bloodborne viruses such as hepatitis B and C, cytomegalovirus, and human immunodeficiency virus.
4. Transfusion also exposes the dialysis patient to a wide range of HLA antigens, resulting in cytotoxic antibody production, which renders successful renal transplantation less likely by reducing the chances of obtaining a negative cross-match and increasing the risk of acute rejection episodes.

E. Intravenous Iron

In the 1970s, several workers studied the effect of administering aggressive iron supplementation on the anemia associated with renal failure (67,68). Although this practice rarely produced a complete correction of the anemia, it was not unusual to see a rise in hemoglobin of 1–2 g/dL, even in iron-replete patients. It seems that iron supply from the reticuloendothelial stores is a rate-limiting step in the process of erythropoiesis, and bypassing this by providing a readily available supply of exogenous iron can result in a partial boost in the hemoglobin concentration. This practice has been revisited in recent times as an adjuvant treatment to erythropoietin therapy (69). It is now recognized that aggressive IV iron supplementation can enhance the response to erythropoietin and allow reductions in the dosage requirements (70–72), with obvious economic benefits.

F. Erythropoietin Therapy

The advent of recombinant human erythropoietin is without doubt one of the greatest advances in nephrological practice in recent years. It has transformed the management of renal anemia, which previously relied on frequent blood transfusions, with considerable disadvantages for the patient (as detailed above). Several large multicenter trials in the United States (73), Canada (74), Japan, and Europe (75) have confirmed that erythropoietin is a highly effective therapy with few adverse effects.

The rationale for its use was recognized many years ago when it was realized that the major factor causing renal anemia was a relative deficiency of erythropoietin produced by the diseased kidneys. Thus, circulating concentrations of the hormone are almost always inappropriately low for the degree of anemia in chronic renal failure (2). The major breakthrough that allowed theory to become practice came in 1977 when human erythropoietin was isolated and purified from the urine of patients with aplastic anemia (76). This allowed the cloning of the gene for human erythropoietin (77), which was then expressed in a suitable mammalian cell line, making possible for the first time the large-scale synthesis of genetically engineered hormone. Animal studies confirmed its efficacy and relative safety, and clinical trials began in Seattle (78) and London/Oxford (79) towards the end of 1985. It became licensed for use in renal anemia in 1990, and since then several million patients worldwide have received this treatment.

1. Pharmacokinetics

In common with other therapeutic protein hormones such as insulin, recombinant human erythropoietin is inactivated by acid in the stomach, and therefore needs to be given parenterally. The early clinical trials in hemodialysis patients used intravenous erythropoietin administered thrice weekly; since then the intraperitoneal, subcutaneous, and intradermal routes of administration have been investigated (80,81).

After intravenous administration, serum erythropoietin concentrations decay mono-exponentially, with an elimination half-life of approximately 4–11 hours (Fig. 2) (82); some, but not all, authors found that the half-life was shortened with repeated administration (83). The apparent volume of distribution of erythropoietin is about one to two times the plasma volume, and the total body clearance is slower than for other protein hormones such as insulin, glucagon, and prolactin.

The intraperitoneal route was investigated as a potential means of administering erythropoietin to patients on peritoneal dialysis. Following intraperitoneal administration, serum erythropoietin concentrations begin to increase after 1–2 hours and reach a peak at around 18 hours (Fig. 2) (82). However, the peak concentrations are only 2–5% of those obtained with the same intravenous dose, and the bioavailability of intraperitoneal erythropoietin is disappointingly low at 3–8%.

With subcutaneous administration, peak serum concentrations of about 4–10% of an equivalent intravenous dose are obtained at around 12 hours, and thereafter they decay slowly such that concentrations greater than baseline are still present at 4 days (Fig. 2) (81). The bioavailability of subcutaneous erythropoietin is about seven times that of intraperitoneal administration, at around 20–25%, which is, however, low compared with insulin, heparin, or growth hormone.

2. Pharmacodynamics

Based on pharmacokinetic studies, initial dosage regimens for erythropoietin employed thrice-weekly administration. This has remained the most popular dosage frequency for both intravenous and subcutaneous administration, although once-weekly, twice-weekly, and seven-times-weekly (once-daily) dosing have all been used successfully in treating patients with subcutaneous erythropoietin (84). With intravenous erythropoietin, once-weekly administration is inadequate, and twice- or thrice-weekly dosing is required. Many studies have compared the efficacy and erythropoietin dose requirements of intravenous versus subcutaneous

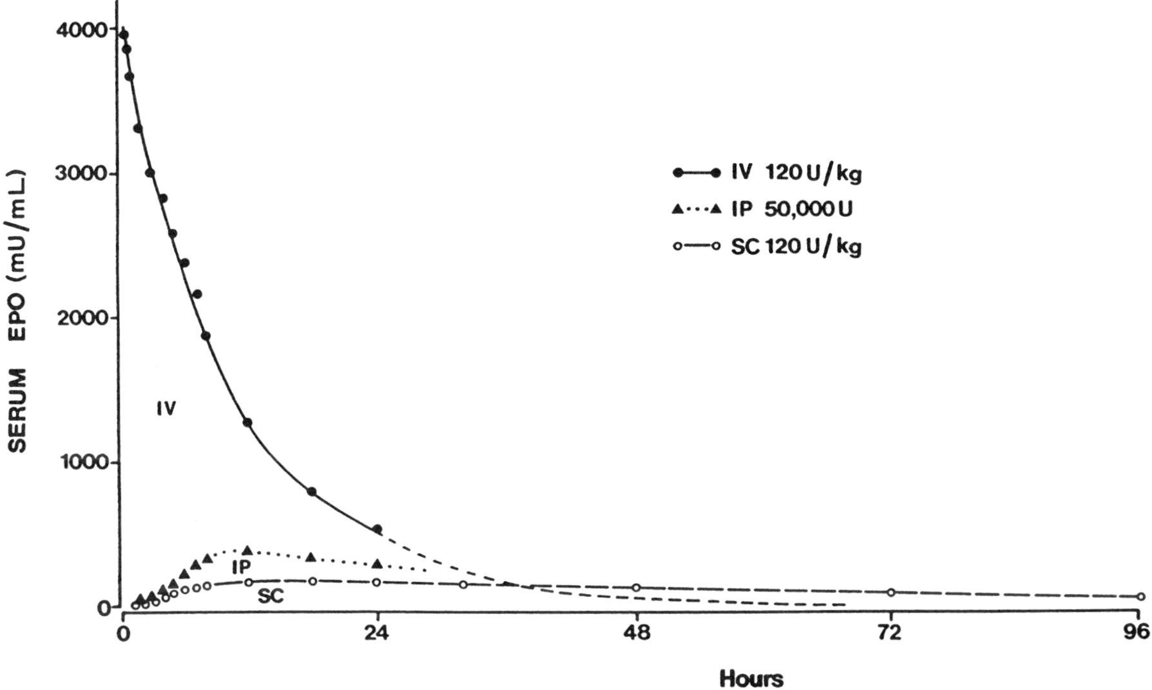

Fig. 2 Pharmacokinetic profiles following a single administration of IV (120 U/kg), IP (50,000 units) and SC (120 U/kg) erythropoietin in 8 stable CAPD patients. (Adapted from Ref. 81.)

administration, and most, but not all, suggest that lower doses may be needed if the subcutaneous route is used.

3. Hematological Effects

Approximately 90–95% of dialysis patients treated with erythropoietin respond with an improvement in their anemia (73). Following commencement of regular therapy, a significant increase in the reticulocyte count of around two to three times baseline is usually evident at 1 week, and an increase in hemoglobin concentration is seen at 2–3 weeks (Fig. 3). The increase is dose-dependent, and most clinicians aim for an increment of not more than 1 g/dL/month in order to minimize the risk of adverse effects. There is currently much controversy regarding the optimum target hemoglobin, but this is often somewhere in the region of 10–12 g/dL and is usually attained after 4–6 months of therapy. Dose reductions may then be necessary to maintain this level thereafter.

The increase in hemoglobin concentration is associated with an increase in red cell count; no significant changes in white cell or platelet counts are usually seen, although a clinically insignificant increase in the platelet count has been documented in a few patients. There is usually a dramatic decline in the serum ferritin concentration and/or the transferrin saturation following commencement of erythropoietin therapy, as large quantities of iron are used up in the manufacture of new red cells (69).

Radioisotopic blood volume studies have confirmed that there is an increase in red cell mass after erythropoietin, which is associated with a compensatory reduction in plasma volume such that the whole blood volume remains unchanged. Ferrokinetic studies indicate that erythropoietin therapy induces a twofold increase in marrow erythropoietic activity, as evidenced by a doubling of marrow and red cell iron turnover (8,85). There is little or no change in mean red cell life span after erythropoietin; thus the increased red cell mass is largely accounted for by the production of greater numbers of red cells, rather than by any change in their survival.

4. Factors Affecting Response to Erythropoietin

Many factors can influence the response to erythropoietin (86). Patients with more severe anemia (hemoglobin <6 g/dL) at the onset of treatment generally require greater doses than those with mild anemia (hemoglobin 6–8 g/dL) (75). Other conditions that may inhibit the response to erythropoietin are summarized in Table 1. All these factors should be considered in any patient failing to respond to treatment, requiring excessive

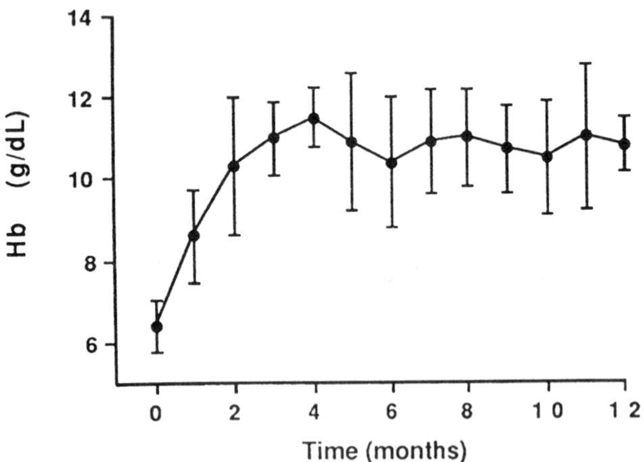

Fig. 3 Hemoglobin response to erythropoietin therapy administered to 10 hemodialysis patients. Results are expressed as means ±SD.

Table 1 Factors Inhibiting Response to Erythropoietin Therapy

Major	Minor
Iron deficiency	Hyperparathyroidism (with marrow fibrosis)
Blood loss	Aluminum toxicity
Infection/Inflammation	Vitamin B_{12}/Folate deficiency
	Hemolysis
	Marrow disorders
	Hemoglobinopathies
	Underdialysis
	Carnitine deficiency
	Poor nutrition
	Obesity/Poor subcutaneous absorption
	ACE inhibitors/Angiotensin II blockers
	? Erythropoietin antibodies

doses of erythropoietin, or losing a previous hemoglobin response. Functional iron deficiency, in particular, has become increasingly apparent in patients on erythropoietin therapy; many individuals who are iron-replete at the start of treatment become deficient under the influence of erythropoietin and require intensive iron supplementation in order to maintain a hemoglobin response (69,87). Dialysis patients often have increased occult gastrointestinal blood loss, partly due to a greater prevalence of gastritis and peptic ulceration, and partly due to an increased bleeding tendency due to both uremic platelet dysfunction and heparin administration during dialysis. The presence of acute or chronic infection, inflammatory disease, or malignancy frequently causes marked inhibition of the response to erythropoietin, even at high doses (86). This is thought to be mediated via suppression of erythropoiesis by other cytokines and growth factors (88) and/or changes in iron metabolism.

5. Secondary Effects of Erythropoietin

a. Cardiovascular System

Long-standing severe anemia has profound effects on the cardiovascular system as detailed above. Many of these effects have been shown to be reversed or improved following erythropoietin therapy (Table 2). The increased cardiac output returns towards normal with correction of the anemia (89), the compensatory hypoxic vasodilatation is reversed (producing an increase in peripheral resistance), and the mean arterial blood pressure increases in 20–30% of patients. There are improvements in oxygen delivery to the myocardium, resulting in a reduction in symptoms of angina and in exercise-induced myocardial ischemia (90,91). Left ventricular mass also decreases progressively following erythropoietin therapy, particularly when this is grossly elevated prior to treatment (90,92,93). This latter finding may have long-term implications for cardiovascular mortality, since left ventricular hypertrophy is an independent determinant of survival in dialysis patients (94). The internal dimensions of the left ventricle in both systole and diastole decrease after erythropoietin therapy, and cardiac size therefore progressively diminishes (92). Finally, there are improvements in exercise physiology following erythropoietin: exercise capacity, maximum oxygen consumption, anaerobic threshold, and carbon monoxide transfer factor have all been shown to increase (90,95).

Table 2 Cardiovascular Effects of Erythropoietin Therapy

↑ Exercise tolerance
Normalization of elevated cardiac output
↑ Peripheral vascular resistance
↑ Blood pressure (30% of patients)
↓ Symptoms of angina
↓ Myocardial ischemia
↓ Left ventricular hypertrophy
↓ Left ventricular internal dimensions
↓ Cardiac size on chest radiograph

Table 3 Noncardiovascular Effects of Erythropoietin Therapy

↑ Quality of life
↑ Brain/Cognitive function
↓ Uremic bleeding tendency
↑ Platelet function
↑ Sexual function
↑ Endocrine function
↑ Immune function
↓ Uremic pruritus

b. Noncardiovascular Effects

The list of secondary effects associated with erythropoietin therapy is ever-increasing (Table 3). Studies on the coagulation and hemostatic pathways, prompted by the early observation of possible increased vascular access thrombosis with erythropoietin, have documented a reduction in bleeding time along with improvements in platelet function, both aggregation and adhesion to endothelium (96). The standard coagulation tests are unaffected by erythropoietin, as are measurements of the coagulation factors. However, a prothrombotic state may develop, possibly contributed to by increased blood viscosity (97), reductions in protein C and protein S levels (98), and increases in thrombin-antithrombin III levels (99), Factor VIII–related activities (100), and plasminogen activator inhibitor-1 production following erythropoietin.

The hematocrit is the major determinant of whole blood viscosity, and thus an erythropoietin-induced increase in red cell mass inevitably causes an increase in blood viscosity. Furthermore, the relationship between hematocrit and blood viscosity is exponential, such that a linear increase in the former results in a disproportionate increase in the latter. Detailed rheological studies have indicated that the increase in blood viscosity occurs solely as a result of the larger quantity of circulating red cells, without any change in plasma viscosity or the rheology of the red cells themselves in terms of their deformability or aggregability (97).

Objective assessments of quality-of-life parameters (101) and of brain and cognitive function (35,102) have also shown improvements following erythropoietin therapy. Patients report subjective improvements in memory, concentration, and other cerebral functions. Electrophysiological studies have shown an increase in amplitude of the P3 component of the brain event–related potential (102), and higher scores in various neuropsychological tests have been recorded. These findings suggest that anemia may be an important factor in the etiology of uremic brain dysfunction.

Impaired sexual function is common in dialysis patients; in females this is manifest by anovulation, amenorrhea, and infertility, while in males impotence, reduced libido, oligospermia, and gynecomastia are often present. Erythropoietin therapy has been shown to improve libido, potency, and sexual performance in males (103,104), and a return of regular menstruation and even pregnancy (105) has been reported in female dialysis patients. These effects may be partly mediated by changes in prolactin or testosterone levels since reductions in the former and increases in the latter have been found following erythropoietin treatment. Other diverse endocrine effects that have been reported in association with erythropoietin include suppressive effects on the renin-angiotensin system, the pituitary-adrenal axis, growth hormone levels, glucagon, gastrin, follicle-stimulating hormone, and luteinizing hormone, while there are reported increases in plasma insulin, parathyroid hormone, and atrial natriuretic peptide (106).

Erythropoietin also appears to have effects on the immune system and is gaining widespread recognition as a physiological regulator of immune function. Levels of circulating cytotoxic antibodies progressively decline in patients receiving erythropoietin therapy (107), and this effect is only partly due to the avoidance of blood transfusion. There is an increase in immunoglobulin production and proliferation of B cells and an enhanced seroconversion response to hepatitis B vaccination (108). Phagocytic function in neutrophils is also increased (109). Uremic pruritus is lessened following commencement of erythropoietin therapy, possibly due to a reduction in plasma histamine concentrations (110). The nutritional status of patients treated with erythropoietin has also been shown to improve.

6. Adverse Effects

Most of the reported complications associated with erythropoietin therapy are thought to be due not to the recombinant product per se, but to the resultant increase in hematocrit and blood viscosity (Table 4). Hypertension is the most common and potentially most worrying adverse effect associated with erythropoietin therapy, occurring in approximately 20–30% of patients treated (111). The risk of developing a significant increase in blood pressure appears to be independent of whether there is a previous history of hypertension, the rate of increase in the hematocrit, or the target hemoglobin achieved. However, most hypertensive prob-

Table 4 Adverse Effects of Erythropoietin Therapy

Hypertension
Seizures/Encephalopathy
Vascular access thrombosis
Clotting of dialysis lines
Hyperkalemia
Myalgia/Influenza-like symptoms
Skin irritation (epoetin alfa only)

lems occur during the acute correction of anemia rather than during the maintenance phase. Interestingly, this side effect of erythropoietin appears to be peculiar to renal patients, being astonishingly rare in nonrenal patients receiving this treatment, such as those with rheumatoid arthritis, etc.

The mechanism of erythropoietin-induced hypertension remains poorly understood, although factors that have been suggested to contribute include an inadequate reversal of the elevated cardiac output of anemia, a relative increase in peripheral resistance as the compensatory hypoxic peripheral vasodilatation of anemia is reversed, an increase in blood viscosity, increased endothelin production, reduced nitric oxide production, and possibly a direct pressor effect of erythropoietin (112). In most instances, blood pressure is easily controlled by fluid removal and the use of standard antihypertensive drugs; it is very rare to have to stop erythropoietin for severe uncontrollable hypertension.

In a number of the early studies there were anecdotal reports of seizures or hypertensive encephalopathy occurring in patients receiving erythropoietin, usually within the first 3 months of treatment (113). The pathogenesis of these adverse effects remains poorly understood, although loss of autoregulation of cerebral blood flow and/or reduced cerebral perfusion may play a part.

Up to 10% of hemodialysis patients treated with erythropoietin develop thrombosis of their vascular access (74,75). This is more common with prosthetic grafts than with native fistulae, and possible pathogenetic factors include an increase in blood viscosity, shortening of the bleeding time, enhanced platelet aggregation and adhesion, a reduction in protein C and protein S levels, an increase in thrombin-antithrombin III levels, enhanced Factor VIII–related activities, and a marginal increase in platelet count in some patients (see above).

Occasionally, patients receiving erythropoietin therapy show an increase in serum potassium, phosphate, and creatinine (73,75) which may be due to enhanced dietary intake and/or reduced dialyzer clearance of these molecules secondary to the increased hematocrit. Heparin requirements for hemodialysis may increase in some patients. Other adverse effects of erythropoietin therapy include transient myalgia or influenza-like symptoms following the first few injections only, and skin irritation around the injection site caused by citrate buffer in one of the formulations of the drug (114). Genuine intolerance to erythropoietin sufficient to warrant stopping treatment is rare, and reports of antibody formation to the recombinant hormone are very rare.

VIII. MANAGING THE PATIENT WITH RENAL ANEMIA: A PRACTICAL APPROACH

There are two major reasons for attempting to correct anemia in renal failure patients. The first is to reverse or improve symptoms associated with anemia, and the second is to arrest or reverse the deleterious effects of long-standing anemia on the heart and other organs, with the aim of improving the cardiovascular morbidity and mortality in dialysis patients (4,5).

In recent times, two separate initiatives in the United States and Europe have developed guidelines to facilitate the optimal management of renal anemia. In the United States, the Dialysis Outcomes Quality Initiative (DOQI) Guidelines were produced under the auspices of the National Kidney Foundation (115), while in Europe the European Best Practice Guidelines have recently been published (116). Both sets of guidelines are fairly similar, with minor differences reflecting variations in clinical practice on either side of the Atlantic (Table 5).

A. Before Starting Erythropoietin Therapy

Before starting a patient on erythropoietin, it is imperative to exclude and reverse (if possible) any other contributory causes to the anemia (117). The most important of these include iron deficiency (if in doubt, a trial of IV iron should be given), blood loss (a clue may be heavy transfusion dependence), and underlying infection or inflammatory disease (sometimes difficult to diagnose, but a raised CRP level may be suggestive).

Screening for hyperparathyroidism, aluminum toxicity, B_{12} and folate deficiency, hemolysis, or an un-

Table 5 Summary of DOQI Guidelines and European Best Practice Guidelines

DOQI guidelines	European best practice guidelines
1. When to initiate the work-up of anemia	1. When to begin the work-up of a patient for the diagnosis of anemia
2. Anemia evaluation	2. Evaluation of anemia in uremic patients
3. Erythropoietin deficiency	3. Diagnosis of the anemia of chronic renal failure
4. Target hematocrit/hemoglobin for epoetin therapy	4. Indications for starting treatment with epoetin
5. Assessment of iron status	5. Target hemoglobin concentration for the treatment of the anemia of chronic renal failure
6. Target iron level	6. Assessing and optimizing iron stores
7. Monitoring iron status	7. Frequency of monitoring iron stores and availability during treatment and follow-up
8. Administration of supplemental iron	8. Administration of supplemental iron
9. Administration of a test dose of IV iron dextran	9. Route of administration of epoetin
10. Oral iron therapy	10. Initial epoetin administration
11. Route of administration of epoetin	11. Monitoring of hemoglobin concentration during epoetin treatment
12. Initial epoetin administration	12. Titration of epoetin dosage
13. Switching from intravenous to subcutaneous epoetin	13. Epoetin dosage perioperatively, during intercurrent illness, and after transplantation
14. Strategies for initiating and converting to subcutaneous epoetin administration	14. Causes of an inadequate response to epoetin treatment
15. Monitoring of hematocrit/hemoglobin during epoetin therapy	15. Management of patients resistant to epoetin
16. Titration of epoetin dosage	16. Red blood cell transfusions in patients with chronic renal failure
17. Inability to tolerate subcutaneous epoetin; IV epoetin dose	17. Possible adverse effects of epoetin treatment: hypertension
18. Intraperitoneal epoetin administration	18. Possible adverse effects of epoetin treatment: access thrombosis
19. Epoetin dosage perioperatively or during intercurrent illness	
20. Causes for inadequate response to epoetin	
21. When to obtain a hematology consultation	
22. Epoetin-resistant patients	
23. Red blood cell transfusions in patients with chronic renal failure	
24. Possible adverse effects related to epoetin therapy: hypertension	
25. Possible adverse effects related to epoetin therapy: seizures	
26. Possible adverse effects related to epoetin therapy: access thrombosis	
27. Possible adverse effects related to epoetin therapy: heparin dose	
28. Possible adverse effects related to epoetin therapy: hyperkalemia	

derlying hemoglobinopathy should be performed if relevant. If there are suggestive abnormalities in the red cell indices or blood film, then a bone marrow should be undertaken to detect such conditions as myelodysplasia, etc.

If the serum ferritin is less than 100 μg/L, the patient should receive one or more top-up infusions of IV iron since the demands for iron after erythropoietin is started will be great, and without iron supplementation the patient will almost certainly have a suboptimal response. The blood pressure should be assessed and antihypertensive medication introduced or intensified as required to ensure a baseline measurement of less than 140/90 if possible.

B. Starting the Patient on Erythropoietin

The optimal dose for treating renal anemia is around 2000 units twice or thrice weekly, given subcutaneously. This is appropriate for both hemodialysis and peritoneal dialysis patients, although in certain instances the IV route may be used for hemodialysis patients (e.g., in patients with a needle phobia or those demonstrating poor compliance). There is some controversy regarding whether the SC route results in lower dose requirements compared with IV administration, with much evidence suggesting that this is the case (118,119). Some studies, however, have shown no difference in dose requirements between IV and SC administration (120,121), but no study has suggested lower doses with the IV route. There is no longer any indication for doses to be calculated per body weight, first because such "fine-tuning" of erythropoiesis is not required, and second because this can potentially result in wastage of incompletely used vials. It has been suggested that hemodialysis patients are slightly more resistant to the effects of erythropoietin than are peritoneal dialysis patients, and hence dosage requirements are higher. This may be so at a population level, but the interindividual variability in erythropoietin sensitivity is so huge that, from a practical point of view, dosage recommendations are no different for hemodialysis or peritoneal dialysis patients. With subcutaneous administration, it is possible to give erythropoietin once weekly using doses such as 4,000 or 10,000 units, but the total dosage requirements are likely to be greater than if the drug is administered as split doses two or three times a week. Once-weekly administration of intravenous erythropoietin is, however, not recommended, since the serum elimination half-life with this route is only around 8 hours.

C. Monitoring the Patient on Erythropoietin

At the start of treatment, patients receiving erythropoietin require fairly close monitoring every 2–4 weeks. As a minimum, the hemoglobin should be measured, there should be an assessment of iron status, and blood pressure should be checked.

1. Hemoglobin

The desired rate of rise in hemoglobin should be of the order of 1 g/dL/month (or 0.25 g/dL/week). Increments lower than this will result in excessively long periods for correction of the anemia, and rates faster than this may compromise patient safety in terms of adverse events. Ideally the hemoglobin should be measured every 2 weeks until some idea of the rate of response is obtained; thereafter it is probably acceptable to monitor this every 3–4 weeks.

2. Iron Status

There has been much controversy over which tests of iron status should be used in patients receiving erythropoietin (69). Many such tests exist, all of which assess different parts of the iron metabolic pathway, and no one single test can be used to give a global picture of iron status. Thus, the serum ferritin gives an approximate indication of iron stores, the transferrin saturation assesses how much iron is circulating in plasma relative to the total iron-binding capacity (transferrin), and the percentage of hypochromic red cells has been advocated as the best means of assessing how much iron is being incorporated into the red cell (122). Opinions differ on the merits of each test, but as an approximate guide it is generally accepted that the serum ferritin should be kept above 100 μg/L, the transferrin saturation above 20%, and the proportion of hypochromic red cells below 10% (69). Other markers of iron status such as the serum transferrin receptor, erythrocyte ferritin, and red cell zinc protoporphyrin levels all have limitations and remain largely research tools.

There are two conditions representing inadequate iron status, namely *absolute* and *functional* iron deficiency. Absolute iron deficiency is present when the total body iron stores are inadequate, as judged by a low serum ferritin. Functional iron deficiency exists when there are ample or even increased iron stores, but these stores are unable to release their iron rapidly enough to satisfy the demands of the bone marrow for erythropoiesis. Both conditions will result in a suboptimal response to erythropoietin and will require aggressive iron supplementation.

Experience over the last decade or so has suggested that administration of oral iron is often inadequate in this context, and intravenous iron is often required. There are several IV iron preparations available for this purpose, of differing molecular weights, degradation kinetics, availability profiles, and adverse effects, and various dosing regimens have been suggested. Frequent "low-dose" administration (20–60 mg every dialysis session) has been advocated in hemodialysis patients, but this is impractical for peritoneal dialysis patients who neither have ready vascular access nor are attending hospital regularly. In this latter group, larger infusions of 300–1000 mg of IV iron can be given every month or so.

3. Blood Pressure

Approximately 20–30% of patients receiving erythropoietin will develop hypertension requiring the initiation or intensification of antihypertensive medication (111). Severe hypertension, resulting in seizures or encephalopathy, which was seen in the early days of erythropoietin use, is now very rare since lower-dosage regimens have been advocated. It is, however, still important to monitor blood pressure every 2–4 weeks, aiming to keep this below 140/90 if possible. Fluid removal on dialysis and/or standard antihypertensive medication may be used for this purpose. It is unusual to have to stop erythropoietin therapy because of hypertensive problems, and this should be avoided if possible. Likewise, there is now little role for venesection in this context.

4. Other Tests

Monitoring of the reticulocyte count allows a rapid and convenient way of assessing marrow erythropoietic activity and may be coupled with the full blood count analysis. Measurements of serum CRP provide a guide to the degree of inflammatory activity (123), which can potentially inhibit the response to erythropoietin. Likewise, monitoring serum PTH may help in assessing the severity of secondary hyperparathyroidism, which can also cause resistance to erythropoietin (23). In patients with homozygous sickle-cell disease, HbS and HbF levels should be measured to reduce the risk of precipitating a sickle-cell crisis with overstimulation of the marrow.

D. Poor Response to Erythropoietin

More than 90% of dialysis patients will respond to erythropoietin with a hemoglobin rise of >1 g/dL/month and an EPO dose of <200 U/kg/week. Patients failing to achieve this hemoglobin response and/or requiring higher doses of EPO are classed as "poor responders," and many causes of resistance to erythropoietin have been identified (86). These include major factors, such as iron deficiency (see above), blood loss, and infection/inflammation, as well as minor factors (as listed in Table 1). Patients with inflammatory disease have increased activation of proinflammatory cytokines, such as IL-1α, TNF-α, and IFN-γ, which have a suppressive effect on erythroid progenitor cell proliferation (88). Hyperparathyroidism has also been shown to inhibit erythropoiesis, although there is some debate about whether this is a direct inhibitory effect of PTH on CFU-E growth or whether this is mediated via increased marrow fibrosis (23). Aluminum toxicity causes a microcytic anemia and erythropoietin resistance by inhibiting heme synthesis and iron utilization (27,28). Vitamin B_{12} and folate deficiencies are much less common than iron deficiency in dialysis patients receiving erythropoietin, but both conditions are easily detected and treated. Hemolysis is often harder to detect, although a clue may be a high reticulocyte count in the absence of any rise in hemoglobin. Marrow conditions causing dyserythropoiesis, such as aplastic anemia or myelodysplastic syndrome, often cause a true resistance to erythropoietin, even at high doses. Likewise, it is very difficult to obtain a rise in hemoglobin in homozygous sickle-cell patients receiving erythropoietin, although the problem here is one of excessive hemolysis since such patients do show evidence of greatly enhanced erythropoiesis as measured by the reticulocyte count and HbS levels. Patients with other hemoglobinopathies such as α-thalassemia trait and β-thalassemia may also show a degree of resistance to erythropoietin, although this is usually not nearly as marked as in sickle-cell disease. More recently, underdialysis has been suggested as a cause of poor response to erythropoietin, and indeed increasing the dialysis prescription improved the hemoglobin response (63). There has been much controversy regarding whether concomitant use of ACE inhibitors confers some resistance to erythropoietin therapy, with studies both for and against this proposal. A recent controlled study by Albitar et al. (124), however, did show higher dose requirements of EPO in patients receiving enalapril compared with nifedipine or placebo (Fig. 4).

There are clearly economic, as well as clinical, consequences of treating patients who respond poorly to erythropoietin. Escalating doses may be used with little therapeutic gain, and high costs may be incurred with little to shown in return.

E. Adjuvant Therapies

Several substances have been found to enhance the response to erythropoietin therapy, and many of these have been the subject of clinical study. These include IV iron, folic acid, vitamin B_{12}, vitamin B_6, ascorbic acid, vitamin D, L-carnitine, androgens, and other cytokines/growth factors.

The evidence that IV iron can augment the response to EPO is really now quite persuasive (70–72). It was not surprising to discover that, in iron-deficient patients, administration of IV iron enhanced the hemoglobin response, but that it did so in seemingly iron-replete patients was unexpected. There are now many

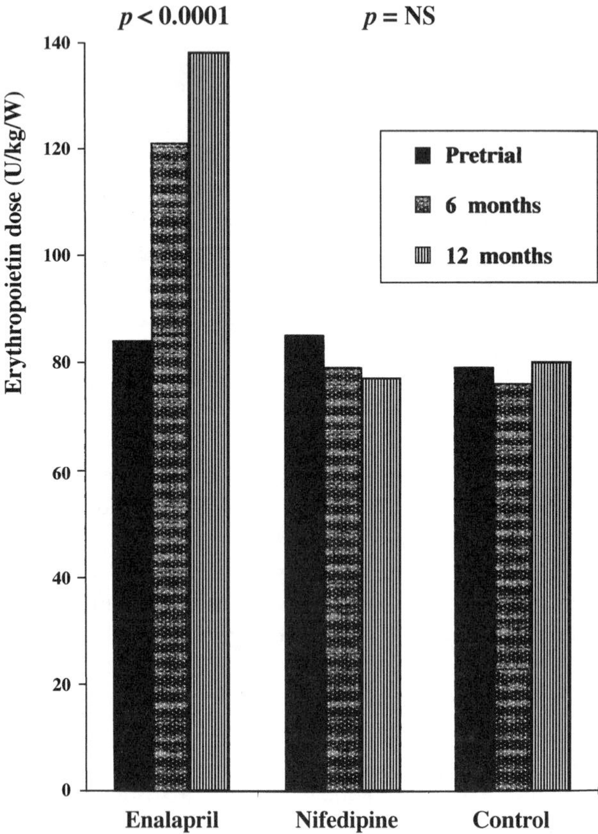

Fig. 4 Erythropoietin dose requirements before, after 6 months, and after 12 months of therapy in patients receiving enalapril and nifedipine, compared with control subjects. Results are expressed as means ±SD for each group. (Taken from Ref. 124, used with permission.)

studies providing supportive evidence for this, showing either improvements in hemoglobin, reductions in EPO dose requirements, or both. Two randomized prospective controlled studies, one in the correction phase of EPO therapy and the other in the maintenance phase, recruited only patients who had a serum ferritin >100 μg/L, and both showed significant enhancement of the response to EPO (70,71).

Folic acid deficiency is much less common than iron deficiency in patients receiving EPO. Pronai et al. (125), however, found that the response to erythropoietin could be enhanced by folic acid supplementation (10 mg/day) in patients who had a high MCV, even when folate levels were normal.

There has been one case report of vitamin B_{12} deficiency causing resistance to erythropoietin, which was reversed by B_{12} administration (126). The same authors, however, monitored B_{12} levels in a cohort of 30 dialysis patients and found no further evidence of B_{12} deficiency. Vitamin B_6 is a low molecular weight substance that is lost in the dialysate, especially during high-flux dialysis. Deficiency of this vitamin in red cells can occur even when plasma B_6 levels are normal. Mydlik et al. (127) showed recently that vitamin B_6 requirements increase with erythropoietin therapy, and patients can develop EPO resistance due to B_6 deficiency. The use of high-dose intravenous ascorbic acid in hemodialysis patients on EPO with iron overload was first suggested by Gastaldello et al. (128), who treated four such patients. This has been followed up by a controlled study comparing IV iron and IV ascorbic acid in iron-overloaded hemodialysis patients with functional iron deficiency (129). IV iron had no effect, but the hemoglobin increased in the patients given IV ascorbic acid, possibly due to mobilization of iron from the stores in the reticuloendothelial system. Two studies have similarly reported enhancement of the hemoglobin response to EPO by high-dose IV vitamin D (25,26). Whether this is due to partial correction of secondary hyperparathyroidism or whether there is a direct effect of vitamin D on erythroid progenitor cells remains unclear. Carnitine levels have been shown by Kooistra et al. (130) to be inversely correlated with EPO dose requirements, and carnitine deficiency is known to exacerbate renal anemia. Labonia (131) performed a placebo-controlled study of IV carnitine supplementation in hemodialysis patients on EPO. After 6 months of follow-up, patients on carnitine showed a significant reduction in EPO dose, whereas there was no change in the placebo group (Fig. 5). Androgen therapy was used to treat renal anemia in the 1970s (60,65), and two mechanisms are believed to be responsible for its effect on erythropoiesis. First, it acts by enhancing endogenous erythropoietin production, and second, it increases the sensitivity of the erythroid progenitor cells to EPO. Several studies have shown that it is possible to potentiate the response to EPO therapy by coadministration of androgens such as nandrolone decanoate (Fig. 6) (132,133). Although this may be used to good effect in countries with limited financial resources, the side effects of androgens such as virilization and hepatic damage prevent their more widespread adoption into clinical practice. Finally, two animal studies of erythropoiesis have suggested that it is possible to boost the response to erythropoietin by simultaneous treatment with other cytokines/growth factors. Brox et al. (134), using a mouse model, have reported a synergistic effect of insulin-like growth factor-1 (IGF-1) and EPO on erythropoiesis, whereas similar results were obtained by coadministration of interleukin-3 (IL-3) and EPO in rabbits (135).

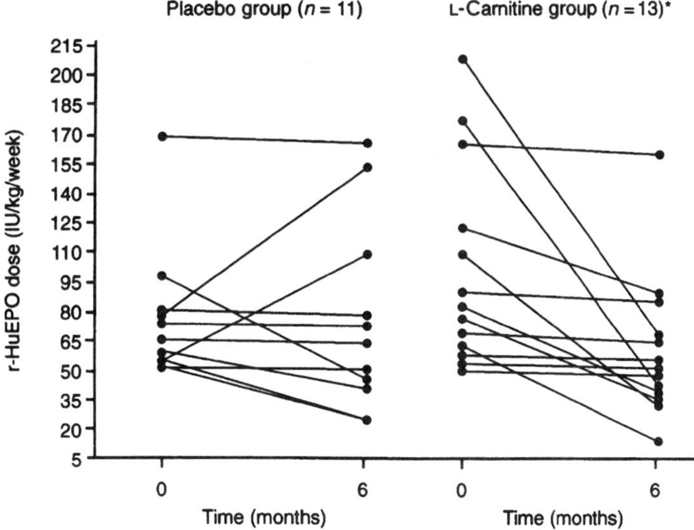

Fig. 5 Effect of 6 months of treatment with L-carnitine or placebo on erythropoietin dose requirements. There was a significant fall in EPO dosages in the L-carnitine-treated patients (*$p < 0.02$). (Adapted from Ref. 131, used with permission.)

F. Target Hemoglobin

Probably *the* most controversial issue in the management of renal anemia at the present time is what target hemoglobin to aim for in patients treated with EPO. In the early clinical trials (78,79), a subnormal target hemoglobin of around 10–12 g/dL was set, and clinical practice has remained largely unchanged over the last decade. Some clinicians have, however, pondered over why we aim for incomplete correction of the anemia in dialysis patients. There are probably several reasons for this: (a) this was the historical target hemoglobin from the first clinical trials of EPO, (b) concerns over possible increased adverse events with a higher hemoglobin, (c) no strong evidence of increased benefit in terms of morbidity and mortality with a normal hemoglobin, and (d) the increased costs of aiming for normalization of hemoglobin. Eschbach et al. (136),

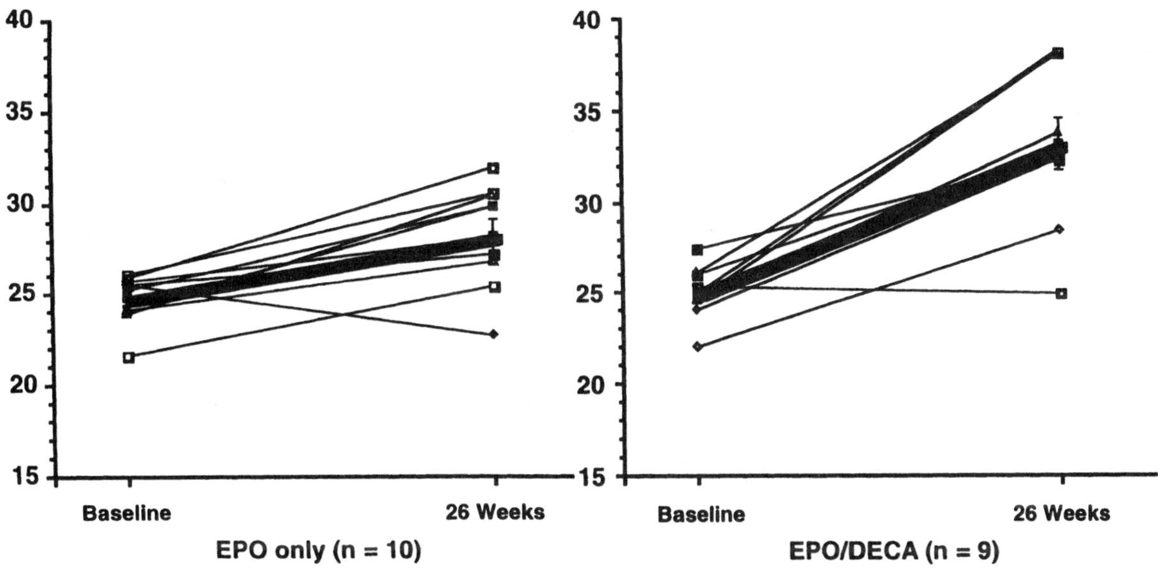

Fig. 6 Hematocrit responses in patients receiving erythropoietin alone compared with those receiving erythropoietin and nandrolone decanoate (DECA). The bold lines represent mean values. (Taken from Ref. 133, used with permission.)

however, studied the effect of normalizing hematocrit in 13 patients already receiving EPO therapy and found beneficial effects in terms of exercise capacity, quality of life, and cardiac hypertrophy, with no serious adverse events. There is also circumstantial evidence to suggest that, in dialysis patients, the higher the hematocrit, the better the quality of life (137) and the lower the incidence of cardiac disease (3); indeed, dialysis patients with spontaneously normal hemoglobin concentrations do the best of all.

The recent publication of the U.S. Normal Hematocrit Cardiac Study (138) has, however, confused the issue. The hypothesis was that there would be a reduced cardiovascular morbidity and mortality in hemodialysis patients aiming for normalization of hematocrit. Two treatment arms were chosen: one group aiming for a normal hematocrit (42%), the other aiming for a conventional hematocrit around 30%. This large multicenter study recruited 1265 patients, but the trial was aborted prematurely when it became apparent that a positive benefit from normalization of hematocrit could not be obtained, and indeed there was even a tendency to show a deleterious effect with an increased mortality in this group of patients (Fig. 7). Unfortunately, the results are not as clear-cut as they might at first seem (139). First, the patients recruited to this study were "high-risk cardiac" patients; second, the increased mortality was not due to the higher hematocrit per se (and indeed in a post hoc analysis there was an inverse relationship between hematocrit and mortality independent of treatment); third, the higher mortality was not due to the higher EPO doses; fourth, the normal hematocrit group had significantly higher doses of intravenous iron; and fifth, the increased mortality was *not* due to cardiovascular causes (as might have been expected), but rather due to an increased incidence of infections. Thus, it is impossible to draw firm conclusions from this study for the general dialysis population receiving EPO.

Two further multicenter studies have sought to investigate this issue, both as yet unpublished. The recently completed Scandinavian study recruited 420 patients, randomizing half to a normal hemoglobin and the other half to a conventional target hemoglobin. A large number of measurements and assessments have been performed to ascertain whether there are additional benefits of aiming for a normal hemoglobin, and the results are eagerly awaited. Preliminary analyses, however, have not confirmed the excess mortality seen in the U.S. multicenter study. The Canadian multicenter study of 140 patients has a similar study design, and one of the major endpoints is to examine cardiac function by echocardiography at the two levels of hematocrit. Before drawing firm conclusions regarding target hemoglobin in patients receiving erythropoietin, we should await the full publication of these latter two studies.

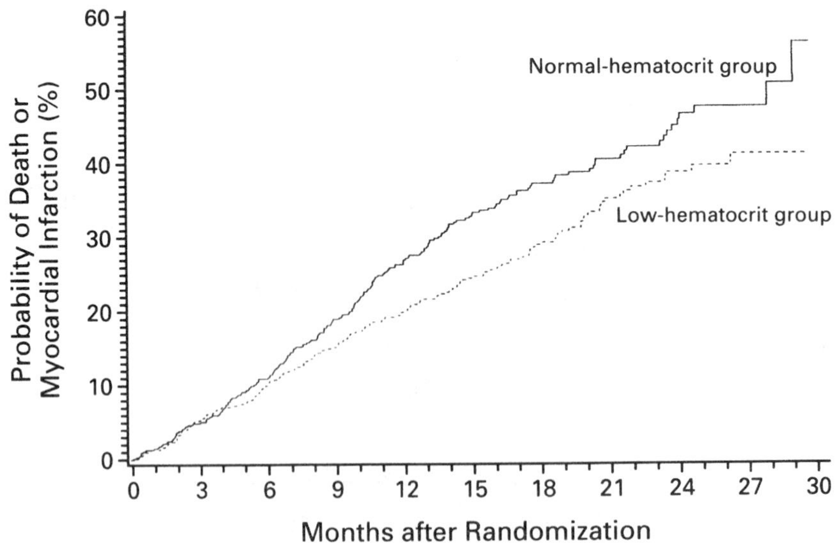

Fig. 7 Survival curves for probability of death or non-fatal myocardial infarction in patients aiming for a normal hematocrit (42%) compared with those maintained at a conventional hematocrit (around 30%) in the US Normal Hematocrit Cardiac Study. (Taken from Ref. 138, used with permission.)

IX. THE FUTURE

We have come a long way with erythropoietin therapy over the last decade. Different formulations have appeared, including prefilled syringes, multidose vials, multidosing "pens," and changes in buffering agents. Generic erythropoietin will be available in some countries of the world around the year 2004. In the last few years, however, at least three new strategies for erythropoietic stimulation have been proposed or developed: (a) novel erythropoiesis stimulating protein (NESP), (b) erythropoietin-mimetic peptides (e.g., EMP1), and (c) HCP inhibitors.

A. Novel Erythropoiesis Stimulating Protein

NESP is a hyperglycosylated analog of erythropoietin, which differs from native human erythropoietin by the substitution of five amino acids and the addition of two extra N-linked sialic acid–containing carbohydrate side chains. It was previously recognized that the sialic acid content of erythropoietin was essential for its metabolic stability in vivo, and this led to the generation of a hypothesis that the addition of extra sialic acid residues might result in a slower metabolic clearance of the glycoprotein. A new molecule called NESP was therefore synthesized by recombinant DNA technology, and initial animal studies confirmed the longer elimination half-life in vivo. The first pharmacokinetic study in humans was conducted at the end of 1996 (140), and this showed that the half-life of NESP was three times longer than that of epoetin alfa (25.3 vs. 8.5 hours). The expectation, therefore, was that NESP might be able to be given less frequently than the thrice-weekly dosing schedule used for epoetin therapy, and this is currently being investigated in several clinical studies. Preliminary data from the first two studies have suggested that there is no difference in once-weekly and thrice-weekly dosing of NESP in hemodialysis and peritoneal dialysis patients, and the efficacy and side-effect profile of NESP seem very similar to that seen with epoetin therapy (141). At the time of this writing, no antibodies to NESP have been detected out of a total of several hundred patients treated thus far. This new agent is in Phase 3 of its clinical development program, and there is much hope that it will become a licensed therapeutic agent within the next couple of years.

B. Erythropoietin-Mimetic Peptides

The search is already underway for erythropoietin mimetics that bind to the erythropoietin receptor and have the same functional properties. This could lead to orally active substances, which would be more convenient to administer and perhaps simpler to produce. A family of peptides has already been discovered that demonstrates erythropoietin-mimetic activity both in vitro and in vivo (142). A member of this peptide family, EMP1 (erythropoietin-mimetic peptide 1), has been identified by phage display technology. EMP1 is a cyclic 20-amino-acid peptide that shares the same functional properties of erythropoietin, although its amino acid sequence is completely unrelated to that of epoetin. In vitro, it induces the proliferation of cells that have a functional erythropoietin receptor, but not their parental cells. In vivo, EMP1 has been shown to be active in two mouse models of erythropoiesis. EMP1 competes with radiolabeled erythropoietin for the erythropoietin receptor and promotes the stabilization and crystallization of this receptor (142). Although EMPs are not orally active, they may form the template by which a small mimetic molecule could be designed, and thus the concept of an orally active erythropoietin mimetic could become a reality over the next decade.

C. HCP Inhibitors

Erythropoietin mediates its effects by binding to its receptor on erythroid progenitor cells, thus initiating the JAK-STAT signal transduction cascade (143). Hematopoietic cell phosphatase (HCP or SHP-1) negatively regulates this pathway by dephosphorylating JAK-2 (144). In theory, inhibitors of HCP would augment the action of erythropoietin. Thus, HCP inhibitors might cause responsive cells to become hypersensitive to erythropoietin, allowing lower doses of epoetin to be used. Such molecules could potentially be used in conjunction with erythropoietin therapy or perhaps as therapeutic agents on their own.

X. CONCLUSIONS

Prior to the late 1980s, the management of renal anemia was deeply unsatisfactory, and many dialysis patients had to rely on repeated blood transfusions. The advent of recombinant human erythropoietin, however, transformed the situation, and several million patients worldwide have experienced the secondary benefits of having their anemia corrected. We have learned a great deal about how to use the genetically engineered hormone most effectively, with particular attention to such issues as iron monitoring and supplementation. There is currently interest in other adjuvant therapies, which may be used in combination with EPO, and indeed other erythropoietic substances are being developed for clinical use. Thus, although the last decade has seen great advances in this field, we can yet look forward to the next decade with much hope and optimism.

ACKNOWLEDGMENT

I am most grateful to my secretary, Christine Mitchell, for her hard work and patience in typing this manuscript.

REFERENCES

1. Bright R. Cases and observations illustrative of renal disease accompanied with the secretion of albuminous urine. Guy's Hosp Rep 1836; 1:338–379.
2. Caro J, Brown S, Miller O, Murray T, Erslev AJ. Erythropoietin levels in uremic nephric and anephric patients. J Lab Clin Med 1979; 93:449–458.
3. Foley RN, Parfrey PS, Harnett JD, Kent GM, Murray DC, Barre PE. The impact of anemia on cardiomyopathy, morbidity, and mortality in end-stage renal disease. Am J Kidney Dis 1996; 28:53–61.
4. Möcks J, Franke W, Ehmer B, Quarder O, Scigalla P. Epoetin therapy reduces mortality? Clinical trials in 3111 HD patients show a decreased cardiovascular risk. Nephrology 1997; 3(suppl 1):S308.
5. Locatelli F, Conte F, Marcelli D. The impact of haematocrit levels and erythropoietin treatment on overall and cardiovascular mortality and morbidity—the experience of the Lombardy Dialysis Registry. Nephrol Dial Transplant 1998; 13:1642–1644.
6. Radtke HW, Claussner A, Erbes PM, Scheuermann EH, Schoeppe W, Koch KM. Serum erythropoietin in chronic renal failure: relationship to degree of anaemia and excretory renal function. Blood 1979; 54:877–884.
7. Eschbach JW. The anemia of chronic renal failure: pathophysiology and the effects of recombinant erythropoietin. Kidney Int 1989; 35:134–148.
8. Cotes PM, Pippard MJ, Reid CDL, Winearls CG, Oliver DO, Royston JP. Characterization of the anaemia of chronic renal failure and the mode of its correction by a preparation of human erythropoietin (r-HuEPO). An investigation of the pharmacokinetics of intravenous r-HuEPO and its effect on erythrokinetics. Q J Med 1989; 70:113–137.
9. Charles G, Lundin AP, Delano BG, Brown C, Friedman EA. Absence of anemia in maintenance hemodialysis. Int J Artif Org 1981; 4:277–279.
10. Salahudeen AK, Keavey PM, Hawkins T, Wilkinson R. Is anaemia during continuous ambulatory peritoneal dialysis really better than during haemodialysis? Lancet 1983; ii:1046–1049.
11. Maggiore Q, Navalesi R, Biagni M. Comparative studies on uraemic anaemia in polycystic kidney disease and in other renal disease. Proc Eur Dial Transplant Assoc 1986; 4:264–269.
12. Chandra M, Miller ME, Garcia JF, Mossey RT, McVicar M. Serum immunoreactive erythropoietin levels in patients with polycystic kidney disease as compared with other hemodialysis patients. Nephron 1985; 39:26–29.
13. Eckardt EU, Mollmann M, Neumann R, Brunkhorst R, Burger HU, Lonnemann G, Scholz H, Keusch G, Buchholz B, Frei U. Erythropoietin in polycystic kidneys. J Clin Invest 1989; 84:1160–1166.
14. Shaloub RJ, Uma R, Kim VV, Goldwasser E, Kark JA, Antoniou LD. Erythrocytosis in patients on long-term hemodialysis. Ann Intern Med 1982; 97:686–690.
15. Naets JP, Garcia JF, Tousaaint G, Buset M, Waks D. Radioimmunoassay of erythropoietin in chronic uraemia or anephric patients. Scand J Haematol 1986; 37: 390–394.
16. Fried W. The liver as a source of extrarenal erythropoietin production. Blood 1972; 40:671–677.
17. Thevenod F, Radtke HW, Grützmacher P, Vincent E, Koch KM, Fassbinder W. Deficient feedback regulation of erythropoiesis in kidney transplant patients with polycythemia. Kidney Int 1983; 24:227–232.
18. Nielsen OJ, Thaysen JH. Erythropoietin deficiency in acute renal failure. Lancet 1989; i:624–625.
19. Chandra M, Clemons GK, McVicar MI. Relation of serum erythropoietin production in chronic renal failure. J Pediatr 1988; 113:1015–1021.
20. Wallner SF, Ward HP, Vautrin R, Alfrey AC, Mishell J. The anemia of chronic renal failure: in vitro response of bone marrow to erythropoietin. Proc Soc Exp Biol Med 1975; 149:939–944.
21. Wallner SF, Kurnick JE, Ward HP, Vautrin R, Alfrey AC. The anemia of chronic renal failure and chronic diseases: in vitro studies of erythropoiesis. Blood 1976; 47:561–569.
22. Meytes D, Bogin E, Ma A, Dukes PP, Massry SG. Effect of parathyroid hormone on erythropoiesis. J Clin Invest 1981; 67:1263–1269.
23. Rao DS, Shih M-S, Mohini R. Effect of serum parathyroid hormone and bone marrow fibrosis on the response to erythropoietin in uremia. N Engl J Med 1993; 328:171–175.
24. Barbour GL. Effect of parathyroidectomy on anemia in chronic renal failure. Arch Intern Med 1979; 139: 889–891.
25. Albitar S, Genin R, Fen-Chong M, Serveaux MO, Schohn D, Chuet C. High-dose alfacalcidol improves anaemia in patients on haemodialysis. Nephrol Dial Transplant 1997; 12:514–518.

26. Goicoechea M, Vazquez MI, Ruiz MA, Gomez-Campdera F, Perez-Garcia R, Valderrabano F. Intravenous calcitriol improves anemia and reduces the need for erythropoietin in hemodialysis patients. Nephron 1998; 78:23–27.
27. Touam M, Martinez F, Lacour B, Bourdon R, Zingraff J, Di Giulio S, Drueke T. Aluminium-induced, reversible microcytic anemia in chronic renal failure: clinical and experimental studies. Clin Nephrol 1983; 19: 295–298.
28. Praga M, Andres A, de la Serna J, Ruilope LM, Nieto J, Estenoz J, Millet VG, Arnaiz F, Rodicio JL. Improvement of anaemia with desferrioxamine in haemodialysis patients. Nephrol Dial Transplant 1987; 2: 243–247.
29. Brozovich B, Cattell WR, Cottrall MF, Gwyther MM, McMillan JM, Malpas JS, Salsbury A, Trott NG. Iron metabolism in patients undergoing regular dialysis therapy. Br Med J 1971; 1:695–698.
30. Hampers CL, Streiff R, Nathan DG, Snyder D, Merrill JP. Megaloblastic hematopoiesis in uremia and in patients on long-term hemodialysis. N Engl J Med 1967; 276:551–554.
31. Shaw AB. Haemolysis in chronic renal failure. Br Med J 1967; 2:213–216.
32. Orringer EP, Mattern WD. Formaldehyde-induced hemolysis during chronic hemodialysis. N Engl J Med 1976; 294:1416–1420.
33. Mayer G, Thum J, Graf H. Anaemia and reduced exercise capacity in patients on chronic haemodialysis. Clin Sci 1989; 76:265–268.
34. Richardson TQ, Guyton AC. Effects of polycythemia and anemia on cardiac output and other circulatory factors. Am J Physiol 1959; 197:1167–1170.
35. Nissenson AR. Epoetin and cognitive function. Am J Kidney Dis 1992; 20(suppl 1):21–24.
36. Lindsay RM, Moorthy AV, Koens F, Linton AL. Platelet function in dialyzed and non-dialyzed patients with chronic renal failure. Clin Nephrol 1975; 4:52–57.
37. Livio M, Marchesi D, Remuzzi G, Gotti E, Mecca G, De Gaetano G. Uraemic bleeding: role of anaemia and beneficial effect of red cell transfusions. Lancet 1982; ii:1013–1015.
38. Moia M, Mannucci PM, Vizzotto L, Casati S, Cattaneo M, Ponticelli C. Improvement in the haemostatic defect of uraemia after treatment with recombinant human erythropoietin. Lancet 1987; ii:1227–1229.
39. Lusvarghi E. Hematopoiesis in renal failure patients. J Nephrol 1994; 8:79–86.
40. Lusvarghi E, Mauri C, Senter M, et al. Granulocytopoiesis in patients on regular dialysis treatment (kinetics by 75-Se-Seleniomethionine). Minerva Nefrol 1982; 29:205–210.
41. Paul JL, Roch-Arveiller M, Man NK, Loung N, Moatti N, Raichvarg D. Influence of uremia on polymorphononuclear leukocytes oxydative metabolism in end-stage renal disease and dialyzed patients. Nephron 1991; 57:428–432.
42. Lucchi L, Cappelli G, Acerbi MA, Spattini A, Lusvarghi E. Oxidative metabolism of polymorphonuclear leukocytes and serum opsonic activity in chronic renal failure. Nephron 1989; 51:44–50.
43. Gibbon R, Martines O, Lim V, Garovoy MR. Defective antigen presentation in uremia. Kidney Int 1986; 31:232.
44. Haniki Z, Cichocki T, Komoroswka Z, Sulowicz W, Smolenki O. Some aspects of cellular immunity in untreated and maintenance hemodialysis patients. Nephron 1979; 23:273–275.
45. Roccatello D, Mazzucco G, Coppo R, et al. Functional changes of monocytes due to dialysis membranes. Kidney Int 1989; 35:622–631.
46. Pertosa G, Marfella C, Tarantino EA, et al. Involvement of peripheral blood monocytes in haemodialysis: in vivo induction of tumor necrosis factor alpha, interleukin 6 and beta 2-microglobulin. Nephrol Dial Transplant 1991; S2:18–23.
47. Taccone-Gallucci M, Giardini O, Ausiello C, Piazza A, Casciani CU. Vitamin E supplementation in hemodialysis patients: effects on peripheral blood mononuclear cells lipid peroxydation and immune response. Clin Nephrol 1986; 25:81–86.
48. Montgomerrie JG, Kalmanson GM, Guze LB. Renal failure and infection. Medicina 1968; 47:1–4.
49. Wakabayashi Y, Sugimoto M, Ishiyama T, et al. Studies on T-cell colony formation in chronic renal failure (CRF) patients. Clin Nephrol 1989; 32:270–275.
50. Beaurain G, Naret C, Marcon L, et al. In vivo T cell preactivation in chronic uremic hemodialyzed and non-hemodialyzed patients. Kidney Int 1989; 36:636–644.
51. Alexiewics JM, Gaciong Z, Klinger M, Linker-Israeli M, Pitts TO, Massry SG. Evidence of impaired T cell function in hemodialysis patients: potential role for secondary hyperparathyroidism. Am J Nephrol 1990; 10:495–501.
52. Osanloo EO, Berlin BS, Popli S, et al. Antibody response to influenza vaccination in patients with chronic renal failure. Kidney Int 1978; 14:614–618.
53. Benigni A, Boccardo P, Galbusera M, et al. Reversible activation defect of the platelet glycoprotein IIb-IIIa complex in patients with uremia. Am J Kidney Dis 1993; 22:668–676.
54. Caster U, Bessler H, Malachi T, Zevin D, Djaldetti M, Levi J. Platelet count and thrombopoietic activity in patients with chronic renal failure. Nephron 1987; 45: 207–210.
55. Lusvarghi E, Curci G, Sacchi E, et al. Evaluation of platelet kinetics in chronic renal failure (conservative and regular dialysis treatment). Hematologica 1979; 64:747–758.
56. Taccone-Gallucci M, Lubrano R, Del Principe D, et al. Platelet lipid peroxidation in hemodialysis patients:

effects of vitamin E supplementation. Nephrol Dial Transplant 1989; 4:975–978.
57. Barradas MA, Fonseca VA, Gill DS, et al. Intraplatelet serotonin, beta-thromboglobulin, and histamine concentrations and thromboxane A2 synthesis in renal disease. Am J Clin Pathol 1991; 96:504–511.
58. Mannucci PM, Remuzzi G, Pusinieri F, et al. Deamino-8-D-arginine vasopressin shortens the bleeding time in uremia. N Engl J Med 1983; 308:8–12.
59. Livio E, Mannucci PM, Viganò G, et al. Conjugated estrogens for the management of bleeding associated with renal failure. N Engl J Med 1986; 315:731–735.
60. Koch KM, Patyna WD, Shaldon S, Werner E. Anemia of the regular hemodialysis patient and its treatment. Nephron 1974; 12:405–419.
61. Summerfield GP, Gyde OHB, Forbes AMW, Goldsmith HJ, Bellingham AJ. Haemoglobin concentration and serum erythropoietin in renal dialysis and transplant patients. Scand J Haematol 1983; 30:389–400.
62. Maiorca R, Cancarini G, Manili L, Brunori G, Camerini C, Strada A, Feller P. CAPD is a first class treatment: results of an eight-year experience with a comparison of patient and method survival in CAPD and hemodialysis. Clin Nephrol 1988; 30(suppl 1): S3–S7.
63. Ifudu O, Feldman J, Friedman EA. The intensity of hemodialysis and the response to erythropoietin in patients with end-stage renal disease. N Engl J Med 1996; 334:420–425.
64. Alexanian R, Vaughn WK, Ruchelman MW. Erythropoietin excretion in man following androgens. J Lab Clin Med 1967; 70:777–785.
65. Eschbach JW, Adamson JW. Improvement in the anemia of chronic renal failure with fluoxymesterone. Ann Intern Med 1973; 78:527–532.
66. Neff MS, Goldberg J, Slifkin RF, Eiser AR, Calamia V, Kaplan M, Bacz A, Gupta S, Mattoo N. A comparison of androgens for anemia in patients on hemodialysis. N Engl J Med 1981; 304:871–875.
67. Carter RA, Hawkins JB, Robinson BHB. Iron metabolism in the anaemia of chronic renal failure: effects of dialysis and of parenteral iron. Br Med J 1969; 3: 206.
68. Strickland ID, Chaput de Saintonge DM, Boulton FE, Francis B, Roubikova J, Waters JI. The therapeutic equivalence of oral and intravenous iron in renal dialysis patients. Clin Nephrol 1977; 7:55–57.
69. Macdougall IC. Monitoring of iron status and iron supplementation in patients treated with erythropoietin. Curr Opin Nephrol Hypertens 1994; 3:620–625.
70. Macdougall IC, Tucker B, Thompson J, Tomson CRV, Baker LRI, Raine AEG. A randomized controlled study of iron supplementation in patients treated with erythropoietin. Kidney Int 1996; 50:1694–1699.
71. Fishbane S, Frei GL, Maesaka J. Reduction in recombinant human erythropoietin doses by the use of chronic intravenous iron supplementation. Am J Kidney Dis 1995; 26:41–46.
72. Sunder-Plassmann G, Hörl WH. Importance of iron supply for erythropoietin therapy. Nephrol Dial Transplant 1995; 10:2070–2076.
73. Eschbach JW, Downing MR, Egrie JC, Browne JK, Adamson JW. USA multicenter clinical trial with recombinant human erythropoietin. Contrib Nephrol 1989; 76:160–165.
74. Canadian Erythropoietin Study Group. Association between recombinant human erythropoietin and quality of life and exercise capacity of patients receiving haemodialysis. Br Med J 1990; 300:573–578.
75. Sundal E, Kaeser U. Correction of anaemia of chronic renal failure with recombinant human erythropoietin: safety and efficacy of one year's treatment in a European multicentre study of 150 haemodialysis-dependent patients. Nephrol Dial Transplant 1989; 4:979–987.
76. Miyake T, Kung CK-H, Goldwasser E. Purification of human erythropoietin. J Biol Chem 1977; 252:5558–5564.
77. Lin FK, Suggs S, Lin CH, Browne JK, Smalling R, Egrie JC, Chen KK, Fox GM, Martin F, Stabinsky Z, Badrawi SM, Lai PH, Goldwasser E. Cloning and expression of the human erythropoietin gene. Proc Natl Acad Sci USA 1985; 82:7580–7585.
78. Eschbach JW, Egrie JC, Downing MR, Browne JK, Adamson JW. Correction of the anemia of end-stage renal disease with recombinant human erythropoietin. N Engl J Med 1987; 316:73–78.
79. Winearls CG, Oliver DO, Pippard MJ, Reid C, Downing MR, Cotes PM. Effect of human erythropoietin derived from recombinant DNA on the anaemia of patients maintained by chronic haemodialysis. Lancet 1986; ii:1175–1178.
80. Boelaert JR, Schurgers ML, Matthys EG, Belpaire FM, Daneels RF, De Cre MJ, Bogaert MG. Comparative pharmacokinetics of recombinant erythropoietin administered by the intravenous, subcutaneous and intraperitoneal routes in continuous ambulatory peritoneal dialysis patients. Perit Dial Int 1989; 9:95–98.
81. Macdougall IC, Roberts DE, Neubert P, Dharmasena AD, Coles GA, Williams JD. Pharmacokinetics of recombinant human erythropoietin in patients on continuous ambulatory peritoneal dialysis. Lancet 1989; i: 425–427.
82. Macdougall IC, Roberts DE, Coles GA, Williams JD. Clinical pharmacokinetics of epoetin (recombinant human erythropoietin). Clin Pharmacokinet 1991; 20: 99–113.
83. Egrie JC, Eschbach JW, McGuire T, Adamson JW. Pharmacokinetics of recombinant human erythropoietin administered to hemodialysis patients. Kidney Int 1988; 33:262.

84. Macdougall IC. Treatment of renal anemia with recombinant human erythropoietin. Curr Opin Nephrol Hypertens 1992; 1:210–219.
85. Macdougall IC, Davies ME, Hutton RD, Cavill I, Lewis NP, Coles G, Williams JD. The treatment of renal anaemia in CAPD patients with recombinant human erythropoietin. Nephrol Dial Transplant 1990; 5: 950–955.
86. Macdougall IC. Poor response to erythropoietin: practical guidelines on investigation and management. Nephrol Dial Transplant 1995; 10:607–614.
87. Van Wyck DB, Stivelman JC, Ruiz J, Kirlin LF, Katz MA, Ogden DA. Iron status in patients receiving erythropoietin for dialysis associated anemia. Kidney Int 1989; 35:712–716.
88. Means RT, Krantz SB. Progress in understanding the pathogenesis of the anemia of chronic disease. Blood 1992; 80:1639–1647.
89. Teruel JL, Pascual J, Jiménez M, et al. Hemodynamic changes in hemodialyzed patients during treatment with recombinant human erythropoietin. Nephron 1991; 58:135–137.
90. Macdougall IC, Lewis NP, Saunders MJ, Cochlin DL, Davies ME, Hutton RD, Fox KAA, Coles GA, Williams JD. Long-term cardiorespiratory effects of amelioration of renal anaemia by erythropoietin. Lancet 1990; 335:489–493.
91. Wizemann V, Kaufmann J, Kramer W. Effect of erythropoietin on ischemia tolerance in anemic hemodialysis patients with confirmed coronary artery disease. Nephron 1992; 62:161–165.
92. Löw-Friedrich I, Grützmacher P, März W, Bergmann M, Schoeppe W. Therapy with recombinant human erythropoietin reduces cardiac size and improves heart function in chronic hemodialysis patients. Am J Nephrol 1991; 11:54–60.
93. Pascual J, Teruel JL, Moya JL, Liano F, Jimenez-Mena M, Ortuno J. Regression of left ventricular hypertrophy after partial correction of anemia with erythropoietin in patients on hemodialysis: a prospective study. Clin Nephrol 1991; 35:280–287.
94. Silberberg JS, Barre PE, Prichard SS, Sniderman AD. Impact of left ventricular hypertrophy on survival in end-stage renal disease. Kidney Int 1989; 36:286–290.
95. Mayer G, Thum J, Cada EM, Stummvoll HK, Graf H. Working capacity is increased following recombinant human erythropoietin treatment. Kidney Int 1988; 34: 525–528.
96. Viganò G, Benigni A, Mendogni D, Mingardi G, Mecca G, Remuzzi G. Recombinant human erythropoietin to correct uremic bleeding. Am J Kidney Dis 1991; 18:44–49.
97. Macdougall IC, Davies ME, Hutton RD, Coles GA, Williams JD. Rheological studies during treatment of renal anaemia with recombinant human erythropoietin. Br J Haematol 1991; 77:550–558.
98. Macdougall IC, Davies ME, Hallett I, et al. Coagulation studies and fistula blood flow during erythropoietin therapy in haemodialysis patients. Nephrol Dial Transplant 1991; 6:862–867.
99. Taylor JE, McLaren M, Henderson IS, Belch JJF, Stewart WK. Prothrombotic effect of erythropoietin in dialysis patients. Nephrol Dial Transplant 1992; 7: 235–239.
100. Huraib S, Al-Momen AK, Gader AMA, Mitwalli A, Sulimani F, Abu-Aisha H. Effect of recombinant human erythropoietin (rHuEpo) on the hemostatic system in chronic hemodialysis patients. Clin Nephrol 1991; 36:252–257.
101. Keown PA. Quality of life in end-stage renal disease patients during recombinant human erythropoietin therapy. Contrib Nephrol 1991; 88:81–86.
102. Marsh JT, Brown WS, Wolcott D, et al. rHuEPO treatment improves brain and cognitive function of anemic dialysis patients. Kidney Int 1991; 39:155–163.
103. Schaefer RM, Kokot F, Wernze H, Geiger H, Heidland A. Improved sexual function in hemodialysis patients on recombinant erythropoietin: a possible role for prolactin. Clin Nephrol 1989; 31:1–5.
104. Bommer J, Kugel M, Schwöbel B, Ritz E, Barth HP, Seelig R. Improved sexual function during recombinant human erythropoietin therapy. Nephrol Dial Transplant 1990; 5:204–207.
105. Gladziwa U, Dakshinamurty KV, Mann H, Siebert HG. Pregnancy in a dialysis patient under recombinant human erythropoietin. Clin Nephrol 1992; 37:215.
106. Kokot F, Wiecek A, Grzeszczak W, Klepacka J, Klin M, Lao M. Influence of erythropoietin treatment on endocrine abnormalities in haemodialyzed patients. Contrib Nephrol 1989; 76:257–272.
107. Bárány P, Fehrman I, Godoy C. Long-term effects on lymphocytotoxic antibodies and immune reactivity in haemodialysis patients treated with recombinant human erythropoietin. Clin Nephrol 1992; 37:90–96.
108. Sennesael JJ, Van Der Niepen P, Verbeelen D. Treatment with recombinant human erythropoietin increases antibody titers after hepatitis B vaccination in dialysis patients. Kidney Int 1991; 40:121–128.
109. Veys N, Vanholder R, Ringoir S. Correction of deficient phagocytosis during erythropoietin treatment in maintenance hemodialysis patients. Am J Kidney Dis 1992; 19:358–363.
110. De Marchi S, Cecchin E, Villalta D, Sepiacci G, Santini G, Bartoli E. Relief of pruritus and decreases in plasma histamine concentrations during erythropoietin therapy in patients with uremia. N Engl J Med 1992; 326:969–974.
111. Macdougall IC. Adverse effects of erythropoietin in chronic renal failure. Prescribers' J 1992; 32:40–44.
112. Raine AEG, Roger SD. Effects of erythropoietin on blood pressure. Am J Kidney Dis 1991; 18(suppl 1): 76–83.

113. Edmunds ME, Walls J, Tucker B, Baker LR, Tomron CR, Ward M, Cummingham-Moore R, Winesolo C. Seizures in haemodialysis patients treated with recombinant human erythropoietin. Nephrol Dial Transplant 1989; 4:1065–1069.
114. Granolleras C, Leskopf W, Shaldon SE. Experience of pain after subcutaneous administration of different preparations of recombinant human erythropoietin: a randomised double-blind crossover study. Clin Nephrol 1991; 36:294–298.
115. NKF-DOQI Work Group. NKF-DOQI clinical practice guidelines for the treatment of anemia of chronic renal failure. Am J Kidney Dis 1997; 30(suppl 3): S192–S240.
116. Working Party for European Best Practice Guidelines. European Best Practice Guidelines for the management of anaemia in patients with chronic renal failure. Nephrol Dial Transplant 1999; 14(suppl 5):1–50.
117. Macdougall IC. How to get the best out of r-HuEPO. Nephrol Dial Transplant 1995; 10(suppl 2):85–91.
118. Bommer J, Barth H-P, Zeier M, Mandelbaum A, Bommer G, Ritz E, Reichel H, Novack R. Efficacy comparison of intravenous and subcutaneous recombinant human erythropoietin administration in hemodialysis patients. Contrib Nephrol 1991; 88:136–143.
119. Eidemak I, Friedberg MO, Ladefoged SD, Lokkegaard H, Pedersen E, Skielboe M. Intravenous versus subcutaneous administration of recombinant human erythropoietin in patients on haemodialysis and CAPD. Nephrol Dial Transplant 1991; 7:526–529.
120. Barclay PG, Fischer ER, Harris DCH. Interpatient variation in response to subcutaneous versus intravenous low dose erythropoietin. Clin Nephrol 1993; 40:277–280.
121. Taylor JE, Belch JJF, Fleming LW, Mactier RA, Henderson IS, Stewart WK. Erythropoietin response and route of administration. Clin Nephrol 1994; 41:297–302.
122. Macdougall IC, Cavill I, Hulme B, Bain B, McGregor E, McKay P, Sanders E, Coles GA, Williams JD. Detection of functional iron deficiency during erythropoietin treatment: a new approach. Br Med J 1992; 304:225–226.
123. Bárány P, Divino Fliho JC, Bergstrom J. High C-reactive protein is a strong predictor of resistance to erythropoietin in hemodialysis patients. Am J Kidney Dis 1997; 29:565–568.
124. Albitar S, Genin R, Fen-Chong M, Serveaux M-O, Bourgeon B. High dose enalapril impairs the response to erythropoietin treatment in haemodialysis patients. Nephrol Dial Transplant 1998; 13:1206–1210.
125. Pronai W, Riegler-Keil M, Silberbauer K, Stockenhuber F. Folic acid supplementation improves erythropoietin response. Nephron 1995; 71:395–400.
126. Zachee P, Chew SL, Daelemans R, Lins RL. Erythropoietin resistance due to vitamin B_{12} deficiency. Case report and retrospective analysis of B_{12} levels after erythropoietin treatment. Am J Nephrol 1992; 12: 188–191.
127. Mydlik M, Derzsiova K, Zemberova E. Metabolism of vitamin B_6 and its requirement in chronic renal failure. Kidney Int 1997; 51(suppl):S56–S59.
128. Gastaldello K, Vereerstraeten A, Nzame-Nze T, Vanherweghem JL, Tielemans C. Resistance to erythropoietin in iron-overloaded haemodialysis patients can be overcome by ascorbic acid administration. Nephrol Dial Transplant 1995; 10(suppl 6):44–47.
129. Tarng D-C, Huang T-P. A parallel comparative study of intravenous iron versus intravenous ascorbic acid for erythropoietin-hyporesponsive anaemia in haemodialysis patients with iron overload. Nephrol Dial Transplant 1998; 13:2867–2872.
130. Kooistra MP, Struyvenberg A, van Es A. The response to recombinant human erythropoietin in patients with the anemia of end-stage renal disease is correlated with serum carnitine levels. Nephron 1991; 57:127–128.
131. Labonia WD. L-carnitine effects on anemia in hemodialyzed patients treated with erythropoietin. Am J Kidney Dis 1995; 26:757–764.
132. Ballal SH, Domoto DT, Polack DC, Marciulonis P, Martin KJ. Androgens potentiate the effects of erythropoietin in the treatment of anemia of end-stage renal disease. Am J Kidney Dis 1991; 17:29–33.
133. Gaughan WJ, Liss KA, Dunn SR, et al. A 6-month study of low-dose recombinant human erythropoietin alone and in combination with androgens for the treatment of anemia in chronic hemodialysis patients. Am J Kidney Dis 1997; 30:495–500.
134. Brox AG, Zhang F, Guyda H, Gagnon RF. Subtherapeutic erythropoietin and insulin-like growth factor-1 correct the anemia of chronic renal failure in the mouse. Kidney Int 1996; 50:937–943.
135. Macdougall IC, Allen DA, Cavill I, Baker LRI, Raine AEG. Interleukin-3 potentiates the effect of erythropoietin in a uraemic anaemic animal model. Nephrol Dial Transplant 1994; 9:1032.
136. Eschbach JW, Glenny R, Robertson T, Guthrie M, Rader B, Evans R, Chandler W, Davidson R, Easterling T, Denney J, Schneider G. Normalizing the hematocrit in hemodialysis patients with EPO improves quality of life and is safe. J Am Soc Nephrol 1993; 4: 425.
137. Moreno F, Valderrabano F, Aracil FJ, Perez R. Influence of haematocrit on quality of life of haemodialysis patients. Nephrol Dial Transplant 1994; 9:1034.
138. Besarab A, Kline Bolton W, Browne JK, Egrie JC, Nissenson AR, Okamoto DM, Schwab J, Goodkin DA. The effects of normal as compared with low hematocrit values in patients with cardiac disease who are receiving hemodialysis and epoetin. N Engl J Med 1998; 339:584–590.

139. Macdougall IC, Ritz E. The Normal Haematocrit Trial in dialysis patients with cardiac disease: Are we any the less confused about target haemoglobin? Nephrol Dial Transplant 1998; 13:3028–3031.
140. Macdougall IC, Gray SJ, Elston O, Breen C, Jenkins B, Browne J, Egrie J. Pharmacokinetics of novel erythropoiesis stimulating protein compared with epoetin alfa in dialysis patients. J Am Soc Nephrol 1999; 10:2392–2395.
141. Macdougall IC, on behalf of the UK NESP Study Group. Novel Erythropoiesis Stimulating Protein (NESP) for the treatment of renal anaemia. J Am Soc Nephrol 1998; 9:258A.
142. Wrighton NC, Farrell FX, Chang R, Kashyap AK, Barbone FP, Mulcahy LS, Johnson DL, Barrett RW, Jolliffe LK, Dower WJ. Small peptides as potent mimetics of the protein hormone erythropoietin. Science 1996; 273:458–463.
143. Darnell JE, Kerr IA, Stark GR. Jak-STAT pathways and transcriptional activation in response to IFNs and other extracellular signaling proteins. Science 1994; 264:1415–1421.
144. Klingmüller U, Lorenz U, Cantley LC, et al. Specific recruitment of SH-PTP1 to the erythropoietin receptor causes inactivation of JAK2 and termination of proliferative signals. Cell 1995; 80:729–738.

17

Coagulation Problems in Dialysis Patients

Paola Boccardo
Mario Negri Institute for Pharmacological Research, Bergamo, Italy

Giuseppe Remuzzi
Azienda Ospedaliera, Ospedali Riuniti di Bergamo, and Mario Negri Institute for Pharmacological Research, Bergamo, Italy

Abnormal bleeding has long been recognized as a common and potentially serious complication of acute and chronic renal failure of different etiologies. Since the first review in 1907 of this association between uremia and abnormal bleeding, the clinical manifestations of uremic bleeding have been well described (1–4). The hemorrhagic tendency has been attributed to abnormalities of primary hemostasis, in particular platelet dysfunction and impaired platelet/vessel wall interaction.

The introduction of dialysis and the modern management of renal failure have definitively reduced the incidence of severe hemorrhages. Ecchymoses, epistaxis, and gastrointestinal bleeding are the most common manifestation seen today: subdural hematoma occurs only occasionally, in 5–15% of hemodialysis patients, while hemopericardium and subcapsular hematoma of the liver are less frequent (5). Nevertheless, bleeding remains a potentially dangerous complication, particularly in case of trauma or surgical or invasive procedures.

I. CAUSES OF UREMIC BLEEDING

A. Platelet Abnormalities

In the past 20 years, research has clarified in part the nature of bleeding time. Uremic bleeding is likely to be the result of multiple pathogenetic factors (Table 1), but abnormal platelet function and endothelial dysfunction appear to be of predominant importance in its development. Impaired platelet-platelet and platelet–vessel wall interactions result in a prolonged bleeding time, still the best available marker of clinical bleeding (6–8). It depends on the platelet number, vascular integrity, activity of von Willebrand factor, and hematocrit and thus gives an excellent overall assessment of primary hemostasis (7). A review of the literature on the diagnostic and clinical utility of this test concluded that it is of value in renal failure, and its use to monitor bleeding in this setting is recommended (9). A recent study compared the usefulness of the modified Ivy bleeding time on the forearm (arm bleeding time) with that in the thigh (thigh bleeding time) as an indicator of hemostatic competence during surgical treatment in patients with uremia (10). The arm bleeding time was significantly longer than the thigh time, and there was no correlation between the two methods. Moreover, prolonged, excessive perioperative bleeding was observed in three patients whose thigh bleeding time was significantly prolonged (>8 min, up to 26.5 min) but whose arm bleeding time was normal. These authors concluded that thigh bleeding time is a better indicator of hemostatic competence during surgery for patients with uremia (10).

The platelet count in uremia usually falls within the normal range (11,12), and thrombocytopenia severe enough to cause bleeding is very rare (3,13). Hemodialysis may cause or aggravate mild thrombocytope-

Table 1 Causes of Uremic Bleeding

Platelet abnormalities
Subnormal dense granule content
Reduction in intracellular ADP and serotonin
Impaired release of the platelet α-granule protein and β-thromboglobulin
Enhanced intracellular cAMP
Abnormal mobilization of platelet Ca^{2+}
Abnormal platelet arachidonic acid metabolism
Abnormal ex vivo platelet aggregation in response to different stimuli
Defective cyclooxygenase activity
Abnormality of the activation-dependent binding activity of GP IIb-IIIa
Uremic toxins, especially parathyroid hormone
Abnormal platelet-vessel wall interactions
Abnormal platelet adhesion
Increased formation of vascular PGI_2
Altered von Willebrand factor
Anemia
Altered blood rheology
Erythropoietin deficiency
Abnormal production of nitric oxide
Drug treatment
β-Lactam antibiotics
Third-generation cephalosporins
Nonsteroidal anti-inflammatory drugs

nia, but the effect is transient (14). Platelet function is impaired: among acquired platelet dysfunctions, low levels of intracellular serotonin and adenosine diphosphate (ADP) (15,16), high levels of intracellular cyclic adenosine monophosphate (AMP) (17), a defective cyclooxygenase activity, and an abnormal mobilization of Ca^{2+} in response to stimulation (18) play a major role in the pathogenesis of uremic bleeding. Elevation in platelet cyclic AMP (17) and abnormal Ca^{2+} mobilization (18) suggest the possibility that parathyroid hormone (PTH) plays a role in uremic platelet dysfunction (19,20). Although PTH has been shown to inhibit platelet aggregation in vitro, there is no correlation between serum concentrations of intact PTH or PTH fragments and bleeding time (21), suggesting that elevated PTH in patients with renal failure is not likely to play a major role in the uremic platelet defect.

Impaired platelet aggregation in response to different stimuli (22–26) and defective platelet thromboxane A_2 (TxA_2) production (27,28) in response to endogenous and exogenous stimuli, not correctable by thrombin (28), have also been reported in uremia. In a subpopulation of uremic patients, irreversible platelet aggregation does not occur in response to platelet-activating factor (29,30): this abnormality, independent of plasma factor(s), is probably due to the reduced capacity of the platelets to form TxA_2 in response to platelet-activating factor. Experimental data have suggested that the bleeding tendency in uremia is associated with excessive formation of nitric oxide (NO) (31), an endogenous vasoactive molecule that also inhibits platelet function (32,33). Thus prolonged bleeding time completely normalizes by giving uremic rats *N*-monomethyl-L-arginine, a competitive inhibitor of NO synthesis. In patients with chronic renal failure, defective platelet aggregation is associated with increased platelet NO synthesis (34). The same study also found significantly higher plasma levels of L-arginine, the substrate of NO synthesis, in uremic patients compared with healthy volunteers, probably due to an activation of inducible nitric oxide forming enzyme.

Fibrinogen, von Willebrand factor (vWF), and their receptors, glycoprotein (GP) Ib and the GPIIb-IIIa complex, play a vital role in normal hemostasis, by initiating and mediating the formation of platelet thrombi at site of vascular injury (35). The activation-dependent receptor function of the GPIIb-IIIa complex is defective in uremia, as shown by decreased binding of both vWF and fibrinogen to stimulated platelets (36). While the number of GPIIb-IIIa receptors expressed on the platelet membrane is normal, their activation is impaired. In contrast, the vWF binding to gpIb is normal. Removal of substances present in uremic plasma markedly improved the GPIIb-IIIa defect, suggesting that dialyzable toxic substances are probably a major component of the altered platelet function in uremia.

The contribution of "uremic toxins" to bleeding diathesis and to functional platelet abnormalities has been extensively investigated, but with conflicting results. The evidence that several dialyzable toxins, e.g., urea, creatinine, phenol, phenolic acids, or guanidinosuccinic acid, may be involved in the genesis ot the uremic platelet is not compelling (37–39). Guanidinosuccinic acid, which accumulates in uremic plasma, inhibits the second wave of platelet aggregation to ADP when added to normal platelet-rich plasma (38). Phenol and phenolic acids, at the concentrations found in uremic plasma, also impair primary aggregation to ADP (37). Then reducing the blood levels of these compounds, the abnormal hemostasis of patient with renal failure is partially corrected. However, no correlation has been found between bleeding time or platelet adhesion and the serum level of the dialyzable metabolites that mainly accumulate in uremia (39).

B. Abnormal Platelet–Vessel Wall Interactions

Platelet adherence to foreign surfaces is significantly impaired in nonthrombocytopenic patients with uremia (3,39,40), but this does not fully explain the prolonged bleeding time (39–41). Studies of platelet adhesion, using a perfusion chamber system, have demonstrated a defective platelet adhesion to vascular subendothelium (42,43).

Increased vascular formation of prostacyclin (PGI_2), a potent vasodilator and inhibitor of platelet function, was demonstrated in uremic patients (44,45) and blood vessels from rats with experimentally induced uremia (46,47). Furthermore, plasma from uremic patients contains increased amounts of a factor that stimulates vascular PGI_2 (48). This could be PTH, since it has been shown to increase urinary excretion of the PGI_2 metabolite, 6-keto-prostaglandin F_{1a} (49). In an investigation of vWF and platelet adhesion using blood from uremic patients with bleeding tendency, evidence was found of both platelet and plasma abnormalities (42).

Von Willebrand factor, a molecule present in the circulation as multimers of different molecular weight, interacting with specific thrombocyte receptors, promotes platelet adhesion and aggregation to subendothelial collagen. Quantitative and qualitative abnormalities of the vWF may alter the platelet–vessel wall interaction and contribute to the hemorrhagic tendency of uremia (50). Functional and structural studies of vWF in uremia have given conflicting results. Some authors reported elevated vWF antigen levels but reduced ristocetin cofactor activity in uremic patients (51). However, other investigators have reported increased vWF functional activity (52–54). The platelet vWF multimeric structure appears to be normal (55,56).

Both cryoprecipitate (55), a plasma derivative rich in factor VIII and vWF, and desmopressin (56), a synthetic derivative of antidiuretic hormone that releases autologuous vWF from storage sites, raise the vWF concentration in plasma and significantly shorten the bleeding time of uremic patients. This suggests that a functional defect in the vWF-platelet interaction may indeed play a role in the abnormal hemostasis of these patients.

C. Anemia

Platelet adhesion and aggregation in flowing systems (57,58) are markedly potentiated by red blood cells. Erythrocytes enhance platelet function by releasing ADP (59), by inactivating PGI_2 (60), and by increasing platelet–vessel wall contact by displacing platelets away from the axial flow and toward the vessel wall (57). The independent role of anemia in the bleeding tendency of uremia has been extensively investigated. A significant negative correlation was found between bleeding time and packed cell volume (PCV) in 52 patients receiving chronic hemodialysis (61). The bleeding time was longer than 270 seconds in 90% of patients with PCV less than 30% but in only 45% of patients with PCV greater than 30%. Despite a shorter bleeding time, a significant negative correlation between hematocrit and bleeding time was still demonstrable in 15 nonuremic anemic patients. These results were subsequently confirmed by other studies (62,63), which found that anemia was the main determinant of the prolonged bleeding time in uremic patient. Uremic bleeding time has been shortened and symptomatic hemostatic improvement has been achieved by treatment with rHuEPO (64,65). In one randomized study (66), the bleeding time became normal in all patients receiving erythropoietin as hematocrits increased from 27 to 32%. Thus, partial correction of anemia was sufficient to correct defective primary hemostasis in uremia.

II. CONSEQUENCES OF THE BLEEDING TENDENCY IN UREMIA

Gastrointestinal bleeding occurs with greater frequency and higher mortality in uremic patients than in the general population (67,68). Upper gastrointestinal bleeding is the second leading cause of death in acute renal failure (69). The most common causes of bleeding are peptic ulcers, hemorrhagic esophagitis, gastritis, duodenitis, and gastric telangiectasias (70–72). Angiodysplasia with gastrointestinal bleeding has been observed in the stomach, duodenum, jejunum, and colon (73,74). This abnormality, affecting the microcirculation of the gastrointestinal mucosa and submucosa, occurs most often in hemodialysis patients (75). Finally, dialysis patients suffering from human immunodeficiency virus nephropathy may have specific lesions such as Kaposi's sarcoma, cytomegalovirus colitis, and non-Hodgkin's lymphoma (76) that contribute to gastrointestinal bleeding. Although now rare, hemorrhagic pericarditis with cardiac tamponade can occur in uremia (77,78). The clinical features of this condition include normal cardiac shadow, increased jugular venous distention with hypotension, shortness of breath, and a pericardial friction rub. Deaths caused by hemorrhagic pericarditis have been reported to be as high as 3–5% among dialysis patients (79,80).

Subdural hematoma reportedly occurs in 5–15% of hemodialysis patients (81). It usually overlies the frontal or parietal lobe and is bilateral in approximately 15% of cases. Headache, vomiting, seizures, hypertension, drowsiness, confusion, and coma are usual symptoms. Head trauma, hypertension, and systemic anticoagulation are risk factors (81). Prognosis is at least partly related to the stage of diagnosis, and the mortality rate may be as high as 90% in patients requiring emergency surgery.

Anticoagulation during dialysis may be a major risk factor in causing bleeding in patients with fibrinous pleuritis (82,83). Spontaneous retroperitoneal bleeding is a rare complication in patients having chronic hemodialysis (84,85). Trauma, anticoagulation, and the presence of polycystic kidneys are predisposing factors. The symptoms and signs include sudden onset of pain in the abdomen, flank, back, or hip, with an associated drop in blood pressure. The hematocrit drops in the absence of any obvious blood loss. Computed tomography is useful in the diagnosis of retroperitoneal bleeding.

Spontaneous subcapsular hematoma of the liver is now a recognized complication in uremia (86). Typically patients have right upper quadrant pain, fever, and sometimes elevated bilirubin and alkaline phosphatase levels accompanied by a falling hematocrit.

Intraocular hemorrhage can also occur in uremia, and spontaneous hyphema has been reported during dialysis (87). There is no visual loss and the hemorrhage generally resolves without any therapy. Intraocular bleeding with only temporary visual loss has also been reported in a large percentage of transplantation and dialysis patients after cataract surgery.

Uremic patients may be at an increased risk of bleeding complications caused by drug treatment. The risk of bleeding associated with the accumulation of β-lactam antibiotics in uremia has been highlighted (88). Four mechanisms have been proposed: drug-induced thrombocytopenia (rare), platelet dysfunction, suppression of synthesis of vitamin K–dependent coagulation factors, and delayed fibrin polymerization. β-Lactam antibiotics apparently act by perturbing platelet membrane function and by interfering with ADP receptors (89,90). The prolonged bleeding time and the abnormal platelet aggregation are related to the dose and duration of treatment and are promptly reversible after discontinuation. Third-generation cephalosporins may also inhibit platelet function and may lead to marked disturbance of blood coagulation (91,92).

Risk of bleeding in uremic patients is also associated with aspirin given to prevent vascular access thrombosis (93) or platelet activation on dialysis membranes (94). The beneficial effect of aspirin on vascular access thrombosis can be achieved with a moderate dose of 160 mg/d, which inhibits platelet thromboxane A_2 generation without affecting vascular PGI_2 formation (93). However, a moderate dose of aspirin may prolong the bleeding time to a greater extent in uremic than in control subjects (95,96). This difference appeared not to be related to increased susceptibility of cyclooxygenase in uremic platelets. Furthermore, a temporal dissociation was found in uremic patients between the prolongation of bleeding time and inhibition of serum thromboxane B_2 generation after aspirin. Indeed, aspirin seems to have two distinct inhibitory effects on platelet function in uremia: a transient effect, which interferes with one of the determinants of bleeding time, and a lasting effect due to the irreversible blocking of platelet cyclooxygenase (96). However, the prolongation of bleeding time caused by aspirin may explain the frequency of gastrointestinal bleeding in uremic patients (97,98). Thus the use of aspirin for uremic patients treated with rHuEPO to prevent thrombotic complications associated with an increasing hematocrit is highly questionable.

III. THERAPEUTIC STRATEGIES

The approach to uremic bleeding must be considered in two contexts: the prevention of bleeding in patients at high risk because of invasive procedures or surgery and the treatment of patients with active bleeding. The strategy depends on the urgency of the situation, the severity of uremia, and the previous therapy employed (Table 2).

A. Dialysis

Dialysis improves platelet functional abnormalities and reduces but does not eliminate the risk of hemorrhage (99). Hemodialysis per se can also contribute to platelet dysfunction and bleeding by inducing platelet–artificial surface interactions. Heparin may also present a problem. It is the most frequently used anticoagulant to prevent the extracorporeal circuit coagulation, but its administration may result in systemic anticoagulation for several hours and thus may enhance the risk of serious bleeding in hemodialysis patients. Few studies have addressed the delicate balance of filter coagulation and patient hemorrhage. However, a recent report on 78

Table 2 Therapeutic Strategies for Uremic Bleeding

Treatment	Indication	Dosage	Effect		
			Start	Peak	End
Blood or RBC transfusion	Prophylaxis of bleeding in high-risk patients with anemia	According to the severity of anemia	PCV = 28–32%		Related to RBC life span
Recombinant human erythropoietin	Prophylaxis of bleeding in high-risk patients with anemia	50–150 U/kg i.v.	PCV = 28–32%		
Cryoprecipitate[a]	Acute bleeding episodes	10 bags	1 hour	4–12 hours	24–36 hours
Desmopressin[b]	Acute bleeding episodes	0.3 μg/kg i.v.[c] 0.3 μg/kg s.c. 3.0 μg/kg intranasal	1 hour	2–4 hours	6–8 hours
Conjugated estrogens	Major surgery or when long-lasting effect is required	0.6 mg/kg/day i.v. infusion for 5 consecutive days	6 hours	5–7 days 21–30 days	
Transdermal 17β-estradiol[d]	Prophylaxis of bleeding in high–risk patients; treatment of clinical bleeding	50–100 μg/24 h every 3.5 days for 2 months	24 hours[e]	17 days	n.a.[f]

[a]Not recommended, because not uniformly observed favorable effect.
[b]Loses efficacy when repeatedly administered.
[c]Added to 50 ml saline and infused over 30 min.
[d]Estrogen patch on a poorly folliculated area of the torso.
[e]Onset of action of topical estrogen quite variable.
[f]Data not available.

hemodialyzed patients showed that the occurrence of filter coagulation or hemorrhages was not correlated with the administered dose of heparin (100).

"Regional" heparinization has been used to minimize the effects of systemic anticoagulation (101–103). Heparin is given by constant infusion into the inlet line of the dialyzer. Simultaneously, protamine sulfate is infused into the outlet port before the blood returns to the patient. Even this schedule of heparin administration, however, may be associated with a high incidence of bleeding. This is because of the high dose needed to maintain adequate regional anticoagulation, the bleeding complications induced by protamine, or heparin rebound (104).

As an alternative, frequent injections of low-dose heparin can be given during dialysis to maintain a lower and more constant level (105). Usually, heparin at 40–50 IU/kg is given at the beginning of hemodialysis, followed by 60% of the initial dose after 1 and 2 hours, and 30% of the initial dose after 3 hours (105). The whole blood activated partial thromboplastin time is measured hourly and should be maintained at 1.5–2 times the basal value.

Citrate anticoagulation has been developed as an alternative to unfractionated heparin anticoagulation in hemodialysis patients with a high bleeding risk. Anticoagulation is achieved by infusion of trisodium citrate into the blood line before, and infusion of calcium into the blood line after the dialyzer, in combination with a calcium-free dialysate. Some comparative trials have been performed, demonstrating that this procedure may be safe and more effective than others in preventing hemorrhages episodes in patients at high risk of bleeding and that it is indicated for hemodialysis patients with an active or recently active bleeding focus (106–108). Serious and documented complications of citrate anticoagulation involve citrate intoxication, hyperaluminemia, hyperammonemia, hypernatremia, and profound metabolic alkalosis (109,110). Recently Flanigan et al. suggested that the regional citrate anticoagulation is simplified by using standard dialysate with a hypertonic rather than an isotonic citrate infusion and serious and dangerous complications are further evaded by adjusting the dialysate bicarbonate to 25–30 mmol/L or substituting a mixture of citric acid and trisodium-citrate (111).

Patients at high risk of bleeding can also use a membrane such as ethylene–vinyl alcohol copolymer hollow-fiber dialysis membrane that does not require systemic anticoagulation with heparin, provided blood flow is maintained at greater than 200 mL/min (112). Double access must be available, with separate needles for arterial and venous return, and blood products must be administered into a different intravenous line.

Low molecular weight heparin has been proposed as an alternative to unfractionated heparin in patients on chronic hemodialysis or hemofiltration who are at high risk of bleeding (113). These data need careful evaluation in controlled clinical trials before low molecular weight heparin can be used in routine hemodialysis. Newer anticoagulants, such as hirudin and dermatan sulfate, have been used in dose-finding studies in hemodialysis, although long term experience is lacking. Hirudin, originally derived from the salivary glands of the medicinal leech, *Hirudo medicinalis*, is a potent anticoagulant: recombinant protein is a strong direct inhibitor of thrombin, independent of antithrombin or heparin cofactor II, that blocks the active center of thrombin by forming a tight stoichiometric complex.

Recently hirudin has been investigated in two dose-finding studies in hemodialysis (114,115). In the former, Vanholder et al. demonstrated that a single dose of 0.08 mg/kg was sufficient to prevent clot formation in 20 stable hemodialyzed patients without causing bleeding complications (114). The latter compared the efficacy of dialysis with heparin to that of dialysis with recombinant hirudin in 11 patients with chronic renal failure on maintenance hemodialysis. Dialysis was therefore equally effective (115). Both studies reported significantly shorter activated partial thromboplastin time compared with standard heparin. A clear disadvantage of hirudin is the variably prolonged half-life, which makes drug accumulation inevitable when hirudin is routinely used during subsequent hemodialysis.

Dermatan sulfate has recently been proposed (116,117) as an alternative to heparin since it causes less bleeding than heparin in animal models. The lower hemorrhagic property may be due to its reduced effect on platelets (118). Short-term clinical studies have been conducted in hemodialysis for chronic renal failure, testing fixed intravenous doses of dermatan sulfate against individualized heparin regimens (117,119,120). Dermatan sulfate suppressed both visible clot formation in the dialysis circuit and the generation of plasma markers of coagulation and platelet activation during the procedure (119–122). It also induced a moderate prolongation of activated partial thromboplastin time (APTT) (120–122). These effects were related to dermatan sulfate doses and plasma concentrations, which followed linear pharmacokinetics (119,120–122). Effective doses ranged from 6 to 10 mg/kg body weight per dialysis session, depending on the type of dialyzer and duration of the procedure (119–122). Recently a comparative short-term clinical study has been performed on 10 hemodialyzed patients (123). Dermatan sulfate dose can be individually titrated to suppress clot formation during hemodialysis as efficiently as does individualized heparin. Individual titration may be facilitated by injecting approximately 60% of the total dose as a bolus and the remaining as a continuous infusion and by monitoring APTT response. These findings confirm that dermatan sulfate is a suitable alternative to heparin for anticoagulation in hemodialysis, but long-term comparative trials are warranted (123).

In the search for real alternatives to heparin, antiplatelet drugs such as sulfinpyrazone, adenosine, and PGE_1 have been used for regional infusion during extracorporeal circulation (124,125) but appear to have no advantage over heparin. Aspirin and dipyridamole analogs reduce fibrin and cellular deposition on the filter membrane, but increase the risk of gastrointestinal bleeding (94,126).

PGI_2 shows some promise as an alternative (127–129). Given as a continuous infusion during the dialysis session at a mean dose of 5 ng/kg/min, PGI_2 completely inhibited platelet aggregation without causing bleeding (127). However, the use of PGI_2 is associated with adverse reactions such as headache, flushing, tachycardia, and chest and abdominal pain, which require careful hemodynamic monitoring and physician supervision (130–132). Thus, the use of PGI_2 should be limited to patients at high risk of hemorrhage.

Another possibility investigated as an alternative to systemic anticoagulation in patients at high risk of bleeding is hemodialysis without anticoagulant, using saline flushes. This method is only successfully 70–90% of the time and inevitably leads to a subclinical disseminated intravascular coagulopathy (133,134).

Peritoneal dialysis, when applicable, avoids the risk of bleeding associated with heparin or anticoagulants. Table 3 summarizes the dialysis strategies for bleeding patients.

B. Correction of Anemia

Uremic patients are often severely anemic and the severity of anemia appears to be related to the extent of the prolongation of bleeding time (62–64). Chronic renal failure patients with prolonged bleeding time consistently benefited from red cell transfusions. The beneficial effect was independent of changes in platelet function tests or in the level of vWF-related properties (62,63).

The cloning of the human erythropoietin gene (132,135) has provided recombinant human erythropoietin for clinical use. This treatment reverses the anemia of uremics, eliminating their dependency on transfusions (64,136–138). The progressive increase in hematocrit was accompanied by a significant decrease in the bleeding time (65,66,138). No consistent changes were found in platelet number, platelet aggregability, or platelet thromboxane A_2 formation (65,138). Only one study (139) observed a significant increase in the levels of vWF and ristocetin cofactor activity.

Since complete correction of renal anemia carries the risk of hypertension, encephalopathy, thrombosis, and hyperkalemia, it was suggested that partial correction of anemia was sufficient to overcome the defective primary hemostasis in uremia (66). In this study, 20 dialysis patients with prolonged bleeding time ($\geq$15 min) were randomly allocated to receive erythropoietin or no specific treatment. Erythropoietin was given intravenously at the dose of 50 U/kg three times a week; every 4 weeks the dose was increased by 25 U/kg until bleeding time became normal. An erythropoietin dosage of 150–300 U/kg/week increased PCV to between 27 and 32% and normalized bleeding times in all patients (Fig. 1). A significant negative correlation was found between PCV and bleeding time (66).

Partial correction of anemia (hematocrit 28–30%) either by red blood cell transfusions or by the use of recombinant human erythropoietin, thus appears to merit a major part in the overall strategy for preventing and controlling abnormal bleeding in uremics.

C. Cryoprecipitate and Desmopressin

Cryoprecipitate is a plasma derivative rich in vWF, fibrinogen, and fibronectin that has traditionally been used in the treatment of hemophilia A, von Willebrand's disease, hypofibrinogenemia, and dysfibrinogenemia. Cryoprecipitate corrects prolonged bleeding in uremic patients within 4–12 hours, and the effect lasts 24 to 36 hours (55). The mechanism of action of cryoprecipitate is not known. It seems to be unrelated to the protein infusion itself or to changes in platelet aggregation. A small rise in platelet levels of fibrinogen and vWF-related properties were the only changes noted after cryoprecipitate infusion. Different preparations of cryoprecipitate, however, had different effects on bleeding time (140).

The poor reproducibility of the results and the risk of disease transmission prompted the search for alternatives. Desmopressin (1-deamino-8-D-arginine vasopressin), a synthetic derivative of the antidiuretic hormone, induces the release of autologous vWF from storage sites (141). In a randomized, double-blind, crossover trial desmopressin given intravenously at a

Table 3 Dialysis Strategies for Bleeding Patients

Treatment	Patients	Strategy	Risk/Benefit
Heparin	Stable hemodialyzed patients	Systemic injection	No correlation of heparin dose and filter coagulation or hemorrhages Risk of systemic anticoagulation
		Regional heparinization[a]	No systemic anticoagulation
		Frequent injection of low-dose[b] heparin	Lower risk of systemic anticoagulation
Low molecular weight heparin		Single bolus at the start or a divided dose regimen[c]	Alternative to unfractionated heparin Risk of systemic anticoagulation
Trisodium citrate	High-risk patients or those with an active or recently bleeding focus	Regional citrate hemodialysis[d]	Alternative to heparin anticoagulation Citrate intoxication Hyperaluminemia Hyperammoniemia Metabolic alkalosis
		Regional hypertonic citrate infusion with dialysate bicarbonate to 25–30 mmol/L	Less dangerous metabolic complications
Hirudin	Stable hemodialyzed patients	Single dose (0.08 mg/kg)	Variably prolonged half-life
Dermatan sulfate	Stable hemodialyzed patients	6–10 mg/kg body wt per dialysis session[e]	Alternative to heparin
Antiplatelet agents	Stable hemodialyzed patients	Regional infusion of sulfinpyrazone, adenosine, or PGE1	No advantage versus heparin
		Aspirin, dipyridamole analog	Increased risk of gastrointestinal bleeding
		Prostacyclin[f]	Headache, flushing, tachycardia, chest and abdominal pain
Special dialysis membrane	High-risk patients for bleeding	Ethylene-vinyl alcohol copolymer hollow-fiber membrane[g]	No systemic anticoagulation with heparin required
Hemodialysis without anticoagulation	High-risk patients for bleeding	Saline flushes	Subclinical disseminated intravascular coagulopathy Only successful 70–90%

[a] Constant infusion of heparin in the inlet line of dialyzer and simultaneously of protamine sulfate into the outlet port.
[b] 40–50 IU/kg at beginning, 60% of initial dose after 1 and 2 hours, and 30% after 3 hours. Whole blood APTT 1.5–2 times over basal value.
[c] 2/3 of the dose at the start and 1/3 after 2.5 hours. Dose adapted to hematocrit and duration of dialysis session.
[d] Trisodium citrate solution infused into the arterial line of the dialyzer (initial: ≤10 mmol/L at rate of 0.34 mmol/100 mL blood flow, adjusted to an activated CT of 200–220 s); calcium-free dialysate; calcium infusion into the blood line after the dialyzer.
[e] Individual titration: 60% of the total dose as a bolus, and the remaining as continuous infusion (monitor APTT response).
[f] At dose of 5 ng/kg/min.
[g] Blood flow >200 mL/min.

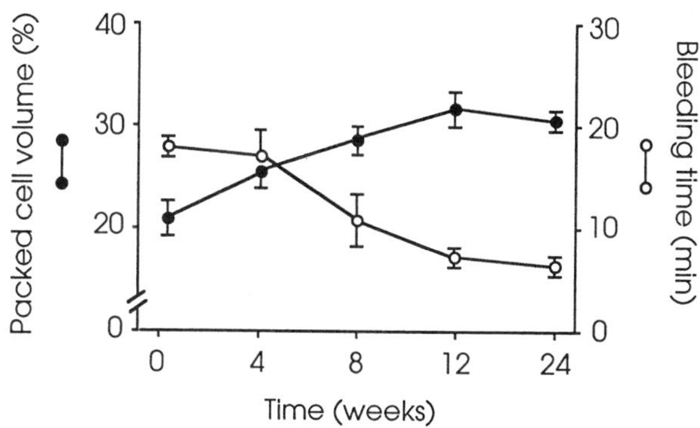

Fig. 1 Effect of recombinant human erythropoietin therapy on packed cell volume and bleeding time in uremic patients.

dose of 0.3 μg/kg body weight in 50 mL of physiological saline over a period of 30 minutes temporarily corrected the prolonged bleeding time in patients with chronic renal failure (56) without appreciable side effects. The shortening of bleeding time was significant one hour after the end of the infusion, and the effect lasted 6–8 hours, after which bleeding time returned to basal values (Fig. 2). Desmopressin loses its efficacy when repeatedly administered (142). This has been ascribed to depletion of vWF storage sites or negative feedback exerted by high circulating vWF levels on further release. Desmopressin can also be given by the intranasal route (143,144), which is well tolerated and quite safe. At 10–20 times the intravenous dose, intranasal desmopressin (3 μg/kg) shortens the prolonged bleeding time (143,144) and decreases clinical bleeding. Desmopressin has also been given subcutaneously (145) in the same dose used for intravenous administration. Peak responses are achieved after a 30- to 90-minute delay when the subcutaneous route is used. Adverse effects include facial flushing, mild transient headache, nausea, abdominal cramps, and mild tachycardia. In one case report an elderly uremic patient with atherosclerosis suffered a stroke immediately after desmopressin infusion (146). Nonetheless, desmopressin is useful in the treatment of bleeding and in the prevention of bleeding during surgery or invasive procedures.

D. Conjugated Estrogens

The anecdotal observation of diminished gastrointestinal bleeding in uremic patients treated with conjugated estrogens and the improved hemostasis in von Willebrand's disease during pregnancy led to investigations of the effect of estrogens on bleeding tendency in uremia (147–149). One oral dose of 25 mg of conjugated estrogen preparation normalizes bleeding time for 3–10 days with no apparent ill effects (147). A controlled study showed that conjugated estrogens given intravenously at the cumulative dose of 3 mg/kg divided over 5 consecutive days produced a long-lasting reduction in the bleeding time in uremics. The estrogens were safe and well tolerated. The therapeutic activity could apparently not be ascribed to an effect on vWF multimeric structure, platelet aggregation in response to dif-

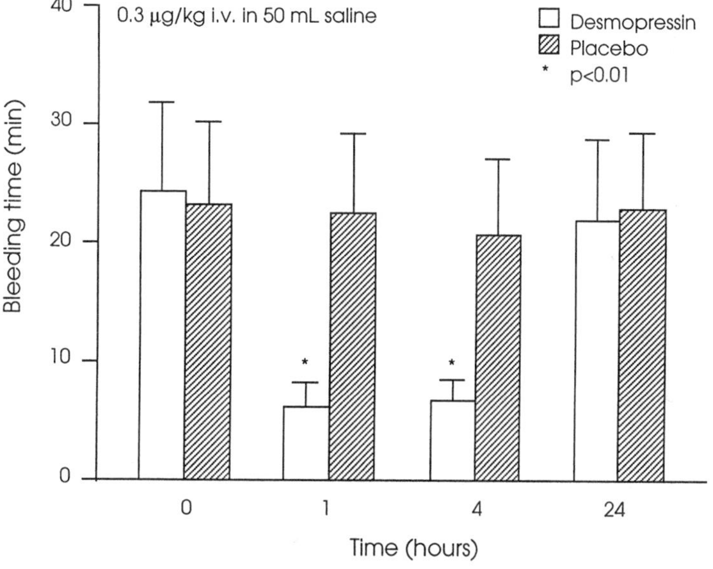

Fig. 2 Effect of desmopressin or placebo on bleeding time in uremic patients.

ferent stimuli (ADP, arachidonic acid, calcium ionophore A23187), or platelet TXB_2 generation. At least 0.6 mg/kg estrogen was needed to reduce bleeding time (149), and four or five infusions spaced 24 hours apart were needed to reduce the bleeding time by at least 50%. Recently the use of transdermal estradiol in treating uremic bleeding has been demonstrated easy, safe, and effective (150). Estrogen transdermally administered improves hemostasis and reduces bleeding time in patients with renal insufficiency: shortening of bleeding time was seen in all patients within a 17-day period of administration, with the most rapid effect seen within 24 hours (150). This product, which contains only the active fraction of the total estrogen present in intravenous or oral preparations, is less expensive than intravenous therapy and avoids the potential complications of first-pass hepatic metabolism seen with oral estrogen therapy. Estrogen normalize the prolonged bleeding time in the experimental rat model of chronic uremia (151). This effect is antagonized by giving the animals L-arginine, the precursor of nitric oxide, suggesting that estrogens exert their hemostatic effect by interfering with the NO synthesis pathway. Thus, estrogens may be a reasonable alternative to cryoprecipitate or desmopressin in the treatment of uremic bleeding, especially when a long-lasting effect is required.

REFERENCES

1. Riesman D. Hemorrhages in the course of Bright' disease with special reference to the occurrence of a hemorrhagic diathesis of nephritic origin. Am J Med Sci 1907; 134:709.
2. Gross R, Nieth H, Mammen E. Blutungsbereitschaft und Gerrinungstörungen bei Uramie. Klin Woschr 1958; 36:107.
3. Larsson SO. On coagulation and fibrinolysis in renal failure. Scand J Haematol 1971; 15:1.
4. Rabiner SF. Bleeding in uremia. Med Clin North Am 1972; 56:221.
5. Watson AJ, Gimenez LF. The bleeding diathesis of uremia. Semin Dial 1991; 4:86–93.
6. Steiner RW, Coggins C, Carvalho ACA. Bleeding time in uremia: a useful test to assess clinical bleeding. Am J Hematol 1979; 7:107–117.
7. Lind SC. Prolonged bleeding time. Am J Med 1984; 77:305–312.
8. Kumar R, Ansell JE, Conaso RT, Duykin D. Clinical trial of a new bleeding time device. Am J Clin Pathol 1978; 70:642–645.
9. Burns ER, Lawrence C. Bleeding time: a guide to its diagnostic and clinical utility. Arch Pathol Lab Med 1989; 113:1219–1224.
10. Liu YK, Goldstein DM, Arora K, Woo D, Ferris FZ, Marcum SG, Garrison RN, Amin M. Thigh bleeding time as a valid indicator of hemostatic competency during surgical treatment of patients with advanced renal disease. Surg Gynecol Obstet 1991; 172:269–274.
11. Lindsay RM, Moorthy AV, Koens F, Linton AL. Platelet function in dialyzed and non-dialyzed patients with chronic renal failure. Clin Nephrol 1975; 4:52–57.
12. Eknoyan G, Wacksman SJ, Glueck HI, Will JJ. Platelet function in renal failure. N Engl J Med 1969; 280: 677–681.
13. Gafter U, Bessler H, Malachi T, Zevin D, Djaldetti M, Levi J. Platelet count and thrombopoietic activity in patients with chronic renal failure. Nephron 1987; 45: 207–210.
14. Lindsay RM, Prentice CR, Davidson JF, Burton JA, McNicol GP. Hemostatic changes during dialysis associated with thrombus formation on dialysis membranes. Br Med J 1972; 4:454.
15. Di Minno G, Martinez J, McKean M, De La Rosa J, Burke JF, Murphy S. Platelet dysfunction in uremia. Multifaceted defect partially corrected by dialysis. Am J Med 1985; 79:552–559.
16. Eknoyan G, Brown CH. Biochemical abnormalities of platelets in renal failure. Evidence for decreased platelet serotonin, adenosine diphosphate and Mg-dependent adenosine triphosphatase. Am J Nephrol 1981; 1: 17–23.
17. Vlachoyannis J, Schoeppe W. Adenylate cyclase activity and cAMP content of human platelets in uremia. Eur J Clin Invest 1982; 12:379–381.
18. Ware JA, Clark BA, Smith M, Salzman EW. Abnormalities of cytoplasmic Ca^{2+} in platelets from patients with uremia. Blood 1989; 73:172–176.
19. Remuzzi G, Benigni A, Dodesini P, Schieppati A, Livio M, Poletti G, Mecca G, de Gaetano G. Parathyroid hormone inhibits human platelet function. Lancet 1981; 2:1321–1323.
20. Benigni A, Livio M, Dodesini P, Schieppati A, Panigada M, Mecca G, de Gaetano G, Remuzzi G. Inhibition of human platelet aggregation by parathyroid hormone: Is cyclic AMP implicated? Am J Nephrol 1985; 5:243–247.
21. Viganò G, Gotti E, Comberti E, Giangrande A, Trevisan R, Remuzzi G. Hyperparathyroidism does not influence the abnormal primary haemostasis in patients with chronic renal failure. Nephrol Dial Transplant 1989; 4:971–974.
22. Rabiner SF. Uraemic bleeding. In: Spaet TH, ed. Progress in Hemostasis and Thrombosis. New York: Grune & Stratton, 1972: 233–250.
23. Remuzzi G, Benigni A, Dodesini P, Schiepapti A, Gotti E, Livio M, Mecca G, Dondi MB, de Gaetano

G. Platelet function in patients on maintenance hemodialysis: depressed or enhanced? Clin Nephrol 1982; 17:60–63.
24. Zicker MB. Biological aspects of heparin action. Heparin and platelet function. Fed Proc 1977; 36:47–49.
25. Di Minno G, Martinez J, McKean ML, De La Rosa J, Burke JF, Murphy S. Platelet dysfunction in uremia. Multifaceted defect partially corrected by dialysis. Am J Med 1985; 79:552–559.
26. Evans EP, Branch RA, Bloom AL. A clinical and experimental study of platelet function in chronic renal failure. J Clin Pathol 1987; 25:745–753.
27. Smith MC, Dunn MJ. Impaired platelet thromboxane production in renal failure. Nephron 1981; 29:133–137.
28. Remuzzi G, Benigni A, Dodesini P, Schieppati A, Livio M, de Gaetano G, Day JS, Smith WL, Pinca E, Patrignani P, Patrono C. Reduced platelet thromboxane formation in uremia. Evidence for a functional cyclooxygenase defect. J Clin Invest 1983; 71:762–768.
29. Macconi D, Viganò G, Bisogno G, Galbusera M, Orisio S, Remuzzi G, Livio M. Defective platelet aggregation in response to platelet-activating factor in uremia associated with low platelet thromboxane A2 generation. Am J Kidney Dis 1992; 19(4):318–325.
30. Livio E, Benigni A, Remuzzi G. Coagulation abnormalities in uremia. Semin Nephrol 1985; 5(2):82–90.
31. Remuzzi G, Perico N, Zoja C, Corna D, Macconi D, Viganò G. Role of endothelium-derived nitric oxide in the bleeding tendency of uremia. J Clin Invest 1990; 86:1768–1771.
32. Ignarro LJ. Endothelium-derived nitric oxide: actions and properties. Fed Am Soc Exp Biol J 1988; 3:31–36.
33. Radomski MW, Palmer RMJ, Moncada S. The role of nitric oxide and cGMP in platelet adhesion to vascular endothelium. Biochem Biophys Res Comm 1987; 148: 1482–1489.
34. Noris M, Benigni A, Boccardo P, Aiello S, Gaspari F, Todeschini M, Figliuzzi M, Remuzzi G. Enhanced nitric oxide synthesis in uremia: implications for platelet dysfunction and dialysis hypotension. Kidney Int 1993; 44:445–450.
35. Schmitt GW, Moake JL, Rudy CK, Vicks SL, Hamburger RJ. Alterations in hemostatic parameters during hemodialysis with dialyzers of different membrane composition and flow design. Am J Med 1983; 83: 411–418.
36. Benigni A, Boccardo P, Galbusera M, Monteagudo J, De Marco L, Remuzzi G, Ruggeri ZM. Reversible activation defect of the platelet glycoprotein IIb-IIIa complex in patients with uremia. Am J Kidney Dis 1993; 22:668–676.
37. Rabiner SF, Molinas F. The role of phenol and phenolic acid on the thrombocytopathy and defective platelet aggregation of patients with renal failure. Am J Med 1970; 49:346–351.
38. Horowitz HI, Stein IM, Cohen BD, White JG. Further studies on the platelet inhibiting effect of guanidinosuccinic acid and its role in uremic bleeding. Am J Med 1970; 49:336–340.
39. Remuzzi G, Livio M, Marchiaro G, Mecca G, de Gaetano G. Bleeding in renal failure: altered platelet function in chronic uraemia only partially corrected by haemodialysis. Nephron 1978; 22:347–353.
40. Rabiner SF. Bleeding in uremia. Med Clin North Am 1972; 56:221–223.
41. Eknoyan G, Wacksman SJ, Glueck HI, Will JJ. Platelet function in renal failure. N Engl J Med 1969; 280: 677–681.
42. Castillo R, Lozano T, Escolar G, Revert L, Lopez J, Ordinas A. Defective platelet adhesion on vessel subendothelium in uremic patients. Blood 1986; 65:337–342.
43. Escolar G, Cases A, Bastida E, Garrido M, Lopez J, Revert L, Castillo R, Ordinas A. Uremic platelets have a functional defect affecting the interaction of von Willebrand factor with glycoprotein IIb-IIa. Blood 1990; 76:1336–1340.
44. Remuzzi G, Cavenaghi AE, Mecca G, Donati MB and De Gaetano G. Prostacyclin-like activity and bleeding in renal failure. Lancet 1977; 2:1195–1197.
45. Remuzzi G, Marchesi D, Livio M, Schieppati A, Mecca G, Donati MB, de Gaetano G. Prostaglandins, plasma factors and haemostasis in uraemia. In: Remuzzi G, Mecca G, De Gaetano G, eds. Hemostasis, Prostaglandins and Renal Disease. New York: Raven Press, 1980: 273–281.
46. Leithner CH, Winter M, Sibauer K, Wagner O, Pinggera W, Sinzinger H. Enhanced prostacyclin availability of blood vessels in uraemic humans and rats. In: Robinson RHB, Hawkins JB, eds. Dyalysis Transplantation Nephrology. Proceeding of the 15th Congress of European Dialysis and Transplant Association. Tunbridge Wells: Pitman Medical, 1978: 418–422.
47. Zoja C, Viganò G, Bergamelli A, Benigni A, De Gaetano G, Remuzzi G. Prolonged bleeding time and increased vascular prostacyclin in rats with chronic renal failure: effects of conjugated estrogens. J Lab Clin Med 1988; 112:380–386.
48. Defreyn G, Vergara Dauden M, Machin SJ, Vermylen J. A plasma factor in uraemia which stimulates prostacyclin release from cultured endothelial cells. Thromb Res 1980; 19:695–699.
49. Saglikes Y, Massry SG, Iseki K, Nadles JL, Campese VM. Effect of PTH on blood pressure and response to vasoconstrictor agonists. Am J Physiol 1985; 248: F674–F681.
50. Gordge MP, Neild GH. Platelet function in uraemia. Platelets 1991; 2:115–123.

51. Kazatchkine N, Sulta V, Caen JP, Bartiery J. Bleeding in uremia: a possible cause. Br Med J 1976; 2:612–615.
52. Hermann RP, Marshall LR, Hurst PE. Bleeding in renal failure: a possible cause. Br Med J 1977; 1:1601–1602.
53. Remuzzi G, Livio M, Roncaglioni MC, Mecca G, Donati MB and De Gaetano G. Bleeding in renal failure: Is von Willebrand factor implicated? Br Med J 1977; 2:359–361.
54. Warrell RP Jr, Hultin MB, Coller BS. Increased factor VIII/von Willebrand factor antigen and von Willebrand factor activity in renal failure. Am J Med 1979; 66:226–228.
55. Janson PA, Jubelirer SJ, Weinstein MJ, Deykin D. Treatment of bleeding tendency in uremia with cryoprecipitate. N Engl J Med 1980; 303:1319–1322.
56. Mannucci PM, Remuzzi G, Pusinieri F, Lombardi R, Valsecchi C, Mecca G, Zimmerman TS. Deamino-8-D-arginine vasopressin shortens the bleeding time in uremia. N Engl J Med 1983; 308:8–12.
57. Turnitto WT, Weiss HT. Red blood cells: their dual role in thrombus formation. Science 1980; 207:541–543.
58. Sakariassen KS, Bollhuid PA, Sixma JJ. Platelet adherence to sub-endothelium of human arteries in pulsatile and steady flow. Thromb Res 1980; 19:547–559.
59. Gaarder A, Jonsen J, Lland S, Hellem A, Owren PS. Adenosine diphosphate in red cells as a factor in the adhesiveness of human blood platelets. Nature 1961; 192:531–532.
60. Willems C, Stel HV, van Aken WG, van Mourik JA. Binding and inactivation of prostacyclin (PGI_2) by human erythrocytes. Br J Haematol 1983; 54:43–52.
61. Livio M, Gotti E, Marchesi D, Mecca G, Remuzzi G, De Gaetano G. Uraemic bleeding: role of anemia and beneficial effect of red cell transfusions. Lancet 1982; 2:1013–1015.
62. Fernandez F, Goudable C, Sie P, Ton-That H, Durand D, Suc JM, Boneu B. Low hematocrit and prolonged bleeding time in uraemic patients: effect of red cell transfusions. Br J Haematol 1985; 59:139–148.
63. Aznar-Salatti J, Hernandez R, Anton P, Cases A, Escolar G, Ordinas A. Serum obtained from uraemic patients modifies the reactivity towards platelets of extracellular matrices produced by endothelial cells (abstr). VIth International Symposium on the Biology of Vascular Cells 1990; 1:57.
64. Gordge MP, Leaker BR, Patel A, Oviasu E, Cameron JS, Neild GH. Recombinant human erythropoietin corrects uraemic bleeding without causing intravascular haemostatic activation. Thromb Res 1990; 57:171–182.
65. Moia M, Mannucci PM, Vizzotto L, Casati S, Cattaneo M, Ponticelli C. Improvement in the haemostatic defect of uraemia after treatment with recombinant human erythropoietin. Lancet 1987; 2:1227–1229.
66. Viganò G, Benigni A, Mendogni D, Mingardi G, Mecca G, Remuzzi G. Recombinant human erythropoietin to correct uremic bleeding. Am J Kidney Dis 1991; 1:44–49.
67. Eiser AR. Gastrointestinal bleeding in maintenance dialysis patients. Semin Dial 1988; 1:198–202.
68. Dinoso VP Jr, Murthy SN, Saris AL, Clearfield HR, Lyons P, Nickey WA, Simonian S. Gastric and pancreatic function in patients with end-stage renal disease. J Clin Gastroenterol 1982; 4:321–324.
69. Kleinknecht D, Jungers P, Chanard J, Barbanel C, Ganeval D. Uremic and non-uremic complications in acute renal failure. Evaluation of early and frequent dialysis on prognosis. Kidney Int 1972; 1:190–196.
70. Shepherd AM, Stewart WK, Wormsley KG. Peptic ulceration in chronic renal failure. Lancet 1973; 1:1357–1359.
71. Margolis DM, Saylor JL, Geisse G, De Schryver-Kecskemeti K, Harter HR, Zuckerman GR. Upper gastrointestinal disease in chronic renal failure: a prospective evaluation. Arch Int Med 1978; 138:1214–1217.
72. Dave PB, Romeu J, Antonelli A, Eiser AR. Gastrointestinal telangiectasias: a source of bleeding in patients receiving hemodialysis. Arch Int Med 1984; 144: 17810–1783.
73. Boley SJ, Sammartano R, Adams A. On the nature and aetiology of vascular ecstasias of the colon. Degenerative lesions of aging. Gastroenterology 1977; 72: 652–660.
74. Zuckerman GR, Cornette GL, Clouse RE, Harter HR. Upper gastrointestinal bleeding in patients with chronic renal failure. Ann Int Med 1978; 138:1214–1217.
75. Cunningham JT. Gastric telangiectasis in chronic hemodialysis patients: a report of six cases. Gastroenterology 1981; 81:1131–1133.
76. Dorothy CC. Gastrointestinal bleeding in dialysis patients. Nephron 1993; 63:132–139.
77. Kumar S, Lesch M. Pericarditis in renal disease. Prog Cardiovasc Dis 1980; 22:357–369.
78. Rutsky EA, Rostand SG. Treatment of uraemic pericarditis and pericardial effusion. Am J Kidney Dis 1987; 10:2–8.
79. Comty CM, Shapiro FL. Cardiac complications of regular dialysis therapy. In: Maher J, ed. Replacement of Renal Function by Dialysis. Dordrecht: Kluwer Academic Publishers, 1983:33–70.
80. Drueke T, Le Pailleur C, Zingraff J, Jungers P. Uraemic cardiomyopathy and pericarditis. Adv Nephrol Necker Hosp 1980; 9:33–70.
81. Bechar M, Lakke JP, van der Hem GK, Beeks JW, Penning L. Subdural hematoma during long term hemodialysis. Arch Neurol 1972; 26:513–516.
82. Berger HW, Rammohan G, Neff MS. Uraemic pleural effusion: a study in 14 patients on chronic dialysis. Ann Int Med 1975; 82:362–364.

83. Galen MA, Steinberg SM, Lowrie FG. Hemorrhagic pleural effusion in patients undergoing chronic dialysis. Ann Int Med 1975; 82:359–361.
84. Bhasin HK, Dana CL. Spontaneous retroperitoneal hemorrhage in chronically hemodialyzed patients. Nephron 1978; 22:322–327.
85. Milutinovich J, Follette WC, Scribner BH. Spontaneous retroperitoneal bleeding in patients on chronic hemodialysis. Ann Int Med 1977; 86:189–192.
86. Borra S, Kleinfeld M. Subscapular liver hematoma in a patient on chronic hemodialysis. Ann Int Med 1980; 93:574–575.
87. Slusher MM, Hamilton RW. Letter: spontaneous hyphema during hemodialysis. N Engl J Med 1975; 293: 561.
88. Andrassy K, Ritz E. Uremia as a cause of bleeding. Am J Nephrol 1985; 5:313–319.
89. Fass RJ, Copelan EA, Brandt JT, Moeschberger ML, Ashton JJ. Platelet-mediated bleeding caused by broad-spectrum penicillins. J Infect Dis 1987; 155: 1242.
90. Shattil S, Bennett J, McDonough M, Turnbull J. Carbenicillin and penicillin G inhibit platelet function in vitro by impairing the interaction of agonists with the platelets surface. J Clin Invest 1980; 65:329–337.
91. Bang N, Tessler S, Heidenreich R, Marks C. Effects of moxolactan on blood coagulation and platelet function. Rev Infect Dis 1982; 4:S546–S554.
92. Bechtold H, Andrassy K, Jahnchen E, Koderisch J, Koderisch H, Weilemann LS, Sonntag HG, Ritz E. Evidence for impaired hepatic Vitamin K metabolism in patients treated with N-methyl-thiotetrazole cephalosporin. Thromb Haemost 1984; 51:358–361.
93. Harter HR, Burch JW, Majerus PW, Stanford N, Delmez JA, Anderson CB, Weerts CA. Prevention of thrombosis in patients on hemodialysis by low dose of aspirin. N Engl J Med 1979; 301:577–579.
94. Lindsay RM, Ferguson D, Prentice CR, Burton JA, McNicol GP. Reduction of thrombus formation on dialyser membranes by aspirin and RA233. Lancet 1972; 2:1287–1290.
95. Livio M, Benigni A, Viganò G, Mecca G, Remuzzi G. Moderate doses of aspirin and risk of bleeding in renal failure. Lancet 1986; 1:414–416.
96. Gaspari F, Viganò G, Orisio S, Bonati M, Livio M, Remuzzi G. Aspirin prolongs bleeding time in uremia by a mechanism distinct from platelet cyclooxygenase inhibition. J Clin Invest 1987; 79:1788–1797.
97. Zuckerman GR, Cornette GL, Clouse RE, Harter HR. Upper gastrointestinal bleeding in patients with chronic renal failure. Ann Intern Med 1985; 102:588–592.
98. Boyle JM, Johnston B. Acute upper gastrointestinal hemorrhage in patients with chronic renal disease. Am J Med 1983; 75:409–412.
99. Remuzzi G, Marchesi D, Livio M, Cavenaghi AE, Mecca G, Donati MB, de Gaetano G. Altered platelet and vascular prostaglandin-generation in patients with renal failure and prolonged bleeding times. Thromb Res 1978; 13:1007–1015.
100. van de Wetering J, Westendorp RGJ, van der Hoeven JG, Stolk B, Feuth JDM, Chang PC. Heparin use in continuous renal replacement procedures: the struggle between filter coagulation and patient hemorrhage. J Am Soc Nephrol 1996; 7:145–150.
101. Gordon LA, Somon ER, Rukes JM, Richards V, Perkins HA. Studies in regional heparinization. N Engl J Med 1956; 255:1063–1066.
102. Maher JF, Lapierre L, Schreiner GE, Geiger M, Westervelt JB. Regional heparinization for hemodialysis. N Engl J Med 1963; 268:451–456.
103. Lindholm DD, Murray JS. A simplified method of regional heparinization during hemodialysis according to a predetermined dosage formula. Trans Am Soc Artif Int Organs 1964; 10:92–97.
104. Blaufox MD, Hampers CL, Merril JP. Rebound anticoagulation occurring after regional heparinization for hemodialysis. Trans Am Soc Artif Int Organs 1966; 12:207–209.
105. Lohr YW, Schwab S. Minimizing hemorrhagic complications in dialysis patients. J Am Soc Nephrol 1991; 2:961–975.
106. Lowr JV, Slussher S, Diederich D. Safety of regional citrate hemodialysis in acute renal failure. Am J Kidney Dis 1989; 2:104–407.
107. Flanigan MJ, Von Brecht J, Freeman RM, Lim VS. Reducing the hemorragic complications of hemodialysis: a controlled comparison of low-dose heparin and citrate anticoagulation. Am J Kidney Dis 1987; 9:147–153.
108. Janssen JFM, Deegens JK, Kapinga TH, Beukhof JR, Huijgens PC, van Loenen AC, van der Meulen J. Citrate compared to low molecular weight heparin anticoagulation in chronic hemodialysis patients. Kidney Int 1996; 49:806–813.
109. Silverstein FJ, Oster JR, Perez GO, Materson BJ, Lopez Ra, Al-Reshaid K. Metabolic alkalosis induced by regional citrate hemodialysis. ASAIO Trans 1989; 35: 22–25.
110. Kelleher SP, Schulman G. Severe metabolic alkalosis complicating regional citrate hemodialysis. Am J Kidney Dis 1987; 9:235–236.
111. Flanigan MJ, Pillsbury L, Sadewasser G, Lim VS. Regional Hemodialysis Anticoagulation: Hypertonic Trisodium citrate or Anticoagulant Citrate Dextrose A. Am J Kidney Dis 1996; 27.4:519–524.
112. Tolkoff-Rubin NE, Nardini J, Fang LST, Rubin RH. Successful hemodialysis of patients at high risk of hemorrhage using the ExVal dialyzer. Dial Transplant 1986; 15:125–126.
113. Liungser B. A low molecular heparin fraction as an anticoagulant during hemodialysis. Clin Nephrol 1985; 25:15–20.

114. Vanholder RC, Camez AA, Veys NM, Sovia Y, Mirshahi M, Soria C, Ringoir S. Recombinant hirudin: a specific thrombin inhibiting anticoagulant for hemodialysis. Kidney Int 1994; 45:1745–1749.
115. van Wijk V, Badenhorst PN, Luus HG, Kotze HF. A comparison between use of recombinant hirudin and heparin during hemodialysis. Kidney Int 1995; 48: 1338–1343.
116. Nurmohamed MT, Hoek JA, Ten Cate JW, Krediet RT, Büller HR. A randomized cross-over study comparing the efficacy and safety of two dosages dermatan sulfate and standard heparin in six chronic hemodialysis patients. Br J Haematol 1990; 76(suppl):23.
117. Ryan KE, Lane DA, Flynn A, Ireland H, Boisclair M, Shepperd J, Curtis JR. Antithrombotic properties of dermatan sulphate (MF 701) in hemodialysis for chronic renal failure. Thromb Haemost 1992; 68:563–569.
118. Fernandez F, van Ryn J, Ofosu F, Hirsh J, Buchanan MR. The haemorragic and antithrombotic effects of dermatan sulphate. Br J Haematol 1986; 64:309–317.
119. Lane DA, Ryan K, Ireland H, Ryan K, Ireland H, Curtis JR, Nurmohamed MT, Krediet RT, Roggekamp MC, Stevens P, ten Cate JW. Dermatan sulphate in haemodialysis. Lancet 1992; 339:334–335.
120. Nurmohamed MT, Knipscheer HC, Stevens P, Krediet RT, Roggekamp MC, Berckmans RJ, ten Cate JW. Clinical experience with a new anticoagulant (dermatan sulphate) in chronic hemodialysis patients. Clin Nephrol 1993; 39:166–171.
121. Gianese F, Nurmohamed MT, Imbimbo BP, Buller HR, Berckmans RJ, Ten Cate JW. The pharmacodynamics of dermatan sulphate MF 701 during haemodialysis for chronic renal failure. Br J Clin Pharmacol 1993; 35:335–339.
122. Nurmohamed MT, Knipscheer HC, Gianese F, Büller HR, Stevens P, Roggekamp MC, ten Cate JW. No clinically relevant accumulation of dermatan sulfate (DS) during chronic use in hemodialysis (abstr). Thromb Haemost 1993; 69:1118.
123. Boccardo P, Melacini D, Rota S, Mecca G, Boletta A, Casiraghi F, Gianese F. Individualized anticoagulation with dermatan sulphate for haemodialysis in chronic renal failure. Nephrol Dialysis Transpl 1997; 12: 2349–2354.
124. Dawson A, Lawinski C, Weston M. Sulfinpyrazone as a method of keeping dialysis membranes clean. In: Frost TH, ed. Technical aspects of Renal Disease. Bath: Pitman Press, 1978.
125. Shaarshmidt BF, Martin JS, Shapiro CG. The use of calcium chelating agents and prostaglandin E_1 to eliminate platelet and white blood cell losses resulting from hemoperfusion through charcoal albumin, aragose gel and neural and neutral and cation exchange resus. J Lab Clin Nephrol 1985; 24:15–20.
126. Morring K, Sinn H, Schuler HW. Comparative evaluation of iatrogenic sources of blood loss during maintenance dialysis. In Proceedings of the 13th Congress of European Dialysis and Transplant Association. Tunbridge Wells: Pitman Medical, 1976:223.
127. Turney JH, Fewell MR, Williams LC, Person V, Weston MJ. Platelet protection and heparin sparing with prostacyclin during regular therapy. Lancet 1980; 2: 219–222.
128. Arze RS, Ward MK. Prostacyclin safer than heparin in haemodialysis. Lancet 1981; 2:50.
129. Zusman RM, Rubin RH, Cato AE, Cocchetto DM, Crow JW, Tolkoff-Rubin N. Hemodialysis using prostacyclin instead of heparin as the sole antithrombotic agent. N Engl J Med 1981; 304:934–939.
130. Swartz RD, Flamenbaum W, Dubrow A, Hall JC, Crow JW, Cato A. Epoprostenol (PGI, prostacyclin) during high risk hemodialysis: preventing further bleeding complications. J Clin Pharmacol 1988; 28: 818–825.
131. Dubrow A, Flamenbaum W, Mittman N, Hall J, Zinn T. Safety and efficacy of epoprostenol (PGI_2) versus heparin in hemodialysis. Trans Am Soc Artif Int Organs 1984; 30:52–54.
132. Jacons J, Shoemaker C, Ruderdorf R. Isolation and characterization of genomic and cDNa clones of human erythropoietin-rich plasma in vivo. J Clin Invest 1984; 74:434–441.
133. Ward DM, Mehta RL. Extracorporeal management of acute renal failure patients at high risk of bleeding. Kidney Int 1993; 41:S237–S244.
134. Sanders PW, Taylor H, Curtis JJ. Hemodialysis without anticoagulation. Am J Kidney Dis 1985; 5:32–35.
135. Lin FK, Suggs S, Lin CH. Cloning and expression of the human erythropoietin gene. PNAS USA 1985; 82: 7580–7584.
136. Winearls CG, Oliver DO, Pippard MJ, Reid C, Downing MR, Coter PM. Effect of human erythropoietin derived from recombinant DNA on the anaemia of patients maintained by chronic hemodialysis. Lancet 1986; 2:1175–1178.
137. Eschbach JW, Egrie JC, Downing MR, Browne JK, Adamson JW. Correction of the anemia and end-stage renal disease with recombinant human erythropoietin: results of a phase I and II clinical trial. N Engl J Med 1987; 316:73–78.
138. Zwaginga JJ, Ijsseldijk MJW, de Groot PG, Kooistra M, Vos J, van-Es A, Koomans HA, Struyvenberg A, Sixma JJ. Treatment of uraemic anemia with recombinant erythropoietin also reduces the defects in platelet adhesion and aggregation caused by uraemic plasma. Thromb Haemost 1991; 66:638–647.
139. Suraib S, Al-Momen AK, Gader AMA. Effect of recombinant human erythropoietin in chronic hemodialysis patients. Thromb Haemost 1989; 61:117.
140. Triulzi DJ, Blumberg N. Variability in response to cryoprecipitate treatment for hemostatic defects in uremia. Yale J Biol Med 1990; 63:1–7.

141. Mannucci PM, Ruggeri ZM, Pareti FI, Capitanio A. 1-Deamino-8D-arginine vasopressin: a new pharmacological approach to the management of haemophilia and von Willebrand's disease. Lancet 1977; 1:869–872.
142. Canavese C, Salomone M, Mangiarotti G, Calitri V. Reduced response of uraemic bleeding time to repeated doses of desmopressin. Lancet 1985; 1:867–868.
143. Shapiro MD, Kelleher SP. Intranasal deamino-8-D-arginine vasopressin shortens the bleeding time in uremia. Am J Nephrol 1984; 4:260–261.
144. Rydzewski A, Rowinski M, Mysliwiec M. Shortening of the bleeding time after intranasal administration of 1-deamino-8-D-arginine vasopressin to patients with chronic anemia. Folia Haematol Int Mag Klin Morphol Blut Forsch 1986; 113:823–830.
145. Viganò G, Mannucci PM, Lattuada A, Harris A, Remuzzi G. Subcutaneous desmopressin (DDAVP) shortens the bleeding time in uremia. Am J Hematol 1989; 31:32–35.
146. Byrnes JJ, Larcada A, Moake JL. Thrombosis following desmopressin for uremic bleeding. Am J Hematol 1988; 28:63–65.
147. Liu YK, Kosfeld RE, Marcum SG. Treatment of uraemic bleeding with conjugated oestrogen. Lancet 1984; 2:887–890.
148. Livio M, Mannucci PM, Vigano GL, Mingardi G, Lombardi R, Mecca G, Remuzzi G. Conjugated estrogens for the management of bleeding associated with renal failure. N Engl J Med 1986; 315:731–735.
149. Viganò G, Gaspari F, Locatelli M, Pusineri F, Bonati M, Remuzzi G. Dose-effect and pharmacokinetics of estrogens given to correct bleeding time in uremia. Kidney Int 1988; 34:853–858.
150. Sloand JA, Schiff MJ. Beneficial effect of low-dose transdermal estrogen on bleeding time and clinical bleeding in uremia. Am J Kidney Dis 1995; 26:22–25.
151. Zoja C, Noris M, Corna D, Viganò G, Perico N, de Gaetano G, Remuzzi G. L-Arginine, the precursor of nitric oxide, abolishes the effect of estrogens on bleeding time in experimental uremia. Lab Invest 1991; 65: 479–483.

18

Arthropathies and Bone Diseases in Hemodialysis and Peritoneal Dialysis Patients

Alkesh Jani, Steven Guest, and Richard A. Lafayette
Stanford University Medical Center, Stanford, California

I. INTRODUCTION

Renal osteodystrophy refers to a collection of bone disorders that affect virtually all patients with end-stage renal disease (ESRD). The term originally described osteitis fibrosa cystica, a high bone-turnover state. In the 1970s, however, it was recognized that excessive aluminum exposure could cause osteomalacia and a low bone-turnover state referred to as adynamic bone disease. It is now recognized that patients may be affected by a combination of these disorders and that mild forms exist. The frequency and pathological findings for each of these disorders are listed in Table 1.

This chapter will describe the clinical and pathological features of the bone disorders collectively referred to as renal osteodystrophy. The additive role that metabolic acidosis may play in these disorders is discussed in a separate section.

II. OSTEITIS FIBROSA CYSTICA

The most common form of renal osteodystrophy is osteitis fibrosa cystica (OFC). This lesion is defined by specific changes in bone architecture, including:

1. Bone marrow fibrosis
2. A parathyroid hormone (PTH)–stimulated increase in the number and activity of osteoclasts
3. An increase in osteoid and nonlamellar bone which defines OFC as a high-turnover bone disease

OFC is typically asymptomatic until end-stage renal disease (ESRD), when bone pain and fractures may occur. However, as discussed in the next section, the changes that result in OFC generally start well before dialysis is initiated.

A. Pathophysiology of OFC

OFC is due to secondary hyperparathyroidism. The primary event is phosphate retention, which typically occurs when the GFR falls below normal. PTH-dependent enhanced urinary phosphate excretion maintains serum phosphorus levels in the normal range, until the GFR falls below 30 mL/min (2). Phosphate loading in rats with varying degrees of renal failure results in an elevated serum PTH due to reduced calcium levels and a coincident reduction in calcitriol (3,4). Elevated serum phosphate itself may also directly stimulate PTH secretion. Conversely, phosphate restriction in dogs with renal insufficiency prevents the development of secondary hyperparathyroidism despite worsening renal function (5). PTH functions to maintain serum calcium and phosphate within normal range. In early renal failure, its release should therefore be seen as an appropriate response. PTH maintains calcium-phosphorus ($Ca\text{-}PO_4$) homeostasis in three ways:

Special thanks to Henry Jones, M.D., Professor Emeritus, Radiology, Stanford University School of Medicine, Stanford, California.

Table 1 Frequency and Pathological Findings

Disease	Frequency (%)	Cause	Pathology
Osteitis fibrosa cystica	50	Secondary hyperparathyroidism	Bone marrow fibrosis Resorption/Remodeling
Osteomalacia	7	Aluminum deposition	Increased osteoid
Mixed disease	13	Secondary hyperparathyroidism and aluminum deposition	Mixed features
Mild disease	3	Early secondary hyperparathyroidism	Increased remodeling
Adynamic bone disease	27	Aluminum deposition	Hypocellularity and no remodeling

Source: Adapted from Ref. 1.

1. It reduces proximal tubule phosphate reabsorbtion from 75–80% to 15% (6).
2. It increases the activity of osteoclasts, resulting in an increase in the serum calcium (4).
3. It promotes the 1 hydroxylation of 25-hydroxy cholecalciferol, resulting in active vitamin D.

As renal failure progresses, excretion of phosphate decreases further, as does production of vitamin D. The resulting hypocalcemia allows for uninhibited PTH secretion and parathyroid gland hyperplasia. Increased osteoclast activity ensues, resulting in bone resorption. Bone marrow fibrosis is thought to occur when stimulated bone marrow mesenchymal cells differentiate into secretory fibroblast-like cells (1).

B. Laboratory Findings/Investigations

1. Serum Calcium

Serum calcium levels are typically low in patients with ESRD and secondary hyperparathyroidism. However, spuriously low values can result from plasma samples or stored serum samples because of adsorption of calcium to the tube or precipitation within the sample. Errors can be reduced if samples are measured expeditiously and if serum is used rather than plasma. Parathyroid cells in uremic patients have decreased sensitivity to calcium. Therefore, a greater serum calcium is needed to inhibit secretion of PTH. A consensus conference on use of calcitriol in dialysis patients with hyperparathyroidism (7) recommended that serum calcium should be maintained at approximately 10–11.5 mg/dL.

2. Serum Phosphorus

Phosphorus is primarily an intracellular anion, and efflux of phosphorus from this compartment to the extracellular space is slow. Consequently, phosphate is poorly cleared by dialysis (~25–30% the clearance of urea). This problem may be exacerbated by the use of recombinant human erythropoeitin, which increases hemocrit and therefore reduces the amount of plasma cleared by the dialyzer (8). The recommended dietary phosphate intake in normal individuals is 800 mg/day (9), while dialysis removes 250–350 mg of the anion per session. Most dialysis patients, therefore, remain in positive phosphate balance without additional therapy.

3. Serum Alkaline Phosphate

Antigenically different forms of alkaline phosphatase are produced by the liver, intestine, kidney, and placenta. Skeletal origin can be confirmed by checking for the specific isoenzyme. In bone, alkaline phosphatase is found anchored to osteoblast cell membranes (10). [In contrast, acid phosphatase is anchored to osteoclast membranes (11).] Increased osteoblastic activity, as occurs with bone remodeling, will lead to an elevation in serum levels of alkaline phosphatase. Serum bone alkaline phosphatase has been found to correlate with the extent of bone osteoblast surface and volume of fibrosis (12). Serum bone alkaline phosphatase can be a useful clinical indicator of the extent of OFC. Levels greater than 20 ng/mL are very suggestive of high-turnover bone disease (13), whereas decreasing values can indicate a response to therapy. Rising serum levels usually indicate progression of OFC, even if the increase is seen within the normal range. However, it is important to note that many patients with abnormal bone architecture have normal levels of alkaline phosphatase (14).

4. Serum PTH

Mature PTH is an 84-amino-acid protein made by the chief cells of the parathyroid glands. The biological activity of PTH resides in the N terminus (amino acids

1–34), while the midportion and C terminus are inactive. The liver cleaves the mature hormone into N-terminal fragments as well as C-terminal fragments. The latter accounts for most of the circulating PTH in the serum of patients with renal failure, as it is cleared mainly by the kidney and has a longer half-life. Since N-terminal and C-terminal fragments can accumulate in renal failure, intact PTH levels should be measured to avoid overestimation of the serum level. Immunoradiometric (IRMA) and immunochemiluminometric (ICMA) assays employ specific two-site antibodies to measure intact hormone and are the preferred tests in patients with renal failure.

In dialysis patients, bone marrow fibrosis does not typically occur until PTH levels exceed 250 pg/mL, and severe OFC is seen with levels greater than ~500 pg/mL. However, PTH levels below 120 pg/mL are more likely to be associated with adynamic bone disease (15). These observations suggest that the ideal serum PTH in a patient with ESRD is not known, and serial serum measurements are required to prevent undertreatment or overvigorous suppression of PTH.

C. Radiological Findings of OFC

Radiological abnormalities indicative of secondary hyperparathyroidism are seen in ~50% of patients with renal failure, and these patients invariably have increased resorption on bone biopsy. Subperiosteal resorption is the most widely recognized finding of OFC and occurs most commonly in the phalanges and hands (Fig. 1). Resorption can also be seen at the distal ends of the clavicles, as well as in the pelvis, ribs, and mandible. Skull x-rays in these patients are often described as having a "salt-and-pepper" appearance, indicating widespread mottling (Fig. 2). This is due to alternating areas of increased cortical resorption and enhanced trabecular density. Other typical findings include erosion of the tufts of the terminal phalanx, cyst formation (Fig. 3), and osteosclerosis. Fig. 4 demonstrates the "Rugger-Jersey" spine of secondary hyperparathyroidism.

D. Indications for Bone Biopsy

As noted previously, serum alkaline phosphatase and PTH levels are useful as correlates of disease severity. They are poor indicators, however, of the type of renal osteodystrophy present. The gold standard for establishing a diagnosis is bone biopsy, but the indications for undertaking this procedure are controversial. Biopsies are generally performed for two indications: (1) to assess the extent of aluminum accumulation prior to therapy with desferoxamine, and (2) to diagnose adynamic bone disease in patients who are symptomatic, with a serum PTH level of <100 pg/mL. Whether a biopsy should be performed on a patient with a serum PTH between 150 and 450 pg/mL is unclear. An alternative approach would be to assume that this most likely represents early OFC and to empirically start calcium supplements, phosphate binders, and, if indicated (i.e., if serum PTH > 400 pg/mL), calcitriol.

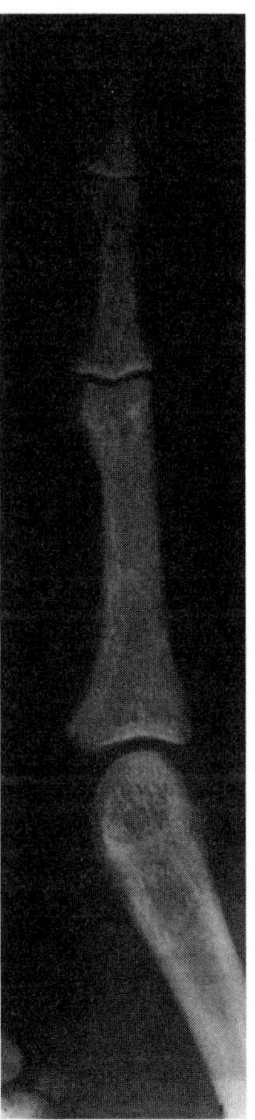

Fig. 1 Subperiosteal resorption and distal phalangeal tuft erosions in a dialysis patient with secondary hyperparathyroidism.

E. Treatment of Osteitis Fibrosa Cystica

1. The Predialysis Patient

Slatopolsky et al. demonstrated that dietary phosphate restriction could entirely prevent the development of secondary hyperparathyroidism in dogs (5). Correction of serum phosphate to 4.5–5.5 mg/dL in children with moderate renal insufficiency (GFR = 45 ± 4 mL/min/1.73 m^2) has been shown to improve hypocalcemia,

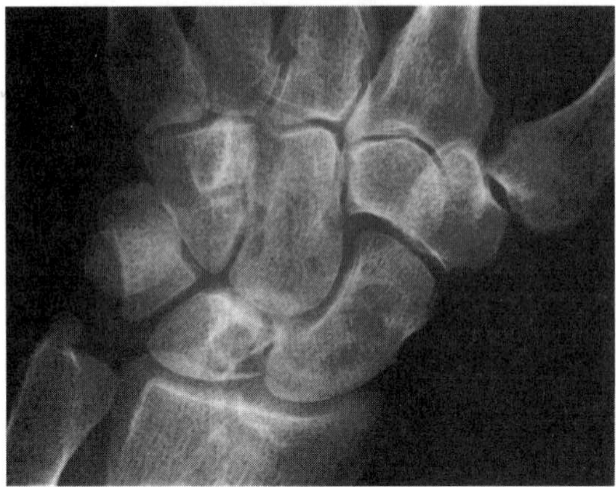

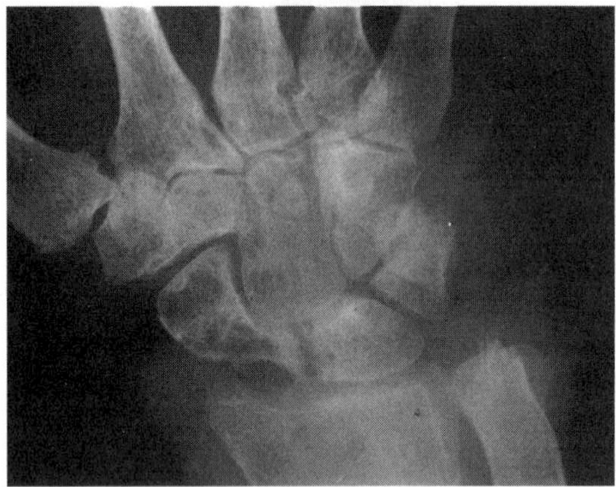

Fig. 2 Cyst formation in the carpal bones and distal phalanges in a patient with dialysis-related amyloidosis.

hyperparathyroidism, and calcitriol deficiency (16). Similar effects can be seen with calcitriol therapy. Szabo et al. demonstrated that administration of 1,25-$(OH)_2$ vitamin D_3 could prevent but not cause, regression of parathyroid cell proliferation in experimental uremia (17). The primary limitation to the use of calcitriol in predialysis patients is the development of hypercalcemia, which could hasten progression to ESRD. Hypercalcemia is seen primarily with doses of ≥ 1 μg/day. A reduction of serum PTH with improvement of renal osteodystrophy has been shown to occur with as little as 0.25 μg/day of calcitriol (18). These studies suggest that secondary hyperparathyroidism can be effectively prevented by control of serum phosphate and judicious use of calcitriol. Serial monitoring of serum calcium levels is important in this setting to avoid hypercalcemia and its potential complications. It should be noted, however, that predialysis patients require a greater serum PTH to maintain a normal osteoblast surface than dialysis patients (16). This study implies that PTH resistance is severe in predialysis patients and has led a reviewer to suggest withholding calcitriol therapy unless serum PTH levels are greater than 400 pg/mL (19). More studies of this patient population are needed to confirm these initial observations, but based on present findings it would seem prudent to actively treat predialysis patients in the hope of preventing the development of OFC.

Treatment recommendations for the predialysis patient are as follows:

Serial monitoring of serum phosphorus as the GFR falls below 30 mL/min.

Dietary phosphorus restriction and, if necessary, use of phosphate binders once serum phosphorus rises above 5.5 mg/dL.

Institution of low-dose calcitriol (0.25 μg/day) therapy if intact serum PTH levels rise above 400 mg/dL, with close monitoring to prevent hypercalcemia. (Data from ESRD patients suggest this therapy is unlikely to be effective if serum phosphorus is not controlled first.)

2. The Dialysis Patient

Slatopolsky et al. recently demonstrated that high phosphate directly stimulated posttranscriptional PTH secretion in tissue culture (20). As with predialysis patients, the first step in management of bone disease in the dialysis population is to control serum phosphate. The following is a discussion of the treatment options available to achieve this goal as well as the other biochemical abnormalities of secondary hyperparathyroidism.

a. Control of Dietary Phosphate

Phosphorus is particularly abundant in proten-rich foods and cereals. Approximately half of the dietary phosphorus in the United States comes from milk, meat, poultry, and fish. Significantly greater amounts of phosphorus are found in processed cheese and meat than in their natural counterparts. Dialysis patients should ideally be restricted to less than 800 mg/day of phosphorus. This is difficult to achieve since many dialysis patients are already malnourished, and limiting phosphate intake could further limit their protein intake. This problem can be partially offset by increasing the proportion of dietary protein with high biological value, such as meat and eggs. Phosphorus-rich food with low biological value, such as dairy products, colas, and processed foods, should obviously be avoided. These measures can help reduce serum phosphorus lev-

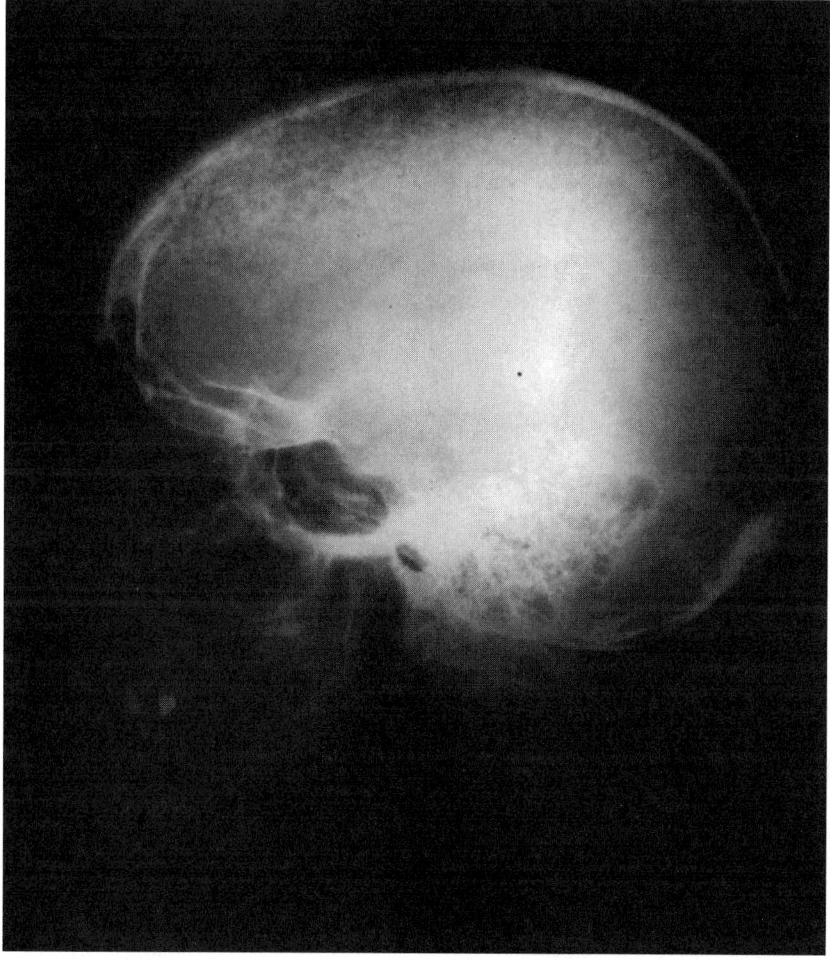

Fig. 3 Skull x-ray demonstrating typical "salt and pepper" appearance caused by hyperparathyroidism.

els, but almost invariably dialysis patients will require medication to achieve this goal.

The treatment recommendation is as follows:

Maintain patients on a diet of ≤800 mg/day of phosphorus, derived from high–biological value protein.

b. Phosphate Binders

Several types of phosphate binders are currently available. All act by forming insoluble complexes with dietary phosphorus, which is then excreted in the stool. The binders differ significantly, however, with respect to their side effects.

Magnesium-containing phosphate binders, such as magnesium hydroxide, are infrequently used because of their propensity to cause potentially serious hypermagnesemia. Furthermore, these agents are effective cathartics, resulting in decreased patient compliance.

For many years, aluminum-containing phosphate binders were the phosphate binders of choice. During the 1970s, it was discovered that an accumulation of aluminum, from either the binding agents or the dialysis water supply, could cause bone disease (1). Consequently, binders containing calcium have largely replaced these agents. Aluminum salts also have additional disadvantages (see below).

Slatopolsky et al. demonstrated that hyperphosphatemia could be controlled in ~70% of dialysis patients using calcium carbonate (21). This agent requires an acid medium to function effectively and is therefore not as useful in patients treated with H_2 blockers. Calcium acetate, however, binds phosphorus more effectively, and its use is not limited by intestinal pH. Both agents

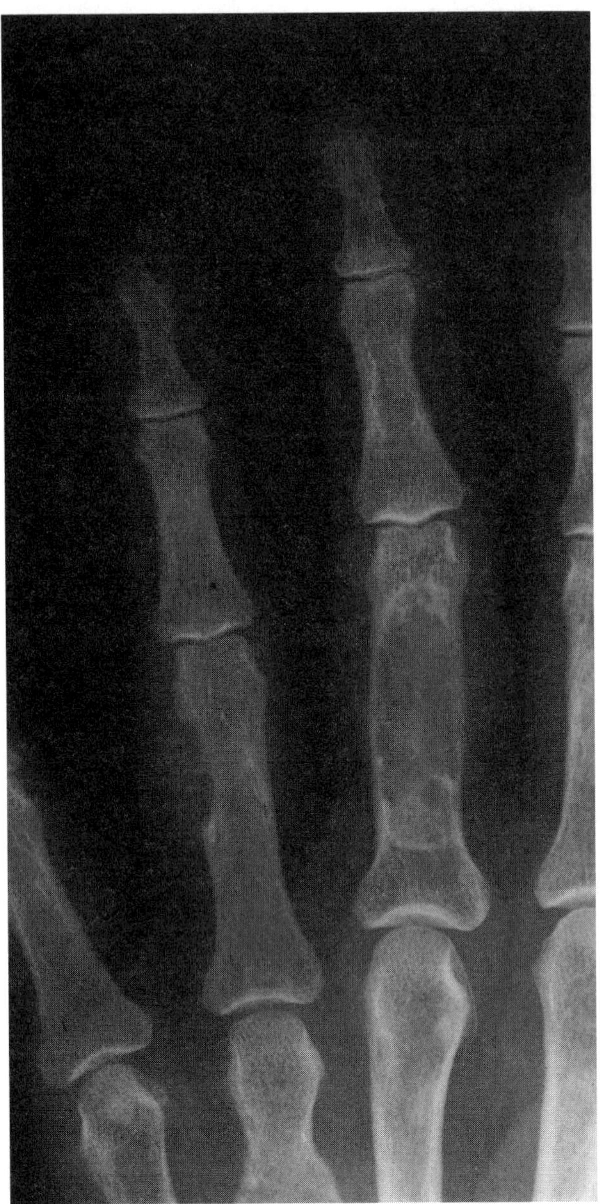

Fig. 4 Severe cystic changes affecting the phalangeal bones of a dialysis patient with secondary hyperparathyroidism.

bind dietary phosphorus and are therefore given with food. If taken between meals they can serve as a calcium supplement since they are relatively well absorbed. The primary side effect of this class of binders is hypercalcemia. Metastatic calcification can occur if the Ca-PO_4 product is >70, and in this setting the binder should be discontinued. An aluminum salt can be used temporarily in this situation. Once the calcium-phosphorus (Ca-PO_4) product decreases, the calcium salt can be started again in addition to a "low" dialysate calcium of 2.5 mg/dL (see below).

Treatment recommendations are as follows:

Use calcium binders as the agents of choice. Avoid magnesium-based binders.

Aim for a serum calcium level of >10 mg/dL and a serum phosphate level of <5.5 mg/dL.

Use binders with meals to most efficiently limit phosphate absorption.

Avoid hypercalcemia (serum calcium > 11.5 mg/dL) and a Ca-PO_4 product of >70. Should this occur, switch temporarily to an aluminum-based binder, and consider a lower dialysate calcium.

Use calcium acetate in patients with H_2 blockers or patients who have achlorhydria.

c. *New Phosphorus-Binding Agents*

Cross-linked poly(allylamine hydrochloride), or Renagel, is a phosphate binder that does not contain magnesium, aluminum, or calcium. It binds preferentially to trivalent anions such as phosphate and citrate and has no gastrointestinal absorption. Renagel also binds bile acids and increases their excretion. In normal human volunteers, Renagel given in doses of 2.5 and 5 g three times a day significantly reduced urinary phosphate excretion compared to placebo. Mean serum phosphorus and calcium levels did not differ between treatment and placebo groups. Subjects treated with 1, 2.5, and 5 g of Renagel also had significant reductions of 15–25% in total cholesterol from baseline. This effect was ascribed to bile acid–binding properties (22). Chertow et al. (23) found that Renagel, 3.5 g per day, significantly reduced serum phosphorus (6.6 ± 2.1 mg/dL to 5.4 ± 1.5 mg/dL) over 2 weeks of treatment. Serum cholesterol was also significantly reduced (from 173 ± 37 to 149 ± 32 mg/dL) when compared to placebo-treated patients. LDL levels were also significantly reduced, but HDL levels remained unchanged. Goldberg et al. (24) evaluated Renagel in 48 hemodialysis patients over an 8-week period. Renagel was dosed to achieve serum phosphorus control. The mean daily dosage was approximately 4.5 g and varied directly with dietary phosphate intake. Renagel produced significantly lower serum phosphorus at the end of the treatment period, and the mean reduction in serum phosphorus was 1.4 mg/dL.

d. *Calcitriol Therapy*

Activated vitamin D_3 suppresses PTH synthesis directly, although the exact mechanism for this effect is uncertain. Calcitriol causes decreased PTH mRNA concentration in cultured bovine cells (25). The levels of vitamin D_3 typically start to fall when the GFR drops below 30 mL/min (26) and ESRD is characterized as a calcitriol-deficient state. In uremic patients, vitamin D_3 receptor binding (27) and receptor density (28) within the parathyroid gland are reduced, especially in areas of nodular hyperplasia, which are more apt to develop in hyperplastic glands (29). These observations provide the rationale for use of calcitriol in patients with ESRD and secondary hyperparathyroidism.

Calcitriol is given either orally or intravenously. Continuous calcitriol refers to daily oral therapy, while intermittent therapy denotes pulse therapy, usually given at the end of dialysis. Controversy exists as to which route of administration and which schedule is superior. Initial observations suggested that pulse intravenous therapy was better than pulse oral therapy, because much higher peak serum levels are obtained with the former (30). However, other studies have failed to show that this effect causes better suppression of PTH (31) or that either route has a greater tendency to hypercalcemia. At this time there are insufficient data to suggest that one route is better than the other. The literature regarding continuous versus pulse therapy is also contradictory, with some investigators able to suggest a difference (32) between the two modes of administration, while others could not. The question is somewhat moot, since most dialysis units prefer to employ pulse intravenous therapy because of convenience, reimbursement issues, and to ensure patient compliance.

Not all patients respond successfully to calcitriol therapy. Felsenfeld suggests that high PTH and hyperphosphatemia identify patients who will have a poor response to therapy (19). Consensus conference guidelines from the American Society of Nephrology annual meeting in 1994 suggest that all patients with a serum PTH > 200 pg/mL be treated with IV calcitriol (7). Furthermore, mild to moderate hyperparathyroidism, defined as a PTH of 200–600 pg/mL in asymptomatic patients, should be treated with an initial dose of 0.5–1 μg/dialysis. Moderate to severe hyperparathyroidism, with serum PTH levels of 600–1200 pg/mL, should be started on 2–4 μg/dialysis. This dose was found by Cannella et al. (33) to control the hyperparathyroidism of patients with a mean serum PTH of 900 pg/mL. However, Quarles et al. (31) were not able to reproduce these findings in patients with serum PTH > 900 pg/mL using similar doses of calcitriol. Hyperphosphatemia was well controlled in the former study, whereas patients in the latter group required much higher doses of phosphate binders. As noted, patients who have uncontrolled hyperphosphatemia are unlikely to have an optimal response to calcitriol. A markedly elevated serum PTH does not preclude controlling secondary hyperparathyroidism with calcitriol. Dressler et al. (34) showed that severe hyperparathyroidism, defined as a PTH > 1200 pg/mL, can be controlled using a mean dose of 4 μg/dialysis. Six patients required a mean maximum dose of 8 μg/dialysis. These findings suggest that such patients may have nodular hyperplasia and relative vitamin D resistance.

The ultimate aim of therapy is to achieve a PTH two to three times the upper limit of normal, or ~130–190 pg/mL. As stated, bone marrow fibrosis is not typically seen until serum PTH exceeds ~200 pg/mL. Normalization and stabilization of serum bone alkaline phosphatase (or total alkaline phosphatase) should parallel the fall in PTH.

As mentioned, the most frequent side effects of calcitriol therapy are hypercalcemia and hyperphosphatemia. Calcitriol should not be used unless the serum phosphate level is <6 mg/dL. Hyperphosphatemia can both reduce the efficacy of calcitriol and put the patient at increased risk of metastatic calcification.

Treatment recommendations include the following:

Control hyperphosphatemia (aim for level of <6 mg/dL) before initiating calcitriol therapy.

For a PTH of 200–600 pg/mL, start calcitriol at a dose of 0.5–1.0 μg/dialysis.

For a PTH of 600–1200 pg/mL, start calcitriol at a dose of 2–4 μg/dialysis.

For a PTH of >1200 pg/mL, use calcitriol at a dose of 4–8 μg/dialysis *only* if hyperphosphatemia is well controlled.

Aim for a PTH of ~130–190 pg/mL. Avoid oversuppression of parathyroid gland activity.

Follow serum calcium levels in anticipation of hypercalcemia.

e. *Concentration of Dialysate Calcium*

Dialysate calcium usually varies between 2.5 and 3.5 mEq/L in hemodialysis and 1 and 1.75 mmol/L in peritoneal dialysis solutions. The "correct" concentration of dialysate calcium should be determined for each individual patient based on his or her calcium balance. The goal should be to induce positive calcium balance, suppress PTH secretion, and at the same time prevent the attendant effects of hypercalcemia, namely extraosseous calcification. Early reports suggested that a positive calcium balance could be achieved with 2.5 mEq/L hemodialysate calcium concentration (35).

More recent studies have shown that use of a 2.5 mEq/L solution can cause an increase in serum PTH levels over the long term. However, the authors found that this effect could be reversed with 1-α-hydroxyvitamin D (36). Use of a 2.5 mEq/L calcium solution would be reasonable in patients with a low PTH who are taking calcium-based phosphate binders and calcitriol. These patients should be monitored for increases in PTH. Dialysate solutions containing 3 and 3.5 mEq/L, on the other hand, do cause a positive calcium balance and result in suppression of PTH (37). In these patients care must be taken to avoid hyperalcemia and extraosseous calcification.

Weinrich et al. (38) compared the use of a 2.0 mEq/L CAPD bath with a standard 3.5 mEq/L bath. The low-calcium bath resulted in significantly lower serum calcium and less need for aluminum binders. However, severe hyperparathyroidism occurred in 23% of the patients in this group, compared to 10.3% in the patients using the standard calcium bath. Thus, as with hemodialysis patients, use of lower dialysate calcium concentration in CAPD patients must be carried out judiciously and with close monitoring of serum PTH.

Treatment recommendations are as follows:

Tailor dialysate calcium concentrations to ensure a positive calcium balance and suppression of PTH secretion, while avoiding hypercalcemia.

Use calcium-based phosphate binders and calcitriol if a dialysate concentration of 2.5 mEq/L is employed. Be vigilant for changes in serum PTH.

Follow serum calcium and Ca × PO_4 product when using dialysate calcium concentrations of >3.0 mEq/L.

f. Parathyroidectomy

Parathyroidectomy is typically reserved for severe secondary hyperparathyroidism with debilitating OFC, untreatable pruritis, severe persistent hypercalcemia despite medical therapy, calciphylaxis, or severe extraosseous calcification. Adynamic bone disease can mimic OFC and be worsened by parathyroidectomy. One should, therefore, confirm that the serum PTH is severely elevated (typically > 1000 pg/mL, although there are no absolute values) prior to surgery.

III. ALUMINUM-INDUCED BONE DISEASE

Aluminum gels have been widely used as phosphate-binding agents. The aluminum-phosphate complex was originally thought to be excreted as an insoluble complex in stool, with little gastrointestinal absorbtion. However, absorption of aluminum was subsequently demonstrated in both normal (39) and dialysis-dependent subjects (40). Aluminum toxicity was then implicated as a cause of encephalopathy, anemia, debilitating muscle and joint pain, and renal osteodystrophy.

The primary sources of aluminum are phosphate-binding gels and local water supplies. Aluminum in dialysate water enters the serum readily and becomes highly protein bound (90%), limiting the degree to which dialysis can remove aluminum from plasma (41). Water purification systems utilizing reverse osmosis, deionization, and demineralization can effectively prevent aluminum intoxication from dialysate water. Aluminum antacids have for the most part been supplanted by calcium-containing phosphate binders. Aluminum-based gels are still used, however, when hypercalcemia and high–calcium-phosphate products preclude the use of calcium-containing binders.

A. Manifestations of Aluminum Toxicity

Aluminum toxicity results in a variety of systemic effects, including neurotoxicity, renal osteodystrophy, anemia and bone and muscle pain. Alfrey et al. (40) showed that patients with dialysis-associated encephalopathy have significantly greater gray-matter aluminum deposition than normal controls or dialysis patients without dementia. The majority of patients who develop encephalopathy have been on dialysis for 3–7 years. The clinical features of this syndrome include focal seizures, dementia, myoclonus, asterixis, and dysarthria. Abnormal EEG patterns of generalized slowing punctuated by bursts of delta wave activity may precede the clinical findings by 3–6 months (41).

Aluminum causes two forms of renal osteodystrophy: osteomalacia and adynamic bone disease (42). The more prevalent form is osteomalacia, which is characterized by an increase in osteoid volume and decreased rate of bone turnover. In contrast, the adynamic form results in a loss of osteoid volume and diminished tetracycline uptake. Andress et al. (43) demonstrated that aluminum deposition occurred more quickly in hemodialysis patients with type 1 diabetes as compared to nondiabetic hemodialysis patients. Decreased serum PTH and a low rate of bone turnover in diabetics (44) may account for the more aggressive disease seen in this population. A similar form of accelerated deposition is seen in patients with aluminum-induced bone disease after parathyroidectomy.

Patients with evidence of aluminum-induced bone disease often complain of debilitating muscle and bone disease. These symptoms are typically unresponsive to therapy with vitamin D but may respond to therapy with deferoxamine (45).

Aluminum toxicity also causes a microcytic anemia that does not respond to therapy with iron. How aluminum affects hematopoesis is unclear. Cannata et al. (42) theorized that aluminum might interfere with iron uptake both in the gastrointestinal tract and in red blood cells.

B. Diagnosis of Aluminum-Induced Bone Disease

The gold standard for diagnosis of aluminum-induced osteodystrophy is bone biopsy, which typically reveals extensive accumulation of aluminum at the mineralization front (46). Due to the invasive nature of this procedure, surrogate markers of aluminum deposition in bone have been investigated.

Serum aluminum levels do not consistently reflect bone deposition or symptoms related to aluminum toxicity (47). Aluminum is ubiquitous, and contamination makes accurate serum measurements difficult. Furthermore, iron balance can affect serum aluminum, regardless of the concentration in bone. Iron overload may reduce serum aluminum, even in the presence of extensive bone deposition (48). Conversely, patients with iron deficiency may have increased serum aluminum concentrations independent of body aluminum burden (46). Despite these difficulties, some investigators suggest that patients with markedly elevated serum levels (>40–75 μg/L) and persistent aluminum consumption will most likely develop bone disease or encephalopathy. These authors therefore recommend monitoring of serum aluminum levels every 3–4 months (49).

The deferoxamine stimulation test has been used to predict the presence of aluminum-induced osteodystrophy. Deferoxamine (DFO) is a chelating agent that releases aluminum from body stores and complexes with it in the serum. Malluche et al. (45) found serum aluminum levels to be consistently increased by DFO stimulation in 12 patients with aluminum deposition in bone. However, 4 out of 10 without aluminum deposition also had equivalent or greater stimulated increases in serum aluminum. The authors concluded that the deferoxamine test could not be used to accurately diagnose aluminum deposition. D'Haese et al. (50) used a low-dose DFO test (5 mg/kg) in combination with serum iPTH levels to detect the presence of aluminum-related bone disease. They found that a DFO-stimulated increase in serum aluminum of 50 μg/L above baseline and a serum iPTH threshold of <150 mg/L had a sensitivity of 87% and a specificity of 95% in detecting aluminum-related bone disease.

C. Treatment of Aluminum-Induced Bone Disease

DFO can also be used for the treatment of aluminum-induced bone disease. Malluche et al. (45) used a regimen of 14.25 mg/kg three times a week for hemodialysis patients and 85 mg/kg per week for peritoneal dialysis patients. Treatment was given for up to 10 months and resulted in reduced muscle and joint pain by 2–4 weeks together with decreased serum aluminum levels, reduced or absent bone aluminum, and an increase in osteoblastic/osteoclastic activity. Hypotension, anemia, visual disturbances, and cataract formation were not encountered during the study. Adverse reactions to DFO have been reported, however. The most serious reaction is the development of severe and sometimes fatal fungal infections. Boelaert et al. (51) reported 59 cases of mucormycosis occurring in dialysis patients. Known risk factors such as diabetes, liver disease, neutropenia, splenectomy, and steroid use were present in only 30% of the patients. However, treatment with DFO was a historical feature in 78% of the subjects. Dosage ranged from 0.3 to 7.4 g/week, and patients were treated for a mean of 10 months (3 weeks to 36 months). Twenty percent of the infected received doses of <1.5 g/week. The course of the infection was fulminant, with death occurring an average 12 ± 6.6 days after the first sign of infection. Twenty-two infected patients were treated with amphotericin B, of whom only 8 survived. Culture results were available in 36% of the cases and always revealed the genus *Rhizopus*. The mechanism by which DFO predisposes to mucor is unclear. It appears that the iron-chelate of DFO may inhibit the fungistatic properties of serum and stimulate growth by increasing fungal iron uptake (52).

DFO therapy can also cause acute hearing and visual loss. These complications were reported in thirteen of 89 non-dialysis patients treated with DFO for transfusion dependent Thalassemia. A further 27 patients were found to have an abnormal visual evoked response, as well as abnormal ophthalmologic, and audiologic assessments. A small number of patients recovered with cessation of DFO therapy. The doses used in this group ranged from 95–123 mg/kg/day (53). This report illustrates the need for baseline and serial audiovisual exams in all patients receiving DFO.

These reports led Barata et al. (54) to treat patients with lower doses of DFO (5 mg/kg once a week for 6 months). This regimen produced markedly lower baseline and stimulated serum aluminum levels and a significant increase in serum iPTH and mean corpuscular volume. In patients known to have a stimulated serum aluminum level of >300 mg/dL, the authors took the precaution of administering the drug 5 hours before dialysis. This limited exposure to circulating DFO-iron complexes, while still providing the same chelation. High-flux polysulfone hemodialyzers allow for substantially increased removal of DFO-aluminum complexes compared to conventional membranes (55).

Diagnosis and treatment recommendations are as follows:

- Serum aluminum levels should be obtained in all patients every 4 months.
- Bone biopsy in the gold standard for diagnosing aluminum-related bone disease.
- Bone biopsy should be considered in patients who are symptomatic and have increasing serum aluminum levels.
- The low-dose DFO test in combination with serum iPTH measurements may diagnose the presence of aluminum-related bone disease.
- Limited exposure to aluminum can be ensured by avoidance of aluminum-containing gels and careful water treatment.
- Low-dose regimens (e.g., 5 mg/kg once a week for 6 months) of DFO should be used to treat aluminum-related bone disease.
- High-flux polysulfone hemodialyzers should be used when DFO therapy is started to maximize clearance of DFO-aluminum complexes.
- Baseline and serial audiovisual exams are suggested for the duration of therapy.

IV. DIALYSIS-RELATED AMYLOIDOSIS

β_2-Microglobulin was first identified as the major protein in dialysis-associated amyloidosis in 1985 (56). This form of amyloidosis is now recognized as unique because of its predilection for bones and joints, with relatively little systemic involvement. β_2-Microglobulin amyloidosis typically manifests in patients who have been dialyzed for extended periods. Laurent et al. (57) found that carpal tunnel syndrome was rare in patients dialyzed less than 5 years, but ubiquitous in patients dialyzed longer than 18 years. Dialysis-associated amyloidosis appears to occur with equal prevalence in hemodialysis and peritoneal dialysis populations when matched for age and duration of dialysis (58).

Approximately 200 mg of β_2-microglobulin is formed per day in uremic patients (59). This is normally degraded by proteases in the renal tubular epithelium (60). Absent glomerular filtration leads to decreased metabolism and markedly elevated levels. No correlation exists, however, between the serum level of β_2-microglobulin and the severity of dialysis-associated amyloidosis (61).

A. Clinical Manifestations

The lesions of dialysis-associated amyloidosis are usually confined to the musculoskeletal system. Zingraff et al. (62) identified the sterno-clavicular joint as the region most commonly affected by β_2-microglobulin deposition. Another commonly affected location is the shoulder, often in conjunction with deposition in the carpal tunnel (Fig. 5). Chary-Valckenaere et al. (63) found that carpal tunnel syndrome was caused predominately, but not exclusively, by β_2-microglobulin deposition. Amyloid deposition correlated with arthralgia and long-term dialysis. Flexor tenosynovitis and carpal bone erosion also occurred more frequently in patients with a histological diagnosis of amyloidosis. Recurrence of carpal tunnel syndrome occurred only in those patients with β_2-microglobulin deposition (63). Amyloid deposition can also occur in tendons and cause trigger finger, flexor tendon contracture, and spontaneous tendon rupture (64). Fatal cervical spondyloarthropathy has been reported in patients on dialysis for extended periods of time (65). Ohashi et al. (66) found that the C4-C7 region was particularly susceptible to β_2-microglobulin deposition and postulated that severe mechanical stress accelerated cervical amyloidosis. Although uncommon, systemic deposits of β_2-microglobulin can occur, usually in the heart, lungs, gastrointestinal tract, and blood vessels. These deposits are usually of no consequence (67) but can result in dire complications such as intestinal infarction (68).

B. Diagnosis

Radiographic features of dialysis-associated amyloidosis include subchondral cysts (Fig. 6), soft tissue masses, replacement of normal bone by amyloid deposits, and fractures. X-rays can underestimate the extent of β_2-microglobulin deposition and are, at best, a screening test during the initial work-up. CT scan and MRI more accurately define the extent of the lesion (69). Radionuclide bone scans tend to be nonspecific,

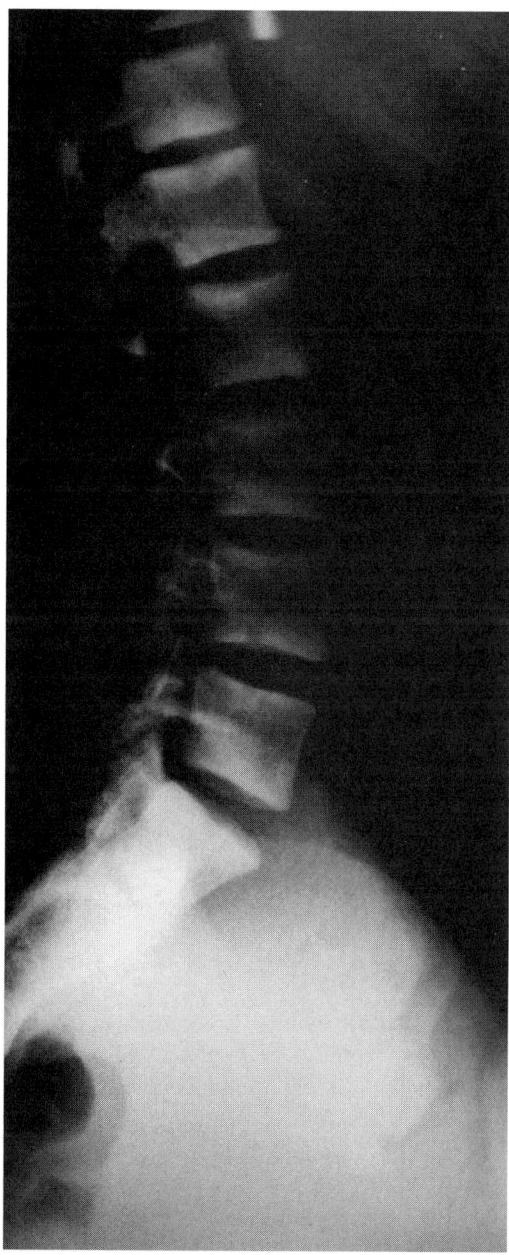

Fig. 5 Wide bands of calcification at the vertebral cortical end plates resulting in the "Rugger-Jersey" spine of secondary hyperparathyroidism.

and it is difficult to determine whether positive scans reveal joint involvement by amyloidosis or some other synovitides. Definitive diagnosis can only be made by histological examination of tissue obtained from the involved joint. As with all amyloidoses, Congo red staining produces apple-green birefringence under polarized light. Anti-β_2-microglobulin antibodies can differentiate dialysis-related amyloid from other forms. Dialysis-related amyloid can also be differentiated from AA or AL amyloidosis by the electron-microscopic appearance of the fibrils.

C. Treatment

High-flux dialyzers remove β_2-microglobulin more efficiently than conventional dialyzers (70). Indeed, dialysis with regenerated cellulose membranes increases serum β_2-microglobulin by 10–15%. In contrast, serum β_2-microglobulin is reduced by 8% using polycarbonate membranes and by 53% with polysulfone membranes (71). The superior removal is due to both increased membrane permeability and biocompatibility (72). Dialyzer reuse has no significant effect on β_2-microglobulin removal (70). Treatment should therefore be aimed at maximizing removal of β_2-microglobulin with high-flux membranes and vigilance for signs and symptoms of amyloidosis in long-term dialysis patients.

Renal transplantation appears to prevent further deposition of β_2-microglobulin, assuming stable graft function. Bardin et al. (73) found that joint symptoms were significantly improved after transplantation. The size and number of subchondral bone erosions did not improve, however, and destructive arthropathy was seen to worsen in some patients (73).

Patients on dialysis for longer than 5 years should be periodically assessed for signs of cervical spondyloarthropathy, joint destruction and carpal tunnel syndrome.
Amyloidosis should be considered in long-term hemodialysis patients complaining of musculoskeletal pain, persistent gastrointestinal symptoms, or cervical radiculopathy.
Patients should be treated with high-flux, biocompatible membranes.

V. METABOLIC ACIDOSIS AND BONE DISEASE

By the 1960s the clinical entities of proximal and distal renal tubular acidosis (RTA) were recognized. Untreated distal RTA was associated with hypercalcemia and hypercalciuria. The source of the elevated calcium levels was presumably acidosis-triggered bone demineralization. Children with RTA were often below the first percentile in height. Yet, with alkalinization, calcium loss in urine decreased and growth in height accelerated to the 37th percentile (74,75). These early observations in children suggested that chronic metabolic acidosis had adverse effects on bone.

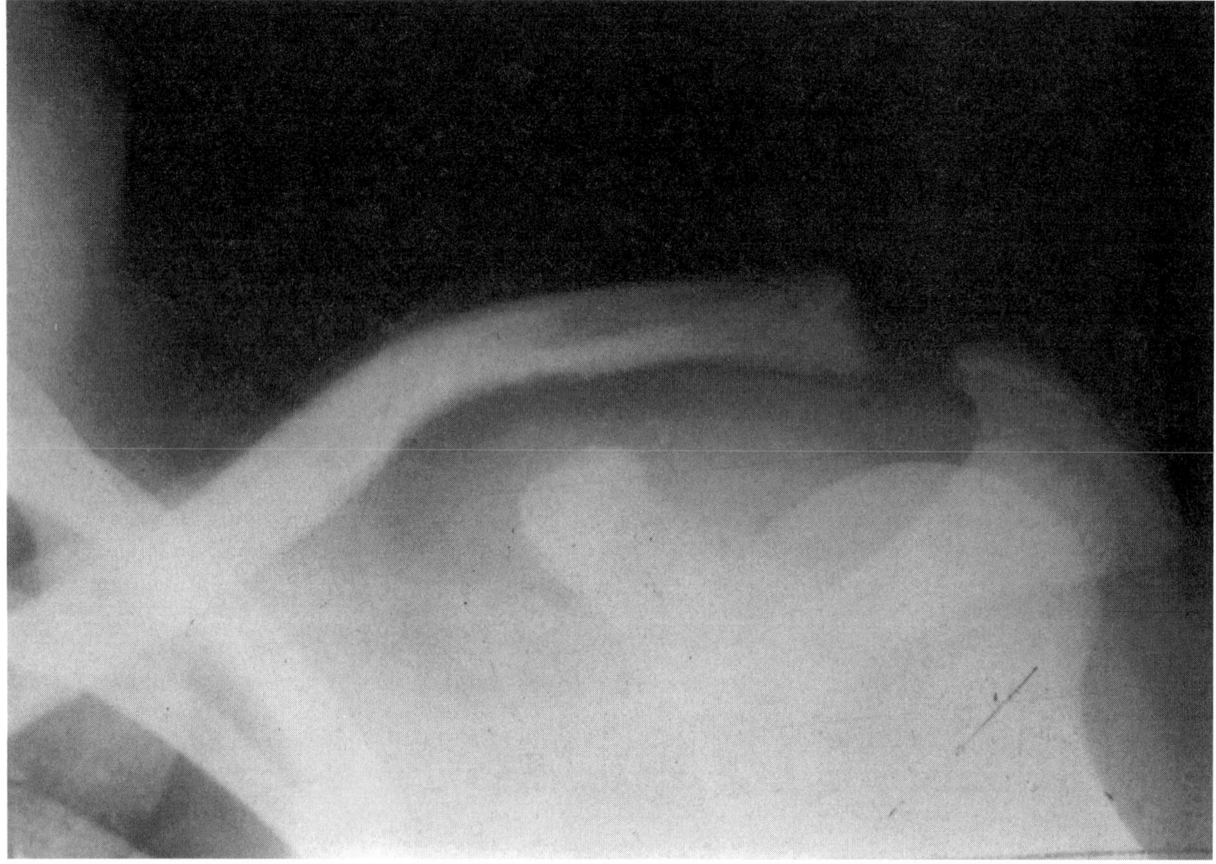

Fig. 6 Widening and loss of definition of the acromioclavicular joint by dialysis-related amyloidosis.

Besides children with RTA, chronic metabolic acidosis (CMA) is most commonly encountered in the patient with renal insufficiency. Metabolic acidosis usually begins when the glomerular filtration rate falls below 30 mL/min and is present in most patients with ESRD. Dialysis treatments often do not correct CMA. Price and Mitch showed that the large majority of chronic hemodialysis patients have serum bicarbonate levels below 24 mEq/L (76). Many internists and nephrologists consider low serum bicarbonate an unavoidable sequelae to renal failure, and as a consequence CMA is often untreated. The lessons learned from children with RTA may also apply to the renal population with chronic metabolic acidosis.

A. Direct Effects of Metabolic Acidosis on Bone

Metabolic acidosis has been shown to affect both the organic and mineral phases of bone. The organic phase of bone consists of cellular components—mainly osteoclasts and osteoblasts and connective tissue such as collagen. Osteoclasts are the principal bone-resorbing cells derived from hematopoietic precursors, possibly from the monocyte-macrophage family. These cells attach to bone and create a compartment between the cell and bone matrix in which H^+ ions are secreted to create a markedly acidic local environment. The H^+-ATPase responsible for this acidification is functionally similar to the renal H^+-ATPase involved in renal tubular acidification. This acidic interface dissolves bone mineral, allowing hydrolytic enzymes to resorb the bone matrix. Teti et al. demonstrated that acidosis stimulates the formation of osteoclast podosomes, which increase attachment areas between the osteoclast and bone surface (77). This increased adhesion is the initial step in acidosis-driven osteoclastic bone resorption. Additionally, Arnett and Dempster, using rat osteoclasts on cortical bone slices, found an increased depth and number of resorption pits after the osteoclasts were exposed to acidic media (78).

Metabolic acidosis also affects osteoblastic function, inhibiting the expression of immediate early genes, alkaline phosphatase activity, and reducing collagen synthesis (79,80). Bushinsky demonstrated a 23% inhibition of osteoblastic collagen synthesis, which leads to a reduction in bone matrix for eventual mineralization (80). Additionally, acidosis may affect the proportion of serum phosphate in the trivalent form, which is essential for mineralization (82).

Taken as a whole, it is clear that in CMA osteoclastic function is augmented with increased bone resorption and osteoblastic new bone formation is diminished. These cellular responses to acidosis facilitate the release of bone carbonate for buffering but may eventually lead to bone demineralization.

The mineral phase of bone also contributes to buffering of an acidic pH. Mineral bone is made predominantly of a highly substituted hydroxyapatite $[Ca_{10}(PO_4)_6(OH)_2]$, in which cations such as Na^+ and K^+ can substitute for Ca^{2+}. Likewise, anions such as HCO_3^- or carbonate can substitute for PO_4^{2-} or OH^-.

In response to acidosis, the excess H^+ can substitute for Na^+ or K^+ in a cation-for-cation exchange on mineral bone surface. This was demonstrated by Bushinsky, who incubated mice calvaria in acidic media and noted a rise in media Na^+ content and a slow rise in the pH of the acidic media (83). The incubated bone was shown to release surface sodium cations even after bone osteoclasts were specifically inhibited by calcitonin. This suggests a direct physicochemical change in mineral bone, independent of the cellular changes discussed above. In addition to direct H^+ binding, mineral bone has been shown to release carbonate independent of osteoclast activity. Approximately a third of mineral bone carbonate exists in a labile pool that can be released in response to acidosis (84). This labile pool serves as a reservoir for alkali. In chronic acidosis, there is eventual depletion of this reservoir of calcium carbonate, and this is one of the most notable changes in uremic osteodystrophy. Pellegrino and Biltz studied bone fragments from 22 uremic patients (85). In patients with long-standing uremia, the 37% of total bone carbonate normally existing in the labile pool was completely depleted with a resultant decrease in bone density.

Therefore, the mineral phase of bone reacts to acidosis by physicochemical exchange of H^+ for Na^+ or K^+ and release of carbonate from a calcium carbonate reservoir. While these are seemingly adaptive responses to acidosis, the overall changes in mineral bone can result in worsened osteodystrophy.

Metabolic acidosis has also been shown to affect vitamin D metabolism. The conversion of $25(OH)D_3$ to active $1,25(OH)_2D_3$ is dependent on 1-alpha-hydroxylase activity in the renal tubule. Lee et al. (86), using a model of vitamin D–deficient animals, demonstrated that metabolic acidosis led to decreased conversion to active $1,25(OH)_2D_3$ (86). They further demonstrated that if acidosis was corrected by carbonate infusion, the serum levels of $1,25(OH)_2D_3$ significantly increased. Others, using direct assays of proximal tubule activity, have shown downregulation of enzyme activity during metabolic acidosis (87). These observations suggest that altered vitamin D metabolism in metabolic acidosis could contribute to renal osteodystrophy. Further work is needed in this area, as other researchers have found variable vitamin D activity in acidosis (88,89).

Metabolic acidosis may also affect parathyroid hormone activity. Bichara et al. noted that rats made acidotic during HCl loading responded with a rise in serum immunoreactive PTH (90). Wills speculated that increased PTH activity during metabolic acidosis evolved to allow increased bone resorption providing increased amounts of buffer base and increased renal phosphate clearance (91). Interestingly, the rise in PTH level seen in acidosis occurs despite increases in plasma ionized calcium concentration. In the hemodialysis population, it has been shown that acidosis decreases the sensitivity of the parathyroid glands to calcium (92). Therefore, for optimal parathyroid tissue response to ionized calcium levels, metabolic acidosis must be corrected.

It becomes apparent that metabolic acidosis, left untreated, can affect bone composition and bone cell metabolism. When these changes are combined with underlying secondary hyperparathyroidism, there can be an additive effect on overall bone cell function. Indeed, Bushinsky and Nilsson (93) studied the effects of parathyroid hormone and acidosis on osteoblastic and osteoclastic function. They noted that acidosis combined with increased PTH had a greater effect on bone cell function than either condition alone. They suggested that uremic osteodystrophy may be the result of the additive effects of secondary hyperparathyroidism and untreated acidosis (93).

B. Treatment Strategies

Chronic metabolic acidosis is more notable in the population treated by intermittent dialysis modalities. In a study of 690 thrice-weekly hemodialysis patients, the large majority exhibited plasma bicarbonate values well below the normal values of 24 mmol/L (94). In another study, 41% of 129 hemodialysis patients had predialysis bicarbonate values of less than 21 mmol/L, and 17% had values less than 19 mmol/L (95).

Peritoneal dialysis, however, has been more effective in normalizing serum bicarbonate. In 19 CAPD patients, 24-hour total acid production was compared with total alkali gained from the dialysate, gastrointestinal alkali absorption, and urinary excretion of acid (96). Total acid production was identical to total alkali gain and thus patients demonstrated true acid-base balance.

In 1984, Van Stone advocated oral administration of alkali to hemodialysis patients with CMA (96). Eight weeks of oral sodium citrate therapy improved the serum bicarbonate levels without adversely affecting blood pressure or increasing 3-day interdialytic weight gains. Citrate-containing compounds, however, augment intestinal absorption of aluminum, especially with the co-administration of aluminum-containing phosphate binders; this is undesirable since aluminum may accumulate and worsen bone disease in ESRD patients. Sodium bicarbonate could be an alternative to citrate, but it often induces gastrointestinal side effects and also represents an added sodium load. Calcium carbonate, used as a phosphate binder, has been shown to increase the serum bicarbonate concentration (97). However, calcium carbonate used in sufficient quantities to normalize the serum bicarbonate presents a risk of hypercalcemia.

Oettinger and Oliver approached the problem of CMA by advocating an increase in the dialysate bicarbonate concentration. They studied the effect of a high-bicarbonate dialysate (42 mmol/L) in 38 hemodialysis patients and found that it corrected predialysis acidosis in 75% (98). Similarly, Williams et al. described, in a double-blind crossover trial, improved control of acidosis with a 40 mmol/L bicarbonate dialysate (99). The higher bicarbonate dialysates were considered safe and well tolerated with normalization of the predialysis arterial pH.

The ideal regimen for correcting CMA in the hemodialysis population may be a combination of increased dialysate bicarbonate concentrations combined with daily doses of oral alkali. The long-term effect of these treatment strategies on bone composition requires further study.

REFERENCES

1. Hruska KA, Teitelbaum SL. Renal osteodystrophy. N Engl J Med 1995; 333:166–174.
2. Schrier RW, Gottschalk CW. Diseases of the Kidney. 5th ed. Boston: Little, Brown, and Company, 1993: 2611.
3. Almadden Y, Canalejo A, Hernandez A, Ballesteros E, Garcia-Navorro S, Torres A, Rodriguez M. Direct effect of phosphorus hormone secretion from whole rat parathyroid gland in vitro. J Bone Miner Res 1996; 11:970–976.
4. Rodriguez M, Almadden Y, Hernandez A, Torres A. Effect of phosphate on the parathyroid gland: direct and indirect? Curr Opin Nephrol Hypertens 1985; 5:321–328.
5. Slatopolsky E, Caglar S, Pennell JP, Taggart DD, Canterbury JM, Reiss E, Bricker NS. On the pathogenesis of hyperparathyroidism in chronic renal insufficiency in the dog. J Clin Invest 1971; 50:492–499.
6. Slatopolsky E, Robson AM, Elkan I, Bricker NS. Control of phosphate excretion in uremic man. J Clin Invest 1968; 47:1865–1874.
7. Fernandez E, Llach F. Guidelines for the dosing of intravenous calcitriol in dialysis patients with hyperparathyroidism. Nephrol Dial Transplant 1996; 11(suppl 3): 96–101.
8. Lim VS, Flanigan MJ, Fangman J. Effect of hematocrit on solute removal during high efficiency hemodialysis. Kidney Int 1990; 37:1557–1562.
9. NRC Committee on Dietary Allowances. Food and Nutrition Board. National Research Council: Recommended Dietary Allowances. 10th rev. ed. Washington, DC: National Academy Press, 1989:184–187.
10. Gomez BJ, Ardakani S, Ju J, Jenkins D, Cerelli MJ, Daniloff GY, Kung VT. Monoclonal antibody assay for measuring bone-specific alkaline phosphatase activity in serum. Clin Chem 1995; 41:1560–1566.
11. Taylor AK, Lueken SA, Libanati C, Baylink DJ. Biochemical markers of bone turnover for the clinical assessment of bone metabolism. Rheum Dis Clin North Am 1994; 20:589–607.
12. Jarava C, Armas JR, Salgueira M, Palma A. Bone alkaline phosphatase isoenzyme in renal osteodystrophy. Nephrol Dial Transplant 1996; 11(suppl 3):43–46.
13. Urena P, Hruby M, Ferreira A, Ang KS, de Vernejoul MC. Plasma total versus bone alkaline phosphatase as markers of bone turnover in hemodialysis patients. J Am Soc Nephrol 1996; 7:506–512.
14. Pierides AM, Skillen AW, Ellis HA. Serum alkaline phosphatase in azotemic and hemodialysis osteodystrophy: a study of isoenzyme patterns, their correlation with bone histology, and their changes in response to treatment with 1alpha OHD3 and 1,25(OH)2D3. J Lab Clin Med 1979; 93:899–909.
15. Torres A, Loranzo V, Hernandez D, Rodriguez JC, Concepcion MT, Rodriguez AP, Hernandez A, de Bonis E, Darias E, Gonzalez-Posada JM, Losada M, Rufino M, Felsenfeld AJ, Rodriguez M. Bone disease in predialysis, hemodialysis, and CAPD patients: evidence of a

better bone response to PTH. Kidney Int 1995; 47: 1434–1442.
16. Portale AA, Booth BE, Halloran BP, Morris RC Jr. Effect of dietary phosphate on circulating concentrations of 1,25-dihydroxyvitamin D and immunoreactive parathyroid hormone in children with moderate renal insufficiency. J Clin Invest 1984; 73:1580–1589.
17. Szabo A, Merke J, Bier E, Mall G, Ritz E. 1,25$(OH)_2$ vitamin D3 inhibits parathyroid cell proliferation in experimental uremia. Kidney Int 1989; 35:1049–1053.
18. Baker LRI, Abrams SML, Roe CJ, Faugere M-C, Fanti P, Suayati Y, Malluche HH. 1,25$(OH)_2D_3$ administration in moderate renal failure: a prospective double-blind trial. Kidney Int 1989; 35:661–669.
19. Felsenfeld AJ. Considerations for the treatment of secondary hyperparathyroidism in renal failure. J Am Soc Nephrol 1997; 8:995–1004.
20. Slatopolsky E, Delmez JA. Pathogenesis of secondary hyperparathyroidism. Nephrol Dial Transplant 1996; 11(suppl 3):130–135.
21. Slatopolsky E, Weerts C, Lopez-Hilker S, Norwood K, Zink M, Windus D, Delmez J. Calcium carbonate as a phosphate binder in patients with chronic renal failure undergoing dialysis. N Engl J Med 1986; 315:157–161.
22. Burke SK, Slatopolsky EA, Goldberg DI. RenaGel, a novel calcium- and aluminium-free phosphate binder, inhibits phosphate absorption in normal volunteers. Nephrol Dial Transplant 1997; 12:1640–1644.
23. Chertow GM, Burke SK, Lazarus M, Stenzel KH, Wombolt D, Goldberg D, Bonventre JV, Slatopolsky E. Poly[allylamine hydrochloride] (RenaGel): a noncalcemic phosphate binder for the treatment of hyperphosphatemia in chronic renal failure. Am J Kidney Dis 1997; 29:66–71.
24. Rosenbaum DP, Holmes-Farley SE, Mandevlle MP, Goldberg DI. Effect of RenaGel, a non-absorbable, cross-linked, polymeric phosphate binder, on urinary phosphorus excretion in rats. Nephrol Dial Transplant 1997; 12:961–964.
25. Silver J, Russell J, Sherwood LM. Regulation by vitamin D metabolites of messenger ribonucleic acid for preproparathyroid hormone in isolated bovine parathyroid cells. Proc Natl Acad Sci USA 1985; 82:4270–4273.
26. Rose BD. Clinical Physiology of Acid-Base and Electrolyte Disorders. New York: McGraw-Hill Inc., 1984.
27. Korkor AB. Reduced binding of [^{3}H]1,25-dihydroxyvitamin D_3 in the parathyroid glands of patients with renal failure. N Engl J Med 1987; 316:1573–1577.
28. Fukuda N, Tanaka H, Tominaga Y, Fukagawa M, Kurokawa K, Seino Y. Decreased 1,25-dihydroxyvitamin D3 receptor density is associated with a more severe form of parathyroid hyperplasia in chronic uremic patients. J Clin Invest 1993; 92:1436–1443.
29. Fukagawa M, Fukuda N, Yi H, Kurokowa K, Seino Y. Resistance of parathyroid cell to calcitriol as a cause of parathyroid hyperfunction in chronic renal failure. Nephrol Dial Transplant 1995; 10:316–319.
30. Slatopolsky E, Weerts C, Thielan J, Horst R, Harter H, Martin JK. Marked suppression of secondary hyperparathyroidism by intravenous administration of 1,25-dihydroxycholecalciferol in uremic patients. J Clin Invest 1984; 74:2136–2143.
31. Quarles LD, Yohay DA, Carroll BA, Sprotzer CE, Minda SA, Bartholomay D, Lobaugh B. Prospective double-blind placebo controlled trial of pulse oral versus intravenous calcitriol treatment of hyperparathyroidism in ESRD. Kidney Int 1994; 45:1710–1721.
32. Reichel H, Szabo A, Uhl J, Persian S, Schmutz A, Schmidt-Gayk H, Ritz E. Intermittent versus continuous administration of 1,25-dihydroxyvitamin D_3 in experimental renal hyperparathyroidism. Kidney Int 1993; 44: 1259–1265.
33. Cannella G, Bonucci E, Rolla D, Ballanti P, Moriero E, de Grandi R, Augeri C, Claudiani F, Di Maio GD. Evidence of healing of secondary hyperparathyroidism in chronically dialzyed uremic patients treated with long-term intravenous calcitriol. Kidney Int 1994; 46:1124–1132.
34. Dressler R, Laut J, Lynn RI, Ginsberg N. Long-term high dose intravenous calcitriol therapy in end-stage renal disease patients with severe secondary hyperparathyroidism. Clin Nephrol 1995; 43:324–331.
35. Hou SH, Zhao J, Ellman CF, Hu J, Griffin Z, Speigel DM, Bourdeau JE. Calcium and phosphorus fluxes during hemodialysis with low calcium dialysate. Am J Kidney Dis 1991; 18:217–224.
36. Argiles A, Kerr PG, Canaud B, Flavier JL, Mion C. Calcium kinetics and the long-term effects of lowering dialysate calcium concentration. Kidney Int 1993; 43: 630–640.
37. Johnson WJ. Optimum dialysate calcium concentration during maintenance hemodialysis. Nephron 1976; 17: 241–258.
38. Weinrich T, Ritz E, Passlick-Deetjen J. Long-term dialysis with low-calcium solution (1.0 mmol/L) in CAPD: effects on bone mineral metabolism. Collaborators of the Multicenter Study Group. Perit Dial Int 1996; 16:260–268.
39. Kaehny WD, Hegg AP, Alfrey AC, Gastrointestinal absorption of aluminum from aluminum-containing antacids. N Engl J Med 1977; 296:1389–1390.
40. Alfrey AC, LeGendre GR, Kaehny WD. The dialysis encephalopathy syndrome. Possible aluminum intoxication. N Engl J Med 1976; 294:184–188.
41. Slatopolsky E. The interaction of parathyroid hormone and aluminum in renal osteodystrophy. Kidney Int 1987; 31:842–854.
42. Cannata Andia JB. Aluminum toxicity: its relationship with bone and iron metabolism. Nephrol Dial Transplant 1996; 11(suppl 3):69–73.
43. Andress DL, Kopp JB, Norma AM, Coburn JW, Sherrard DJ. Early deposition of aluminum in bone in dia-

betic patients on hemodialysis. N Engl J Med 1987; 316:292–296.
44. Vincenti F, Arnaud SB, Recker R, Genant H, Amend W, Feduska NJ, Salvatierra O. Parathyroid and bone response of the diabetic patient to uremia. Kidney Int 1984; 25:677–682.
45. Malluche HH, Smith AJ, Abreo K, Faugere M-C. The use of deferoxamine in the management of aluminum accumulation in bone in patients with renal failure. N Engl J Med 1984; 311:140–144.
46. D'Haese PC, Couttenye M-M, De Broe ME. Diagnosis and treatment of aluminum bone disease. Nephrol Dial Transplant 1996; 11(suppl 3):74–79.
47. Chazan JA, Abuelo JG, Blonsky SL. Plasma aluminum levels (unstimulated and stimulated): clinical and biochemical findings in 185 patients undergoing chronic hemodialysis for 4 to 95 months. Am J Kidney Dis 1989; 13:284–289.
48. Landeghem GF, D'Haese PC, Lamberts LV, Djukanovic L, Pejanovic S, Goodman WG, De Broe ME. Low serum aluminum values in dialysis patients with increased bone aluminum levels. Clin Nephrol 1998; 50:69–76.
49. Winney RJ, Cowie JF, Robson JS. The role of plasma aluminum in the detection and prevention of aluminum toxicity. Kidney Int 1986; 29:S91–S95.
50. D'Haese PC, Couttenye MM, Goodman WG, Lemoniatou E, Digenis P, Sotornik I, Fagalde A, Barsoum RS, Lamberts LV, De Broe ME. Use of the low-dose desferrioxamine test to diagnose and differentiate between patients with aluminium-related bone disease, increased risk for aluminium toxicity, or aluminium overload. Nephrol Dial Transplant 1995; 10:1874–1884.
51. Boelaert JR, Fenves AZ, Coburn JW. Deferoxamine therapy and mucormycosis in dialysis patients: report of an international registry. Am J Kidney Dis 1991; 18: 660–667.
52. Boelaert JR, de Locht M, Van Cutsem J, Kerrels V, Cantinieaux B, Verdonck A, Van Landuyt HW, Schneider Y-J. Mucormycosis during deferoxamine therapy is a siderophore-mediated infection. In vitro and in vivo studies. J Clin Invest 1993; 91:1979–1986.
53. Olivieri NF, Buncic R, Chew E, Gallant T, Harrison RV, Keenan N, Logan W, Mitchell D, Ricci G, Skarf B, Taylor M, Freedman MH. Visual and auditory neurotoxicity in patients receiving subcutaneous deferoxamine infusion. N Engl J Med 1986; 314:869–873.
54. Barata JD, D'Haese PC, Pires C, Lamberts LV, Simões J, De Broe ME. Low-dose (5 mg/kg) desferrioxamine treatment in acutely aluminium-intoxicated haemodialysis patients using two drug administration schedules. Nephrol Dial Transplant 1996; 11:125–132.
55. Molitoris BA, Alfrey AC, Alfrey PS, Miller NL. Rapid removal of DFO-chelated aluminum during hemodialysis using polysulfone dialyzers. Kidney Int 1988; 34: 98–101.
56. Gejyo F, Yamada T, Odani S, Nakagawa Y, Arakawa M, Kunitomo T, Kataoka H, Suzuki M, Hirasawa Y, Shirahama T, et al. A new form of amyloid protein associated with chronic hemodialysis was identified as beta 2-microglobulin. Biochem Biophys Res Commun 1985; 129:701–706.
57. Laurent G, Calemard E, Charra B. Dialysis related amyloidosis. Kidney Int 1991; 39:1012–1019.
58. Jadoul M, Garbar C, Vanholder R, Sennesael J, Michael C, Robert A, Noel H, van Ypersele de Strihou C. Prevalence of histological beta2-microglobulin amyloidosis in CAPD patients compared with hemodialysis patients. Kidney Int 1998; 54:956–959.
59. Odell RA, Slowiaczek P, Moran JE, Schindhelm K. Beta 2-microglobulin kinetics in end-stage renal failure. Kidney Int 1991; 39:909–919.
60. Carone FA, Peterson DR, Oparil S, Pullman TN. Renal tubular transport and catabolism of proteins and peptides. Kidney Int 1979; 16:271–278.
61. Gejyo F, Odani S, Yamada T, Honma N, Saito H, Suzuki Y, Nakagawa Y, Kobayashi H, Maruyama Y, Hirasawa Y, et al. Beta 2-microglobulin: a new form of amyloid protein associated with chronic hemodialysis. Kidney Int 1986; 30:385–390.
62. Zingraff J, Noël LH, Bardin T, Kuntz D, Dubost C, Drüeke T. Beta-2 microglobulin amyloidosis: a sternoclavicular joint biopsy study in hemodialysis patients. Clin Nephrol 1990; 33:94–97.
63. Chary-Valckenaere I, Kessler M, Mainard D, Schertz L, Chanliau J, Champigneulle J, Pourel J, Gaucher A, Netter P. Amyloid and non-amyloid carpal tunnel syndrome in patients receiving chronic renal dialysis. J Rheumatol 1998; 25:1164–1170.
64. Kurer MH, Baillod RA, Madgwick JC, Musculoskeletal manifestations of amyloidosis. A review of 83 patients on haemodialysis for at least 10 years. J Bone Joint Surg 1991; 73:271–276.
65. Allard JC, Artze ME, Porter G, Ghandur-Mnaymneh L, de Velasco R, Pérez GO. Fatal destructive cervical spondyloarthropathy in two patients on long-term dialysis. Am J Kidney Dis 1992; 19:81–85.
66. Ohashi K, Hara M, Kawai R, Ogura Y, Honda K, Nihei H, Mimura N. Cervical discs are most susceptible to beta 2-microglobulin amyloid deposition in the vertebral column. Kidney Int 1992; 41:1646–1652.
67. Noël LH, Zingraff J, Bardin T, Atienza C, Kuntz D, Drüeke T. Tissue distribution of dialysis amyloidosis. Clin Nephrol 1987; 27:175–178.
68. Choi HS, Heller D, Picken MM, Sidhu GS, Kahn T. Infarction of intestine with massive amyloid deposition in two patients on long-term hemodialysis. Gastroenterology 1989; 96:230–234.
69. Drüeke TB. Dialysis-related amyloidosis. Nephrol Dial Transplant 1998; 13(suppl 1):58–64.
70. DiRaimondo CR, Pollak VE. Beta 2-microglobulin kinetics in maintenance hemodialysis: a comparison of conventional and high-flux dialyzers and the effects of dialyzer reuse. Am J Kidney Dis 1989; 13:390–395.

71. Flöge J, Granolleras C, Bingel M, Deschodt G, Branger B, Oules R, Koch KM, Shaldon S. Beta 2-microglobulin kinetics during haemodialysis and haemofiltration. Nephrol Dial Transplant 1987; 1:223–228.
72. Hakim RM, Wingard RL, Husni L, Parker RA, Parker TF. The effect of membrane biocompatibility on plasma beta 2-microglobulin levels in chronic hemodialysis patients. J Am Soc Nephrol 1996; 7:472–478.
73. Bardin T, Lebail-Darné JL, Zingraff J, Laredo JD, Voisin MC, Kreis H, Kuntz D. Dialysis arthropathy: outcome after renal transplantation. Am J Med 1995; 99:243–248.
74. McSherry E, Morris RC. Attainment and maintenance of normal stature with alkali therapy in infants and children with classic renal tubular acidosis. J Clin Invest 1978; 61:509–527.
75. Nash MA, Torrado AD, Greifer I, et al. Renal tubular acidosis in infants and children. Pediatrics 1972; 80: 738–748.
76. Price SR, Mitch WE. Metabolic acidosis and uremic toxicity: protein and amino acid metabolism. Semin Nephrol 1994; 14:232–233.
77. Teti A, Blair HC, Schlesinger P, Grano M, Zambonin-Zallone A, Kahn AJ, Teitelbaum SL, Hruska KA. Extracellular protons acidify osteoclasts, reduce cytosolic calcium, and promote expression of cell-matrix attachment structures. J Clin Invest 1989; 84:773–780.
78. Arnett TR, Dempster DW. Affect of pH on bone resorption by rat osteoclast in vitro. Endocrinology 1986; 119:119–124.
79. Frick KK, Jiang L, Bushinsky DA. Acute metabolic acidosis inhibits the induction of osteoblastic egr-1 and type I collagen. Am J Physiol 1997; 272:C1450–C1456.
80. Bushinsky DA. Stimulated osteoclastic and suppressed osteoblastic activity in metabolic but not respiratory acidosis. Am J Physiol 1995; 268:C80–C88.
81. Krieger NS, Sessler NE, Bushinsky DA. Acidosis inhibits osteoblastic and stimulates osteoclastic activity in vitro. Am J Physiol 1992; 162:F442–F448.
82. Cochran M, Nordin BEC. Role of acidosis in renal osteomalacia. Br Med J 1969; ii:276–279.
83. Bushinsky DA, Levi-Setti R, Coe FL. Ion microprobe determination of bone surface elements: effects of reduced medium pH. Am J Physiol 1986; 250:F1090–F1097.
84. Bushinsky DA. The contribution of acidosis to renal osteodystrophy. Kidney Int 1995: 47:1816–1832.
85. Pellegrino ED, Biltz RM. The composition of human bone in uremia. Medicine 1965; 44:397–418.
86. Lee SW, Russell J, Avioli LV. 25-hydroxy-cholecalciferol conversion to 1,25-dihydroxy-cholecalciferol: Conversion impaired by systemic metabolic acidosis. Science 1977; 195:994–996.
87. Kawashima H, Kraut JA, Kurokawa K. Metabolic acidosis suppresses 25-hydroxyvitamin D_3-1-alpha-hydroxylase in the rat kidney. J Clin Invest 1982; 70:35–140.
88. Cunningham J, Bikle DD, Avioli LV. Acute but not chronic, metabolic acidosis disturbs 25-hydroxyvitamin D3 metabolism. Kidney Int 1984; 25:47–52.
89. Krapf R, Vetsch R, Vetsch W, Hulter HN. Chronic metabolic acidosis increased the serum concentration of 1,25-dihydroxyvitamin D in humans by stimulating its production rate. J Clin Invest 1992; 90:2456–2463.
90. Bichara M, Mercier O, Borensztein P, Paillard M. Acute metabolic acidosis enhances circulating parathyroid hormone, which contributes to the renal response against acidosis in the rat. J Clin Invest 1990; 86:430–443.
91. Wills MR. Fundamental physiological role of parathyroid hormone in acid-based homeostasis. Lancet 1970; ii:802–804.
92. Graham KA, Hoenich NA, Tarbit M, Ward MK, Goodship THJ. Correction of acidosis in hemodialysis patients increases the sensitivity of the parathyroid glands to calcium. J Am Soc Nephrol 1997; 8:627–631.
93. Bushinsky DA, Nilsson EL. Additive effects of acidosis and parathyroid hormone on osteoblastic and osteoclastic function. Am J Physiol 1995; 269:C1364–C1370.
94. Bergstrom J, Lindholm B. Nutrition and adequacy of dialysis: How do hemodialysis and CAPD compare? Kidney Int 1993; 43:S39–S50.
95. Uribarri J, Buquing J, Oh MS. Acid-base balance in chronic peritoneal dialysis patients. Kidney Int 1995; 47:269–273.
96. Van Stone JC, Oral base replacement in patients on hemodialysis. Ann Intern Med 1984; 101:199–201.
97. Makoff DL, Gordon A, Franklin SS, et al. Chronic calcium carbonate therapy in uremia. Arch intern Med 1969; 123:15–21.
98. Oettinger CE, Oliver JC. Normalization of uremic acidosis in hemodialysis patients with a high bicarbonate dialysis. J Am Soc Nephrol 1993; 3:1804–1807.
99. Williams AJ, Dittmer ID, McArley A, Clarke J. High bicarbonate dialysate in haemodialysis patients: effects on acidosis and nutritional status. Nephrol Dial Transplant 1997; 12:2633–2637.

19

Acid–Base Problems in Hemodialysis and Peritoneal Dialysis

F. John Gennari
University of Vermont College of Medicine, Burlington, Vermont

Mariano Feriani
S. Bartolo Hospital, Vicenza, Italy

I. INTRODUCTION

Despite major advances in renal replacement therapy over the last 20 years, mild to moderate metabolic acidosis remains a persistent finding in patients receiving dialysis treatments. In this chapter we review the evidence that acidosis has deleterious effects and then turn to the factors influencing acid-base homeostasis during peritoneal dialysis and hemodialysis. The final sections of the chapter are devoted to strategies to improve serum bicarbonate concentration ([HCO_3^-]) in individuals receiving dialysis therapy and to providing guidelines for recognizing the presence of superimposed acid-base disturbances in this specialized population.

II. METABOLIC ACIDOSIS AS A UREMIC TOXIN

Metabolic acidosis is a characteristic feature of chronic renal insufficiency and is also present in most patients receiving renal replacement therapy for end-stage renal disease (1,2). On average, serum [HCO_3^-] is reduced by 6 mEq/L in patients with even mild to moderate renal insufficiency (glomerular filtration rate approximately 15–50 mL/min) (2). Irrespective of the nature of the underlying disease, this acid-base disturbance always reflects an impairment in renal acid excretion and, in many instances, impaired renal HCO_3^- reabsorption as well (3–5). Most patients with end-stage renal disease receiving hemodialysis therapy and many patients receiving peritoneal dialysis therapy have a persistent metabolic acidosis. As discussed below, experimental studies in animals and human subjects have demonstrated that metabolic acidosis has adverse effects on physiological functions in several organ systems.

A. Cardiovascular Function

Cardiac function is affected both directly and indirectly by metabolic acidosis. In vitro studies of cardiac muscle contractility show a depressant effect of acidosis, manifested by a decrease in myocardial response to circulating catecholamines (6). This depressant effect reflects the influence of intracellular pH on contractile proteins. Intracellular acidification also depresses the response of myocardium to calcium and decreases the performance of ischemic muscle. These effects may be due to the displacement of calcium by hydrogen ions at critical binding sites (7). Depression of cardiac contractile force, however, is not clinically apparent unless arterial pH is less than 7.20 (7).

A lower pH and [HCO_3^-] during a hemodialysis session are correlated with the number and severity of cardiac arrhythmias (8). In comparison with dialysis against an HCO_3^--containing bath (which more rapidly increases pH and [HCO_3^-] during treatment), dialysis with an acetate-containing bath increases the frequency and severity of arrhythmias. The ameliorating effect of rapid correction of metabolic acidosis is associated with a higher intracellular potassium concentration (measured in erythrocytes) (8). Whether the beneficial effect is related to the improvement in acid-base status or is the result of the removal of acetate from the bath, however, is uncertain.

B. Bone Disease

The calcium carbonate contained in bone is a potentially important buffer reservoir in the defense against chronic metabolic acidosis. The specific role of this buffer source in long-term metabolic acidosis, however, remains an area of controversy (4,9). Release of calcium from bone clearly occurs in response to acute and short-term chronic acid loading both in experimental animals and in humans (10,11). In vitro experiments using neonatal mouse calvariae have shown that incubation in an acid medium causes a net efflux of calcium in a dose-dependent fashion (12). With acute exposure to acid, the calcium loss is a physicochemical process (12,13), whereas with sustained exposure it is cell mediated. The response to sustained exposure is due to an increase in osteoclast activity and decrease in osteoblast activity (14). Of note, the release of calcium from bone is greater for any given pH with metabolic acidosis (i.e., when bath $[HCO_3^-]$ is reduced) than with respiratory acidosis (15).

In normal human subjects, ammonium chloride administration leads to urinary calcium losses, and these losses are correlated with retention of the administered acid (10). Discontinuation of the acid load does not result in complete correction of the calcium losses, suggesting that acidosis over time can produce irreversible bone calcium losses. These same investigators and others have demonstrated a small but significant daily positive acid balance and a corresponding daily calcium loss in patients with chronic renal insufficiency and mild stable metabolic acidosis (3,4). The problem with these seemingly straightforward observations is that bone calcium stores are insufficient to buffer retained acid for longer than 6 months to one year (4,9). Even if the contribution of calcium carbonate to buffering was only half as large as measured, major bone problems should be present in all patients with renal failure and metabolic acidosis. However, the bone disease seen in renal failure is more closely related to disordered parathyroid hormone function than to acidemia. A major issue is whether patients with chronic renal insufficiency or failure are in acid balance. Unfortunately, acid balance is difficult to measure, and small errors could lead to false conclusions. In patients with chronic renal insufficiency, the issue is unresolved. Patients receiving renal replacement therapy, however, appear to be in acid balance, that is, they are not continually retaining acid (see below) (1,16).

The relationship between metabolic acidosis, parathyroid hormone (PTH) dysfunction, and metabolic bone disease is also complex and somewhat controversial. In experimental animals, acute induction of metabolic acidosis stimulates PTH secretion (17), but whether secretion of this hormone remains increased with sustained acidosis is unclear. The data in support of such an effect comes from patients receiving chronic hemodialysis therapy. In one controlled prospective study, patients with serum $[HCO_3^-]$ restored to normal by adding more HCO_3^- to the bath solution had a smaller increase in PTH levels over an 18-months period of observation when compared to a group of patients with no correction of acidosis (18). Strikingly, correction of acidosis not only decreased bone turnover in high-turnover, that is, hyperparathyroid, osteodystrophy (documented by bone biopsies and osteocalcin measurements) but also improved bone turnover in low-turnover bone disease (unrelated to hyperparathyroidism). In a second study, correction of acidosis in hemodialysis patients improved the sensitivity of PTH to changes in serum calcium concentration (19).

In patients receiving peritoneal dialysis, the use of a low-calcium (1.25 mmol/L) dialysate with a higher lactate concentration (40 mmol/L) is associated with a fall in plasma PTH levels (20). The authors postulated that this beneficial outcome was a consequence of better control of serum phosphate due to increased supplementation with calcium carbonate. It is interesting to note, however, that serum $[HCO_3^-]$ was higher in the low-calcium bath group in this study. It is conceivable that serum PTH decreased because of the improvement in acid-base status rather than from any effect on serum phosphate.

C. Protein Metabolism

Numerous studies in humans and in experimental animals have shown that metabolic acidosis promotes protein catabolism (21–30). This catabolic process appears to be dependent on stimulation of glucocorticoid secretion and is directly attributable to acidosis as opposed to other effects of chronic renal insufficiency (21,22). Acidosis-induced protein degradation is associated with increased rates of branched-chain amino acid (BCAA) oxidation (23). In humans with end-stage renal disease, net uptake by muscle of branched-chain amino acids is directly correlated with steady-state serum $[HCO_3^-]$

(29). In acidotic rats, plasma and muscle BCAA levels are low and the activity of branched-chain keto acid dehydrogenase is increased, leading to an increase of BCAA breakdown (23). In normal human subjects given ammonium chloride to induce metabolic acidosis, albumin synthesis is inhibited and negative nitrogen balance develops within 7 days (31). This effect is associated with a suppression of insulin-like growth factor, free thyroxine, and tri-iodothyronine, and it is possible that these changes are contributing factors to the catabolic state.

Clinical studies have demonstrated that correction of uremic acidosis improves nitrogen balance (25) and decreases protein degradation (26,32–34). In patients with chronic renal insufficiency ingesting a protein-restricted diet, plasma levels of urea and uric acid are significantly reduced when acidosis is corrected (27). Correction of metabolic acidosis with bicarbonate supplementation in patients with chronic renal insufficiency reduces skeletal muscle protein catabolism, measured by urinary 3-methylhistidine excretion, improving the effect of protein restriction on nitrogen balance (28). In both hemodialysis and peritoneal dialysis patients, correction of metabolic acidosis (increasing serum [HCO_3^-] from 17–18 to 25–26 mEq/L) decreases protein degradation significantly (33,34). Despite the acute effects of acidosis on albumin synthesis described above, sustained normalization of serum [HCO_3^-] in hemodialysis patients has no effect on serum albumin concentration (35).

The mechanisms responsible for the catabolic effect of acidosis are uncertain. Insulin is known to decrease whole-body protein degradation (36) and acidosis impairs insulin-mediated glucose metabolism (37). In addition to acidosis, chronic renal insufficiency is itself associated with insulin resistance (38). It is therefore possible that acidosis in chronic renal failure patients both impairs insulin-mediated glucose uptake and the action of insulin to inhibit protein breakdown.

Mitch et al. (39) have proposed that metabolic acidosis is an example of the adaptive, or trade-off, response to uremia. Acidosis increases the production of glucocorticoids, and they act to stimulate protein turnover. This response is beneficial if renal function is normal because the catabolic effect of glucocorticoids stimulates the synthesis of glutamine, providing the substrate for renal ammonium production and thereby facilitating renal acid excretion. In patients with renal insufficiency, this response becomes maladaptive because the combination of acidosis and increased glucocoritcoids stimulate catabolic pathways, but renal acid excretion cannot increase. As a result, metabolic acidosis and the associated catabolic state persist. Thus if protein intake falls, as commonly occurs in patients with chronic renal insufficiency, the ability to conserve muscle mass is impaired and lean body weight loss is accelerated.

D. Summary of Toxic Effects of Metabolic Acidosis

In most of the studies cited above, the term "metabolic acidosis" is defined by a lower than normal serum [HCO_3^-]. When measured, arterial pH is often within the normal range or only very slightly reduced because of adaptive hypocapnia (see Table 1). Nonetheless, this

Table 1 Steady-State Acid-Base Status: Peritoneal Dialysis versus Standard Hemodialysis

PD[a]			HD[b]					
N	[Total CO_2] (mEq/L)	Ref.	N	[HCO_3] (mEq/L)	[Total CO_2] (mEq/L)	pH	PCO_2 (mmHg)	Ref.
25	27.4 ± 3.3	50	10	18.9 ± 2.5	—	7.37 ± .09	33 ± 2.5	64
8	26.0 ± 3.3	51	16	19.8 ± 1.2	—	7.37 ± .02	36 ± 1.9	63
20	26.3 ± 2.5	94	10	20.2[e]	—	7.40 ± .04	33 ± 1.2	69
8	28.8 ± 3.0	47	22	—	21.4 ± 2.4	—	—	94
17	24.0 ± 3.1	1	38	—	19.0 ± 3.1	—	—	87
31	23.9 ± 4.0[c]	50	44	—	20.3 ± 2.0	—	—	1
Mean[d]	26.4 ± 3.0		Mean[d]	19.7 ± 1.9	20.1 ± 2.5			

[a]CAPD with bath [lactate] = 40 mM, venous blood values.
[b]HD with HCO_3^--containing bath ([HCO_3^-] = 35 or 36 mEq/L, acetate = 3–4 mM), arterial blood values (obtained from A-V fistulas).
[c]Bath [lactate] = 35 mM.
[d]Weighted by # of observations. For CAPD only bath [lactate] = 40 mM included.
[e]Calculated from mean pH and PCO_2. Means ± SD.

type of metabolic acidosis probably worsens metabolic bone disease and, even when only mild, has detrimental effects on skeletal muscle metabolism. More severe metabolic acidosis, associated with a reduction in pH, impairs cardiovascular function. In the search for "uremic toxins," metabolic acidosis is the one factor that clearly has been demonstrated to be toxic. Given this information, it seems prudent to try to correct this acid-base disorder in patients with renal failure. In the next section, we examine in more detail the acid-base characteristics of the techniques currently used for renal replacement, and why the most commonly used technique, hemodialysis, fails to restore serum [HCO_3^-] to normal levels.

III. ACID-BASE HOMESTASIS IN END-STAGE RENAL DISEASE

Maintenance of a normal serum [HCO_3^-] and pH requires day-to-day replenishment of the alkali consumed in neutralizing the acids produced by endogenous metabolic processes and the alkali lost in the urine and stool (Fig. 1). In patients with functioning kidneys, alkali stores are replenished by renal acid excretion, a process that generates new HCO_3^- in the body. In patients without functioning kidneys, alkali replenishment is accomplished by the addition of either HCO_3^- itself or a metabolic precursor of this anion, such as lactate or acetate. Regardless of the type of renal replacement therapy, however, a new equilibrium almost certainly develops, once the amount of dialysis and the alkali concentration of the dialysis bath are fixed, in which steady-state serum [HCO_3^-] is determined primarily by endogenous acid production (1,16).

A. General Principles of Acid Balance

During renal replacement therapy, the rate of net alkali addition during treatment is dependent on the transmembrane concentration gradient for [HCO_3^-]. Thus, when extracellular [HCO_3^-] is lower, net alkali addition will be greater during any given treatment, and when extracellular [HCO_3^-] is higher, less alkali will be added. With hemodialysis using a HCO_3^--containing bath, the transmembrane concentration gradient regulates the amount of HCO_3^- added. With peritoneal dialysis using a lactate-containing bath or with hemodialysis using an acetate-containing bath, the transmembrane gradient regulates the amount of HCO_3^- lost into the bath and therefore net alkali addition. In all patients receiving renal replacement therapy, the prevailing pH and [HCO_3^-] are determined by the characteristics of the dialysis treatment and by endogenous acid production. Because the bath concentration and dialysance of HCO_3^- and its precursors (lactate or acetate) are fixed once the dialysis prescription is set, the only variable component of these determinants is endogenous acid production. Given these fixed and unvarying alkali replacement conditions, it is not surprising that steady-state serum [HCO_3^-] varies as a function of endogenous acid production much more than in in-

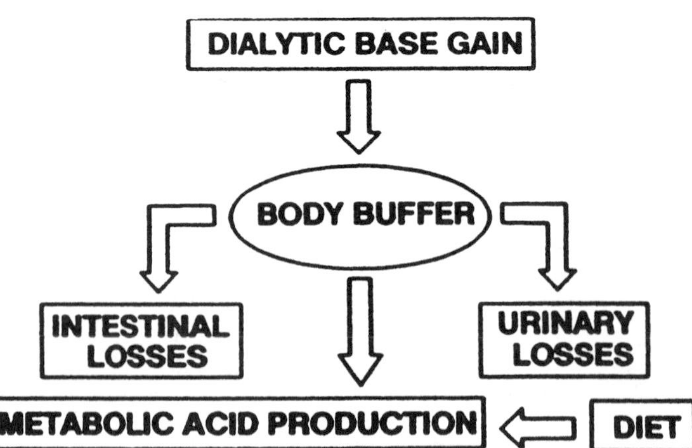

Fig. 1 Schematic representation of acid-base homeostasis in end-stage renal disease. Body buffer stores are depleted by titration of acids produced by metabolism, a component that is determined by diet and by intestinal and any urinary alkali losses. Repletion of body buffer stores occurs as a result of alkali added during dialysis. (From Ref. 43.)

dividuals with functioning kidneys, who can vary acid excretion in response to variations in acid production.

The implication of this analysis is that the acids produced by body metabolism do not continually accumulate in patients with end-stage renal disease receiving dialysis treatment. If true, then continued consumption of bone buffers by retained H^+ should not be occurring. The deleterious effects of chronic metabolic acidosis described earlier are still likely to be evident, however, because they appear to be related more to the prevailing serum $[HCO_3^-]$ and pH than to the state of acid balance.

B. Peritoneal Dialysis

With the exception of experimental studies using bicarbonate (see below) (40–46), lactate is used in peritoneal dialysis bath solutions to accomplish the goal of replenishing the HCO_3^- consumed in buffering acid production. In order to generate new HCO_3^- from absorbed lactate, this organic anion must be taken up by cells with an associated H^+ and metabolized either to CO_2 and water or to some neutral substance such as glucose. During a typical 6-hour equilibration with a standard peritoneal dialysis solution, approximately 75% of the lactate is absorbed and essentially all the absorbed lactate is metabolized to generate new HCO_3^- (47). Metabolism of absorbed lactate occurs primarily in hepatocytes and is not rate limited at the usual amounts delivered during peritoneal dialysis. The lactate in peritoneal dialysis solutions is racemic, containing both d- and l-lactate (48,49). Cellular metabolic processes can only utilize l-lactate, and this ion species is readily metabolized. Absorbed d-lactate is slowly converted to l-lactate in the body, allowing for metabolism to occur. Only minor accumulation of d-lactate occurs in peritoneal dialysis patients, and, at the concentrations measured, it has no apparent toxic effects (49). Bath solutions contain lactate in a concentration of either 35 or 40 mEq/L, the latter being the most commonly used because it results in a higher steady-state venous [total CO_2] (50,51). Although the average value for venous [total CO_2] falls within the normal range (see Table 1), it should be emphasized that 40–50% of patients receiving peritoneal dialysis have steady-state values below the lower limit of normal (50). In addition, when arterial $[HCO_3^-]$ has been measured, the average values are slightly lower than normal in patients using either 35 or 40 mM lactate as an alkali source in their bath solution (43).

Clearly, a more straightforward way to replace body HCO_3^- stores would be to add this anion directly, rather than using lactate. Bath solutions containing only lactate have an acid pH (less than 6.0), and it has been postulated that this acidity may damage the peritoneal membrane (40). The addition of HCO_3^- to the solution solves this problem, but unfortunately it causes calcium carbonate to precipitate unless PCO_2 can be kept high enough to prevent pH from rising to greater than 7.60. This technical problem has been solved by using a split bag, with the bicarbonate solution kept in one compartment and the calcium-containing solution kept in the other (40–42). The two compartments are mixed just prior to infusing the solution into the peritoneum, where the prevailing PCO_2 is high enough to maintain pH in a physiological range. Bicarbonate-containing peritoneal dialysis solutions have been tested in small groups of patients and have been shown to be well tolerated with no adverse effects, when compared to lactate-containing solutions (40–45). In patients with infusion pain, the use of HCO_3^--containing bath solutions significantly reduces symptoms as compared to a standard lactate bath (46). Given the theoretical and practical benefits of HCO_3^- as an alkali source for peritoneal dialysis, it is likely to replace lactate in the future. In addition, by adjusting the concentration of bicarbonate in the solution, one can maintain serum $[HCO_3^-]$ and pH at truly optimal levels (44) (see Table 2).

C. Measurements of Acid-Base Homeostasis

To gain an understanding of acid-base homeostasis in patients receiving chronic ambulatory peritoneal dialysis, Uribarri and colleagues carried out acid balance studies using measurements of blood and peritoneal fluid (47). These workers showed that 75% of the lactate contained in the bath solution was absorbed and generated new HCO_3^- during a standard 6-hour dwell. They also demonstrated that dialysate $[HCO_3^-]$ was 80% of plasma $[HCO_3^-]$ at the end of the dwell time. Based on these measurements, they calculated that net alkali delivery from the dialysis therapy was 31 mEq/day. Acid production measured from sulfate and organic anion excretion was 52 mEq/day, equivalent to $0.84 \times$ protein catabolic rate corrected for body weight (a value closely similar to the theoretical value of 0.77). The difference between acid production and alkali delivered by dialysis, however, was totally accounted for by net alkali absorbed from the gastrointestinal tract. Thus, patients receiving peritoneal dialysis were in day-to-day acid balance, as would be predicted from the analysis presented earlier. Of interest, acid production from metabolism of sulfur-containing amino acids was lower than in individuals with normal renal func-

Table 2 Improving Steady-State Serum [HCO_3^-] in End-Stage Renal Disease: Techniques and Results

N	Duration (months)	Renal therapy	[HCO_3^-] (mEq/L) Baseline	Treatment	Technique used	Ref.
12	2	HD	17.0	21.1	Bath unchanged Sodium citrate 1 mEq/kg/day and 25 mEq per liter of fluid retained	90
11	18	HD	15.6	24.0	↑ Bath [HCO_3^-] to 40–48 mEq/L	18
38	3	HD	19.0	24.8	↑ Bath [HCO_3^-] to 39 mEq/L	87
8	1	HD	18.6	25.3	↑ Bath [HCO_3^-] to 40 mEq/L	19
6	1	HD	18.5	24.8	↑ Bath [HCO_3^-] to 40 mEq/L + $NaHCO_3$ 24 mEq/day in 2 pts	33
16	4	HD	16.7	20.3	↑ Bath [HCO_3^-] to 40 mEq/l + $NaHCO_3$ 1 mEq/Kg/Day[b]	35[a]
7	1	CAPD	19.3	26.2	Bath unchanged $NaHCO_3$ 24–36 mEq/day	34[c]
9	1	CAPD[d]	22.0	25.9	↑ Bath [HCO_3^-] from 34 to 39 mEq/L	44

HD = Standard hemodialysis, [HCO_3^-] values are all predialysis; CAPD = continuous ambulatory peritoneal dialysis.
[a]Only patients with pre-dialysis [HCO_3^-] ≤ 18 mEq/L studied.
[b]Oral $NaHCO_3$ needed in 13 of 16 patients in addition to bath adjustment.
[c]Only patients with serum [HCO_3^-] < 22 mEq/L studied, venous [total CO_2].
[d]CAPD with HCO_3^--containing bath.

tion, and organic acid production was higher. To date, there is no good explanation of the sulfate data, but the increased organic acid production is very likely related to the unregulated loss of organic anions into the dialysis solution. Unregulated organic anion loss is also an important issue in hemodialysis (see later).

In addition to being in acid balance, patients receiving standard ambulatory peritoneal dialysis therapy (four to five exchanges/day) have normal or near-normal values for [HCO_3^-] (Table 1). Although considerable data exist concerning acid-base values in patients receiving ambulatory peritoneal dialysis, there is little information with regard to the effect of overnight cycling peritoneal dialysis on acid-base status. Informal observations show no significant effect of this modification in therapy on acid-base status, but it is too early to tell. To the extent that HCO_3^- and lactate have differing convection and/or diffusion rates across the peritoneal membrane, then decreasing the dwell time of each exchange could alter net alkali delivery. Although metabolic acidosis (defined by a serum [HCO_3^-] below the lower limit of normal) occurs in a significant fraction of patients receiving peritoneal dialysis, the problem if of less concern than in patients receiving hemodialysis who, with rare exception, have sustained metabolic acidosis. This issue is discussed further below.

D. Hemodialysis

1. Alkali Delivery

a. Standard Hemodialysis

When hemodialysis was first developed as a renal replacement therapy, HCO_3^- was used as the sole alkali source. To prevent precipitation of calcium in the bath, a gas mixture containing 5% CO_2 was continuously bubbled through the bath during the entire treatment (52,53). In 1964, Mion and coworkers substituted the bicarbonate precursor acetate for HCO_3^- to avoid having to bubble PCO_2 through the bath and showed that reasonable alkali addition occurred (54). Because it simplified bath preparation, acetate quickly became the universal buffer source for hemodialysis from the 1960s through the late 1980s. A bath acetate concentration of 37 mEq/L was used most commonly, a value empirically settled upon that balanced optimum alkali addition against minimum acetate side effects.

The use of acetate as the sole buffer source for alkali delivery created the same bidirectional process (acetate in and HCO_3^- out during the treatment) that exists for peritoneal dialysis. However, given the rapid rates of transfer during hemodialysis, the magnitude of the HCO_3^- loss is much greater than in peritoneal dialysis. For example, at a blood flow rate of only 200 mL/min, almost 1000 mmol of acetate are added and over 800 mmol of HCO_3^- are lost during a 4-hour dialysis treatment (16,55,56). The new HCO_3^- generated by acetate metabolism during treatment, in fact, is almost immediately lost into the bath during the treatment. The increase in serum [HCO_3^-] that occurs with acetate dialysis (3–4 mEq/L with each treatment) happens only after the treatment is stopped and the residual acetate is metabolized (16,55,56). This increase is clearly insufficient to restore serum [HCO_3^-] to normal levels, given daily acid production, and patients receiving acetate dialysis have an average predialysis serum [HCO_3^-] of only approximately 18 mEq/L (16,55). Thus, although they may be in acid balance, they have a persistent metabolic acidosis with an average blood pH of 7.34 (16).

Another problem with acetate dialysis is that the dialysis membrane serves as an adjunct lung for CO_2 removal. The rapid loss of CO_2 into the bath during hemodialysis decreases ventilatory drive and contributes to dialysis-induced hypoxia (57,58). Finally, acetate accumulation, due to delivery outstripping the body's ability to metabolize this anion, causes vasodilation and hypotension (55,59–63). As blood flow rates have increased and dialysis membranes with increased clearance rates for low molecular weight substances have been developed, the likelihood of symptoms from acetate accumulation increased (63). With the advent of aggressive dialysis using high-efficiency and high-flux membranes, the use of acetate as the sole buffer in the bath solution became untenable because of the high probability of its accumulation during treatment and the inevitable development of patient symptoms.

The problem of acetate toxicity was solved in the mid-1980s by the reintroduction of HCO_3^- as the main buffer source in hemodialysis bath solutions (62,64,65). Calcium precipitation was easily prevented by two modifications. First, HCO_3^--containing solution was added to the rest of the bath solution only seconds before its delivery to the membrane (similar to the approach used for HCO_3^--containing peritoneal dialysis solutions). Second, a small amount of acetic acid (4 mEq/L) was added to the non-HCO_3^- portion of the bath concentrate. This acid reacts with the HCO_3^- when the two solutions are combined, generating new CO_2 in the final bath solution. In the most commonly used mixture, the HCO_3^- concentrate is diluted to a [HCO_3^-] of 39 mEq/L. This alkali reacts with the 4 mEq/L of acetic acid when the two solutions are mixed to produce a final [HCO_3^-] of 35 mEq/L and an acetate concentration of 4 mEq/L in the bath solution. The reaction of acetic acid and HCO_3^- generates 4 mmol/L of CO_2, which, at a temperature of 37°C, produces a PCO_2 of 133 mmHg, assuring an acid pH in the mixture. When this solution flows across the dialysis membrane, PCO_2 in the bath rapidly falls as CO_2 is added to the blood (66). The added CO_2 has no significant effect on arterial PCO_2 because it is trivial in relation to CO_2 production by metabolic processes in the body and is rapidly excreted by the lungs. The presence of CO_2 in the bath also removes the problem of CO_2 loss and hypoventilation that occurred with the acetate-containing bath solution.

The bath solution delivers not only 35 mEq/L of HCO_3^-, but also an additional alkali source in the 4 mEq/L of acetate it contains. The acetate, now stripped of its H^+, diffuses into the blood and is metabolized to create additional HCO_3^-. Studies quickly demonstrated that hemodialysis using this HCO_3^--containing bath solution increased steady-state predialysis serum [HCO_3^-] by approximately 3 mEq/L and decreased patient symptoms significantly, as compared to an acetate bath (62,65,67–69). As a result, acetate-based hemodialysis was gradually replaced, and by the early 1990s virtually all standard hemodialysis was carried out using a HCO_3^--containing bath.

b. *Sorbent Cartridge Hemodialysis*

Another mode of alkali delivery, which removes the need for large volumes of bath solution, is a technique that regenerates HCO_3^- from the enzymatic cleavage of urea to ammonium and carbonate (70). This system centers on a cartridge containing a sorbent that removes the newly generated ammonium ions from the bath and adds H^+, converting CO_3^- into HCO_3^-. The HCO_3^- produced by this process is insufficient to provide all the alkali needed, and as a result substantial acetate has to be added to the solution (70). The amount added can be varied, but during a typical treatment the bath composition is approximately 50% HCO_3^- and 50% acetate. Unfortunately, by its nature the sorbent cartridge technique can produce uncontrollable variations in bath alkali composition and severe acidosis can develop if it malfunctions (71). Because of this problem and the limited production of cartridges, sorbent regenerative hemodialysis is now rarely used.

c. *Hemofiltration*

This technique utilizes the principle of convection rather than diffusion for renal replacement therapy. A high-permeability membrane is used with no bath, and a large volume of fluid is rapidly ultrafiltered during a standard treatment. The alkali lost during this procedure (as well as the fluid) is replaced by a postfilter intravenous solution containing alkali or an alkali precursor such as acetate. The use of intravenous acetate for alkali replacement during hemofiltration increases serum [HCO_3^-] more effectively than does the acetate added from the bath during standard acetate hemodialysis (72–74). The difference—about 2–3 mEq/L at the end of the treatment—is due either to more effective metabolism of acetate or to less HCO_3^- lost during the treatment (74). With hemofiltration using an acetate solution, however, serum [HCO_3^-] falls dramatically during the first hour, suggesting a lag between HCO_3^- loss and acetate metabolism at the beginning of the treatment (73). Feriani and coworkers proposed that a HCO_3^--containing solution be developed as replacement fluid for hemofiltration, using the same technique they employed for peritoneal dialysis fluid (75). Recently such a solution has been developed commercially. Using this solution, Santoro and coworkers found a direct correlation between replacement fluid [HCO_3^-] and end-treatment serum [HCO_3^-], and they proposed a mathematical model to predict acid-base outcome with hemofiltration (76). Hemofiltration is now used only rarely for chromic renal replacement therapy. Its use is confined in most centers to the treatment of acute renal failure, using a technique with much lower ultrafiltration rates (see below).

d. *Hemodiafiltration*

This technique is a modification of hemodialysis in which a dialysis membrane with high permeability is used to ultrafilter large volumes of fluid during the treatment. Using this technique, toxins are removed primarily by convection rather than by diffusion, but, unlike hemofiltration, a dialysis bath solution is employed. When first introduced, an acetate-containing bath was used (77), but this solution has now been replaced by a HCO_3^--containing bath in most centers (78,79). Because of the high rate of ultrafiltration, a postfilter replacement solution is required. Both lactate- and HCO_3^--containing solutions have been used for fluid replacement. Feriani and coworkers have shown that, despite the presence of HCO_3^- in the bath, the flux of this ion is still from the patient to the bath unless serum [HCO_3^-] drops to less than 17.5 mEq/L, because of the high ultrafiltration rates achieved (78). Thus, much of the replacement alkali is lost during the procedure, limiting the increase in serum [HCO_3^-] that can be achieved.

e. *Acetate-Free Biofiltration*

A variant of hemodiafiltration, called acetate-free biofiltration, uses a dialysis bath containing no alkali or alkali precursor (79,80). Instead, all the alkali is provided by a postfilter $NaHCO_3$ solution. This technique removes all exposure to acetate and, using a sufficiently high concentration of HCO_3^- in the postfilter solution, one can raise end-dialysis serum [HCO_3^-] to high levels (80). Nonetheless, predialysis serum [HCO_3^-] with this form of therapy is no different than in other forms of hemodialysis (79,80), and thus it provides no advantage other than the removal of all acetate from the procedure.

f. *Continuous Venovenous Hemofiltration*

This technique is only used for short-term renal replacement therapy in an intensive care setting (81). As its name implies, it is a continuous therapy, ultrafiltering for as long as the treatment is continued. It utilizes a high-permeability membrane, but the rates of ultrafiltration are slower than in intermittent hemofiltration or hemodiafiltration because of the lower blood flow rates used. The ultrafiltration rate ranges from 1000 to 1500 mL/h, a level at which intravenous alkali replacement can easily overcome HCO_3^- losses. The most common replacement solution used is Ringer's lactate, which contains 40 mEq/L of lactate. Alternatively, solutions can be mixed to provide varying amount of $NaHCO_3^-$ as needed to adjust serum [HCO_3^-]. A normal serum [HCO_3^-] can easily be achieved by monitoring the level and adjusting the replacement solution as needed during treatment.

2. Acid-Base Homeostasis

During hemodialysis with HCO_3^--containing bath, the amount of HCO_3^- added from the bath to the patient is dependent on the dialysance of this anion (a function of blood and dialysate flow rate and of the surface area and permeability of the dialysis membrane used), the transmembrane concentration gradient, and the rate of ultrafiltration (1,16,67). The bath [HCO_3^-] is essentially fixed by the high dialysate flow rate and by the absence of any recirculation, as are the permeability and surface area of the dialyzer (with the exception of any minor changes in permeability that occur with multiple reuses). Thus the concentration of HCO_3^- in the blood traversing the membrane is the main variable factor that determines the net movement of this anion during the dialysis treatment. The serum [HCO_3^-] at the onset of dialysis sets the initial rate of HCO_3^- transfer. This value is determined by three factors: (a) the equilibrium value for serum [HCO_3^-] at the end of the previous treatment, (b) the rate of endogenous acid production in the interdialytic period, and (c) the amount of fluid retention. These factors interact with the dialysis treatment itself in a self-regulating fashion because the lower the predialysis [HCO_3^-], the greater the initial rate of HCO_3^- transfer across the membrane. This self-correction results in a steady-state predialysis serum [HCO_3^-] that persists as long as the rate of endogenous acid production and the rate of fluid retention between treatments remains stable and the net amount of HCO_3^- added during each treatment is the same.

The total amount of HCO_3^- added during each treatment depends not only on the serum [HCO_3^-] at the start of the treatment but also on the rate of change during the course of the treatment. To the extent that the added HCO_3^- is retained in the extracellular compartment, it will increase serum [HCO_3^-] and reduce the transmembrane concentration gradient. The rapid addition of HCO_3^- to the body fluids elicits a characteristic buffer response that is well described in experiments in animals and humans (1,16,67,82–85). This response includes not only the release of H^+ from nonbicarbonate buffers, but also metabolic production of organic acids. In patients with end-stage renal disease, the response (measured before a dialysis treatment) is similar to that observed in individuals with normal renal function and results in an apparent space of distribution of the added alkali that is equivalent to approximately 50% of body weight (85). What is not known is the magnitude of the organic acid response to HCO_3^- loading during a hemodialysis treatment when rapid fluxes are occurring.

In theory, production of new organic acids has the capacity for almost unlimited consumption of newly added HCO_3^-, and the generation rate of these acids may be augmented during dialysis (1). The organic anions produced by this reaction are rapidly removed by the dialysis process, moreover, and the loss of these anions is equivalent to alkali loss. Organic anion loss may be as high as 100 mEq during an uncomplicated dialysis treatment (1,59,67,86). During the initial part of a hemodialysis treatment, serum [HCO_3^-] increases rapidly, but little further increase occurs during the latter half (Fig. 2) (1,66). The total increase in serum [HCO_3^-] during a standard 4-hour dialysis treatment is

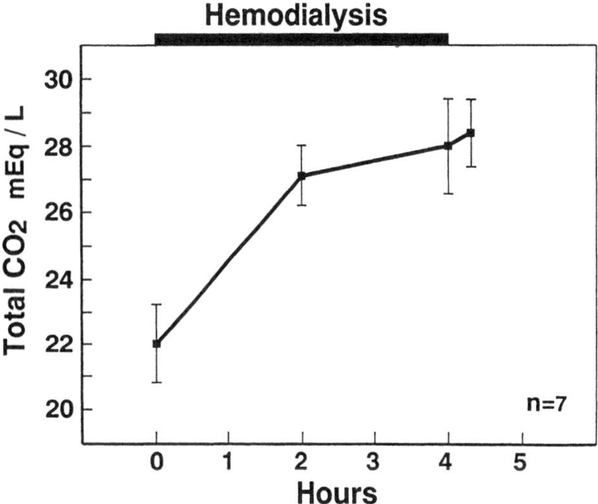

Fig. 2 Pattern of change in serum [total CO_2] during and immediately following a 4-hour hemodialysis treatment using a high-flux dialysis membrane in 7 nondiabetic patients. Vertical lines represent ±1 SE. (From Ref. 100.)

only approximately 6 mEq/L (1,66), and the response is quite variable from patient to patient. In patients with low blood pressures or severe cramps, serum [HCO_3^-] actually has been observed to fall during a standard hemodialysis treatment, presumably due to a major increase in organic acid production (1). Thus, an important factor determining steady-state predialysis serum [HCO_3^-] is the individual organic acid response to the acute addition of alkali during each hemodialysis session.

3. Determinants of Steady-State Serum [HCO_3^-]

Patients receiving intermittent renal replacement therapy do not have a stable serum [HCO_3^-] and pH from day to day, as do individuals with normal renal function or patients receiving a continuous renal replacement therapy such as peritoneal dialysis. As discussed above, serum [HCO_3^-] increases rapidly during the 3- to 4-hour treatment and then decreases gradually in the interval between treatments, reaching its nadir just before the next treatment. The serum [HCO_3^-] concentrations shown in Table 1 for hemodialysis patients reflect the lowest steady-state values, not the integrated level over time. In fact, the values obtained will vary depending on whether they are obtained after the longest interval between treatments (2 days) or after only a 1-day interval. Nonetheless, maneuvers to increase their nadir values to normal levels have beneficial effects on bone and muscle metabolism (see above) (18,19,33).

To assist in thinking about how to improve the acid-base state in patients receiving hemodialysis, it is useful to understand the factors contributing to the low predialysis serum [HCO_3^-]. The first factor is the end-dialysis [HCO_3^-]. Patients who are dialyzed with a standard HCO_3^--containing bath have postdialysis values that range from 25 to 30 mEq/L (Fig. 2) (1,66,87). Several investigators have modeled the process of HCO_3^- transfer to the patient during treatment, and some have advocated individualizing the [HCO_3^-] in the bath to achieve the optimal result in a given patient (88). It is clear that adjustments in bath [HCO_3^-] can achieve the desired level of predialysis serum [HCO_3^-] (see below and Table 2). Less attention has been paid to altering the factors that contribute to the decline in serum [HCO_3^-] between treatments. The two major factors are the rate of endogenous acid production and the amount of fluid retained (without additional alkali) between treatments. Fluid retention without associated alkali simply dilutes the existing alkali stores and thereby lowers serum [HCO_3^-]. Assuming a distribution of retained acid equivalent to 50% of body weight (see earlier) and a weight gain of 2 kg between treatments, one can estimate the influence of a reasonable range of acid production rates on predialysis serum [HCO_3^-] (1). The results of such an analysis, shown in Table 3, indicate that predialysis serum [HCO_3^-] can vary by as much as 6 mEq/L over a range of acid-production rates from 40 to 120 mEq/day. This theoretical analysis is supported indirectly by observations demonstrating a significant inverse correlation between normalized protein catabolic rate and predialysis serum [HCO_3^-] (85). A similar theoretical analysis, holding acid production constant at 60 mEq/day, indicates that variations in fluid retention between 0 and 6 L between treatments can have a large impact on predialysis serum [HCO_3^-] (Table 3). The latter analysis is supported by experimental observations showing that differences in fluid retention of only 1 L can change predialysis serum [HCO_3^-] by more than 1 mEq/L (89). In patients receiving a continuous form of renal replacement therapy, such as peritoneal dialysis, these effects of fluid retention do not occur. Alkali is added continuously, automatically adjusting serum [HCO_3^-] for any changes in extracellular volume.

Table 3 Calculated Effect of Changes in Net Acid Production or in Fluid Retention on Predialysis Serum [HCO_3^-][a]

Net acid production (mEq/day)	Fluid retention[b] (L)	Predialysis [HCO_3^-] (mEq/L)
40	2	23.4
80	2	20.4
120	2	17.3
60	0	23.1
60	3	21.3
60	6	19.8

Assumptions: Wt = 70 Kg; postdialysis serum [HCO_3^-] = 28 mEq/L; HCO_3^- buffer space = 0.5 × body weight.

[a]Predialysis serum [HCO_3^-] after long interval between hemodialysis treatments (68 h).

[b]Liters retained during interval between treatments.

4. Clinical Studies of Correction of Acidosis

Table 2 summarizes the studies in which interventions have been undertaken to increase serum [HCO_3^-] in patients receiving renal replacement therapy. With the exception of two of these studies, one each of hemodialysis and peritoneal dialysis, this goal was achieved primarily by changing bath [HCO_3^-]. Lefebvre and coworkers increased predialysis serum [HCO_3^-] from 15.6 to 24 mEq/L in patients receiving hemodialysis by increasing bath [HCO_3^-] from 33 to as high as 48 mEq/L (18). No untoward effects were noted with this marked increase in dialysate [HCO_3^-]. By contrast, Oettinger and Oliver and Graham and colleagues increased predialysis serum [HCO_3^-] to average values of 23–25 mEq/L after only a 3–5 mEq/L increase in bath [HCO_3^-] (19,87). In a second study by Graham and colleagues, an oral bicarbonate supplement was needed in two of six patients, in addition to increasing bath [HCO_3^-], to raise predialysis serum [HCO_3^-] to the same levels (33). Brady and Hasbargen studied patients preselected for a low predialysis serum [HCO_3^-] and found they had to give large amounts of supplemental $NaHCO_3$, in addition to increasing bath [HCO_3^-], to raise predialysis serum [HCO_3^-] to a reasonable level (35). The reasons for these differing requirements are unclear, but in all likelihood they relate to differences in endogenous acid production in the populations studied. Correction of acidosis was achievable in patients receiving peritoneal dialysis using a HCO_3^--containing bath by increasing bath [HCO_3^-] from 34 to 39 mEq/L (44). Van Stone made no changes in bath composition but instead gave sizable sodium citrate supplements to patients receiving hemodialysis and was able to increase predialysis serum [HCO_3^-] notably (90). Weight gain between treatments, however, was increased in the citrate-treated patients. Graham and colleagues demonstrated that much more modest alkali supplements

Table 4 Management of Low Serum [HCO_3^-] in Patients with End-Stage Renal Disease

1. Evaluate the cause
   a. Measure pre- and postdialysis serum [HCO_3^-]
   b. Assess weight gain between treatments
   c. Assess diet/catabolic state
2. Intervene
   a. Modify dialysis treatment to minimize organic acid production
   b. Minimize interdialytic weight gain
   c. Reduce sulfur-containing amino acids in diet
   d. Use $NaHCO_3$ supplements or alter bath [HCO_3^-]

could easily correct metabolic acidosis in a group of patients receiving peritoneal dialysis who were preselected because of low serum [HCO_3^-] values (34).

5. Approach to Correcting Acidosis

The first step in management of a patient with end-stage renal disease with a low serum [HCO_3^-] is to evaluate its cause (Table 4). From the foregoing discussion, it is apparent that this evaluation should include measurement of serum [HCO_3^-] pre- and postdialysis to assess whether the level is increasing as expected. If the value does not increase by at least 4 mEq/L, then attention should be addressed to the events occurring during the dialysis treatment itself. Increasing bath [HCO_3^-] is unlikely to help in this setting. Modifying the treatment in ways that avoid hypotension (e.g., sodium modeling or nonlinear ultrafiltration) could improve net alkali addition during treatments. If postdialysis serum [HCO_3^-] is in the appropriate range (26–30 mEq/L), then attention should be directed at the interdialytic period. Modification of diet and controlling fluid intake could correct the problem without any other intervention (see Table 3). If these interventions are not possible, predialysis serum [HCO_3^-] can be raised by increasing bath [HCO_3^-] (Table 2). Oral alkali supplementation ($NaHCO_3$) should be effective regardless of whether the problem is due to excess alkali consumption during dialysis or to a high rate of acid production, but it carries the risk of increased fluid retention between treatments (90).

IV. RECOGNITION OF SUPERIMPOSED ACID-BASE DISORDERS

In addition to assuring that patients receiving renal replacement therapy have optimal serum [HCO_3^-] levels, it is important to recognize the presence of superimposed acid-base disorders. For metabolic disorders, this task is straightforward because serum [total CO_2] is routinely measured. A sudden deviation of more than 3 mEq/L in either direction from the usual value indicates the presence of a new metabolic acid-base disorder. Respiratory acid-base disorders are more difficult to uncover because arterial pH and PCO_2 are not routinely measured. In patients with functioning fistulas, blood samples from the fistulas can easily provide the necessary information because fistula blood is equivalent to arterial blood (16,91). Such measurements should be obtained if one suspects a ventilatory problem or if serum [HCO_3^-] deviates markedly from the usual value. Because the ventilatory response to changes in serum [HCO_3^-] in patients with end-stage renal disease is not different than in individuals with normal renal function (16,59,62,67,92,93), one can use the following empirical formulas to estimate the expected PCO_2 for any given level of serum [HCO_3^-] (94–96):

For serum [HCO_3^-] 24 mEq/L or less:

$$PCO_2\,(\text{mmHg}) = 40 - 1.3 \times (24 - [HCO_3^-]) \quad (1)$$

For serum [HCO_3^-] > 24 mEq/L:

$$PCO_2\,(\text{mmHg}) = 40 + 0.7 \times ([HCO_3^-] - 24) \quad (2)$$

It should be emphasized that these formulas represent only approximations. One should not conclude that the PCO_2 is abnormally high or low unless it deviates from the calculated value by more than 5 mmHg. If the measured value does deviate by more than 5 mmHg from the calculated value, then a separate respiratory acid-base disorder is likely to be present (see below). The diagnosis of each of the four cardinal acid-base disorders is discussed below.

A. Metabolic Acidosis

In patients with end-stage renal disease, a superimposed metabolic acidosis is heralded by a fall in serum [HCO_3^-] of greater than 3 mEq/L from the usual value. In these patients, the spectrum of causes is narrower than in patients with functioning kidneys (Table 5). One need not, for example, consider renal causes. Given the high fraction of dialysis patients who have diabetes mellitus, it is not surprising that the most common cause of a new metabolic acidosis is diabetic ketoacidosis. In these patients, the fall in serum [HCO_3^-] should be matched by an increase in anion gap ($[Na^+] - \{[HCO_3^-] + [Cl^-]\}$), because the newly produced ketoanions are not lost in the urine. Toxin in-

Table 5 Causes of Worsening Metabolic Acidosis in End-Stage Renal Disease

Increase in anion gap	No increase in anion gap
Endogenous causes	Gastrointestinal alkali loss (e.g., diarrhea, pancreatic drainage)
Diabetic ketoacidosis	
Lactic acidosis	
Alcoholic ketoacidosis	Bath alkali replacement with NaCl
Toxin ingestions	Ammonium chloride ingestion
Methyl alcohol	Use of NaCl replacement fluid during continuous hemofiltration
Ethylene glycol	
Salicylates	
Paraldehyde	
Increased endogenous acid production	Dilutional
Diet-induced	Salt and water retention
Catabolic states	

gestions will produce the same electrolyte pattern. In patients who become more catabolic, the increase in endogenous acid production will also reduce serum [HCO_3^-]. Much more rarely, metabolic acidosis occurs as a result of gastrointestinal alkali losses due to diarrhea or from pancreatic drainage. In this setting the anion gap should not increase from its usual level. One should remember that the anion gap in hemodialysis patients is normally higher than in individuals with functioning kidneys (1,16,94).

B. Metabolic Alkalosis

In patients with end-stage renal disease, a new metabolic alkalosis is heralded by an increase in serum [HCO_3^-] of >3 mEq/L (95,96). Because such a change often results in a serum [HCO_3^-] within the normal range, this acid-base disorder may not be recognized until a much larger increase in serum [HCO_3^-] has occurred (97). Even a small increase in serum [HCO_3^-] above the usual value that occurs without a change in dialysis prescription, however, is associated with an increase in mortality (98). Thus one should be aware of this acid-base disorder. The diagnostic spectrum is again narrower than in patients with functioning kidneys. In patients with end-stage renal disease, metabolic alkalosis is generated by HCl losses from the gastrointestinal tract or by the addition of excess alkali. Because these patients have no way to excrete the excess alkali generated by HCl losses or alkali addition, the disorder is sustained independent of extracellular volume or body chloride stores. Renal causes, that is, "chloride-resistant" forms of metabolic alkalosis, need not be considered. In addition, hypokalemia is not a component of metabolic alkalosis in end-stage renal disease because no renal K^+ losses occur. When confronted with an elevated serum [HCO_3^-], one need only consider whether gastrointestinal acid loss is occurring or search for the source of new alkali (95,96).

C. Respiratory Acidosis

Carbon dioxide retention is a serious complication in patients with end-stage renal disease because the normal renal adaptive mechanisms to protect systemic pH cannot operate. A patient with functioning kidneys and sustained hypercapnia develops an increase in serum [HCO_3^-] that ameliorates the resultant acidosis. For example, if the PCO_2 is maintained at 55 mmHg, serum [HCO_3^-] will rise by approximately 5 mEq/L and pH will only fall to 7.37. In renal failure no such adaptation occurs. Serum [HCO_3^-] is determined by the same interplay between dialysis prescription and endogenous acid production as in patients with normal alveolar ventilation. Thus, at the same PCO_2 (55 mmHg), a patient with end-stage renal disease will have no change in serum [HCO_3^-], and if it is maintained at 20 mEq/L, arterial pH will fall to 7.18 (95). Thus, unless the hypercapnia can be corrected, long-term survival on dialysis is unlikely.

D. Respiratory Alkalosis

As is the case for respiratory acidosis, no renal adaptive response occurs to respiratory alkalosis in patients with end-stage renal disease. As a result, severe and sustained alkalemia can occur when primary hyperventilation develops (95,99). Respiratory alkalosis has many causes, including central nervous system diseases such as stroke and tumors, sepsis, particularly due to gram-negative organisms, and hepatic failure (95). Recognition of the presence of this disorder, diagnosing it with appropriate blood gas measurements, and treating the underlying cause are critical for patient survival.

E. Mixed Acid-Base Disorders

It is important to remember that, on occasion, more than one acid-base disorder can be present (95). For example, a patient can have a mixed metabolic and respiratory acidosis if the serum [HCO_3^-] is decreased and the ventilatory response is inadequate. These disorders can be identified by obtaining measurements of arterial PCO_2 and pH and by using the formulas presented earlier. The importance of identifying more than one disorder is that treatment needs to be directed at both disorders (95). In the example cited above, attention needs to be paid to improving ventilation as well as adding alkali to improve serum [HCO_3^-].

V. SUMMARY

Extensive experimental and clinical evidence indicates that metabolic acidosis worsens metabolic bone disease and is detrimental to skeletal muscle metabolism in patients with renal failure. It appears that even a mild degree of metabolic acidosis can be considered to be a "uremic toxin." Alkali replacement during dialysis therapy is directed at minimizing the effects of this toxin. When dialysis treatment is initiated, a new acid-base equilibrium develops that is determined primarily by the interplay between the specific dialysis prescription and acid production by the patient. Regardless of the type of dialysis therapy used, serum bicarbonate concentration in the new steady-state is set at a level at which metabolic acid production is balanced by the alkali gained from dialysis fluids and acid retention no longer continues. Despite the ability to provide large amounts of alkali (or alkali precursors) during dialysis therapy, serum bicarbonate concentration in patients receiving peritoneal dialysis is often lower than normal, and predialysis bicarbonate concentration in most hemodialysis patients is notably lower than normal. In addition, because of the fixed and unvarying conditions of the dialysis prescription in terms of alkali delivery, serum bicarbonate concentration varies more in patients with end-stage renal disease than in individuals with normal renal function. Given the evidence that even mildly reduced values for serum bicarbonate concentration have deleterious effects, efforts should be undertaken to understand the causes for metabolic acidosis in patients receiving renal replacement therapy. These causes include the patient's dialysis prescription (including the type of dialysis provided), their response to acute alkali addition during the treatment, the rate of endogenous acid production (i.e., diet), and the rate of fluid retention between treatments for those receiving intermittent hemodialysis. Superimposed acid-base disturbances can also occur in dialysis patients, and these should be recognized and treated when present.

REFERENCES

1. Gennari FJ. Acid-base homeostasis in end-stage renal disease. Sem Dial 1996; 9:404–411.
2. Widmer B, Gerhardt RE, Harringon JT, Cohen JJ. Serum electrolyte and acid-base composition: the influence of graded degrees of chronic renal failure. Arch Intern Med 1979; 139:1099–1102.
3. Litzow JR, Lemann J, Lennon EJ. The effect of treatment of acidosis on calcium balance in patients with chronic azotemic renal disease. J Clin Invest 1967; 46: 280–286.
4. Uribarri J, Douyon H, Oh MS. A re-evaluation of the urinary parameters of acid production and excretion in patients with chronic renal acidosis. Kidney Int 1995; 47:624–627.
5. Schwartz WB, Hall PW, Hays RM, Relman AS. On the mechanism of acidosis in chronic renal disease. J Clin Invest 1959; 38:39–45.
6. Marsiglia JC, Cingolani HE, Gonzales NC. Relevance of beta receptor blockade to the negative inotropic effect induced by metabolic acidosis. Cardiovasc Res 1973; 7:336–343.
7. Harrington JT, Cohen JJ. Metabolic acidosis. In: Cohen JJ, Kassirer JP, eds. Acid Base. Boston: Little, Brown, 1982:121–225.
8. Fantuzzi S, Caico S, Amatruda O, et al. Hemodialysis-associated cardiac arrhythmias: a lower risk with bicarbonate? Nephron 1991; 58:196–200.
9. Oh MS. Irrelevance of bone buffering to acid-base homeostasis in chronic metabolic acidosis. Nephron 1991; 59:7–10.
10. Lemann J, Litzow JR, Lennon EJ. The effects of chronic acid loads in normal man: Further evidence for the participation of bone mineral in the defense against chronic metabolic acidosis. J Clin Invest 1966; 45:1608–1614.
11. Barzel US, Jowsey J. The effects of chronic acid and alkali administration on bone turnover in adult rats. Clin Sci 1969; 36:517–521.
12. Goldhaber P, Rabadjija L. H^+ stimulation of cell-mediated bone resorption in tissue culture. Am J Physiol 1987; 253:E90–98.

13. Bushinsky DA, Lechleider RJ. Mechanism of proton-induced bone calcium release: calcium carbonate dissolution. Am J Physiol 1987; 253:F998–F1005.
14. Krieger NS, Sessler NE, Bushinsky DA. Acidosis inhibit osteoblastic and stimulates osteoclastic activity in vitro. Am J Physiol 1992; 262:F442–448.
15. Bushinsky DA, Sessler NE, Krieger NS. Greater unidirectional calcium efflux from bone during metabolic, compared with respiratory, acidosis. Am J Physiol 1992; 262:F425–F431.
16. Gennari FJ. Acid-base balance in dialysis patients. Kidney Int 1985; 28:678–688.
17. Bichara M, Mercier O, Borensztein P, Paillard M. Acute metabolic acidosis enhances circulating parathyroid hormone, which contributes to the renal response against acidosis in the rat. J Clin Invest 1990; 86:430–443.
18. Lefebvre A, de Verneoul MC, Gueris J, Goldfarb B, Graulet AM, Morieux C. Optimal correction of acidosis changes progression of dialysis osteodystrophy. Kidney Int 1989; 36:1112–1118.
19. Graham KA, Hoenich NA, Tarbit M, Ward MK, Goodship THJ. Correction of acidosis in hemodialysis patients increases the sensitivity of the parathyroid glands to calcium. J Am Soc Nephrol 1997; 8:627–631.
20. Hutchison AJ, Freemont AJ, Boulton HF, Gokal R. Low calcium dialysis fluid and oral calcium carbonate in CAPD. A method of controlling hyperphosphatemia whilst minimizing aluminum exposure and hypercalcaemia. Nephrol Dial Transplant 1992; 7:1219–1225.
21. May RC, Kelly RA, Mitch WE. Mechanisms for defects in muscle protein metabolism in rats with chronic uremia: Influence of metabolic acidosis. J Clin Invest 1987; 79:1099–1103.
22. May RC, Kelly RA, Mitch WE. Metabolic acidosis stimulates protein degradation in rat muscle by a glucocorticoid-dependent mechanism. J Clin Invest 1986; 77:614–621.
23. Hara Y, May RC, Kelly RA, Mitch WE. Acidosis, not azotemia, stimulates branched-chain amino acid catabolism in uremic rats. Kidney Int 1987; 32:808–814.
24. Mitch WE, Clark AS. Specificity of the effects of leucine and its metabolites on protein degradation in skeletal muscle. Biochem J 1984; 222:579–586.
25. Papadoyannakis NJ, Stefanidis CJ, McGeown M. The effect of the correction of metabolic acidosis on nitrogen and protein balance of patients with chronic renal failure. Am J Clin Nutr 1984; 40:623–627.
26. Reaich D, Channon SM, Scrimgeour CM, Daley SE, Wilkinson R, Goodship THJ. Correction of acidosis in humans with CRF decreases protein degradation and amino acid oxidation. Am J Physiol 1993; 265:E230–235.
27. Jenkins D, Burton PR, Bennet SE, Baker F, Walls J. The metabolic consequences of the correction of acidosis in uraemia. Nephrol Dial Transpl 1989; 4:92–95.
28. Williams, B, Hattersley J, Layward E, Walls J. Metabolic acidosis and skeletal muscle adaptation to low protein diets in chronic uremia. Kidney Int 1991; 40: 779–786.
29. Bergström J, Alvestrand A, Fürst P. Plasma and muscle free amino acids in maintenance hemodialysis patients without protein malnutrition. Kidney Int 1990; 38:108–114.
30. Garibotto G, Russo R, Sofia A, et al. Skeletal muscle protein synthesis and degradation in patients with chronic renal failure. Kidney Int 1994; 45:1432–1439.
31. Ballmer PE, McNurlan MA, Hulter HN, Anderson SE, Garlick PJ, Krapf R. Chronic metabolic acidosis decreases albumin synthesis and induces negative nitrogen balance in humans. J Clin Invest 1995; 95:39–45.
32. Stein A, Baker F, Larratt C, Bennett S, Harris K, Feehally J, Walls J. Correction of metabolic acidosis and protein catabolic rate in PD patients. Perit Dial Int 1994; 14:187–189.
33. Graham KA, Reaich D, Channon SM, et al. Correction of acidosis in hemodialysis decreases whole-body protein degradation. J Am Soc Nephrol 1997; 8:632–637.
34. Graham KA, Reaich D, Channon SM, Downie S, Gilmour E, Passlick-Deetjen J, Goodship THJ. Correction of acidosis in CAPD decreases whole-body protein degradation. Kidney Int 1996; 49:1396–1400.
35. Brady JP, Hasbargen JA. Correction of metabolic acidosis and its effect on albumin in chronic hemodialysis patients. Am J Kidney Dis 1998; 31:35–40.
36. Fukagawa NK, Minaker KL, Rowe JW, et al. Insulin-mediated reduction of whole body protein breakdown. Dose-response effects on leucine metabolism in postabsorptive men. J Clin Invest 1985; 76:2306–2311.
37. Defronzo RA, Beckles AD. Glucose intolerance following chronic metabolic acidosis in man. Am J Physiol 1979; 236:E328–334.
38. Defronzo RA, Alvestrand A, Smith D, Hendler R, Hendler E, Wahren J. Insulin resistence in uremia. J Clin Invest 1981; 67:563–568.
39. Mitch WE, Price SR, May RC, Jurkovitz C, England BK. Metabolic consequences of uremia: extending the concept of adaptive responses to protein metabolism. Am J Kidney Dis 1994; 23:224–228.
40. Feriani M. Buffers: Bicarbonate, lactate and pyruvate. Kidney Int 1996; 50(suppl 56):S75–S80.
41. Feriani M, Biasioli S, Borin D, et al. Bicarbonate buffer for CAPD solution. Trans Am Soc Artif Intern Organs 1985; 31:668–671.
42. Feriani M, Dissegna D, La Greca G, Passlick-Deetjen J. Short term clinical study with bicarbonate containing peritoneal dialysis solution. Perit Dial Int 1993; 13:296–301.

43. Feriani M. Adequacy of acid base correction in continuous ambulatory peritoneal dialysis patients. Perit Dial Int 1994; 14(suppl 3):S133–S138.
44. Feriani M, Carobi C, La Greca G, Buoncristiani U, Passlick-Deetjen J: Clinical experiences with a bicarbonate buffered (39 mmol/L) peritoneal dialysis solution. Perit Dial Int 1997; 17:17–21.
45. Coles GA, Gokal R, Ogg C, et al. A randomized controlled trial of a bicarbonate and a bicarbonate/lactate containing dialysis solution in CAPD. Perit Dial Int 1997; 17:48–5.
46. Mactier RA, Sprosen TS, Gokal R, et al. Bicarbonate and bicarbonate/lactate peritoneal dialysis solutions for the treatment of infusion pain. Kidney Int 1998; 53:1061–1067.
47. Uribarri J, Buquing J, Oh MS. Acid-base balance in chronic peritoneal dialysis patients. Kidney Int 1995; 47:269–273.
48. Graham KA, Reaich D, Goodship THJ. Acid-base regulation in peritoneal dialysis. Kidney Int 1994; 46(suppl 48):S47–S50.
49. Yasuda T, Ozawa S, Shiba C, et al. D-lactate metabolism in patients with chronic renal failure undergoing CAPD. Nephron 1993; 63:416–422.
50. Nolph KD, Prowant B, Serkes KD, et al. Multicenter evaluation of a new peritoneal dialysis solution with a high lactate and a low magnesium concentration. Perit Dial Bull 1983; 3:63–65.
51. Mandelbaum JM, Heistand ML, Schardin KE. Six months' experience with PD-2 solution. Dial Transplant 1983; 12:259–260.
52. Murphy WP, Swan RC, Walter CW, Weller JM, Merrill JP. Use of an artificial kidney. III: Current procedures in clinical hemodialysis. J Lab Clin Med 1952; 40:436–444.
53. Brandon JM, Nakamoto S, Rosenbaum JL, Franklin M, Kolff WJ. Prolongation of survival by periodic prolonged hemodialysis in patients with chronic renal failure. Am J Med 1962; 33:538–544.
54. Mion CM, Hegstrom RM, Boen ST, Scribner BH. Substitution of sodium acetate for sodium bicarbonate in the bath fluid for hemodialysis. Trans Am Soc Artif Intern Organs 1964; 10:110–113.
55. Tolchin N, Roberts JL, Hayashi J, Lewis EJ. Metabolic consequences of high mass-transfer hemodialysis. Kidney Int 1977; 11:361–378.
56. Gennari FJ. Comparative physiology of acetate and bicarbonate alkalinization. In: Cummings NB, Klahr S, eds. Chronic Renal Disease. New York: Plenum, 1985:453–461.
57.. Dolan MJ, Whipp BJ, Davidson WD, Weitzman RE, Wasserman K. Hypopnea associated with acetate hemodialysis: carbon dioxide-flow-dependent ventilation. N Engl J Med 1981; 305:72–75.
58. Hunt JM, Chappell TR, Henrich WL, Rubin LJ. Gas exchange during dialysis. Am J Med 1984; 77:255–260.
59. Vreman HJ, Assomull VM, Kaiser BA, Blaschke TF, Weiner MW. Acetate metabolism and acid-base homeostasis during hemodialysis: influence of dialyzer efficiency and rate of acetate metabolism. Kidney Int 1980; 18(suppl 10):S62–S74.
60. Kveim M, Nesbakken R. Utilization of exogenous acetate during hemodialysis. Trans Am Soc Artif Intern Organs 1975; 21:138–143.
61. Graefe U, Milutinovich J, Folette WC, Vizzo JE, Babb AL, Scribner BH. Less dialysis-induced morbidity and vascular instability with bicarbonate in dialysate. Ann Intern Med 1978; 88:332–336.
62. Hakim RM, Pontzer M, Tilton D, Lazarus JM, Gottlieb MN. Effects of acetate and bicarbonate dialysate in stable chronic dialysis patients. Kidney Int 1985; 28:535–540.
63. Vinay P, Prud'homme M, Vinet B, et al. Acetate metabolism and bicarbonate generation during hemodialysis: 10 years of observation. Kidney Int 1987; 31: 1194–1204.
64. Man NK, Fournier G, Thireau P, Gaillard JL, Funck-Brentano JL. Effect of bicarbonate-containing dialysate on chronic hemodialysis patients: a comparative study. Artif Organs 1982; 6:421–425.
65. Ward RA, Wathen RL, Williams TE. Effects of long-term bicarbonate hemodialysis on acid-base status. Trans Am Soc Artif Intern Organs 1982: 28:295–298.
66. Symreng T, Flanigan MJ, Lim VS. Ventilatory and metabolic changes during high efficiency hemodialysis. Kidney Int 1992; 41:1064–1069.
67. Gotch FA, Sargent JA, Keen ML. Hydrogen ion balance in dialysis therapy. Artif Organs 1982; 6:388–395.
68. Ward RA, Wathen RL, Williams TE, Harding GB. Hemodialysate composition and intradialytic metabolic, acid-base and potassium changes. Kidney Int 1987; 32:129–135.
69. Henrich WL, Woodard TD, Meyer BD, Chappell TR, Rubin LJ. High sodium bicarbonate and acetate hemodialysis: Double blind crossover comparison of hemodynamic and ventilatory effects. Kidney Int 1983; 24:240–245.
70. Bahnsen M, Broch Møller B, Christiansen E, et al. The REDY system. Experiments and experiences. Scand J Urol Nephrol 1976; (suppl 30):5–38.
71. Brezis M, Brown RS. An unsuspected cause for metabolic acidosis in chronic renal failure: sorbent system hemodialysis. Am J Kidney Dis 1985; 6:425–427.
72. Bosch JP, Lauer A. Acid-base balance in hemofiltration. In: Henderson LW, Quellhorst EA, Baldamus CA, Lysaght MJ, eds. Hemofiltration. Berlin: Springer-Verlag, 1986:147–154.
73. Schaefer K, Ryzlewicz T, Sandri M, von Bernewitz S, von Herrath D. Acid-base balance and pulmonary function in hemofiltration. Int J Artif Organs 1983; 6: 43–47.

74. Kishimoto T, Yamamoto T, Yamamoto K, et al. Acetate kinetics during hemodialysis and hemofiltration. Blood Purif 1984; 2:81–87.
75. Feriani M, Biasioli S, Fabris A, et al. Calcium and bicarbonate containing solutions for peritoneal dialysis and hemofiltration. In: Nosè Y, Kjellstrand C, Ivanovich P, eds. Progress in Artificial Organs. Cleveland: ISAO Press, 1986:277–281.
76. Santoro A, Ferrari G, Bolzani R, Spongano M, Zucchelli P. Regulation of base balance in bicarbonate hemofiltration. Int J Artif Organs 1994; 17:27–36.
77. Leber HW, Wizemann V, Goubeand G, Rawer P, Schütterle G. Simultaneous hemofiltration/hemodialysis: an effective alternative to hemofiltration and conventional hemodialysis in the treatment of uremic patients. Clin Nephrol 1978; 9:115–121.
78. Feriani M, Ronco C, Biasoli S, Bragantini L, La Greca G. Effect of dialysate and substitution fluid buffer on buffer flux in hemodiafiltration. Kidney Int 1990; 39: 711–717.
79. Movilli E, Camerini C, Zein H, et al. A prospective comparison of bicarbonate dialysis, hemodiafiltration, and acetate-free biofiltration in the elderly. Am J Kid Diseases 1996; 27:541–547.
80. Santoro A, Ferrari G, Spongano M, Badiali F, Zucchelli P. Acetate-free biofiltration: a viable alternative to bicarbonate hemodialysis. Artif Organs 1989; 13: 476–485.
81. Forni LG, Hilton PJ. Continuous hemofiltration in the treatment of acute renal failure. N Engl J Med 1997; 336:1303–1309.
82. Adrogué HJ, Brensilver J, Cohen JJ, Madias NE. Influence of steady-state alterations in acid-base equilibrium on the fate of administered bicarbonate in the dog. J Clin Invest 1983; 71:867–883.
83. Singer RB, Clark JK, Barker ES, Crosley AP, Elkinton JR. The acute effects in man of rapid intravenous infusion of hypertonic sodium bicarbonate solution. I. Changes in acid-base balance and the distribution of the excess buffer base. Medicine 1955; 34:51–95.
84. Fernandez PC, Cohen RM, Feldman GM. The concept of bicarbonate distribution space: the crucial role of body buffers. Kidney Int 1989; 36:747–752.
85. Uribarri J, Zia M, Mahmood J, Marcus RA, Oh MS. Acid production in chronic hemodialysis patients. J Am Soc Nephrol 1998; 9:114–120.
86. Ward RA, Wathen RL, Williams TE, Harding GB. Hemodialysate composition and intradialytic metabolic, acid-base and potassium changes. Kidney Int 1987; 32:129–135.
87. Oettinger CW, Oliver JC. Normalization of uremic acidosis in hemodialysis patients with a high bicarbonate dialysate. J Am Soc Nephrol 1993; 3:1804–1807.
88. Thews O. Model-based decision support system for individual prescription of the dialysate bicarbonate concentration in hemodialysis. Int J Artif Organs 1992; 15:447–455.
89. Fabris A, LaGreca G, Chiaramonte S, et al. The importance of ultrafiltration and acid-base status in a dialysis population. Trans Am Soc Artif Intern Organs 1988; 34:200–201.
90. Van Stone JC. Oral base replacement in patients on hemodialysis. Ann Intern Med 1984; 101:199–201.
91. Santiago-Delpin EA, Buselmeier TJ, Simmons RL, Najarian JS, Kjellstrand CM. Blood gases and pH in patients with artificial arteriovenous fistulas. Kidney Int 1972; 1:131–133.
92. Cohen E, Liu K, Batlle DC. Patterns of metabolic acidosis in patients with chronic renal failure: impact of hemodialysis. Int J Artif Organs 1988; 11:440–448.
93. Bushinsky DA, Coe FL, Katzenberg C, Szidon JP, Parks JH. Arterial P_{CO_2} in chronic metabolic acidosis. Kidney Int 1982; 22:311–314.
94. Gennari FJ, Rimmer JM. Acid-base disorders in end-stage renal disease: Part I. Sem Dial 1990; 3:81–85.
95. Gennari FJ, Rimmer JM. Acid-base disorders in end-stage renal disease: Part II. Sem Dial 1990; 3:161–165.
96. Rimmer JM, Gennari FJ. Metabolic alkalosis. J Intensive Care Med 1987; 2:137–150.
97. Gennari FJ. A normal serum bicarbonate level in a woman receiving chronic hemodialysis. Sem Dial 1991; 4:59–61.
98. Lowrie EG, Lew NL. Death risk in hemodialysis patients: the predictive value of commonly measured variables and an evaluation of death rate differences between facilities. Am J Kidney Dis 1990; 15:458–482.
99. Kenamond TG, Graves JW, Lempert KD, Moss AH, Whittier FC. Severe recurrent alkalemia in a patient undergoing continuous cyclic peritoneal dialysis. Am J Med 1986; 81:548–550.
100. Gennari FJ. Acid-base considerations in end-stage renal disease. In: Henrich WL, ed. Principles and Practice of Dialysis. 2d ed. Baltimore: Williams and Wilkins, 1999:341–356.

20

Infectious Problems in Dialysis Patients

Raymond C. Vanholder and Renaat Peleman
University Hospital of Gent, Gent, Belgium

I. INTRODUCTION

Infectious diseases remain among the major morbid events in patients affected by uremia, both in those who have not yet reached end-stage renal disease (ESRD) as well as in those dialyzed or transplanted. Because of the special conditions that are at stake in dialysis [hemodialysis (HD), as well as continuous ambulatory peritoneal dialysis (CAPD)], whereby various protective mechanisms of the immune system are affected, infection is especially problematic in dialyzed patients. In addition, infectious diseases may provoke both acute and chronic renal failure, which in turn may necessitate dialysis. In this chapter, infectious diseases complicating dialysis will be reviewed. The main complications reviewed in this chapter are listed in Table 1.

II. ETIOLOGY OF INCREASED RISK FOR INFECTION

A. Breakdown of Cutaneous Protective Barriers

Dialysis necessitates the introduction of an access device, either into the bloodstream (HD) or into the peritoneal cavity (CAPD). In HD, the safest access site is provided by the endogenous arteriovenous fistula, because it consists of vascular material and the skin is only perforated by needles or cannulas at the moment of dialysis. Nevertheless, this act of cannulation carries the risk of entry of bacteria into the blood stream. The risk of infection is directly correlated to the number of cannulation procedures, and in case of access problems with repetitive cannulation attempts, the risk increases significantly.

When foreign material is introduced, this risk becomes even higher, as bacteria have an affinity for this material (see Sec. II.B). Therefore, polytetrafluoroethylene (PTFE) vascular graft systems and central vein dialysis catheters carry a substantially greater infectious risk than arteriovenous fistulae (1,2).

In addition, for all dialysis procedures the access must be connected to the extracorporeal circuit, and these manipulations may further increase the risk for infection. The dialysis procedure as such may inhibit immune function (see Sec. II.F), both acutely and chronically (3). An acute inhibition may occur immediately after the vascular access has been connected to the extracorporeal circuit (4). If bacteria are introduced, the performance of the immune system is at its weakest at that moment.

For central vein catheter dialysis, either intermittent or continuous catheterization may be used. For continuous catheterization, either stiff small-bore catheters (polyurethane or teflon) can be used for a relatively short period of time (maximum 6–8 weeks), or soft large-bore catheters (silicone) can be used for longer periods (up to several months to years). Because the soft large-bore catheters are tunneled during the introduction procedure and because they contain a protective cuff, the incidence of infection per application period will be significantly lower compared to the stiffer variants (1,5) (soft: 2.16 events/100 patient-months; stiff: 10.0 events/100 patient-months).

The same holds true for peritoneal dialysis: the risk of infection via the access system is substantial, espe-

Table 1 Main Infectious Complications of Dialysis

Bacteremia
CAPD peritonitis
Catheter sepsis
Cytomegalovirus infection
Endocarditis
Fungal infections
Hepatitis
Infection of vascular access (AV fistula, PTFE graft, central vein catheter)
Osteomyelitis
Transfer bacteria from contaminated dialysate reused dialyzers
Tuberculosis
Tunnel infection of catheter insertion site

cially as the number of manipulations per unit of time is more frequent than for HD (currently 28/3 >9 times more frequent). In addition, whereas in HD germs may enter the blood directly when they are introduced in the circulation, in PD the germs enter the peritoneal cavity, where immune active cells and solutes are diluted and suppressed continuously.

The introduction of bacteria through the access tunnel is inhibited by Dacron cuffs. In addition, various structural modifications have been introduced in the access systems for PD in the hope of reducing the number of infectious complications (6). Whether these modifications actually significantly reduce the infectious risk remains a matter of debate. For twin-bag systems, it has been demonstrated that the incidence of infection is lower when compared to single-bag systems, but the purchase cost of twin-bag systems is higher (7). This effect is, however, largely compensated for by the lower hospitalization costs for infection (7).

On the other hand, the manipulations at the moment of the connection of the dialysate have been simplified and optimized, decreasing the risk for infection. As such, exit site and tunnel infections have become the major source of peritonitis in the CAPD population (6,8).

B. Affinity of Bacteria for Foreign Materials

Bacteria have a special affinity for artificial devices and synthetic materials (9,10). Factors enhancing this affinity are surface roughness and electrostatic charge.

In every condition where artificial access systems are used for dialysis purposes, infection may become a major problem (1,11,12). Once bacterial contamination enters these systems, bacteria may easily stick to the polymer materials and to the fibrin sheath that covers them.

Modification of the surface of catheters may be of help in coping with this problem. A silver coating has been applied and was claimed to decrease infectious risks (13). Well-controlled studies are, however, lacking regarding this issue.

Bonding of the surface with antibiotics may be another way to prevent infectious overgrowth. In a study by Kamal et al. (14), bonding with cefazolin decreased the risk for catheter infection. It is conceivable that the antibiotic gradually disappears from the surface, so that at a certain point the constitution of the catheter is not different from an unbonded variant. It is, however, never certain when this return to the original condition happens. It should also be stressed that the few studies of catheters bonded with antibiotics were undertaken in indications other than dialysis. Catheters may be maintained for a much longer period in the dialysis setting than in other conditions, whereas shear conditions are much more preponderant; therefore, the loss of antibiotic during long-term application is a possibility that certainly should be taken into consideration.

C. Affinity of Bacteria for Endogenous Materials

Bacteria also show affinity for the patient's own tissue, especially if it is damaged. A common example is endocarditis, which occurs more readily if the heart valves are affected by stenosis or other structural alterations (15). Endocarditis is especially a risk in patients undergoing catheter dialysis because of the closeness of the catheter tip to the heart valves (16). Another preferential site of metastatic infection is the bone. In principle, however, any tissue can be affected by metastatic infectious disease; this risk is markedly enhanced by the immune deficiency of the uremic patient (see Sec. II.F).

D. Contamination of Water

Dialysis cannot be performed without the use of water in the preparation of dialysate. This water may be contaminated in its original state as tap water, before any treatment. In addition, germs may be added in water-treatment systems, and they may also be present in the electrolyte concentrate that is added to the tap water to pursue the final "ideal" corrective electrolyte composition.

These bacteria may enter the blood stream through small cracks in the structure of the dialysis membrane.

In addition, bacteria shed endotoxins, which as a whole or after degradation may penetrate the pores of the membrane (17). There is a specific risk for membranes with larger pores, although small-pore cellulosic membranes have been shown to allow transfer of pyrogenic or endotoxin fragments as well (18,19). These endotoxins have been related to an enhanced immune response and inflammatory changes. Hence, dialysate contamination should be avoided by applying appropriate water-purification methods (preferably reversed osmosis) and sterile concentrates (in bags, not in containers). Regular control should be undertaken to check and eventually correct this contamination.

For hemodiafiltration, on-line preparation of the reinfusion fluid from the dialysate has been promoted as a more economic way to apply this strategy (20). Most studies indicate that such a system is safe. There may, however, be exceptional and sudden events of failure, and if this is the case life-threatening complications may ensue.

With CAPD, the problem of dialysate contamination is less important, as there are virtually no dialysis units where PD dialysate is directly prepared. In earlier years, contamination, especially with atypical mycobacteria, was demonstrated in units preparing their own peritoneal dialysate for intermittent PD on the spot (21). This procedure has for the most part been abandoned. Water contamination may also infect dialyzers during reuse procedures, if sterilization is inadequate, allowing direct entry of bacteria into the blood stream, leading to acute sepsis (21,23).

E. Opsonization Defect

Opsonins, such as complement and immunoglobulins, attach to the outer wall of bacteria, thereby increasing the speed and the intensity of the phagocytic destruction. The quality of opsonins may be altered during uremia, e.g., as a result of modification by advanced glycosylation end products (AGEs). Very few data, if any, however, point to a decreased quality of serum opsonins in ESRD.

In CAPD, immunoglobulins may be diluted in the peritoneal cavity, resulting in a local decrease of the immune response (24,25). This dilution is maximal when fresh dialysate has been instilled in the peritoneum but remains present at the end of the dwell time (26).

The production of immunoglobulins may be depressed in uremia. This is of clinical importance with regard to the vaccination for hepatitis B, which may be inefficient in a substantial proportion of the patients, and may necessitate an increase in the vaccine dose and the number of vaccinations before a protective response is obtained (27). Some studies claim that the response can be increased by administering immune-stimulating agents, but this issue remains debatable, whereas such medication is not always safe as far as complications are concerned.

F. Decreased Immune Defense

Four factors with a possible impact on immune function are continuously present in all dialyzed patients: the bio(in)compatibility of dialysis, retention of uremic toxins, the time since the start of dialysis, and the presence of other diseases, related to the development of renal failure, which as such may affect immune function.

1. Bio(in)compatibility

The term bio(in)compatibility covers an extended number of reactions that occur when the body or body organs come into contact with foreign material (28,29). Several factors may have an influence on the immune system. Attention has been paid to complement activation, which in turn activates the white blood cells.

Some dialyzers have the capacity to activate complement more than others. This is especially the case for cuprophane (30), whereas other cellulosic membranes (e.g., hemophan) cause less complement activation than cuprophane. On the other hand, there may also be differences in complement-activating capacity among the synthetic membranes. Therefore, the earlier distinction between cellulosic dialyzers, considered to be less biocompatible towards the complement system, and synthetic dialyzers, considered to be more biocompatible, is not correct. It has been suggested that the natural cytotoxic response of leukocytes towards bacteria might be blunted upon activation on dialysis membranes, as has been demonstrated for cuprophane (31). Such a blunted response occurs both acutely with each dialysis session and chronically after the serial application of several dialyses, and it is present not only for markers of leukocyte respiratory burst activity (3), but also for the expression of surface molecules and adhesion molecules on the cell membrane (32). In addition, the leukocyte count also drops during the first minutes of cuprophane dialysis.

As a clinical consequence there should be an increased incidence of infectious diseases in relation to the dialyzer membrane. Several studies have addressed this problem and indicated that infectious morbidity and mortality are more prominent with cuprophane dialysis. However, the design of these studies does not allow definite conclusions to be drawn (3,33–36).

CAPD also has a suppressive effect on the immune system, at least in the peritoneal cavity. First, cells and solutes involved in the immune response or its stimulation are diluted and washed away on a regular basis. Furthermore, the presence of glucose, lactate, and an acid pH in the dialysate might have a deleterious effect on the response of immune cells. Alternative osmotic agents (amino acids, polyglucose) and/or alternative buffers (bicarbonate) may be a better choice in this respect but are more expensive and/or can be used for only one of the four or five exchanges per day (37). Not only the fresh instilled dialysate but also the dwell fluid drained from the peritoneal cavity has an immunosuppressive effect (26). This can be related, at least in part, to uremic solutes diffusing into the dialysate during the dialysis process.

The question has been raised whether overnight cycler dialysis might alter immune capacity in the peritoneal cavity, as dilution might be more important when compared to traditional CAPD, whereas on the other hand the maintenance of an empty abdomen or only one exchange during the daytime may have a beneficial effect (38); infection is certainly not prevented entirely with cycler dialysis (39).

The clinical consequence of increased immune suppression in the peritoneal cavity is peritonitis. Whether the incidence of peritoneal infection is lower with certain types of dialysate and/or peritoneal dialysis still remains unclear.

2. Uremic Toxicity

The progression of renal failure is characterized by the accumulation of compounds that may affect various biochemical functions. The immune function has been shown to be affected by different solutes, such as parathormone, *p*-cresol, and various peptides (40–42). Most of these compounds are, however, not or only incompletely removed by the current dialysis procedures. Removal patterns might also be different among membranes and/or dialysis strategies. Further studies are required to gain more insight into the impact of the nature of the dialyzer membrane on the incidence of infectious disease.

3. Time Since Start of Dialysis

Changes in polymorphonuclear function occur during long-term dialysis. Some authors observed a severe depression of the phagocytic response during the first weeks after the start of dialysis (3). The functional capacity improved once dialysis treatment was prolonged (43), as had also been demonstrated earlier, using the skin window test as an index of macrophage functional capacity (44).

This functional improvement over time may be attributed to the development of compensatory mechanisms. Patients on long-term dialysis have higher serum levels of interleukin-1 than their not-yet-dialyzed counterparts (45).

4. Other Diseases Causing Immune Deficiency

Several diseases causing immune deficiency can be accompanied by renal failure. This is the case for alcoholism (IgA nephropathy), cirrhosis (IgA nephropathy, hepato-renal syndrome), hepatitis B (membranous nephropathy), malignancy (obstructive nephropathy), diabetes mellitus, myeloma, or lymphoma. In addition, chronic renal failure may also be complicated by diseases such as cancer and hepatitis, providing an additional weakening of the immune system. Splenectomy enhances the infectious rate in kidney transplant patients, but risk for infection returns to normal once these patients are on dialysis again (46). Finally, some renal diseases may necessitate the administration of drugs with an inhibitory effect on the immune function (e.g., corticosteroids and other immunosuppressive agents as well as antibiotics such as cotrimoxazole, tetracycline, rifampicin, ampicillin, and gentamicin) (47).

Diabetic patients are at increased risk for the incidence of infectious disease. Diabetes mellitus has become one of the major causes of ESRD leading to dialysis, and the prevalence of diabetes as a primary cause of renal failure is still increasing. Diabetes is an extra source of immune deficiency, superimposed on the uremic mechanisms. This condition increases the risk for serious opportunistic infections, such as fungal disease, in addition to the fact that several barrier functions work insufficiently. Finally, these patients are also prone to vascular occlusion, and infection of ischemic diabetic lesions is one of the leading causes of morbidity and even mortality in this population. Focal infections (e.g., of access systems) also tend to metastasize more easily throughout the body.

G. Associated Diseases

Many diseases associated with renal failure are by themselves a cause of local infection of the kidney and/or the urinary tract. Such diseases include polycystic kidney disease, nephrolithiasis, urinary tract infection, urinary tract obstruction, reflux, and papillary necrosis. These local infections may become systemic and disseminate throughout the body. Other associated disorders that occur frequently in renal failure, such as vascular ulcers of the limbs (48) or pulmonary edema, are prominent causes of infection.

H. Carriage of Bacteria or Viruses

A substantial number of dialysis patients are nasal or intestinal carriers of *Staphylococcus aureus*, which enhances the risk of infection of the access site or of the peritoneum in patients on HD and CAPD, respectively (8). Nasal carriers of *S. aureus* have a significantly higher incidence of staphylococcal infections than noncarriers. Methicillin-resistant *S. aureus* (MRSA) nasal carriage in patients undergoing CAPD is also associated with an increased risk of CAPD-related infections in comparison with methicillin-sensitive *S. aureus* (MSSA) nasal carriers and noncarriers (49). Screening for MRSA should be performed on a regular basis, the frequency being determined by local circumstances. Check-up for carrier state in dialysis patients for MRSA should be performed in all patients at least once every 3 months, and samples should be collected from nose, skin, and rectum.

Two recent studies have demonstrated that health-care staff screening may be helpful in well-defined outbreaks on surgical and intensive care wards in hospitals with a low prevalence of MRSA where the initial investigation of the patients does not reveal a source (50,51). In hospitals where the care of MRSA-colonized patients is common, staff are constantly exposed to the organism and some degree of colonization is inevitable. In any case, the screening of staff yields fewer benefits than screening patients.

Carriership can be eliminated by local intranasal antibiotic treatment (e.g., mupirocin). It has been demonstrated that the eradication of the nasal carriage of *S. aureus* in hemodialysis and CAPD patients is associated with a significant reduction in the incidence of infections. The topical application of the drug should not be performed continuously but at given intervals (e.g., for 5 days every month or one day a week) (52). Such strategies help to reduce the number of infectious and peritonitis episodes as well as prevent the development of bacterial resistance to mupirocin.

The problem of carriership of glycopeptide-resistant enterococci (GRE) emerged only recently (53) and is potentially dangerous for patients who are at the same time also contaminated with MRSA, since the transfer of genetic material may result in a strain resistant to both methicillin and vancomycin. This hypothesis was recently proven in a dialysis patient who was infected with so-called VISA (vancomycin intermediately resistant *S. aureus*) (54). Whether a regular screening should be applied as well for GRE remains open for discussion. The incidence of MRSA in the dialysis population has increased in many countries to 15% or more (55) in a population that is already highly susceptible to *S. aureus* carriage (56,57). No convincing data exist for GRE, but it should be taken into account that GRE-carriership is consistently present even in the normal healthy population (58,59).

The question should be raised whether carriers of MRSA and GRE need to be isolated in the dialysis unit. Whereas there is not much debate that this should be the case for MRSA, the options are less clear with regard to GRE. Therefore, it seems wise to separate GRE carriers from other patients as well.

Hepatitis B and C carriership implies a potential risk for patient-to-patient transmission. Here also isolation is indicated (60). The consequence of this trend towards isolation is that at least five subgroups have to be created in the HD population: patients with GRE, MRSA, and hepatitis B and C and noncarriers. Such strategies pose a major practical problem for the dialysis units.

The problems of carriership and risks for infection by multiresistant germs have provoked a debate about the choice of antibiotic in dialysis patients, especially if staphylococcal infection is presumed. This issue will be discussed below (see Sec. III.A).

I. Malnutrition

Malnourishment undoubtedly causes a defect of immune function and decreases the defense mechanisms against infection (61,62). The prevalence of malnutrition is often underestimated, but once it is addressed in the appropriate way, a substantial proportion of the dialyzed population appears to be malnourished (63,64).

Malnourishment can be the consequence of underdialysis, as suggested by the direct correlation between parameters of dialysis adequacy (Kt/V) and of food intake (PCR) (65). Apart from pursuing optimal dialysis adequacy, oral or intravenous complementary alimentation might equally be of help.

J. Anemia

Red blood cells deliver oxygen to all tissues, enabling metabolic activity. This is also the case for cells of the immune system. Renal anemia, at least in chronic renal failure, has been demonstrated to affect immune function: correction of renal anemia by administration of erythropoietin results in an improvement of various parameters of immune function (66–69). Although this effect has at least in part been attributed to an improvement of the iron status (66), studies performed in patients without iron overload, whereby body iron reserves were maintained constant, still indicated an improvement of immune function (67). Therefore, anemia per se does play a role as well.

K. Iron Overload

Increased iron reserves result in immune dysfunction and an increased risk for infection. Dialysis patients are at risk for iron overload due to the administration of iron, blood transfusions, and hemolysis, although the prevalence has been reduced by the introduction of erythropoietin. High serum ferritin, as an index of iron overload, has been related to disturbed phagocytosis (70,71) and increased incidence of bacteremia (72). Therapy with desferrioxamine is potentially immunosuppressive by itself. Specific disease states, such as mucormycosis, have been associated with this form of therapy (73).

L. Deficiencies

Iron, zinc, aluminum, fibronectin, and vitamin deficiencies may all be responsible for immune dysfunction. Not only is the active vitamin D compound $1,25(OH)_2$ vitamin D_3, or calcitriol, produced insufficiently by the failing kidneys due to a deficiency of $1\text{-}\alpha$-hydroxylase, but the uremic status also creates a condition of relative resistance to vitamin D due to the retention of uremic solutes (74,75). Although vitamin D is best known to affect bone status and Ca^{2+} metabolism, it also has a substantial effect on immune function, in which case it acts like a cytokine (76).

M. Drugs

Various drugs, especially antibiotics (47), may affect the immune system in a positive or a negative way. Some of them are reviewed in Table 2. Also, immunosuppressive agents, used in the treatment of immune-mediated disorders and to prevent rejection after transplantation, are strong immune-suppressors. Current therapeutic approaches for ESRD patients, such as erythropoietin and vitamin D analogs, also have immune-modulating properties (see Secs. II.J and II.L).

Table 2 Drugs with Potential Influence on Immune Function

	Positive	Negative
Antibiotics	Amphotericin B Cefodizime Cefoxitin Clindamycin Imipenem	Ampicillin Cefotaxime Cotrimoxazole Gentamicin Rifampicin Tetracycline
Immunomodulators	Interferons	Antithymocyte globulin Corticosteroids Cyclosporine Cytostatics FK506 OKT3
Varia	Erythropoietin	

III. CAUSATIVE MICROORGANISMS

A. Bacterial Infection

1. Incidence

Several publications address the issue of the incidence of bacterial infection in renal failure (Table 3). A fair interpretation of these studies remains difficult due to the heterogeneity of parameters used (hospitalization, morbidity, mortality) and the differences in study duration, population, definition, and diagnosis of infectious diseases. The figures are probably underestimated, since patients may be hospitalized because of infection but die from a different cause (e.g., cardiac arrest, ARDS).

Table 3 Morbidity and Mortality Due to Infection

% of patients developing infection	% of patients dying from infection	Ref.
20.0	19.8	78
—	13.7	82
7.8	15.9	79
—	19.0	84
—	36.0	80
25.4	—	62
32.6	29.0	81

Data collected more than 20 years ago pointed to an infectious mortality in the order of 40% (77). Patient population and treatment modalities were, however, too different from the ones presently used to allow an extrapolation to today's conditions.

In 1977 Keane et al. evaluated the causes of death in a total group of 111 fatalities in a dialysis unit: infection was a cause of death in approximately 30% of these patients (78). An identical analysis by the same authors in 1989 confirmed this tendency (79). Mailloux et al. found an overall mortality due to infection of 36% (80). The study covered a time period of more than 10 years, mortality being higher in the early 1970s than in the 1980s. Infectious mortality risk was markedly higher in patients below the age of 60. In a more recent publication by Fernandez et al., death together with hospitalization due to infections ranged up to 32.6% (81) in patients treated according to current rules defining adequate dialysis.

Churchill et al., in the Canadian Hemodialysis Morbidity Study, undertook a 1.5-year prospective cohort study in 18 HD centers covering approximately 500 patients (62). In this group 25.4% patients had at least one infectious event (excluding local vascular access infections). In total, 164 infectious events were observed in 126 patients, including 34 septic episodes. Low serum albumin and nonendogenous vascular access systems imposed an extra risk.

In a 6-year comparative study on technique survival between CAPD and HD, Maiorca et al. observed a mortality due to infection of approximately 15%, similarly distributed among both treatment modalities (82). According to the same authors, mortality due to peritonitis alone in CAPD patients ranged between 7 and 10% (83). In a paper by Higgins, sepsis accounted for 19% of deaths (84). Morbidity due to infectious diseases was especially high in subgroups with additional risk factors (diabetes mellitus, multiple myeloma, immunosuppression, polycystic kidney disease, reflux nephropathy). In patients treated with prednisolone and azathioprine and/or cyclophosphamide, the infectious mortality was 62.5%.

Even today, with all modern acquirements of optimized intensive care, diagnostic procedures, dialysis, and anti-infectious treatment, bacterial infection remains a major cause of hospitalization and death in the hemodialyzed population. This is of critical importance, in view of the approximately 600,000 patients treated worldwide by maintenance hemodialysis. This impact would be even more striking when considering patients with pre-ESRD (nondialyzed) and with acute renal failure as well. It is therefore beyond any doubt that immune deficiency influences survival and life quality of uremics and that all aims should be pursued to optimize this immune function.

2. Responsible Organisms

The vast majority of causative bacterial species are gram positive: 84.1% in vascular access–related bacteremia, 90% in bacteremia of unknown origin, and 48.6% in non–access-related bacteremia—overall 75.0% (78). Among these, staphylococcal species play a predominant role (75.3%). Disseminated *S. aureus* bacteremia carries a substantial mortality and occurs especially in patients with a history of prior staphylococcal infection or carriage, local access trauma, hematoma, and diabetes mellitus.

3. Specific Conditions

All vascular access systems for HD may become infected due to their frequent manipulation and the perforation of the protective skin barrier (see Sec. II.A). The risk increases with the number of manipulations (e.g., number of fistula punctures), with the presence of structural abnormalities in the access system, and with the use of foreign material for the creation of an access site (2). The most frequent cause of infection is staphylococcal infection. Therefore, antistaphylococcal antibiotic treatment should be the first choice if infection of unknown origin is detected in HD patients, with eventual adaptations according to the antibiogram. The first choice should be a glycopeptide, even when considering the increasing incidence of GRE: the possibility that the infection of unknown origin in the dialysis patient is caused by staphylococcal species is high in contrast to other infected populations, where this chance is much more restricted; in addition, the risk that the responsible germ is methicillin resistant is substantial. Glycopeptides should be replaced by methicillin or related antibiotics once the antibiogram demonstrates that the infection is caused by a methicillin-sensitive germ (85).

In view of the affinity of bacteria for foreign material, the risk of access infection is the least pronounced for endogenous arteriovenous fistulae and much more for vascular grafts (PTFE) and central vein catheters (86). Removal of catheters or of vascular grafts might be necessary to cope with infection. For soft large-bore catheters of the Hickman-Broviac or Tesio type, it is worthwhile to try an antibiotic treatment first.

In view of the proximity of the heart valves to the catheter tip, catheter infection often results in endocarditis, a disease that is sometimes hard to diagnose.

Transesophageal echocardiography is the preferred diagnostic tool. In case of persistent infection, the valve may need to be removed.

In the case of tunnel infection, a local antibiotic unguent (e.g., mupirocin), systemic antibiotic treatment, or ultimately catheter withdrawal may be necessary. Preventive measures may include frequent replacement of covering sterile dressings (ideally once weekly) and local treatment of staphyloccal nasal carriership.

For a detailed discussion of CAPD peritonitis, see Chapter 11 in this volume.

B. Viral Infection

The most frequent and most morbid viral infections in dialyzed patients are associated with hepatitis—hepatitis A, B, C, and G and cytomegalovirus infection (see Chapter 38). It should be stressed that not only patients but also staff personal are at risk for these hepatic infections, because both groups reside in the same reservoirs (87). They should be protected by hygienic measures and active vaccination programs, when applicable.

Apart from these, the most morbid viral problem in the dialyzed population involves the acquired immunodeficiency syndrome (AIDS). Since the original description of the AIDS in 1981, a broad spectrum of renal manifestations has been recognized (88). Although initial reports provided little evidence that major renal complications occurred frequently in AIDS patients, more recent reports suggest important renal and electrolyte disorders in up to as many as 50% of patients infected with the human immunodeficiency virus (HIV) (88,89). An extended description of these renal disorders falls outside the scope of this chapter, but acute tubular necrosis, various secondary parenchymal renal lesions, as well as a specific variant of focal and segmental glomerulosclerosis [HIV-associated nephropathy (HIVAN)] have been reported (88,89). The nephrological impact of AIDS, as well as its epidemiology in dialysis units, is discussed in detail in Chapter 37 of this volume.)

C. Tuberculosis

Infection with *Mycobacterium tuberculosis* occurs with increased frequency in patients with host defense failure, especially of cellular immunity. The incidence of tuberculosis is increased up to 15 times in HD patients when compared to the overall population (90). Geographical, racial, and social differences explain the wide range of variation in the absolute incidence from less than 1% (62) to more than 10% (91,92) in regions where tuberculosis is endemic. Symptoms of dialysis-associated tuberculosis may be nonspecific (91,92) (e.g., low-grade fever, anorexia, and weight loss). The value of skin tests is difficult to estimate because they can be negative due to suppressed cellular immunity. Extrapulmonary tuberculosis, especially the miliary form, occurs frequently (91,92). Thus, a high index of suspicion, especially in specific ethnic and immigrant populations, is necessary to facilitate prompt diagnosis. This early diagnosis, appropriate long-term antituberculous treatment, and prevention of malnutrition by adequate dialysis strategies and sufficient food supply are the prerequisites to reduce the mortality of dialysis-associated tuberculosis (90). Mycobacterial PD peritonitis is exceptional but extremely morbid and should be suspected in the case of persistent biochemical peritonitis in spite of repeated negative cultures (93).

D. Fungal Infections

Nosocomial candidemia has become an important infection not only because of an increasing incidence but also because of its high fatality rate (94) (57% in the general population). In HD patients the clinical setting in which *Candida* species evolve from their commensal relation with the human host into destructive pathogens can be defined as situations with exposure to broad-spectrum antibiotics, systemic steroids and other immunosuppressive treatment, cytotoxic chemotherapy, a status of overall immune suppression, and use of indwelling intravascular cannulas or catheters (94).

Fungal infection is relatively frequent in CAPD patients compared to HD patients due to an enhanced risk for fungal peritonitis, most frequently caused by *Candida albicans* (83). Even with intraperitoneal and additional systemic antifungal treatment, most patients with fungal CAPD infection will fail to respond unless the Tenckhoff catheter is removed (83).

Special attention has been focused on mucormycosis, an opportunistic infection caused by fungi of the Mucorales order (mainly of the genus *Rhizopus*). This infection may present itself as a rhinocerebral, pulmonary, gastrointestinal, cutaneous, or widely disseminated infection with high fatality rate (86%) (73). In more than 50% of cases the diagnosis is made on postmortem examination. Chronic liver disease, the administration of corticosteroids or antibiotics, metabolic acidosis, diabetes mellitus, splenectomy, and hematological diseases have been implicated as possible predisposing factors in ESRD. Furthermore, desferrioxamine as a chelator of aluminum or iron seems to play a major pathogenetic role (see Sec. II.K).

Fungal peritonitis is characterized by a high morbidity (95) and often necessitates catheter withdrawal and intensive antifungal therapy.

IV. CONCLUSIONS

Infectious diseases remain frequent in dialysis patients, either as a cause or as a consequence of renal failure. Nevertheless, the incidence of infectious disease has not changed substantially during the last few years, probably because preventive measures are not applied vigorously enough, but also because more and more seriously ill patients survive longer and longer on dialysis.

A number of preventive measures, as summarized in Table 4, can be taken to reduce this incidence. To avoid the migration of pathogens through the cutaneous barrier, as well as the fixation of these microorganisms on the foreign material, vascular access systems should be composed as much as possible of endogenous material. When catheters are applied, soft catheters for long-term use should be preferred. Repeated punctures and other manipulations of the access system increase the infectious risk. Dialysate contamination should be prevented by the appropriate treatment of tap water and the use of sterile, pharmacologically treated concentrate. Non–complement activating dialyzers for HD and non–glucose-containing dialysate solutions for peritoneal dialysis might reduce the risk for immune depression due to bioincompatibility. Optimal solute removal should be pursued. Carriers of morbid microorganisms should be isolated. Specific carriership for *S. aureus* should be treated by topic unguents. Malnutrition and iron overload should be avoided by the appropriate measures. Drugs with a negative impact on the immune system should be administered only if they are strictly indicated.

If all these precautions are taken into account, infectious risks might be reduced in spite of opposite trends such as progressively increasing resistance to antibiotics and increasing age and invalidity of the population with ESRD.

Table 4 Potential Measures to Improve Immune Function and Prevent Infection in Dialyzed Patients

Problem	Measure
Breakdown of cutaneous barrier	Avoid foreign material
	Soft long-term catheters
	Avoid surreptitious manipulations
Affinity bacteria for foreign material	Avoid foreign material
Contamination of water	Appropriate water treatment
	Sterile concentrate
Bioincompatibility	Non–complement-activating dialyzers (HD)
	Alternative osmotic agents (PD)
Uremic toxicity	Optimal adequacy of removal
Carriership	Local unguents
	Isolation of patients
Malnutrition	Optimal adequacy of removal
	Complementary alimentation
Iron overload	Avoid extra sources of iron
	Desferrioxamine
	Erythropoietin
Deficiencies	Substitute
Drugs	Avoid drugs with negative impact
	Prefer drugs with positive impact

REFERENCES

1. Vanholder R, Hoenich N, Ringoir S. Morbidity and mortality of central venous catheter hemodialysis: a review of 10 years' experience. Nephron 1987; 7:274–279.
2. Fan PY, Schwab SJ. Vascular access: concepts for the 1990s. J Am Soc Nephrol 1992; 3:1–11.
3. Vanholder R, Ringoir S, Dhondt A, Hakim R. Phagocytosis in uremic and hemodialysis patients: a prospective and cross sectional study. Kidney Int 1991; 39: 320–327.
4. Vanholder R, Dell'Aquila R, Jacobs V, Dhondt A, Veys N, Waterloos MA, Van Landschoot N, Van Biesen W, Ringoir S. Depressed phagocytosis in hemodialyzed patients: in vivo and in vitro mechanisms. Nephron 1993; 63:409–415.
5. De Meester J, Vanholder R, De Roose J, Ringoir S. Factors and complications affecting catheter and technique survival with permanent single-lumen dialysis catheters. Nephrol Dial Transplant 1994; 9:678–683.
6. Piraino B. A review of *Staphylococcus aureus* exit-site and tunnel infections in peritoneal dialysis patients. Am J Kidney Dis 1990; 16:89–95.
7. Harris DCH, Yuill EJ, Byth K, Chapman JR, Hunt C. Twin- versus single-bag disconnect systems: infection rates and cost of continuous ambulatory peritoneal dialysis. J Am Soc Nephrol 1996; 7:2392–2398.

8. Luzar MA. Exit-site infection in continuous ambulatory peritoneal dialysis: a review. Perit Dial Int 1991; 11: 333–340.
9. Cowan MM, Taylor KG, Doyle RJ. Role of sialic acid in the kinetics of streptococcus sanguis adhesion to artificial pellicle. Infect Immun 1987; 55:1552–1557.
10. MacIntyre Campbell K, Johnson CM. Identification of *Staphylococcus aureus* binding proteins to isolated porcine cardiac valve cells. J Lab Clin Med 1990; 115: 217–223.
11. Vanholder R, Lameire N, Verbanck J, van Rattinghe R, Kunnen M, Ringoir S. Complications of subclavian catheter hemodialysis: a 5 year prospective study in 257 consecutive patients. Int J Artif Organs 1982; 5:297–303.
12. Kherlakian GM, Roedersheimer LR, Arbough JJ, Newmark KJ, King LR. Comparison of autologous fistula versus expanded polytetrafluoroethylene graft fistula for angioaccess in hemodialysis. Am J Surg 1986; 152: 238–242.
13. Bambauer R, Mestres P, Pirrung KJ, Sioshansi P. Scanning electron microscopic investigation of catheters for blood access. Artif Organs 1994; 18:272–275.
14. Kamal GD, Pfaller MA, Rempe LE, Jebson PJR. Reduced intravascular catheter infection by antibiotic bonding. JAMA 1991; 265:2364–2368.
15. Fernicola DJ, Roberts WC. Clinicopathologic features of active infective endocarditis isolated to the native mitral valve. Am J Cardiol 1993; 71:1186–1197.
16. Watanakunakorn C, Burkert T. Infective endocarditis at a large community teaching hospital, 1980–1990. Medicine 1993; 72:90–102.
17. Bommer J, Ritz E. Water quality—a neglected problem in hemodialysis. Nephron 1987; 46:1–6.
18. Lonnemann G. Dialysate bacteriological quality and the permeability of dialyzer membranes to pyrogens. Kidney Int 1993; 43(suppl 41):S-195–S-200.
19. Lonnemann G, Krautzig S, Koch KM. Quality of water and dialysate in haemodialysis. Nephrol Dial Transplant 1996; 11:946–949.
20. Canaud B, Nguyen QV, Argiles A, Polito C, Polascheoo HD, Mion C. Hemodiafiltration using dialysate as substitution fluid. Artif Organs 1987; 11:188–190.
21. Band JD, Ward JI, Fraser DW, Peterson NJ, Silcox VA, Good RC, Ostroy PR, Kennedy J. Peritonitis due to *Mycobacterium chelonei*-like organism associated with intermittent chronic peritoneal dialysis. J Infect Dis 1981; 145:9–17.
22. Bolan G, Reingold AL, Carson LA, Silcox VA, Woodley CL, Hayes PS, Hightower AW, McFarland L, Brown JW, Petersen NJ, Favero MS, Good RC, Broome CV: Infections with *Mycobacterium chelonei* in patients receiving dialysis and using processed hemodialyzers. J Infect Dis 1985; 152:1013–1019.
23. Vanholder R, Van Haecke E, Ringoir S. Pseudomonas septicemia due to deficient disinfectant mixing during reuse. Int J Artif Organs 1992; 15:19–24.
24. Peterson PK, Matzke G, Keane WF. Current changes in the management of peritonitis in patients undergoing continuous peritoneal dialysis. Rev Infect Dis 1987; 9: 604–612.
25. Gordon DL, Rice JL, Avery VM. Surface phagocytosis and host defence in the peritoneal cavity during continuous ambulatory peritoneal dialysis. Eur J Clin Microbiol Infect Dis 1990; 9:191–197.
26. Vanholder R, Lameire N, Waterloos MA, Van Landschoot N, De Smet R, Vogeleere P, Lambert MC, Vijt D, Ringoir S. Disturbed host defense in the peritoneal cavity during CAPD: characterization of responsible factors in dwell fluid. Kidney Int 1996; 50:643–652.
27. Rapicetta M. Hepatitis B vaccination in dialysis centres: advantages and limits. Nephron 1992; 61:284–286.
28. Ringoir S, Vanholder R. An introduction to biocompatibility. Artif Organs 1986; 10:20–27.
29. Vanholder R, Ringoir S. Bioincompatibility: an overview. Int J Artif Organs 1989; 12:356–365.
30. Hakim RM, Breilatt J, Lazarus JM, Port FK. Complement activation and hypersensitivity reactions to dialysis membranes. N Engl J Med 1984; 311:878–882.
31. Himmelfarb J, Hakim RM. Biocompatibility and risk of infection in haemodialysis patients. Nephrol Dial Transplant 1994; 9(suppl 2):138–144.
32. Dhondt AW, Vanholder RC, Waterloos MA, Glorieux GL, Ringoir SMG. Leukocyte CD14 and CD45 expression during hemodialysis: polysulfone versus cuprophane. Nephron 1996; 74:342–348.
33. Levin NW, Zasuwa G, Dumler F. J Am Soc Nephrol 1991; 2:335 (abstr).
34. Hornberger JC, Chernew M, Petersen J, Garber AM. A multivariate analysis of mortality and hospital admissions with high-flux dialysis. J Am Soc Nephrol 1992; 3:1227–1237.
35. Hakim RM, Wingard RL, Parker RA, Vanholder R, Husni L, Parker TF. J Am Soc Nephrol 1994; 5:443 (abstr).
36. Schiffl H, Lang M, König A, Strasser T, Haider MC, Held E. Biocompatible membranes in acute renal failure: prospective case-controlled study. Lancet 1994; 344:570–572.
37. Vanholder RC, Lameire NH. Osmotic agents in peritoneal dialysis. Kidney Int 1986; 50(suppl 56):S86–S91.
38. Kohli HS, Arora P, Kher V, Gupta A, Sharma RK, Bhaumik SK. Daily peritoneal dialysis using a surgically placed Tenckhoff catheter for acute renal failure in children. Renal Fail 1995; 17:51–56.
39. Ponferrada LP, Prowant BF, Rackers JA, Pickett B, Satalowich R, Khanna R, Twardowski ZJ, Nolph KD. A cluster of gram-negative peritonitis episodes associated with reuse of HomeChoice cycler cassettes and drain lines. Perit Dial Int 1996; 16:636–638.
40. Vanholder R, Ringoir S. Infectious morbidity and defects of phagocytic function in end-stage renal disease: a review. J Am Soc Nephrol 1993; 3:1541–1554.

41. Vanholder R, De Smet R, Waterloos MA, Van Landschoot N, Vogeleere P, Hoste E, Ringoir S. Mechanisms of the uremic inhibition of phagocyte reactive species production: characterization of the role of p-cresol. Kidney Int 1995; 47:510–517.
42. Hörl WH, Haag-Weber M, Georgopoulos A, Block LH. Physicochemical characterization of a polypeptide present in uremic serum that inhibits the biological activity of polymorphonuclear cells. Proc Natl Acad Sci USA 1990; 87:6353–6357.
43. Vanholder R, Van Biesen W, Ringoir S. Contributing factors to the inhibition of phagocytosis in hemodialyzed patients. Kidney Int 1993; 44:208–214.
44. Ringoir S, Van Looy L, Van de Heyning P, Leroux-Roels G. Impairment of phagocytic activity of macrophages as studied by the skin window test in patients on regular dialysis treatment. Clin Nephrol 1975; 4: 234–236.
45. Herbelin A, Urena P, Nguyen AT, Zingraff J, Descamps-Latscha B. Influence of first and long-term dialysis on uraemia-associated increased basal production of interleukin-1 and tumor necrosis factor alpha by circulating monocytes. Nephrol Dial Transplant 1991; 6:349–357.
46. Shofer FS, London WT, Lyons P, Simonian SJ, Burke JF, Jarrell BE, Grossman RA, Barker CF. Adverse effect of splenectomy on the survival of patients with more than one kidney transplant. Transplantation 1986; 42: 473–478.
47. Van Vlem B, Vanholder R, De Paepe P, Vogelaers D, Ringoir S. Immunomodulating effects of antibiotics: literature review. Infection 1996; 24:275–291.
48. Johnson BL, Glickman MH, Bandyk DF, Esses GE. Failure of foot salvage in patients with end-stage renal disease after surgical revascularization. J Vasc Surg 1995; 22:280–286.
49. Wenzel RP, Perl TM. The significance of nasal carriage of *Staphylococcus aureus* and the incidence of postoperative wound infection. J Hosp Infect 1995; 31: 13–24.
50. Cox RA, Conquest C. Strategies for the management of healthcare staff colonized with epidemic methicillin-resistant *Staphylococcus aureus*. J Hosp Infect 1997; 35:117–127.
51. Lessing MPA, Jordens JZ, Bowler ICJ. When should healthcare workers be screened for methicillin-resistant *Staphylococcus aureus*? J Hosp Infect 1996; 34:205–210.
52. Boelaert JR, Van Landuyt HW, De Baere YA, Deruyter MM, Daneels RF, Schurgers ML, Matthys EG, Gordts BZ. *Staphylococcus aureus* infections in haemodialysis patients: pathophysiology and use of nasal mupirocin for prevention. J Chemother 1995; 7(suppl 3):49–53.
53. Montecalvo MA, Shay DK, Patel P, Tacsa L, Maloney SA, Jarvis WR, Wormser GP. Bloodstream infections with vancomycin-resistant enterococci. Arch Intern Med 1996; 156:1458–1462.
54. Hiramatsu K. Reduced susceptibility of *Staphylococcus aureus* to vancomycin. Japan, 1996. Am J Infect Control 1997; 25:405–407.
55. Lye WC, Leong SO, Lee EJC. Methicillin-resistant *Staphylococcus aureus* nasal carriage and infections in CAPD. Kidney Int 1993; 43:1357–1362.
56. Kirmani N, Tuazon CU, Murray HW, Parrish AE, Sheagren JN. *Staphylococcus aureus* carriage rate of patients receiving long-term hemodialysis. Arch Intern Med 1978; 138:1657–1659.
57. Sewell CM, Clarridge J, Lacke C, Weinman EJ, Young EJ. Staphylococcal nasal carriage and subsequent infection in peritoneal dialysis patients. JAMA 1982; 248: 1493–1495.
58. Chadwick PR, Chadwick CD, Oppenheim BA. Report of a meeting on the epidemiology and control of glycopeptide-resistant enterococci. J Hosp Inf 1996; 33: 83–92.
59. Vandamme P, Vercauteren E, Lammens C, Pensart N, Ieven M, Pot B, Leclercq R, Goossens H. Survey of enterococcal susceptibility patterns in Belgium. J Clin Microbiol 1996; 34:2572–2576.
60. Shusterman N, Singer I. Infectious hepatitis in dialysis patients. Am J Kidney Dis 1987; 9:447–455.
61. Redmond HP, Shou J, Kelly CJ, Schreiber S, Miller E, Leon P, Daly JM. Immunosuppressive mechanisms in protein-calorie malnutrition. Surgery 1991; 110:311–317.
62. Churchill DN, Taylor DW, Cook RJ, LaPlante P, Barre P, Cartier P, Fay WP, Goldstein MB, Jindal K, Mandin H, McKenzie JK, Muirhead N, Parfrey PS, Posen GA, Slaughter D, Ulan RA, Werb R. Canadian hemodialysis morbidity study. Am J Kidney Dis 1992; 19:214–234.
63. Cianciaruso B, Brunori G, Kopple JD, Traverso G, Panarello G, Enia G, Strippoli P, De Vecchi A, Querques M, Viglino G, Vonesh E, Maiorca R. Cross-sectional comparison of malnutrition in continuous ambulatory peritoneal dialysis and hemodialysis patients. Am J Kidney Dis 1995; 26:475–486.
64. Madore F, Wuest M, Ethier JH. Nutritional evaluation of hemodialysis patients using an impedance index. Clin Nephrol 1994; 41:377–382.
65. Lindsay RM, Spanner E, Heidenheim P, Kortas C, Blake PG. PCR, Kt/V and membrane. Kidney Int 1993; 43(suppl 41):S268–S273.
66. Boelaert JR, Cantinieaux BF, Hariga CF, Fondu PG. Recombinant erythropoietin reverses polymorphonuclear granulocyte dysfunction in iron-overloaded dialysis patients. Nephrol Dial Transplant 1990; 5:504–507.
67. Veys N, Vanholder R, Ringoir S. Correction of deficient phagocytosis during erythropoietin (EPO) treatment in maintenance haemodialysis patients. Am J Kidney Dis 1992; 19:358–363.
68. Sennesael JJ, Van der Niepen P, Verbeelen DL. Treatment with recombinant erythropoietin increases anti-

body titers after hepatitis B vaccination in dialysis patients. Kidney Int 1991; 40: 121–128.
69. Collart FE, Dratwa M, Wittek M, Wens R. Effects of recombinant human erythropoietin on T lymphocyte subsets in hemodialysis patients. Trans Am Soc Artif Intern Organs 1990; 36:M219–M223.
70. Flament J, Goldman M, Waterlot Y, Dupont E, Wybran J, Vanherweghem JL. Impairment of phagocyte oxidative metabolism in hemodialyzed patients with iron overload. Clin Nephrol 1986; 25:277–230.
71. Cantinieaux B, Boelaert J, Hariga C, Fondu P. Impaired neutrophil defense against *Yersinia enterocolitica* in patients with iron overload who are undergoing dialysis. J Lab Clin Med 1988; 111:524–528.
72. Boelaert JR, Daneels RF, Schurgers ML, Matthys EG, Gordts BZ, Van Landuyt HW. Iron overload in haemodialysis patients increases the risk of bacteraemia: a prospective study. Nephrol Dial Transplant 1990; 5: 130–134.
73. Boelaert JR, Fenves AZ, Coburn JW. Deferoxamine therapy and mucormycosis in dialysis patients: report of an international registry. Am J Kidney Dis 1991; 18: 660–667.
74. Hsu CH, Vanholder R, Patel S, De Smet R, Sandra P, Ringoir SMG. Subfractions of uremic plasma ultrafiltrate inhibit calcitriol metabolism. Kidney Int 1991; 40: 868–873.
75. Patel SR, Ke HQ, Vanholder R, Koenig RJ, Hsu CH. Inhibition of calcitriol receptor binding to vitamin D response elements by uremic toxins. J Clin Invest 1995; 96:50–59.
76. Manolagas SC, Yu X, Girasole G, Bellido T. Vitamin D and the hematopoietic tissue: a 1994 update. Sem Nephrol 1994; 14:129–143.
77. Blagg CR, Hickman RO, Eschbach JW, Scribner BH. Home hemodialysis: six years' experience. N Engl J Med 1970; 283:1126–1131.
78. Keane WF, Shapiro FL, Raij L. Incidence and type of infections occurring in 445 chronic hemodialysis patients. Trans Am Soc Artif Intern Organs 1977; 23: 41–47.
79. Keane WF, Maddy MF. Host defenses and infectious complications in maintenance hemodialysis patients. In: Maher JF, ed. Replacement of Renal Function by Dialysis. 3rd ed. Kluwer Academic, Dordrecht: Kluwer Academic, 1989:865–880.
80. Mailloux LU, Bellucci AG, Wilkes BM, Napolitano B, Mossey RT, Lesser M, Bluestone PA. Mortality in dialysis patients: analysis of the causes of death. Am J Kidney Dis 1991; 18:326–335.
81. Fernandez JM, Carbonell ME, Mazzuchi N, Petruccelli D. Simultaneous analysis of morbidity and mortality factors in chronic hemodialysis patients. Kidney Int 1992; 41:1029–1034.
82. Maiorca R, Vonesh E, Cancarini GC, Cantaluppi A, Manili L, Brunori G, Camerini C, Feller P, Strada A. A six-year comparison of patient and technique survivals in CAPD and HD. Kidney Int 1988; 34:518–524.
83. Maiorca R, Cancarini GC, Brunori G, Camerini C, Manili L. Morbidity and mortality of CAPD and hemodialysis. Kidney Int 1993; 43(suppl 40):S-4–S-15.
84. Higgins RM. Infections in a renal unit. Quart J Med 1989; 70:41–51.
85. Lameire N, Vogelaers D, Verschraegen G, Veys N. Vancomycin resistant enterococci—a threat to the nephrologist on the horizon? Glycopeptide-resistant enterococci and the ICDC-recommendations for a limited use of glycopeptides. Nephrol Dial Transplant 1996; 11: 2402–2406.
86. Cheesbrough JS, Finch RG, Burden RP. A prospective study of the mechanisms of infection associated with hemodialysis catheters. J Infect Dis 1986; 154:579–589.
87. Jovanovich JF, Saravolatz LD, Arking LM. The risk of hepatitis B among select employee groups in an urban hospital. JAMA 1983; 250:1893–1894.
88. Glassock RJ, Cohen AH, Danovitch G, Parsa KP. Human immunodeficiency virus (HIV) infection and the kidney. Ann Intern Med 1990; 112:35–49.
89. Seney FD, Burns DK, Silva FG. Acquired immunodeficiency syndrome and the kidney. Am J Kidney Dis 1990; 16:1–13.
90. Belcon MC, Smith EKM, Kahana LM, Shimizu AG. Tuberculosis in dialysis patients. Clin Nephrol 1982; 17:14–18.
91. Mitwalli A. Tuberculosis in patients on maintenance dialysis. Am J Kidney Dis 1991; 18:579–582.
92. Hussein MM, Bakir N, Roujouleh H. Tuberculosis in patients undergoing maintenance dialysis. Nephrol Dial Transplant 1990; 5:584–587.
93. Hakim A, Hisam N, Reuman PD. Environmental mycobacterial peritonitis complicating peritoneal dialysis: three cases and review. Clin Infect Dis 1993; 16:426–431.
94. Wey SB, Mori M, Pfaller MA, Woolson RF, Wenzel RP. Risk factors for hospital-acquired candidemia. A matched case-control study. Arch Intern Med 1989; 149:2349–2353.
95. Tapson JS, Mansy H, Freeman R, Wilkinson R. The high morbidity of CAPD fungal peritonitis—description of 10 cases and review of treatment strategies. Quart J Med 1986; 61:1047–1053.

21

Immune Dysfunction in Hemodialysis and Peritoneal Dialysis Patients

Walter H. Hörl
University of Vienna, Vienna, Austria

I. INTRODUCTION

Infectious complications are frequent in uremic patients. Several decades ago Montgomerie et al. (1) reported on an increased incidence of pulmonary infections, wound infections, peritonitis, urinary tract infections, septicemia, and infections of the gastrointestinal tract in renal failure patients. Bacterial infections were found to be the most common cause for hospitalization and the second most common cause of death in hemodialysis patients (2).

In a more recent study, Mailloux et al. (3) identified causes of death in 222 out of 532 maintenance dialysis patients who survived at least 90 days and were monitored during a 16-year period. The causes of death, in order of frequency, were infections (36%), withdrawal (21%), cardiac failure (15%), sudden death (10%), vascular (8%), and other (9%). The risk of cardiac death increased from 5.6% in 1970–1973 to 25.6% in 1982–1985. There was a decrease in deaths due to infections from 44.4% (1970–1973) to 21.6% (1982–1985). Patients entering dialysis below the age of 41 years had a higher death rate from infection as compared with the other causes of death in this dialysis patient population. Himmelfarb and Hakim (4) summarized most large series published between 1977 and 1989 and examined mortality related to infection in hemodialysis patients. There was an infectious mortality rate between 13.1% and 35.7% in hemodialysis patients. Hoen et al. (5) followed up 607 adult hemodialysis patients from 13 dialysis centers prospectively for 6 months in an attempt to appraise the current risk factors for bacterial infections. One hundred and eighteen patients (19.4%) had developed at least one bacterial infection during the study period. Previous history of bacterial infection, type of angioaccess device (catheter versus native fistula), and elevated serum ferritin level (greater versus lower than 500 μg/L) were found to be significant and independent risk factors for bacterial infection (5). In a recent multicenter prospective cross-sectional study, catheters, especially long-term implanted catheters, were found to be the leading risk factor of bacteremia in chronic hemodialysis patients (6). Bacterial infections are also common in peritoneal dialysis patients.

The recent Annual Data Report of the U.S. Renal Data System indicates that infection accounts for almost a quarter of all deaths in the 20- to 44-year age group, but only 17% and 14% of deaths in the 45- to 64-year and 65 and older age groups, respectively. Septicemia makes up more than 75% of the infection category (7). Over 7 years of follow-up, 11.7% of 4005 hemodialysis patients and 9.4% of 913 peritoneal dialysis patients had at least one episode of septicemia. Among hemodialysis patients, low serum albumin, temporary vascular access, and dialyzer reuse were also associated with increased risk. Among peritoneal patients, white race and having no health insurance at dialysis initiation were also risk factors (8).

These data indicate that microbial antigens are a major risk for end-stage renal disease patients undergoing hemodialysis and peritoneal dialysis therapy. Impairment of the host defense is primarily responsible for

Table 1 Components of Impaired Host Defense in Uremia

Polymorphonuclear leukocytes
Lymphocytes
T cells
B cells
Antigen-presenting cells (e.g., monocytes)

the susceptibility to infections. The components of impaired host defense in uremia are summarized in Table 1.

II. METHODS FOR EVALUATING IMMUNE DYSFUNCTION

Methods for evaluating immune dysfunction in uremic patients include metabolic and functional parameters of polymorphonuclear leukocytes (PMNL) as well as expression of several adhesion molecules and neutrophil apoptosis (Table 2). CD11a is identical to LFA-1 (leukocyte function–associated antigen), CD11b is identical to CR3 (complement receptor type 3) or MAC-1 (macrophage/monocyte adhesion complex-1, macrophage differentiation antigen), CD45 is identical to LCA (leukocyte common antigen), CD54 is identical to ICAM-1 (intercellular adhesion molecule-1), and CD62L is identical to L-selectin.

Tables 3–5 summarize the methods for evaluation of T-cell, B-cell, and monocyte function in uremic patients.

Table 2 Methods for Evaluating Immune Dysfunction: Polymorphonuclear Leukocytes in Uremic Patients

Metabolic parameters
Glucose uptake
ATP formation
Glycolytic response
Oxygen consumption
Functional parameters
Migration
Chemotaxis
Degranulation
Reactive oxygen production
Intracellular killing of bacteria
Phagocytosis
Expression of adhesion molecules (e.g., CD11a, CD11b, CD45, CD54, CD62L, CD66b)
Neutrophil apoptosis

Table 3 Methods for Evaluating Immune Dysfunction: T Cells in Uremic Patients

T-cell proliferative responsiveness to stimulation with lectins (phytohemagglutinin, concanavalin A), recall antigens, alloantigens, or anti-CD3 antibody
Measurement of cytokine synthesis (e.g., interleukin-2, interferon-gamma) following mitogenic stimulation (ELISA, intracellular staining and flow cytometric analysis, polymerase chain reaction)
T-cell adhesion to extracellular matrix
Surface receptor expression (e.g., T-cell receptor, CD3)
Cytotoxicity assays ($CD8^+$)
Expression of activation associated molecules/markers (MHC II, CD25) for cellular activation following stimulation with phytohemagglutinin, concanavalin A, anti-CD3 mAb
T-cell help ($CD4^+$) for immunoglobulin production by B cells
In vivo cutaneous responsiveness to recall antigens

III. NATURE OF IMMUNE DYSFUNCTION IN UREMIA

Immune dysfunction in uremia is caused by the accumulation of low and high molecular weight uremic toxins (e.g., *p*-cresol, guanidino compounds, oxidation products, granulocyte inhibitory proteins) (Table 6).

Several compounds present in uremic serum have been isolated and characterized that inhibit the activity of PMNLs. Of the known uremic retention solutes, *p*-cresol dose-dependently depresses whole blood respiratory burst activity at concentrations encountered in patients with end-stage renal disease (9).

Masuda et al. (10) investigated membrane fluidity, an important feature in regulating functional proteins on the membrane of PMNLs. They found that membrane fluidity of PMNLs was significantly lower in uremic patients during the predialysis period compared to healthy subjects. Membrane fluidity was normal after hemodialysis treatment. Fractionating the sera of

Table 4 Methods for Evaluating Immune Dysfunction: B Cells in Uremic Patients

a) B-cell proliferation in response to mitogenic stimulation (e.g., pokeweed mitogen)
b) Immunoglobulin production following stimulation with pokeweed mitogen
c) In vivo responsiveness to vaccination (e.g., against hepatitis B virus)

Table 5 Methods for Evaluating Immune Dysfunction: Monocytes in Uremic Patients

a) Measurement of T-cell response to monocyte antigen presentation/costimulation
b) Expression of adhesion/costimulatory molecules (e.g., LFA-3, B7, ICAM-1)
c) Measurement of secretion of proinflammatory cytokines (interleukin-1, interleukin-6)

uremic patients by Sephadex G-25 column chromatography, a low molecular weight fraction responsible for the decreased membrane fluidity was demonstrated (10).

Jörstad and Viken (11) cultured human mononuclear phagocytes in plasma from uremic patients and found a decreased digestive ability of 25.5%. Creatinine, urea, and methylguanidine in concentrations higher than those usually measured in plasma from uremic patients were not responsible for this effect. Separation of uremic plasma into fractions of different molecular sizes indicated that substances in uremic plasma responsible for the impaired function of human mononuclear phagocytes cultured in vitro consisted of molecules of a molecular weight higher than 10,000 daltons (12). The factors in uremic plasma inhibiting phagocytosis of *Candida albicans* could not be removed by means of conventional hemodialysis with cuprophane or polyacrylonitrile membranes. However, hemofiltrates of uremic plasma produced by the polyacrylonitrile membranes caused a significant inhibition of phagocytes while cuprophane hemofiltrates did not (13). Porter et al. (14) studied PMNL function of patients with end-stage renal failure before and 3 months after starting continuous ambulatory peritoneal dialysis (CAPD). They found impaired killing of *Staphylococcus epidermidis* before treatment, which was corrected by CAPD therapy. It was suggested that a dialyzable toxin is involved in PMNL inhibition (14).

Several peptides accumulate in renal failure and interfere with specific cellular functions. One granulocyte inhibitory protein (GIP I) that has been isolated and characterized is responsible for the PMNL dysfunction in uremia. The polypeptide inhibits the uptake of deoxyglucose, chemotaxis, oxidative metabolism, and intracellular bacterial killing by PMNLs (15). GIP I shows homology with light-chain proteins (16). A second granulocyte inhibitory protein (GIP II) was subsequently isolated from plasma ultrafiltrates obtained from hemodialysis patients. It also interferes with PMNL functions. GIP II displays homology with β_2-microglobulin. GIP II inhibits in vitro O_2^- production by PMNL as well as glucose uptake stimulated by phorbol ester. In contrast, GIP I inhibits formyl-methionyl-leucyl-phenylalanine (FMLP)–mediated PMNL functions (17). Intact β_2-microglobulin does not influence these granulocyte parameters. GIP II, the peptide with homology to β_2-microglobulin, stimulates interleukin-1β (IL-1β) and IL-6 production by cultured human mononuclear cells. This effect is comparable to that of AGE-modified β_2-microglobulin. Intact β_2-microglobulin was without effect on cytokine production (18). Both proteins (GIP I and II) were also isolated and characterized from peritoneal effluents of CAPD patients. The effluents inhibited the identical PMNL properties (19).

A PMNL degranulation inhibiting protein (DIP I) was purified from plasma ultrafiltrates obtained from patients undergoing regular hemodialysis therapy. DIP I is identical with angiogenin and inhibits spontaneous as well as stimulated PMNL degranulation (20). A polyclonal antibody to human recombinant angiogenin abolishes the inhibitory effect of the isolated protein upon PMNL. The same but diminished effect is induced by the disulfide C^{39}-C^{92} containing tryptic angiogenin fragment, indicating a new, biologically active site of angiogenin that is different from the sites responsible for the angiogenetic activity of the protein (20). Plasma angiogenin levels are significantly elevated in hemodialysis and CAPD patients (21). A second degranulation inhibiting protein (DIP II) was isolated from human plasma ultrafiltrate by a three-step purification method (ion-exchange chromatography, gelfiltration, affinity chromatography). The protein was identified as complement factor D by means of sequence analysis. Complement factor D caused a dose-dependent decrease of stimulated lactoferrin degranulation to a value of 34% of stimulated controls (22). Serum of healthy donors contains factor D in low concentrations (1–2 μg/mL), whereas this level can be increased 10-fold in serum of dialysis patients (23).

Kappa and lambda light-chain protein monomers and dimers were isolated from high-flux dialyzer ultrafiltrates of hemodialysis patients and from peritoneal

Table 6 Nature of Immune Dysfunction Uremia

Accumulation of low and high molecular weight uremic toxins (e.g., *p*-cresol, granulocyte inhibitory proteins)
Advanced glycation end products (AGEs)
Oxidation products
Guanidino compounds

effluents of CAPD patients. All these proteins inhibit in vitro glucose uptake and chemotaxis of PMNLs at nanomolar concentrations (24). Light chains of immunoglobulins (Ig) are produced by B cells slightly in excess of Ig heavy chains (25). Therefore, a small amount of light chains exists in free form in the serum, i.e., not as part of an intact Ig (26). Solling (27) found an up to fivefold increase in the level of free Ig light chains in sera from patients with severely reduced kidney function. Wakasugi et al. (28) observed a significantly increased level of free light chains in sera after the start of hemodialysis therapy.

By applying three different chromatographic methods, a chemotaxis inhibiting peptide was isolated from the peritoneal effluent of peritoneal dialysis patients. In an in vitro assay this peptide inhibits the chemotactic movement of polymorphonuclear leukocytes in a concentration-dependent, nonreversible manner, and therefore belongs to the group of uremic toxins. Amino acid sequencing showed that the isolated peptide has the same amino-terminal sequence as ubiquitin. The peptide also related with anti-ubiquitin antibodies in a Western blot experiment but had a more acidic isoelectric point than ubiquitin. By using affinity chromatography, anti-ubiquitin antibody–binding fractions were isolated from all peritoneal dialysis and hemodialysis patients investigated. These fractions, containing the same acidic band, also significantly inhibited PMNL chemotaxis. Ubiquitin per se had no effect on PMNL chemotaxis. It was concluded that a modified form of ubiquitin was isolated and that this modification was responsible for its inhibitory effect (29).

Table 7 summarizes the granulocyte inhibitory proteins isolated and characterized so far from high-flux dialyzer ultrafiltrates and peritoneal effluents of uremic patients.

Table 7 Granulocyte Inhibitory Proteins Isolated from Patients on Hemodialysis and CAPD

1. Granulocyte inhibitory protein I (80% homology to the KAPPA and 40% homology to the LAMBDA light chain sequence, MW 28,000 daltons)
2. Granulocyte inhibitory protein II (homology to beta$_2$-microglobulin, MW 9,500 daltons)
3. Degranulation-inhibiting protein I (identical to angiogenin, MW 14,400 daltons)
4. Degranulation-inhibiting protein II (identical to complement factor D, MW 24,000 daltons)
5. Immunoglobulin light chains (KAPPA mono- and dimers, LAMBDA mono- and dimers)
6. Chemotaxis-inhibiting protein (modified ubiquitin, MW 8,500 daltons)

Table 8 Factors Associated with Alterations in Immune Dysfunction

Malnutrition
Inadequate dialysis
Iron overload
Increased intracellular calcium due to secondary hyperparathyroidism
Calcitriol deficiency
Deficiency of vitamins and trace elements
Vascular access (e.g., catheters)
Immunosuppressive therapy
Resistance to erythropoietin
Bioincompatible membranes
Dialyzer reuse

Centoroglo et al. (30) investigated the contribution of apoptosis to neutrophil dysfunction in uremia. Compared with normal neutrophils, uremic neutrophils demonstrated greater apoptosis in the presence of autologous plasma. Compared with normal neutrophils exposed to heterologous normal plasma, those exposed to heterologous uremic plasma exhibited higher apoptosis rates, lower stimulated superoxide production, and a lower phagocytosis index. It was concluded that uremic neutrophils undergo accelerated in vitro apoptosis. Uremic plasma also accelerates apoptosis of normal neutrophils (30).

IV. FACTORS ASSOCIATED WITH ALTERATIONS IN IMMUNE DYSFUNCTION

Factors associated with alterations in immune dysfunction of end-stage renal disease patients are presented in Table 8.

A. Malnutrition

A substantial number of end-stage renal disease patients develops malnutrition (31,32). Spontaneous protein intake decreases parallel with the reduction of renal function (33). The reduced caloric intake and the loss of vitamins, trace elements, and micronutrients during dialysis therapy contribute not only to malnutrition but also to the enhanced risk of infection. Briggs et al. (34) compared lymphocyte and granulocyte function in zinc-treated and zinc-deficient hemodialysis patients. Zinc therapy may improve impaired cell-mediated immunity in these patients. It has been shown that a low serum albumin is associated with an increased risk of infection (35). A low serum albumin may be the result of malnutrition, but more probably low serum albumin is a negative acute phase protein (36,37). Nevertheless, malnutrition causes inhibition of various aspects of immune function (38,39). Very-low-energy all-protein reducing diets are associated with a decrease in circulating leukocyte numbers and an ineffective in vitro response of mononuclear cells to various mitogens (40).

B. Renal Anemia, Iron Overload

Iron deficiency is the most common cause of hyporesponsiveness to recombinant human erythropoietin (r-HuEPO) in patients with end-stage renal disease. However, high-dose iron therapy may enhance the risk of iron overload associated with a higher frequency of infectious complications (41–43). Multiple dysfunctions of the PMNL have been described in iron-overloaded patients (44–49). In a recent study (49), healthy subjects (group I) were compared with intravenous (i.v.) r-HuEPO and i.v. iron-saccharate–treated regular hemodialysis patients who were subdivided into three groups as follows: patients with serum ferritin of >100 and <350 μg/L (group II), patients with ferritin of <60 μg/L (group III), and patients with ferritin of >650 μg/L but transferrin saturation of <20% (group IV). PMNL parameters (phagocytosis, intracellular killing of bacteria, oxidative metabolism, glucose uptake, intracellular calcium) for each group were compared with those of multitransfused, iron-overloaded primary hematological patients (group V) and those of patients suffering from hereditary hemochromatosis (group VI). Compared to PMNLs obtained from healthy subjects, group II hemodialysis patients showed mild inhibition of phagocytosis but significant inhibition of intracellular killing of bacteria. Oxidative burst of PMNLs from group II patients was also significantly reduced after stimulation in vitro. Impairment of PMNLs was markedly aggravated in group IV patients. The PMNL defect of group IV patients was comparable to group V and group VI patients with normal renal function, suggesting a direct inhibitory effect of iron (49).

Boelaert et al. (48) showed that PMNL dysfunction of iron-overloaded hemodialysis patients is, at least in part, related to the accumulation of iron into the neutrophils. An improvement of impaired phagocytosis was found in parallel with a decrease of serum ferritin during r-HuEPO therapy for more than one year. Iron staining of PMNL was initially positive and became negative under r-HuEPO treatment (48). Veys et al. (50) found a correction of deficient phagocytosis during r-HuEPO treatment in patients undergoing regular hemodialysis treatment. Granulocyte CO_2 production in response to stimuli is correlated to the hematocrit (51). R-HuEPO therapy normalizes the composition of the lymphocyte subpopulation and improves response upon vaccination as well as cytokine and immunoglobulin production (52,53).

C. Impairment of PMNL Function by Increased Cytosolic Calcium

Chronic renal failure is a state of increased calcium burden of cells, and this abnormality plays a major role in the genesis of many manifestations of the uremic syndrome (54). A large body of evidence indicates that the state of secondary hyperparathyroidism is responsible for the elevation of cytosolic calcium $[Ca^{2+}]_i$ (55). An increased entry of calcium into cells by parathyroid hormone and an inhibition of mitochondrial oxygen consumption and phosphorylation with a consequent decrease in PMNL ATP content are suggested as mechanisms for this effect of parathyroid hormone. The reduction in ATP would impair the function of the calcium pumps and reduce the extrusion of calcium out of the PMNLs, resulting in a sustained rise of their $[Ca^{2+}]_i$. This process would continue until a steady state is achieved with higher resting levels of $[Ca^{2+}]_i$ and lower ATP content.

Intracellular calcium plays an important role in neutrophil function and metabolism. Increased cytosolic calcium is associated with several alterations of PMNL function (56), e.g., impaired phagocytosis (57), decreased glucose uptake (58,59), inhibition of glycogen metabolism (58,59), and decreased oxygen consumption (60). Normalization of cytosolic calcium by treatment with the calcium channel blockers verapamil (56,59) or nitrendipine (58) resulted in improved PMNL function without influencing the elevated plasma parathyroid hormone level. Kiersztejn et al. (60) demonstrated an improvement of decreased O_2 consumption of PMNLs from humans with chronic renal failure by verapamil and of PMNLs from rats with chronic renal failure by parathyroidectomy. Lowering of parathyroid hormone by 1,25-dihydroxyvitamin D_3 therapy also resulted in normalization of cytosolic calcium and improvement of stimulated glucose uptake of PMNLs from hemodialysis patients (58). Another mechanism for elevated cytosolic calcium in PMNLs of hemodialysis patients is the activation of PMNLs by membrane material (61) during hemodialysis treatment.

This increase of $[Ca^{2+}]_i$, however, can also be inhibited by calcium channel blockers (62).

D. PMNL Function and Hemodialysis Treatment

There is clear evidence that each dialysis session triggers neutrophil activation, mainly through the generation of activated complement components following the contact of neutrophils with bioincompatible dialysis membranes (63). This is evidenced by the overexpression of adhesion molecules (CD11/CD18) (64) contributing to the sequestration of neutrophils in the lung (65), generation of highly reactive oxygen species (66–73), and release of PMNL granular enzymes (74,75). Rosenkranz et al. (76) evaluated the contribution of reactive oxygen intermediate formation for receptor modulation on neutrophils by the cellulosic dialyzer membrane cuprophane. CD11b and CD66b upregulation on neutrophils and a downregulation of L-selectin were seen, whereas expression of CD11a remained unaltered. It was concluded that, in addition to the alternative pathway of complement, a C5-dependent mechanism probably activated by neutrophil-derived reactive oxygen intermediate leads to receptor modulation and subsequent generation of the well-known side effects of bioincompatible dialyzer membranes.

Phagocyte function with different stimuli is suppressed during dialysis with complement-activating cuprophane membranes. In contrast, PMNL activity remains unaltered during hemodialysis with other, non–complement-activating dialyzer membranes, like polysulfone. In a prospective study Vanholder et al. (70) found at every evaluation moment during the first 12 weeks after start of hemodialysis that the glycolytic response and the reactive oxygen production were substantially lower in patients treated with cuprophane compared with polysulfone. These authors concluded that complement-activating cuprophane suppresses phagocytotic response both acutely and chronically. Himmelfarb et al. (71) found that there was less granulocyte reduced oxygen species production in response to *Staphylococcus aureus* during hemodialysis with complement-activating membrane compared with non–complement-activating membranes. Decreased responsiveness to *S. aureus* during the dialysis procedure is the result of increased granulocyte reduced oxygen species production during hemodialysis with complement-activating membranes. In agreement with these results, Rosenkranz et al. (73) found significantly more pronounced production of reactive oxygen intermediates by PMNLs during hemodialysis with cuprophane compared with polysulfone membranes. It is therefore conceivable that membrane-related complement stimulation decreases the ability of the white blood cell to respond when it is really necessary (77).

Intracellular antioxidant PMNL enzymes of hemodialysis and CAPD patients were measured by Shurtz-Swirski et al. (78). In both groups of patients superoxide dismutase and glutathione peroxidase were significantly reduced, whereas catalase activity was significantly augmented. It was concluded that this impairment in antioxidant enzyme activity, involved in the respiratory burst and phagocytosis, may contribute to the understanding of the reduced bactericidal ability of PMNL activity found in these patients. In contrast, studies of Ward and McLeish (79) clearly demonstrate that PMNLs exist in a primed state in chronic renal insufficiency patients without dialysis therapy.

It has been demonstrated that adhesion of leukocytes to endothelial cells is of fundamental importance in inflammatory processes (80–82). Selectins are responsible for the initial rolling interaction with the vascular endothelium (83), whereas firm adhesion of leukocytes to endothelial cells is dependent on the β_2-integrins (80). Adherence of PMNLs to the vascular endothelium at the site of infection is followed by transmigration across the vascular wall, chemotaxis toward bacteria, phagocytosis of bacteria, and killing of ingested bacteria by reactive oxygen metabolites and lysosomal enzymes. The transition to a low L-selectin and high Mac-1 expression on granulocytes during cuprophane hemodialysis, resulting in a decreased ratio between L-selectin and Mac-1 on granulocytes, may impair the defense against infection in hemodialysis patients, particularly when cellulosic membranes are used (84). A retrospective clinical study suggests that the type of dialyzer membrane influences susceptibility to infection (85).

E. Bioincompatibility of Peritoneal Dialysis Solutions

Infectious complications of peritoneal dialysis therapy are related to exit site infection (86), tunnel infection (87), and peritonitis (88). These complications may be caused by the nonphysiological composition of the peritoneal dialysis solutions and by the catheter entering the peritoneal cavity through the skin barrier. Peritoneal host defense mechanisms are repeatedly exposed to dialysis solutions of unphysiological composition, which may compromise peritoneal immune cell function. Bioincompatibility of the peritoneal dialysate (low pH, high glucose and lactate concentration, increased osmolality) suppresses bactericidal activity of leukocytes. There is a negative impact of peritoneal effluent dialysis fluid on multiple functions of phagocytic cells (89). Peritoneal dialysate inhibits IL-6 and TNF-α release by mononuclear leukocytes (90). Exposure to conventional dialysis fluid impairs the cytokine response by activated leukocytes, whilst the use of bicarbonate-buffered solutions containing 1.0% amino acids or 1.5% glucose results in improved biocompatibility (91). It has been shown that peritoneal macrophages obtained from patients suffering from a high incidence of peritonitis are insensitive to the cytokine effect of calcitriol (92).

PMNLs obtained from peripheral blood of healthy volunteers and from the peritoneal effluent of CAPD patients with acute peritonitis were incubated in fresh CAPD dialysates or control buffer. Incubation in fresh solutions for peritoneal dialysis severely depressed leukotriene release from both cell populations. These results indicate that dialysate exposure could contribute to the impairment of host defense early in the CAPD cycle (93). Exposure of human peritoneal mesothelial cells to peritoneal dialysis fluid (pH 5.2) resulted in a time-dependent increase of cytotoxicity (94). The study of Liberek at al. (95) demonstrates that not only the acidic pH but also the high osmolality and high glucose concentration of the peritoneal dialysis fluid cause inhibition of phagocyte function.

F. Lymphocytes and Monocytes

There in a large amount of clinical evidence for the existence of profound defects of the specific immune system represented by lymphocytes and monocytes in renal failure patients.

After performing the first human renal allografts, Hume et al. (96) in 1957 found a prolonged functional allograft survival exceeding the time that was expected from the experience with allograft survival in normal dogs. Extended survival of skin allografts was demonstrated by Dammin et al. (97) in uremic patients. Patients with chronic renal failure showed markedly decreased cutaneous responsiveness to a broad panel of antigens (98–105). Allotransfer of lymphocytes from uremic patients into normal individuals by intradermal injection caused fewer inflammatory reactions than allotransfer of lymphocytes from normal subjects (106). The immune deficiency of uremic patients is further underlined by the high occurrence of active tuberculosis in dialysis units. Several authors (107,108) found a 6- to 16-fold incidence in comparison to nonuremic populations. The tuberculin skin reaction often remains negative (109–112).

Despite decreased antibody response to distinct antigens, immunoglobulin levels in dialysis patients have been reported to be normal (97,105). However, Nolph et al. (113) found low titers of autoantibodies against ENA and native DNA in 25% of dialysis patients, while Mayet et al. (114) demonstrated a high incidence of low titers of autoantibodies against cytoskeletal components. These data may indicate low-grade polyclonal B-cell activation in dialysis patients.

G. T Lymphocytes

Lymphocyte counts were found to be decreased in uremic patients by Toraine et al. (115). However, a recent publication (116) reported normal lymphocyte counts and normal $CD4^+/CD8^+$ ratio in end-stage renal failure not to be influenced by the dialysis procedure (117). T lymphocytes from uremic patients display an impaired blastogenic response to mitogens and allogenic lymphocytes (reviewed in Ref. 118). These effects are more pronounced in the presence of autologous serum, and uremia markedly reduces the proliferative response to normal T cells (119), suggesting the involvement of circulating inhibitory substances (120). Another hypothesis for the mechanism of defective T-cell response is that monocytes could be involved directly (121) or via blood transfusion and iron overload (122).

A reduced costimulatory signaling by accessory cells is involved in the pathogenesis of the cellular immune defect in dialysis patients. Impaired expression of B7 molecules on monocytes leads to reduced signaling to the molecule CD28 on T cells (123). Vitamin E has an enhancing effect on lymphocyte proliferation after activation by lectins (124), and oral supplementation improves cell-mediated immunity in the elderly (125,126). Only one large double-blind trial in healthy elderly persons did not find any improvement in T-cell functional parameters although plasma tocopherol levels increased by 51% (127).

Defective proliferation of T cells is associated with lowered IL-2 and interferon-gamma production, which was recently confirmed at the level of gene expression (128). Normalization of proliferation can be obtained by adding exogenous recombinant IL-2 to the culture (117,119). Characteristic of the immune system dysregulation in uremia is that, despite the presence of an impaired response to most pathogens, T cells from dialysis patients show clear signs of activation. This is manifested by an increased expression of the P55 receptor for IL-2 and by the presence of elevated circulating levels of the soluble form of IL-2R (129). Descamps-Latscha et al. (130) suggested that the paradoxical coexistence of a deficiency and an activation state in the T cell could be caused by an increased consumption of IL-2 by its own receptor, leading to its decreased bioavailability in mounting the T-cell response. Recent studies on the antigen T-cell receptor in uremic patients suggested that the blunted T-cell response to antigen is due to downregulation of the T-cell receptor/CD3 antigen receptor complex in the uremic milieu (115).

Mechanisms that play a role in the impaired T-cell function are uremic toxins, hyperparathyroidism, and dialysis treatment per se. Donati et al. (120) clearly demonstrated the effect of uremic serum on both phenotypic and functional signs of T-cell activation. Increased T-cell proliferative response to phytohemagglutinin stimulation was found in peripheral blood mononuclear cell cultures obtained from uremic rats with hyperparathyroidism compared to normal rats or after parathyroidectomy (131,132). Zaoui et al. (133) and Degiannis et al. (134) investigated the effect of dialysis membranes on T-cell function and found that dialysis with complement-activating membranes induces upregulation of the expression of interleukin-2 receptor, which can be reversed by dialysis with more biocompatible membranes.

H. B Lymphocytes

Great interest has been focused on determining whether B-lymphocyte activation contributes to the acquired immunodeficiency in uremic patients. Despite the fact that hemodialysis patients can develop abnormal antibody response (113,114,135), controversial data exist on the functional status of B cells (117,136). Since most studies have involved pokeweed mitogen, where the action is T-cell dependent (reviewed in Ref. 118), it is often unclear whether there is only a defect in the cooperation between T and B cells or whether there exists aberrant B-lymphocyte function per se. Descamps-Latscha reported in several reviews (130,137,138) that B cells from uremic patients produce large amounts of IgM and IgG in the absence of stimulation. The same authors (reviewed in Ref. 130) demonstrated elevated plasma levels of the soluble form of the low-affinity Fc receptor of IgG (CD23), which is predominantly expressed on activated B cells and is considered as a multifunctional cytokine. Furthermore, it is suggested that high circulating levels of CD23 are associated with an increased expression and shedding of CD23 by uremic B cells, supporting the hypothesis of an activated B-cell state in uremia (134). One possible mechanism of B-cell dysfunction in uremic patients may be the elevated parathyroid hormone. In both healthy controls and uremic patients Alexiewicz et al. (139) found inhibition of *S. aureus*–induced B-cell proliferation in the presence of 1-84 parathyroid hormone. There is also evidence that parathyroid hormone inhibits immunoglobulin production by cultured B cells (140).

I. Monocytes

There are only a few reports on the state and function of monocytes in uremic patients (reviewed in Ref. 141). Like neutrophils, monocytes undergo predialytic activation associated with depressed chemotactic, phagocytic, and bactericidal capacities (141). In view of the task of monocytes to present antigens to T cells, it has been suspected that there is a decrease in this capacity. This has been recently confirmed in a study by Ruiz et al. (142) demonstrating a marked impaired monocyte Fc receptor function in long-term hemodialyzed patients. Controversial studies exist on the monocyte/macrophage-mediated suppressor activity on lymphocyte response. Tsakolos et al. (143) found that the monocyte-dependent reduction in the T-cell proliferative response can be corrected by replacing autologous uremic monocytes by normal allogeneic monocytes. Other studies have failed to demonstrate that monocytes decrease T-cell IL-2 production (144).

Alterations in the function of immunocompetent cells include dysregulation of cytokine production. During contact of blood with dialyzer membranes, activation of mononuclear cells occurs (145). There is also reduced excretion and metabolism of cytokines in end-stage renal disease patients. High levels of IL-6 correlate with impaired clinical immune status (123). Advanced glycation endproduct pentosidine is associated with monocyte activation in renal failure (146). Girndt et al. (147) showed that high levels of proinflammatory IL-6 in hemodialysis patients are due to an increased number of monocytes producing this cytokine. IL-6 production per cell remains unchanged. The elevated levels of the anti-inflammatory cytokine IL-10, however, are the result of an increased synthesis per cell (147). Kimmel et al. (148) conducted a prospective, cross-sectional, observational multicenter study of urban hemodialysis patients to determine the contribution of immunological factors to patient survival. Two hundred and thirty patients entered the study. After an almost 3-year mean follow-up period, increased IL-1, TNF-α, IL-6, and IL-13 levels were significantly associated with increased relative mortality risk, while higher levels of IL-2, IL-4, IL-5, IL-12, T-cell number and function, and CH50 were associated with improved survival. Higher levels of circulating proinflammatory cytokines are associated with mortality, while immune parameters reflecting improved T-cell function are associated with survival in ESRD patients treated with hemodialysis, independent of other medical risk factors (148).

It has been shown that calcitriol regulates not only mineral metabolism but also cytotoxic cells and biosynthesis of immunoglobulins, gamma-interferon, granulocyte/macrophage colony-stimulating factor, tumor necrosis factor, HLA-DR, as well as the differentation of malignant cells and monocytes (149,150). Glorieux et al. (151) evaluated the effect of uremic ultrafiltrate (UUF) on basal and calcitriol-induced membrane-bound CD14 expression of monocytes. CD14 is a 55-kDa glycoprotein expressed on the surface of mature monocytes and macrophages and acts as a receptor for the complexes of lipopolysaccharide and lipopolysaccharide-binding protein. UUF suppressed both basal and calcitriol-induced CD14 expression. Similar effects were demonstrated with uric acid, xanthine, and hypoxanthine. It was concluded that UUF contains factors that impair calcitriol-activated function of monocytes (151).

J. Impaired Efficacy of Vaccinations

The clinical state of immunodeficiency in chronic renal failure patients is characterized by impaired efficacy of vaccinations. Vaccination responses have been shown to be suboptimal to hepatitis B, influenza, or pneumococcus (152–154). The typical course of hepatitis B infection in dialysis patients is mild, prolonged, and anicteric with only moderate elevation of liver enzymes. The majority of patients are not able to eliminate the virus and acquire chronic HBs antigenemia (155,156). Seroconversion after hepatitis B vaccination is markedly decreased (157–161), but lower and more rapidly decreasing antibody titers are found after vaccination with influenca (152,162,163) and pneumococcal vaccine in dialysis patients (154).

In the study of Köhler et al. (153) only 50–60% of the dialysis patients developed anti-HBs antibodies after three vaccinations, and titers were lower than in healthy controls. It has been shown that this immunodeficiency is already present in end-stage renal disease patients before initiation of chronic renal replacement therapy (164,165). IL-2 injection 4 hours after vaccination (166) or multiple intradermal applications of the vaccine (167) have been recommended to improve the response rate after hepatitis B vaccination. A new recombinant hepatitis B vaccine caused a seroconversion rate of 65% after the third and 71% after the fourth vaccination in 17 nonresponders (anti-HBs titer = 0) and 4 low responders (anti-HBs titer $\leq$5 IU/mL) with chronic renal failure (168). Caillat-Zucman et al. (169) reevaluated the genetic factors that may explain the variations in response to hepatitis B vaccine in hemodialysis patients. These authors demonstrated a negative correlation of DR 2 with nonresponse to hepatitis B. These results indicate an important role of HLA-linked immune response gene controlling the humoral response to HBs antigen.

Tetanus immunization and its association to hepatitis B vaccination in renal disease patients have been analyzed by Girndt et al. (170). Only 11 of 20 (55%) chronic renal failure patients and 16 of 23 (69%) in the dialysis group had a protective antibody response after triple vaccination. All control patients with essential hypertension and normal kidney function as well as six of seven renal transplant patients seroconverted. The response to tetanus toxoid was highly associated with the response to a previously administered vaccination against hepatitis B. The antibody concentrations after vaccination were lower in all renal patient groups compared to the patients with essential hypertension (170).

Kreft et al. (171) analyzed the immunity to diphtheria of 228 hemodialysis patients and the efficiency of single versus triple vaccination against diphtheria. The overall protection rate against diphtheria was 22%. After triple immunization, only 35% of the hemodialysis patients developed protective antibody concentration 6 months after the third vaccination. A single vaccination caused protective titers 12 months later in 41% of the patients (171).

V. CONCLUSION

Chronic uremia, particularly if associated with malnutrition, results in profound alterations of the immune system. PMNL functions such as chemotaxis, oxidative metabolism, phagocytic activity, degranulation, intracellular killing, or the carbohydrate metabolism are inhibited by low and high molecular weight inhibitors. Hemodialysis treatment with bioincompatible membranes results in further impairment of PMNL function. On the other hand, effective detoxification is a prerequisite for improved PMNL activity of these patients.

Iron overload in i.v. iron–treated end-stage renal disease patients and accumulation of intracellular calcium in patients with secondary hyperparathyroidism result in deactivation of neutrophils.

Uremia is characterized by the coexistence of B-cell, T-cell, and monocyte activation and deactivation, the so-called paradox of uremia.

REFERENCES

1. Montgomerie JZ, Kalmanson GM, Guze LB. Renal failure and infection. Medicine (Baltimore) 1968; 47: 1–32.
2. Nsouli KA, Lazarus JM, Schoenbaum SC, Gottlieb MN, Lowrie EG, Shocair M. Bacteremic infection in hemodialysis. Arch Intern Med 1979; 139:1255–1258.
3. Mailloux LU, Bellucci AG, Wilkes BM, Napolitano B, Mossey RT, Lesser M, Bluestone PA. Mortality in dialysis patients: analysis of the causes of death. Am J Kidney Dis 1991; 18:326–335.
4. Himmelfarb J, Hakim RM. Biocompatibility and risk of infection in haemodialysis patients. Nephrol Dial Transplant 1994; 9(suppl 2):138–144.
5. Hoen B, Kessler D, Hestin D, Mayeux D. Risk factors for bacterial infections in chronic haemodialysis adult patients: a multicentre prospective survey. Nephrol Dial Transplant 1995; 10:377–381.
6. Hoen B, Paul-Dauphin A, Hestin D, Kessler M. EPIBACDIAL: a multicenter prospective study of risk factors for bacteremia in chronic hemodialysis patients. J Am Soc Nephrol 1998; 9:869–876.
7. U.S. Renal Data System. USRDS 1998 annual data report. Am J Kidney Dis 1998; 32(suppl 1):S81–S88.
8. Powe NR, Jaar B, Furth SL, Hermann J, Briggs W. Septicemia in dialysis patients: incidence, risk factors and prognosis. Kidney Int 1999; 55:1081–1090.
9. Vanholder R, De Smet R, Waterloos MA, Van Landschoot N, Vogeleere P, Hoste E, Ringoir S. Mechanisms of uremic inhibition of phagocyte reactive species production: characterization of the role of p-cresol. Kidney Int 1995; 47:510–517.
10. Masuda M, Komiyama Y, Murakami T, Murata K. Decrease of polymorphonuclear leukocyte membrane fluidity in uremic patients on hermodialysis. Nephron 1990; 54:36–41.
11. Jörstad S. Viken KE. Inhibitory effects of plasma from uraemic patients on human mononuclear phagocytes cultured in vitro. Acta Pathol Microbiol Scand C 1977; 85:169–177.
12. Jörstad S, Kvernes S: Uraemic toxins of high molecular weight inhibiting human mononuclear phagocytes cultured in vitro. Acta Pathol Microbiol Scand C 1978; 86:221–226.
13. Jörstad S, Smeby LC, Wideroe TE, Berg KJ. Transport of uremic toxins through conventional hemodialysis membranes. Clin Nephrol 1979; 12:168–173.
14. Porter CJ, Burden RP, Morgan AG, Daniels I, Fletcher J. Impaired polymorphonuclear neutrophil function in end-stage renal failure and its correction by continuous ambulatory peritoneal dialysis. Nephron 1995; 71: 133–137.
15. Hörl WH, Haag-Weber M, Georgopoulos A, Block LH. Physicochemical characterization of a polypeptide present in uremic serum that inhibits the biological activity of polymoprhonuclear cells. Proc Natl Acad Sci USA 1990; 87:6353–6357.
16. Haag-Weber M, Mai B, Cohen G, Hörl WH. GIP and DIP: a new view of uraemic toxicity. Nephrol Dial Transplant 1994; 9:346–347.
17. Haag-Weber M, Mai B, Hörl WH. Isolation of a granulocyte inhibitory protein from uraemic patients with homology of beta$_2$-microglobulin. Nephrol Dial Transplant 1994; 9:382–388.
18. Beimler J, Schaefer RM, Haag-Weber M, Hörl WH. Effect of granulocyte inhibiting proteins from uremic patients on mononuclear cell cytokine production. (submitted for publication)
19. Haag-Weber M, Mai B, Hörl WH. Impaired cellular host defense in peritoneal dialysis by two granulocyte inhibitory proteins. Nephrol Dial Transplant 1994; 9: 1769–1773.
20. Tschesche H, Kopp C, Hörl WH, Hempelmann U. Inhibition of degranulation of polymorphonuclear leukocytes by angiogenin and its tryptic fragment. J Biol Chem 1994; 269:30274–30280.
21. Schuraldienst S, Oberpichler A, Tschesche H, Hörl WH. Angiogenin: a novel inhibitor of neutrophil lactoferin release during extracorporeal circulation. J Am Soc Nephrol (in press).
22. Balke N, Holtkamp U, Hörl WH, Tschesche H. Inhibition of degranulation of human polymorphonuclear leukocytes by complement factor D. FEBS Lett 1995; 371:300–302.
23. Volanakis JE, Barnum SR, Giddens M, Galla JH. Renal filtration and catabolism of complement protein D. N Engl J Med 1985; 312:395–399.
24. Cohen G, Haag-Weber M, Mai B, Deicher R, Hörl WH. Effect of immunoglobulin light chains from hemodialysis and CAPD patients on PMNL functions. J Am Soc Nephrol 1995; 6:1592–1599.
25. Hannam-Harris AC, Gordon J, Smith JL. Immunoglobulin synthesis by neoplastic B lymphocytes: free light chain synthesis as a marker of B cell differentiation. J Immunol 1980; 125:2177–2181.
26. Peterson PA, Berggard I. Urinary immunoglobulin components in normal tubular and glomerular proteinuria: quantities and characteristics of free light chains, IgG, IgA, and Fc-gamma fragment. Eur J Clin Invest 1971; 1:255–264.

27. Solling K. Free light chains of immunoglobulins. Scand J Clin Lab Invest 1981; 157(suppl 1):1–83.
28. Wakasugi K, Sasaki M, Suzuki M, Azumo N, Nobuto T. Increased concentratons of free light chain lambda in sera from chronic hemodialysis patients. Biomater Artif Cells Immobilization Biotechnol 1991; 19:97–109.
29. Cohen G, Rudnicki M, Hörl WH. Isolation of modified ubiquitin as a neutrophil chemotaxis inhibitor from uremic patients. J Am Soc Nephrol 1998; 9:451–456.
30. Cendoroglo M, Jaber BL, Balakrishnan VS, Perianayagam M, King AJ, Pereira BJG. Neutrophil apoptosis and dysfunction in uremia. J Am Soc Nephrol 1999; 10:93–100.
31. Young GA, Kopple JD, Lindholm B, Vonesh EF, De Vecchi A, Scalamogna A, Castelnova C, Oreopoulos DG, Anderson GH, Bergström J. Nutritional assessment of continuous ambulatory peritoneal dialysis patients: an international study. Am J Kidney Dis 1991; 17:462–471.
32. Morgenstern A, Winkler J, Narkis R, Zilverman S, Lipa R, Boner G, Morduchowicz G. Adequacy of dialysis and nutritional status in hemodialysis patients. Nephron 1994; 66:438–441.
33. Ikizler TA, Greene JH, Wingard RL, Parker RA, Hakim RM. Spontaneous dietary protein intake during progression of chronic renal failure. J Am Soc Nephrol 1995; 6:1386–1391.
34. Briggs WA, Pedersen MM, Mahajan SK, Sillix DH, Prasad AS, McDonald FD. Lymphocyte and granulocyte function in zinc-treated and zinc-deficient hemodialysis patients. Kidney Int 1982; 21:827–832.
35. Churchill DN, Taylor W, Cook RJ, LaPlante P, Barre P, Cartier P, Fay WP, Goldstein MB, Jindahl K, Mandin H. Canadian hemodialysis morbidity study. Am J Kidney Dis 1992; 19:214–234.
36. Kaysen GA, Rathore V, Shearer GC, Depner TA. Mechanisms of hypoalbuminemia in hemodialysis patients. Kidney Int 1995; 48:510–516.
37. Bergström J, Heimbürger O, Lindholm B, Qureshi AR. Elevated serum C-reactive protein is a strong predictor of increased mortality and low serum albumin in hemodialysis (HD) patients (abstr). J Am Soc Nephrol 1995; 6:596.
38. Villa ML, Ferrario E, Bergamasco E, Bozzetti F, Cozzaglio L, Clerici E. Reduced natural killer cell activity and IL-2 production in malnurished cancer patients. Br J Cancer 1991; 63:1010–1014.
39. Redmond HP, Shou J, Kelly CJ, Schreiber S, Miller E, Leon P, Daly JM. Immunosuppressive mechanisms in protein-caloric malnutrition. Surgery 1991; 110: 311–317.
40. Field CJ, Gougeon R, Marliss EB.Changes in circulating leukocytes and mitogen responses during very-low-energy all-protein reducing diets. Am J Clin Nutr 1991; 54:123–129.
41. Seifert A, von Herrath D, Schaefer K. Iron overload but not treatment with desferrioxamine favours the development of septicemia in patients on maintenance haemodialysis. Q J Med 1987; 65:1015–1024.
42. Tielemans C, Lenclud C. Respective role of hemosiderosis and desferrioxamine therapy in the risk from infection of hemodialysis patients. Q J Med 1988; 68: 573–574.
43. Boelaert JR, Daneels RF, Schurgers ML, Matthys EG, Gordts BZ, Van Landuyt HW. Iron overload in haemodialysis patients increases the risk of bacteraemia: a prospective study. Nephrol Dial Transplant 1990; 5: 130–134.
44. Van Asbeck BS, Marx JJ, Struyvenberg A, van Kats JH, Verhoef J. Effect of iron (III) in the presence of various ligands on the phagocytic and metabolic activity of human polymorphonuclear leukocytes. J Immunol 1984; 132:851–856.
45. Waterlot Y, Cantinieaux B, Hariga-Muller C, de Maertelaere-Laurent E, Vanhergweghem JL, Fondu P. Impaired phagocytic activity of neutrophils in patients receiving haemodialysis: the critical role of iron overload. Br Med J 1985; 291:501–504.
46. Flament J, Goldman M, Waterlot Y, Dupont E, Wybran J, Vanherweghem JL. Impairment of phagocyte oxidative metabolism in hemodialyzed patients with iron overload. Clin Nephrol 1986; 25:227–230.
47. Cantinieaux B, Boelaert J, Hariga C, Fondu P. Impaired neutrophil defense against Yersinia enterocolitica in patients with iron overload who are undergoing dialysis. J Lab Clin Med 1988; 111:524–528.
48. Boelaert JR, Cantinieaux BF, Hariga CF, Fondu PG. Recombinant erythropoietin reverses polymorphonuclear granulocyte dysfunction in iron-overloaded dialysis patients. Nephrol Dial Transplant 1990; 5:504–517.
49. Patruta SI, Edlinger R, Sunder-Plassmann G, Hörl WH. Neutrophil impairment associated with iron therapy in hemodialysis patients with functional iron deficiency. J Am Soc Nephrol 1998: 9:655–663.
50. Veys N, Vanholder R, Ringoir S. Correction of deficient phagocytosis during erythropoietin treatment in maintenance hemodialysis patients. Am J Kidney Dis 1992; 19:358–363.
51. Vanholder R, Van Biesen W, Ringoir S. Contributing factors to the inhibition of phagocytosis in hemodialyzed patients. Kidney Int 1993; 44:208–214.
52. Collart FE, Dratwa M, Wittek M, Wens R. Effects of recombinant human erythropoietin to T lymphocyte subsets in hemodialysis patients. Trans Am Soc Artif Intern Organs 1990; 36:M219–223.
53. Sennesael JJ, Van der Niepen P, Verbeelen DL. Treatment with recombinant erythropoietin increases antibody titers after hepatitis B vaccination in dialysis patients. Kidney Int 1991; 40:121–128.
54. Massry SG, Fadda GZ. Chronic renal failure is a state

of cellular calcium toxicity. Am J Kidney Dis 1993; 21:81–86.
55. Massry SG, Smogorzewski M. Mechanisms through which parathyroid hormone mediates its deleterious effect on organ function in uremia. Semin Nephrol 1994; 14:219–231.
56. Shurtz-Swirski R, Shkolnik T, Shasha SM. Parathyroid hormone and the cellular immune system. Nephron 1995; 70:21–24.
57. Alexiewicz JM, Smogorzewski M, Fadda GZ, Massry SG. Impaired phagocytosis in dialysis patients: studies on mechanisms. Am J Nephrol 1991; 11:102.
58. Haag-Weber M, Mai B, Hörl WH. Normalization of enhanced neutrophil cytosolic free calcium of hemodialysis patients by 1,25-dihydroxyvitamin D_3 or calcium channel blocker. Am J Nephrol 1993; 13:467–472.
59. Hörl WH, Haag-Weber M, Mai B, Massry SG. Verapamil reverses abnormal $[Ca^{2+}]_i$ and carbohydrate metabolism of PMNL of dialysis patients. Kidney Int 1995; 47:1741–1745.
60. Kiersztejn M, Smogorzewski M, Thanakitcharu P, Fadda GZ, Massry SG. Decreased O_2 consumption by PMNL from humans and rats with CRF: role of secondary hyperparathyroidism. Kidney Int 1992; 42: 602–609.
61. Haag-Weber M, Hörl WH. Effect of biocompatible membranes on neutrophil function and metabolism. Clin Nephrol 1994; 42(suppl 1):S31–S36.
62. Haag-Weber M, Mai B, Hörl WH. Effect of hemodialysis on intracellular calcium in human polymorphonuclear neutrophils. Miner Electrolyte Metab 1992; 18:151–155.
63. Descamps-Latscha B, Herbelin A. Long-term dialysis and cellular immunity: a critical survey. Kidney Int 1993; 43(suppl 41):S135–S142.
64. Himmelfarb J, Zaoui P, Hakim R. Modulation of granulocyte LAM-1 and MAC-1 during dialysis—a prospective, randomized controlled trial. Kidney Int 1992; 41:388–395.
65. Craddock PR, Fehr J, Dalmasso AP, Brigham KL, Jacob HS. Hemodialysis leukopenia: pulmonary vascular leukostasis resulting from complement activation by dialyser cellophane membrane. J Clin Invest 1977; 59:879–888.
66. Nguyen AT, Lethias C, Zingraff J, Herbelin A, Naret C, Descamps-Latscha B. Hemodialysis membrane-induced activation of phagocyte oxidative metabolism detected in vivo and in vitro within microamounts of whole blood. Kidney Int 1985; 28:158–167.
67. Kuwahara T, Markert M, Wauters JP. Neutrophil oxygen radical production by dialysis membranes. Nephrol Dial Transplant 1988; 3:661–665.
68. Hirabayashi Y, Kobayashi T, Nishikawa A, Okazaki H, Aoki T, Takaya J, Kobayashi Y. Oxidative metabolism and phagocytosis of polymorphonuclear leukocytes in patients with chronic renal failure. Nephron 1988; 49:305–312.
69. Himmelfarb J, Lazarus M, Hakim R. Reactive oxygen species production by monocytes and polymorphonuclear leukocytes during dialysis. Am J Kidney Dis 1991; 17:271–276.
70. Vanholder R, Ringoir S, Dhondt A, Hakim R. Phagocytosis in uremic and hemodialysis patients: a prospective and cross sectional study. Kidney Int 1991; 39:320–327.
71. Himmelfarb J, Ault KA, Holbrook D, Leeber DA, Hakim RM. Intradialytic granulocyte reactive oxygen species production: a prospective, crossover trial. J Am Soc Nephrol 1993; 4:178–186.
72. Cristol JP, Canaud B, Rabesandratana H, Gaillard I, Serre A, Mion C. Enhancement of reactive oxygen species production and cell surface markers expression due to haemodialysis. Nephrol Dial Transplant 1994; 9:389–394.
73. Rosenkranz AR, Templ E, Traindl O, Heinzl H, Zlabinger GJ. Reactive oxygen product formation by human neutrophils as an early marker for biocompatibility of dialysis membranes. Clin Exp Immunol 1994; 98:300–305.
74. Hörl WH, Steinhauer HB, Schollmeyer P. Plasma levels of granulocyte elastase during hemodialysis: effects of different dialyzer membranes. Kidney Int 1985; 28:791–796.
75. Haag-Weber M, Schollmeyer P, Hörl WH. Granulocyte activation during haemodialysis in the absence of complement activation: inhibition by calcium channel blockers. Eur J Clin Invest 1988; 18:380–385.
76. Rosenkranz AR, Körmoczi GF, Thalhammer F, Menzel EJ, Hörl WH, Mayer G, Zlabinger GJ. Novel D5-dependent mechanism of neutrophil stimulation by bioincompatible dialyzer membranes. J Am Soc Nephrol 1999; 10:128–135.
77. Vanholder R, Van Loo A, Dhondt AM, De Smet R, Ringoir S. Influence of uraemia and haemodialysis on host defence and infection. Nephrol Dial Transplant 1996; 11:593–598.
78. Shurtz-Swirski R, Mashiach E, Kristal B, Shkolnik T, Shasha SM. Antioxidant enzymes activity in polymorphonuclear leukocytes in chronic renal failure. Nephron 1995; 71:176–179.
79. Ward RA, McLeish KR. Polymorphonuclear leukocyte oxidative burst is enhanced in patients with chronic renal insufficiency. J Am Soc Nephrol 1995; 5:1697–1702.
80. Springer TA. Adhesion receptors of the immune system. Nature 1990; 346:425–434.
81. Arnaout MA. Structure and function of the leukocyte adhesion molecules CD11/CD18. Blood 1990; 75: 1037–1050.
82. Arnaout MA. Leukocyte adhesion molecules deficiency: its structural basis, pathophysiology and im-

plications for modulating the inflammatory response. Immunol Rev 1990; 114:145–180.
83. Lawrence MB, Springer TA. Leukocytes roll on a selectin at physiologic flow rates. Distinction from and prerequisite for adhesion through integrins. Cell 1991; 65:859–873.
84. Thylén P, Fernvik E, Lundahl J, Hed J, Jacobson SH. Cell surface receptor modulation on monocytes and granulocytes during clinical and experimental hemodialysis. Am J Nephrol 1995; 15:392–400.
85. Hornberger JC, Chernew M, Petersen J, Garber AM. A multivariate analysis of mortality and hospital admissions with high-flux dialysis. J Am Soc Nephrol 1992; 3:1227–1237.
86. Vychytil A, Lorenz M, Schneider B, Hörl WH, Haag-Weber M. New strategies to prevent *Staphylococcus aureus* infections in peritoneal dialysis patients. J Am Soc Nephrol 1998; 9:669–676.
87. Vychytil A, Lorenz M, Schneider B, Hörl WH, Haag-Weber M. New criteria for management of catheter infections in peritoneal dialysis patients using ultrasonography. J Am Soc Nephrol 1998; 9:290–296.
88. Report of the Working Party of the British Society for Antimicrobial Chemotherapy. Diagnosis and management of peritonitis in CAPD. Lancet 1987; 1:845–849.
89. Vanholder R, Lameire N. Waterloos MA, Van Landschoot N, De Smet R, Vogeleere P, Lambert MC, Vijt D, Ringoir S. Disturbed host defense in peritoneal cavity during CAPD: characterization of responsible factors in dwell fluid. Kidney Int 1996; 50:643–652.
90. Jörres A, Topley N, Steenweg L, Müller C, Köttgen E, Gahl GM. Inhibition of cytokine synthesis by peritoneal dialysate persists throughout the CAPD cycle. Am J Nephrol 1992; 12:80–85.
91. Jörres A, Gahl GM, Ludat K, Frei U, Passlick-Deetjen J. In vitro biocompatibility evaluation of a novel bicarbonate-buffered amino-acid solution for peritoneal dialysis. Nephrol Dial Transplant 1997; 12:543–549.
92. Levy R, Klein J, Rubinek T, Alkan M, Shany S, Chaimovitz C. Diversity in peritoneal macrophage response of CAPD patients to 1,25 dihydrovitamin D3. Kidney Int 1990; 37:1310–1315.
93. Jörres A, Jörres D, Topley N, Gahl GM, Mahiout A. Leukotriene release from peripheral and peritoneal leukocytes following exposure to peritoneal dialysis solutions. Nephrol Dial Transplant 1991; 6:495–501.
94. Witowski J, Topley N, Jörres A, Liberek T, Coles GA, Williams JD. Effect of lactate-buffered peritoneal dialysis fluids on human peritoneal mesothelial cell interleukin-6 and prostaglandin synthesis. Kidney Int 1995; 47:282–293.
95. Liberek T, Topley N, Jörres A, Coles GA, Gahl GM, Williams JD. Peritoneal dialysis fluid inhibition of phagocyte function: effects of osmolality and glucose concentration. J Am Soc Nephrol 1993; 3:1508–1515.
96. Hume DM, Merrill JP, Miller BF, Thorn GW. Experiences with renal homotransplantation in the human: report of nine cases. J Clin Invest 1955; 34:327–382.
97. Dammin GJ, Couch NP, Murray JE. Prolonged survival of skin homografts in uremic patients. Ann NY Acad Sci 1957; 64:967–976.
98. Kirkpatrick CH, Wilson WEC, Talmage DW. Immunologie studies in human organ transplantation. J Exp Med 1964; 119:727–742.
99. Buchanan WW, Klinenberg JR, Seegmiller JE. The inflammatory response to injected microcrystalline monosodium urate in normal, hyperuricemic, gouty and uremic subjects. Arthritis Rheum 1965; 8:361–367.
100. Huber H, Pastner D, Dittrich P, Braunsteiner H. In vitro reactivity of human lymphocytes in uraemia. A comparison with the impairment of deleayed hypersensitivity. Clin Exp Immunol 1969; 5:75–82.
101. Boulton-Jones JM, Vick R, Cameron JS, Black PJ. Immune responses in uremia. Clin Nephrol 1973; 1:351–360.
102. Selroos O, Pasternack A, Virolainen M. Skin test sensitivity and antigen-induced lymphocyte transformation in uraemia. Clin Exp Immunol 1973; 14:365–370.
103. Sengar DP, Rashid A, Harris JE. In vitro cellular immunity and in vivo delayed hypersensitivity in uremic patients maintained on hemodialysis. Int Arch Allergy Appl Immun 1974; 47:829–838.
104. Touraine JL, Touraine F, Revillard JP, Brochier J, Traeger J. T-lymphocytes and serum inhibitors of cell-mediated immunity in renal insufficiency. Nephron 1975; 14:195–208.
105. McIntosh J, Hansen P, Ziegler J, Penny R. Defective immune and phagocytic functions in uraemia and renal transplantation. Int Archs Allergy Appl Immun 1976; 51:544–559.
106. Bridges JM, Nelson SD, Mcgeown MG. Evaluation of lymphocyte transfer test in normal and uraemic subjects. Lancet 1964; i:581–584.
107. Papadimitriou M, Memmos D, Metaxas P. Tuberculosis in patients on regular haemodialysis. Nephron 1979; 24:53–57.
108. Pradhan RP, Katz LA, Nidus BD, Matalon R, Eisinger RP. Tuberculosis in dialyzed patients. JAMA 1974; 229:798–800.
109. Lundin AP, Adler AJ, Berlyne GM, Friedman EA. Tuberculosis in patients undergoing maintenance haemodialysis. Am J Med 1979; 67:597–602.
110. Rutsky EA, Rostand SG. Myobacteriosis in patients with chronic renal failure. Arch Intern Med 1980; 140: 57–61.
111. Sasaki S, Akiba T, Suenaga M, Tomura S, Yoshiyama N, Nakagawa S, Shoji T, Sasaoka T, Takeuchi J. Ten years' survey of dialysis-associated tuberculosis. Nephron 1979; 24:141–145.
112. Andrew OT, Schoenfeld PY, Hopewell PC, Humphreys MH. Tuberculosis in patients with end-stage renal disease. Am J Med 1980; 68:59–65.

113. Nolph KD, Husted FC, Sharp GC. Antibodies to nuclear antigens in patients undergoing long-term hemodialysis. Am J Med 1976; 60:673–676.
114. Mayet WJ, Wandel E, Hermann E, Dumann H, Köhler H. Antibodies to cytoskeletal components in patients undergoing long-term hemodialysis detected by a sensitive enzyme-linked immunosorbent assay (ELISA). Clin Nephrol 1990; 33:272–278.
115. Touraine JL, Touraine F, Revillard JP, Brochier J, Traeger J. T-lymphocytes and serum inhibitors of cell mediated immunity in renal insufficiency. Nephron 1975; 14:195–208.
116. Donati D, Degiannis D, Homer L, Gastaldi L, Raskova J, Raska K. Immune deficiency in uremia: interleukin-2 production and responsiveness and interleukin-2 receptor expression and release. Nephron 1991; 58:268–275.
117. Chatenoud L, Dugas B, Beaurain G, Touam M, Drueke T, Vasquez A, Galanaud P, Bach JF, Delfraissy JF. Presence of preactivated T cells in hemodialyzed patients: their possible role in altered immunity. Proc Natl Acad Sci USA 1986; 83:7457–7461.
118. Chatenoud L, Heberlin A, Beaurain G, Descamps-Latscha B. Immune deficiency of the uremic patient. Adv Nephrol 1990; 19:259–274.
119. Beaurain G, Naret C, Marcon L, Grateau G, Drueke T, Ureña P, Nelson DL, Bach JF, Chatenoud L. In vivo T cell preactivation in chronic uremic hemodialyzed and non-hemodialyzed patients. Kidney Int 1989; 36: 636–644.
120. Donati D, Degiannis D, Raskova J, Raska K JR. Uremic serum effects on peripheral blood mononuclear cell and purified T-lymphocyte responses. Kidney Int 1992; 42:681–689.
121. Meuer SC, Hauer M, Kurz P, Meyer zum Büschenfelde KH, Köhler H. Selective blockade of the antigen-receptor-mediated pathway of T cell activation in patients with impaired primary immune responses. J Clin Invest 1987; 80:743–749.
122. Keown P, Descamps-Latscha B. In vitro suppression of cell mediated immunity by ferroproteins and ferric salts. Cell Immunol 1983; 80:257–266.
123. Girndt M, Köhler H, Schiedhelm-Weick E, Meyer zum Büschenfelde KH, Fleischer B. T-cell activation defect in hemodialysis patients: evidence for a role of the B7/CD28 pathway. Kidney Int 1993; 44:359–365.
124. Calder PC, Newsholme EA. Influence of antioxidant vitamins on fatty acid inhibition of lymphocyte proliferation. Biochem Mol Biol Int 1993; 29:175–183.
125. Meydani SN, Meydani M, Blumberg JB, Leka-LS, Silber G, Loszewski R, Thompson C, Pedrosa MC, Diamond RD, Stollar BD. Vitamin E supplementation and in vivo immune response in healthy elderly subjects. A randomized controlled trial. JAMA 1997; 277: 1380–1386.
126. Beharka A, Redican S, Leka L, Meydani SN. Vitamin E status and immune function. Methods Enzymol 1997; 282:247–263.
127. De Waart FG, Portengen L, Doekes G, Verwaal CJ, Kok FJ. Effect of 3 months vitamin E supplementation on indices of the cellular and humoral immune response in elderly subjects. Br J Nutr 1997; 78:761–774.
128. Gerez L, Madar L, Shkolnik T, Kristal B, Arad G, Reshes A, Steinberger A, Ketzinel M, Sayar D, Shasha S. Regulation of interleukin-2 and interferon-gamma gene expression in renal failure. Kidney Int 1991; 40: 266–272.
129. Walz G, Kunzendorf U, Josimovic-Alasevic O, Preuschoff L, Schwarz A, Keller F, Asmus G, Offermann G, Diamantstein T, Distler A. Soluble interleukin-2 receptor and tissue polypeptide antigen serum concentrations in end-stage renal failure. Nephron 1990; 56: 157–161.
130. Descamps-Latscha B, Herbelin A, Nguyen AT, Zingraff J, Jungers P, Chatenaud L. Immune system dysregulation in uremia. Sem Nephrol 1994; 14:253–260.
131. Lewin E, Ladefoged J, Brandi L, Olgaard K. Parathyroid hormone dependent T cell proliferation in uremic rats. Kidney Int 1993; 44:379–384.
132. Alexiewicz JM, Gaciong Z, Klinger M, Linker-Israeli M, Pitts TO, Massry SG. Evidence of impaired T cell function in hemodialysis patients: potential role for secondary hyperparathyroidism. Am J Nephrol 1990; 10:495–501.
133. Zaoui P, Green W, Hakim RM. Hemodialysis with cuprophane membrane modulates interleukin-2 receptor expression. Kidney Int 1991; 39:1020–1026.
134. Degiannis D, Czarnecki M, Donati D, Homer L, Eisinger RP, Raska K JR, Raskova J. Normal T lymphocyte function in patients with end-stage renal disease hemodialyzed with "high-flux" polysulphone membranes. Am J Nephrol 1990; 10:276–282.
135. Rumpf KW, Seubert S, Seubert A, Lowitz HD, Valentin R, Rippe H, Ippen H, Scheler F. Association of the ethylene-oxide induced IgE antibodies with symptoms in dialysis patients. Lancet 1985; 2:1385–1387.
136. Raskova J, Ghobrial J, Czerwinski DK, Shea SM, Eisinger RP, Raska K JR. B cell activation and immunoregulation in end-stage renal disease patients receiving hemodialysis. Arch Int Med 1987; 147:89–93.
137. Descamps-Latscha B, Chatenoud L. T cells and B cells in chronic renal failure. Semin Nephrol 1996; 16: 183–191.
138. Descamps-Latscha B. The immune system in end-stage renal disease. Curr Opin Nephrol Hypert 1993; 2:883–891.
139. Alexiewicz JM, Klinger M, Pitts TO, Gaciong Z, Linker-Israeli M, Massry SG. Parathyroid hormone inhibits B cell proliferation: implications in chronic renal failure. J Am Soc Nephrol 1990; 1:236–244.

140. Gaciong Z, Alexiewicz JM, Pitts TO, Linker-Israeli M, Shulman I, Massry SG. Effect of parathyroid hormone (PTH) on immunoglobulin (Ig) production in normals and in chronic renal failure (CRF) patients (abstr). Proc Am Soc Nephrol 1988; 20:45.
141. Gibbons RA, Martinez OM, Garovoy MR. Altered monocyte function in uremia. Clin Immunol Immunopathol 1990; 56:66–80.
142. Ruiz P, Gomez F, Schreiber AD. Impaired function of macrophage Fc gamma receptors in end stage renal disease. N Engl J Med 1990; 322:717–722.
143. Tsakolos ND, Theoharides TC, Hendler ED, Goffinet J, Dwyer JM, Whisler RL, Askenase PM. Immune defects in chronic renal impairment: evidence for defective regulation of lymphocyte response by macrophages from patients with chronic renal impairment on hemodialysis. Clin Exp Immunol 1986; 63:218–227.
144. Alevy YG, Slavin RG. Immune response in experimentally induced uremia. II. Suppression of PHA response in uremia is mediated by an adherent, Ia-negative and indomethacin insensitive suppressor cell. J Immunol 1981; 126:2007–2010.
145. Schindler R, Linnenweber S, Schulze M. Geneexpression of interleukin-1β during hemodialysis. Kidney Int 1993; 43:712–721.
146. Friedlander MA, Witko-Sarsat V, Nguyen AT, Wu YC, Labrunte M, Verger C, Jungers P, Descamps-Latscha B. The advanced glycation endproduct pentosidine and monocyte activation in uremia. Clin Nephrol 1996; 46:379–382.
147. Girndt M, Sester U, Kaul H, Köhler H. Production of proinflammatory and regulatory monokines in hemodialysis patients shown at a single-cell level. J Am Soc Nephrol 1998; 9:1689–1696.
148. Kimmel PL, Phillips TM, Simmens SJ, Peterson RA, Weihs KL, Alleyne S, Cruz I, Yanovski JA, Veis JH. Immunologic function and survival in hemodialysis patients. Kidney Int 1998; 54:236–244.
149. Manolagas SC, Yu X-P, Girasole G, Bellido T. Vitamin D and the hematolymphopoietic tissue: a 1994 update. Semin Nephrol 1994; 14:129–143.
150. Lemire JM. Immunomodulatory role of 1,25-dihydroxyvitamin D_3. J Cell Biochem 1992; 49:26–31.
151. Glorieux G, Hsu CH, De Smet R, Dhondt A, Van Kaer J, Vogeleere P, Lameire N, Vanholder R. Inhibition of calcitriol-induced monocyte CD14 expression by uremic toxins: role of purines. J Am Soc Nephrol 1998; 9:1826–1831.
152. Cappel R, Van Beers D, Liesnard C, Dratwa M. Impaired humoral and cell-mediated immune responses in dialyzed patients after influenza vaccination. Nephron 1983; 33:21–25.
153. Köhler H, Arnold W, Renschin G, Dormeyer HH, Meyer zum Büschenfelde KH. Active hepatitis B vaccination of dialysis patients and medical staff. Kidney Int 1984; 25:124–128.
154. Nikoskelainen J, Koskela M, Forsström J, Kasanen M, Leinonen M. Persistence of antibodies to pneumococcal vaccine in patients with chronic renal failure. Kidney Int 1985; 28:672–677.
155. London WT, DiFiglia M, Sutnick AI, Blumberg BS. An epidemic of hepatitis in a chronic-hemodialysis unit. Australia antigen and differences in host responses. N Engl J Med 1969; 281:571–578.
156. Nordenfelt E, Landholm T, Dahlquist E. A hepatitis epidemic in a dialysis unit. Occurrence and persistence of Australia antigen among patients and staff. Acta Pathol Microbiol Scand Microbiol Immunol B 1970; 78:692–700.
157. Crosnier J, Jungers P, Couroucé AM, Laplanche A, Benhamou E, Degos F, Lacour B, Prunet P, Cerisier Y, Guesry P. Randomised placebo-controlled trial of hepatitis B surface antigen vaccine in French hemodialysis units. I. Medical staff. Lancet 1981; i:455–459.
158. Crosnier J, Jungers P, Couroucé AM, Laplanche A, Benhamou E, Degos F, Lacour B, Prunet P, Cerisier Y, Guesry P. Randomized placebo-controlled trial of hepatitis B surface antigen vaccine in french hemodialysis units. II. Hemodialysis patients. Lancet 1981; i:797–800.
159. Stevens CE, Alter HJ, Taylor PE, Zang EA, Harley EJ, Szmuness W. Hepatitis B vaccine in patients receiving hemodialysis. Immunogenicity and efficacy. N Engl J Med 1984; 311:496–501.
160. De Graeff PA, Dankert J, de Zeeuw D, Gips CH, van der Hem GK. Immune response to two different hepatitis B vaccines in haemodialysis patients: a 2-year follow-up. Nephron 1985; 40:155–160.
161. Albertoni F, Battilomo A, Di Nardo V, Franco E, Ippolito G, Marinucci G, Perucci CA, Petrosillo N, Sommella L. Evaluation of a region-wide hepatitis B vaccination program in dialysis patients: experience in an Italian region. Nephron 1991; 58:180–183.
162. Versluis DJ, Beyer WE, Masurel N, Diderich PP, Kramer P, Weimar W. Intact humoral immune response in patients on continuous ambulatory peritoneal dialysis. Nephron 1988; 49:16–19.
163. Beyer WE, Noordzij TC, Kramer P, Diderich PP, Op den Hoek CT, Janssen J, Masurel N, Weimar W. Effect of immunomodulator thymopentin on impaired seroresponse to influenza vaccine in patients on haemodialysis. Nephron 1990; 54:296–301.
164. Bommer J, Rambausek M, Ritz E. Vaccination against hepatitis B in patients with renal insufficiency. Proc Eur Dial Transplant Assoc Eur Ren Assoc 1985; 21: 300–305.
165. Duman H, Meuer S, Meyer zum Büschenfelde KH, Köhler H. Hepatitis B vaccination and interleukin 2 receptor expression in chronic renal failure. Kidney Int 1990; 38:1164–1168.
166. Köhler H, Dumann H, Meyer zum Büschenfelde KH,

Meuer S. Secondary immune deficiency in renal failure exemplified by hepatitis B vaccination. Klin Wochenschr 1988; 66:865–872.

167. Ono K, Kashiwagi S. Complete seroconversion by low-dose intradermal injection of recombinant hepatitis B vaccine in hemodialysis patients. Nephron 1991; 58:47–51.

168. Haubitz M, Ehlerding G, Beigel A, Heuer U, Hemmerling AE, Thoma HA. Clinical experience with a new recombinant hepatitis B vaccine in previous nonresponders with chronic renal insufficiency. Clin Nephrol 1996; 45:180–182.

169. Caillat-Zucman S, Giminez JJ, Albouze G, Lebkiri B, Naret C, Jungers P, Bach JF. HLA genetic heterogeneity of hepatitis B vaccine response in hemodialyzed patients. Kidney Int 1993; 43:S157–S160.

170. Girndt M, Pietsch M, Köhler H. Tetanus immunization and its association to hepatitis B vaccination in patients with chronic renal failure. Am J Kidney Dis 1995; 26:454–460.

171. Kreft B, Klouche M, Kreft R, Kirchner H, Sack K. Low efficiency of active immunization against diphtheria in chronic hemodialysis patients. Kidney Int 1997; 52:212–216.

22

Nutritional Complications in Chronic Hemodialysis and Peritoneal Dialysis Patients

T. Alp Ikizler
Vanderbilt University Medical Center, Nashville, Tennessee

Jonathan Himmelfarb
Maine Medical Center, Portland, Maine

I. INTRODUCTION

Despite substantial improvements in the science and technology of renal replacement therapy (RRT), the morbidity and mortality of patients with end-stage renal disease (ESRD) remains excessively high (1–4). Among the many factors that adversely affect patient outcome, protein-calorie malnutrition has been shown to be highly associated with increased morbidity and mortality in the chronic dialysis patient population (5–8). Chronic uremia per se as well as chronic dialysis therapy may predispose the ESRD patient to multiple nutritional complications and hence protein-calorie malnutrition (Table 1). In this chapter we will attempt to define the importance of nutrition to the outcome of chronic hemo- and peritoneal dialysis patients and explore the possible mechanisms that cause and/or promote poor nutritional status in these patients, with a specific emphasis on their special dietary requirements. We will discuss measures to prevent malnutrition in stable chronic dialysis patients as well as several treatment options in patients who are already malnourished. We will finally discuss the clinically important aspects of vitamins and trace elements in chronic dialysis patients.

II. INDICES OF NUTRITIONAL STATUS

Before discussing the extent and importance of malnutrition, it is essential to discuss the indices of nutritional status that are utilized in chronic dialysis patients. Although practical methods to assess nutritional status are imperative, the appropriate interpretation of nutritional markers in ESRD patients remains a challenge. The nutritional state of patients with multiple different diseases is routinely monitored by using various anthropometric and biochemical indices. Although a significant relationship has been established between the nutritional state of the patients and the various markers, the variance of the association is quite large and ESRD patients are no exception. Further, several markers utilized for nutritional purposes are influenced by many nonnutritional factors, especially in chronic dialysis patients. We shall briefly mention the important clinical aspects of several nutritional indices. A list of commonly used indices of malnutrition in chronic dialysis patients is depicted in Table 2.

A. Biochemical Markers

In chronic dialysis patients, relatively simple biochemical measures reflecting the visceral protein stores, such as serum albumin, creatinine, and blood urea nitrogen (BUN), as well as more complex and not readily available parameters such as transferrin, prealbumin, and insulin-like growth factor-1 (IGF-1) have been proposed as nutritional indices (9–12). Serum albumin is probably the most extensively examined nutritional index in almost all patient populations, probably due to its easy availability and strong association with out-

Table 1 Nutritional Complications of Renal Disease

Decreased protein and calorie intake (anorexia)
Increased protein catabolism and energy expenditure
Metabolic and hormonal abnormalities
Impaired vitamin/trace element homeostasis
Impaired lipid profile (? increased cardiovascular risk)
Impaired quality of life/rehabilitation

come, especially in ESRD patients. Studies have shown that serum albumin concentrations are closely affected by the level of dietary protein intake. In fact, low serum albumin concentrations are usually accompanied by other markers of malnutrition in multiple studies with different patient populations including ESRD patients and have been accepted as one of the most consistent markers of chronic protein-calorie malnutrition (9,13–17). These observations have led to the general concept that an abnormal serum albumin concentration by itself is usually sufficient to diagnose protein-energy malnutrition in ESRD patients. However, it should be kept in mind that serum albumin concentration may also be affected by many other co-existing problems in addition to malnutrition. Specifically, serum albumin is a negative acute-phase reactant, and its serum concentration decreases sharply in response to stress and inflammation and thus may not necessarily reflect the changes in nutritional status in acutely ill patients. Conditions that promote an acute-phase response such as infection and/or trauma can induce prompt and significant decreases in serum albumin concentrations. In this context, the decrease in serum albumin concentrations closely reflects the degree of illness and inflammation, rather than the overall nutritional status (18,19). Finally, serum albumin concentration in chronic dialysis patients is also affected by other nonnutritional factors, such as external losses, intra- and extravascular fluid shifts, and other illnesses, (e.g., liver disease). Therefore, to the extent that serum albumin reflects malnutrition, it should be considered as a late index of nutritional status changes.

Table 2 Indices of Malnutrition in Chronic Dialysis Patients

1) Biochemical parameters
    - Serum albumin concentrations <4.0 g/dL
    - Serum transferrin concentrations <200 mg/dL
    - Serum IGF-1 concentrations <200 ng/mL
    - Serum prealbumin concentrations <20 mg/dL or an apparent decreasing trend
    - Abnormally low plasma and muscle essential amino acid concentrations
    - Inappropriately low serum creatinine and BUN concentrations
2) Anthropometric measures
    - Continuous decline in body weight or low % ideal body weight (<85%)
    - Abnormal skinfold thickness, midarm muscle circumference and/or muscle strength
3) Body composition analysis
    - Abnormally low % of lean body mass by bioelectrical impedance analysis and/or DEXA
    - Low total body nitrogen and/or nitrogen index (observed nitrogen/predicted nitrogen)
4) Dietary assessment
    - Protein catabolic rate <1.0 g/kg/d
    - Dietary protein intake <1.0 g/kg/d by dietary recall

In addition to serum albumin, BUN and serum creatinine concentrations are also considered simple biochemical markers of nutritional status. BUN is a metabolic end-product of dietary protein intake, and serum creatinine is a reflection of the total body muscle mass. The advantages of these simple markers are that they are easily available and cheap to measure. They also accurately reflect recent protein and calorie intake in most chronic dialysis patients. Finally, both indices are associated with mortality in large surveys in ESRD patients. However, concentrations of both BUN and serum creatinine are altered due to renal failure and are also determined by the dose of dialysis, which makes their interpretation as nutritional indices more complicated. Further, they primarily reflect short-term dietary protein intake.

Estimation of dietary protein intake (DPI) by different methods can also be used as a simple marker of overall nutritional status in the stable ESRD patient. Although dietary recall is a direct and simple measure of DPI, several studies have shown that this method lacks accuracy in estimating the actual intake of patients, even in experimental settings (20). Therefore, other means of measuring DPI, such as protein catabolic rate (PCR) calculations in dialysis patients, have been suggested as useful methods to estimate protein intake (21). However, these indirect estimations of DPI are valid only in stable patients in neutral nitrogen balance, and may easily overestimate the actual intake in catabolic patients where endogenous protein breakdown may lead to a high urea nitrogen appearance. More recently, there has been an active debate whether formulas used to measure PCR are mathematically linked to Kt/V or PCR is an independent nutritional parameter since they both make use of postdialysis BUN values. The lack of correlation between PCR and other nutritional markers such as serum albumin in most but not all studies suggests that the former is likely. Therefore, the indirect estimation of DPI and nutritional status should be evaluated with caution.

Several more complex biochemical markers are also utilized for assessment of nutritional status in ESRD patients. Serum transferrin is a transport protein with a smaller body pool. Its concentrations are affected by dietary protein intake and it has a shorter half-life (8–9 days) compared to serum albumin, which makes it more advantageous as an early indicator of visceral serum protein concentrations. It is readily available in most chronic dialysis units, and serum concentrations below 200 mg/dL have been suggested as an indicator of poor nutrition. However, its concentrations are also affected by iron stores and usually do not correlate with other proteins with shorter half-life (e.g., prealbumin). Since the introduction of erythropoietin for treating anemia of renal disease, the prevalence of iron deficiency may be increased in this patient population, making serum transferrin a less reliable indicator of nutritional status.

Serum prealbumin is a promising nutritional marker due to its short half-life of 1–2 days and measurable response to nutritional supplementation (11,22). It is also a serum transport protein (transports thyroxine and retinol-binding protein) and has a smaller body pool. Its concentrations are closely and rapidly effected by dietary nutrient (especially energy) intake and body protein stores. It has been shown as a powerful predictor of mortality in ESRD patients, and its concentrations correlate well with other nutritional indices (23). However, its main route of excretion is the kidneys, and serum concentrations of prealbumin may be falsely elevated in patients with minimal renal function (e.g., chronic renal failure). While prealbumin concentration is not particularly useful in patients with progressive chronic renal failure, it is probably most useful in chronic dialysis patients with stable, albeit markedly reduced renal function. For the same reason, the lower threshold of prealbumin that is associated with nutritional depletion has not been identified in ESRD patients. Nevertheless, an apparent decline in both transferrin and/or prealbumin concentrations should suggest inadequate nutrient intake.

Serum concentration of IGF-1 has also been suggested as a nutritional marker in ESRD patients, due to its nutrient dependency and shorter half-life (12–15 hours) (15,24,25). IGF-1 is a growth factor that is structurally related to insulin and is produced primarily by the liver. It is released constantly, and 95% is bound to binding proteins. Therefore, daily variations in its concentration are small. Indeed, multiple studies have shown that IGF-1 concentrations are more informative than the traditional markers such as serum albumin and transferrin, showed a better correlation with simultaneously evaluated body composition measurements, and reflected the changes in dietary protein and calorie intake more precisely. Since serum IGF-1 concentration is significantly influenced by dietary protein and energy intake, it is reasonable to expect relatively rapid changes in serum IGF-1 concentrations with changes in nutrient intake. Several recent reports suggest that IGF-1 is also a reliable nutritional marker in renal failure patients. As is the case for serum prealbumin, the concentration of IGF-1 at which malnutrition is significant is not established in chronic renal failure patients. Our current experience is that serum IGF-1 concentrations below 200 ng/mL are usually associated with other signs of poor nutrition. Most recent data have also suggested that longitudinal changes in serum IGF-1 concentrations can prospectively predict the changes in other nutritional parameters, specifically serum albumin concentrations in chronic dialysis patients (26). However, it should also be kept in mind that its concentrations are altered due to renal failure and liver disease and are dependent on binding proteins and growth hormone. Finally, its diagnostic accuracy as well as its association with outcome in ESRD patients is not fully validated in large-scale studies.

B. Body Composition Analysis

In addition to serum protein concentrations, analysis of body composition is another important tool for assessment of nutritional status in ESRD patients. A list of these methods with their relationship to malnutrition is depicted in Table 2. The simplest, but unfortunately the least reliable, technique uses anthropometric studies. This relatively easy but largely subjective test is a readily available method that may be tried as a confirmatory analysis in any patient with suspected protein-energy malnutrition. However, there are more reliable and accurate methods of body composition analysis, such as prompt neutron activation analysis which measures total body nitrogen content, and dual-energy x-ray absorptiometry (DEXA), which is also reported to be useful in ESRD patients (27). These measurements require expensive equipment and are only available in specialized centers, and their validity must be confirmed with further studies. A promising method of nutritional assessment is bioelectrical impedance analysis (BIA), which has been proposed as an accurate and reproducible measure of body composition in various patient populations including ESRD patients (28). Although this method provides a good correlation of total body water and lean body mass in normal subjects, the variation in ESRD patients may be large. This is partly because BIA does not detect acute changes in body composition. Therefore, for consistency and accuracy it is suggested that the measurements be done predialysis or 30 minutes postdialysis in hemodialysis (HD) patients. Several other issues that have not been clarified are the validity of the results in moderately or severely malnourished ESRD patients and its usefulness in prospective studies. Finally, body composition can also be estimated by creatinine kinetics, which correlates well with other lean body mass measurements.

Subjective global assessment is a recently proposed method to evaluate the nutritional status of chronic dialysis patients (29). It was originally designed for general surgery patients but is being utilized for renal failure patients also. Its advantage is that it includes objective data (disease state, weight changes), several manifestations of poor nutritional status, and the clinical judgment of the involved physician. Its limitations are the reliance on clinical judgment and the inability to tailor a specific nutritional intervention. Its use as a standard nutritional tool is yet to be determined.

In summary, an optimal assessment of malnutrition should rely on multiple indices of nutritional status simultaneously. These indices have several advantages as well as disadvantages, as listed in Table 3. In order to maximize the accuracy of the nutritional assessment, the methods should comprise several biochemical measures such as a combination of serum albumin, transferrin, or prealbumin as well as an analysis of body composition using either BIA or DEXA, if available. Subjective global assessment can also be utilized in combination with these methods. Multiple markers used in this manner can simultaneously reflect both somatic tissue status from body composition analysis and visceral protein status from serum proteins.

III. EXTENT OF MALNUTRITION IN ESRD PATIENTS

Virtually every study that has evaluated the nutritional status of ESRD patients has reported some degree of malnutrition in this population. The prevalence of malnutrition has been estimated to range from approximately 20 to 50% in different ESRD patient populations using the above-mentioned parameters. Lowrie and Lew reported serum albumin concentrations of less than 3.7 g/dL in 25% of their patient population, which included more than 12,000 HD patients (7). Similar findings with regard to serum albumin are found in a recent report by the Health Care Financing Administration (30). In an analysis of all networks in the United States, 53% of the chronic hemodialysis patients are reported to have a serum albumin concentration between 3.5 and 3.9 g/dL and 22% of the patients had a serum albumin concentration of 3.4 g/dL and below. An analysis of the National Cooperative Dialysis Study (NCDS) patient population revealed insufficient dietary protein and energy intake in a notable proportion of patients (approximately 23%), as well as reductions in body fat and muscle stores in up to 40% of the study population (20). Several smaller studies have shown evidence of malnutrition ranging between 45 and 60% of their patient populations using either a single or combined indices of malnutrition (10,12,31,32).

Analysis of body composition with different techniques has also shown evidence of malnutrition in chronic dialysis patients (33,34). In fact, Rayner et al. reported that body protein depletion was detected in up to 26% of their patients who were considered to be nutritionally normal by other indices of nutrition (35). Another recent report by Pollock et al. (36) suggested that 76% of their chronic dialysis patient population had a nitrogen index lower than the predicted value (observed nitrogen/predicted normal nitrogen) when analyzed with prompt neutron activation analysis, which measures total body nitrogen.

Malnutrition appears to be even more prevalent in CAPD patients. A recent multicenter international study reported severe to moderate malnutrition in 40% of the CAPD patients as evaluated by subjective nutritional assessment (29). Several studies have confirmed the high prevalence of poor nutritional status in this patient population (32,37,38). Cianciaruso et al. reported the extent of malnutrition in CAPD patients (42.3%) to be higher than in their CHD population (30.8%) (39).

IV. FACTORS AFFECTING THE NUTRITIONAL STATUS OF ESRD PATIENTS

Considering the magnitude of the problem, one can predict that multiple factors play important roles in the evolution of malnutrition in ESRD patients (Fig. 1). Many of these factors act simultaneously in the progression from suboptimal nutrition to apparent malnutrition. A list of these factors is shown in Table 4. When considering these factors, it is also important to remem-

Table 3 Advantages and Disadvantages of Nutritional Indices

Advantages	Disadvantages
Biochemical parameters	
Serum albumin	
Easy to measure Good predictor of outcome	Negative acute phase reactant Long (20 days) half-life
Serum transferrin	
Readily available	Dependent on iron stores Negative acute phase reactant Half-life of 8–9 days
Serum prealbumin	
Good predictor of outcome Good response to nutritional support	Excreted by the kidney and falsely elevated in renal failure Negative acute phase reactant
Serum IGF-1	
Good association with other markers Short half-life	Not readily available for clinical use Not validated in large scale studies
Body Composition Techniques	
Anthropometric measures	
Useful if followed longer time	Crude marker Operator dependent Large variations in measurements
Bioelectrical impedance analysis	
Easy to measure Good predictor of outcome	Affected by fluid status Not clinically validated in large studies
DEXA	
Good association with other methods	Affected by fluid status Expensive Not readily available Operator dependent
Dietary assessment	
Protein catabolic rate	Related to short-term dietary intake Not well established association with other nutritional markers
Dietary Recall	Unreliable
Subjective Global Assessment	
Includes objective data (disease state, weight changes)	Heavy reliance on the clinical judgment Inability to tailor a specific nutritional intervention

ber the fact that the basic nutritional requirements are substantially altered in chronic dialysis patients.

A. Protein Requirements

In general, the "minimal" daily protein requirement is one that maintains a neutral nitrogen balance and prevents malnutrition; this has been estimated to be a daily protein intake of approximately 0.6 g/kg in healthy individuals, with a "safe level" of protein intake equivalent to the minimal requirement plus 2 "standard deviations," or approximately 0.75 g/kg/d (40,41). This suggested intake of protein for normal individuals does not necessarily apply to ESRD patients, who may require higher levels due to concurrent abnormalities. Indeed, it has been shown that for chronic dialysis patients a protein intake of 1.4 g/kg/d is needed to maintain a positive or neutral nitrogen balance during nondialysis days, and even this intake may not be adequate for dialysis days (42). There are very few other studies that have systematically evaluated the actual protein requirements of dialysis patients (43). Nevertheless, a minimum of 1.2 g/kg/d is suggested as safe level of dietary protein intake for both chronic hemo- and peritoneal dialysis patients based on several metabolic balance studies (44). These suggested levels of

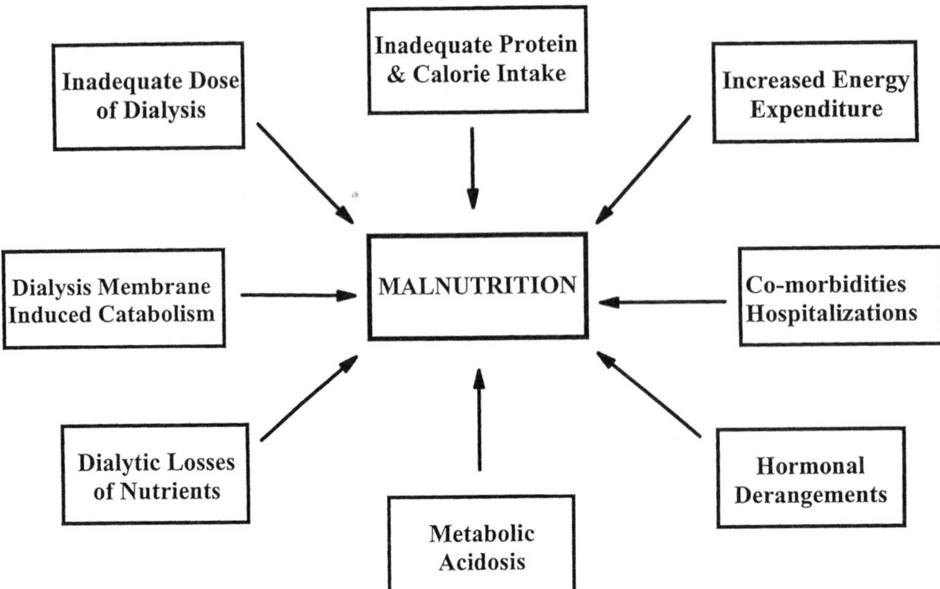

Fig. 1 Factors causing malnutrition in chronic dialysis patients.

DPI are clearly much higher (almost twofold) than the normal population, and there are a number of identified factors that actually increase the requirement of protein intake in dialysis patients.

B. Energy Requirements

The minimum energy requirements of chronic dialysis patients are less well defined. This requirement is dependent on the resting energy expenditure (REE), the activity level of the patient, and other ongoing illnesses. Several earlier studies on this issue reported that REE was not different between normal healthy controls and chronic renal failure patients either prior to or after initiation of RRT (45–47). However, more recent studies have reported that REE is actually higher in CHD patients, especially after adjusting REE for fat-free mass where the majority of energy expenditure occurs, even on nondialysis days, compared to age-, sex-, and body mass index–matched normal controls (48). Interestingly, this higher level of REE was further increased during the hemodialysis procedure when nutrient losses and catabolism are at maximum. This increase in REE during nondialysis periods as well as hemodialysis may comprise an additional increase of 10–20% of REE compared to normal individuals. However, the cause of this increased REE in CHD patients is not well defined.

Although there are not many earlier studies with regard to the resting energy expenditure in PD patients, a recent study conducted in one of our laboratories indicated that REE of PD patients is also comparably increased as in CHD patients (49). The same study also showed that the REE of CRF patients who are not undergoing dialysis was actually lower than predicted. This finding suggests that the uremic milieu induced by end-stage renal disease rather than the dialysis modality is responsible for abnormally increased REE in chronic dialysis patients.

Table 4 Factors Associated with the Nutritional Status of Chronic Dialysis Patients

Increased protein and energy requirements
Losses of nutrients (amino acids and/or proteins)
Increased resting energy expenditure
Decreased protein and calorie intake
Frequent hospitalizations
Inadequate dialysis dose
Co-morbidities (Diabetes mellitus, GI diseases, ongoing inflammatory response)
Medications
Increased Catabolism/Decreased Anabolism
Dialysis induced catabolism
Bioincompatible hemodialysis membranes
Amino acid abnormalities
Metabolic acidosis
Hormonal derangements
Hyperparathyroidism
Insulin and growth hormone resistance

With the available information, a minimum energy intake of 30–35 kcal/kg/d is usually suggested for chronic dialysis patients. This energy intake is for stable patients, and at the time of concurrent illnesses, especially if they require hospitalizations, this intake may be increased.

C. Nutrient Losses

Hemodialysis has long been considered a catabolic process, and inevitable losses of nutrients during HD is an important component of dialysis-related catabolism. Early studies by Kopple et al. and Wolfson et al. documented a loss of 5–8 g of free amino acids during each hemodialysis session using low-flux dialyzers (50,51). With the use of larger-pore membranes, the so-called high-flux membranes, these losses further increase by 30% compared to low-flux membranes due to the larger surface area of the membranes and the higher blood flows used (52). Simultaneous changes in plasma amino acid concentrations suggested that these patients catabolized approximately 25–30 g of body protein to compensate for these losses.

Losses of proteins and amino acids into the dialysate fluid have long been identified as a catabolic factor in PD patients. Several studies have reported a loss of 5.5–11.8 g of proteins into the dialysate daily (53). A large amount of these losses consists of albumin, along with immunoglobulins as well as amino acids. Free amino acid losses have been estimated to be in the range of 1.7–3.4 g per day according to different studies (54). Most importantly, during episodes of peritonitis, these losses of proteins and amino acids increase substantially (53). The generally lower serum albumin concentrations, as well as several abnormalities in plasma amino acid profiles seen in PD patients, are presumed to be a result of these inevitable losses. Nevertheless, the continuous unavoidable loss of nutrients repetitively predisposes the chronic dialysis patients to negative nitrogen balance, especially in the presence of inadequate intake.

Conversely, the amount of energy intake, at least indirectly, is relatively higher in PD patients due to the absorption of glucose from the dialysate fluid. This absorption usually provides energy in the range of 5–20 kcal/kg/d in many patients and is possibly the explanation for the relatively lower resting energy expenditure levels observed in some studies (55). Unfortunately, this absorption of glucose may also predispose these patients to further anorexia due to the development of satiety, in addition to the feeling of fullness related to the fluid in the peritoneal cavity. The extensive presence of protein malnutrition in these patients, in spite of this increased energy consumption, is probably related to their inadequate intake of dietary protein since protein intake affects nitrogen balance more profoundly than does overall energy intake (56).

D. Decreased Dietary Nutrient Intake

One of the most significant clinical indicators of advanced uremia is an apparent decrease in appetite. Although not studied in detail, it has been generally thought that anorexia worsens as the renal failure progress. Even though there has been a clear association between decreased dietary protein intake (DPI) and outcome in chronic dialysis patient, the mechanism by which this apparent decline in DPI occurs is not clear-cut. In a recent report it was suggested that accumulation of a low molecular weight (<5 kDa) substance isolated from uremic plasma ultrafiltrate and normal urine may be a potential marker of this decreased food intake in uremia, since it induces a dose-dependent suppression of appetite after injection into otherwise normal rats (57).

Decreased dietary nutrient intake may also be related to factors other than accumulation of toxins. Indeed, in a recent report, it was suggested that the actual daily protein and energy intake of CHD patients admitted to a regular ward is at perilously low levels (0.55 ± 0.33 g/kg/d) and that simultaneous calculations of PCR by urea kinetics revealed a negative nitrogen balance in 80% of these hospitalized patients (58). Serum albumin concentrations showed a significant decrease with hospitalizations in the same patients. Therefore, frequent hospital admissions may also be an insidious and important cause of poor dietary intake in chronic dialysis patients (59).

E. Dose of Dialysis

One of the most important factors that affects the nutritional status of dialysis patients is the dose of dialysis. The results of the NCDS, where an association between lower protein intake and higher time-averaged urea concentrations was observed, suggested a relationship between underdialysis and anorexia (20). More recently, Lindsay and Spanner have hypothesized that PCR is dependent on the type and the dose of dialysis (60). In a study of 55 HD patients, they were able to show a significant linear relationship between Kt/V and PCR. Moreover, the attempts to increase DPI of these patients by dietary counseling were unsuccessful unless the dose of dialysis was first increased. Of note, their data further suggested that the type of dialysis membrane used also affected the nature of the relationship between the dose of dialysis and PCR. Specifically, lower dialysis doses were needed to obtain a specific PCR when a biocompatible membrane was used in comparison to a cellulosic membrane. Bergstrom and Lindholm have also reported a significant linear relationship between Kt/V and PCR, all consistent with anorexia related to underdialysis (61). However, these retrospective and/or cross-sectional studies did not definitively show a cause-and-effect relationship between dose of dialysis and nutrition.

In a further study of their patient population, Lindsay and coworkers prospectively analyzed the effects of increasing the dialysis dose in a group of patients with PCR values of <1 g/kg/d (62). Their results showed that PCR increased significantly in the group of patients whose Kt/V values were increased, whereas there was no change in PCR values in the group of patients whose Kt/V values remained the same. In studies by Acchiardo et al. and Burrowes et al. significant increases in serum albumin concentrations were demonstrated in chronic HD patients when their dose of dialysis was increased to adequate levels (63,64). In the study by Burrowes and coworkers (64), a significant increase in serum albumin levels was observed in a cohort of chronic HD patients when they were dialyzed adequately. Serum albumin levels increased from 3.13 ± 0.24 to 3.51 ± 0.41 g/dL (p <0.001) in 30 newly initiated HD patients when they were dialyzed with a Kt/V of 1.37 ± 0.17. Similar increases were seen in patients who were transferred from other units and in patients who received intradialytic parenteral nutrition. Likewise, Acchiardo and coworkers (63) also reported increase in serum albumin (3.2 ± 0.1 to 3.8 ± 0.1 g/dL) in conjunction with a decrease in mortality (12%) when the dialysis dose is increased in 416 patients (1.09 ± 0.1 to 1.44 ± 0.3). Recently, Hakim et al. performed a prospective 4-year study in which the dose of dialysis was increased intentionally to 1.33 (measured by delivered Kt/V) in 130 CHD patients (65). They observed that when the nutritional parameters of patients with yearly average double-pool Kt/V values below 0.86 and above 1.21 were identified, statistically significant differences were found between serum albumin, transferrin, and PCR measurements.

It has been suggested that the relationship between dose of dialysis and nutrition, as measured by Kt/V and PCR, respectively, is actually a mathematical artifact and not a metabolic response reflecting better nutrition. In this respect, in a recent large cross-sectional study by Owen et al., no statistically significant relationship between serum albumin and dose of dialysis was seen (6). Thus, the question of whether the decreased PCR truly reflects a deterioration of nutritional status of these patients has become a subject of debate that has not yet been resolved. Nevertheless, the changes in PCR and serum albumin concentrations over time are probably not artifactual.

Similar conclusions with regard to the dose of dialysis are reported in CAPD patients in several studies. Lindsay et al. have hypothesized the same association between dose of dialysis and dietary protein intake in CAPD patients (62). Bergstrom and Lindholm have also reported similar findings with regard to their dialysis patients, with the additional observation that CAPD patients required a lower dialysis dose as compared to HD patients to achieve a given dietary protein intake (61). They have postulated that better removal of middle molecules, which are thought to be the causal factor in the anorexia associated with uremia, is the explanation for this relationship.

An important report on this issue is the cross-sectional analysis of an international study on the nutritional status of CAPD patients. In this study, a higher incidence of malnutrition was observed in patients who were treated with CAPD for longer than 3 months compared to patients who were treated less than 3 months, suggesting that as residual renal function decreases (a major contributor to total clearance in PD patients), indices of malnutrition become more evident (29). Keshaviah also suggested that as residual renal function declines in CAPD patients, PCR also decreases (66). Lameire et al. and Teehan et al. reported higher survival rates and better nutritional markers with higher Kt/V (67,68). Although several etiological factors have been postulated, it is not yet well established by which mechanisms underdialysis causes decreased protein and calorie intake.

Most recently, the results of the CANUSA study were published and suggested a positive relationship between adequacy of dialysis and nutritional status in CAPD patients (69). It was reported that decreasing serum albumin concentrations and worsening nutrition according to subjective global assessment were predictive of worsening mortality and increasing hospitalizations. A further analysis of the data showed that the estimates of adequacy of dialysis and nutritional status are positively correlated in these patients (70). Importantly, an improvement in the nutritional parameters was observed within the first 6 months of initiation of peritoneal dialysis, whereas during the remainder of the study (months 6–18), when there was a decrease in residual renal function, these parameters actually worsened. Although not conclusive, this information supports the critical role of residual renal function on multiple outcome measures in peritoneal dialysis patients.

All the available evidence in ESRD patients therefore confirm the close association between dialysis dose and nutrition. It is important to note, however, that the specific level of optimal dose of dialysis, after which no further improvement in nutritional status is observed, has not yet been established. Several prospective studies are underway to evaluate this question.

Specific co-morbid conditions can also facilitate the development of malnutrition in chronic dialysis patients. Patients with renal failure secondary to diabetes mellitus, which is the leading cause of ESRD in United States, have a higher incidence of malnutrition as compared to patients who are not diabetic. The etiology of this observation is probably multifactorial. Diabetic patients are likely to be more prone to malnutrition because of associated gastrointestinal symptoms such as gastroparesis, nausea and vomiting, bacterial overgrowth in the gut, pancreatic insufficiency, as well as high occurrence of nephrotic syndrome and related complications (24).

Depression, which is commonly seen in ESRD patients, is also associated with anorexia. In addition, chronic renal failure patients are usually prescribed a large number of medications, particularly sedatives, phosphate binders, and iron supplements, which are also associated with gastrointestinal complications. Finally, the socioeconomic status of the patients, their lack of mobility, as well as their age are other predisposing factors in the development of malnutrition in ESRD patients.

F. Biocompatibility

Another well-defined—at least experimentally—cause of inappropriate protein catabolism in dialysis patients is the contact between blood and foreign material during hemodialysis, i.e., the effects of bioincompatibility (71). It is now well established that the type of dialysis membrane used affects the protein metabolism in CHD patients. In studies by Gutierrez et al. (72) and Ikizler et al. (52), bioincompatible membranes that vigorously activate the complement system also induce net protein catabolism as compared to dialysis membranes, which do not activate this inflammatory response. Although both membranes induce net protein catabolism due to amino acid losses observed during hemodialysis, this catabolism is more intense with bioincompatible membranes (52) and can be observed even at 6 hours after initiation of dialysis in normal subjects (73). Using leucine turnover studies, Lim et al. were unable to show any adverse effects of dialysis with bioincompatible membranes on protein metabolism in CHD patients (74). However, their study did not evaluate protein metabolism in the period following the termination of dialysis when an increase in amino acid flux was demonstrated in normal subjects (73).

The effect of hemodialysis membranes on nutritional aspects of CHD patients was further supported clinically by Lindsay and Spanner (60). These investigators established a link between PCR, a putative marker of DPI in stable CHD patients, with the modality and the dose of dialysis. They further suggested that at a given dialysis dose, patients dialyzed with a biocompatible dialysis membrane had a higher PCR compared to patients dialyzed with a bioincompatible membrane.

The mechanism by which the biocompatibility and activation of the complement pathway enhances protein catabolism is not clear. Production of cytokines, such as interleukin-1 (IL-1) and tumor necrosis factor-alpha (TNF-α), may induce muscle protein degradation and excess amino acid release (75,76). In studies by Gutierrez et al. (72), the release of amino acids during dialysis with bioincompatible membranes was most prominent at 6 hours after the initiation of hemodialysis, a time period consistent with activation of monocytes and subsequent release of cytokines followed by their action on muscle cells (77). Complement activation has been shown to result in increased transcription of TNF-α, and in a recent study by Canivet and coworkers increased serum TNF-α concentrations were reported in CHD patients dialyzed with a complement-activating membrane (78).

Several experimental and cross-sectional studies have highlighted the catabolic and anorectic effects of bioincompatible membranes (72,79). However, it is still not clearly established whether long-term use of biocompatible membranes per se can improve the nutritional markers in CHD patients. In fact, the first evidence that supports the argument that biocompatible hemodialysis membranes favorably impact on the nutritional status of CHD patients was recently reported by our laboratory (26). In a prospective randomized study of 159 new hemodialysis patients randomized to either a low-flux biocompatible membrane or a low-flux bioincompatible membrane, we measured the effects of biocompatibility on several nutritional parameters, including estimated dry weight, serum albumin, and IGF-1 over 18 months. Our results showed that the biocompatible group had a mean increase in their dry weight of 4.36 ± 8.57 kg at the end of the study, whereas no change in mean weight was observed in the bioincompatible group. In addition, the biocompatible group had an earlier (6 months vs. 12 months) and more marked increase in serum albumin concentrations compared to the bioincompatible group, as well as consistently higher IGF-1 values. In fact, recent reports from the USRDS have suggested that use of bioincompatible membranes are associated with increased risk of death in comparison to biocompatible membranes (80). Whether altered nutritional status plays a role in this process is not clear. However, a recent analysis of cause of death in these two groups of patients dialyzed with biocompatible versus bioincompatible membranes highlighted the significant increase of infection-related deaths in the bioincompatible group (81). It is possible that poor nutritional status may increase the prevalence of infectious episodes in patients dialyzed with bioincompatible membranes and eventually increase the risk of death. Nevertheless, further studies are required to evaluate the cause-and-effect relationship between these factors.

V. AMINO ACID ABNORMALITIES IN CHRONIC DIALYSIS PATIENTS

Chronic dialysis patients have well-defined abnormalities in their plasma and, to a lesser extent, in their muscle amino acid profiles. Commonly, essential amino acid (EAA) concentrations are low and nonessential amino acid concentrations (NEAA) are high. The etiology of this abnormal profile is multifactorial. The progressive loss of renal tissue where metabolism of several amino acids takes place is an important factor that alters the plasma concentrations. Specifically, glycine and phenylalanine concentrations are elevated and serine and tyrosine concentrations are decreased. Since histidine concentrations are also decreased due to decreased synthesis, histidine is considered to be an EAA in renal failure patients. Plasma and muscle concentrations of branched-chain amino acids (BCAAs)—valine, leucine, and isoleucine—are reduced in chronic dialysis patients. Among BCAAs, valine displays the greatest reduction. In contrast, plasma citrulline, cystine, aspartate, methionine, and both 1- and 3-methylhistidine levels are increased.

The overall decrease in EAA concentrations suggests that protein malnutrition is an additional factor in abnormal amino acid profiles. However, certain abnormalities occur even in the presence of adequate dietary nutrient intake indicating that uremic milieu or other conditions have an additional effect on amino acid profiles. Indeed, it has been suggested that metabolic acidosis, which is commonly seen in uremic patients, plays an important role in increased oxidation of BCAAs. Further, there is a direct relationship between predialysis plasma bicarbonate concentrations and intracellular valine concentrations. Although there are no specific interventions other than adequate dietary nutrient intake for correction of abnormal amino acid profiles, treatment of metabolic acidosis may be a potential maneuver to improve at least BCAA concentrations.

VI. METABOLIC AND HORMONAL DERANGEMENTS

Multiple metabolic and hormonal abnormalities related to the loss of renal tissue as well as renal function become apparent in chronic dialysis patients. Metabolic acidosis, which commonly accompanies progressive renal failure, also promotes malnutrition by increased protein catabolism. Detailed experimental in vitro and animal model studies suggest that muscle proteolysis is stimulated by an ATP-dependent pathway involving ubiquitin and proteasomes during metabolic acidosis (82,83). It has been reported that metabolic acidosis lasting 7 days induced with high doses of NH_4Cl (4.2 mmol/kg) significantly reduced albumin synthesis and induced negative nitrogen balance in otherwise healthy subjects (84). It has also been shown that correction of metabolic acidosis actually improves muscle protein turnover in a small number of CHD and/or CAPD patients (85,86). Two recent studies in CHD and PD patients also showed improvements in antrophometric measurements and body weight (87,88). However, several other cross-sectional as well as prospective studies showed no difference in nutritional parameters, most importantly in serum albumin, in chronic dialysis patients (89,90). Therefore, although the evidence suggests that correction of metabolic acidosis may be nutritionally beneficial in chronic dialysis patients, large-scale studies are still warranted in this respect.

Several hormonal derangements including insulin resistance, increased glucagon concentrations, and secondary hyperparathyroidism are also implicated as factors in the development of malnutrition in chronic renal failure (83,91). A postreceptor defect in insulin responsiveness of tissues is the most likely cause of insulin resistance and associated glucose intolerance in uremia (92). However, it is not clear to what extent this defect affects protein metabolism in CRF. It has also been suggested that hyperparathyroidism usually seen in chronic renal failure is, at least in part, responsible for this decreased tissue responsiveness to insulin via in-

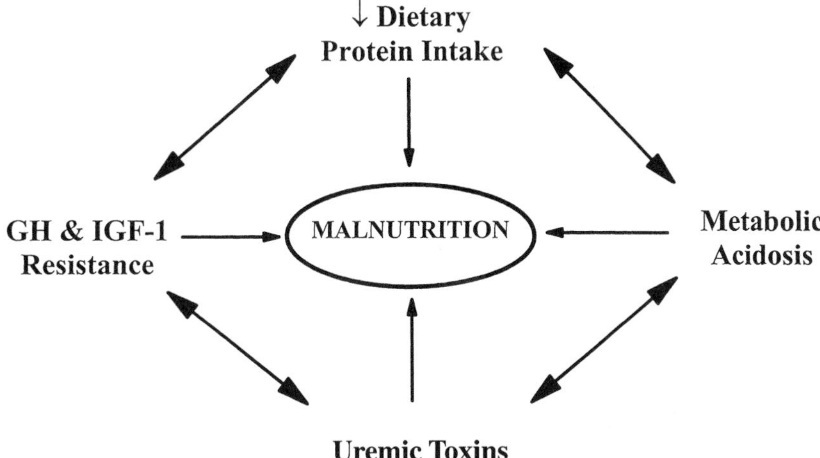

Fig. 2 Potential relationship between malnutrition, uremic toxins, decreased dietary protein intake, and hormonal and metabolic derangements in chronic dialysis patients. GH: growth hormone; IGF-1: insulin-like growth factor 1.

hibition of insulin secretion by pancreatic β cells (91,93). Increased concentrations of parathyroid hormone have also been implicated as a catabolic factor that promotes protein metabolism in uremia by enhancing amino acid release from muscle tissue (94). Finally, there are several abnormalities in thyroid hormone profiles of uremic patients, characterized by low thyroxine and triiodothyronine concentrations (95). These changes resemble the changes seen in prolonged malnutrition in other patient populations (96), and it has been suggested that the thyroid hormone profile of malnutrition (97) and possibly of renal failure is a maladaptative response to decreased energy intake in an effort to preserve overall energy balance.

More recently, abnormalities in growth hormone and IGF-1 axis have been suggested as an important factor in the development of malnutrition in uremic patients (98). Growth hormone is the major promoter of growth in children and exerts several anabolic actions in adults, such as enhancement of protein synthesis, increased fat mobilization and increased gluconeogenesis, with IGF-1 as the major mediator of these actions (99–101). Although plasma concentrations of growth hormone actually increase during the progression of renal failure, probably due to its reduced clearance, recent evidence suggests that uremia per se is associated with the development of resistance to growth hormone action at cellular levels (102). In experimental settings, uremia is characterized by reduced hepatic growth hormone receptor mRNA as well as hepatic IGF-1 mRNA expression (103,104). This blunted response would be expected to attenuate the anabolic actions of these hormones. Interestingly, these abnormalities can also be observed with decreased food intake, as well as in experimental metabolic acidosis (105). Clinically, metabolic acidosis and decreased dietary protein and energy intake are also associated with decreased IGF-1, although it is not clear which is the primary response and which is the secondary effect (84,106,107). Thus, the current evidence suggests an interesting, as yet ill-defined interrelationship between these hormonal, metabolic, and nutritional factors, which are involved in the evolution of malnutrition in chronic dialysis patients (Fig. 2). With this information, use of anabolic growth factors such as recombinant growth hormone and recombinant human insulin-like growth factor 1 at pharmacological doses have been proposed as potential interventions for treatment of chronic dialysis patients who are already malnourished in spite of prevention strategies (see below).

VII. THE EFFECT OF MALNUTRITION OF MORBIDITY AND MORTALITY

A number of studies have documented the increased mortality and morbidity in ESRD patients suffering from malnutrition (8,24). This direct relationship between poor nutrition and outcome is also observed in patient populations other than ESRD, particularly in acutely ill and elderly patients (16,18,108). A recent study by Herrmann and colleagues (14) of more than 15,000 hospitalized patients suggested that serum albumin concentrations on admission strongly predicted death, length of stay, and readmission. Specifically, patients with serum albumin less than 3.4 g/dL on admission had 10% higher in-hospital mortality as compared to patients with serum albumin higher than 3.5 g/dL.

It is interesting to note that in the ESRD patient, malnutrition is rarely documented as a cause of death. Nevertheless, there is a body of evidence to suggest that the nutritional status of ESRD patients plays a major role in the outcome of these patients. In fact, the first apparent indication of suboptimal nutrition and related poor outcome in ESRD patients came from the analysis of the NCDS results. In this well-known comprehensive study of 262 CHD patients divided into four groups, the patient group with the lowest PCR, which presumably reflects the DPI in stable CHD patients, had the highest treatment failure and dropout rate (5). In addition, this group of patients had the highest death rate following the termination of the study. This observation was later confirmed in a study by Acchiardo et al., who suggested that CHD patients with a PCR below 0.63 g/kg/d had a higher mortality and hospitalization rate compared to patients with PCR above 0.93 g/kg/d (109).

The most comprehensive study on this issue was reported by Lowrie and Lew (7). In their cross-sectional analysis of more than 12,000 CHD patients, they identified serum albumin concentration as the most powerful indicator of mortality. The risk of death in patients with serum albumin concentration below 2.5 g/dL was close to 20-fold compared to patients with serum albumin of 4.0–4.5 g/dL, which is considered to be the reference range. When compared to this reference range, even serum albumin values of 3.5–4.0 g/dL resulted in a 2-fold increase in the relative risk of death. It is important to note that this latter value of albumin is in the range of "normal" for many laboratories. Therefore, a small difference in serum albumin concentrations, even when it is in the "normal" range, may adversely affect the relative mortality risk in CHD patients. In addition to serum albumin, Lowrie and Lew were able to define a close relationship between mortality and other biochemical markers of nutrition. Specifically, low BUN and serum cholesterol concentrations, indicators of low protein and energy intake, as well as low serum creatinine, an indicator of decreased muscle mass, were also associated with increased risk of death in this patient population. In a recent report, they also included anion gap and percent of ideal body weights of these patients as other significant predictors of death and suggested that four out of the six most significant predictors of death in CHD patients, namely serum creatinine, albumin, anion gap, and percent ideal body weight, were nutritional factors (110). These observations by Lowrie and Lew were later confirmed by many other studies in multiple patient populations and have highlighted the association of serum albumin with morbidity and mortality (6,111–113).

Several nutritional parameters other than serum albumin have also been associated with increased risk of death, including serum transferrin, prealbumin, and IGF-1, as well as total lymphocyte counts and abnormal plasma amino acid profiles (7,16,114–116). However, most of these studies were performed in smaller study populations, and their validity, or relationship to serum albumin, remains to be determined.

Similar observations can be made in CAPD patients. Several studies reported that serum albumin was the best predictor of death and a strong predictor of hospitalization days (68,117,118). Most recently, Lowrie et al. reported their findings for death risk predictors among 1522 peritoneal dialysis patients (119). In this regard, it is important to note that the relative risk of death for patients with low serum albumin was the same for CHD and PD patients, suggesting that peritoneal losses of albumin does not mitigate against serum albumin as a prognostic factor of the patient's mortality. Avram et al. reported the independent association of serum albumin, prealbumin, and creatinine with increased risk of death in their patient population who were followed up to 7 years (120). The importance of initial nutritional parameters including serum albumin with regard to subsequent survival were also reported by the large multicenter CANUSA study (69).

VIII. STRATEGIES FOR TREATMENT OF MALNUTRITION IN ESRD PATIENTS

A list of measures to prevent and/or to treat malnutrition in different stages of ESRD is presented in Table 5.

A. Conventional Nutritional Therapy

Considering the catabolic nature associated with chronic dialysis, it is clear that attempts to encourage patients to maintain an adequate protein and calorie intake must be provided to chronic dialysis patients. It is a common experience that most of these patients continue their predialysis diets while on chronic RRT. It is the nephrologist's responsibility to ensure that the dietary protein and calorie intake of these patients fulfill the increased requirements after initiation of dialysis. Repetitive comprehensive dietary counseling by

Table 5 Interventions to Prevent and/or Treat Malnutrition

Nutritional counseling to encourage increased intake
Appropriate amount of dietary protein (>1.2 g/kg/d) and calorie (>30 kcal/kg/d)
Optimal dose of dialysis (Kt/V >1.4 or URR >70%)
Use of biocompatible dialysis membranes
Oral nutritional supplements
Intradialytic parenteral nutritional supplements for hemodialysis patients; amino acid dialysate for peritoneal dialysis patients
Enteral nutritional supplementation (PEG tube)
Growth factors (experimental):
Recombinant human growth hormone
Recombinant human insulin-like growth factor–1

an experienced dietitian is an important factor in improving dietary intake as well as detecting early signs of malnutrition. Similar efforts should be spent not only in outpatient settings, but also during hospitalizations of these patients. Hospitalized patients should be closely followed by experienced renal dietitians during their frequent and at times long hospital admissions, since, as mentioned above, these patients have even lower dietary protein and calorie intake.

Aggressive dietary counseling to improve nutritional status may be unsuccessful in optimizing the dietary intake in some malnourished dialysis patients (121). For these patients other forms of supplementation such as enteral [including oral protein, amino acid tablets and energy supplementation (122–124), nasogastric tubes (91), percutaneous endoscopic gastroscopy or jejunostomy tubes (125)] and intradialytic parenteral nutrition (IDPN)) are suggested. Only a limited number of studies evaluating the effects of enteral supplementation in malnourished ESRD patients are available (123,124,126,127). Furthermore, most of these studies are not controlled and are small in scope, and the degree of success is variable. Therefore, for the nephrologist it is usually a challenge to determine whether an enteral form of supplementation is effective or not and when to try further, relatively expensive measures such as IDPN.

Several recent reports have emphasized the effective use of IDPN as a potential therapeutic intervention in malnourished chronic dialysis patients (128). This mode of treatment has been advocated after a trial of enteral nutritional supplementation. The early studies by Heidland and Kult, as well as several subsequent studies, reported positive effects of intradialytic infusions of nutrients on several nutritional parameters (17,129). In contrast, several other studies were not able to show any benefit of IDPN (130,131). Importantly, all these studies had drawbacks in their designs and patient populations, and therefore no definitive conclusions could be made. Cano et al. reported improvements in multiple nutritional parameters with IDPN in a group of 26 malnourished CHD patients (132). In a retrospective analysis of more than 1500 CHD patients treated with IDPN, Chertow et al. reported a decreasing risk of death with the use of IDPN, particularly in patients with serum albumin concentrations below 3.5 g/dL and serum creatinine concentrations below 8 mg/dL (133). They were able to show substantial improvements in these parameters following use of IDPN. These findings suggested that this mode of treatment is probably most useful in patients with moderate to severe malnutrition.

Studies using amino acid dialysate (AAD) in CAPD patients have also provided conflicting results. In studies that suggested benefit from AAD, serum transferrin and total protein concentrations increased and plasma amino acid profiles tended towards normal with one or two exchanges of AAD (134,135). On the other hand, an increase in BUN concentrations associated with exacerbation of uremic symptoms as well as metabolic acidosis remain as complications of AAD (134–136). Kopple et al. reported significant short-term improvements in nitrogen balance studies as well as serum total protein and transferrin concentrations in 19 malnourished CAPD patients treated with AAD (137). In a study, in abstract form, Jones et al. reported significant improvements in serum albumin and prealbumin concentrations in malnourished CAPD patients, particularly in those who had serum albumin concentrations within the lowest tertile (138). These results are consistent with the reports in CHD patients suggesting that these interventions are probably most useful in patients with severe malnutrition.

In summary, the available evidence suggests that IDPN and AAD may be useful in the treatment of malnourished chronic dialysis patients and offers an alternative method of nutritional intervention in a group of dialysis patients in whom oral or enteral intake cannot be maintained. However, most of the studies evaluating IDPN are retrospective, uncontrolled, and short-term. Furthermore, there is no clear data to prove that aggressive nutritional supplementation through the gastrointestinal tract is actually inferior to parenteral supplementation in dialysis patients. Until a controlled study comparing various forms of nutritional supplementation in similar patient groups is completed, one should be cautious in choosing extremely costly nutritional interventions; thus, there is an urgent need to initiate prospective studies to evaluate the long-term effects of IDPN and compare it to different forms of enteral nutrition.

B. Experimental Nutritional Therapies

As previously mentioned, growth hormone and its major mediator IGF-1 have several anabolic properties. With the availability of recombinant forms of these agents, recombinant human growth hormone (rhGH) has been utilized in multiple patient populations at pharmacological doses to promote net anabolism (101). Consequently, with the recognition of alterations in growth hormone–IGF-1 axis in ESRD patients, rhGH has been proposed as a potential anabolic agent in this patient population (139). Several animal studies have suggested that rhGH induces a net anabolic action in uremic rats and also improves food utilization (140). Furthermore, a preliminary short-term study in CHD patients by Ziegler et al. demonstrated a decrease of predialysis BUN concentrations by approximately 25% and a significant reduction in net urea generation and PCR with rhGH administration (141). In a subsequent study by our laboratory where rhGH was given to seven malnourished HD patients in association with IDPN, the combination of IDPN with rhGH resulted in significant improvements in serum albumin, transferrin, and IGF-1 concentrations (142).

Similar net anabolic actions of rhGH have also been observed in CAPD patients. In a controlled prospective study by Ikizler et al., rhGH treatment was shown to induce a substantial (29%) decrease in net urea generation in 10 CAPD patients (143). Interestingly, these changes were associated with concurrent statistically significant decreases in serum potassium and phosphorus concentrations, as well as an increase in serum creatinine concentrations, suggestive of a net anabolic process in muscle mass. In a subsequent analysis of amino acid (AA) profiles of the same patients, the net anabolic processes induced by rhGH reflected a shift in AA metabolism towards peripheral muscle tissues (54). Other studies in abstract form also suggested consistent results with rhGH administration in CAPD patients (144).

Since IGF-1 is the major mediator of growth hormone action, recombinant human IGF-1 has also been proposed as an anabolic agent. Preliminary nitrogen balance studies in CAPD patients are consistent with this hypothesis, however the side effect profile of this agent, at least as observed in CRF patients, may impede its widespread use at this time (145). Interestingly, the combined utilization of these agents in healthy subjects seems to provide the most efficient anabolic action with the least side effect profile (146). It is yet unknown whether the long-term use of these agents in malnourished CHD and CAPD patients would result in improved nutritional parameter and hence in better outcome. Nevertheless, such studies should be encouraged in these patient populations.

IX. VITAMIN AND TRACE ELEMENT REQUIREMENTS

A. Vitamins

The status of many vitamins is altered in chronic dialysis patients, and both decreased as well as increased concentrations can be found in these patients. A list of vitamins with their relevance to chronic dialysis patients is depicted in Table 6. We will briefly discuss the clinically important vitamins below. Vitamin A concentrations are usually elevated in chronic dialysis patients and even small amounts lead to excessive accumulation. There have been several reports on vitamin A toxicity in chronic dialysis patients and therefore it should not be supplemented in these patients. The vitamin E level in chronic dialysis patients is not well defined, and there have been reports of increased, decreased, and unchanged concentrations. Therefore, it is not clear whether vitamin E supplementation is required in chronic dialysis patients. However, there have not been any studies reporting adverse effects of vitamin E supplementation, with several short-term studies reporting improved lipid peroxidation. Vitamin K supplementation is usually not recommended in chronic dialysis patients unless they are at high risk for developing deficiency such as during prolonged hospitalizations with poor dietary intake. Vitamin D metabolism and renal bone disease are discussed in detail in another section of this book.

The serum concentrations of any of the water-soluble vitamins are reported to be low in chronic dialysis patients mainly due to decreased dietary intakes and increased clearances by diffusion during hemodialysis. The use of daily multivitamin prescriptions that are specifically designed for renal failure patients usually alleviate these low concentrations. Nevertheless, it is important to recognize that the daily requirements of vitamin B_6, folic acid, and ascorbic acid are usually higher in chronic dialysis patients and that their levels may be followed for patients at risk such as ones that require prolonged hospitalizations. Furthermore, the ef-

Table 6 Vitamins and Trace Elements in Chronic Dialysis Patients

Vitamin[a]	Function	Clinical syndrome	Requirements
A[b] (=/↑)	Vision, immune resp.	CNS toxicity, ↑ Ca^{2+}	None
E[b] (=/↑/↓)	Antioxidant	None	Not Clear
K[b] (=/↓)	Coagulation	↑ PT, bleeding	None
B_1 (=)	Coenzyme	Beriberi (rare)	1–5 mg/day[c]
B_2 (=/↑)	Oxidation-reduction	None	1.2–1.7 mg/day[c]
B_6 (=/↓)	Coenzyme	↑ Hyperoxalemia, hyperhomocysteinemia ↓ Decreased immune response	10 mg/day[c]
B_{12} (=)	Myelin synthesis Folic acid metabolism	Pernicious Anemia	2 μg/day[c]
C (=/↓)	Antioxidant Collagen synthesis	↑ Hyperoxalemia ↓ Scurvy	60 mg/day[c]
Folic acid (=/↓)	DNA synthesis	Anemia (macrocytic)	1–5 mg/day
Niacin (=/↑)	Enzymatic reactions	Pellegra	13–19 mg/day[c]
Biotin (=/↑)	CO_2 carrier, coenzyme	Depression, dermatitis, muscle pain	30–100 μg/day[c]
Pentothenic acid (=/↓)	Synthesis of fatty acids, cholesterol, amino acids	Retarded growth (animals), fatigue	4–7 mg/day[c]

Trace element	Normal serum levels[a]	Possible toxic effects[d]
Aluminum	1.0–6.0 μg/L (↑)	↑ Encephalopathy, osteomalacia
Arsenic	0.09–5.49 μg/L (↑)	↑ Cancer, anemia
Cadmium	<0.20 μg/L (↑)	↑ Cancer, osteomalacia
Cobalt	0.04–0.40 μg/L (↑)	↑ Heart failure
Copper	0.98–1.07 μg/L (=/↑)	↑ Fever, myocardial infarction ↓ Pancytopenia, ischemic Herat disease
Iron	0.79–1.63 mg/L (↑)	↑ Hepatotoxicity, cardiac ischemia ↓ Anemia
Mercury	0.55–2.10 μg/L (↑)	↑ Hypertension
Selenium	0.081–0.185 mg/L (=/↓)	↓ Cardiomyopathy, cancer, anemia, immune dysfunction
Zinc	0.69–1.21 mg/L (↓)	↓ Sexual dysfunction, decreased taste and smell acuity

[a]Arrows in parenthesis indicate the levels reported in chronic dialysis patients.
[b]Lipid soluble.
[c]RDA recommendation.
[d]Arrows indicate levels associated with toxicity/deficiency.

fects of high-flux and high-efficiency dialyzers on water-soluble vitamins are not clearly defined.

B. Trace Elements

The concentrations of most of the trace elements are mainly dependent on the degree of renal failure. Although there is an extensive list of trace elements that may have altered concentrations in body fluids in chronic dialysis patients, only a few of these compounds are thought to be important in this patient population. Mostly the serum concentrations of trace elements are increased with the exception of selenium and zinc. A list of trace elements with their relevance to chronic dialysis patients is depicted in Table 6. We will briefly discuss the clinically important trace elements below.

Serum aluminum concentration is an important consideration in chronic dialysis patients since elevated levels have been shown to be associated with *dialysis dementia* as well as aluminum-related bone disease. The first reports on aluminum intoxication were recognized in CHD patients who were dialyzed with untreated water sources. These untreated water resources usually occur in areas where soil is rich in minerals and/or in industrial areas where environmental precautions are not employed vigorously. This scenario is mostly eliminated in developed countries, but the risk still continues in many developing countries. Another source of aluminum is the use of phosphate binders that contain aluminum hydroxide. In chronic dialysis patients with poor control of phosphate intake, prolonged use may be a risk for aluminum intoxication, therefore these patients' aluminum concentrations should be monitored carefully and frequently. A serum aluminum concentration below 40 μg/L is the desired level in chronic dialysis patients. Finally, concomitant use of aluminum-containing phosphate binders and citrate-containing preparations is contraindicated since citrate increases aluminum absorption and predisposes that patient to acute aluminum intoxication.

Selenium deficiency has been associated with cardiovascular disease through increased peroxidative damage to the cells. Decreased concentrations of selenium have also been observed in chronic dialysis patients probably secondary to inadequate dietary intake. However, whether selenium supplementation to correct concentrations would be beneficial is not well defined. Similarly, low concentrations of zinc have been reported in chronic dialysis patients. Zinc deficiency is associated with impotence and anorexia. However, the beneficial effects of supplemental zinc therapy have not been confirmed in dialysis patients.

Other metabolic complications seen in renal failure such as lipid disturbances, vitamin D metabolism, and disorders in carnitine homeostasis are discussed in detail in other chapters in this book.

ACKNOWLEDGMENTS

This work is partly supported by NIH Grant No. DK-45604–06 and FDA Grant No. FD-R-000943–04.

REFERENCES

1. United States Renal Data System. Excerpts from United States Renal Data System 1995 Annual Data Report. Am J Kidney Dis 1995; 26(suppl 2):S69–S84.
2. Fenton S, Desmeules M, Copleston P, Arbus G, Froment D, Jeffery J, Kjellstrand C. Renal replacement therapy in Canada: a report from the Canadian Organ Replacement Register. Am J Kidney Dis 1995; 25: 134–150.
3. Teraoka S, Toma H, Nihei H, Ota K, Babazono T, Ishikawa I, Shinoda A, Maeda K, Koshikawa S, Takahashi T, et al. Current status of renal replacement therapy in Japan. Am J Kidney Dis 1995; 25:151–164.
4. Mallick NP, Jones E, Selwood N. The European (European Dialysis and Transplantation Association-European Renal Association) Registry. Am J Kidney Dis 1995; 25:176–187.
5. Parker TFI, Laird NM, Lowrie EG. Comparison of the study groups in the national cooperative dialysis study and a description of morbidity, mortality, and patient withdrawal. Kidney Int 1983; 23(suppl 13):S42–S49.
6. Owen WF Jr, Lew NL, Liu Y, Lowrie EG, Lazarus JM. The urea reduction ratio and serum albumin concentrations as predictors of mortality in patients undergoing hemodialysis. N Engl J Med 1993; 329: 1001–1006.
7. Lowrie EG, Lew NL. Death risk in hemodialysis patients: the predictive value of commonly measured variables and an evaluation of death rate differences between facilities. Am J Kidney Dis 1990; 15:458–482.
8. Kopple JD. Effect of nutrition on morbidity and mortality in maintenance dialysis patients. Am J Kidney Dis 1994; 24:1002–1009.
9. Blumenkrantz MJ, Kopple JD, Gutman RA, Chan YK, Barbour GL, Roberts C, Shen FH, Gandhi VC, Tucker CT, Curtis FK, Coburn JW. Methods for assessing nutritional status of patients with renal failure. Am J Clin Nutr 1980; 33:1567–1585.
10. Young GA, Swanepoel CR, Croft MR, Hobson SM, Parsons FM. Anthropometry and plasma valine, amino acids, and proteins in the nutritional assessment of hemodialysis patients. Kidney Int 1982; 21:492–499.
11. Cano N, Feinandez JP, Lacombe P, Lankester M, Pascal S, Defayolle M, Labastie J, Saingra S. Statistical selection of nutritional parameters in hemodialysis patients. Kidney Int 1987; 32(suppl 22):S178–S180.
12. Jacob V, Carpentier JEL, Salzano S, Naylor V, Wild G, Brown CB, El Nahas AM. IGF-1, a marker of undernutrition in hemodialysis patients. Am J Clin Nutr 1990; 52:39–44.
13. Anderson CF, Wochos DN. The utility of serum albumin values in the nutritional assessment of hospitalizede patients. Mayo Clin Proc 1982; 57:181–184.
14. Herrmann FR, Safran C, Levkoff SE, Minaker KL. Serum albumin level on admission as a predictor of death, length of stay, and readmission. Arch Intern Med 1992; 152:125–130.
15. Sullivan DH, Carter WJ. Insulin-like growth factor I as an indicator of protein-energy undernutrition among metabolically stable hospitalized elderly. J Am Coll Nutr 1995; 13:184–191.
16. Verdery RB, Goldberg AP. Hypocholesterolemia as a predictor of death: a prospective study of 224 nursing home residents. J Gerontol 1994; 46:M84–90.
17. Guarnieri G, Faccini L, Lipartiti T, Raniew F, Spangaro F, Guintrni D, Toigo G, Dewdi F, Berguier-Vldali F, Raimondi A. Simple methods for nutritional assessment in hemodialyzed patients. Am J Clin Nutr 1980; 33:1598–1607.
18. Law MR, Morris JK, Wald NJ, Hale AK. Serum albumin and mortality in the BUPA study. British United

Provident Association. Int J Epidemiol 1994; 23: 38–41.
19. O'Keefe SJ, Dicker J. Is plasma albumin concentration useful in the assessment of nutritional status of hospital patients? Eur J Clin Nutr 1988; 42:41–45.
20. Schoenfeld PY, Henry PR, Laird NM, Roxe DM. Assessment of nutritional status of the National Cooperative Dialysis Study population. Kidney Int 1983; 23:80–88.
21. Hakim RM, Lazarus JM. Initiation of dialysis. J Am Soc Nephrol 1995; 6:1319–1328.
22. Waterlow JC. Metabolic changes. In: Waterlow JC, ed. Protein-Energy Malnutrition. London: Edward Arnold, 1992:83.
23. Avram MM, Goldwasser P, Erroa M, Fein PA. Predictors of survival in continuous ambulatory peritoneal dialysis patients: the importance of prealbumin and other nutritional and metabolic markers. Am J Kidney Dis 1994; 23:91–98.
24. Hakim RM, Levin N. Malnutrition in hemodialysis patients. Am J Kidney Dis 1993; 21:125–137.
25. Sanaka T, Shinobe M, Ando M, Hizuka N, Kawaguchi H, Nihei H. IGF-I as an early indicator of malnutrition in patients with end-stage renal disease. Nephron 1994; 67:73–81.
26. Parker TF III, Wingard RL, Husni L, Ikizler TA, Parker RA, Hakim RM. Effect of the membrane biocompatibility on nutritional parameters in chronic hemodialysis patients. Kidney Int 1996; 49:551–556.
27. Ikizler TA, Hakim RM. Nutrition in end-stage renal disease. Kidney Int 1996; 50:343–357.
28. Chertow GM, Lowrie EG, Wilmore DW, Gonzales J, Lew NL, Ling J, Leboff MS, Gottlieb MN, Huang W, Zebrowski B, College J, Lazarus JM. Nutritional assessment with bioelectrical impedance analysis in maintenance hemodialysis patients. J Am Soc Nephrol 1995; 6:75–81.
29. Young GA, Kopple JD, Lindholm B, Vonesh EF, Devecchi A, Scalamogna A, Castelnova C, Oreopoulos DG, Anderson GH, Bergstrom J, Dichiro J, Gentile D, Nissenson A, Sakhrani L, Brownjohn AM, Nolph KD, Prowant BF, Algrim CE, Martis L, Serkes KD. Nutritional assessment of continuous ambulatory peritoneal dialysis patients: an international study. Am J Kidney Dis 1991; 17:462–471.
30. Health Care Financing Administration. Opportunities to improve care for adult in-center hemodialysis patients. 1994.
31. Thunberg BJ, Swamy A, Cestera RVM. Cross-sectional and longitudinal measurements in maintenance hemodialysis patients. Am J Clin Nutr 1981; 34:2005–2009.
32. Marckmann P. Nutritional status and mortality of patients in regular dialysis therapy. J Intern Med 1989; 226:429–432.
33. Biasioli S, Petrosino Z, Cavalli L, Zambello A, Cesaro A, Fazion S. Bioelectrical impedance for the assessment of body composition of dialyzed patients [letter]. Clin Nephrol 1989; 31:274–275.
34. Stenver DI, Gotfredsen A, Hilsted J, Nielsen B. Body composition in hemodialysis patients measured by dual-energy x-ray absorptiometry. Am J Nephrol 1995; 15:105–110.
35. Rayner HC, Stroud DB, Salamon KM, Strauss BJ, Thomson NM, Atkins RC, Wahlqvist ML. Anthropometry underestimates body protein depletion in haemodialysis patients. Nephron 1991; 59:33–40.
36. Pollock CA, Ibels LS, Ayass W, Caterson RJ, Waugh DA, Macadam C, Pennock Y, Mahony JF. Total body nitrogen as a prognostic marker in maintenance dialysis. J Am Soc Nephrol 1995; 6:82–88.
37. Heimburger O, Bergstrom J, Lindholm B. Maintenance of optimal nutrition in CAPD. Kidney Int 1994; 46(suppl 48): S39–S46.
38. Lindholm B, Alvestrand A, Furst P, Bergstrom J. Plasma and muscle free amino acids during continuous ambulatory peritoneal dialysis. Kidney Int 1989; 35:1219–1226.
39. Cianciaruso B, Brunori G, Kopple JD, Traverso G, Panarello G, Enia G, Strippoli P, De Vecchi A, Querques M, Viglino G, Vonesh E, Maiorca R. Cross-sectional comparison of malnutrition in continuous ambulatory peritoneal dialysis and hemodialysis patients. Am J Kidney Dis 1995; 26:475–486.
40. Maroni BJ. Nutritional requirements of normal subjects and patients with renal insufficiency. In: Jacobson HR, Striker GE, Klahr S, eds. The Principles and Practice of Nephrology. Philadelphia: BC Decker, 1991:708.
41. Young VR. Nutritional requirements of normal adults. In: Mitch WE, Klahr S, eds. Nutrition and the Kidney. Boston: Little, Brown and Company, 1993:1.
42. Borah MF, Schoenfeld PY, Gotch FA, Sargent JA, Wolfson M, Humphreys MH. Nitrogen balance during intermittent dialysis therapy of uremia. Kidney Int 1978; 14:491–500.
43. Bergstrom J, Furst P, Alvestrand A, Lindholm B. Protein and energy intake, nitrogen balance and nitrogen losses in patients treated with continuous ambulatory peritoneal dialysis. Kidney Int 1993; 44:1048–1057.
44. Blumenkrantz MJ, Kopple JD, Moran JK, Coburn JW. Metabolic balance studies and dietary protein requirements in patients undergoing continuous ambulatory peritoneal dialysis. Kidney Int 1982; 21:849–861.
45. Schneeweiss B, Graninger W, Stokenhuber F, Druml W, Ferenci P, Eichinger S, Grimm G, Laggner AN, Lenz K. Energy metabolism in acute and chronic renal failure. Am J Clin Nutr 1990; 52:596–601.
46. Monteon FJ, Laidlaw SA, Shaib JK, Kopple JD. Energy expenditure in patients with chronic renal failure. Kidney Int 1986; 30:741–747.
47. Olevitch LR, Bowers BM, Deoreo PB. Measurement of resting energy expenditure via indirect calorimetry

among adult hemodialysis patients. J Renal Nutr 1994; 4:192–197.

48. Ikizler TA, Wingard RL, Sun M, Harvell J, Parker RA, Hakim RM. Increased energy expenditure in hemodialysis patients. J Am Soc Nephrol 1996; 7:2646–2653.
49. Neyra RN, Chen K, Sun M, Shyr Y, Hakim RM, Ikizler TA. Resting energy expenditure and energy balance in chronic renal failure, peritoneal dialysis and hemodialysis patients (abstr). J Am Soc Nephrol 1997; 8:223A.
50. Kopple JD, Swendseid ME, Shinaberger JH, Umezawa CY. The free and bound amino acids removed by hemodialysis. Trans Am Soc Artif Int Organs 1973; 19:309–313.
51. Wolfson M, Jones MR, Kopple JD. Amino acid losses during hemodialysis with infusion of amino acids and glucose. Kidney Int 1982; 21:500–506.
52. Ikizler TA, Flakoll PJ, Parker RA, Hakim RM. Amino acid and albumin losses during hemodialysis. Kidney Int 1994; 46:830–837.
53. Kopple JD, Hirschberg R. Nutrition and peritoneal dialysis. In: Mitch WE, Klahr S, eds. Nutrition and the Kidney. Boston: Little, Brown and Company, 1993: 290.
54. Ikizler TA, Wingard RL, Flakoll PJ, Schulman G, Parker RA, Hakim RM. Effects of recombinant human growth hormone on plasma and dialysate amino acid profiles in CAPD patients. Kidney Int 1996; 50:229–234.
55. Lindholm B, Bergstrom J. Nutritional management of patients undergoing peritoneal dialysis. In: Nolph KD, ed. Peritoneal Dialysis. Dordrecht: Kluwer Academic Publishers, 1989:230.
56. Bursztein S, Elwyn DH, Askanazi J, Kinney JM, Kvetan V, Rothkopf MM, Weissman C. Nitrogen balance. In: Bursztein S, Elwyn DH, Askanazi J, Kinney JM, eds. Energy Metabolism, Indirect Calorimetry, and Nutrition. Williams and Wilkens, 1989:85.
57. Anderstam B, Mamoun AH, Sodersten P, Bergstrom J. Middle-sized molecule fractions isolated from uremic ultrafiltrate and normal urine inhibit ingestive behavior in the rat. J Am Soc Nephrol 1996; 7:2453–2460.
58. Ikizler TA, Greene JH, Wingard RL, Hakim RM. Nitrogen balance in hospitalized chronic hemodialysis patients. Kidney Int 1996; 50(suppl 57):S53–S56.
59. Sanders HN, Narvarte J, Bittle PA, Ramirez G. Hospitalized dialysis patients have lower nutrient intakes on renal diet than on regular diet. J Am Dietet Assoc 1991; 91:1278–1280.
60. Lindsay RM, Spanner E. A hypothesis: the protein catabolic rate is dependent upon the type and amount of treatment in dialyzed uremic patients. Am J Kidney Dis 1989; 132:382–389.
61. Bergstrom J, Lindholm B. Nutrition and adequacy of dialysis. How do hemodialysis and CAPD compare? Kidney Int 1993; 43(suppl 40):539–550.
62. Lindsay R, Spanner E, Heidenheim P, Lefebure J, Hodsman A, Baird J, Allison M. Which comes first, Kt/V or PCR—chicken or egg? Kidney Int 1992; 42(suppl 38):S32–S37.
63. Acchiardo SR, Moore L, Smith SO, Burk LB, Smith SJ, Will K. Increased dialysis prescription improved nutrition (abstr). J Am Soc Nephrol 1995; 6:571.
64. Burrowes DD, Lyons TA, Kaufman AM, Levin NW. Improvement in serum albumin with adequate hemodialysis. J Renal Nutr 1993; 3:171–176.
65. Hakim RM, Breyer J, Ismail N, Schulman G. Effects of dose of dialysis on morbidity and mortality. Am J Kidney Dis 1994; 23:661–669.
66. Keshaviah P. Urea kinetic and middle molecule approaches to assessing the adequacy of hemodialysis and CAPD. Kidney Int 1993; 43(suppl 40):S28–S38.
67. Lameire NH, Vanholder R, Veyt D, Lambert M, Ringoir S. A longitudinal, five year survey of kinetic parameters in CAPD patients. Kidney Int 1992; 42:426–432.
68. Teehan BP, Schleifer CR, Brown JM, Sigler MG, Raimondo J. Urea kinetic analysis and clinical outcome on CAPD. A five year longitudinal study. Adv Perit Dial 1990; 6:181–185.
69. Canada-USA (CANUSA) Peritoneal Dialysis Study Group. Adequacy of dialysis and nutrition in continuous peritoneal dialysis: association with clinical outcomes. J Am Soc Nephrol 1996; 7:198–207.
70. Churchill DN. Adequacy of peritoneal dialysis: How much dialysis do we need? Kidney Int 1997; 48:S2–S6.
71. Hakim RM. Clinical implications of hemodialysis membrane biocompatibility. Kidney Int 1993; 44:484–494.
72. Gutierrez A, Alvestrand A, Wahren J, Bergstrom J. Effect of in vivo contact between blood and dialysis membranes on protein catabolism in humans. Kidney Int 1990; 38:487–494.
73. Gutierrez A, Bergstrom J, Alvestrand A. Protein catabolism in sham-hemodialysis: the effect of different membranes. Clin Nephrol 1992; 38:20–29.
74. Lim VS, Bier DM, Flanigan MJ, Sum-Ping ST. The effect of hemodialysis on protein metabolism: a leucine kinetic study. J Clin Invest 1993; 91:2429–2436.
75. Flores EA, Bistrian BA, Pomposelli JJ, Dinarello CA, Blackburn GL, Istfan NW. Infusion of tumor necrosis factor/cachectin promoted catabolism in the rat. J Clin Invest 1989; 83:1614–1622.
76. Himmelfarb J, Hakim RM. Biocompatibility and risk of infection in hemodialysis patients. Nephrol Dial Transplant 1994; 9:138–144.
77. Himmelfarb J, Lazarus JM, Hakim RM. Reactive oxygen species production by monocytes and polymor-

phonuclear leukocytes during dialysis. Am J Kidney Dis 1991; 17:271–276.

78. Canivet E, Lavaud S, Wong T, Guenounou M, Willemin JC, Potron G, Chanard J. Cuprophane but not synthetic membrane induces in serum tumor necrosis factor-alpha levels during hemodialysis. Am J Kidney Dis 1994; 23:41–46.
79. Lindsay RM, Spanner E, Heidenheim P, Kortas C, Blake PG. PCR, Kt/V, and membrane. Kidney Int 1993; 43(suppl 41):S268–S273.
80. Hakim RM, Held PJ, Stannard DC, Wolfe RA, Port FK, Daugirdas JT, Agodoa L. Effects of the dialysis membrane on mortality of chronic hemodialysis patientss. Kidney Int 1994; 50:566–570.
81. Bloembergen WE, Port FK, Hakim RM, Stannard D, Wolfe RA, Agodoa LYC, Held PJ. The relationship of dialysis membrane and cause-specific mortality in chronic hemodialysis patients (abstr) Kidney Int 1996; 50:557–565.
82. May RC, Kelly RA, Mitch WE. Mechanisms for defects in muscle protein metabolism in rats with chronic uremia: the influence of metabolic acidosis. J Clin Invest 1987; 79:1099–1103.
83. Mitch WE, Walser M. Nutritional therapy of the uremic patient. In: Brenner BM, Rector FC, eds. The Kidney. Philadelphia: Saunders, 1991:2186.
84. Ballmer PE, McNurlan MA, Hulter HN, Anderson SE, Garlick PJ, Krapf R. Chronic metabolic acidosis decreases albumin synthesis and induces negative nitrogen balance in humans. J Clin Invest 1995; 95:39–45.
85. Graham KA, Reaich D, Channon SM, Downie S, Gilmour E, Passlick-Deetjen J, Goodship TH. Correction of acidosis in CAPD decreases whole body protein degradation. Kidney Int 1996; 49:1396–1400.
86. Graham KA, Reaich D, Channon SM, Downie S, Goodship THJ. Correction of acidosis in hemodialysis decreases whole body protein degradation. J Am Soc Nephrol 1997; 8:632–637.
87. Williams AJ, Dittmer ID, McArley A, Clarke J. High bicarbonate dialysate in hemodialysis patients: effects on acidosis and nutritional status. Nephrol Dial Transplant 1997; 12:2633–2637.
88. Walls J. Effect of correction of acidosis on nutritional status in dialysis patients. Miner Electrolyte Metal 1997; 23:234–236.
89. Brady JP, Hasbargen JA. Correction of metabolic acidosis and its effect on albumin in chronic hemodialysis patients. Am J Kidney Dis 1998; 31:35–40.
90. Uribarri J. Moderate metabolis acidosis and its effects on nutritional parameters in hemodialysis patients. Clin Nephrol 1997; 48:238–240.
91. Bergstrom J. Nutritional requirements of hemodialysis patients. In: Mitch WE, Klahr S, eds. Nutrition and the Kidney. Boston: Little Brown, 1993:263.
92. Defronzo RA, Alvestrand A, Smith D, Hendler R, Hendler E, Wahren J. Insulin resistance in uremia. J Cin Invest 1981; 67:563–568.
93. Mak RHK, Bettinelli A, Turner C, Haycock GB, Chantler C. The influence of hyperparathyroidism on glucose metabolism in uremia. J Clin Endocrinol Metab 1985; 60:229–233.
94. Garber AJ. Effects of parathyroid hormone on skeletal muscle protein and amino acid metabolism in the rate. J Clin Invest 1983;71:1806–1821.
95. Kaptein EM, Fainstein EI, Massry SG. Thyroid hormone metabolism in renal disease. Contrib Nephrol 1982; 33:122–135.
96. Waterlow JC. Endocrine changes in severe PEM. In: Waterlow JC, ed. Protein-energy Malnutrition. London: Edward Arnold, 1992:112.
97. Waterlow JC. Metabolic adaptation to low intakes of energy and protein. Ann Rev Nutr 1986; 6:495–526.
98. Krieg JRJ, Santos F, Chan JCM. Growth hormone, insulin-like growth factor and the kidney. Kidney Int 1995; 48:321–336.
99. Chwals WJ, Bistrian BR. Role of exogenous growth hormone and insulin-like growth factor 1 in malnutrition and acute metabolic stress. a hypothesis. Crit Care Med 1991; 19:1317–1322.
100. Wilmore DW. Catabolic illness: strategies for enhancing recovery. N Engl J Med 1991; 325:695.
101. Kaplan SL. The newer uses of growth hormone in adults. Advance Int Med 1993; 38:287–301.
102. Veldhuis JD, Johnson ML, Wilkowski MJ, Iranmanesh A, Bolton WK. Neuroendocrinee alterations in the somatotrophic axis in chronic renal failure. Acta Paediatr Scand 1991; 379:12–22.
103. Chan W, Valerie KC, Chan JCM. Expression of insulin-like growth factor-1 in uremic rats. Growth hormone resistance and nutritional intake. Kidney Int 1993; 43:790–795.
104. Tonshoff B, Eden S, Weiser E, Carlsson B, Robinson IC, Blum WF, Mehls O. Reduced hepatic growth hormone (GH) receptor gene expression and increased plasma GH binding protein in exerpimental uremia. Kidney Int 1994; 45:1085–1092.
105. Challa A, Chan W, Krieg RJ, Jr., Thabet MA, Liu F, Hintz RL, Chan JC. Effect of metabolis acidosis on the expression of insulin-like growth factor and growth hormone receptor. Kidney Int 1993; 44:1224–1227.
106. Underwood LE, Clemmons DR, Maes M, D'Ercole AJ, Ketelslegers JM. Regulation of somatomedin-C/insulin-like growth factor I by nutrients. Hormone Research 1986; 24:166–176.
107. Thissen JP, Ketelslegers JM, Underwood LE: Nutritional regulation of the insulin-like growth factors. Endocrinol Rev 1994; 15:80–101.
108. Horber FF, Hoppeler H, Herren D, Claassen H, Howald H, Gerber C, Frey FJ. Altered skeletal muscle ultrastructure in renal transplant patients on prednisone. Kidney Int 1986; 30:411–416.
109. Acchiardo SR, Moore LW, Latour PA. Malnutrition as the main factor in morbidity and mortality of hemo-

dialysis patients. Kidney Int 1983; 24(suppl 16): S199–S203.
110. Lowrie EG, Huang WH, Lew NL, Liu Y. The relative contribution of measured variables to death risk among hemodialysis patients. In: Friedman EA, ed. Death on Hemodialysis. Amsterdam: Kluwer Academic Publishers, 1994:121.
111. Churchill DN, Taylor DW, Cook RJ, et al. Canadian hemodialysis morbidity study. Am J Kidney Dis 1992; 19:214–234.
112. Iseki K, Kawazoe N, Fukiyama K. Serum albumin is a strong predictor of death in chronic dialysis patients. Kidney Int 1993; 44:115–119.
113. Collins AJ, Ma JZ, Umen A, Keshaviah P. Urea index and other predictors of hemodialysis patient survival. Am J Kidney Dis 1993; 23:272–282.
114. Goldwasser P, Michel MA, Collier J, Mittman N, Fein P, Gusik SA, Avran MM. Prealbumin and lipoprotein(a) in hemodialysis: Relationships with patient and vascular access survival. Am J Kidney Dis 1993; 22: 215–225.
115. Goldwasser P, Mittman M, Antignani A, Burrel D, Michel M, Collier T, Avram MM. Predictors of mortality on hemodialysis. J Am Soc Nephrol 1993; 3: 1613–1622.
116. Oksa H, Ahonen K, Pasternack A, Marnela KM. Malnutrition in hemodialysis patients. Scand J Urol Nephrol 1991; 25:157–161.
117. Blake PG, Flowerdew G, Blake RM, Orepoulos DG. Serum albumin in patients on continuous ambulatory peritoneal dialysis: Predictors and correlations with outcomes. J Am Soc Nephrol 1993; 3:1501–1507.
118. Rocco MV, Jordan JR, Burkart JM. The efficacy number as a predictor of morbidity and mortality in peritoneal dialysis patients. J Am Soc Nephrol 1993; 4: 1184–1191.
119. Lowrie EG, Huang WH, Lew NL. Death risk predictors among peritoneal dialysis and hemodialysis patients: a preliminary comparison. Am J Kidney Dis 1995; 26:220–228.
120. Avram MM, Mittman N, Bonomini L, Chattopadhyay J, Fein P. Markers for survival in dialysis: a seven-year prospective study. Am J Kidney Dis 1995; 26: 209–219.
121. Compher C, Mullen JL, Barker CF. Nutritional support in renal failure. Surg Clin North Am 1991; 71: 597–608.
122. Hecking E, Port FK, Brehm H, Zobel R, Brandl M, Prellwitz W, Opferkuch W, Keim HJ, Kohler H. A controlled study on the value of oral supplementation with essential amino acids and keto analogues in chronic hemodialysis. Proc Dial Transplant Forum 1977; 7:157–161.
123. Hecking E, Kohler H, Zobel R, Lemmel EM, Mader H, Opferkuch W, Prellwitz W, Keim HJ, Muller D. Treatment with essential amino acids in patients on chronic hemodialysis: a double blind cross-over study. Am J Clin Nutr 1978; 31:1821–1826.
124. Tietze IN, Pedersen EB. Effect of fish protein supplementation on aminoacid profile and nutritional status in haemodialysis patients. Nephrol Dial Transplant 1991; 6:948–954.
125. Ponsky JL. Percutaneous endoscopic stomas. Surg Clin North Am 1989; 69:1227–1236.
126. Allman MA, Stewart PM, Tiller DJ, Horvath JS, Duggin GG, Truswell AS. Energy supplementation and the nutritional status of hemodialysis patients. Am J Clin Nutr 1990; 51:558–562.
127. Mastroiacovo P, Pace V, Sagliaschi G. Amino acids for dialysis patients. Clin Ther 1993; 15:698–704.
128. Ikizler TA, Wingard RL, Hakim RM. Interventions to treat malnutrition in dialysis patients: the role of the dose of dialysis, intradialytic parenteral nutrition, and growth hormone. Am J Kidney Dis 1995; 26:256–265.
129. Heidland A, Kult J. Long-term effects of essential amino acids supplementation in patients on regular dialysis treatment. Clin Nephrol 1975; 3:234–239.
130. Foulkes CJ, Goldstein DJ, Kelly MP, Hunt JM. Indications for the use of intradialytic parenteral nutrition in the malnourished hemodialysis patient. Renal Nutr 1991; 1:23–33.
131. Wolfson M. Use of intradialytic parenteral nutrition in hemodialysis patients [editorial; comment]. Am J Kidney Dis 1994; 23:856–858.
132. Cano N, Labastie-Coeyrehourq J, Lacombe P, Stroumza P, Costanzo-Dufetel JD, Durbec J-P, Coudray-Lucas C, Cynober L. Perdialytic parenteral nutrition with lipids and amino acids in malnourished hemodialysis patients. Am J Clin Nutr 1990; 52:726–730.
133. Chertow GM, Ling J, Lew NL, Lazarus JM, Lowrie EG. The association of intradialytic parenteral nutrition with survival in hemodialysis patients. Am J Kidney Dis 1994; 24:912–920.
134. Bruno M, Bagnis C, Marangella M, Rovera L, Cantaluppi A, Linari F. CAPD with an amino acid dialysis solution: a long-term, cross-over study. Kidney Int 1989; 35:1189–1194.
135. Arfeen S, Goodship THJ, Kirkwood A, Ward MK. The nutritional/metabolic and hormonal effects of 8 weeks of continuous ambulatory peritoneal dialysis with a 1% amino acid solution. Clin Nephrol 1990; 33:192–199.
136. Young GA, Dibble JB, Hobson SM, Tompkins L, Gibson J, Turney JH, Brownjohn AM. The use of an amino-acid-based CAPD fluid over 12 weeks. Nephrol Dial Transplant 1989; 4:285–292.
137. Kopple JD, Bernard D, Messana J, Swartz R, Bergstrom J, Lindholm B, Lim V, Brunori G, Leiserowitz M, Bier DM, Stegink LD, Martis L, Boyle CA, Serkes KD, Vonesh E, Jones MR. Treatment of malnourished CAPD patients with an amino acid based dialysate. Kidney Int 1995; 47:1148–1157.

138. Jones MR, Hagen T, Vonesh E, Moran J. Use of a 1.1% amino acid (AA) dialysis solution to treat malnutrition in peritoneal dialysis (PD) patients (abstr). J Am Soc Nephrol 1995; 6:580.
139. Kopple JD. The rationale for the use of growth hormone or insulin-like growth factor-1 in adult patients with renal failure. Min Electrolyte Metab 1992; 18: 269–275.
140. Mehls O, Ritz E, Hunziker EB, Eggli P, Heinrich U, Zapf J. Improvement of growth and food utilization by human recombinant growth hormone in uremia. Kidney Int 1988; 33:45–52.
141. Ziegler TR, Lazarus JM, Young LS, Hakim R, Wilmore DW. Effects of recombinant human growth hormone in adults receiving maintenance hemodialysis. J Am Soc Nephrol 1991; 2:1130–1135.
142. Schulman G, Wingard RL, Hutchinson RL, Lawrence P, Hakim RM. The effects of recombinant human growth hormone and intradialytic parenteral nutrition in malnourished hemodialysis patients. Am J Kidney Dis 1993; 21:527–534.
143. Ikizler TA, Wingard RL, Breyer JA, Schulman G, Parker RA, Hakim RM. Short-term effects of recombinant human growth hormone in CAPD patients. Kidney Int 1994; 46:1178–1183.
144. Kang DH, Lee SW, Kim HS, Choi KH, Lee HY, Han DS. Recombinant human growth hormone (rhGH) improves nutritional status of undernourished adult CAPD patients (abstr). J Am Soc Nephrol 1994; 5: 494.
145. Peng S, Fouque D, Kopple J. Insulin-like growth factor-1 causes anabolism in malnourished CAPD patients (abstr). J Am Soc Nephrol 1993; 4:414.
146. Kupfer SR, Underwood LE, Baxter RC, Clemmons DR. Enhancement of the anabolic effects of growth hormone and insulin-like growth factor I by use of both agents simultaneously. J Clin Invest 1993; 91: 391–396.

23

Nutritional Problems, Including Vitamins and Trace Elements and Continuous Renal Replacement Therapy Treatments

Wilfred Druml
University of Vienna, Vienna, Austria

I. INTRODUCTION

Patients with acute renal failure (ARF) are specifically prone to the development of metabolic problems and complications during nutritional therapy. This fact is due to (a) the complex metabolic alterations associated with renal breakdown and the underlying disease process and (b) the pronounced metabolic impact induced by renal replacement therapies and especially the continuous treatment modalities (continuous renal replacement therapy, or CRRT), which have gained wide acceptance in the therapy of the ARF in many intensive care units (1–3).

Nutritional complications may result from an inappropriate intake of nutrients relative to the ability to metabolize substrates. Patients with ARF not only have an obvious reduction in tolerance to fluids and electrolytes, derangements of fluid, and electrolyte balance, but additionally have specific metabolic alterations associated with acute renal breakdown, which compromise the tolerance to many nutritional substrates. An absolute/relative deficient intake of nutrients can occur due to the omission of substrates that may become conditionally essential during ARF or of nutrients that are lost during renal replacement therapies. On the other hand, an excess of nutrients may result from an absolute increase in the amount given or a relative excess greater than the metabolic capacity.

Because of this increase in the risk of metabolic disturbances during nutritional therapy, patients with ARF require more frequent metabolic monitoring than other patient groups in order to avoid the development of sometimes life-threatening complications. The frequency of testing will be determined by the metabolic stability of the patient and the presence of additional complications/organ dysfunctions besides ARF.

In this chapter information relevant to the understanding of metabolic alterations induced by ARF and/or CRRT and potential problems arising from nutritional interventions is summarized. This knowledge is necessary not only to avoid the development of complications and side effects during nutritional therapy but also to define adapted nutritional regimens in the face of complex metabolic disturbances.

In the first two sections, the metabolic alterations characteristic for ARF and the metabolic impact induced by CRRT are analyzed; in the last section the potential problems and complications occurring during the provision of nutritional substrates are summarized. It must be stressed at this point that ARF is often a complication of sepsis, trauma, or multiple organ failure, therefore it is difficult to ascribe specific metabolic alterations to ARF. Metabolic changes in most patients will be determined by—besides the acutely uremic state—the underlying disease process, by associated complications such as severe infections and additional organ dysfunctions and, last but not least, by the type and intensity of renal replacement therapy.

II. METABOLIC ALTERATIONS IN ACUTE RENAL FAILURE

A. Energy Metabolism

In animal experiments, ARF is associated with decreased oxygen consumption even when hypothermia and acidosis are corrected ("uremic hypometabolism"). In contrast, in the clinical setting oxygen consumption is increased by approximately 20% in ARF (4,5). However, this appears to be mediated by the underlying disease process and not by the acute uremic state. Energy expenditure was increased in septic patients with ARF but was normal in nonseptic subjects (4). Remarkably, in patients with multiple organ failure, oxygen consumption was significantly higher in subjects without impairment of renal function than in those with associated ARF (6).

Taken together these data indicate that a clinically well-controlled uremic state (by hemodialysis or hemofiltration) exerts little if any influence on energy metabolism and, that in contrast to many other acute disease processes, ARF may rather decrease than augment energy expenditure.

B. Amino Acid and Protein Metabolism

A hallmark of metabolic alterations in ARF is excessive protein catabolism and sustained negative nitrogen balance (7,8). Hypercatabolism results in excessive release of amino acids from skeletal muscle, but there is also defective muscular utilization of amino acids for protein synthesis (9). Amino acids are redistributed to the liver: hepatic extraction of amino acids from the circulation, gluconeogenesis (and ureagenesis), and protein synthesis (acute phase protein secretion) are all increased (10). Moreover, amino acid transport across the cell membrane is impaired in ARF (11) (Table 1).

As a consequence of these metabolic alterations, imbalances in amino acid pools in plasma and in the intracellular compartment occur in ARF. A typical plasma amino acid pattern is present and the elimination of amino acids from the intravascular space is altered, which increases the risk of inducing imbalances of plasma amino acids and associated complications during nutritional therapy (12,13).

Endocrine factors (e.g., release of catabolic hormones, hyperparathyroidism), suppression of growth factors, circulating proteases, release of inflammatory mediators (e.g., tumor necrosis factor, interleukins), and catabolism stimulated by renal replacement therapy all can contribute to accelerated protein breakdown in ARF (7,14). A major catabolic factor is insulin resistance, which interrupts the normal control of protein turnover. In muscle, both insulin-mediated stimulation of protein synthesis and inhibition of protein degradation is depressed in ARF. Moreover, metabolic acidosis has been identified as an important factor that stimulates protein breakdown (15). Nitrogen loss in ARF is augmented further by the type and frequency of renal replacement therapy and when stressful factors such as infection, trauma, sepsis, or thermal injury are present. Last but not least, and of major relevance in the clinical

Table 1 Basic Metabolic Alterations in Acute Renal Failure

	Clinical finding	Underlying mechanisms	Proposed causes
Protein and amino acid metabolism	Hypercatabolism Loss of lean body mass	Activation of muscular protein catabolism, depression of muscular protein synthesis, augmentation of hepatic gluconeogenesis/ureagenesis/protein synthesis, altered amino acid transport and metabolism, decreased renal peptide catabolism	Insulin resistance Inflammatory mediators Acidosis Catabolic hormones Growth factor resistance Release of proteases Substrate deficiencies Loss of substrates (dialysis)
Carbohydrate metabolism	Hyperglycemia	Peripheral insulin resistance (postreceptor defect) + augmented hepatic gluconeogenesis	Stress hormones Cytokines (TNFα) Hyperparathyroidism Acidosis
Lipid metabolism	Hypertriglyceridemia	Inhibition of lipolysis increased hepatic triglyceride secretion?	Inhibitor of lipoprotein lipase Cytokines?

Source: Adapted from Ref. 2.

situation, is inadequate nutritional support, which may potentiate loss of lean body mass (16).

Protein and amino acid metabolism in ARF is also affected by impairment of multiple metabolic functions of the kidney itself (17). The loss of kidney function can render several amino acids, such as tyrosine, arginine, serine, and cysteine, indispensable (18,19). In addition, the kidney is an important organ of protein degradation. Multiple peptides are filtered and catabolized at the tubular brush border, and the constituent amino acids are reabsorbed and recycled into the metabolic pool. In renal failure, catabolism of peptides such as peptide hormones but also of those dipeptides, which are increasingly used in nutritional support (tyrosine-containing dipeptides, glutamin-containing dipeptides), is retarded (20). As one consequence, insulin requirements decrease in diabetic patients after development of ARF (21).

C. Carbohydrate Metabolism

ARF is commonly associated with hyperglycemia. The major cause of elevated blood glucose concentrations is periphereal insulin resistance (Table 1). Plasma insulin concentration is elevated, maximal insulin-stimulated glucose uptake by skeletal muscle is decreased by 50%, and muscular glycogen synthesis is impaired (22).

A second feature of glucose metabolism in ARF is accelerated hepatic gluconeogenesis mainly from conversion of amino acids released during protein catabolism. Hepatic extraction of amino acids, their conversion to glucose, and urea production are all increased in ARF (10).

In healthy subjects, hepatic gluconeogenesis from amino acids is readily and completely suppressed by exogenous glucose infusion. In contrast, in acute disease states, such as sepsis but also ARF, hepatic glucose formation can only be decreased but not halted by substrate supply (23,24). This has important implications for nutritional support in ARF patients: Protein catabolism cannot be suppressed by provision of nutritional substrates alone, and thus, for future advances alternative means of preserving lean body mass must be identified.

D. Lipid Metabolism

Profound alterations of lipid metabolism occur in patients with ARF (Table 1). The triglyceride content of plasma lipoproteins, especially very low density lipoproteins (VLDL) and low density lipoproteins (LDL), is increased, while total cholesterol and in particular high density lipoproteins (HDL) are decreased (25). The major cause of lipid abnormalities in ARF is impairment of lipolysis. The activities of both lipolytic systems—peripheral lipoprotein lipase and hepatic triglyceride lipase—are decreased to less than 50% of normal (26). However, oxidation of free fatty acids released from triglycerides is not impaired in patients with ARF (27).

The nutritional consequence of impaired lipolysis in ARF is delayed elimination of intravenously infused lipid emulsions because fat particles of artificial fat emulsions for parenteral nutrition are degraded similarly to endogenous VLDL. Elimination half-life is doubled, and the clearance of conventional fat emulsions is reduced by more than 50% (25). Thus, the risk of inducing hypertriglyceridemia during parenteral nutrition including lipid emulsions is increased in patients with ARF.

III. METABOLIC EFFECTS AND POTENTIAL COMPLICATIONS ON METABOLISM DURING CRRT

A. Heat Loss

Hemofiltration systems without warming equipment for the substitution fluid CRRT induce a heat loss in the patient (Table 2). Depending on the fluid turnover, this can account for as much as 750 kcal/day, which has to be considered in the calculation of energy requirements of the patient. This will usually result in a decrease in body temperature. In several clinical conditions this treatment-induced hypothermia can be a desired effect (such as in hyperpyrectic states or in multiple organ failure associated with cardiovascular instability). The

Table 2 Metabolic Effects of Continuous Renal Replacement Therapies

Renal replacement plus:
Heat loss
Loss of substrates (amino acids, water-soluble vitamins)
Excessive supply of substrates (glucose, lactate)
Elimination of short chain peptides (hormones, mediators)
Adsorption of substances (endotoxin, complement factors)
Induction of an inflammatory reaction
Induction of electrolyte derangements, metabolic alkalosis

reduction of body temperature can reduce oxygen consumption and may also reduce the extent of protein catabolism. Moreover, it has been convincingly shown that a decrease in blood temperature during hemofiltration is a major factor responsible for improvement of cardiovascular stability (28).

Thus, CRRT can contribute to a reduction of oxygen consumption in clinical states associated with hypermetabolism and may help to optimize the relationship between oxygen consumption (fall in VO_2 by reduction of body temperature) and oxygen delivery (DO_2). However, if intravascular volume is depleted by vigorous dehydration (such as was advocated in the treatment of ARDS), continuous hemofiltration can result in a fall in DO_2 and actually may deteriorate the VO_2/DO_2 relationship.

Potentially, the therapy-associated heat loss may also generate untoward effects by blunting the metabolic response to injury and may also impair immunocompetence. Therefore, several modern hemofiltration machines include a heating system that can warm the substitution fluid as required.

B. Glucose Balance

The substitution fluids used in CRRT should contain glucose in a concentration of 100–180 mg/dL in order to maintain a zero glucose balance. The use of glucose-free solutions does not contribute—as sometimes mistakingly assumed—to an improvement in the metabolic control in patients with impaired glucose utilization (such as in most patients with acute disease states). This will simply result in a glucose loss accounting for 40–80 g/day (depending on the filtration volume), which must be compensated for by an activation of endogenous gluconeogenesis, mainly from amino acids (thus promoting protein breakdown). In this case, the glucose loss during the use of glucose-free solutions has to be considered in evaluating the energy balance of the patient and must be replaced by nutritional therapy.

On the other hand, substitution fluid with high glucose concentrations (such as CAPD solutions used for CRRT by some centers) will result in a massive glucose uptake and induce major metabolic disturbances by the high glucose load and should thus no longer be used (29).

C. Lactate and/or Acetate Intake

Most available substitution solutions for CRRT contain lactate as an organic anion. Unfortunately, DL-lactate is still in use in several countries, and this should be replaced by the physiological L-lactate because of potential toxic side effects. Acetate-containing solutions are restricted to special indications; the infusion of large amounts of acetate is associated with well-documented side effects in intensive care patients (e.g., vasodilation, reduction of myocardial contractility, aggravation of cardiovascular instability).

Depending on the filtered volume and the amount of fluid replacement, respectively, the organism is confronted with a potentially relevant if not excessive amount of lactate. This may account for more than 2000 mmol/day and can equal the endogenous lactate formation rate during physiological conditions (~100 mmol/h in healthy subjects).

This lactate load can gain clinical relevance either in disease states in which lactate utilization is impaired (such as in acute or chronic liver failure) or in any clinical condition associated with increased lactate formation (e.g., circulatory instability, septic shock, or hypoxic states). In these situations any CRRT using lactate-containing solutions will increase plasma lactate concentrations, and thus lactate and/or acetate should be replaced by bicarbonate. Bicarbonate-buffered substitution fluids for CRRT have become available in several countries.

Recent evidence suggests that hyperlactemia induced by exogenous lactate infusion may present more than just a changed laboratory value and can assume pathophysiological relevance. Several negative side effects such as an impairment of myocardial contractility, inhibition of endogenous lactate metabolism, and aggravation of insulin resistance have been reported (30,31). Furthermore, it was suggested that lactate-containing substitution fluids may promote protein catabolism (32). The clinically acceptable elevation of blood lactate level during therapy remains to be defined but might range from 3 to 4 mmol/L.

Both lactate and acetate are energy-yielding substrates, which are metabolized in the tricarboxylic acid cycle and generate bicarbonate. Little is known about the impact of these compounds on energy metabolism in the critically ill. The lactate load may correspond to an caloric intake of up to 500 kcal, which should be considered in calculating the energy balance of patients.

D. Electrolyte Disturbances

Most available substitution fluids used in CRRT were originally designed for intermittent hemofiltration in chronic renal failure patients. The use of these solutions can induce pronounced electrolyte disturbances in patients with ARF. Inadequate sodium concentration for replacement of large quantities of plasma water (usually with a higher sodium concentration) will result in a negative sodium balance and hyponatremia in a considerable fraction of patients. Most solutions do not contain phosphate and can aggravate hypophosphatemia, which is frequently present in patients with ARF. Similarily, because these solutions are free of magnesium, a negative balance is induced by CRRT.

E. Loss of Substrates

Water-soluble molecules with low molecular weight and low protein binding, such as amino acids or water-soluble vitamins, are readily filtered, resulting in a considerable loss of several nutritional substrates during CRRT. During postdilutional hemofiltration, this loss is proportional to the filtered volume and the plasma concentration of the substrate and can thus be easily estimated.

In the case of amino acids, this loss accounts for the average amino acid plasma concentration multiplied by the filtered volume (AA loss/day (g) = 0.25 × 1/day). During continuous hemodialysis diffusive clearance of amino acids is also high, and it is more difficult to estimate the actual loss. Depending on filtrate volume/day and/or dialysate flow, amino acid elimination will account for 6–15 g AA per day during CRRT (33,34).

Thus, during CRRT there is an obligatory loss of amino acids, however nutritional therapy including amino acids does not increase this elimination substantially. The endogenous clearance of amino acids is up to 100 times higher than the filtration clearance, and consequently, amino acid infusions using clinically relevant infusion rates (1.0–1.5 g AA/kg/day) have a minimal effect on plasma concentrations and do not augment loss of amino acids (35). However, any exaggerated intake of amino acids (some authors used up to 2.25 g AA/kg/day) will also considerably increase the therapy-induced amino acid elimination (36). The dependence of amino acid losses on plasma concentrations exerts a smoothing effect on the plasma amino acids profile, particularly if unbalanced amino acid solutions are used for nutritional support.

When designing a nutritional program this obligatory loss of substrates must be considered in the estimation of nitrogen requirements. Amino acid supply should be increased by approximately 0.2 g AA/kg/day to compensate for these CRRT-associated losses.

F. Elimination of Peptides

Convective transport during hemofiltration is characterized by a near linear clearance of molecules up to a molecular weight defined by the pore size of the filtration membrane. This "cut-off" of the commonly used filtration membranes ranges between 20 and 40 kDa. Obviously, the convective clearance extends not only to "bad molecules" (mediators), which are implicated in the evolution of several disease states, such as sepsis, ARDS, SIRS and MODS, but also to other short-chain peptides, such as many hormones (37).

For discussion of the pathophysiological relevance of the elimination of a substance by hemofiltration, the endogenous turnover must be taken into account. Even if a compound is filtered with a sieving coefficient of 1.0, the eliminated amount is negligible when the endogenous turnover rate is high (as for most mediators and hormones). For example, extracorporeal extraction rate of catecholamines is high, but this does not affect plasma concentration or the need for exogenous catecholamine infusion, nor does it impair cardiovascular stability (38). Similarily, insulin has excellent filtration properties, but glucose intolerance is not aggravated and insulin requirements are not increased during CRRT.

G. Adsorption of "Mediators" and/or Endotoxin on the Artificial Membrane

The elimination of substances during CRRT is caused not only by filtration/diffusion but also by adsorption of proteins (hormones, interleukins, complements factors, and other potential mediators) and, possibly, also of endotoxins at the membrane (39). A "protein coating" contributes to an improvement of biocompatibility of the membrane. When assessing the clinical relevance of these mechanisms, it must be considered that any potential effect is of limited duration. After saturation of the membrane, adsorption decreases sharply so that certainly after 8 hours of treatment, no further effectivity is to be expected. This indicates that if an adsorptive property of the membrane is a therapeutically desired effect, the filters must be regularly replaced (maximum filter time 12 h ?).

H. Bioincompatibility: Activation of an Inflammatory Reaction

Any extracorporeal circuit induces obligatory phenomena of bioincompatibility by blood membrane interactions (40). The contact of blood with artificial surfaces will induce an activation of several biological cascade systems (e.g., coagulation factors, complement, kinins) and stimulation of cellular factors (platelets, polymorphonuclear cells, monocytes, basophils). For these reasons nonsynthetic, poorly biocompatible membrane materials such as cuprophane should not be used in intensive care patients with ARF (41).

Membranes used in CRRT are composed of synthetic materials characterized by a high biocompatibility. Nevertheless, prolonged and continuous interaction for many days, even weeks, between blood components and the membrane will result in low-grade activation of various biological systems. There are indications that CRRT may cause a chronic inflammatory reaction, but these phenomena have not been systematically investigated during CRRT (42).

IV. NUTRITIONAL PROBLEMS ARISING FROM THE PROVISION OF SUBSTRATES

A. Energy Substrates: Untoward Effects of Hyperalimentation

There is overwhelming evidence that patients with acute disease processes should not receive more calories than can be utilized (i.e. oxidized). Any excess caloric intake must be stored in the body, which essentially means that the substrates provided must be converted to fat (43). This liponeogenesis takes place within hepatocytes, but lipid particles cannot be exported from the liver, resulting in fatty infiltration of the liver.

The side effects and complications associated with calorie overfeeding are manyfold (Table 3). Besides the fatty infiltration of the liver, which can impair hepatic function and can even progress to liver failure, surplus calories increase oxygen consumption as well as body temperature (substrate-induced thermogenesis) and stimulate catecholamine secretion (nutritional stress) (44). Moreover, liponeogenesis is associated with an exaggerated release of carbon dioxide, which may result in respiratory failure in patients with compromised respiratory reserve (45). Calorie overfeeding beyond actual energy requirements impairs survival in animal experiments (46).

It is generally accepted that a normocaloric energy supply should be followed in artificial nutrition, which should be oriented to the actual needs of the patient. Earlier recommendations for provision of as much as 50 kcal/day originate from a time where individual energy requirements were grossly overestimated (47).

Table 3 Side Effects and Complications of Energy Intake Above Requirements

Induction of nutritional stress reaction
Fatty infiltration of the liver
Increase in body temperature
Increase in CO_2 production and respiratory work
Activation of protein breakdown
Decreased survival (animal experiments)

As individual energy expenditure can only rarely be measured directly in the clinical setting (either by indirect calorimetrie or by using a Swan-Ganz catheter), formulas have to be used to estimate individual needs. There is good evidence that energy requirements in an ARF patient with sepsis but also multiple organ dysfunction syndrome rarely exceed 25–30% above basic requirements (4–6). Thus in 90% of the patients an energy supply of 130% of basic energy expenditure (BEE) as estimated by the Harris-Benedict equation will be sufficient.

1. Carbohydrates

Glucose should be used as the main energy substrate because it can be utilized by all organs even under hypoxic conditions. Glucose infusions in patients with ARF, however, are associated with several potential problems. Since ARF impairs glucose tolerance, exogenous insulin is frequently necessary to maintain normoglycemia. One should keep in mind that exogenous insulin does not improve oxidative glucose disposal. Moreover, when glucose intake is increased above 5 g/kg of body weight per day, it will not be used for energy but will promote lipogenesis with fatty infiltration of the liver and excessive carbon dioxide production and hypercapnia (48).

It must be recognized that hyperglycemia is not to be neglected as it is associated with several serious side effects (Table 4), among which are fatty infiltration of the liver, glycation of plasma proteins such as immu-

Table 4 Disadvantages and Complications of Hyperglycemia

Aggravation of tissue injury/tubular dysfunction
Fatty infiltration of the liver
Impairment of immunocompetence
Activation of proteolysis
Stimulation of CO_2 production
Inhibition of gastrointestinal motility

noglobulins, aggravation of tissue injury and tubular dysfunction (49,50). Moreover, hyperglycemia impairs enteral nutrition by inhibition of intestinal motility (51).

The most suitable means of providing the energy requirements in critically ill patients is not glucose or lipids, but glucose *and* lipids. Thirty to 50% of non-protein calories should consist of lipids (52,53). Carbohydrates, including fructose, sorbitol, or xylitol, which are available in some countries, should be avoided because of potential adverse metabolic effects such as an increase in renal oxygen consumption.

2. Lipid Emulsions

Advantages of intravenous lipids include a high specific energy content, a low osmolality, provision of essential fatty acids but also of phospholipids to prevent deficiency syndromes, a lower frequency of hepatic side effects, and reduced carbon dioxide production, especially relevant in patients with respiratory failure. Lipid emulsions provide an excellent nutritional substrate even in critically ill patients with various organ dysfunctions and sepsis. These disease states are associated with both enhanced lipid oxidation and secondary insulin resistance (54). At clinically relevant infusion rates, the elimination of emulsion particles, triglyceride hydrolysis, and oxidation of released free fatty acids is adequate, also in the presence of pulmonary insufficiency, septicemia, hepatic and/or renal failure (54).

The changes in lipid metabolism associated with ARF increase the risk of inducing side effects but nevertheless should not prevent the use of lipid emulsions in these patients. Because of impaired elimination of lipid particles from the blood stream, the amount infused should be adjusted to meet the patient's capacity to utilize lipids. Usually 1 g fat/kg of body weight per day will not substantially increase plasma triglycerides, so that about 20–25% of energy requirements can be met (55).

Lipids should not be administered to patients with hyperlipidemia (plasma triglycerides > 400 mg/dL), activated intravascular coagulation, acidosis (pH < 7.20), impaired circulation, or hypoxemia. Potential side effects occur mainly during excessive infusion rates (short-term infusions of 500 mL 20% lipid emulsions were common practice in the past) and/or impaired clearance from the blood stream. These problems include induction of hyperlipidemia, a lipid overload syndrome, which may be associated with deposits of lipid particles mainly in the pulmonary vasculature, which may aggravate intravascular coagulation activation and, most importantly, affect reticuloendothelial clearance function and thus immunocompetence of the organism. With modern low infusion rates over prolonged periods and if plasma triglycerides levels are maintained below 400 mg/dL, these complications are rarely seen.

Parenteral lipid emulsions usually contain long-chain triglycerides, mostly derived from soybean oil. Recently fat emulsions containing a mixture of long- and medium-chain triglycerides have been introduced for intravenous use. Proposed advantages include faster elimination from the plasma due to a higher affinity for the lipoprotein lipase enzyme, complete, rapid, and carnitine-independent metabolism, and a triglyceride-lowering effect. The use of medium-chain triglycerides does not promote lipolysis, and the elimination of both types of fat emulsions is equally retarded in ARF (26).

B. Amino Acid Solutions and Protein Intake

1. Optimal Nitrogen Intake

The relationship between nitrogen intake and protein catabolism presents a U-shaped curve: an insufficient intake will augment endogenous protein catabolism; conversely, any excessive intake will simply convert surplus amino acids into urea. An optimal intake will combine minimal endogenous protein breakdown and urea production with maximal protein synthesis (24). The optimal intake of protein or amino acids is influenced more by the nature of the illness causing ARF and the extent of protein catabolism and the type and frequency of renal replacement therapy than by renal dysfunction per se.

The few studies that attempted to define the optimal requirements for protein or amino acids in ARF suggest that in nonhypercatabolic patients and in the recovery phase of ARF, a protein intake of about 1.0–1.2 g/kg of body weight per day is required to achieve a positive nitrogen balance (2). There is agreement that in hypercatabolic critically ill patients with ARF on CRRT, nitrogen requirements are higher. In these subjects provision of 1.5 g of amino acids or protein per kg of body weight per day is more effective in reducing nitrogen losses than lower rates of nitrogen intake (56–58).

Again, it must be emphasized that hypercatabolism cannot be overcome by increasing protein or amino acid intake to more than 1.3–1.5 g/kg of body weight per day. Any exaggerated protein intake as high as >2 g kg as recommended in some studies (36), will simply stimulate the formation of urea and other nitrogenous waste products and may aggravate uremic complications. Moreover, this practice will also augment amino acid losses during CRRT.

2. Type of Amino Acid Solutions

Side effects and complications of amino acid/protein intake beyond the absolute amount of nitrogen may be associated with deficiencies or toxic effects of certain amino acids. It may also induce an amino acid imbalance syndrome, which may be associated with various adverse effects on protein metabolism. This spectrum of potentially life-threatening side effects can be demonstrated with solutions of essential amino acids (EAA) only (Table 5). These solutions are suboptimal and can cause serious complications and should not be used in patients with ARF. They are deficient in various amino acids which become conditionally indispensable in patients (e.g., histidine, arginine, tyrosine, serine, cysteine) (1,2,18). Arginine-free amino acid solutions can cause hyperammonemia, acidosis, and coma (59). The content of other amino acids such as methionine and phenylalanine is excessive, with pronounced rises in plasma concentrations during infusion again entailing the potential of inducing toxic effects. Furthermore, the unbalanced composition together with metabolic alterations characteristic for patients with ARF and the required high infusion rates can result in excessive imbalances of plasma amino acid concentrations (1).

Table 5 Side Effects and Complications Associated with Unbalanced/Incomplete Amino Acid Solutions

Amino acid deficiencies: conditionally indispensable (e.g., histidine, arginine, tyrosine, serine, cysteine)
Amino acid toxicities: excessive amino acid content (e.g., methionine)
Amino acid requirements higher than suggested in the past: the required high infusion rates can unmask the unbalanced composition of amino acid solutions
Alterations in amino acid metabolism caused by ARF (and/or hypercatabolism) can result in serious imbalances of plasma amino acid concentrations during infusion
Infusion of more than 0.8 g exclusively essential amino acids/kg/day induces an imbalance syndrome and will simply lead to conversion of infused amino acids to waste products
Use of essential amino acids to synthesize nonessential amino acids has no obvious metabolic advantage and wastes energy
Complete amino acid mixtures adapted to the metabolic alterations in the critically ill patient with ARF may improve plasma amino acid pattern and net nitrogen retention

These data suggest that solutions containing exclusively EAA should no longer be used in critically ill patients with ARF. Mixtures including both EAA, nonessential amino acids (NEAA), and those amino acids that might become conditionally essential in ARF ("nephro" solutions), either in standard or in special proportions, should be preferred for nutritional support in patients with ARF (1,2).

Because of the low water solubility of tyrosine, dipeptides containing tyrosine (such as glycyl-tyrosine) are contained in modern "nephro" solutions as a tyrosine source (19,20). One should be aware of the fact that the amino acid analog *N*-acetyl tyrosine, previously frequently used as tyrosine source, cannot be converted into tyrosine in humans and might even stimulate protein catabolism (19).

Despite considerable investigation, there is not persuasive evidence that amino acid solutions enriched in branched-chain amino acids will exert any clinically significant anticatabolic effect. These solutions entail the risk of inducing an amino acid imbalance syndrome. Studies conduced so far have not demonstrated any advantage for these mixtures regarding nitrogen balance or concentrations of plasma proteins as compared to standard solutions (60).

Glutamine, an amino acid that traditionally was termed nonessential, has been suggested to exert important metabolic functions in regulating nitrogen metabolism and to support immunological functions and preserve gastrointestinal barrier. It may thus become conditionally indispensable in catabolic illness (61). Glutamine supplementation to animals with postischemic ARF decreased survival rate (62). However, this may not reflect the clinical situation where obviously any excess nitrogen will be removed during renal replacement therapy. A recent study suggested that fewer critically ill patients died with ARF when glutamine supplementation was administered (63). Since free glutamine is not stable in aequous solutions, glutamine-containing dipeptides are used as a glutamine source in parenteral nutrition (61). It must be recognized that the utilization of dipeptides is in part dependent on intact renal function and that renal failure may impair hydrolysis (64). Side effects beyond the increased nitrogen load (and rise of plasma ammonia in the presence of hepatic failure) have not been reported during infusions of glutamine-containing dipeptides.

It has been suggested that amino acids infused before or during ischemia or nephrotoxicity may enhance tubular damage and accelerate loss of renal function (65). In part, this "therapeutic paradox" from amino acid alimentation in ARF is related to the increase in metabolic work for transport processes when the oxygen supply is limited, which may aggravate ischemic injury (66). Similar observations have been made with excess glucose infusion during renal ischemia (67). During the insult phase of ARF, the "ebb phase" immediately after trauma, shock, major surgery, etc., any excess nutritional intake should be avoided. Infusion of modern adapted amino acid solution raises plasma amino acids levels marginally, eliminates concentration peaks, and limits the likelihood of these side effects.

Amino acids may also have protective potential. Glycine and, to a lesser degree, alanine limit tubular injury in ischemic and nephrotoxic models of ARF (68). Arginine (possibly by producing nitric oxide) reportedly acts to preserve renal perfusion and tubular function in both nephrotoxic and ischemic models of ARF, whereas inhibitors of nitric oxide synthase exert an opposite effect (69).

Table 6 Causes of Electrolyte Disturbances in Patients with Acute Renal Failure

Hyperkalemia
Decreased renal elimination
Increased release during catabolism:
(2.38 mmol/g N)
(0.36 mmol/g glycogen)
Decreased cellular uptake/increased release:
Uremic intoxication, septicemia
Drugs (ß-blockers, digitalis glycosides, ACE inhibitors)
Metabolic acidosis (0.6 mmol/L rise of K^+/0.1 decrease in pH)
Hyperphosphatemia
Decreased renal elimination
Increased release from bone
Increased release during catabolism
(2 mmol/g N)
Decreased cellular uptake/utilization and/or increased release from cells

C. Electrolytes

Because of the high interindividual differences in and the rapid intraindividual changes of electrolyte requirements during the course of disease, no standardized recommendations can be made for electrolyte supplementation. Electrolyte requirements are highly variable in patients with ARF and must be given as required according to the monitoring of electrolyte balance and plasma concentrations. Certainly, patients with ARF are the group of subjects with the highest risk of developing electrolyte derangements.

1. Potassium

Hyperkalemia is frequently observed in patients with ARF. Elevation of plasma potassium is caused not only by impaired renal excretion of the electrolyte but also by increased cellular release during accelerated protein catabolism and altered distribution between intra- and extracellular spaces (Table 6). Several factors contribute to a decrease of cellular uptake of potassium, e.g., the uremic state per se, acidosis, drugs such as digitalis glycosides or beta-blocking agents. Thus, the potassium tolerance of the organism is impaired and the rise in plasma potassium level is augmented during exogenous infusion. However, with modern infusion therapy and nutritional support, excessive hyperkalemia rarely is seen and in less than 5% of the cases, hyperkalemia presents the major indication for initiation of extracorporeal therapy (70).

It must be noted, however, that many patients with ARF may have a decreased serum potassium concentration on presentation. Infusion of glucose and/or amino acids causes a shift of potassium and phosphate into the cells, and thus nutritional support with low electrolyte contents may induce hypokalemia in a considerable number of patients (70). Potassium depletion may aggravate tissue injury and the severity of metabolic disturbances in ARF (71).

2. Phosphate

Serum phosphate may increase in uremic patients, not only because of impaired renal excretion, but also because of increased release from cells during catabolism, enhanced gastrointestinal adsorption, decreased metabolic utilization, and augmented mobilization from bone (Table 6). Thus, the type of underlying disease and the degree of hypercatabolism will also determine the occurrence and extent of electrolyte abnormalities. Hyperphosphatemia per se may predispose to the development of ARF, and in some cases of tumor lysis syndrome excessive release of phosphate from cells is the leading cause of renal shutdown by intrarenal precipitation of calcium phosphate (72).

However, in ARF decreased plasma phosphate levels are common and, in fact, in 20% of patients may present with hypophosphatemia on admission (70). Furthermore, during the diuretic phase of ARF (especially after renal transplantation), during phosphate-free CRRT, during artificial nutritional support with low phosphate contents, hypophosphatemia may develop in a considerable number of patients during the further course of disease (73). Even if hyperphosphatemia was present on admission, hypophosphatemia developed during phosphate-free nutritional therapy within several days (74). Phosphate depletion increases the risk initiation and maintenance of ARF (75).

If phosphate is added to "all-in-one" solutions, organic phosphates (glycero-phosphate, glucose-1-phosphate) must be used to avoid incompatibilities with other ions in the solution. Divalent ions (calcium, magnesium) can impair the stability of fat emulsions and should be used with caution in lipid-containing nutrition solutions (76).

3. Calcium

The majority of patients with ARF are hypocalcemic usually with a diminution of both protein-bound and ionized fractions. The causes of hypocalcemia are only partially understood, but hypoalbuminemia, hyperphosphatemia, citrate anticoagulation, a reduced formation of 1,25$(OH)_2$ vitamin D_3 with reduced calcium adsorption from the gastrointestinal tract, and potentially skeletal resistance to the calcemic effect of parathyroid hormone all may contribute (77).

If calcium supplements are added to all-in-one solution—similar to phosphate supplementation—organic compounds such as calcium gluconate must be used to avoid precipitation of calcium salts (76).

Hypercalcemia may develop with high dialysate calcium concentrations, immobilization, acidosis, and/or hyperparathyreoidism because parathyroid hormone is also elevated in ARF (78). In ARF caused by rhabdomyolysis, persistent elevations of serum calcitriol may result in a rebound hypercalcemia during the diuretic phase (79). Acute hypercalcemia per se can cause ARF by inducing acute nephrocalcinosis, arterial calcifications, and interstitial nephritis.

4. Magnesium

Elevations of serum magnesium are rarely encountered in patients with ARF. Symptomatic hypermagnesemia may only develop during increased magnesium intake and/or infusion. Hypomagnesemia, on the other hand, may be seen more frequently, such as during use of magnesium-free substitution fluids for hemofiltration, during citrate anticoagulation, in the presence of associated gastrointestinal disorders, and during the diuretic phase of ARF, especially after renal transplantation (80). Moreover, several nephrotoxic drugs such as cisplatin, aminoglycosides, and amphotericin B may cause renal magnesium wasting. In transplant recipients treated with cyclosporine, hypomagnesemia was seen in up to 100% of patients in several case series (81).

D. Micronutrients

1. Vitamins

Serum levels of water-soluble vitamins are decreased in patients on CRRT mainly because of losses induced by renal replacement therapy, but systematic information on vitamin metabolism in ARF is limited (82,83). In addition, nutritional status before hospital admission and the type, severity, and duration of underlying disease determine vitamin body stores.

Depletion of thiamine (vitamin B_1) during CRRT and inadequate exogenous supplementation may result in perturbations in energy metabolism and lactic acidosis (84). A routine supplementation of additional thiamine should be performed in intensive care patients and especially those with liver disease.

On the other hand, the potential of inducing toxic effects during overdosage is low for water-soluble vitamins. An exception is vitamin C, an excess supply of which should be avoided. Ascorbic acid is metabolized via oxalic acid, and any exaggerated intake may induce a secondary oxalosis and initiate or retard resolution of ARF (85).

Fat-soluble vitamins are obviously not eliminated by renal replacement therapy. Nevertheless, with the exception of vitamin K, body stores of these vitamins are depleted in patients with ARF (78). On the other hand, the risk of inducing toxic effects have rarely been reported with the exception of vitamin K and vitamin A.

Activation of vitamin D_3 is—as in chronic renal failure—decreased in patients with ARF. Plasma levels of 25-hydroxyvitamin D and 1,25-dihydroxyvitamin D plasma levels are profoundly depressed (77,78). Whether—as in patients with chronic renal failure—active vitamin D metabolites should be supplemented in patients with ARF remains to be shown.

Vitamin K pools are mostly normal or even elevated in patients with ARF (78). With additional exogenous vitamin K supplementation, toxic effects may occur; high-dose vitamin K administration was implicated as the cause of a prolonged nonoliguric ARF in a renal transplant recipient (86). Vitamin K deficiency is much less frequent and has been mainly reported in patients receiving certain antibiotics that may reduce intestinal vitamin K production. The prolonged plasma half-life of the drug in the presence of the ARF might contribute to vitamin depletion (87).

In experimental ARF (and patients with chronic renal failure), hepatic release of retinol and retinol-binding protein is increased concomitant with the decreased renal breakdown of the transport protein, resulting in elevated vitamin A plasma levels. In contrast, in patients with ARF, associated or not with multiple organ dysfunctions, a severe depression of plasma concentrations of both retinol and the vitamin A precursor β-carotene was seen (78,88).

Similarly (and in contrast to findings in chronic renal failure), plasma and intraerythrocyte concentrations of vitamin E (α-tocopherol) are decreased in patients with both isolated ARF and ARF and associated MODS (78,88).

2. Trace Elements

With supplementation of trace elements, one should keep in mind the possibility of inducing toxic effects because during parenteral administration in ARF, both main regulatory functions in trace element homeostasis —intestinal absorption and renal excretion—are circumvented (89). Moreover, it must be recognized that due to the high protein binding, trace elements losses are negligible during renal replacement therapy and thus CRRT does not increase trace element requirements in critically ill patients (90).

Nevertheless, available information on trace element metabolism in ARF is limited and somewhat contradictory. The cause and stage of underlying disease and type of tissue in which the concentration of an element is measured must be considered in the interpretation of specific findings and, in fact, may be more relevant than the acutely uremic state per se (91).

Many of the reported findings such as decreases in plasma concentrations of iron, zinc, and selenium or increases in copper levels might present unspecific alterations within the spectrum of "acute phase reaction" and do not necessarily reflect disturbances of external trace element balance (deficiency or toxicity states) but may be the consequence of alterations in tissue distribution (92). Geographic and therapeutic factors such as the content of tap water, type of therapy, and especially the highly variable contamination of infusion/dialysis/hemofiltration fluids with trace elements may profoundly affect tract element balance (93).

Selenium concentrations in plasma and erythrocytes have been found to be decreased in patients with chronic as well as acute renal failure (88,90). Selenium deficiency has been implicated in accelerated lipid peroxidation, impaired immune function, and cardiomyopathy. In critically ill patients, selenium administration not only replenished selenium stores and improved various aspects of antioxidative system, but also reduced the development of renal dysfunction and improved prognosis (94). Similarly, it was suggested that zinc requirements may be increased in critically ill patients, particularly in those with gastrointestinal disease (91,92).

Several vitamins and trace elements are components of the nonenzymatic oxygen radical scavenger system. A profoundly reduced antioxidant status has been found in patients with MODS and associated ARF (88). In the rat model of ARF, antioxidant deficiency of the organism (decreased vitamin E and/or selenium status) exacerbates an ischemic renal injury, worsens the course of disease, and increases mortality (95). In turn, administration of antioxidants can attenuate tissue injury in experimental ARF (96). These data support the concept of a crucial role of reactive oxygen species and peroxidation of lipid membrane components in initiating and/or mediating tissue injury.

V. CONCLUSION

Acute renal dysfunction is associated not only with the obvious disturbances of water and electrolyte metabolism and acid base balance but also with a complex pattern of specific alterations of amino acid, carbohydrate, and lipid metabolism. In addition, in the critically ill patient with ARF, the metabolic environment will be determined by the acute disease state per se ("systemic inflammatory response syndrome") and, most importantly, by the underlying disease process and/or associated organ dysfunctions and/or complications, such as severe infections. Moreover, the type and intensity of renal replacement therapy and especially modern CRRT will exert a major impact on nutrient requirements and metabolism. These complex metabolic alterations render patients with ARF with/without CRRT extremely susceptible to development of side effects and complications of nutritional interventions. In any patient with ARF, this broad pattern of metabolic alteration must be taken into account to define an optimal nutritional program, to increase the efficiency of nutritional therapy, to correct existing and avoid the development or aggravation of metabolic disturbances, and to avoid complications during nutrition and renal replacement therapy.

REFERENCES

1. Druml W. Nutritional support in acute renal failure. In: Mitch WE, Klahr S, eds. Nutrition and the Kidney. Boston: Little Brown, 1998: 314–345.

2. Druml W, Mitch WE. Metabolic abnormalities in acute renal failure. Semin Dialysis 1996; 9:484–490.
3. Druml W. Metabolic aspects of continuous renal replacement therapies. Kidney Int 1999; 56(suppl 72): S56–S61.
4. Schneeweiß B, Graninger W. Stockenhuber F, Druml W. Ferenci P, Eichinger S, Grimm G, Laggner AN, Grimm G. Energy metabolism in acute and chronic renal failure. Am J Clin Nutr 1990; 52:596–601.
5. Bouffard Y, Viale JP, Annat G, Delafosse B, Guillaume C, Motin J. Energy expenditure in the acute renal failure patient mechanically ventilated. Intens Care Med 1987; 13:401–406.
6. Soop M, Forsberg E, Thörne A, Alvestrand A. Energy expenditure in postoperative multiple organ failure with acute renal failure. Clin Nephrol 1989; 31:139–143.
7. Druml W. Protein metabolism in acute renal failure. Miner Electrolyte Metab 1998; 24:47–54.
8. Mitch WE. Amino acid release from the hindquarter and urea appearance in acute uremia. Am J Physiol 1981; 241:E415–E419.
9. Clark AS, Mitch WE. Muscle protein turnover and glucose uptake in acutely uremic rats. J Clin Invest 1983; 72:836–845.
10. Fröhlich J, Schölmerich J, Hoppe-Seyler G, Maier KP, Talke H, Schollmeyer P, Gerok W. The effect of acute uremia on gluconeogenesis in isolated perfused rat livers. Eur J Clin Invest 1974; 4:453–458.
11. Maroni BJ, Haesemeyer RW, Kutner MH, Mitch WE. Kinetics of system A amino acid uptake by muscle: effects of insulin and acute uremia. Am J Physiol 1990; 258:F1304–F1310.
12. Druml W, Bürger U, Kleinberger G, Lenz K, Laggner AN. Elimination of amino acids in acute renal failure. Nephron 1986; 42:62–67.
13. Druml W, Fischer M, Liebisch B, Lenz K, Roth E. Elimination of amino acids in renal failure. Am J Clin Nutr 1994; 60:418–423.
14. Wilmore DW. Catabolic illness; strategies for enhancing recovery. N Engl J Med 1991; 325:695–702.
15. Mitch WE, May RC, Maroni BJ, Druml W. Protein and amino acid metabolism in uremia: influence of metabolic acidosis. Kidney Int 1989; 36(suppl 27):S205–S207.
16. Mault JR, Bartlett RH, Dechert RE, Clark SF, Schwartz RD. Starvation: a major contributor to mortality in acute renal failure. Trans Am Soc Artif Intern Organs 1983; 29:390–394.
17. Mitch ME, Chesney RW. Amino acid metabolism by the kidney. Miner Electrolyte Metab 1983; 9:190–202.
18. Laidlaw SA, Kopple JD. Newer concepts of indispensable amino acids. Am J Clin Nutr 1987; 46:593–605.
19. Druml W, Roth E, Lenz K, Lochs H, Kopsa H. Phenylalanine and tyrosine metabolism in renal failure. Kidney Int 1989; 36 (suppl 27):S282–S286.
20. Druml W, Lochs H, Roth E, Hübl W, Balcke P, Lenz K. Utilisation of tyrosine dipeptides and acetyl-tyrosine in normal and uremic humans. Am J Physiol 1991; 260: E280–E285.
21. Naschitz JE, Barak C, Yeshurun D. Reversible diminished insulin requirement in acute renal failure. Postgrad Med J 1983; 59:269–271.
22. May RC, Clark AS, Goheer MA, Mitch WE. Specific defects in insulin-mediated muscle metabolism in acute uremia. Kidney Int 1985; 28:490–497.
23. Cianciaruso B, Bellizzi V, Napoli R, Sacca L, Kopple JD. Hepatic uptake and release of glucose, lactate and amino acids in acutely uremic dogs. Metabolism 1991; 40:261–290.
24. Shaw JFH, Wildbore M, Wolfe RR. Whole body protein kinetics in severely septic patients: the response to glucose infusion and total parenteral nutrition. Ann Surg 1987; 205:288.
25. Druml W, Fischer M, Sertl S, Schneeweiss B, Lenz K, Widhalm K. Fat elimination in acute renal failure: Long chain versus medium chain triglycerides. Am J Clin Nutr 1992; 55:468–472.
26. Druml W, Zechner R, Magometschnigg D, Lenz K, Kleinberger G, Laggner AN, Kostner G. Post-heparin lipolytic activity in acute renal failure. Clin Nephrol 1985; 23:289–293.
27. Adolph M, Eckart J, Metges C, Neeser G, Wolfram G. Oxidative utilization of lipid emulsions in septic patients with and without acute renal failure. Clin Nutr 1995; 14 (suppl 2):35A.
28. VanKuijk WHM, Hillion D, Saoiu C, Leunissen KML. Critical role of the extracorporeal blood temperature in the hemodynamic response during hemofiltration. JASN 1997; 8:949–955.
29. Monaghan R, Watters JM, Clancey SM, Moulton SB, Rabin EZ. Uptake of glucose during continuous arteriovenous hemofiltration. Crit Care Med 1993; 21: 1159–1163.
30. Yatani A, Fujiono T, Kinoshita K, Goto M. Excess lactate modulates ionic currents and tension components in frog atrial muscle. J Mol Cell Cardiol 1981; 13:147–161.
31. Lovejoy J, Newby FD, Gebhart SSP, DiGirolamo M. Insulin resistance in obesity is associated with elevated lactate levels and diminished lactate appearance following intravenous glucose and insulin. Metabolism 1992; 41:22–27.
32. Olbricht CJ, Huxman-Nägeli D, Koch KM. Harnstoffgeneration bei kontinuierlicher arteriovenöser Hämofiltration (CAVH) mit Laktat- und Bikarbonat-Lösungen. Nieren Hochdruckkrankh 1992; 21:410A.
33. Davies SP, Reaveley DA, Brown EA, Kox WJ. Amino acid clearances and daily losses in patients with acute renal failure treated by continuous arteriovenous hemodialysis. Crit Care Med 1991; 19:1510–1515.
34. Davenport A, Robert NB. Amino acid losses during continuous high-flux hemofiltration in the critically ill patient. Crit Care Med 1989; 17:1010–1015.

35. Druml W. Nutritional considerations in the treatment of acute renal failure in septic patients. Nephrol Dial Transplant 1994; 9 (suppl4):219–223.
36. Frankenfeld DC, Badellino MM, Reynolds N, Wiles CE, Siegel JH, Goodarzi S. Amino acid loss and plasma concentration during continuous hemofiltration. JPEN 1993; 17:551–561.
37. Druml W. Prophylactic use of CRRT in patients with normal renal function. Am J Kidney Dis 1996; 28 (suppl 3):S-114–120.
38. Bellomo R, McGrath B, Boyce N. In vivo catecholamine extraction during continuous hemodiafiltration in inotrope-dependent patients Trans Am Soc Intern Organs 1991; 37:324–325.
39. Gasche Y, Pascual M, Suter PM, Favre H, Chevrolet JC, Schifferli JA. Complement depeletion during haemofiltration with polyacrylonitrile membranes. Nephrol Dial Transplant 1996; 11:117–119.
40. Gutierrez A, Alvestrand A, Bergström J. Membrane selection and muscle protein catabolism. Kidney Int 1992; 42 (suppl.38):S-86–S-90.
41. Himmelfarb J, Tolkoff R, Chandran P, Parker RA, Wingard RL, Hakim R. A multicenter comparison of dialysis membranes in the treatment of acute renal failure requiring dialysis. J Am Soc Nephrol 1998; 9:257–266.
42. Riegel W. Ziegenfuss T, Rose, Bauer M, Marzi I. Influence of venovenous hemofiltration on posttraumatic inflammation and hemodynamics. Contrib Nephrol 1995; 116:56–61.
43. Burke JF, Wolfe RR, Mullany CJ, Mathews DE, Bier DM. Glucose requirements following burn injury. Ann Surg 1979; 190:274–285.
44. Nordenström J, Jeevanadam M, Elwyn DH, Carpentier YA, Askanazi J, Robin A, Kinney JM. Increasing glucose intake during parenteral nutrition increases norepinephrine excretion in trauma and sepsis. Clin Physiol 1981; 1:525–534.
45. Askenazi J, Elwyn DH, Silberberg PA, Rosenbaum SH, Kinney JM. Respiratory distress secondary to a high carbohydrate load. Surgery 1980; 87:596–598.
46. Alexander JW, Gonce SJ, Miskell PW. A new model for studying nutrition in peritonitis. The adverse effect of overfeeding. Ann Surg 1989; 209:334–340.
47. Spreiter SC, Myers BD, Swenson RS. Protein-energy requirements in subjects with acute renal failure receiving intermittent hemodialysis. Am J Clin Nutr 1980; 33: 1433–1437.
48. Wolfe RR, Allsop JR, Burke JF. Glucose metabolism in man: response to intravenous glucose infusion. Metabolism 1979; 28:210–220.
49. Flakoll PJ, Hill JO, Abumrad NN. Acute hyperglycemia enhances proteolysis in normal man. Am J Physiol 1993; 265:E715–E721.
50. Hennessey PJ, Black CT, Andrassy RJ. Nonenzymatic glycosylation of immunoglobulinG impairs complement fixation. JPEN 1991; 15:60–64.
51. Björnsson ES, Urbanavicius V, Eliasoson B, Attval S, Smith U. Effects of hyperglycemia on interdigestive gastrointestinal motility in humans. Scand J Gastroenterol 1994; 29:1096–1104.
52. Bresson JL, Bader B, Rocchiccioli F, Mariotti A, Ricour C, Sachs C, Rey J. Protein-metabolism kinetics and energy-substrate utilization in infants fed parenteral solutions with different glucose-fat ratios. Am J Clin Nutr 1991; 54:346–350.
53. Schneeweiß B, Graninger W, Ferenci P, Druml W, Ratheiser K, Steger G, Grimm G, Schurz B, Laggner AN, Siostrzonek P, Lenz K. Short term energy balance in patients with infections: Carbohydrate-based versus fat-based diets. Metabolism 1992; 41:125–130.
54. Druml W, Fischer, M, Ratheiser K. Utilization of intravenous lipids in critically ill patients with sepsis without and with hepatic failure. JPEN 1998; 22:
55. Druml W, Laggner AN, Lenz K, Balcke P. Kleinberger G, Schmidt P. Lipid metabolism and lipid utilization in renal failure. Infusionstherapie 1983; 10:206–212.
56. Kierdorf H, Kindler J, Sieberth HG. Nitrogen balance in patients with acute renal failure treated by continuous arteriovenous hemofiltration. Nephrol Dial Transplant 1986; 1:72.
57. Chima CS, Meyer L, Hummell AC, Bosworth C, Heyka R, Paganini EP, Werynski A. Protein catabolic rate in patients with acute renal failure on continuous arteriovenous hemofiltration and total parenteral nutrition. JASN 1993; 3:1516–1521.
58. Macias WL, Alaka KJ, Murphy MH, Miller ME, Clark WR, Mueller BA. Impact of nutritional regimen on protein catabolism and nitrogen balance in patients with acute renal failure. JPEN 1996; 20:56–62.
59. Grazer RE, Sutton JM, Friedstrom S, McMarron FD. Hyperammoniemic encephalopathy due to essential amino acid hyperalimentation. Arch Int Med 1984; 144: 2278–2279.
60. Kierdorf HP. The nutritional management of acute renal failure in the intensive care unit. New Horizons 1995; 3:699–707.
61. Fürst P, Stehle P. The potential use of dipeptides in clinical nutrition. Nutr Clin Pract 1993; 8:106–114.
62. Imai E, Yamanoto S, Isaka Y, Fukuhara Y, Fujii Y, Kikuchi T, Tanaka T, Kamada T, Ueda N. Delay of recovery from renal ischemic injury by administration of glutamine. JASN 1991; 2:648A.
63. Griffiths RD, Jones CJ, Palmer TEA. Six-month outcome of critically ill patients given glutamine-supplemented parenteral nutrition. Nutrition 1997; 13:295–302.
64. Hübl W, Druml W, Roth E, Lochs H. Importance of liver and kidney for the utilization of glutamine-containing dipeptides in man. Metabolism 1994; 43:1104–1107.
65. Zager RA, Venkatachalam MA, Potentiation of ischemic renal injury by amino acid infusion. Kidney Int 1983; 24:620–625.

66. Brezis M, Rosen S, Spokes K, Silva P, Epstein FH. Transport-dependent anoxic cell injury in the isolated perfused rat kidney. Am J Pathol 1984; 116:327–341.
67. Moursi M, Rising CL, Zelenock GB, D'Alecy LG. Dextrose administration exacerbates acute renal ischemic damage in anesthestized dogs. Arch Surg 1987; 122:790–794.
68. Heyman SN, Rosen S, Silva P, Spokes K, Egorin MJ, Epstein FH. Protective action of glycine in cisplatin nephrotoxicity. Kidney Int 1991; 40:273–279.
69. Schramm L, Heidbreder E, Lopau K, Schaar J, Zimmermann J, Harlos J, Teschner M, Ling H, Heidland A. Influence of nitric oxide on renal function in toxic renal failure in the rat. Miner Electrolyte Metab 1996; 22: 168–177.
70. Druml W. Lax F, Grimm G, Schneeweiss B, Lenz K, Laggner AN. Acute renal failure in the elderly 1975–1990. Clin Nephrol 1994; 342–349.
71. Hörl WH, Schaefer RM, Haag M, Heidland A. Acute uremia following dietary potassium depletion. Mineral Electrolyte Metab 1986; 12:218–225.
72. Haas M, Öhler L, Watzke H, Böhmig G, Prokesch R, Druml W. The spectrum of acute renal failure in tumor lysis syndrome. Nephrol Dial Transpl. In Press.
73. Lumlertgul D, Harris DCH, Burke TJ, Schrier RW. Detrimental effects of hypophosphatemia on the severity and progression of ischemic acute renal failure. Mineral Electrolyte Metab 1986; 12:204–209.
74. Kleinberger G, Gabl F, Gaßner A, Lochs H, Pall H, Pichler M. Hypophosphatemia during parenteral nutrition in patients with renal failure. Wien Klin Wochenschr 1978; 90:169–172.
75. Kurtin P, Kouba J. Profound hypophosphatermia in the course of acute renal failure. Am J Kidney Dis 1987; 10:346–349.
76. Druml W. Global quality assurance in parenteral nutrition. Clin Nutr 1996; 15:39–40.
77. Pietrek J, Kokot F, Kuska J. Serum 25-hydroxyvitamin D and parathyoid hormone in patients with acute renal failure. Kidney Int 1978; 13:178–185.
78. Druml W, Schwazenhofer M, Apsner R, Hörl WH. Fat soluble vitamins in acute renal failure. Miner Electrolyte Metab 1998; 24:220–226.
79. Akmal M, Bishop JE, Telfer, N, Norman AW, Massry SG. Hypocalcemia and hypercalcemia in patients with rhabdomyolysis with and without acute renal failure. J Clin Endocrinol Metab 1986; 63:137–142.
80. Al-Ghamdi SMG, Cameron ECC, Sutton RAL. Magnesium deficiency: pathophysiologic and clinical overview. Am J Kidney Dis 1994; 24:737–752.
81. Shaah GM, Kirschenbaum MA. Renal magnesium wasting associated with therapeutic agents. Min Electrolyte Metab 1991; 17:58–64.
82. Story DA, Ronco C, Bellomo R. Trace element and vitamin concentrations and losses in critically ill patients treated with continuous venovenous hemofiltration. Crit Care Med 1999; 27:220–223.
83. Fortin MC, Amyot SL, Geadah D, Leblanc M. Serum concentrations and clearances of folic acid and pyridoxal-5-phosphate during venovenous continuous renal replacement therapy. Intensive Care Med 1999; 25: 594–598.
84. Madl Ch, Kranz A, Liebisch B, Traindl O, Lenz K, Druml W. Lactic acidosis in thiamine deficiency. Clin Nutr 1993; 12:108–111.
85. Friedmann AL, Chesney RW, Gilbert EF, Gilchrist KW, Latorraca R, Segar WE. Secondary oxalosis as a complication of parenteral nutrition in acute renal failure. Am J Nephrol 1983; 3:248–252.
86. Chung YC, Huang MT, Chang CN, Lee PH, Lee CS, Huang TW. Prolonged nonoliguric acute renal failure associated with high-dose vitamin K administration in a renal transplant recipient. Transplant Proc 1994; 26: 2129–2131.
87. Lipsky JJ. Vitamin K deficiency. J Intensive Care Med 1992; 7:328–336.
88. Metnitz PGH, Fischer M, Bartnes S, Steltzer H, Lang Th, Druml W. Impact of acute renal failure on antioxidant status in patients with multiple organ failure. Acta Anaesthesiol Scand 2000; 43:236–240.
89. Besunder JB, Smith PG. Toxic effects of electrolyte and trace mineral administration in the intensive care unit. Crit Care Clin 1991; 7:659–693.
90. König JS, Fischer M, Bulant E, Tiran B, Elmadfa I, Druml W. Antioxidant status in patients on chronic hemodialysis therapy: impact of parenteral selenium supplementation. Wien Klin Wochenschr 1997; 109:13–19.
91. Okada A, Takagi Y, Nezu R, Sando K, Shenkin A. Trace element metabolism in parenteral and enteral nutrition. Nutrition 1995; 11:106–113.
92. Shenkin A. Trace elements and inflammatory response: implications for nutritional support. Nutrition 1995; 11: 100–105.
93. Jetton MM, Sullivan JF, Burch RE. Trace element contamination of intravenous solutions. Arch Int Med 1976; 136:782–784.
94. Angstwurm MW, Schottdorf J, Schopohl J, Gaerner R. Selenium replacement in patients with severe systemic inflammatory response syndrome improves clinical outcome. Crit Care Med 1999; 27:1807–1813.
95. Nath KA, Paller MS. Dietary deficiency of antioxydants exacerbates ischemic injury in the rat kidney. Kidney Int 1990; 38:1109–1117.
96. Zurovsky Y, Gispaan I. Antioxidants attenuate endotoxin-induced acute renal failure in rats. Am J Kidney Dis 1995; 25:51–57.

24

Endocrine and Sexual Problems in Adult and Pediatric Hemodialysis and Peritoneal Dialysis Patients

Ahmed Mahmoud, Frank H. Comhaire, Margarita Craen, and Jean Marc Kaufman
University Hospital of Gent, Gent, Belgium

I. GROWTH RETARDATION IN CHILDREN WITH CHRONIC RENAL FAILURE

Growth impairment and retardation of sexual development are common and serious complications of chronic renal insufficiency (CRI) and chronic renal failure (CRF). Growth velocity decreases significantly when glomerular filtration is lower than 50 mL/min/1.73 m^2. With the more widespread use of long-term peritoneal dialysis, hemodialysis, and transplantation, many children survive to adulthood. Growth rate normalization is occasionally achieved, but catch-up growth is only rarely observed. Even with optimal therapeutic intervention, the adult stature is often markedly diminished.

The pathogenesis of impaired growth in CRI and CRF is complex. Possible factors contributing to growth retardation are early onset of CRI, anorexia, and malnutrition with altered protein, lipid, and carbohydrate metabolism and deficient energy utilization. Acidosis, accumulation of uremic toxins, renal anemia, renal osteodystrophy, and decreased end-organ response to endogenous hormones are major causes of growth impairment.

Growth is mostly affected during the years when rapid growth is expected, namely the first 2 years of life and at puberty. During the first 2 years of life, congenital and hereditary nephro-uropathies are diagnosed and the consecutive malnutrition intervenes by decreasing the synthesis and expression of insulin-like growth factor I (IGF-I) (1, 2). Puberty is delayed and the pubertal peak height velocity is diminished. Obviously, children who develop CRI from an acquired renal disease that occurs after they have reached or nearly reached their growth potential are unlikely to experience any significant growth failure.

A. Growth Hormone

The basal level of serum growth hormone (GH) and the stimulated GH secretion are increased in CRF as a result of hypophyseal GH hypersecretion in uremia as well as a greatly reduced metabolic clearance of GH (3).

Growth retardation in children with CRF despite elevated GH levels indicates a peripheral insensitivity to the action of GH (4). One possible molecular mechanism is a reduced density of GH receptors in GH target organs. The circulating high-affinity GH-binding protein (GHBP) reflects GH receptor expression because it is derived from the extracellular domain of the GH receptor by proteolytic cleavage. In CRF serum GHBP concentrations are below the mean of controls matched for age and gender (4). These low GHBP levels represent a quantitative tissue GH receptor deficiency. GH exerts its action by stimulating the production of hepatic IGF-I synthesis and by its direct effect on target tissues (5). In uremia, IGF-I serum concentrations are falsely reported to be reduced to about 50% of normal values, as measured by radioimmunoassay (RIA) or radioreceptorassay (RRA) (1, 2). These erroneous results are related to the increase of the IGF-binding protein (IGFBP) concentration in uremia, which interferes with the assay (1). When IGF-I is separated from the binding protein (by acid chromatography), a normal IGF-I serum concentration is found. On the other hand, there is a reduction of IGF-I secretion in CRF.

In uremia, the bioactivity of IGF-I is reduced. The discrepancy between the normal serum concentration of IGF-I and the reduced IGF-I bioactivity indicates the presence of IGF inhibitors. $IGFBP_3$ is the most important circulating transport protein. Small molecular subunits of $IGFBP_3$, which are normally eliminated from the circulation by glomerular filtration, accumulate in renal failure (2). The excess of IGFBP and their subunits in uremia leads to a markedly increased IGF-binding capacity and a reduced amount of free (bioactive) IGF-I.

The recommended guideline of recombinant human growth hormone (rhGH) therapy in children and adolescents with chronic renal failure, with or without dialysis, is daily subcutaneous injection of rhGH at a dose of 4 U/m^2 or 0.15 U/kg.

B. Thyroid Hormone

Abnormalities in some thyroid function tests have been reported in children and adolescents with renal failure (6). These alterations depend on the pre- or pubertal status of the patient, the degree of chronic renal insufficiency or end-stage renal disease, and the type of treatment (conservative, hemodialysis, peritoneal dialysis, transplantation). The kidney plays a role in the metabolism and clearance of thyroid hormones, thyroid-stimulating hormone (TSH), and thyrotropin-releasing hormone (TRH).

Serum total thyroxine (T_4), and total triiodothyronine (T_3) have been found to be either low or normal in CRF. Some of the possible mechanisms responsible for the low T_4 and low T_3 are a moderate reduction of T_4 secretion by the thyroid gland, reduced extrathyroidal (renal) conversion of T_4 to T_3, reduced secretion of TSH by the pituitary gland relative to the low levels of circulating thyroid hormones, and impaired secretion of TRH.

Unbound or free thyroxine (FT_4) and unbound or free triiodothyronine (FT_3) may be normal in serum. Concentrations of the specific serum-binding proteins, thyroxine-binding protein (TBG) and thyroxin-binding prealbumin (TBPA), are low in prepubertal patients with CRF in comparison with appropriate control subjects. Because thyroxine and triiodothyronine circulate mostly bound to TBG, TBPA, and albumin, a decrease in the concentration of thyroid hormones may be associated with changes in the degree of binding on the serum proteins. Some uremic factors can alter TBG binding or displace T_4 and T_3 from TBG. These effects might be the result of hemodialysis or peritoneal dialysis.

In pubertal patients with CRF, serum TBG and TBPA are not decreased in comparison with appropriate control subjects. Basal TSH levels are in the normal range in CRF, but the TSH response to TRH can be blunted with a prolonged curve.

There is a high incidence of goiter in patients undergoing hemodialysis, which is attributed to removal of iodine during dialysis or to the presence of goitrogens in patients with uremia.

C. Puberty

The quality of the pubertal growth spurt is dependent not only on a physiological increase of endogenous GH secretion but also on the gonadal steroid hormones. In patients with CRF, pubertal growth failure may be the consequence of a complex dysregulation. The disturbance of GH-dependent prepubertal baseline growth continues during puberty. The growth-stimulating effect of the gonadal hormones causes a pubertal growth spurt of normal amplitude but shortened duration. Gonadal hormone–mediated acceleration of skeletal maturation is not affected. The combination of normal gonadal hormone effects and impaired GH efficacy leads to an irreversible loss of growth potential.

In prepubertal boys with CRF, the secretory reserve of the Leydig cells reveals a subclinical reduction, most marked in patients on hemodialysis, and improving partially after transplantation. In pubertal boys with CRF, the function of the Leydig cells seems to be maintained. Subnormal plasma estrogen levels are found in prepubertal girls with CRF. Estrogen levels are most affected in girls on hemodialysis. In pubertal girls with severe renal function deterioration, estradiol increases insufficiently. After successful transplantation, even if it is performed after several years of dialysis, estradiol concentrations increase. As expected from the high incidence of anovulatory cycles in postmenarche girls with CRF, progesterone levels during the menstrual cycle are frequently low.

Increased concentration of luteinizing hormone (LH) and follicle-stimulating hormone (FSH) are found before and during puberty in CRF. The combination of raised gonadotropin levels and low to normal concentrations of gonadal hormones suggests a partially compensated hypergonadotrophic hypogonadism.

However, there are several complicating factors to consider. The metabolic clearance of LH and FSH is reduced in proportion to the severity of renal failure. On the other hand, the concentration of certain biologically inactive peptide fragments and hormone subunits (e.g., the α-subunit of LH and FSH) are disproportionately increased, and this can lead to false high values if the specificity of the assay is inadequate (7). Finally, stimulation tests of the pituitary gonadotrophin secretion using gonadotrophin-releasing hormone (GNRH or LHRH) showed delayed and reduced secretion of gonadotrophins in prepubertal and pubertal patients with CRF.

II. EVALUATION OF THYROID FUNCTION

End-stage renal disease (ESRD) is accompanied by alterations in the regulation of the hypothalamo-pituitary-thyroid axis and by changes in the plasma protein binding and metabolism of thyroid hormones, which should be taken into account when exploring the functional status of the thyroid hormonal axis. Moreover, evaluation of thyroid function may be complicated by pharmacological agents frequently used in these patients and by a relatively high prevalence of malnutrition and a variety of nonrenal nonthyroidal illnesses (8).

A. Serum Thyrotropin Levels

Metabolic clearance of serum thyrotropin (TSH) is reduced by about 40% in ESRD (9). Whereas basal TSH serum levels are normal in a majority of ESRD patients receiving chronic hemodialysis, observations of a reduced TSH pulse amplitude, of a blunting of the TSH diurnal rhythm with diminished or absent nocturnal rise (10,11), and of a diminished TSH response upon stimulation with thyrotropin-releasing hormone (TRH) (12–15) indicate the existence of subtle alterations of the neuro-endocrine regulation of TSH secretion.

Measurement of serum TSH with a highly sensitive assay, i.e. a second-generation (sensitivity limit of 0.1–0.2 mU/L) or third-generation (sensitivity limit 0.01–0.02 mU/L) assay, is now commonly used as the first-line diagnostic test for detection of thyroid dysfunction in unselected patient populations, with elevated values suggesting the possibility of primary hypothyroidism, while maximally suppressed TSH levels are compatible with the existence of a thyrotoxicosis. Mean basal TSH levels tend to be somewhat higher in euthyroid ESRD patients as compared to healthy controls, and although TSH levels are within the normal range in a majority of the patients, slightly elevated basal serum TSH levels (<10 mU/L) is not an uncommon finding in euthyroid ESRD patients, whether or not they are receiving chronic hemodialysis (16,17). More markedly elevated TSH serum levels (>10 mU/L) in euthyroid ESRD patients is a less common finding ($\leq$1%), lower TSH levels usually being found on repeat testing in the same subjects (8,17). Transient elevation of serum TSH can also be observed during recovery from acute nonthyroidal illnesses of nonrenal origin, and an increased serum TSH level can certainly not be regarded as a specific marker of primary hypothyroidism in a general hospital population. Indeed, in hospitalized patients a serum TSH above 20 mU/L may be due, with equal frequency, to either a nonthyroidal illness or to primary hypothyroidism, the former being by far the most frequent cause of more limited increases of serum TSH (<20 mU/L) in a hospital population (18). The transient TSH elevation in nonthyroidal illnesses is usually accompanied by normal or rising thyroid hormone levels, while sick patients with primary hypothyroidism usually present with consistently increased TSH together with permanently decreased total T_4, free T_4 index, and free T_4 as estimated by the equilibrium dialysis techniques (17–20).

ESRD has not been reported to be associated with suppressed serum TSH levels in euthyroid patients (8,16). However, it should be remembered that suppressed serum TSH is not an uncommon finding in nonthyroidal illnesses, especially in the most severely ill, and it is then usually associated with reduced total serum thyroid hormone concentrations (21). In hospitalized patients, nonthyroidal illnesses are more frequently than thyrotoxicosis the cause of serum TSH levels below 0.1 mU/L as measured with use of a second-generation TSH assay, and are responsible for over a quarter of the TSH values below 0.01 mU/L encountered in this population when using a third-generation assay (18,22).

It has been reported that, besides abnormalities in serum TSH levels, euthyroid ESRD patients also have markedly increased circulating levels of free α-subunit, the common subunit of TSH and the gonadotropins (7).

B. Serum T_4 Levels

Even though ESRD is accompanied by alterations in neuro-endocrine regulation of TSH secretion and although there are also indications for an altered thyroid responsiveness to TSH stimulation in these patients (14), steady-state thyroidal production rates for T_4 have been found to be normal (13,23). Nevertheless, serum total T_4 concentrations as well as estimates of serum free T_4 may be reduced in euthyroid ESRD patients who do or do not receive dialysis therapy; these abnormalities are possibly related in part to concurrent malnutrition and nonthyroidal illnesses (8,17). The reduced total serum T_4 concentrations observed in euthyroid ESRD patients are secondary to a decrease of the concentration of protein-bound T_4, whereas low values for estimates of serum free T_4 are essentially method-related spurious results (8).

Serum albumin concentrations may be reduced in ESRD patients, but the serum levels of transthyretin (prealbumin) are usually maintained and concentrations of T_4-binding globulin (TBG) are commonly normal or even increased (24–27). Rather than by consequence of changes in carrier protein concentrations, low total serum T_4 concentrations in ESRD are explained by the presence of inhibitors of T_4 binding to serum carrier proteins in the circulation of euthyroid uremic patients. These T_4-binding inhibitors may include increased concentrations of hippuric acid, indoxyl sulfate, and 3-carboxy-4-methyl-5-propyl-2-furanpropanoic acid (CPMF) as well as increased levels of cytokines, such as interleukin-1b, tumor necrosis factor-α and interleukin-6 (21,28–31). Binding of T4 to the carrier proteins may be further inhibited by drugs such as heparin and nonsteroidal anti-inflammatory drugs (32,33). Hemodilution may be another factor contributing to low total serum T_4 values, and in chronic peritoneal dialysis protein loss, in particular loss of TBG, may also play a role besides the presence of T_4-binding inhibitors (34).

Alterations of T_4 protein binding are not expected to affect free circulating T_4 concentrations in steady-state situations. In fact, in ESRD patients both the T_4 production rates and the conversion rates of T_4 to reverse T_3 (rT_3) are normal (25,35), so that free T_4 serum concentrations can be expected to be normal as is the case in nonrenal nonthyroidal illnesses. However, estimates of serum free T_4 levels in patients with nonthyroidal illnesses are plagued by methodological problems, and all of the various available methods for estimation of free T_4 concentrations, with the exception of the direct equilibrium dialysis method, may produce spurious results (36,37). Low free T_4 index values are observed in an substantial proportion of ESRD patients with low serum total T_4 concentrations. Inhibition by patient serum components of the in vitro T_4 binding to solid matrices in the applied assays may be one of the mechanisms involved (17,37,38). A variety of methods for direct estimation of free T_4, such as the one-step labeled T_4 analog immunoassays, the one-step labeled T_4 antibody immunoassays, some two-step immunoextraction assays, and the tracer equilibrium dialysis method, show protein-bound T_4 dependency of the observed values for free T_4 (39,40). These assays tend to underestimate free T_4 serum concentrations in subjects with decreased T_4 binding to carrier proteins, including euthyroid ESRD patients with low total serum T_4 concentrations (8,25,36,37).

Transient elevation of serum free T_4 is not uncommon in mild nonrenal nonthyroidal illnesses, possibly as a consequence of decreased T_4 clearance, but this is seldom the case in ESRD patients, due to the severity of their illness and to malnutrition (8).

C. Serum T_3 Levels

Decreased total and free T_3 serum concentrations, a frequent finding in nonrenal nonthyroidal illnesses, is also observed in as many as two thirds of patients with ESRD (17). This is the consequence of reduced peripheral conversion of T_4 to T_3 (13,23,35). The decrease of T_4 to T_3 conversion may result from interference with tissue T_4 uptake and subsequent deodination by circulating CMPF, hippuric acid, and indoxyl sulfate in uremic patients (30) but may also be related to malnutrition and concurrent nonrenal nonthyroidal illnesses (17) and to the effect of increased circulating concentrations of cytokines such as interleukin-1b and tumor necrosis factor-α (31). Reduced T_3 serum concentrations in ESRD patients is not associated with clinical hypothyroidism (41), which may be explained by increased tissue availability of T_3 nuclear receptor proteins as reported in euthyroid ESRD patients on chronic hemodialysis or CAPD therapy (42).

D. Serum Reversed T_3 Levels

Total serum rT_3 concentrations are usually normal in euthyroid ESRD patients, in contrast with the elevated rT_3 levels seen in most subjects with nonrenal nonthyroidal illnesses and low serum T_3 (25,35). In ESRD, conversion of T_4 to rT_3 and rT_3 clearance rates are normal, but rT_3 fractional transfer rates from serum to the tissue compartments are increased (25,35).

E. Influence of Therapy

Comparison of hormone concentrations before and after a hemodialysis session may show a limited and transient correction of the decreased thyroid hormone levels, possibly related to reduction of hemodilution, partial epuration of inhibitors of T_4 binding to carrier proteins, and transient increase of free hormone fractions resulting from administration of heparin (27,43). However, thyroid function tests are usually not normalized by either chronic hemodialysis or CAPD treatment, with no essential differences between the effects of these two types of treatment (17,27,34,44–46). Nevertheless, lower TBG and albumin levels in patients under CAPD (34,45) might result in a slightly higher prevalence of low total serum T_4 concentrations.

Partial correction of anemia by administration of erythropoietin does not consistently result in an improvement of the abnormalities in thyroid function tests observed in ESRD (15,47). A report including a limited number of subjects receiving intermittent peritoneal dialysis therapy has suggested that zinc supplementation may normalize some thyroid function abnormalities in these patients (48).

F. Conclusions and Practical Implications for the Diagnosis of Thyroid Dysfunction

From the foregoing discussion it is clear that abnormal results of routine thyroid testing in ESRD patients are more frequently the consequence of functional adaptation, alterations in serum protein binding of thyroid hormones, and method-dependent spurious findings related to the nonthyroidal disease state rather than the reflection of clinically significant thyroid dysfunction. It is, therefore, important for the clinician to be familiar with the type of results frequently obtained in ESRD patients and the type of assays used in a particular clinical laboratory. Obviously, the high prevalence of abnormal results of thyroid function tests in ESRD patients complicates the diagnosis of subtle thyroid abnormalities, but careful interpretation of these tests in conjunction with a thorough clinical evaluation will usually allow for a correct diagnosis of suspected thyroid dysfunction.

The prevalence of primary hypothyroidism is increased in ESRD patients as compared to the general population, which may be explained by the characteristics of ESRD patients (e.g., the higher prevalence of primary hypothyroidism in ESRD patients with insulin-dependent diabetes mellitus) and possibly by a role of increased circulating levels of anorganic iodine resulting from a markedly reduced clearance (49), even if ESRD patients are under chronic hemodialysis or CAPD treatment. The diagnosis of primary hypothyroidism can be confirmed by the finding of a serum TSH persistently elevated above 20 mU/L with concurrent persistent decrease of total and free serum T_4 concentrations (8).

The frequency of hyperthyroidism in ESRD patients is probably not different from that in the general population. The diagnosis can usually be confirmed by finding a maximally surpressed TSH (<0.1 mU/L with a second-generation assay or <0.01 mU/L with a third-generation assay) together with increased values for total serum T_4 concentrations and free T_4 estimates. On the other hand, total and free serum T_3 levels may not necessarily be increased in ESRD patients with mild to moderate hyperthyroidism. When results of in vitro thyroid function testing in ESRD patients do not allow for definitive conclusions, repeat testing after a few weeks is often helpful.

III. SEXUAL DYSFUNCTION AND INFERTILITY

Reduced sexual activity and interest has consistently been reported in both males and females on dialysis. Fertility is diminished, and both factors may reduce the well-being and quality of life of these patients. The reasons for these disturbances are complex. Recent developments, however, have improved the therapeutic possibilities.

A. Male

1. Sexual Dysfunction

Sexual dysfunction is reported in 50–80 % of men with chronic renal failure (CRF) (50–55). After starting dialysis, sexual function usually does not improve, and, in fact, about 35% of the patients develop sexual dysfunction. On the other hand, adaptation to the sexual deficit is possible (51,56). The incidence of sexual dysfunction was not different when patients on hemodialysis or peritoneal dialysis were compared (53).

It has been suggested that sexual dysfunction in men on hemodialysis or peritoneal dialysis was not so much due to erectile failure but largely to loss of sexual interest (libido), subjectively ascribed to fatigue (50).

Many factors may be involved in the pathogenesis of sexual problems in men with CRF, including psychological, hormonal, neurological, vascular, nutritional, and drug-related factors.

a. *Mechanisms of Male Sexual Dysfunction*

Age In normal men, age is the variable most strongly associated with erectile dysfunction and impotence (57). Some studies indicate that the unfavorable effect of age on gonadal function and potency is more pronounced in uremic patients (58,59). In one study, an age of greater than 40 years was the only factor deleterious to potency (59).

Psychological Factors Dialysis patients not having intercourse were found to have a poorer quality of life and higher degree of depression and anxiety than patients having intercourse more than two times per month (60). Dialysis patients were more depressed and experienced more marital difficulties than patients who had received transplants (61). Although patients treated by dialysis may appear to have more reasons to be depressed than nondialysis patients, depression itself has not been found to be correlated with erectile dysfunction (62). This stands in contrast to findings by Feldman et al. (57) that anger and depression were clearly related to sexual dysfunction. It is not clear, however, whether the psychological changes are the cause or rather the result of the sexual problems.

Hormonal Causes Studies indicate sexual dysfunction in CRF/dialysis patients to be associated with low serum concentrations of total and free testosterone (63,64), hyperprolactinemia (11,54,65,66), hyperoestrogenemia (67,11,54), and elevated serum LH levels (63,64). These hormonal changes are common findings among men with renal failure. Patients on hemodialysis may show further decrease of plasma testosterone (63). In contrast, testosterone levels were significantly higher in patients treated by continuous ambulatory peritoneal dialysis, but the incidence of sexual dysfunction was not different from patients treated by hemodialysis (53).

Some studies assign an important role to the excess blood levels of parathormone in the genesis of the hypotestosteronemia (68). In dialyzed patients secondary hyperparathyroidism is alleged to further decrease serum testosterone concentration (69). The effect of excess parathormone on serum testosterone levels would be mediated through the accumulation of calcium in the testes, reducing the synthesis and release of testosterone (68). According to this hypothesis, ketoanalogs may restore low serum testosterone secretion by correcting parathormone levels without, however, improving pituitary dysregulation (69).

Vascular Factors Cavernous artery occlusive disease was found in 78% of uremic patients studied by Kaufman et al. (70). The most likely pathophysiology of the penile vascular impairment in these patients includes renal failure–associated atherosclerosis, which occurs independently of the presence of known systemic atherosclerotic risk factors. Also, renal failure–associated hypoxia may change the contractile (smooth muscle) and structural (collagen/elastin) components of the erectile tissue (70). Corporeal veno-occlusive dysfunction is also commonly found in these patients (70), but this may be secondary to the deficient arterial blood supply rather than being the primary pathogenic mechanism of erectile insufficiency. In another study, vasculogenic impotence was identified in no more than 6% of patients (53). These remarkable differences in frequency of detected vascular deficit probably results from differences in diagnostic techniques and accuracy.

Also, hypertension and/or its treatment has been shown to be associated with erectile dysfunction. Interruption of both hypogastric arteries during renal transplantation may be, but is not necessarily, related to impotence (59).

Drugs Patients with uremia are commonly treated with drugs that may cause sexual dysfunction including antihypertensives, antiemetics, and psychotropic drugs (71). The latter two are known to induce hyperprolactinemia and may suppress testosterone production.

Neuropathy Several studies suggest that impairment of the autonomic nervous system may play an important role in the genesis of erectile abnormalities in patients with uremia (72,73). Better sexual function is reported in patients with the lowest degree of neuropathy (74). The same study indicated that sexual dysfunction was not related to other medical factors (74).

b. *Therapy for Male Sexual Dysfunction*

The influence of dialysis mode (hemodialysis vs. peritoneal dialysis), dialysis adequacy, and the use of erythropoietin (EPO) on the likelihood of sexual inadequacy among patients on dialysis has been evaluated in several studies, but these come to sometimes contradictory conclusions so that the impact of such influences remains largely unknown (75).

Renal Transplantation The impairment of testicular function seen in advanced uremia is not reversible by maintenance hemodialysis, and it may even deteriorate further (63,76,77). In contrast, after successful transplantation, steroidogenesis usually became almost normal, sexual potency improved, and spermatogenesis showed a striking though not always complete recovery (51,63,76). Early renal transplantation may delay or prevent the development of the penile vasculopathy (70) and uremic neuropathy. In addition, impaired prolactin regulation in uremia will probably be reversed by successful renal transplant (78).

Zinc Therapy Mahajan et al. (79,80) have suggested that sexual function improved significantly in patients receiving oral zinc but not during administration of placebo. This finding was not confirmed by Rodger et al. (81).

Prolactin-Lowering Agents Treatment with prolactin-lowering medication, namely Pergolide, showed no benefit over administration of placebo in the treatment of uremic patients with sexual impotence and hyperprolactinemia, in spite of decreasing serum prolactin (81). Improvement of sexual function following bromocriptin treatment has, however, been reported provided that pretreatment serum testosterone concentration was above the lower end of the normal range. Side effects of bromocriptin intake were relatively common, limiting the use of this medication (82,83).

Testosterone and Anabolic Steroids The correction of biochemical hypogonadism in the male dialysis population using testosterone uncommonly restores sexual function to normal (53,84). At the other hand, meta-analysis of published papers suggests that anabolic steroids improve the nutritional status, anemia, and sexual function of uremic men (85). If testosterone is given, it is preferable to administer an oral preparation without "first-pass" effect on the liver such as testosterone undecanoate (Andriol, Organon, Oss, The Netherlands) or one of the transdermal systems such as Andractim gel, Testoderm, or Androderm patches. Parenteral treatment with testosterone esters (Testosterone oenantate, Testoviron depot, Schering, Berlin, Germany; Sustanon, Organon, Oss, The Netherlands) should not be recommended because these require repeated intramuscular injections.

Vacuum Tumescence Therapy Vacuum tumescence therapy corrects penile erectile dysfunction in most patients (84). This treatment is not invasive and is relatively convenient, and it can be successful in the majority of patients. However, the artificial nature of the procedure sometimes meets with psychological resistance from either partner, and some users experience local discomfort.

Intracavernosal Injection of Vasoactive Drugs Intracavernosal self-injection of papaverine, possibly in combination with fentolamine, or of prostaglandin E1 (Caverject, Upjohn), either alone or in combination with the former drugs, was shown to be effective, well accepted, and tolerated by kidney transplant patients and posed no apparent risks (86). Also, the pure alphalytic drug moxicylite (Icavex, Asta Medica, Mérignac/Bordeaux, France; Erecnos, Fournier, Garches, France) can be used for intracavernosal injection. The latter seems to have some advantages over the former, since it virtually never provokes priapism and causes little or no pain at the site of injection. Also, fibrosis of the cavernous smooth muscles is less likely to occur with moxicylite than with other drugs.

Recombinant Human Erythropoietin Data indicate that recombinant human EPO therapy shows a beneficial effect on sexual function in dialysis patients, in addition to correcting anemia and improving physical, social, and mental functioning (87–91). Therapy with EPO may result in a significant increase in serum concentration of testosterone (92,93) even without suppressing hyperprolactinemia or hyperestrogenemia (93). The observed increase of testosterone levels in the internal spermatic vein, in the absence of any effect on gonadotropin secretion, suggests that EPO might act directly on Leydig cell function (94). Others have reported that improvement of erectile function was associated with a decrease in serum prolactin levels, sometimes without significant changes in serum testosterone concentration (90,92,95,96). Some of the beneficial effects of EPO may be mediated through an increase of the hematocrit level improving oxygenation (91) or, possibly, through a direct trophic action (15).

Breathing-Coordinated Exercise Breathing-coordinated exercises have been reported to improve the quality of life in hemodialysis patients including enhanced sexual activity (97), but this approach has not been substantiated further.

Oral Phosphodiesterase Inhibitor The new "wonder drug" Sildenafil (Viagra, Pfizer, New York) exerts an inhibitory effect on the phosphodiesterase isoenzyme 5, causing enhanced rigidity and longer-lasting erection. In contrast to treatment with intracavernosal injection or vacuum aspiration, erection results from physiological erotic stimulation. Patients experience erection after Sildenafil intake as more natural and pleasurable than when the former techniques are used. Sildenafil has been reported successful in cases with either psychogenic impotence or organic causes, both vascular and neurogenic (98). So far, there have been no reports on treatment with this medication in men with renal failure or during dialysis.

Penile Prosthesis Due to concern about the patient's immunocompromised status, penile prostheses have not been recommended for patients on dialysis or for renal transplant recipients. However, a recent study indicates that penile prostheses can be successfully implanted without excessive risk of infection in patients with erectile dysfunction resulting from end-stage renal disease when other treatment modalities have failed (99).

2. Male Infertility

a. *Mechanisms of Male Infertility*

In male dialysis patients, spermatogenesis is impaired (75). Azoospermia, severe oligozoospermia, and decreased sperm viability are common. Especially when FSH is elevated, sperm deficiency is usually severe (63, 76). Maintenance hemodialysis has no effect, or it may exert a deleterious influence on sperm concentration (63,100,101). In these patients testicular histology shows hypospermatogenesis, maturation arrest, or germ cell aplasia (63,76). Also, the rete testis may present cystic transformation (102). Studies in rats suggest chronic renal failure to also have adverse effects on the overall sperm fertilizing capacity (103).

Many investigators believe that these defects represent primary gonadal damage by uremic toxins (80,104), probably via impairing the activity of the enzyme 17β-hydroxysteroid-dehydrogenase. A derangement of the peripheral conversion of steroids, however, cannot be excluded. Increased estradiol secretion by patients with renal failure has been described, and this may interfere with steroid biosynthesis. The coexistence of central neuroendocrine disorders in the regulation of gonadotropin secretion has been proposed (104).

b. *Treatment of Male Infertility*

After successful transplantation semen quality and testicular histology may show a striking improvement, sometimes reaching complete recovery of spermatogenesis (63,76) with restoration of fertility (76,101,105). Cyclosporin A does not seem to adversely affect fertility in renal transplant patients (106).

Studies on zinc therapy give contradictory results, and it may (79) or may not cause significant improvement in sperm characteristics (81).

Stimulation of Leydig cell function by human chorionic gonadoropin (hCG) during 4 months did not improve fertility (107), neither were there any significant changes in sperm counts after pergolide administration (81). The effect of clomiphene citrate on spermatogenesis in dialysis patients is inconclusive because either improvement or deterioration may occur (108). This is similar to observations in men with idiopathic oligozoospermia and may be related to the combined antiestrogenic and slightly estrogenic activity of this drug. So far, there are no data on the use of the pure antiestrogen tamoxifen in the treatment of male infertility associated with renal failure.

Present-day assisted reproductive technology, especially in vitro fertilization (IVF) with intracytoplasmic sperm injection (ICSI), offers new hope for subfertile men with severely impaired semen quality.

B. Female

A detailed description of problems of women in dialysis is given in Chapter 40.

1. Female Sexual Dysfunction

Loss of sexual interest often is subjectively ascribed to fatigue and was also found in women on hemodialysis or peritoneal dialysis (50). Women on maintenance hemodialysis report a reduction in their sexual desire and the frequency of intercourse, and their ability to reach orgasm was found to be significantly decreased. Sexual activity ended at an earlier age compared to a control group (109). Patients with hyperprolactinemia reported lower frequencies of intercourse and fewer orgasms than normoprolactinemic ones (109).

2. Female Infertility

The major reproductive consequence of chronic renal failure in women on hemodialysis is a severe impairment in ovulatory function (110). The normal estradiol-stimulated LH surge does not occur, resulting in anovulation (75). Amenorrhea and other menstrual disturbances are common (104). Despite these hurdles to conception, women on dialysis can spontaneously conceive, and pregnancy has been reported in 1–7% of women on dialysis in survey studies (75).

3. Treatment of Female Sexual Dysfunction and Infertility

EPO therapy may improve sexual function (95) and restore menstruation (90,96). Recovery of fertility is a benefit of renal transplantion and should be included as a possible advantage in discussions with young women when choosing between dialysis and transplantation for the treatment of renal failure (111).

On the one hand, adequate counseling on contraception after transplantation is imperative in order to avoid unwanted pregnancies and to delay parenthood for at least 1 year (112). Premature delivery is a major problem in these patients and can be avoided by maintaining adequate graft function and controlling hypertension and infections (112). Follow-up of the post-transplant pregnancy indicated a significant increase in serum creatinine concentration from the prepregnancy level and that the long-term graft survival of those with a pregnancy was shorter than in the control patients (113). Ovarian hyperstimulation may precipitate renal failure (114) and must be avoided in these women.

Finally, some preliminary and anecdotal reports suggest that treatment with Sildenafil may facilitate the occurrence of orgasm in some anorgasmic women. Up to now, no studies are available on this subject in patients with renal failure.

C. The Roles of Hyperprolactinemia and Cortisol in Sexual Dysfunction and Infertility

1. Hyperprolactinemia

Hyperprolactinemia is a common finding in ESRD patients and has been considered an expression of the endocrine dysfunction of the hypothalamus (115). Also, reduced clearance of prolactin has been held responsible in these patients. Hemodialysis may or may not reduce prolactin levels, but renal transplantation does. Hyperprolactinemia affects sexual function of both males and females and causes menstrual and ovulatory disturbances.

Attempts to correct hyperprolactinemia by dopaminergic agents such as bromocryptine and lisuride have been reported to be less efficient among patients with ESRD than in other patients (83,116), but there is no published data on the use of the newest dopaminergic drug cabergoline. One of the problems caused by dopaminergic agents is the occurrence of hypotension, limiting their dosage particularly among patients on hemodialysis.

2. Cortisol

Cortisol is converted to cortisone by 17β-hydroxysteroid dehydrogenase, which presumably occurs in part in the liver, but the major site of conversion is the kidney (117). The enzyme appears to reside mainly in the proximal convoluted tube and pars recta, and plasma cortisone concentration and the urinary excretion of cortisone metabolites progressively decrease with increasing renal impairment. Renal failure has, however, little effect on plasma cortisol levels, provided these are measured by highly specific assays. Indeed, retained cortisol metabolites may interfere with some of the older radioimmunoassays, yielding falsely elevated values in serum (118).

REFERENCES

1. Blum WF. Insulin-like growth factors (IGFs) and IGF binding proteins in chronic renal failure: evidence for reduced secretion of IGFs. Acta Paediatr Scand 1991; 79(suppl 3):24–31.
2. Blum WF, Ranke MB, Kietzmann K, Tonshoff B, Metils O. Growth hormone resistance and inhibition of somatomedin activity by excess of insulin-like growth factor binding protein in uremia. Pediatr Nephrol 1991; 5:539–544.
3. Santos F, Orejas G, Rey C, Garcia Vicente S, Malagas S. Growth hormone metabolism in uremia. Child Nephrol Urol 1991; 11:130–133.
4. Tonshoff B, Cronin MJ, Reicbert M, Haffner D, Wingen AM, Blum WF, Mehls O, Ratsch I, Michelis KK, Kapogiannis T, Lennert T, Jun GF, Gellert S, Tulassay T, Sallay P, Von Lilien T, Querfeld U, Von Wendt Goknur MA, Bonzel KE. Reduced concentration of serum growth hormone (GH)- binding protein in children with chronic renal failure: correlation with GH insensitivity. J Clin Endocrinol Metabol 1997; 82:1007–1013.
5. Flyvbjerg A. The growth hormone/insulin-like growth factor axis in the kidney: aspects in relation to chronic renal failure. J Pediatr Endocrinol 1994; 7:85–92.
6. Castellano M, Turconi A, Chaler E, Maceiras M, Rivarola MA, Belgorosky A. Thyroid function and serum thyroid binding proteins in prepubertal and pubertal children with chronic renal insufficiency receiving conservative treatment, undergoing hemodialysis, or receiving care after renal transplantation. J Pediatr 1996; 128:784–790.
7. Medri G, Carella C, Padmanabhan V, Rossi CM, Amato G, De Santo NG, Beitins IZ, Beck-Peccoz P. Pituitary glycoprotein hormones in chronic renal failure: evidence for an uncontrolled alpha-subunit release. J Endocrinol Invest 1993; 16:169–174.
8. Kaptein EM. Thyroid hormone metabolism and thyroid diseases in chronic renal failure. Endocr Rev 1996; 17:45–63.
9. Beckers C, Machiels J, Soyez C, Cornette C. Metabolic clearance rate and production rate of thyroid stimulating hormone in man. Horm Metab Res 1971; 3:34–40.
10. Bartalena L, Pacchiarotti A, Palla R, Antonangeli L, Mammoli C, Monzani F, De Negri F, Panichi V, Mar-

tino E, Baschieri L, Pinchera A. Lack of nocturnal serum thyrotropin (TSH) surge in patients with chronic renal failure undergoing regular maintenance hemofiltration: a case of central hypothyroidism. Clin Nephrol 1990; 34:30–34.

11. Wheatley T, Clark PM, Clark JD, Holder R, Raggatt PR, Evans DB. Abnormalities of thyrotrophin (TSH) evening rise and pulsatile release in haemodialysis patients: evidence for hypothalamic- pituitary changes in chronic renal failure. Clin Endocrinol (Oxf) 1989; 31: 39–50.
12. Czernichow P, Dauzet MC, Boyer M, Rappaport R. Abnormal TSH, PRL, and GH response to TSH releasing factor in chronic renal failure. J Clin Endocrinol Metab 1976; 43:630–637.
13. Lim SL, Fang VS, Katz AI, Refetoff S. Thyroid dysfunction in chronic renal failure: a study of the pituitary-thyroid axis and peripheral turnover kinetics of thyroxine and triiodothyronine. J Clin Invest 1977; 60: 522–534.
14. Ramirez G, O'Neill W, Jubiz W, Bloomer HA. Thyroid dysfunction in uremia: evidence for thyroid and hypophyseal abnormalities. Ann Intern Med 1976; 84: 672–676.
15. Ramirez G, Bittle PA, Sanders H, Bercu BB. Hypothalamo-hypophyseal thyroid and gonadal function before and after erythropoietin therapy in dialysis patients. J Clin Endocrinol Metab 1992; 74:517–524.
16. Hardy MJ, Ragbeer SS, Nascimento L. Pituitary-thyroid function in chronic renal failure assessed by a highly sensitive thyrotropin assay. J Clin Endocrinol Metab 1988; 66:233–236.
17. Kaptein EM, Quion-Verde H, Chooljian CJ, Tang WW, Friedman PE, Rodriquez HJ, Massry SG. The thyroid in end-stage renal disease. Medicine (Baltimore) 1988; 67:187–197.
18. Spencer CA, Eigen A, Shen D, Duda M, Qualls S, Weiss S, Nicoloff JT. Specificity of sensitive assays of thyrotropin (TSH) used to screen for thyroid disease in hospitalized patients. Clin Chem 1991; 33:1391–1396.
19. Brent GA, Hershman JM. Thyroxine therapy in patients with severe nonthyroidal illnesses and low serum thyroxine concentration. J Clin Endocrinol Metab 1986; 63:1–8.
20. Hamblin PS, Dyer SA, Mohr VS, Le Grand BA, Lim CF, Tuxen DV, Topliss DJ, Stockigt JR. Relationship between thyrotropin and thyroxine changes during recovery from severe hypothyroxinemia of critical illness. J Clin Endocrinol Metab 1986; 62:717–722.
21. Docter R, Krenning EP, de Jong M, Hennemann G. The sick euthyroid syndrome: changes in thyroid hormone serum parameters and hormone metabolism. Clin Endocrinol (Oxf) 1993; 39:499–518.
22. Spencer CA, LoPresti JS, Patel A, Guttler RB, Eigen AD, Shen, Gray D, Nicoloff JT. Applications of a new chemiluminometric thyrotropin assay to subnormal measurement. J Clin Endocrinol Metab 1990; 70:453–460.
23. Kaptein EM. Thyroid hormone metabolism in illness. In: G Hennemann, ed. Thyroid Hormone Metabolism. New York: Marcel-Dekker, 1986:297–333.
24. Hershman JM, Krugman LG, Kopple JD, Reed AW, Azukizawa M, Shinaberger JH. Thyroid function in patients undergoing maintenance hemodialysis: unexplained low serum thyroxine concentration. Metabolism 1978; 27:755–759.
25. Kaptein EM, Feinstein EI, Nicoloff JT, Massry SG. Serum reverse triiodothyronine and thyroxine kinetics in patients with chronic renal failure. J Clin Endocrinol Metab 1983; 57:181–189.
26. Neuhaus K, Baumann G, Walser A, Thoen H. Serum thyroxine, thyroxine-binding proteins in chronic renal failure without nephrosis. J Clin Endocrinol Metab 1975; 41:395–398.
27. Sakurai S, Hara Y, Miura S, Urabe M, Inoue K, Tanikawa T, Yanagisawa M, Iltaka M, Ishii J. Thyroid function before and after maintenance hemodialysis in patients with chronic renal failure. Endocrinol Jpn 1988; 35:865–876.
28. Boelen A, Schiphorst PT MC, Wiersinga WM. Association between serum interleukin-6 and serum 3,5,3′-triiodothyronine in nonthyroidal illness. J Clin Endocrinol Metab 1993; 77:1695–1699.
29. Liewendahl K, Tikanoja S, Mahonen H, Helenius T, Valimaki M, Tallgren LG. Concentrations of iodothyronine in serum of patients with chronic renal failure and other nonthyroidal illnesses; role of free fatty acids. Clin Chem 1987; 33:1382–1386.
30. Lim CF, Bernard BF, de Jong M, Docter R, Krenning EP, Hennemann G. A furan fatty acid and indoxyl sulfate are the putative inhibitors of thyroxine hepatocyte transport in uremia. J Clin Endocrinol Metab 1993; 76:318–324.
31. Pereira BJG, Shapiro L, King AJ, Falagas ME, Strom JA, Dinarella CA. Plasma levels of IL-1B, TNFa and their specific inhibitors in undialyzed chronic renal failure, CAPD and hemodialysis patients. Kidney Int 1994; 45:890–896.
32. Brodersen HP, Korsten FW, Esser PW, Korlings K, Holtkamp W, Larbig D. Release of thyroid hormones from protein-binding sites by low-molecular-weight heparin in hemodialysis patients. Nephron 1997; 75: 366–367.
33. Munro SL, Lim CF, Hall JG, Barlow JW, Craik DJ, Topliss DJ, Stockigt JR. Drug competition for thyroxine binding to transthyretin (prealbumin): comparison with effects on thyroxine-binding globulin. J Clin Endocrinol Metab 1989; 68:1141–1147.
34. Robey C, Schreedhar K, Batuman V. Effects of chronic peritoneal dialysis on thyroid function tests. Am J Kidney Dis 1989; 13:99–103.

35. Faber J, Heaf J, Kirkegaard C, Lumholtz IB, Siersbaek-Nielsen K, Kolendorf K, Friis T. Simultaneous turnover studies of thyroxine 3,5,3′-triiodothyronine, 3,5-, 3,3′- and 3′,5′-diiothyronine, and 3′-monoiodothyronine in chronic renal failure. J Clin Endocrinol Metab 1983; 56:211–217.
36. Kaptein EM. Clinical application of free thyroxine determinations. Clin Lab Med 1993; 13:653–672.
37. Kaptein EM. Thyroid in vitro testing in non-thyroidc illness. Exp Clin Endocrinol 1994; 102:92–101.
37. Melmed S, Geola FL, Reed AW, Pekary AE, Park J, Hershman JM. A comparison of methods for assessing thyroid function in nonthyroidal illness. J Clin Endocrinol Metab 1982; 54:300–306.
38. Oppenheimer JH, Schwartz HL, Mariash CN, Kaiser FE. Evidence for a factor in the sera of patients with nonthyroidal disease which inhibitis iodothyronine binding by solid matrices, serum proteins, and rat hepatocytes. J Clin Endocrinol Metab 1982; 54:757–766.
39. Nelson JC, Wilcox RB, Pandian MR. Dependence of free thyroxine estimates obtained with equilibrium tracer dialysis on the concentration of thyroxine-binding globulin. Clin Chem 1992; 38:1294–1300.
40. Nelson JC, Wiss RM, Wilcox RB. Underestimates of serum free thyroxine (T_4) concentrations by free T_4 immunoassays. J Clin Endocrinol Metab 1994; 79:76–79.
41. Spector DA, Davis PJ, Helderman JH, Bell B, Utiger RD. Thyroid function and metabolic state in chronic renal failure. Ann Intern Med 1976; 85:724–730.
42. Williams GR, Franklyn JA, Neuberger JM, Sheppard MC. Thyroid hormone receptor expression in the "sick euthyroid" syndrome. Lancet 1998; 2:1477–1481.
43. Okabayashi T, Takeda K, Kawada M, Kubo Y, Nakamura S, Chikamori K, Terao N, Hashimoto K. Free thyroxine concentrations in serum measured by equilibrium dialysis in chronic renal failure. Clin Chem 1996; 42:1616–1620.
44. Lim VS, Flanigan MJ, Zavala DC, Freeman RM. Protective adaptation of low serum triiodothyronine in patients with chronic renal failure. Kidney Int 1985; 28: 541–549.
45. Pagliacci MC, Pelicci G, Grignani F, Giammartino C, Fedeli L, Carobi C, Buoncristiani U, Nicoletti I. Thyroid function tests in patients undergoing maintenance dialysis: characterization of the "low-T_4 syndrome" in subjects on regular hemodialysis and continuous abulatory peritoneal dialysis. Nephron 1987; 46:225–230.
46. Ross RJM, Goodwin FJ, Houghton BJ, Boucher BJ. Alteration of pituitary-thyroid function in patients with chronic renal failure treated by haemodialysis or continuous ambulatory peritoneal dialysis. Ann Clin Biochem 1985; 22:156–160.
47. Seyrek N, Paydas S, Sagliker Y. Effect of erythropoietin administration on thyroid functions of the patients undergoing regular hemodialysis. Nephron 1996; 72: 714–715.
48. Arreola F, Paniagua R, Perez A, Diaz-Bensussen S, Junco E, Villalpando S, Exaire E. Effect of zinc treatment on serum thyroid hormones in uremic patients under peritoneal dialysis. Horm Metab Res 1993; 25: 539–542.
49. Beckers C, van Ypersele de Strihou C, Coche E, Troch R, Malvaux P. Iodine metabolism in severe renal insufficiency. J Clin Endocrinol Metab 1969; 29:293–296.
50. Toorians AW, Janssen E, Laan E, Gooren LJ, Giltay EJ, Oe PL, Donker AJ, Everaerd W. Chronic renal failure and sexual functioning: clinical status versus objectively assessed sexual response. Nephrol Dial Transplant 1997; 12:2654–2663.
51. Abram HS, Hester LR, Sheridan WF, Epstein GM. Sexual functioning in patients with chronic renal failure. J Nerv Ment Dis 1975; 160:220–226.
52. Lye WC, Chan PS, Leong SO, van der Straaten JC. Psychosocial and psychiatric morbidity in patients on CAPD. Adv Perit Dial 1997; 13:134–136.
53. Rodger RS, Fletcher K, Dewar JH, Genner D, McHugh M, Wilkinson R, Ward MK, Kerr DN. Prevalence and pathogenesis of impotence in one hundred uremic men. Uremia Invest 1984; 8:89–96.
54. Rodriguez Rodriguez R, Burgos Revilla FJ, Gomez Dosantos V, Galbis Sanjuan F, Navarro Antolin J, Allona Almagro A, Orofino Azcue L. Endocrine changes and sexual dysfunction in kidney transplantation and hemodialysis: comparative study. Actas Urol Esp 1996; 20:697–701.
55. Procci WR, Goldstein DA, Adelstein J, Massry SG. Sexual dysfunction in the male patient with uremia: a reappraisal. Kidney Int 1981; 19:317–323.
56. Procci WR, Martin DJ. Effect of maintenance hemodialysis on male sexual performance. J Nerv Ment Dis 1985; 173:366–372.
57. Feldman HA, Goldstein I, Hatzichristou DG, Krane RJ, McKinlay JB. Impotence and its medical and psychosocial correlates: results of the Massachusetts Male Aging Study. J Urol 1994; 151:54–61.
59. Nghiem DD, Corry RJ, Mendez GP, Lee HM. Pelvic hemodynamics and male sexual impotence after renal transplantation. Am Surg 1982; 48:532–535.
60. Steele TE, Wuerth D, Finkelstein S, Juergensen D, Juergensen P, Kliger AS, Finkelstein FO. Sexual experience of the chronic peritoneal dialysis patient. J Am Soc Nephrol 1996; 7:1165–1168.
61. Glass CA, Fielding DM, Evans C, Ashcroft JB. Factors related to sexual functioning in male patients undergoing hemodialysis and with kidney transplants. Arch Sex Behav 1987; 16:189–207.
62. Foulks CJ, Cushner HM. Sexual dysfunction in the

male dialysis patient: pathogenesis, evaluation, and therapy. Am J Kidney Dis 1986; 8:211–222.

63. Mastrogiacomo I, De Besi L, Zucchetta P, Serafini E, Gasparotto ML, Marchini P, Pisani E, Dean P, Chini M. Effect of hyperprolactinemia and age on the hypogonadism of uremic men on hemodialysis. Arch Androl 1984; 12:235–242.
63. Lim VS, Fang VS. Gonadal dysfunction in uremic men. A study of the hypothalamo- pituitary- testicular axis before and after renal transplantation. Am J Med 1975; 58:655–662.
64. Semple CG, Beastall GH, Henderson IS, Thomson JA, Kennedy AC. The pituitary-testicular axis of uraemic subjects on haemodialysis and continuous ambulatory peritoneal dialysis. Acta Endocrinol (Copenh) 1982; 101:464–467.
65. Mastrogiacomo I, De Besi L, Zucchetta P, Serafini E, La Greca G, Gasparotto ML, Lorenzi S, Dean P. Male hypogonadism of uremic patients on hemodialysis. Arch Androl 1988; 20:171–175.
66. Gura V, Weizman A, Maoz B, Zevin D, Ben-David M. Hyperprolactinemia: a possible cause of sexual impotence in male patients undergoing chronic hemodialysis. Nephron 1980; 26:53–54.
67. Joven J, Villabona C, Rubies-Prat J, Espinel E, Galard R. Hormonal profile and serum zinc levels in uraemic men with gonadal dysfunction undergoing haemodialysis. Clin Chim Acta 1985; 148:239–245.
68. Akmal M, Goldstein DA, Kletzky OA, Massry SG. Hyperparathyroidism and hypotestosteronemia of acute renal failure. Am J Nephrol 1988; 8:166–169.
69. Fioretti P, Melis GB, Ciardella F, Barsotti G, Orlandi MC, Paoletti AM, Giovannetti S. Parathyroid function and pituitary-gonadal axis in male uremics; effects of dietary treatment and of maintenance hemodialysis. Clin Nephrol 1986; 25:155–158.
70. Kaufman JM, Hatzichristou DG, Mulhall JP, Fitch WP, Goldstein I. Impotence and chronic renal failure: a study of the hemodynamic pathophysiology. J Urol 1994; 151:612–618.
71. Bansal S. Sexual dysfunction in hypertensive men. A critical review of the literature. Hypertension 1988; 12:1–10.
72. Campese VM, Procci WR, Levitan D, Romoff MS, Goldstein DA, Massry SG. Autonomic nervous system dysfunction and impotence in uremia. Am J Nephrol 1982; 2:140–143.
73. Sherman FP. Impotence in patients with chronic renal failure on dialysis: its frequency and etiology. Fertil Steril 1975; 26:221–223.
74. Berkman AH, Katz LA, Weissman R. Sexuality and the life-style of home dialysis patients. Arch Phys Med Rehabil 1982; 63:272–275.
75. Schmidt RJ, Holley JL. Fertility and contraception in end-stage renal disease. Adv Ren Replace Ther 1998; 5:38–44.
76. Prem AR, Punekar SV, Kalpana M, Kelkar AR, Acharya VN. Male reproductive function in uraemia: efficacy of haemodialysis and renal transplantation. Br J Urol 1996; 78:635–638.
77. de Vries CP, Gooren LJ, Oe PL. Haemodialysis and testicular function. Int J Androl 1984; 7:97–103.
78. Peces R, Horcajada C, Lopez-Novoa JM, Frutos MA, Casado S, Hernando L. Hyperprolactinemia in chronic renal failure: impaired responsiveness to stimulation and suppression. Normalization after transplantation. Nephron 1981; 28:11–16.
79. Mahajan SK, Abbasi AA, Prasad AS, Rabbani P, Briggs WA, McDonald FD. Effect of oral zinc therapy on gonadal function in hemodialysis patients. A double-blind study. Ann Intern Med 1982; 97:357–361.
80. Mahajan SK, Prasad AS, McDonald FD. Sexual dysfunction in uremic male: improvement following oral zinc supplementation. Contrib Nephrol 1984; 38:103–111.
81. Rodger RS, Sheldon WL, Watson MJ, Dewar JH, Wilkinson R, Ward MK, Kerr DN. Zinc deficiency and hyperprolactinaemia are not reversible causes of sexual dysfunction in uraemia. Nephrol Dial Transplant 1989; 4:888–892.
82. Ramirez G, Butcher DE, Newton JL, Brueggemeyer CD, Moon J, Gomez-Sanchez C. Bromocriptine and the hypothalamic hypophyseal function in patients with chronic renal failure on chronic hemodialysis. Am J Kidney Dis 1985; 6:111–118.
83. Muir JW, Besser GM, Edwards CR, Rees LH, Cattell WR, Ackrill P, Baker LR. Bromocriptine improves reduced libido and potency in men receiving maintenance hemodialysis. Clin Nephrol 1983; 20:308–314.
84. Lawrence IG, Price DE, Howlett TA, Harris KP, Feehally J, Walls J. Correcting impotence in the male dialysis patient: experience with testosterone replacement and vacuum tumescence therapy. Am J Kidney Dis 1998; 31:313–319.
85. Soliman G, Oreopoulos DG. Anabolic steroids and malnutrition in chronic renal failure. Perit Dial Int 1994; 14:362–365.
86. Mansi MK, Alkhudair WK, Huraib S. Treatment of erectile dysfunction after kidney transplantation with intracavernosal self-injection of prostaglandin E1. J Urol 1998; 159:1927–1930.
87. Levin NW. Quality of life and hematocrit level. Am J Kidney Dis 1992; 20:16–20.
88. Sobh MA, Abd el Hamid IA, Atta MG, Refaie AF. Effect of erythropoietin on sexual potency in chronic haemodialysis patients. A preliminary study. Scand J Urol Nephrol 1992; 26:181–185.
89. Trembecki J, Kokot F, Wiecek A, Marcinkowski W, Rudka R. Improvement of sexual function in hemodialyzed male patients with chronic renal failure treated with erythropoietin (rHuEPO). Przegl Lek 1995; 52:462–466.

90. Yeksan M, Tamer N, Cirit M, Turk S, Akhan G, Akkus I, Erkul I. Effect of recombinant human erythropoietin (r-HuEPO) therapy on plasma FT3, FT4, TSH, FSH, LH, free testosterone and prolactin levels in hemodialysis patients. Int J Artif Organs 1992; 15:585–589.
91. Beusterien KM, Nissenson AR, Port FK, Kelly M, Steinwald B, Ware JEJ. The effects of recombinant human erythropoietin on functional health and well-being in chronic dialysis patients. J Am Soc Nephrol 1996; 7:763–773.
92. Suzuki H, Murakami M, Ichihara A, Saruta T. Alterations in sex hormones and sexual function of patients with renal failure treated with recombinant human erythropoietin. Nippon Jinzo Gakkai Shi 1992; 34:79–84.
93. Lawrence IG, Price DE, Howlett TA, Harris KP, Feehally J, Walls J. Erythropoietin and sexual dysfunction. Nephrol Dial Transplant 1997; 12:741–747.
94. Foresta C, Mioni R, Bordon P, Miotto D, Montini G, Varotto A. Erythropoietin stimulates testosterone production in man. J Clin Endocrinol Metab 1994; 78: 753–756.
95. Schaefer RM, Kokot F, Wernze H, Geiger H, Heidland A. Improved sexual function in hemodialysis patients on recombinant erythropoietin: a possible role for prolactin. Clin Nephrol 1989; 31:1–5.
96. Schaefer RM, Kokot F, Kuerner B, Zech M, Heidland A. Normalization of serum prolactin levels in hemodialysis patients on recombinant human erythropoietin. Int J Artif Organs 1989; 12:445–449.
97. Tsai TJ, Lai JS, Lee SH, Chen YM, Lan C, Yang BJ, Chiang HS. Breathing-coordinated exercise improves the quality of life in hemodialysis patients. J Am Soc Nephrol 1995; 6:1392–1400.
98. Goldstein I, Lue TF, Padma-Nathan H, Rosen RC, Steers WD, Wicker PA. Oral sildenafil in the treatment of erectile dysfunction. Sildenafil Study Group. N Engl J Med 1998; 338:1397–1404.
99. Ahuja SK, Krane NK, Hellstrom WJ. Penile prostheses in the management of impotence in patients with end- stage renal disease. J La State Med Soc 1998; 150:32–34.
100. Tourkantonis A, Spiliopoulos A, Pharmakiotis A, Settas L. Haemodialysis and hypothalamo-pituitary-testicular axis. Nephron 1981; 27:271–272.
101. Holdsworth SR, de Kretser DM, Atkins RC. A comparison of hemodialysis and transplantation in reversing the uremic disturbance of male reproductive function. Clin Nephrol 1978; 10:146–150.
102. Nistal M, Santamaria L, Paniagua R. Acquired cystic transformation of the rete testis secondary to renal failure. Human Pathol 1989; 20:1065–1070.
103. Yamamoto Y, Sofikitis N, Miyagawa I. Effects of chronic renal failure on the sperm fertilizing capacity. Urol Int 1997; 58:105–107.
104. Lim VS. Reproductive function in patients with renal insufficiency. Am J Kidney Dis 1987; 9:363–367.
105. Phadke AG, MacKinnon KJ, Dossetor JB. Male fertility in uremia: restoration by renal allografts. Can Med Assoc J 1970; 102:607–608.
106. Haberman J, Karwa G, Greenstein SM, Soberman R, Glicklich D, Tellis V, Melman A. Male fertility in cyclosporine-treated renal transplant patients. J Urol 1991; 145:294–296.
107. Bundschu HD, Rager K, Heller S, Hayduk K, Pfeiffer EH, Luders G, Liebau G. Effects of longterm HCG administration on testicular function in hemodialysis patients. Klin Wochenschr 1976; 54:1039–1046.
108. Lim VS, Fang VS. Restoration of plasma testosterone levels in uremic men with clomiphene citrate. J Clin Endocrinol Metab 1976; 43:1370–1377.
109. Mastrogiacomo I, De Besi L, Serafini E, Zussa S, Zucchetta P, Romagnoli GF, Saporiti E, Dean P, Ronco C, Adami A. Hyperprolactinemia and sexual disturbances among uremic women on hemodialysis. Nephron 1984; 37:195–199.
110. Mantouvalos H, Metallinos C, Makrygiannakis A, Gouskos A. Sex hormones in women on hemodialysis. Int J Gynaecol Obstet 1984; 22:367–370.
111. Hou S. Pregnancy in organ transplant recipients. Med Clin North Am 1989; 73:667–683.
112. Rager K, Bundschu H, Gupta D. The effect of HCG on testicular androgen production in adult men with chronic renal failure. J Reprod Fertil 1975; 42:113–120.
113. Salmela KT, Kyllonen LE, Holmberg C, Gronhagen-Riska C. Impaired renal function after pregnancy in renal transplant recipients. Transplantation 1993; 56: 1372–1375.
114. Elchalal U, Schenker JG. The pathophysiology of ovarian hyperstimulation syndrome—views and ideas. Human Reprod 1997; 12:1129–1137.
115. Handelsman D. Hypothalamic-pituitary gonadal dysfunction in renal failure, dialysis and renal transplantation. Endocr Rev 1985; 6:151–182.
116. Ruilope L, Garcia-Robles R, Paya C, deVilla L, Miranda B, Morales J, Sanch J, Ridicio J. Influence of lisuride, a dopaminergic agonist, on sexual function of male patients with chronic renal failure. Am J Kidney Dis 1985; 3:182–185.
117. Witworth JA, Stewart PM, Burt D, Atherden SM, Edwards CR. The kidney is the major site of cortisone production in man. Clin Endocr 1989; 31:355–361.
118. Ramirez G, Gomez-Sanchez C, Meikle AW, Jubiz W. Evaluation of hypophyseal adrenal axis in patients receiving long term hemodialysis. Arch Intern Med 1982; 142:1448–1452.

25

Dermatological Problems in Dialysis Patients, Including Calciphylaxis

Jean Marie Naeyaert and Hilde Beele
University Hospital of Gent, Gent, Belgium

I. INTRODUCTION

Skin changes are present in numerous patients undergoing maintenance hemodialysis. The findings of Lubach (1) indicate that up to 78% of 64 German patients had some skin changes and more than 50% had hair and/or nail changes (Table I).

This chapter is not intended as an encyclopedic review of all possibly described cutaneous changes in hemodialysis patients. Emphasis is put on the description of cutaneous disorders that are most frequently encountered by the attending physician. Several reviews of cutaneous abnormalities in patients with chronic renal failure have been published (1–3).

II. COLOR CHANGES

The skin of end-stage chronic renal failure (CRF) patients is pale gray or yellow-brown, depending on the skin phototype present before onset of the renal disease. Anemia and urochrome pigment depositions are responsible for this color change (4).

In patients with frank hyperpigmentation, increased levels of poorly dialyzable β-melanocyte–stimulating hormone (β-MSH) have been observed. β-MSH stimulates melanogenesis, leading to increased melanin deposition adding to the already present urochrome pigment deposits (5). Hemosiderosis is also a rare cause for hyperpigmentation in this patient group.

Only two cases of diffuse hypopigmentation have been reported (4,6). A disturbed phenylalanine metabolism was postulated to be important in the pathogenesis.

III. PRURITUS

A. Definition

Itch is defined as the sensation that provokes the desire to scratch. It is a cardinal symptom in many dermatoses. A large number of patients, however, present with itch and no visible skin lesions other than those produced by scratching. This phenomenon, called pruritus, may be a manifestation of numerous systemic disorders. Chronic renal failure, especially when treated with dialysis, is currently the most prevalent underlying systemic disease. Other disorders associated with pruritus are obstructive biliary disease, myeloproliferative disorders (e.g., polycythemia vera, Hodgkin's disease), iron deficency, endocrine disorders, and visceral malignancies (7).

The neurophysiology of pruritus is still poorly understood. Itch and pain sensations are carried along similar pathways: the sensation of itch begins at the free, unmyelinated nerve endings that serve as receptors for different stimuli. The sensation then goes along unmyelinated C fibers, which enter the spinal cord via the dorsal root ganglia and ascend in the spinothalamic tracts. Itch cannot be elicited in regions or subjects insensitive to pain. It is known that the sensation of itch is modified by central processing. Up until now, the

Table 1 Skin, Hair, and Nail Changes in Patients (n = 64) with Chronic Renal Failure Under Maintenance Hemodialysis

Location	Change	Percent
Skin	Hyperpigmentation	78
	Dry skin	73
	Pruritus	67
	Pseudo porphyria cutanea tarda	5
Hair	Hypotrichosis (of trunk, axillae, and/or pubis)	61
	Dry and/or fragile hair	39
	Hair loss (diffuse)	33
Nails	Subungual erythema (including half-and-half nails)	56
	Nail plate fragility	55
	Flattened nails (platonychia)	44
	Spoon nails (koilonychia)	11

Source: Adapted from Ref. 1.

details of this mechanism have not been clearly understood.

Histamine is the classic mediator of itch. Hence, antihistamines are often prescribed in the treatment of itching disorders. On the other hand, antihistamines are not always effective in reducing pruritus. Other molecules such as kallikrein, substance P, serotonin, prostaglandins, etc. may act as primary or potentiating mediators in the pathogenesis of itch (7–9).

B. Prevalence

Pruritus has been reported to be the most common cutaneous symptom in hemodialysis patients. Prevalence rates varying between 37% (10) and 85% (7,11,12) have been cited. The prevalence is higher in female patients on dialysis; patients with pruritus are older than those without (13). In general, the prevalence rates in hemodialysis patients are higher than those mentioned in renal failure in the predialysis era.

Some patients never complain of pruritus until hemodialysis is started (13), whereas others experience relief of their pruritus as soon as they are on hemodialysis. On the other hand, pruritus usually subsides when the patient is transplanted (14,15).

C. Pathophysiology

The pathophysiology of pruritus in patients on dialysis is still somewhat controversial. Abnormalities in calcium and phosphorus metabolism, e.g., hypercalcemia, hyperphosphatemia, raised calcium-phosphate product, and the deposition of calcium in the cutis, are considered to be important in the etio-pathogenesis of pruritus in hemodialysis patients. The relief of complaints experienced by some patients after (sub)total parathyroidectomy favors this hypothesis.

In 1979, Shmunes (16) suggested that hypervitaminosis A may also be related to the extent of the pruritus. Other factors that may be involved in the pathogenesis of pruritus are increased levels of magnesium within the skin, abnormalities in the function of the sweat glands, and the elevated levels of histamine found in uremic patients (17,18). Relief of pruritus and decrease in plasma histamine concentration were observed in a number of patients treated with erythropoietin (19).

Studies on the biocompatibility of components of dialytic circuits and of sterilizing methods (e.g., ethylene oxide) have suggested their possible role in the pathogenesis of intolerance phenomena, which could result in itching. Clinical studies, however, could not show any relationship between pruritus and possible allergens, as tested by patch tests. Therefore, the role of contact allergy in the pathogenesis of pruritus should be questioned (20).

Allergy to heparin has also been mentioned as a pathophysiological mechanism to explain pruritus. Although lesions occur quite often after subcutaneous administration of heparin, skin reactions and/or pruritus due to intravenous administration are very rare (21).

Serum concentrations of di (2-ethylhexyl) phthalate (DEHP), the most commonly used plasticizer in PVC hemodialysis tubings, and its metabolites have been measured in hemodialysis patients before and after hemodialysis. No immediate relationship to the occurrence or intensity of uremic pruritus could be demonstrated (22).

Xeroderma was observed in 73% of CAPD patients and in 72% of patients on hemodialysis. A positive correlation was found between xeroderma and the severity of pruritus, suggesting that xeroderma is important in eliciting pruritus (13). It has been shown that dialysis patients have drier skin than controls, especially patients on peritoneal dialysis. Moreover, pruritic patients had significantly lower hydration than nonpruritic patients (23).

In addition, most patients on hemodialysis take a number of drugs to treat the underlying disease or the complications of chronic renal failure and/or the dialysis treatment. Some of these drugs, such as captopril, indomethacin, nifedipin, prazosin, and ranitidin, may also enhance pruritus (24).

D. Clinical Presentation

The pruritus in chronic renal failure and hemodialysis usually occurs with nonspecific lesions. It is normally generalized but is highly variable in intensity and often paroxysmal (10,25,26).

E. Management

The management of pruritus in patients on hemodialysis relies on several treatment modalities:

1. Patient Education

The patient with itching should be taught that a number of factors may enhance his complaints. Dryness of the skin is probably the most important provoking factor. In a study where 21 patients with dry skin and pruritus were treated with regular emollient use, total disappearance of the itch was seen in 9 patients (23). Lowering the frequency of bathing (to once or twice a week), using bath oil and mild soaps, and the application of emollient creams, at least after bathing, reduce the dryness of the skin and may help to raise the threshold for pruritus. It is also important to keep the room temperature as low as possible and to encourage the use of humidifiers (27).

The patient should try to break the itch-scratch cycle. When the urge to scratch comes, it can be helpful to apply a cool washcloth or to exert pressure on the itching skin region (28). Wool and certain synthetic fabrics, such as polyester, are irritating in a large number of atopic patients, but also in any other patient with an itchy skin.

Increase in cutaneous blood flow enhances every itching condition. Heat, vigorous exercise, and certain foods can increase the blood flow in the skin. Therefore, patients should be taught to avoid overheating their environment and not to overdress, especially at night. They should not exaggerate with physical exercise, especially not on hot summer days. Hot foods, alcohol, and coffee should be avoided.

Stress may also worsen the problem of itch. On the other hand, pruritus has an important, often underestimated role in creating stress. Therefore, specialized help of psychiatrists, clinical psychologists, and social workers may also be useful in the management of pruritus. Dietary adaptations such as low-protein diets in patients with uremic pruritus may be helpful in some of them.

2. Topical Treatment

Whereas topical steroids can be very efficacious in the treatment of numerous itching dermatoses, there is no rationale for using steroid-containing ointments in the treatment of pruritus in hemodialysis patients. Menthol (0.25–2%), phenol (0.5–2%), and camphor (1–3%) may be added to a variety of vehicles for their antipruritic effects.

3. Oral or Intravenous Treatment

Antihistamines are usually ineffective for pruritus caused by systemic disorders, such as renal insufficiency and hemodialysis. The older antihistamines may be helpful because of their sedative effects.

Cholestyramine may be effective in relieving pruritus of renal origin. It presumably acts by binding and removing pruritogenic substances in the gut. Cholestyramine is not universally successful, and it may provoke gastrointestinal side effects (29).

Activated charcoal has been reported to be useful in the treatment of pruritus in patients on hemodialysis. Ten out of 11 patients treated in a double-blind crossover study improved upon treatment with 6 g of oral activated charcoal (30).

Intravenous administration of lidocaine during dialysis is effective in relieving pruritus for up to 24 hours, especially in patients who suffer from pruritus only during dialysis (15). This therapy, however, can cause serious hypotension and cardiac arrythmias.

Other treatments that have been mentioned to be beneficial in the treatment of pruritus in patients on dialysis are heparin (31), cimetidine (32), and lowering the magnesium content of the dialysate (33).

4. Phototherapy

Ultraviolet phototherapy with UVB irradiation is one of the most effective treatments in the control of pruritus related to renal disease, even in the presence of hyperparathyroidism (24,34). UVA, on the other hand, is not effective. Suberythemogenic doses of UVB exposure have to be given. Therapeutic benefit seems to be related to the number of treatment sessions. This results in a quicker response in patients treated with a higher frequency. Improvement usually commences after 4–6 UVB exposures (35). Seventeen out of 155 patients receiving long-term hemodialysis who were rated as having severe pruritus were randomly treated with either UVA or UVB phototherapy, which was administrated three times weekly before hemodialysis. Eight of the nine patients who received UVB phototherapy experienced a significant reduction, or even resolution of their pruritus, within 2 weeks. In contrast, long-wave UVA exposure did not have a significant effect.

The mechanism of action of UVB therapy is not completely clear at this moment. The finding of general improvement following treatment to only one side of the body suggests a systemic effect (10). Phototherapy may inactivate a circulating substance or substances that are responsible for the pruritus. A lowering of the phosphorus level of the skin in patients with pruritus and on hemodialysis treatment has been observed. In a healthy control population, the treatment with UVB radiation did not affect the mineral content of the skin (36).

5. Surgical Treatment (Parathyroidectomy)

In patients with secundary hyperparathyroidism, parathyroidectomy may result in a dramatic relief of itching within 24–48 hours. The results of this treatment are not invariable, and pruritus can recur when patients become hypercalcemic postoperatively (28,37).

IV. CUTANEOUS AGING AND CUTANEOUS MALIGNANCIES

Lesions associated with cutaneous aging have a high incidence in patients with end-stage renal failure on chronic hemodialysis. The large amount of toxins in uremic patients, a defective vitamin D metabolism, changes in the antioxidative homeostasis and failure of the immunosurveillance mechanism have all been mentioned to play a role in the pathogenesis of increased cutaneous aging in patients on hemodialysis (38,39).

Wrinkles are associated with actinic elastosis (40). Altmeyer et al. were the first to report a relation between the intensity of wrinkling and time on dialysis (41). In another study, the degree of wrinkling was related to age but also independently related to time on dialysis (42).

The overall incidence of senile purpura in a hemodialysis population is comparable to the incidence in elderly patients in the general population. In a study of 114 chronically dialyzed patients, the patients with senile purpura were significantly older than those without purpura. The mean age of patients with purpura, however, was lower than the age at which the disease normally appears. The authors suggest that the lower total protein plasma levels and the fragility of the capillaries in hemodialysis could be associated with this finding (42).

Actinic keratoses are seen more often in patients with hemodialysis compared to a control population. In general, actinic keratosis is associated with skin types I or II (43). In a hemodialysis population, however, multivariate analysis could not demonstrate a correlation between phototypes and actinic keratoses, nor between facial wrinkles and actinic keratoses. Moreover, the patients with actinic keratosis had been on hemodialysis for a longer period than patients without such lesions. These findings suggest that hemodialysis may play a distinct role in the development of actinic keratoses (42). Similar findings were reported by Anderson et al., who found an increased actinic damage in patients on hemodialysis in comparison to the general population (44).

The incidence of malignant neoplasms, including skin cancer, is increased in patients on hemodialysis, probably due to the relative immunosuppression (45,46). Recent data of Buccianti et al. showed that in patients on hemodialysis there is an increased risk for primary liver cancer, kidney cancer, thyroid cancer, lymphoma, and multiple myeloma. They did not find a statistically significant increase in skin cancer (47).

Basal cell carcinoma (Fig. 1) and especially squamous cell carcinoma are observed more frequently in every immunosuppressed population. The renal transplant patients are known to have an increased risk of developing skin cancer (48). In this group, the risk increases with the age of the patient, with the amount of previous UV exposure, and with the duration of immunosuppression. Up until now no clear relationship of basal skin carcinoma with the duration of hemodialysis has been demonstrated (42).

V. CONTACT DERMATITIS

A. Introduction

Contact dermatitis may be produced by primary irritants or allergic sensitizers. Primary irritant contact dermatitis is a nonallergic reaction to irritating substances applied on the skin. Any person would react to an irritant if the concentration and duration of the contact were sufficient. Irritants account for the majority of both occupational and nonoccupational contact reaction. Soaps, detergents, and most solvents are typical examples of mild irritants. Repeated and/or prolonged exposure to these products will produce erythema, microvesiculation, and oozing, which may be indistinguishable from allergic contact dermatitis. Chronic exposure results in dry, thickened, and often fissured skin.

Allergic contact dermatitis, on the other hand, is a manifestation of delayed hypersensitivity and is only seen in sensitized individuals who are exposed to the contact allergen. The inflammation proces is initiated by the binding of an allergen to an epidermal protein on or in the neighborhood of Langerhans cells to form a complete antigen. This antigen then reacts with sensitized T lymphocytes (type 4 reaction). These lym-

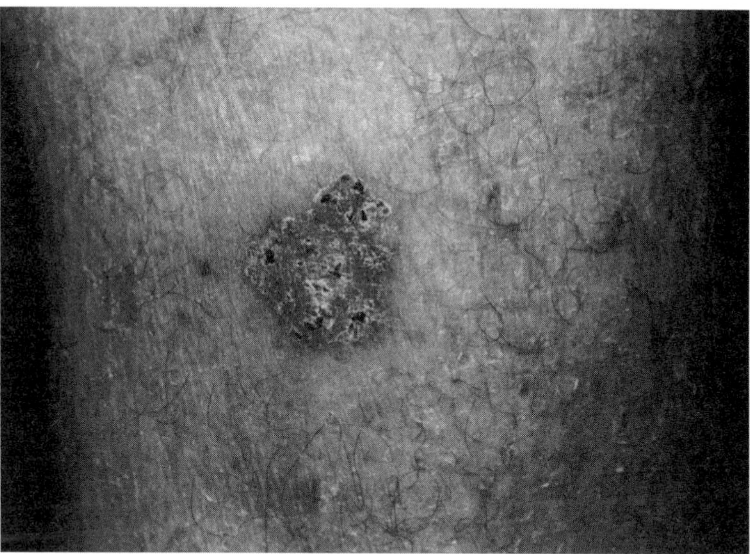

Fig. 1 Superficial basal cell carcinoma on dorsal side of forearm. The surrounding skin is atrophic with dry scaling.

phocytes release lymphokines such as IL-2, which attract an inflammatory infiltrate, consisting of macrophages, neutrophils, basophils, and eosinophils.

In trying to solve a case of suspected contact dermatitis, the patient should be questioned thoroughly about his or her total environment. Depending on the localization of the dermatitis, inquiry must be adapted.

In case of dermatitis at the site of the needle puncture, it is important to inquire as to the topicals used to wash or disinfect the region, the kind of needles used, the kind of gloves worn by the nurses, etc.

Patch testing for contact allergens is essential to identify the specific causative agents of an allergic contact dermatitis. Patch testing can be done with a standard battery containing the more frequently observed contact allergens. Next to this standard battery, it can be interesting to test the products that have been in contact with the skin region where the lesions developed.

On the other hand, there are no clinically useful methods available to evaluate in an objective way patients thought to have an irritant dermatitis. In these cases, history will be essential to identify the causative irritant.

B. Specific Examples of Contact Dermatitis in Hemodialyzed Patients

Using the methods of assessment as described above, some specific examples of contact dermatitis in hemodialyzed patients have been observed and described.

A number of patients suffered from an eczematous dermatitis around the site of the cannula injection. They were found to have a positive reaction for epoxy resin and for the glue used to fix the needle. The manufacturer of the glue used to fix the needles in this type of hemodialysis sets confirmed that the glue contained epoxy resin. Changing the dialysis set to another type not containing epoxy resin resulted in a clearing of the skin problems (49).

In 1976, Penneys and collegues (50) described the appearance of local and widespread dermatitis in four patients undergoing hemodialysis in one particular hemodialysis unit. Analogous problems were not observed in neighboring hemodialysis facilities. All 21 patients were tested, 8 of whom were found to have allergic contact sensitivity to thiuram compounds. These products are used primarily to accelerate the vulcanization of rubber. They are found in rubber but also in a number of fungicides and insecticides. Thirty-two control patients (treated in neighboring hemodialysis units) were also tested, but none were found to be sensitive to thiuram compounds. Thiuram-containing compounds were not used directly in the hemodialysis unit where the dermatitis problem arose. The authors suggested that the sensitization may have followed exposure of the patients, blood to dialysate that had been in contact with rubber-containing components of the dialysis machine (50).

A Dutch group described positive patch test to rubber chemicals (thiuram group and carba group) in a number of hemodialyzed patients who developed a subacute dermatitis of the area surrounding the arteriovenous fistula in the forearm. They suggested that the allergy might be caused by the intermittent contact of the fragile skin of these patients with the rubber gloves used by the nursing staff during the connection and disconnection of the bloodlines with the patients' circulation. However, they could not exclude the possibility that rubber chemicals, incorporated somewhere within the apparatus, dissolve into the extracorporal blood (51).

In 1980, the first report was published of a group of patients suffering from nausea, vomiting, headaches, and palpitation, but not skin lesions, after dialysis with a solution containing nickel leached from a nickel-plated water heater. The authors hypothesized that the systemic toxic reaction to nickel was due to the increased nickel plasma level. In 1984, Olerud and coworkers (53) showed with an in vitro experiment that nickel can be dialyzed into blood from a standard hemodialysis system and that plasma concentrations exceed those of the dialysate solution, even after one single pass of blood over the dialysis membrane. This finding can be explained by the plasma protein binding of nickel in the blood, a phenomenon described by Sunderman et al. (52). The group of Olerud also described the case of a 24-year-old woman who developed pruritic papules and vesicles on the face and the neck after her second treatment session with hemodialysis. She experienced the rash as very comparable with the eruption she previously had after wearing inexpensive jewelry. The rash became worse after each dialysis session, and the patient also developed pruritic lesions on the wrist and the fingers. The dialysis system was checked for potential sources of nickel contamination. The source of the nickel was a stainless steel fitting that came into contact with 6 N hydrochloride during dialysis. The metal fitting was removed from the dialysis system, after which the patient no longer experienced dermatitis (53).

It has also been seen in other situations that systemic contact with nickel can cause cutaneous lesions in a previously sensitized patient (54). Since the population of persons with cutaneous hypersensitivity to nickel is large, especially in females, it seems that the potential exists that presensitized patients are exposed to a subtoxic level of nickel through the dialysis system. When pruritus in uremic patients undergoing dialysis is associated with a dermatitis, distributed in a "jewelry dermatitis" fashion, the above-described cutaneous hypersensitivity to nickel should be considered.

Next to epoxy resin, thiuram compounds and nickel, antiseptic solutions used for disinfection and ethylene oxide used to sterilize membranes have been suggested as possible antigenic substances. In the case of ethylene oxide, it has been suggested that the molecule acts as a hapten and becomes a powerful immunogen after binding with certain proteins. Marshall et al., however, only observed 5 positive prick test results in a group of 86 dialyzed patients. In the study of Rollino et al. in a group of 107 dialysis patients with pruritus, no positive response was observed to membranes sterilized with ethylene oxide tested by patch tests (55).

Sensitization to components of topical medication is not uncommon. Not only the active product, but also components such as preservatives added to prevent bacterial contamination, may act as contact allergen. When an eruption is slow to disappear while being treated with a topical containing corticoids (which would seem to be the appropriate therapy), it is useful to consider the possibility of a contact sensitivity to topical corticosteroids (56).

C. Prevention and Therapy

Preventive measures are very important in the management of contact dermatitis. Once the causative agent of an allergic contact dermatitis is identified, the patient should try to avoid any contact with this agent and also with chemically related products. In the case of irritant dermatitis, it is often very difficult to find a single irritant. Therefore it is important to decrease exposure to household and work irritants, such as soaps, solvents, bleaches, etc. If the primary site of the dermatitis is localized on the hands, it is useful to wear vinyl or plastic gloves. Barrier protective creams and lubricating topicals can also be useful.

The treatment of active dermatitis lesions consists of cold wet dressings when the lesions are oozing. Wet dressings can be soaked with physiological or antiseptic solutions. After vesiculation and exsudation subsides, a topical corticosteroid will help. It is advisable to use a potent corticosteroid for a short time rather than a weaker one that is insufficient to clear the dermatosis. As soon as the active lesions diminish, the corticoids can be tapered carefully. Meanwhile, it is important not to wash the affected region and to use simple hydrating creams (e.g., ureum 5% in cold cream). Only in very severe and/or generalized cases may systemic treatment with corticoids be necessary.

VI. CALCIPHYLAXIS OR THE VASCULAR CALCIFICATION-CUTANEOUS NECROSIS SYNDROME

A. Introduction

Metastatic calcinosis is a common feature of chronic renal failure and results from an increased calcium phosphate product in serum. First described by Virchow in 1855, it is now recognized as being rather common in patients on long-term hemodialysis. The incidence is 20% in patients without hyperparathyroidism, 58% in patients with secondary hyperparathyroidism, and up to 75% in patients with autonomous tertiary hyperparathyroidism. Cutaneous necrosis secondary to metastatic calcification, however, is a rare event. Sixty-two cases have been published, among whom only 3 were children (57,58).

Many authors use the term calciphylaxis in a broad sense to describe the occurrence of cutaneous ulcerations with vascular calcification in a patient with renal failure. Others reserve this term for the most severe form of cutaneous metastatic calcinosis with calcification not limited to the vessels, but disseminated in the cutis and subcutis. This condition carries a mortality rate of about 50%, with death usually arising from secondary sepsis.

In a recent report from the Mayo Clinic, the term "vascular calcification—cutaneous necrosis syndrome (VCCNS)"(55) was proposed as an alternative for "calciphylaxis" (used in a broad sense). This descriptive nomenclature has the advantage of being clear and avoiding confusion. The male-to-female ratio of VCCNS is 1:2, indicating a clear predilection for women since chronic renal failure is more common in men.

B. Pathophysiology

The pathophysiology of vessel and tissue calcification in VCCNS is still unclear. In some cases of chronic renal failure, an elevated calcium-phosphorus product is formed due to secondary or tertiary hyperparathyroidism. Chronic renal insufficiency leads to lowered synthesis of 1,25-dihydroxycholecalciferol, with decreased absorption of calcium from the gut.

Hyperphosphatemia results from decreased renal clearance of phosphate. The resulting lowered serum calcium concentration stimulates the parathyroid gland to secrete parathyroid hormone (PTH), resulting in mobilization of calcium and phosphate from bone and decreased absorption of phosphate from the gut. The overall result is an elevated calcium-phosphate product that causes precipitation of hydroxyapatite crystals in vessel walls and interstitial skin tissue.

There are, however, many cases of VCCNS that have a normal calcium-phosphorus product, and not all patients with an elevated calcium-phosphorus product develop VCCNS. In these patients calciphylaxis as defined by Selye et al. is one of the proposed mechanisms (60). It is a condition of induced systemic hypersensitivity in which tissues respond with local calcification to appropriate challenging agents. Selye et al. performed their experiments in rats sensitized by feeding them a high-phosphate diet, by exogenous vitamin D, or by biochemically induced hyperparathyroidism. The challenging agent could be a metal salt or trauma, and subsequently extravascular calcification developed.

In reports from the last 7 years, attention has been focused on the possible role of coagulation disorders. Inspired by the clinical resemblance of VCCNS to warfarin-induced necrosis, Mehta et al. found lowered functional protein C levels in five patients with VCCNS (61). This could be an important pathogenic event. However, the fact that functional protein C levels remained low with healing of the ulcers suggests that still other factors are important. Kant et al. described two patients on CAPD who developed severe skin necrosis and who had protein S deficiency due to dialysate losses (62). Janigan et al. reported a patient in whom sepsis led to intravascular coagulation (63), and in a French report the presence of a circulating IgG-type anticoagulant molecule with antiprothrombinase activity in one patient was considered to be of importance (64). VCCNS has been described in two AIDS patients, and here also coagulation disorders could be promoting factors (65).

Dereure et al. proposed a framework for the pathogenesis of VCCNS (64). In chronic renal failure there is a high incidence of metastatic calcification of vessel walls. This would predispose these patients to vascular occlusion and/or thrombosis if aggravating factors are present. Coagulation disorders due to infection, dialysis itself, the causative disease of chronic renal failure, renal failure itself, and liver disease form one of those aggravating disorders. The other would be a direct action of PTH on cutaneous vessels with vasospasm and platelet microthrombi due to interaction with endothelial cells.

Although the pathophysiology of VCCNS remains incompletely understood, a growing body of evidence suggests that the pathogenesis is multifactorial.

C. Clinical Presentation

Clinically, VCCNS manifests itself as reticulated ecchymotic plaques on the buttocks, abdomen, and upper and lower extremities that become necrotic and ulcerate (Fig. 2). The lesions can be extremely painful. Characteristically, a livedoid pattern develops. Palpation reveals tender nodules. In severe cases, gangrene of the toes and fingers can develop.

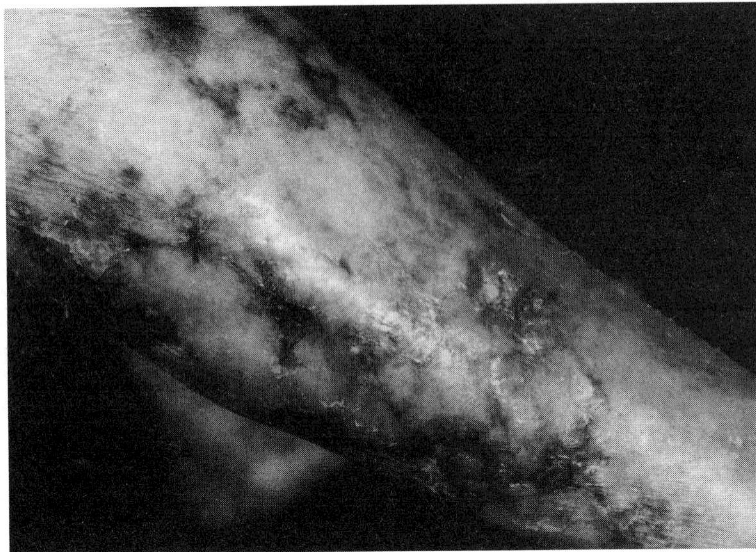

Fig. 2 Vascular calcification-cutaneous necrosis syndrome (VCCNS): livedoid pattern of ecchymotic plaques on lower leg with ulceration.

In many cases, routine radiographies are not sufficiently sensitive to detect calcification of cutaneous vessels, but xeroradiography has been reported to reveal calcification of cutaneous arterioles in patients with VCCNS (66).

D. Pathology

Histologically, a mural calcification of dermal and subcutaneous arterioles and arteries is observed and some vessels are secondarily occluded. Fibrin thrombi can be present in venules. The end result is ischemia with infarction of the skin. Inflammatory changes are usually lacking and in severe cases a stromal calcification is present in dermal and subcutaneous tissues. In some patients a pseudoxanthoma elasticum-like picture is present due to clumping and calcification of elastic fibers (67). A Von Kossa stain is particularly well suited to demonstrate calcium salts as black deposits.

E. Differential Diagnosis

The differential diagnosis includes vasculitis, pyoderma gangraenosum, septic emboli, and warfarin-induced necrosis. Most of these entities can be ruled out by histology. Biopsies should preferably be performed at the edge of and not in an ulcerated area.

F. Therapy

Therapy is difficult and primarily supportive. Obvious biochemical abnormalities will be corrected (uremia, hypercalcemia, hyperphosphataemia, hyperparathyroidism) but will not always result in clinical amelioration, and healing can occur in spite of persisting abnormal values. Parathyroidectomy has given excellent results in some but certainly not all reported patients (57,59,68). Phosphate-binding agents and a low-phosphate diet are prescribed. Exogenous vitamin D sources should be banned.

Ulcerated skin areas should be surgically debrided and secondary sepsis treated promptly and vigorously. The beneficial role of hyperbaric oxygen therapy has been reported (69).

VII. BULLOUS DERMATOSIS OF END-STAGE RENAL DISEASE

A. Introduction

Bullous dermatosis (BD) of end-stage renal disease (ESRD) was first decribed by Gilchrest et al. in 1975 (70). It is frequently coined "pseudo porphyria cutanea tarda" (pseudoPCT) due to its great resemblance to the autosomal dominant disorder of porphyrin metabolism PCT (71,72). In PCT, a decreased activity of uroporphyrinogen decarboxylase (UROD) leads to elevated plasma uroporphyrin levels.

B. Clinical Presentation

BD of ESRD is a disorder predominantly seen in male patients who have been on dialysis for a long time, be it hemodialysis or CAPD. Patients are usually anuric. The disorder is reported to occur in more than 5% of the ESRD patient population (73).

Classically, patients will present with increased skin fragility and bullae on the extensor surface of the hands (Fig. 3). The lesions can be quite painful, and scratching can lead to denudation and subsequent infection. Healing takes place with formation of milium cysts and scars. In contrast to "true" PCT, no sclerodermiform skin changes or hypertrichosis are observed.

C. Etiology and Pathogenesis

The cause of BD of ESRD has been the subject of much debate, especially in view of conflicting data on porphyrin levels in these patients. Recent studies may shed some light on the pathogenesis of this intriguing disorder. Gafter et al. studied a group of 6 patients with BD of ESRD versus 12 ESRD patients without BD and 12 healthy controls (73). They found that plasma uroporphyrins and RBC protoporphyrins were significantly elevated in ESRD patients versus controls. Moreover, both parameters were significantly higher in the BD group versus the group of ESRD patients without BD. Serum aluminum (Al) levels were significantly elevated in patients with BD versus the two other groups. The elevated plasma uroporphyrin levels in ESRD patients are due to the lack of excretion in anuric patients and to the failure to remove them by dialysis. The normal values of UROD in the two ESRD patient groups make this assumption plausible. The elevated red blood cell (RBC) protoporphyrin levels are due to reduced ferrochelatase activity.

Finally, it is known that high serum Al levels may lead to overproduction of porphyrins due to interference with the activity of enzymes in the heme biosynthetic pathway (74). The important role of Al has been suspected in several other reports (75–78).

D. Therapy

Therapy will be aimed at reducing excess porphyrin and Al levels, if present. The latter can be done by giving desferrioxamine or by avoiding the intake of the phosphate-binding agent aluminum hydroxide. The dialysis water should be checked for its Al content.

The patients are sensitive to visible light with a peak sensitivity at 400 nm. Therefore, photoprotective measures should be taken by using protective clothing and broad-spectrum physical sunscreens containing titanium dioxide and/or zinc oxide.

VIII. ACQUIRED PERFORATING DERMATOSIS

A. Introduction

Acquired perforating dermatosis (APD) is present in 5–10% of patients undergoing hemodialysis. The onset of lesions can occur before, during, or after the dialysis period. The literature on perforating disorders is extremely confusing due to the variability of diagnostic criteria used by different authors (78).

Here the term "acquired perforating dermatosis" will be used as the comprehensive term for all perforating skin disorders associated with systemic disorders (79). CRF is a very important disease group in this respect. Others are diabetes mellitus and, less commonly, liver disease and internal malignancy.

Cases of APD have been published as examples of reactive perforating collagenosis, elastosis perforans serpiginosa, and perforating folliculitis. Rapini suggests using the term Kyrle's disease as a synonym for APD (79). Kyrle described the disease named after him in 1916 as hyperkeratosis follicularis et parafollicularis in cutem penetrans (80).

Reactive perforating collagenosis and elastosis perforans serpiginosa are genuine genodermatoses that should be differentiated from APD. They usually start in childhood. The first disorder is not associated with a systemic disease, while the latter is associated in about 40% of cases with other genetic diseases (Down syndrome, Ehlers-Danlos syndrome, osteogenesis imperfecta, pseudoxanthoma elasticum) (81).

B. Clinical Presentation

APD is clinically characterized by the presence of 1–8 mm papules containing a central cone-shaped keratotic plug (Fig. 4). The eruption is classically bilateral and involves the extensor side of the lower extremities but can also occur on the arm, head, and neck area and trunk. Both follicular and nonfollicular lesions are seen. The eruption is usually asymptomatic, although this can be difficult to evaluate due to coexisting pruritus

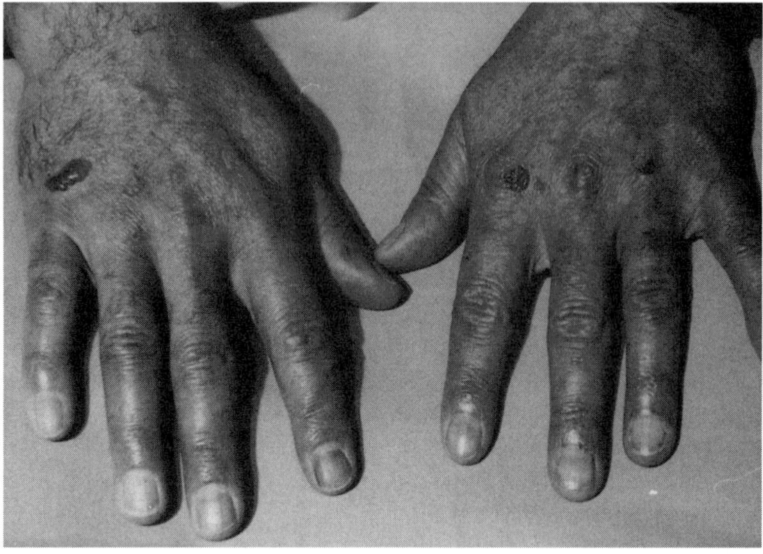

Fig. 3 Bullous dermatosis of end-stage renal disease (BD of ESRD): erosions and intact bulla on dorsal surfaces of both hands.

provoked by the underlying disorder—CRF and hemodialysis in particular.

The Koebner phenomenon (an isomorphic skin reaction in response to trauma) is occasionally positive.

C. Pathology

The histology of APD varies with the stage of evolution of the biopsied lesions (79,81). Basically a hyperkeratotic plug with variable parakeratosis and/or crusting will be observed. In early lesions microabcesses of neutrophils can be present in the epidermis and/or dermis. In later lesions granulomas are present at the base of the lesion. In some cases transepidermal elimination of collagen fibers or elastin fibers can be demonstrated by use of a Masson trichrome resp. Verhoeff-van Gieson stain. Most cases, however, reveal only amorphous débris within the perforation. The perforation site in APD can be at the infundibulum of follicules or at interfollicular epidermal locations.

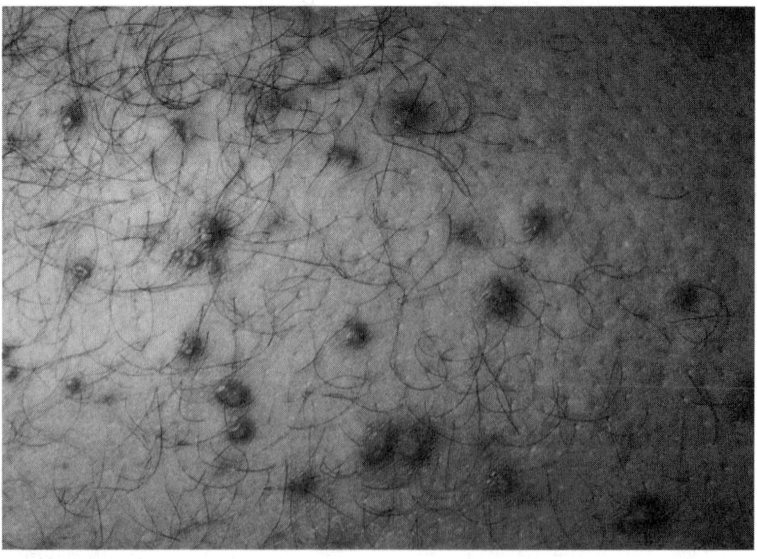

Fig. 4 Acquired perforating dermatosis (APD): 1–8 mm papules with central keratin plug on extensor side of thigh.

D. Pathogenesis

The pathogenesis of APD seems to involve the elimination of some "foreign" or "changed" connective tissue and is the result of a complex interaction between epidermal kinetics and "trapped" elements of the dermis. The term perforating dermatosis is misleading since there is no active perforation but a transepidermal (passive) elimination. A wide variety of provoking factors initiate this process: genetic or acquired abnormalities of connective tissue, deposition of hydroxyapatite or uric acid, scratching due to pruritus, mechanical disruption of follicular epithelium by hair due to repeated friction, diabetic microangiopathy, abnormal vitamin A or D metabolism, and release of neutrophilic enzymes.

E. Differential Diagnosis

APD should be differentiated from other dermatoses more or less frequently encountered in patients with CRF, e.g., prurigo nodularis, folliculitis, insect bites, multiple keratoacanthomas, and dermatofibromas.

F. Therapy

Therapy for APD can be difficult and frustrating. In most patients with CRF, UVB phototherapy will be the treatment of choice, having the advantage that it is also an effective treatment for pruritus. It can be combined with intralesional corticosteroids or, if a large number of lesions is present, with oral retinoids. In some cases destruction (by electrosurgery or CO_2 laser therapy) or excision will prove necessary.

IX. PSEUDO-KAPOSI'S SARCOMA AS A COMPLICATION OF ARTERIOVENOUS FISTULAS

A. Introduction

Pseudo-Kaposi's sarcoma (or acroangiodermatitis) is a self-limited cutaneous disease that occurs in patients with chronic venous insufficiency, congenital arteriovenous (AV) fistulas, paralytic changes, and Klippel-Trenaunay syndrome (82,83). It was first described by Mali in 1965 (84) and is histologically characterized by a marked proliferation of capillaries and fibroblasts with extravasation of red blood cells and hemosiderin deposition in the dermis. Clinically and histologically lesions resemble Kaposi's sarcoma, but clinicopathological correlation, immunohistology, and if necessary DNA-cytometric analysis will lead to a correct diagnosis (83).

B. Pathogenesis and Clinical Presentation

Pseudo-Kaposi's sarcoma is the result of insufficient drainage or overflow of blood, and it is therefore not surprising that it was also reported as a complication of AV fistulas in patients with CRF. Seven cases have been reported up to now in patients with both external Scribner AV shunts and endogenous Cimino-Brescia AV fistulas (82,83).

Clinically, intermittent swelling and cyanosis of the hand and fingers are followed by the appearance of bluish-brown pigmented plaques (Fig. 5). Papulonodules will develop with time, and one of our cases was complicated by the appearance of a large, difficult-healing ulceration (82).

Clinical diagnosis is usually straightforward if one is aware of the existence of this condition. Fistulography and/or Doppler are necessary to reveal the cause of the increased pressure in the vascular bed, distal to the fistula. Skin biopsy can lead to a difficult-healing wound and should only be performed if the clinical diagnosis is uncertain.

C. Therapy

Corrective surgery of the fistula, usually ligation, is the therapy of choice.

X. INFECTIONS

Bencini et al. reported that 23% of patients on hemodialysis had infectious skin lesions, mainly fungal (85). Skin surface pH is higher in hemodialyzed patients than in healthy controls in most areas of the body (except the axilla region). In diabetic patients, the high surface skin pH in intertriginous areas was found to affect host susceptibility to candidal infection (86). The high skin pH in patients on hemodialysis may predispose them to fungal infections.

XI. NAIL CHANGES

Fingernail changes have been observed in a large number of patients on chronic hemodialyis (1,87). In the more typical cases, the fingernails are characterized by a distal red-to-brown coloration that does not fade upon pressure. Proximally, the nails are more pale than expected. This combination has been described as "half-

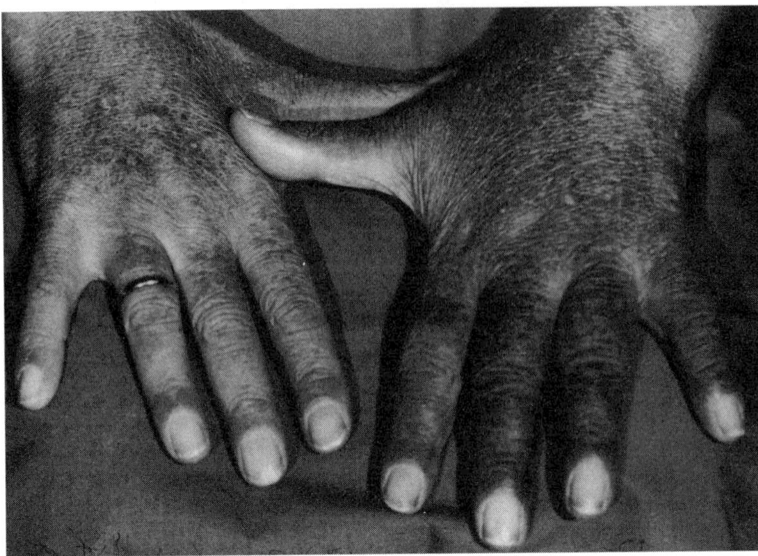

Fig. 5 Pseudo-Kaposi's sarcoma: swelling of the fingers of the left hand with bluish-red discoloration and early multinodular appearance.

and-half nail" or "red and white nails" (Fig. 6). These have been reported in 35% of patients with chronic renal failure and in only 2% of the general hospital population (88). Half-and-half nails have also been observed in patients with AIDS, following chemotherapy, and as an age-related condition (89). In some patients minor color changes were observed only 6 months after the onset of chronic renal failure in both fingernails and toenails. The phenomenon could not be linked with certain types of renal disease (14).

On histological examination, Stewart and Raffle (88) observed melanin granules in the basal layer of the nailbed epidermis, and Leyden and Wood (90) found melanin granules throughout the distal part of the nail plate. The observation of melanin deposits could not be confirmed by Kint et al. (14), who described an increased number of capillaries with thickened walls.

In some patients on chronic hemodialysis, the width and the intensity of the brown distal arch may decrease over a period of months (14). In renal transplant pa-

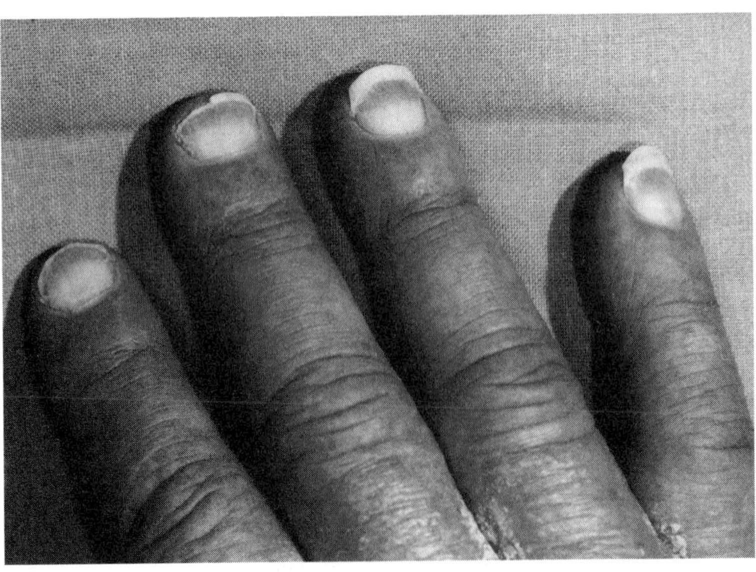

Fig. 6 Half-and-half nails: the proximal part of the nail plate is pale and the lunulae are obscured; the distal part is dull red.

tients, on the other hand, the nail discolorations may resolve 2–3 weeks after renal transplant (12). Splinter hemorrhages of the nail are seen more often in patients on chronic hemodialysis than in a general hospital populations (21,91). Other nail changes that have been observed are striped nails in patients with associated hypoalbuminemia and Beau's lines in patients suffering from an acute disease (21).

XII. HAIR LOSS

Diffuse hair loss was described in up to 33% of patients under maintenance hemodialysis (1). In some patients diffuse alopecia is seen in the early months of hemodialysis and is usually attributed to heparin administration (14). Other potential causes for diffuse alopecia are hypervitaminosis A (92) and hypothyroidism (93).

XIII. OTHER ENTITIES WITH OVERT OR SUBCLINICAL SKIN INVOLVEMENT

Dialysis-related β_2-microglobulin (B2M) amyloidosis manifests clinically as destructive arthropathy, spondylarthropathy, and carpal tunnel syndrome. B2M is deposited in skin but does not form amyloid. This deposition begins early in the course of maintenance dialysis and increases over time but is reversible after succesful renal transplantation. There is no correlation between skin B2M content and the severity of B2M amyloidosis (94). A skin biopsy is of no use in making the diagnosis of B2M amyloidosis.

Cutaneous oxalate deposits have been described in only seven patients with hemodialysis oxalosis. The crystal deposits present clinically as miliary nodules on the fingers, nose, and earlobes (95).

One case of an acrodermatitis enteropathica-like syndrome in a dialysis patient was recently reported (96). This syndrome manifests itself with diffuse alopecia, a pustular dermatitis of the extremities, paronychia, and inflamed mucosae. Low plasma zinc levels confirm the diagnosis, and there is a quick response to oral supplementation of zinc sulfate (2 mg/kg, 3 × dd). The cause for low zinc plasma levels in dialysis patients remains unclear.

Pseudoacanthosis nigricans was observed in one patient, aged 42, with typical papillomatous and warty elevations located under the arms, in the anogenital region, and around the areola mammae. The lesions disappeared after renal transplantation (14).

REFERENCES

1. Lubach D. Dermatologische Veränderungen bei Patienten mit Langzeithämodialyse. Hautarzt 1980; 31:82–85.
2. Becini Pl, Montagnino G, Citterio A, Graziani G, Cristi C, Ponticelli C. Cutaneous abnormalities in uremic patients. Nephron 1985; 40:316–321.
3. Pico MR, Lugo-Somolinos A, Sanchez JL, Burgos-Calderon R. Cutaneous abnormalities in patients with chronic renal failure. Int J Dermatol 1992; 31:860–863.
4. Ben Hmida M, Turki H, Hachicha J, Reygagne P, Rabier D, Zahaf A, Jarraya A. Hypopigmentation in hemodialysis. Dermatology 1996; 192:148–152.
5. Gilkes JJH, Eady RAS, Lesly HR, Munro DD, Moorhead JF. Plasma immunoreactive melanotropic hormones in patients on maintenance hemodialysis. Br Med J 1975; I:656–658.
6. El Matri A, Aïssa F, Ben Abdallah T, Ben Hamida F, Kechrid C, El Gharbi R, Ben Ayed H. Blondissement du système pileux associé à une pseudo-porphyrie cutanée tardive chez un hémodialysé chronique (abstr). Néphrologie 1990; 11:53.
7. Denman ST. A review of pruritus. J Am Acad Dermatol. 1986; 14:375.
8. Gilchrest BA. Pruritus: pathogenesis, therapy and significance in systemic disease states. Arch Intern Med 1982; 142:101–105.
9. Martin J. Pruritus. Int J Dermatol 1985; 24:634–639.
10. Gilchrest BA, Stern RS, Steinman TI. Clinical features of pruritus among patients undergoing maintenance hemodialysis. Arch Dermatol. 1982; 118:154–156.
11. Young AW, Sweeney EW, David DS. Dermatologic evaluation of pruritus in patients on hemodialysis. NY State Med 1973; 73:2670–2674.
12. Lubach D, Strubbe J, Schmidt J. The "half and half nail" phenomenon in chronic hemodialysis patients. Dermatologica 1982; 164:350–353.
13. Balaskas EV, Chu M, Uldall RP, Gupta A, Oreopoulos DG. Pruritus in continuous ambulatory peritoneal dialysis and hemodialysis patients. Peritoneal Dial Int 1992; 13:S527–S532.
14. Kint A, Bussels L, Fernandes M, Ringoir S. Skin and nail disorders in relation to chronic renal failure. Acta Derm Venereol. 1974; 54:137–140.
15. Tapia L. Pruritus on hemodialysis. Int J Dermatol 1979; 18:217–218.
16. Shmunes E. Hypervitaminosis A in a patient with alopecia receiving renal dialysis. Arch Dermatol 1979; 115:882–883.
17. Neiman RS, Bishel MD, Lukes RJ. Uremia and mast cell proliferation. Lancet 1972; 1:959.
18. Mettang T, Fritz P, Weber J, Machleidt C, Hubel E, Kuhlmann U. Uremic pruritus in patients on hemodialysis or continuous ambulatory peritoneal dialysis (CAPD). The role of the plasma histamine and skin mast cells. Clin Nephrol. 1990; 34:136–141.

19. De Marchi S, Cecchin E, Villalta D, Sepiacci G, Santini G, Bartoli E. Relief of pruritus and decreases in plasma histamine concentrations during erythropoietin therapy in patients with uremia. N Engl J Med. 1992; 326:969–974.
20. Rollino C, Goitre M, Piccoli G, Puiatti P, Martina G, Formica M, Quarello F, Bernengo MG. What is the role of sensitization in uremic pruritus? Nephron 1991; 57: 319–322.
21. Boehncke WH, Weber L, Gall H. Tolerance to intravenous administration of heparin and heparinoid in a patient with delayed-type hypersensitivity to heparins and heparinoids. Contact Dermatitis 1996; 35(2):73–75.
22. Mettang T, Thomas S, Kiefer T, Fischer FP, Kuhlmann U, Wodarz R, Rettenmeier AW. Uraemic pruritus and exposure to di (2-ethylhexyl) phthalate (DEHP) in haemodialysis patients. Nephrol Dial Transplant 1996; 11(12):2439–2443.
23. Morton CA, Lafferty M, Hau C, Henderson I, Jones M, Lowe JG. Pruritus and skin hydratation during dialysis. Nephrol Dial Transplant 1996; 11:2031–2036.
24. Gupta AK, Gupta MA, Cardella CJ, Haberman HF. Cutaneous associations of chronic renal failure and dialysis. Int J Dermatol 1986; 25:498–503.
25. Rosen T. Uremic pruritus: a review. Cutis 1979; 23: 790–792.
26. Stahle-Backdahl M. Uremic pruritus: clincal and experimental studies. Acta Derm Venereol 1989; 145:S1–S38.
27. Arndt KA. Pruritus. In: Arndt KA, ed. Manual of Dermatologic Therapeutics. 4th ed. Boston: Little Brown, 1989:115–118.
28. Bernhard JD. Clinical aspects of pruritus. In: Fitzpatrick TB, Eisen AZ, Wolff K, Freedberg IM, Austen KF, eds. Dermatology in General Medicine. 3rd ed. New York: McGraw-Hill, 1987:78–90.
29. Silverberg DS, Iaina A, Reisin E. Cholestyramine in uremic pruritus. Br Med J 1977; 1:752–753.
30. Pederson JA. Relief of idiopathic gneralized pruritus in dialysis patients treated with activated charcoal. Ann Intern Med 1980; 93:446–449.
31. Yatzidis H, Digenis P, Tountas C. Heparin treatment of uremic itching. JAMA 1972; 222:1183.
32. Aubia J, Aguilera J, Llorach I. Dialysis pruritus: effect of cimetidine. J Dialysis 1980; 4:141–145.
33. Graf H, Kovarik J, Stummvoll HK. Disappearance of uremic pruritus after lowering dialysate magnesium concentration. Br Med J 1979; 2:1478–1479.
34. Shultz BC, Roenigk HH. Uremic pruritus treated with ultraviolet light. JAMA 1980; 243:1836–1837.
35. Gilchrest BA. Relief of uremic pruritus with ultraviolet phototherapy. N Engl J Med 1977; 297:136–139.
36. Blachley JD, Blankenship M, Menter A. Uremic pruritus: skin divalent ion content and response to ultraviolet phototherapy. Am J Kidney Dis 1985; 5:237–242.
37. Massry SG, Popovtzer MM, Coburn JW, Makoff DL, Maxwell MH, Kleeman CR. Intractable pruritus as a manifestation of secondary hyperparathyroidism in uremia. Disappearance of itching after subtotal parathyroidectomy. N Engl J Med 1968; 279:697–700.
38. Yaar M, Gilchrest BA. Cellular and molecular mechanisms of cutaneous aging. J Dermatol Surg Oncol 1990; 16:915–922.
39. Schmidtmann S, Müller M, von Baehr R. Changes of antioxidative homeostasis in patients on chronic hemodialysis. Nephrol Dial Transplant 1991; 6(S3):71–74.
40. Kligman AM, Zheng P, Lavker RM. The anatomy and pathogenesis of wrinkles. Br J Dermatol 1985; 113:37–42.
41. Altmeyer P, Kachel HG, Jünger M. Hautveränderungen bei langzeit Dialyse-patienten. Eine klinische Studie. Hautarzt 1982; 33:303–309.
42. Tercedor J, Lopez-Hernandez B, Rodenas JM, Delgado-Rodriguez M, Cerezo S, Serrano-Ortega S. Multivariate analysis of cutaneous markers of aging in chronic hemodialyzed patients. Int J Dermatol 1995; 34:546–550.
43. Griffiths CEM. The clinical identification and quantification of photodamage. Br J Dermatol 1992; 127(S41): 37–42.
44. Anderson CD, Gibson IM, Rossi E. Actinic damage in the skin of patients on hemodialysis for chronic renal failure. Photodermatology 1988; 5:12–24.
45. Lindner A, Farewell VT, Sherrard DJ. High incidence of neoplasia in uremic patients receiving long term dialysis. Nephron 1981; 27:292–296.
46. Inamoto H, Ozaki R, Matsuzaki T. Incidence and mortality pattern of malignancy and factors affecting the risk of malignancy in dialysis patients. Nephron 1991; 59:611–617.
47. Buccianti G, Ravasi B, Cresseri D, Maisonneuve P, Boyle P, Locatelli F. Cancer in patients on renal replacement therapy in Lombardy, Italy. Lancet 1996; 347:59–60.
48. Euvrard S. Cutaneous complications in renal transplant patients. Eur J Dermatol 1991; 1:175–184.
49. Mork NJ. Contact sensitivity from epoxy resin in a hemodialysis seet. Contact Dermatitis 1979; 5:331–332.
50. Penneys NS, Edwards LS, Katsikas JL. Allergic contact sensitivity to thiuram compounds in a hemodialysis unit. Arch Dermatol 1976; 112:811–813.
51. Kruis-De Vries MH, Coenraads PJ, Nater JP. Allergic contact dermatitis due to rubber chemicals in hemodialysis equipment. Contact Dermatitis 1987; 17:303–305.
52. Sunderman FW Jr. Decsy MI, Mc Neely MD. Nickel metabolism in health and disease. Ann NY Acad Sci 1972; 199:312–330.
53. Olerud JE, Lee MY, Uvelli DA, Goble GJ, Babb AL. Presumptive nickel dermatitis from hemodialysis. Arch Dermatol 1984; 12:1066–1068.

54. Samitz MH, Katz SA. Nickel dermatitis from a foreign body in the stomach. Br J Dermatol 1975; 92:287–290.
55. Marshall C, Shimizu A, Smith EKB. Ethylene oxide allergy in a dialysis center: prevalence in hemodialysis and peritoneal dialysis population. Clin Nephrol 1984; 21:346–349.
56. Guin JD. Contact sensitivity to topical corticosteroids. JAAD 1984; 10:773–782.
57. Whittam LR, McGibbon DH, MacDonald DM. Proximal cutaneous necrosis in association with chronic renal failure. Br J Dermatol 1996; 135:778–781
58. Zouboulis CC, Blume-Peytavi U, Lennert T, Stavropoulos PG, Schwarz A, Runkel N, Trautmann C, Orfanos CE. Fulminant metastatic calcinosis with cutaneous necrosis in a child with end-stage renal disease and tertiary hyperparathyroidism. Br J Dermatol 1996; 135:617–622.
59. Dahl PR, Winkelmann RK, Connolly SM. The vascular calcification-cutaneous necrosis syndrome. J Am Acad Dermatol 1995; 33:53–58.
60. Selye H, Gabbiani G, Strebel R. Sensitization to calciphylaxis by endogenous parathyroid hormone. Endocrinology 1962; 71:554–558.
61. Mehta R, Scott G, Sloand JA, Francis CW. Skin necrosis associated with acquired protein C deficiency in patients with renal failure and calciphylaxis. Am J Med 1990; 88:252–257.
62. Kant KS, Glueck HI, Coots MC, Tonne VA, Brubaker R, Penn I. Protein S deficiency and skin necrosis associated with continuous ambulatory peritoneal dialysis. Am J Kidney Dis 1992; 19:264–271.
63. Janigan DT, Morris J, Hirsch D. Acute skin and fat necrosis during sepsis in a patient with chronic renal failure and subcutaneous arterial calcification. Am J Kidney Dis 1992; 20:643–646.
64. Dereure O, Leray H, Barneon G, Canaud B, Mion C, Guilhou JJ. Extensive necrotizing livedo reticularis in a patient with chronic renal failure, hyperparathyroidism and coagulation disorder: regression after subtotal parathyroidectomy. Dermatology 1996; 192:167–170.
65. Cockerell JC, Dolan ET. Widespread cutaneous and systemic calcification (calciphylaxis) in patients with the acquired immunodeficiency syndrome and renal disease. J Am Acad Dermatol 1992; 26:559–562.
66. Lazorik FC, Friedman AK, Leyden JJ. Xeroradiographic observations in four patients with chronic renal disease and cutaneous gangrene. Arch Dermatol 1981; 117:325–328.
67. Nikko AP, Dunningan M, Cockerell CJ. Calciphylaxis with histologic changes of pseudoxanthoma elasticum. Am J Dermatopathol 1996; 18:396–399.
68. Chan YL, Mahony JF, Turner JJ, Posen S. The vascular lesions associated with skin necrosis in renal failure. Br J Dermatol 1983; 109:85–89.
69. Vassa N, Twardowsky ZJ, Campbell J. Hyperbaric oxygen therapy in calciphylaxis-induced skin necrosis in a peritoneal dialysis patient. Am J Kidney Dis 1994; 23:878–881.
70. Gilchrest B, Rowe JW, Mihm MC Jr. Bullous dermatosis of hemodialysis. Ann Intern Med 1975; 83:480–483.
71. Thivolet J, Euvrard S, Perrot H. La pseudo-porphyrie cutanée tardive des hémodialysés. Ann Derm Vénéréol 1977; 104:12–17.
72. Poh-Fitzpatrick MB. Porphyria, pseudo porphyria, pseudo pseudoporphyria...? Arch Dermatol 1986; 122: 403–404.
73. Gafter U, Mamet R, Korzets A, Malachi T, Schoenfeld N. Bullous dermatosis of end-stage renal disease: a possible association between abnormal porphyrin metabolism and aluminium. Nephrol Dial Transplant 1996; 11: 1787–1791.
74. Scharf R, Mamet R, Zimmels Y, Kimchie S, Schoenfeld N. Evidence for the interference of aluminium with bacterial porphyrin biosynthesis. Biometals 1994; 7: 135–141.
75. King J, Day RS, Milne FJ, Bezwoda WR, Viljoen JD, Kramer S. Delayed onset of overt porphyria cutanea tarda in a patient on long-term hemodialysis. SA Med J 1983; 63:743–746.
76. McCarthy JT, Milliner DS, Johnson WJ. Clinical experience with desferrioxamine in dialysis patients with aluminium toxicity. Q J Med 1990; 74:257–276.
77. Yasuda G, Ikeda Y, Satta H, Shionoiri H, Ishii M, Ikezawa Y. Porphyrin metabolism. abnormalities and its treatment in a uremic patient with porphyria cutanea tarda. Nephron 1993; 63:235–236.
78. Sehgal VN, Jain S, Thappa DM, Bhattacharya SN, Logani K. Perforating dermatoses: a review and report of four cases. J Dermatol 1993; 20:329–340.
79. Rapini RP. Perforating disorders. In: Arndt KA, Leboit PE, Robinson JK, Wintroub BU, eds. Cutaneous Medicine and Surgery. Philadelphia: WB Saunders Company, 1996:407–411.
80. Kyrle J. Hyperkeratosis follicularis et parafollicularis in cutem penetrans. Arch Dermatol Syph (Berlin) 1916; 123:466–493.
81. McKee P. Necrobiotic and granulomatous diseases. In: McKee P, ed. Pathology of the Skin. 2d ed. London: Mosby-Wolfe, 1996:12–17.
82. Bogaert AM, Vanholder R, De Roose J, De Keyzer L, Kint A, Matthys E, Ringoir. Pseudo-Kaposi's sarcoma as a complication of Cimino-Brescia arteriovenous fistulas in hemodialysis patients. Nephron 1987; 46:170–173.
83. Landthaler M, Stolz W, Eckert F, Schmoeckel C, Braun-Falco O. Pseudo-Kaposi's sarcoma occurring after placement of arteriovenous shunt. J Am Acad Dermatol 1989; 21:499–505.
84. Mali JH, Kuiper JP, Hamers AA. Acro-angiodermatitis of the foot. Arch Dermatol 1965; 92:515–518.
85. Bencini PL, Montagnino G, Citterio A, Graziani G,

Crosti C, Ponticelli C. Cutaneous abnormalities in uremic patients. Nephron 1985; 40:316–321.
86. Yosipovitch G, Tur E, Morduchowicz G, Boner G. Skin surface pH, moisture and pruritus in hemodialysis patients. Nephrol Dial Transplant 1993; 8:1129–1132.
87. Linsay PG. The half-and-half nail. Arch Intern Med 1967; 119:583–587.
88. Stewart WK, Raffle EJ. Brown nail bed arcs and chronic renal disease. Br Med J 1972; 1:784–786.
89. Thomsen K. Nails, A Manual and Atlas. Copenhagen: FADL Publishers, 1992:25,37.
90. Leyden JJ, Wood MG. The "half-and-half nail." An uremic onychopathy. Arch Dermatol 1972; 105:591–592.
91. Glum M, Aviram A. Splinter hemorrhages in patients receiving regular hemodialysis. JAMA 1978; 239:47–48.
92. Shmunes E. Hypervitaminosis A in a patient with alopecia receiving renal dialysis. Arch Dermatol 1979; 115:882–883.
93. Galambl, Mako J, Renyi-Vamos F, Balogn F. Haarausfall nach chronischer Häinodialyse. Z Urol Nephrol 1984; 77:419–494.
94. Spiegel DM, Costante N, Janiga AM, Haas M, Soltani K. Deposition and removal of cutaneous beta2-microglobulin. Am J Nephrol 1992; 12:330–335.
95. Nakazawa R, Hamaguchi K, Hosaka E, Shishido H, Yokoyama T. Cutaneous oxalate deposition in a hemodialysis patient. Am J Kidney Dis 1995; 25:492–497.
96. Parra E, Campistol JM, Soy D, Deulofeu R. Acrodermatitis enteropathica-like syndrome in a dialysis patient. Nephron 1995; 70:389–390.

26

Hypertension in Dialysis Patients

Steven Fishbane, John K. Maesaka, Muhammed A. Goreja, and Edward A. Kowalski
Winthrop-University Hospital, Mineola, New York

I. INTRODUCTION

Arterial hypertension remains one of the major public health problems of industrialized nations, resulting in a great burden of morbidity, mortality, and cost. Broad educational initiatives and improved treatement options for hypertension have probably been important factors associated with a 52% reduction in the age-adjusted risk of death from cardiovascular disease in the United States between 1968 and 1986 (1). Nonetheless, the attributable risk imposed by hypertension is great, as noted by a fivefold increase in ischemic heart disease in men with mild hypertension in the Framingham Study (2). For patients with end-stage renal disease, hypertension poses a particular problem. It has been estimated that greater than 80% of patients initiating renal replacement therapy are hypertensive (3–6). Many patients remain hypertensive despite dialysis therapy; the 1996 Core Indicators Project found systolic blood pressure greater than 150 mmHg in 53% of hemodialysis patients and 29% of peritoneal dialysis patients (7,8). Several studies utilizing 24-hour ambulatory blood pressure monitoring have confirmed that blood pressure control tends to be poor among dialysis patients. In addition, most of these studies have shown that nighttime blood pressure does not decrease normally in dialysis patients, increasing the overall hypertensive load (9–12). Given the strong link between hypertension and adverse outcomes in nonuremic populations, it would seem highly probable that hypertension plays an important role in the high rates of cardiovascular disease and mortality experienced by dialysis patients (13). The purpose of this chapter shall be to review the complicated subject of hypertension management for patients treated with hemodialysis or peritoneal dialysis.

II. MEASUREMENT OF BLOOD PRESSURE IN DIALYSIS PATIENTS

The measurement of blood pressure and definition of hypertension for patients treated with peritoneal dialysis is fairly straightforward, given these patients' relatively stable volume. It is usually reasonable for patients to check their blood pressure on a daily basis, with a pressure above 150/90 mmHg [this value was used in the HCFA Core Indicators Study for hemodialysis patients (14)] representing inadequately controlled hypertension. Reducing blood pressure below this level may be beneficial, and the target in an individual patient should reflect the patient's existent cardiac risk factors and cormobidity. Measurement of blood pressure in patients on hemodialysis presents a more difficult situation, in that volume removal is distinctly intermittent. This creates a problem because blood pressure may be expected to change considerably from pre- to postdialysis and through the interdialytic period. Studies of blood pressure using ambulatory monitoring for 48-hour periods in hemodialysis patients confirm that this is indeed true (9).

When is the best time to measure blood pressure in hemodialysis patients? Measuring a single predialysis or postdialysis blood pressure is simple to perform, but do either reflect the hypertensive burden during the 48- to 72-hour interdialytic period? Rodby et al. found that ambulatory average blood pressure was not well predicted by either pre- or postdialysis blood pressure (15). This finding is of concern given the fact that most hemodialysis patients have hypertension management guided exclusively by blood pressures measured at dialysis.

Since readings of blood pressure at dialysis are certainly convenient and practical, several other investigators have examined their value. Salem preferred using the predialysis blood pressure in a study of hemodialysis patients, while recognizing that is may be inflated by predialysis overhydration. He used a level of 160/90 mmHg to indicate the presence of hypertension (16). A recent study found, in fact, that predialysis blood pressure readings did correlate significantly with 24-hour ambulatory blood pressure and left ventricular hypertrophy (12). Postdialysis blood pressure ideally reflects the patient's true dry hydration state. However, recent studies indicate that blood pressure rebounds shortly after hemodialysis treatments (9,17,18), making it clear that postdialysis blood pressure probably is not a good correlate of interdialytic hypertensive load in many patients. A study reported by Kooman et al., however, found postdialysis blood pressure actually correlated well with average interdialytic blood pressure (19). Ultimately, 24- or 48-hour ambulatory blood pressure monitoring provides the clearest picture of interdialytic hypertensive load, but the test is impractical to apply. Therefore, given the complexity of the problem and the mixed results from the literature, it is not possible to recommend a specific best practice for monitoring blood pressure control for hemodialysis patients. The predialysis, postdialysis, and interdialytic blood pressures may all be important. The clinician should attempt to maintain both pre- and postdialysis blood pressure below the target level. Occasional ambulatory monitoring could greatly enhance the understanding of the individual patient's hypertensive load. Further research is needed to examine this issue.

III. TARGET BLOOD PRESSURE

The appropriate target value for blood pressure is not clearly defined for dialysis patients. The JNC-V recommended that a systolic pressure above 130 mmHg or a diastolic blood pressure above 85 mmHg is abnormal for the general population (20). This is a level that many believe would be difficult to achieve for hypertensive hemodialysis patients. The Health Care Financing Administration (HCFA) Core Indicators Project used a target of 150/90 mmHg, a level frequently suggested for these patients (14). A value below 150/90 mmHg recorded both pre and postdialysis certainly can increase our comfort that hypertension is not severe or is reasonably well controlled. Of note, however, are data indicating that lowering blood pressure to a significantly lower level (mean arterial pressure below 90 mmHg) resulted in reduced mortality (21). It is likely that the target blood pressure for hemodialysis patients may need to be individualized to reflect the patient's age, cardiac status, history of diabetes or vascular disease, and associated cardiovascular risk factors. In a young healthy hemodialysis patient, a target mean arterial pressure of less than 90 mmHg may be appropriate. Further studies are clearly needed, however, to define target blood pressures for hemodialysis patients.

IV. PATHOGENESIS

The pathogenesis of hypertension in dialysis patients is complex, incompletely understood, and probably multifactorial. Hypertension is common at entrace to end-stage renal disease, present in more than 80% of patients (29), and reported as the second leading cause of end-stage renal disease. Among African Americans hypertension is found to be the most common cause of end-stage renal disease (30). Therefore, hypertension in many patients far predates the onset of dialysis treatment. In these patients the etiology of dialysis-associated hypertension may be related to preexisting pathogenic fators. Dialysis patients are also at risk for many of the same secondary causes of hypertension that nonuremic subjects develop. Specifically, the diagnosis of ischemic nephropathy should not be overlooked in these patients. Renal artery stenosis is underrecognized as a cause of hypertension and as a frequent diagnosis leading to end-stage renal disease (31–34). It is likely that a significant number of patients on dialysis may have undetected renovascular disease contributing to dialysis-associated hypertension. In addition, thyroid disease and pheochromocytoma should be considered as secondary causes of hypertension under appropriate clinical circumstances. The remainder of this section will examine specific factors related to renal disease that may contribute to the pathogenesis of hypertension in dialysis patients.

V. ROLE OF SODIUM AND VOLUME EXCESS AND THE RENIN-ANGIOTENSIN AXIS

Blood pressure reflects the interplay between cardiac output and peripheral vascular resistance, and hypertension is, therefore, always due a maladaptive increase in one or both. Cardiac output is a function of heart rate and left ventricular stroke volume, the latter of which may be increased by several factors, one of which is volume excess. We therefore begin our discussion with an examination of the effect of pervasive hypervolemia experienced by patients with chronic renal failure. Volume expansion has often been stated to be the most important factor in the causation and maintenance of hypertension in the dialysis population (3,21,35–40). Many clinical observations support the important role of volume overload. In several centers, (21,41,41a,b) long, slow hemodialysis treatments (≥24 hours per week) allow for gentle and complete fluid removal to a patient's "true" dry weight. In one of the centers, antihypertensive medications were discontinued in 98% of patients using this dialytic regimen (21). The greater success in blood pressure control with peritoneal dialysis probably also reflects the benefits of gradual, slow ultrafiltration (42). Inadequate removal of excess volume during hemodialysis is also probably a major cause of what has been termed dialysis refractory hypertension (high blood pressure that does not improve with dialytic volume removal) (43). Finally, more than 80% of patients are hypertensive at the initiation of dialysis, and many of these patients normalize their blood pressure after weeks of dialysis and ultrafiltration, consistent with the concept that hypervolemia is the major cause of hypertension in these patients (29).

The mechanisms by which volume excess and inappropriate vasoconstrictgion interact to cause arterial hypertension in uremic patients are complex. In dogs, sodium excess leads to increased cardiac output, followed by a reflex increase in total peripheral vascular resistance due to autoregulation in tissue beds (44). Dialysis patients tend towards volume overload due to the loss of renal excretory function. In many patients the hypervolemia is balanced by a decrease in vascular resistance, and, therefore, blood pressure remains normal. Failure of this compensatory vasodilatation by the peripheral vascular system in the face of volume excess leads to hypertension. An ultimate understanding of hypertension in dialysis patients requires that this secondary vasoconstriction be explained. According to some this may be due to inappropriate elevations of circulating angiotensin II in relation to increased body volume and sodium loading (35,45,46). Even normal plasma concentrations of angiotensin II observed in some dialysis patients may be inappropriately high in the face of volume excess. The importance of the pathogenic role of the renin-angiotensin system in dialysis patients is supported by the effectiveness of bilateral nephrectomy in eliminating hypertension in these patients. While nephrectomy causes several changes in homeostasis, it clearly eliminates the body's main source of renin.

Another factor that may explain the inappropriate vasoconstriction in dialysis patients is the presence of increased secretion of oubain-like inhibitors of vascular smooth muscle Na^+-K^+ ATPase activity, with a resultant increase in peripheral vascular resistance (47–49). Lower pump activity has been noted in hypertensive dialysis patients in association with an inverse relationship between Na^+-K^+ ATPase activity and peripheral vascular resistance (50–53). As a consequence of Na^+-K^+ ATPase pump inhibition, intracellular Na^+ increases (52,54–57) paralleled by increased cytosolic Ca^{2+} in red blood cells (RBCs) (58) and platelets (59,60), resulting in enhanced vascular tone and responsiveness to vasoconstrictive agents (50). The cause of increased production of these oubain-like substances in uremic patients is unclear but may be due to salt and volume excess directly.

Whatever the mechanism of the inappropriate vasoconstriction, removal of excess volume and attainment of true dry weight may result in normalization of blood pressure in most dialysis patients. It must be noted that the degree of volume overload is usually not great enough to lead to frank peripheral edema. The determination of true dry weight is clinically elusive, and there is, therefore, a need for more sophisticated, accurate, and validated methods to determine patients' actual volume status.

VI. SYMPATHETIC ACTIVITY

Increased activity of the sympathetic nervous system could raise blood pressure both by increasing cardiac output and by vasoconstriction. It is difficult in humans to rigorously measure and define activity of the sympathetic system. Assays of plasma catecholamine levels provide only a weak reflection of sympathetic activity. Studies of uremic patients in which plasma norepinephrine levels were measured have yielded varying results. There has been a range of results from very low to very high plasma levels (60a,b). Recording of peroneal nerve electrical discharge has been used as a more direct marker of sympathetic activity (61,62). Converse et al. (61) found that discharge from this nerve was greater in dialysis patients than in controls. The increased nerve activity was associated with increased local vascular resistance, supporting a possible role of the sympathetic system in sustaining inappropriate vasoconstriction in uremic patients. Furthermore, they demonstrated that dialysis patients with their native kidneys intact had greater sympathetic activity than dialysis patients who had undergone bilateral nephrectomy (61). A possible explanation for the increased sympathetic activity involves an excitatory signal arising in the failing kidney (61,63–65) in response to stimulation of chemosensitive renal afferent nerves by either ischemic metabolites or by uremic toxins such as urea. The reflex traverses afferent pathways to the CNS (66), which may result in increased efferent sympathetic tone. A support for this contention comes from the observation that sympathetic activation is not seen in anephric patients (61,66) and by the fact that selective surgical interruption of afferent renal nerves prevents hypertension in experimental renal failure.

VII. ROLE OF ERYTHROPOIETIN

Blood pressure elevation is the primary side effect of treatment with recombinant human erythropoietin (rHuEPO), with an incidence ranging from 10 to 70% (67–70). Multicenter trials have shown an increase in diastolic pressure of more than 10 mmHg or a need to start or increase antihypertensive therapy in 35% of previously hypertensive patients and 44% of previously normotensive patients on dialysis (71–73). The rise in blood pressure during rHuEPO administration usually occurs within the initial 2–16 weeks of treatment, although in some patients the rise in blood pressure is delayed for months. Patients who are at greatest risk are ones whose anemia is corrected rapidly, have preexisting hypertension, have native kidneys in place, have a family history of hypertension, or are treated with a greater total dose of rHuEPO. The risk of hypertension appears to be greater in patients treated with intravenous rather than subcutaneous rHuEPO (74). This may be explained by the fact that subcutaneous administration does not appear to cause an increase in plasma levels of endothelin (75). Factors implicated in the pathogenesis of hypertension in ESRD patients on rHuEPO therapy include increased blood viscosity (76,77), increased blood volume, increased total peripheral resistance secondary to loss of hypoxic vasodilatation (78,79), increased plasma endothelin, increased vascular responsiveness to norepinephrine (75), and a direct vasoconstrictor effect (80).

From a practical standpoint, the hypertensive effect of rHuEPO tends not to be very clinically significant. It is rare for rHuEPO therapy to induce an increase in blood pressure that cannot be easily controlled by adjusting the antihypertensive regimen. The salutary effects of correction of anemia would seem to far outweigh the risk for increased blood pressure. However, among patients with poorly controlled hypertension, the hypertensive risk can be ameliorated by using the subcutaneous route of administration and by co-treating with adjuvant therapy (iron and androgens) to decrease the total rHuEPO dose required.

VIII. ROLE OF DIVALENT IONS AND PARATHYROID HORMONE

Intracellular calcium is raised in the tissues of patients with end-stage renal disease due in part to hyperparathyroidism. Studies have shown that there exists a relationship between increased cellular calcium and blood pressure in essential hypertension (81,82). Increased intracellular calcium may, therefore, contribute to hypertension in dialysis patients. Recent studies lend support to this hypothesis. Raine et al. (83) demonstrated significant correlations between serum parathyroid hormone (PTH) and platelet calcium, platelet calcium and mean arterial blood pressure, and serum PTH and mean arterial blood pressure in chronic renal failure patients. Treatment of a subset of patients with hyperparathyroidism with a vitamin D analog resulted in a decrease in serum PTH, platelet intracellular calcium, and mean arterial blood pressure (83). In another report there was a significant correlation between decreased mean systolic pressure and plasma Ca^{2+} over a period of 9 months following parathyroidectomy (84).

Although increased dietary calcium intake tends to be associated with lower blood pressure, hypercalcemia often causes hypertension. In dialysis patients, hypercalcemia is common as a result of overtreatment with calcium supplements or vitamin D analogs, severe hyperparathyroidism, low-turnover bone disease, or vitamin A toxicity (85). It is interesting that hypercalcemia is more likely to raise blood pressure in the presence of increased serum levels of PTH. This effect appears to be mediated by an increase in systemic vascular resistance rather than by affecting cardiac output (86).

IX. VASCULAR ENDOTHELIUM

Systemic vascular resistance plays a major role in determining blood pressure. Originally, the role of vascular endothelial cells in regulating vascular smooth muscle cell contraction was not recognized. This changed in 1980, when Furchgott and Zawadski demonstrated that acetylcholine-induced vasodilatation was dependent on the presence of the endothelium (87). This effect was believed to be mediated by a secreted substance that relaxes the blood vessel; hence the initial name endothelium-derived relaxation factor (EDRF). This factor has subsequently been more fully characterized and termed nitric oxide (88). Among endothelial-derived constricting factors, the most potent is endothelin, first characterized by Yanagisawa et al. in 1988 (89). It has subsequently become clear that the vascular endothelium releases a number of relaxing and constricting factors that are important regulators of vascular tone. It is likely that these vasoactive peptides play a role in the pathogenesis of hypertension (90,91). The mechanism by which these factors could contribute to the hypertension experienced by patients on dialysis is incompletely understood.

The most extensively studied of the endothelium-derived vasorelaxing factors has been nitric oxide. Concentrations of this substance have been demonstrated to be chronically elevated in hemodialysis patients (92). Nitric oxide is formed from the amino acid L-arginine by the enzyme nitric oxide synthetase. Several forms of this enzyme have been identified and well characterized. Inhibition of this system using N^W L-nitro-L-arginine-methyl ester (L-NAME), has facilitated experiments designed to examine the role of nitric oxide in hypertension. An endogenous compound, asymmetrical dimethyl-L-arginine (ADMA), also inhibits nitric oxide synthesis. This substance appears to accumulate in the blood of uremic patients, perhaps contributing to the predisposition of these patients to be hypertensive (93). However, a recent study reported by Bergstrom et al. (47) casts serious doubt on the hypothesis that accumulated endogenous ADMA plays a significant role in the development of hypertension in dialysis patients. It is still possible that other endogenous inhibitors of NO pathway may play a pathogenic role.

Endothelin has been the most extensively studied vasoconstrictive peptide produced by the vascular endothelium. This substance is produced as three peptide isoforms termed endothelin-1, -2, or -3 (94). Endothelin-1 was linked to the pathogenesis of hypertension by the demonstration of cure of hypertension in two patients with endothelin-producing tumors (95). In one of these patients, recurrence of the tumor resulted again in increased endothelin-1 levels and hypertension. Increased circulating levels of endothelin-1 or -3 have been found in hypertensive patients with chronic renal failure (96–99). Whether the increased serum levels actually play a causative role in hypertension has not been fully defined.

X. OUTCOMES AND TREATMENT OF HYPERTENSION IN DIALYSIS PATIENTS

There has been an extensive literature of studies examining the effect of hypertension on outcomes of dialysis patients. At least nine studies including more than 100 patients have been published since 1982. The methodologies utilized varied widely, as have the results. Seven of the studies have shown a positive association between hypertension and increased risk of death; two studies did not demonstrate this association (Table 1) (4,21–28). A positive correlation was found by Charra et al. (21) with an 85% 10-year survival for patients with mean arterial pressure less than 99 mmHg. In an interesting recent study, Foley et al. (27) followed 432 patients (261 hemodialysis, 171 peritoneal dialysis) for a mean of 41 months. Higher mean arterial blood pressure was associated with an increased risk of left ventricular hypertrophy, left ventricular dilatation, de novo ischemic heart disease, and congestive heart failure. Paradoxically, it was lower rather than high blood pressure that was associated with an increased risk of death. The authors noted that the excess mortality risk among patients with lower blood pressure could best be attributed to the presence of severe congestive heart failure in many of these patients (27).

This issue was explored again recently in a study reported by Zager et al. (27a). These investigators studied 5433 hemodialysis patients for 5 years and found a "U," curve relationship between blood pressure and

Table 1 Relationship Between Hypertension and Cardiovascular Mortality in Renal Failure Patients, Studies of Greater than 100 Patients

n	Prospective/ retrospective	Relation	Ref.
320	R	Positive	4
1453	P	Positive	22
400	R	Positive	23
405	R	Positive	24
445	R	Positive	21
196	P	Negative	25
178	R	Positive	26
432	P	Positive	27
370	R	Negative	28

outcomes. High postdialysis pressures, as measured by systolic >180 mmHg and diastolic >90 mmHg, were associated with a relative risk of cardiovascular mortality of 1.96 and 1.73, respectively ($p < 0.05$). But low blood pressure also was also associated with increased risk, particularly when the pre- or postdialysis systolic pressure was <110 mmHg (27a).

It has been estimated that 85% of patients initiate dialysis with hypertension (4,100) and that at least 60% of these patients have end-organ damage as evidenced by left ventricular hypertrophy (101). There are few reports describing the extent and status of control of hypertension in this patient population. Cheigh et al. (9) utilized 48-hour ambulatory blood pressure measurements to study 53 hemodialysis patients. Using 150/90 mmHg as their target, they concluded that the majority of patients treated for chronic hypertension were not adequately controlled. Raine et al. (102), in a large European study, reported a 70% prevalence of hypertension in their population. Recently, Salem (16) reported the first large epidemiological hypertension study in a U.S. hemodialysis cohort. Of 649 patients studied, using 140/90 mmHg as a basis for stage 1 hypertension, they demonstrated a prevalence of 72%. We recently studied our hemodialysis population and using 150/90 mmHg as evidence for mild hypertension found a prevalence of 77% (103). Table 2 lists several factors that may contribute to the difficulty of hypertension control in dialysis patients. It has been observed that patients on peritoneal dialysis seem to have better blood pressure control than patients treated with hemodialysis (104,105). The 1996 Core Indicators Project found systolic blood pressure greater than 150 mmHg in 53% of hemodialysis patients and 29% of peritoneal dialysis patients (7,8). Lower blood pressure in patients treated with peritoneal dialysis may reflect the modality's gentler method for volume removal, allowing for closer approximation of patients' true dry weight.

The approach to the control of hypertension in dialysis patients should be multidisciplinary. The team should consist of representatives from all four disciplines in the dialysis unit—medical, nursing, social work, and dietary. Members should work closely with each patient with the aim of bringing blood pressure consistently to <150/90 mmHg. We have developed a treatment algorithm that has proven very useful (Table 3). The use of algorithms reduces practice variability, improves education of staff and patients, and eases the implementation of quality improvement initiatives. It is critical at the dialysis unit level to consider hypertension as a core indicator, with the success of the treatment program tracked over time. To standardize monitoring we have developed an index, the hypertension severity index, to serve as the primary outcome measure. The index quantitates blood pressure control on a simple 1–12 scale (103a).

Lifestyle modification is an important foundation on which the treatment paradigm builds. Initial efforts should be targeted at teaching the patient nonmedicinal aspects of hypertension therapy—aerobic exercise, weight loss, avoidance of smoking and ethanol, and dietary modification (Table 4). The beneficial effects of

Table 2 Some Reasons for Lack of Control of Hypertension in Dialysis Patients

1. Providers are satisfied with level of BP and do not strive for better control
2. Not enough attention to lifestyle modification to reduce BP
3. Patient noncompliance with salt and fluid intake
4. Inadequate ultrafiltration during dialysis treatment
5. Inadequate prescription of medications
6. Underlying secondary form of hypertension

Table 3 Algorithm for Blood Pressure Control—HBP (>150/90) on Three Occasions

1a. Discuss nonmedicinal reduction of BP with patient
1b. Estimate dry weight (EDW)
2. Confirm compliance with BP meds
3. Determine Hypertension Severity Index
2a. Attain dry weight
  Decrease EDW by 1/2–1 lb per week until BP < 120/80 postdialysis or until patient has hypotension or cramping:
    if patient on antihypertensives, stop prior to dialysis, and begin to taper dosage
    if uncertain of EDW, use in line Hct determination
2b. Start/Increase meds to maintain BP < 150/90
3. BP not controlled (<150/90) or EDW not attained in 30 days, consider;
    24–48 hour ambulatory blood pressure monitor
    inreasing time on dialysis to facilitate removal of fluid and attainment of dry weight
    discontinuing sodium modeling
    increasing medication therapy
4. If BP remains uncontrolled, consider:
    evaluating for secondary forms of hypertension
    peritoneal dialysis
    bilateral nephrectomy

Note: Patients should be encouraged to monitor blood pressure on nondialysis days. Patients should be encouraged to bring a day's dosage of antihypertensives with them to each dialysis.

Table 4 Nonmedicinal Treatments of Hypertension

Aerobic exercise
Control of salt and fluid intake
Cessation of smoking
Weight reduction
Avoidance of alcohol

aerobic exercise on blood pressure in nondialysis patients are well described (106,107). The exercise tolerance of dialysis patients, however, is in general less than that of age-matched nonuremic subjects. Therefore, exercise programs should be initiated gradually, with stepwise increments in effort over time as the patient's conditioning and confidence improves. Of note, the use of recombinant human erythropoietin (r-HuEPO) has been found to increase the exercise capacity of patients on dialysis (108,109). It is unclear, however, whether there is a specific level of hematocrit at which the ability to exercise is optimized.

The use of tobacco products is well recognized to be one of the strongest correlates for risk of cardiovascular disease and mortality in dialysis patients (110,111). Biesenbach and Zazgornik studied the effect of smoking on survival and found that hemodialyzed diabetic cigarette smokers had higher serum fibrinogen and systolic blood pressure values. In addition, they experienced a greater incidence of myocardial infarctions and a 5-year survival rate significantly reduced compared to nonsmoking subjects (110.)

The mainstay of therapy for the control of hypertension in dialysis patients is adequate fluid removal. The ideal situation for a hemodialysis patient occurs when the patient comes to the dialysis treatment without symptoms or signs of volume excess, normotensive, and having gained less than 1 kg per interdialytic day. Unfortunately, this rarely occurs. Although it is frequently difficult to convince new dialysis patients to eat sufficient amounts of protein, it is well known that many patients on dialysis consume large amounts of fluid. Giovanetti et al. (112) found exaggerated thirst or polydipsia in 213 of 247 (86%) patients studied. They found polydipsia to be most pronounced during the first 4 hours posthemodialysis and postulated that hypernatremia was the most likely cause. Graziani et al. (113) measured serum ADH and angiotensin II levels in normodipsic and polydipsic patients. They found that patients with increased thirst had abnormally high levels of angiotensin II both before and after hemodialysis-induced volume removal. To investigate whether angiotension-converting enzyme (ACE) inhibition would be effective in inhibiting thirst in these patients, Kurayama et al. (114) gave 1 mg of cilazapril at the end of hemodialysis treatments. They reported the interdialytic weight gain to be significantly less in the ACE inhibitor–treated group, suggesting that cilazapril may alleviate dialysis-associated polydipsia. This salutary effect of ACE inhibitors on interdialytic weight gain has subsequently been disputed (115). Nonetheless, it is clear that successful hypertension therapy requires persistent efforts to limit the patient's interdialytic intake of fluid.

If hemodialysis patients begin to experience hypotension or cramping, they are usually assumed to be at dry weight, and the amount of fluid removal is curtailed. Using the technique of slow, deliberate, weekly decreases in dry weight, we have found that many patients are able to adapt to increased volume removal with a stepwise improvement in blood pressure. If uncertainty remains as to whether the patient is at his or her true dry weight, we then use intradialytic hematocrit monitoring (IHM), a noninvasive method to assess plasma volume, to guide further attempts at volume removal (116). It should be noted that there has been significant effort to develop noninvasive tools to determine actual dry weight, such as IHM, plasma ANP levels, bioimpedance plethysmography, and ultrasound measurement of the inferior vena cava diameter. While all are based on sound theoretical constructs, it can be reasonably stated that none has proven to have great clinical utility.

Despite a general consensus on the importance of adequate volume removal to treat hypertension in dialysis patients, it should be noted that some reports in the literature have not demonstrated a link between volume removal and blood pressure. Cheigh et al. (9) found no decline in blood pressure in response to ultrafiltration and suggested that volume excess may not play a role in the maintenance of hypertension for many patients. They hypothesized, however, that an overestimation of dry weight could be responsible. Luik et al. (17) performed a controlled study of 20 hemodialysis patients, measuring dry weight by echography of the vena cava. They failed to find a correlation between interdialytic weight gain and rise in blood pressure and concluded that fluid overload does not play a major role in blood pressure control. In a subsequent report by the same group, individual patients were studied during treatments with small versus large interdialytic weight gains. The large weight gain treatments were not associated with increased blood pressure, attesting to a disconnect between hypertension and volume excess (17a). Salem and Davis (117) measured blood pressure and volume parameters in 434 patients over a one-year period. They found that weight changes were not correlated with significant changes in predialysis blood pressure.

In contrast, we studied three groups of patients: one normotensive, another with blood pressure responsive to hemodialysis fluid removal, and the third with blood pressure refractory to fluid removal. Assays of atrial natriuretic factor were utilized to study volume status. We found inadequate removal of excess fluid to be the major cause of dialysis-associated hypertension, especially in patients whose blood pressure was not responsive to volume removal (43). In perhaps the most convincing report to date, Charra et al. (41) studied 692 hemodialysis patients. Their center in Tassin, France, performs 24 hours of hemodialysis per week, resulting in slow, gentle volume removal allowing for the attainment of true dry weight. Using this regimen, hypertension has been almost eliminated as a problem and survival data is outstanding. They reported that 98% of patients had well-controlled blood pressure within 3 months. The conclusion was that ultrafiltration was the most important determinant of effective blood pressure control.

If blood pressure remains >150/90 mmHg after attaining presumed dry weight and after a trial of lifestyle modification, then therapy with medications should be initiated. Table 5 reviews commonly used antihypertensive drugs and dosing issues involved in their use in patients with end-stage renal disease. Considerations derived from what is known of the pathogenesis of hypertension in dialysis patients would suggest that many different classes of antihypertensive agents might be effective (see above). The inappropriate increase in plasma angiotensin II levels in these patients indicates that ACE inhibitors or angiotensin II receptor antagonists would be effective. Beta- or alpha-adrenergic blocking agents would help to counteract the increase in sympathetic nerve activity. Calcium channel blockers would help reverse the pervasive vasoconstriction that is superimposed on volume overload.

The choice of specific medications is difficult because there are no studies that demonstrate that any one agent is more effective than others in this patient population. Therapeutic decisions often depend on associated medical conditions: e.g., beta-blockers for patients with angina or previous myocardial infarctions or ACE inhibitors for patients with congestive heart failure. The presence of left ventricular hypertrophy (LVH) is a comorbid condition of great clinical relevance to dialysis patients. Echocardiographic studies have demonstrated that LVH is highly prevalent in these patients (101) and clearly linked to adverse outcomes (118). An interesting recent study reported by Cannella et al. demonstrated that one class of medications, ACE inhibitors, had a profound effect on inducing regression of LVH. The use of these antihypertensives was associated with a 27% reduction in left ventricular mass index over a 2-year period, independent of blood pressure-lowering effects (119).

A significant number of patients remain hypertensive despite attempts at ultrafiltration and initial drug therapy. Consideration should be given to revisiting the patient's compliance with the medical regimen, use of ambulatory blood pressure (ABP) monitoring to evaluate the interdialytic hypertensive load (12,120–122), increasing dialysis time to improve volume removal (21,123), discontinuing sodium modeling (123–127), or further additions of drug therapy. Ambulatory blood pressure monitoring is an especially valuable tool to help guide changes in drug therapy. It provides a clear picture of the magnitude of hypertensive burden during the interdialytic period. In many patients, blood pressure recorded during dialysis treatment is not an accurate reflection of overall hypertensive load. Since blood pressure in hemodialysis patients usually peaks predialysis, ABP is valuable for detecting those patients whose blood pressure is due to "white coat hypertension," i.e., their blood pressure is seen to rise as the patient presents to the dialysis unit but is normal at other times. These patients can have medication doses reduced or be taken off medications with little adverse effect but require ABP to be repeated off medications.

The recent increased use of variable sodium baths during hemodialysis has led to a number of studies on the subject. In theory, hypertonic dialysate could prevent osmolar-driven volume shifts from plasma to the cellular space during dialysis. This could facilitate volume removal by preventing the induction of hypotension. If plasma remains hypertonic postdialysis, however, the improved volume removal may be for naught, because increased thirst could lead to greater volume gains between treatments. There is no consensus at present as to whether the practice of sodium modeling is beneficial for improving hypertension treatment. Sang et al. (125) found that interdialytic thirst, blood pressure, and weight gains increased with dialysate sodium ramping (sodium graded from 155 mEq/L at the initiation of dialysis to 140 mEq/L at the end). In contrast, Flanigan et al. (124) demonstrated a decrease in need for blood pressure medications in those patients treated with a variable sodium model. They found, however, that postdialysis target weight tended to in-

Table 5 Antihypertensive Medications

Drug	Half-life (hours)		Normal dose range (mg)	ESRD dose adjustment (%)	Dialysis removal (%)	
	Normal	ESRD			HD	PD
Alpha-adrenergic blockers						
Doxazocin	22	22	1–16	None	None	
Terazosin	11.4–14	11.4–15	1–10	None	10	
Prazosin	2–3	2–3	6–15	None	None	None
Beta-adrenergic blockers						
Atenolol	6–7	>27	25–100	75	50	50
Acebutalol	3–4	Increased	400–800	75	50	
Propranolol	4	4	40–240	None	None	None
Labetalol	6–8	6–8	100–800	None		
Pindolol	3–4	3–4	10–60	None		
Nadolol	16	45	20–240	25–50	>40	
Metoprolol	3–7	3–7	50–200	None	>50	
ACE inhibitors						
Benazepril	10	?	5–40	None	None	
Captopril	2–3	21–32	50–200	25–50	Some	
Fosinopril	12	Increased	20–40	None	Some	Some
Enalapril	11	34–60	5–40	25–50	30	
Ramipril	10	Increased	2.5–20	25–50	Some	
Lisinopril	12	40–50	2.5–40	25–50	50	
Quinapril	2	12	20–80	25		
Calcium channel blockers						
Amlodipine	30–50	30–50	5–10	100		
Diltiazem	3–4.5	Unchanged	120–240	None		
Felødipine	10	Unchanged	2.5–10	None		
Isradipine	10	10–11	5–20	None		
Nicardipine	6	Unchanged	60–120	None		
Nifedipine	2	Unchanged	30–60	None		
Verapamil	8	Unchanged	120–360	None		
Nisoldipine	7–12	Unchanged	20–40	None		
Others						
Clonidine	12–16	41	0.2–0.6	50	5	
Hydralazine	3–7	Increased	75–150		None	None
Minoxidil	2.8–4.2	4.2	5–30	100	Some	Some
Methyldopa	1–2	3–16	500–2000	50	50	30

crease with the use of the sodium model. Therefore, it is not possible at this time to definitively conclude whether sodium modeling is beneficial to most patients. For individual patients with difficult-to-control hypertension, especially when intradialytic symptoms limit volume removal, a trial of modeling is reasonable. Conversely, in a patient treated with variable sodium dialysate who continues to have hypertension and significant weight gains between treatments, the model should be discontinued and the effect evaluated.

Since adequate fluid removal during dialysis remains paramount for effective blood pressure treatment, if hypertension cannot be controlled sufficiently then additional time on dialysis may be necessary. With short dialysis times, interdialytic fluid gain often leads to aggressive ultrafiltration that results in hypotension and cramping. Subsequently, the target weight is adjusted upwards, dry weight is not reached, and hypertension becomes difficult to treat. Increased dialysis time could allow for more complete removal of fluid and an eventual reduction in the need for antihypertensive medications (21,41a,b).

If all the above methods are ineffective and a patient's blood pressure remains uncontrolled, then eval-

Table 6 Principal Secondary Forms of Hypertension in Dialysis Patients

1. Renal (vascular or parenchymal disease)
2. Endocrine (adrenal, thyroid, or parathyroid disease)
3. Drugs (cyclosporin, erythropoietin)
4. Increased cardiac output secondary to thyroid disease or AV fistula

Table 7 Hypertension Severity Index

HSI score	Systolic (mmHg)	HSI score	Diastolic (mmHg)
0	<150	0	<90
1	150–159	1	90–99
2	159–179	2	99–109
3	>179	3	>109

To calculate for an individual dialysis treatment, sum the predialysis systolic and diastolic and postdialysis systolic and diastolic blood pressure scores. The HSI can range from 0 to 12. A patient with predialysis blood pressure of 160/100 mmHg and postdialysis 130/94 mmHG would have an HSI of 5 for that treatment. Ideally, at least 2 weeks of scores should be averaged to evaluate overall blood pressure control.

uation for a secondary cause of hypertension should be considered (Table 6). In addition, thought should be given to changing dialytic modality to peritoneal dialysis (8,105). As a last resort, bilateral nephrectomy may be helpful in patients with severe, refractory hypertension. See Table 7 for the Hypertension Severity Index.

REFERENCES

1. The National Center for Health Statistics. Vital Statistics Report, Final Mortality Statistics, 1986.
2. Kannel WB, Gordon T, Scwartz MJ. Systolic versus diastolic blood pressure and risk of coronary heart disease. The Framingham Study. Am J Cardiol 1971; 27:335–345.
3. Comty C, Rottka H, Sjaldon S. Blood pressure control in patients with end-stage renal failure treated by intermittent hemodialysis. Proc Eur Dial Trans Assoc 1964; 1:209–220.
4. Rostand SG, Kirk KA, Rutsky EA. Relationship of coronary risk factors to hemodialysis associated ischemic heart disease. Kidney Int 1982; 22:304–308.
5. Herrera-Acosta J. Hypertension in chronic renal disease. Kidney Int 1982; 22:702–712.
6. Zucchelli P, Santoro A, Zuccala A. Genesis and control of hypertension in hemodialysis patients. Semin Nephrol 1988; 8:163.
7. HCFA 1995 Annual Report. ESRD Core Indicators Project. Baltimore: Health Care Financing Administration, DHHS, 1996.
8. Rocco MV, Flanagan MJ, Beaver S, et al. Report from the 1995 core indicators for peritoneal dialysis study group. Am J Kidney Dis 1997; 30:165–173.
9. Cheigh JS, Milite C, Sullivan JF, Rubin AL, Stenzel KH. Hypertension is not adequately controlled in hemodialysis patients. Am J Kidney Dis 1992; 19:453–459.
10. Amar J, Vernier I, Rossignol, et al . Influence of nycthermal blood pressure pattern in treated hypertensive patients on hemodialysis. Kidney Int 1997; 51:1863–1866.
11. Luik AJ, Gladziwa U, Kooman JP, et al. Influence of interdialytic weight gain on blood pressure in hemodialysis patients. Blood Purif 1994; 12:259–266.
12. Conlon PJ, Walshe JJ, Heinle SK, et al. Predialysis systolic blood pressure correlates strongly with mean 24-hour systolic blood pressure and left ventricular mass in stable hemodialysis patients. J Am Soc Nephrol 1996; 7:2658–2663.
13. U.S. Renal Data System. USRDS 1997 Annual Data Report. U.S. Department of Health and Human Services. Bethesda, MD: The National Institutes of Health, National Institute of Diabetes and Digestive and Kidney Diseases, 1997.
14. Highlights from the 1996 Core Indicators Project for Hemodialysis Patients. HCFA; Dial Transplant 1997: 188–191.
15. Rodby RA, Vonesh EF, Korbet SM. Blood pressures in hemodialysis and peritoneal dialysis using ambulatory blood pressure monitoring. Am J Kidney Dis 1994; 23:401–411.
16. Salem MM. Hypertension in the hemodialysis population: a survey of 649 patients. Am J Kidney Dis 1995; 26:461–468.
17. Luik AJ, Gladziwa U, Kooman JP, van Hoof JP, de Leeuw PW, van Bortel LM, Leunissen KM. Blood pressure changes in relation to interdialytic weight gain. Contrib Nephrol 1994; 106:90–93.

17a. Luik AJ, van Kuijk WH, Spek J, et al. Effects of hypervolemia on interdialytic hemodynamics and blood pressure control in hemodialysis patients. Am J Kidney Dis 1997; 30:466–474.

18. Acchiardo SR, Burk L, Smith SJ. Automated ambulatory blood pressure monitoring of hemodialysis patients (abstr). J Am Soc Nephrol 1994; 5:555.
19. Kooman JP, Gladziwa U, Bocker G, et al. Blood pressure during the interdialytic period in hemodialysis patients: estimation of representitive blood pressure values. Neprol Dial Transplant 1992; 7:917–923.
20. Joint National Committee on Detection, Evaluation, and Treatment of High Blood Pressure. 5th Report of the Joint National Committee on Detection, Eval-

uation, and treatment of High Blood Pressure. Bethesda: NIH, 1993.

21. Charra B, Calemard E, Ruffet M, Chazot C, Terrat J-C, Vanel T, Laurent G. Survival as an index of adequacy of dialysis. Kidney Int 1992; 41:1286–1291.
22. Degoulet P, Legrain M, Reach I, Aime F, Devries C, Rojas P, Jacobs C. Mortality risk factors in patients treated by chronic hemodialysis. Nephron 1982; 31: 103–110.
23. Ritz E, Ruffman K, Rambausek M, Mall G, Schmidli H. Dialysis hypotension- is it related to diastolic left ventricular malfunction? Nephrol Dial Transplant 1987; 2:293–297.
24. Santiago A, Chazan JA. The cause of death and comorbid factors in 405 chronic hemodialysis patients. Dial Transplant 1989; 18:484.
25. Ritz E, Koch M. Morbidity and mortality due to hypertension in patients with renal failure. Am J Kidney Dis 1993; 21 (suppl 2):113–118.
26. Tomita J, Kimura G, Inoue T, Inenaga T, Sanai T, Kawano Y, Nakamura S, Baba S, Matsuoka H, Omae T. Role of systolic blood pressure in determining prognosis of hemodialyzed patients. Am J Kidney Dis 1995; 25:405–412.
27. Foley RN, Parfrey PS, Harnett JD, Kent GM, Murray DC, Barre PE. Impact of hypertension on cardiomyopathy, morbidity and mortality in end-stage renal disease. Kidney Int 1996; 49:1379–1385.
27a. Zager PG, Nikolic J, Brown RH, et al. "U" curve association of blood pressure and mortality in hemodialysis patients. Kidney Int 1998; 54(2):561–569.
28. Duranti E, Imperiali P, Sasdelli M. Is hypertension a mortality risk factor in dialysis? Kidney Int 1996; 49(suppl 55):S173-S174.
29. Vertas V,Cangiano JL,Berman LB. Hypertension in end-stage renal disease. N Engl J Med 1969; 280: 978–981.
30. U.S. Renal Data System. USRDS 1994 Annual Data Report. Bethesda, MD: National Institute of Diabetes and Digestive and Kidney Diseases, 1994 (NIH Publication No. 94–3176).
31. Appel RG, Bleyer AJ, Reavis, Hansen KG. Renovascular disease in older patients beginning renal replacement therapy. Kidney Int 1995; 48:171–180.
32. Jackobson HR. Ischemic renal disease: an overlooked clinical entity. Kidney Int 1988; 34:729–734.
33. Mailloux JU, Napolitano B, Belluci AG, et al. Renal vascular disease causing end stage renal disease. Incidence, clinical correlates, and outcome: a 20 year clinical experience. Am J Kidney Dis 1994; 24:622–628.
34. Hansen KJ. Prevalance of Ischemic nephropathy in the atherosclerotic population. Am J Kidney Dis 1994; 24:615–621.
35. Zuccchelli P, Santoro A, Zuccala A. Genesis and control of hypertension in hemodialysis patients. Sem Nephrol 1988; 8(2):163.
36. Herrara-Acosta J. Hypertension in chronic renal disease. Kidney Int 1982; 22:702–712.
37. Scribner B. A personalized history of hemodialysis. Am J Kidney Dis 1990; 16:511–519.
38. Piero D, Michelangelo V, Pietro B. Influence of the hydration state on blood pressure values in a group of patients on regular maintenance hemodialysis. Blood Purif 1997; 15:25–33.
39. Koomans HA, Roos, JC. Salt sensitivity of blood pressure in chronic renal failure: evidence for renal control of body fluid distribution in man. Hypertension 1982; 4:190–197.
40. Sulkova S, Valek A. Role of antihypertensive drugs in the therapy of patients on regular dialysis treatment. Kidney Int 1988; 34(suppl 25):S198-S200.
41. Charra B. Control of blood pressure in long slow hemodialysis. Blood Purif 1994; 12:252–258.
41a. Uldall R, Ouwendyk M, Francoeur R, et al. Slow nocturnal home hemodialysis at the Wellesley Hospital. Adv Ren Replace Ther 1996; 3:133–136.
41b. Goldsmith DJ, Covic AC, Venning MC, et al. Ambulatory blood pressure minitoring in renal dialysis and transplant patients. Am J Kidney Dis 1997; 4: 593–600.
42. Cannata JB, Isles CG, Briggs JD, Junor BJ. Comparison of blood pressure control during hemodialysis and CAPD. Nephrol Dial Transplant 1986; 15: 674–679.
43. Fishbane S, Natke E, Maesaka JK. Role of volume overload in dialysis refractory hypertension Am J Kidney Dis 1996; 28;257–261.
44. Coleman TG, Guyton AC. Hypertension caused by salt loading in the dog: III.Onset transients of the cardiac output and other variables. Circ Res 1969; 25:153–160.
45. Mailloux LU, Belluci AG, Napolitano B. The impact of comorbid risk factors at the start of dialysis upon the survival of ESRD patients. ASAIO J 1996; 42: 164–169.
46. Lazarus JM, Hampers CL, Merrill JP. Hypertension in chronic renal failure. Treatment with hemodialysis and nephrectomy. Arch Intern Med 1974; 133:1059–1065.
47. Glatter KA, Graves SW, Hollenberg NK. Sustained volume expansion and (Na-K) ATPase inhibition in chronic renal failure. Am J Hypertension 1994; 7: 1016–1024.
48. Hamlyn JM, Manunta P. Ouabain, digitalis like factors in hypertension. J Hypertens 1992; 10(suppl 7): S99–111.
49. Haddy FJ, Buckalew VM. Endogenous digitalis like factors in hypertension In: Laragh J Brenner BM, eds., Hypertension: Pathophysiology, Diagnosis and

Management. New York: Raven Press, 1995:1055–1067.
50. Boero R, Guarena C, Berto IM. Pathogenesis of arterial hypertensionin chronic uremia. The role of reduced Na-K ATPase activity. J Hypertens 1988; 6(suppl 14):S363-S365.
51. Kresinski JM, Rorive G. Plasma Na-K ATPase inhibitor activity and intrcellular ion during hemodialysis. Int J Artif Organs 1993; 16:23–30.
52. Fervenza F, Hendry BM, Ellory JC. Effects of dialysis and transplantation on red cell sodium pump function in renal failure. Nephron 1989; 53:121–128.
53. Woolfson R, Hilton P, Poston L. Effect of ouabain and low sodium on contractility of human resistance arterial hypertension 1990; 15:583–590.
54. Krzesinski JM, Rorie G. Influence of sodium balance on uremic red blood cell ion transport Nephron 1988; 49:126–131.
55. Cole CH. Decreased ouabain-sensitive adenosine triphophatase activity in the erythrocyte membrane of patients with chronic renal disease. Clin Sci Mol Med 1973; 45775–45784.
56. Kramer HJ. Functional and metabolic studies on red blood cell sodium transport in chronic Uremia. Nephron 1976; 16:344–358.
57. Labonia WK. Effects of L-carnitine on sodium transport in erythrocyte from dialysed uremic patients. Kidney Int 1987; 32:754–759.
58. Gafter U, Levi J. Red blood cell calcium homeostasis in patients with end stage renal disease. J Lab Clin Med 1989; 114:222–231.
59. Moosa A, Greaves M. Elevated platelet-free calcium in uremia. Br J Hematol 1990; 74:300–305.
60. Schiffl H. Correlation of blood pressure in end stage renal disease with platelet cytosolic free calcium concentration. Klin Wochenschr 1990; 68(14):718–722.
60a. Textor SC, Gavras H, Tifft CP, et al. Norepinephrine and renin activity in chronic renal failure. Hypertension 1981; 3:294–299.
60b. Campese VM, Romoff MS, Levitan D, et al. Mechanisms of autonomic nervous system dysfunction in uremia. Kidney Int 1981; 20:246–253.
61. Converse RL, Jackobsen TN, Toto, Fouad-Tarazi F. Sympathetic overactivity in patients with chronic renal failure. N Engl J Med 1992; 327:1912–1917.
62. Hansen J, Victor RG. Direct measurement of sympathetic activity: New insight into disordered blood pressure regulation in chronic renal failure. Curr Opin Neph Hyper 1994; 3:636–643.
63. Recordati G, Moss NG. Renal chemoreceptor. J Auton Nerv Syst 1981; 3:237–251.
64. Dibona GF. The function of renal nerves. Rev Physio Biochem Pharmacol 1982; 4:76–181.
65. Katholi RE. Renal nerves and hypertension: an update. Fed Proc 1985; 44:2846–2850.
66. Katholi RE. Intrarenal adenosine produces hypertension by activating the sympathetic nervous system via the renal veins. J Hypertens 1984; 2:349–359.
67. Winearls CG, Oliver DO, Cotes PM. Effect of human erythropoietin derived from recombinant DNA on the anemia of patients maintained by chronic hemodialysis. Lancet 1986; 301:1175–1178.
68. Eschbach JW, Adamson JW, et al. Correction of the anemia of end stage renal disease with recombinent human erythropoietin. N Engl J Med 1987; 316: 73–78.
69. Raine AEG. Hypertension, blood viscosity and cardiovscular morbidity in renal failure: implications of erythropoietin therapy. Lancet 1988; 316:73–78.
70. Buckner FS, Adamson JW. Hypertension following erythropoietin therapy in anemic hemodialysis patients. Am J Hypertens 1990; 3:947–955.
71. Maschio G. Erythropoietin and systemic hypertension. Nephrol Dial Transplant 1995; 10(suppl 2): 74–79.
72. Eschbach JW, Kelly MR. Treatment of anemia of progressive renal failure with recombinant human erythropoietin. N Engl J Med 1989; 321:158–163.
73. Eschbach JW, Abdulhadi MH. Recombinent human erythropoietin in anemic patients with end stage renal disease. Ann Intern Med 1989; 111:992–1000.
74. Watson AJ, Giminez LF, Cotton S, et al. Treatment of the anemia of chronic renal failure with subcutaneous recombinant human erythropoieitin. Am J Med 1990; 89:432.
75. Hand MF, Haynes WG, Johnstone HA, et al. Erythropoieitin enhances vascular responsiveness to norepinephrine in renal failure. Kidney Int 1995; 48:806.
76. Schaefer RM, Heidland A. Blood rheology and hypertension in hemodialysis patients treated with erythropoietin. Am J Nephrol 1988; 8:449–453.
77. Nonnast-Daniel B, Creutzig A, Kohn K. Effect of treatment with recombinant human erythropoietin on peripheral hemodynamics and oxygenation. Contrib Nephrol 1988; 66:185–194.
78. Verbeelen D, Jonckheer MH. Hemodynamics of patient with renal failure treated with recombinant human erythropoietin. Clin Nephrol 1989; 31:6–11.
79. London GM, Pannier B. Vascular changes in hemodialysis patients in response to recombinant human erythropoietin. Kidney Int 1989; 36:878–882.
80. Heidenreich S, Rahn KH, Zidek W. Direct vasopressor effect of recombinant human erythropoietin on renal resistance vessels. Kidney Int 1991; 39:259–265.
81. Ernie P, Bolli P, Buhler FR. Correlation of platelet Calcium with blood pressure. N Engl J Med 1984; 310:1084–1088.
82. Alexiewicz JM, Campese VM. Effect of dietary sodium intake on intracellular calcium in lymphocytes of salt sensitive hypersensitive patients. Am J Hypertens 1992; 5:536–541.

83. Raine AEG, Bedford L, Simpson AWM, Ashley CC, Ledingha JGG. Hyperparathyroidism, platelet intracellular free calcium and hypertension in chronic renal failure. Kidney Int 1993; 43:700–705.
84. Goldsmith DJA, et al. Blood pressure reduction after parathyroidectomy for secondary hyperparathyroidism: further evidence implicating calcium homeostasis in blood pressure regulation. Am J Kidney Dis 1996; 27:819–825.
85. Fishbane S, Frei GL, Dressler R, Finger M, Silbiger S. Hypervitaminosis A in two hemodialysis patients. Am J Kidney Dis 1995; 25(2):346–349.
86. Iseki K, et al. Effects of hypercalcemia and PTH on blood pressure in normal and renal failure rats. Am J Physiol 1986; 250:F924-F929.
87. Furchgott RF, Zawadski JV. The obligatory role of endothelial cells in the relaxation of arterial smooth muscle cells by acetylcholine. Nature 1980; 299: 373–376.
88. Palmer RMJ, Ferrige JAG, Moncada S. Nitric oxide release accounts for the biologic activity of endothelium-derived relaxation factor. Nature 1987; 327: 524–526.
89. Yanagisawa M, Hurihara M, Kimura S et al. A novel vasoconstrictor peptide produced by vascular endothelial cells. Nature 1988; 332:411–415.
90. Luscher TF. Imbalance of endothelium derived relaxing and contracting factors. Am J Hypertens 1990; 3:317–330.
91. Luscher TF. The endothelium-target and promoter of hypertension. Hypertension 1990; 15:482–485.
92. Madore F, Prud'homme L, Austin JS, Blaise G, Francoeur M, Leveille M, Prud'homme M, Vinay P. Impact of nitric oxide on blood pressure in hemodialysis patients. Am J Kidney Dis 1997; 30:665–671.
93. Vallance P, Leone A, Calver A, Collier J, Moncada S. Accumulation of an endogenous inhibitor of nitric oxide synthesis in chronic renal failure. Lancet 1992; 339:572–575.
94. Luscher TF, Oemar BS, Boulanger CM, Hahn AWA. Molecular and cellular biology of endothelin and its receptors. J Hypertens 1993; 11:7–11.
95. Yokokawa K, Tahara H, et al. Hypertension associated withendothelin secreting malignant hemangioendothelioma. Ann Intern Med 1991; 114:213–215.
96. Shichiri M, Hirata Y, Ando K, et al. Plasma endothelin levels in hypertension and chronic renal failure. Hypertension 1990; 15:493–496.
97. Koyama H, Tabata T, et al. Plasma endothelin levels in patients with uremia. Lancet 1989; 1:991–992.
98. Suzuki N, Matsumoto H, Miyauchi T, et al. Endothelin-3 concentrations in human plasma: the increased concentrations in patients undergoing hemodialysis. Biochem Biophys Res Commun 1990; 169:809–815.
99. Miyauchi T, Masaki T, et al. Plasma concentrations of endothelin 1 and endothelin 3 are altered differently in various pathophysiological conditions in humans. J Cardiovasc Pharmacol 1991; 17(suppl 7): S394–S397.
100. Thomson GE, Waterhouse K, McDonald HP Jr, Friedman EA. Hemodialysis for chronic renal failure. Arch Int Med 1967; 120:153–167.
101. Parfrey PS, Hartnett JD, Griffiths SM, et al. The clinical course of left ventricular hypertrophy in dialysis patients. Nephrol Dial Transplant 1990; 5:39–44.
102. Raine AEG, Margreiter R, Brunner FP, et al. Report on management of renal failure in Europe. Nephrol Dial Transplant 1992; 7(suppl 2):7–35.
103. Kowalski EA, Mittal SK, Trenkle J, et al. Hypertension in a hemodialysis population. (abstr) J Am Soc Nephrol 1997;8:242.
103a. Kowalski EA, Mittal SK, Trenkle J, et al. Hypertension in a hemodialysis population. Clin Nephrol.
104. Canziani ME, Cendroglio M, Saragoca M, et al. Hemodialysis versus continuous ambulatory peritoneal dialysis: effects on the heart. Artif organs 1995; 19(3) 241–244.
105. Saldhana LF, Weiler EW, Gonick HC. Effect of continuous ambulatory peritoneal dialysis on blood pressure control. Am J Kidney Dis 1993; 21(2):184–188.
106. Fagard, RH. The role of exercise in blood pressure control: supportive evidence. J Hypertension 1995; 13:1223–1226.
107. Duncan JJ, Farr JE, Upton SJ, et al. The effects of aerobic exercise on plasma catecholamines and blood pressure in patients with mild essential hypertension. JAMA 1985; 254:2609.
108. Lundin AP, Ackerman MJ, Chesler RM, et al. Exercise in hemodialysis patients after treatment with recombinant human erythropoietin. Nephron 1991; 58: 315–319.
109. Painter P. The importance of exercise training in rehabilitation of patients with end stage renal disease. Am J Kidney Dis 1994; 24(suppl 1):S2–9.
110. Biesenbach G, Zazgornik J. Influence of smoking on the survival rate of diabetic patients requiring hemodialysis. Diabetes Care 1996; 19:(6)625–628.
111. Davis JW, Arnold J, Wiegmann T. Cigarette smoking affects platelets and endothelium in chronic hemodialysis patients. Nephron 1993; 64(3):359–364.
112. Giovanetti S, Barsotti G, Cupristi A, et al. Dipsogenic factors operating in chronic uremics on maintenance hemodialysis. Nephron. 1994; 66(4):413–420.
113. Graziani G, Badalamenti S, Del Bo A, et al. Abnormal hemodynamics and elevated angiotensin II plasma levels in polydipsic patients on regular hemodialysis treatments. Kidney Int 1993; 44 (1):107–114.
114. Kuriyama S, Tomonari H, Sakai O. Effect of cila-

zepril on hyperdipsia in hemodialyzed patients. Blood Purif 1996; 14(1):35–41.

115. Bastani B, Redington J. Lack of efficacy of angiotensin converting enzyme inhibitors in reducing interdialytic weight gain. Am J Kidney Dis 1994; 24(6):907–922.
116. Steuer RR, Leypoldt JK, Cheung AK, et al. Reducing symptoms during hemodialysis by continuously monitoring the hematocrit. Am J Kidney Dis 1996; 27(4):525–532.
117. Salem MM, Davis M. Effects of one year of hemodialysis on weight and blood pressure in 434 patients. Artif Organs 1997; 21(5):402–404.
118. Silverberg JS, Barre PE, Prichard SS, et al. Impact of left ventricular hypertrophy on survival in end-stage renal disease. Kidney Int 1989; 36:286–290.
119. Cannella G, Paoletti E, Delfino R, Peloso G, Rolla D, Molinari S. Prolonged therapy with ACE inhibitors induces a regression of left ventricular hypertrophy of dialyzed uremic patients independently from hypotensive effects. Am J Kidney Dis 1997; 30:659–664.
120. Chazot C, Charra G, Laurent C, et al. Interdialysis blood pressure control by long hemodialysis sessions. Nephrol Dial Transplant 1995; 10:831–837.
121. Mansoor G, White W. Ambulatory blood pressure monitoring in current clinical practice and research. Current Opinion Nephrol Hypertens 1995; (4):531–537.
122. Coomer RW, Schulman G, Breyer JA, Shyr Y Ambulatory blood pressure monitoring in dialysis patients and estimation of mean interdialytic blood pressure. Am J Kidney Dis 1997; 29(5):678–684.
123. Levin A, Goldstein MB. The benefits and side effects of ramped hypertonic sodium dialysis. JASN 1996; (7):242–246.
124. Flanigan MJ, Khairullah QT, Lim VS. Dialysate sodium delivery can alter chronic blood pressure management. Am J Kidney Dis 1997; 29(3):383–391.
125. Sang GL, Kovithavongs C, Ulan R, et al. Sodium ramping in hemodialysis: a study of beneficial and adverse effects. Am J Kidney Dis 1996; 29(5):669–677.
126. Petitclerc T, Trombert JC, Coevert B, et al. Electrolyte modeling: sodium IS dialysate sodium profiling actually useful? Nephrol Dial Transplant 1996; 11(suppl 2):35–38.
127. Movilli E, Camerini C, Viola BF, et al. Volume changes during three different profiles of sodium variation with similar intradialytic sodium indices in chronic hemodialyzed patients. Am J Kidney Dis 1997; 30(1)58–63.

27

Pulmonary Problems in Hemodialysis and Peritoneal Dialysis

Eric E. O. Gheuens and Ronald Daelemans
General Hospital Stuivenberg, Antwerp, Belgium

Marc E. De Broe
University Hospital Antwerp, Antwerp, Belgium

I. INTRODUCTION

Alterations in respiratory function (respiratory drive, lung mechanics, muscle function, and gas exchange) are frequent consequences of uremia. Patients with acute or end-stage chronic renal failure, whether treated by dialysis or not, frequently develop pulmonary complications such as edema, pleural effusion, and infection (1). In addition, hemodialysis treatment itself also affects the pulmonary system. This chapter deals with the dialysis-related pulmonary aspects of patients with renal failure.

II. UREMIC LUNG

Radiologists first described the characteristic butterfly or batwing appearance in anteroposterior x-rays of the lung. The distinctive radiological features are an enlarged vascular pedicle, a "balanced" pulmonary blood flow distribution, an increased pulmonary blood volume, and a central distribution of edema (2). As this entity frequently complicated end-stage renal failure, it was referred to as "uremic lung." Later it was also recognized in other conditions such as acute rheumatic fever and chronic left ventricular failure. Gavelli et al. published a state-of-the-art work concerning radiography of the thoracic manifestations of terminal uremia (3) in which they state that a chest x-ray is not able to accurately discriminate between cardiogenic edema and fluid overload edema.

In patients with chronic renal failure, the pressure forces in the Starling equation often favor secondary pulmonary edema. Hydrostatic pressures in the central circulation may be high because of increased intravascular volume or congestive heart failure or both. Intravascular oncotic pressure may also be low because of hypoproteinemia, predisposing to pulmonary edema at lower hydrostatic pressures (4). For these reasons alone, butterfly infiltrates of pulmonary edema on chest radiograph would be expected. Uremic lung is thus a form of pulmonary edema that can eventually result in fibrotic interstitial changes.

In the early phase the alveolar fibrinous edema fluid and the interlobular septa are very edematous and swollen. Usually the edema fluid is completely absorbed, but in more chronic, persistent cases the exudate organizes and fibrotic changes occur in the interstitium.

The characteristic distribution of the edematous exudate found in uremic lung is largely explained by diversion of flow to more central parts of the lung, which are supplied by the shortest arterial pathway. Indeed, the increased pulmonary venous pressure due to left ventricular failure causes reflex vasoconstriction in the pulmonary arteries, especially of the longer arterial pathways resulting in diversion of the blood flow through more central parts of the lung.

It is now generally agreed that uremic lung is a form of pulmonary edema caused primarily by left ventricular failure and pulmonary engorgement, but a local capillary toxic factor and possibly deficient fibrinolysis may also play a part. This toxic factor, still unknown and most probably the same as involved in the occurrence of uremic pleuritis, increases the permeability of alveolar capillaries resulting in leakage of macromolecular proteins and even red blood cells. Alveolar edemas caused by these lesional factors tend to regress slowly and incompletely, leaving fibrosis (3).

The most important cause of lung edema in dialysis patients is noncompliance with fluid restriction, a rather frequent condition especially in patients with no or negligible residual diuresis. Patients with acute renal failure are also highly susceptible to pulmonary edema. They frequently have decreased plasma oncotic pressure, an increased hydrostatic pressure in pulmonary capillaries because of fluid overload, and changes in alveolar capillaries due to their uremic state.

In contrast to patients with normal renal function, dialysis patients cannot be managed with the classical measures of preload reduction (nitrates, morphine, and diuretics) alone. Treatment of pulmonary edema mainly consists of emergency dialysis with ultrafiltration. Until dialysis therapy can be initiated, supportive measures (oxygen, raising the upper body, nitrates, and morphine) have to be undertaken. Occasionally the patient presents with severe respiratory distress requiring sedation, intubation, and mechanical ventilation. When dialysis cannot be instituted promptly, some authors advocate phlebotomy as an emergency measure (5). Usually symptoms gradually improve from the onset of dialysis over a short period of time (hours).

III. PLEURAL EFFUSION IN DIALYSIS

Richard Bright noted that in patients who died of nephritis "of all the membranes, the pleura has decidedly been most often diseased" (6). Uremic patients have an increased susceptibility to many causes of transsudative or exudative pleural effusions such as congestive heart failure, nephrotic syndrome, salt and water retention, and infection (7). Among the latter, tuberculous pleural effusion in particular should be excluded. In addition, an idiopathic uremic pleural effusion exists.

Idiopathic pleural involvement in uremia and in dialysis patients is due to necrotizing fibrinous inflammation and often results in a serous serosanguineous or even hemorrhagic effusion (8,9). This type of pleural reaction may occur without concomitant overhydration and without apparent cause; gradual spontaneous resolution often occurs, sometimes followed by recurrences (8). One should search carefully for evidence of coexisting pericardial effusion in these cases. A few patients have progressive disease wherein the pleural fluid becomes gelatinous and a thick fibrous peel develops (10,11). Fibrous uremic pleuritis causes progressive restriction of pulmonary function with restricted lung volumes and disabling dyspnea of increasing severity, until relieved by surgical decortication (10).

The etiology and/or pathogenesis of uremic pleuritis remains unknown and has been the subject of numerous speculations (7). It must be emphasized that the finding of hemorrhagic pleural effusion in a uremic patient (dialyzed or not) requires the exclusion of all causes of hemorrhagic pleural effusion before it is concluded to be due to uremia.

In a recent study pleural effusions were present in 28% of predialysis chest radiographs (n = 36), half of which persisted after dialysis and half resolved (12). Pleural effusion is a radiological sign of fluid retention, and prior to any diagnostic testing the patient's dry weight should be reduced. If after appropriate weight reduction the pleural effusion persists, further investigation is warranted. The diagnostic approach to pleural effusions has been recently reviewed (13) and is not different in a dialysis patient compared to the approach in a patient with normal renal function. The chest x-ray is not very sensitive for the detection of pleural effusion until the amount of pleural fluid exceeds 500 ml (14). Nevertheless, in most cases, conventional chest radiography with lateral decubitus views will show the presence and location of pleural effusion. When additional imaging is required to either detect or localize pleural effusion or guide thoracocentesis, ultrasound is the preferred technique for reasons of cost and availability. When more detailed information about the pleural space is required, computerized tomography is superior to ultrasound. In order to determine the specific cause of a pleural effusion, a diagnostic thoracocentesis has to be performed. The differential diagnosis is usually separated into transudates versus exudates, defined by the classical criteria of Light et al. (15). Fluid is considered exudative if it meets one or more of the following criteria: the absolute pleural fluid lactate dehydrogenase (LDH) level is >200 units, the pleural:serum LDH ratio is >0.6, and/or the pleural:serum protein ratio is >0.5. These criteria have a high sensitivity and specificity for the separation of transudates from exudates. Defining an effusion as a transudate limits the differential diagnosis to a low number of disorders and ends the need for further investigation of the effusion itself (Table 1). The differential diagnosis of exudative effusions is much broader (Table 1). Three of the most common causes are pneumonia, malig-

Table 1 Pleural Effusions: Differential Diagnosis of Transudates and Exudates

Transudative effusions	
Congestive heart failure	Atelectasis
Cirrhosis	Myxedema
Nephrotic syndrome	Pulmonary embolism
Peritoneal dialysis	Urinothorax
Exudative effusions	
Malignancy	Other inflammatory
Lung	Pulmonary embolism
Lymphoma	Dressler's syndrome
Mesothelioma	Asbestosis
Metastatic	Uremia
	Trapped lung
Infectious	Radiation therapy
Parapneumonic	Meigs' syndrome
Tuberculous	
Fungal	Lymphatic disease
Viral	Chylothorax
Parasitic	Lymphangiolyomyomatosis
Abdominal abscess	Yellow nail syndrome
Hepatitis	
Noninfectious gastrointestinal	Drug-induced
Pancreatitis	Drug-induced lupus
Esophageal rupture	Nitrofurantoin
Abdominal surgery	Dantrolene
Variceal sclerotherapy	Amiodarone
	Methysergide
Collagen vascular disease	Procarbazine
Lupus erythematosus	Practolol
Rheumatoid arthritis	Bromocriptine
Wegener's granulomatosis	Minoxidil
Churg-Strauss syndrome	Bleomycin
Familial Mediterranean fever	Methotrexate
Sjögren's syndrome	Mitomycin
Immunoblastic lympadenopathy	Trauma
Diseases that can present with transudative or exudative effusions	
Pulmonary embolism (usually exudate)	
Diuresed transudate	

Source: Ref. 13.

nancy, and *Mycobacterium tuberculosis*. Pleural biopsy (needle or thorascoscopic biopsy) for pathology and culture can be helpful in the work-up of an exudative effusion, especially when the cause is still undiagnosed after initial thoracocentesis (14). When after these procedures the diagnosis still has not been established and there are parenchymal abnormalities on chest x-ray or the patient has hemoptoe, a bronchoscopy is the logical next step.

Dialysis patients may also develop pleural effusions directly related to their type of treatment such as a catheter-related superior vena cava obstruction or subclavian venous catheter leak (16). With peritoneal dialysis, a leakage of dialysate through a small, often congenital diaphragmatic defect may result in a rather small pleural effusion relieved by erect posture, up to a massive, usually right-sided hydrothorax within hours to days after starting this type of treatment. It is an unusual complication of CAPD. When it persists or recurrs, surgical correction or alternate forms of dialysis are required.

The diagnosis of pleural effusion related to peritoneal dialysis is fairly simple. Analysis of the fluid usually matches the dialysate, with low protein, low lactic dehydrogenase, but high glucose content. Several techniques can be applied to actually illustrate the transfer of dialysate from the peritoneum to the pleural cavity. Methylene blue can be added to the dialysate and recovered from the pleural fluid. However, this technique is unreliable and can cause chemical peritonitis (17). The intraperitoneal use of radio-isotopes such as technetium 99m-tagged macroaggregated albumin, sulphur colloid, or human albumin is a valid alternative (18–23). Some investigators combine the intraperitoneal instillation of the radiocontrast agent iopamidol with abdominal x-ray and computerized tomography to diagnose noninfectious complications of peritoneal dialysis, including pleuroperitoneal communications (24–26).

Jagasia et al. recently managed three patients with CAPD-induced right hydrothorax secondary to dialysate leakage through a diaphragmatic defect (27). Earlier treatment methods included thoracentesis or tube thoracostomy with chemical pleurodesis and even thoracotomy with attempts to locate and close the communication. The authors used a new approach consisting of video-assisted thoracic surgery and direct talc poudrage. All patients were successfully returned to CAPD; one patient required a repeat procedure after an initial recurrence. Video-assisted thoracic surgery with talc poudrage is an effective and safe procedure with minimal morbidity for management of hydrothorax secondary to CAPD. This procedure allows identification of diaphragmatic defects amenable to repair and talc placement under direct visualization, allowing even distribution of the talc over the inferior surface of the lung.

IV. PULMONARY EMBOLISM

The enhanced tendency for intravascular anticoagulation, seen in the nephrotic syndrome and characterized by renal vein thrombosis (35%) and pulmonary embolism (20%), is a well-known entity (28). However, clinically significant pulmonary embolism is considered to be rare in patients with end-stage renal disease (29). Recent literature reports have identified two possible etiologies for pulmonary embolism specific to hemodialysis patients. Several authors observed the existence of a sheet surrounding the surface of the catheter (30,31). In most instances, the sheet is stripped off during a catheter-replacement procedure and remains in the subcutaneous tunnel or in the vascular bed without causing much clinical discomfort in most patients. Occasionally an episode of cough, dyspnea, hypotension, retrosternal oppression, or hemoptoe after removing the dialysis catheter suggests pulmonary embolism or lung infarction. By means of pulmonary perfusion scintigraphy, Smits et al. found that there is substantial risk of pulmonary embolism in patients undergoing percutaneous intravascular thrombolysis for an occluded hemodialysis graft (32). In 35% of the patients studied, there was evidence of pulmonary embolism resulting from the interventional procedure. However, this rarely resulted in clinical symptoms.

Diagnosis of pulmonary embolism is essentially no different in dialysis patients than in the general population. It is based on clinical suspicion combined with laboratory evaluation (blood gas analysis, D-dimers), electrocardiographic signs, and imaging techniques (echocardiography, ventilation-perfusion scintigraphy, spiral CT scanning, and pulmonary angiography). Pulmonary angiography remains the "gold standard" and is a safe technique when performed by experienced radiologists (33,34).

Treatment of pulmonary embolism consists of supportive measures and prevention of recurrences with unfractionated heparin or low molecular weight heparins, followed by systemic anticoagulation for 6 months. Thrombolytic therapy is only indicated in patients with massive pulmonary embolism, complicated by hypotension in the absence of contraindications to thrombolysis (35).

V. THE LUNG IN CHRONIC RENAL FAILURE

Changes in lung mechanics and lung hemodynamics occur even without overt signs or symptoms in patients with end-stage chronic renal failure. Lee et al. (36) studied the pulmonary function of 55 patients with chronic renal failure, 10 of them undergoing chronic dialysis treatment. These patients had no clinical or radiographic evidence of lung disease.

They found a defect in gas transfer [decrease in carbon monoxide diffusing capacity (DLCO)] due to a reduction in the diffusing capacity across the alveolar capillary membrane, vital capacities were decreased indicative of mild restriction, while forced vital capacity and the ratio of the forced vital capacity in the first second to the vital capacity ruled out obstructive disease. The reduction in carbon monoxide transfer persists after renal transplantation (37). In the recipients of grafts the residual pulmonary volume is significantly reduced.

In addition to these limited observations concerning the functional pulmonary changes in end-stage renal failure (with or without dialysis), there are also some important pathological observations. Soft tissue calcification was identified in 79% of dialysis patients and in 44–60% of nondialysis patients with chronic renal failure (38–40). Lesions were severe in 36% of the dialysis population and were most frequently found in heart, lungs, and stomach. These visceral calcifications are mostly diagnosed postmortem because they tend to be discrete and asymptomatic, although several case reports describe symptomatic pulmonary calcifications in children as well as adults in chronic hemodialysis (41–43).

Serum calcium levels were slightly higher in patients with calcifications, but there was no measurable association with the duration of dialysis, serum phosphorus concentration, calcium × phosphorus product, serum bicarbonate level, or arterial pH. A critical assessment of the role of parathyroid hormone in the pathogenesis of these pulmonary calcifications is still required. Pulmonary clinical symptoms were scarce, and x-ray findings were absent, except in a single patient. Taguchi et al. reported a case of metastatic pulmonary calcification that showed hyperintense signals on T_1-weighted MRI (44). This uncommon MR appearance of calcification due to abnormal calcium metabolism was similar to the MR characteristics of calcification in the brain.

The calcific lesion consisted of deposits occurring as linear bands, occasionally as granular humps in alveolar septal walls. Varying degrees of thickening and fibrosis of the alveolar walls accompanied the deposits. Calcium was found to be frequently located within the walls of pulmonary vessels and smaller bronchi. In general, vascular calcifications in the lungs paralleled those of the pulmonary parenchyma. By x-ray diffraction, a whitlockite crystal pattern $(CaMg)_3\ (PO_4)_2$ with calcium pyrophosphate was predominantly found in these pulmonary calcifications. Jarava and colleagues (45) found pulmonary calcifications, detected by technetium-99m diphosphonate scanning, in 40% of their hemodialysis patients.

Pulmonary function tests showed a close relation between changes in vital capacity, DLCO, and the severity of lung calcifications. However, the limitation of significant abnormalities of vital capacity and diffusion to those patients with most severe histopathological changes suggests that the degree of septal thickening and fibrosis rather than the mere presence of calcium deposits determines the magnitude of the functional changes.

The available biochemical data are not sufficient to evaluate adequately either the cause or the pathogenesis of these metabolic calcifications, fibrosis, and alveolar septal thickening.

Several hypotheses (38) have been put forward, none of which would explain all aspects of this disorder(s). However, the variable degree of secondary hyperparathyroidism present in almost all patients with severe renal failure, whether treated by dialysis or not, has to be taken into account. It remains speculative to link the complement activation that is observed in the majority of patients dialyzed thrice weekly with bioincompatible membranes and is accompanied by an acute inflammatory reaction at the level of the pulmonary microcirculation, with the morphological lung lesions observed in the majority of the patients. No data are available, to date, to suggest a beneficial effect of membrane reuse in prevention and/or treatment of metastatic pulmonary calcifications.

VI. PULMONARY FUNCTION DURING DIALYSIS

A. Pulmonary Function During Hemodialyis

In a study dealing with the long-term survival of regular dialysis, Avram (46) found that 8 out of 11 of these patients over 10 years on dialysis had severe restrictive lung function. The effects of hemodialysis on pulmonary function appear attributable to changes in fluid volume. Dialysis causes an increase in the diffusing capacity (47), a decrease in closing capacity (48), an increase in the ventilation to basilar areas of the lung (47), and, in patients with edema, an increase in vital capacity (49). All these changes can be explained by a decrease in lung water content (50).

It has been hypothesized that patients with chronic renal failure, even in the absence of cardiopulmonary symptoms, accumulate interstitial pulmonary fluid, which is removed by hemodialysis. The presence of subclinical pulmonary edema that was removed by dialysis was elegantly shown in a group of patients with established renal failure by several authors using different technologies such as the indocyanine green (ICG)–heavy water double indicator dilution method, computed tomography, total body plethysmography, and bioelectrical impedance analysis (51–53). This was reflected in significant increases in the total lung capacity and functional residual capacity after dialysis. The decrease in thoracic fluid content during dialysis is partly due to the sudden ultrafiltration-induced hypovolemia leading to a fall in thoracic blood volume, but the variations in lung water cannot be explained by hydrostatic mechanisms alone. The new technique for recording and analyzing continuous measurement of oxygen saturation by pulse oximeter in dialysis patients seems promising for identifying patients at risk for clinically relevant hypoxemia (54).

Bazzi et al. reported a study concerning patients in hemodialysis for a very long time (55). To assess bronchial reactivity, a methacholine inhalation test was performed 2–24 hours after a dialysis session in 19 patients with a dialysis treatment duration of almost 20 years (221 ± 26 months) (group 1) and in 14 patients on dialysis therapy for a shorter time (24 ± 22 months) (group 2); all patients had normal standard pulmonary function test results (group 1: forced vital capacity, 95 ± 13% and forced expiratory volume in one second [FEV_1], 97 ± 17%; group 2: forced vital capacity, 108 ± 11% and FEV_1, 108 ± 9% of expected values). The methacholine provocation dose causing a 20% decrease in FEV_1 was significantly lower than normal in seven (37%) group 1 patients and in only one (7%) group 2 patient; this difference was statistically significant ($p = 0.049$). There were no correlations between bronchial hyperresponsiveness and interdialysis weight gain, left ventricular hypertrophy, diastolic dysfunction (expressed as the ratio between early diastolic filling and filling during atrial contraction), secondary hyperparathyroidism, and iron overload. Therefore, bronchial hyperresponsiveness is present in a substantial percentage of patients on renal replacement therapy of very long duration, but its cause is unknown. No specific studies exist on treatment of this condition specific for dialysis patients.

B. Pulmonary Function During Peritoneal Dialysis

From the time of its introduction, peritoneal dialysis has been associated with significant alterations in pulmonary function and gas exchange (56–59). Atelectasis, pneumonia, purulent bronchitis, chronic pleural effusion, and acute hydrothorax are among the various complications that may occur during peritoneal dialysis (56,60).

In a severely ill patient, the level of consciousness may be diminished, causing impaired cough reflex. Bronchial secretions may pool in the basal atelectic segments, predisposing to purulent bronchitis, pneumonia, or both (60). Pleural effusions, mostly right-sided, are also a well-known complication of CAPD, and massive hydrothorax may rarely occur. In most instances of this complication, peritoneal dialysis must be discontinued. In a few cases successful pleurodesis has been applied (61).

Atelectasis of the basal segments of the lung is considered as the consequence of the upward displacement of the diaphragm following overdistention of the peritoneal cavity with dialysate. The effect on pulmonary function is attributed to the increased intraperitoneal pressure. This leads to an elevated and lengthened diaphragm, a reduced functional residual capacity, possible hypoxemia, and altered respiratory muscle function (58,59). Distention of the abdomen with 2 and 3 L of dialysate causes significant reduction of total lung capacity, vital capacity, functional residual capacity, and PaO_2 and $A\text{-}aO_2$ (alveolar-arterial oxygen gradient) (57,62–64). In patients on chronic peritoneal dialysis, adaptations may occur that limit the reductions in lung volumes and PaO_2 (59,65–67). On the other hand, there is an increase in respiratory muscle strength due to a rightward shift in the force-length relationship of the diaphragm (63,66,67). During periods of peritonitis, however, a 25–30% drop in vital capacity and a 11.7 mmHg drop in PaO_2 was observed (65). The most likely explanation is altered mobility of the diaphragm because of pain.

Casuistic data also showed the presence of a respiratory acidosis in patients with ventilatory limitation. Excess CO_2 production resulted from high glucose loads and was reversed by decreasing the glucose concentration in the dialysate (68).

CAPD may not be tolerated by patients with chronic obstructive pulmonary disease (COPD) because of increased abdominal pressure in the standing position after instillation of peritoneal fluid. Bhatla et al. treated a patient with COPD who had marked distress while on CAPD but was more comfortable with intermittent peritoneal dialysis in the supine position (CIPD) (69). IPD may be the preferred mode of peritoneal dialysis for patients with COPD for whom no alternative treatment exists.

Patients with normal pulmonary function and most patients with minimal obstructive pulmonary disease are capable of tolerating CAPD (63,70). At present, severe obstructive or restrictive pulmonary disease are considered to be relative contraindications to peritoneal dialysis. In special circumstances where tolerance to CAPD needs to be assessed before instillation of a chronic peritoneal catheter, a peritoneal instillation test can provide valuable information (71). In patients with pulmonary disease, sequential measurements of pulmonary function should be useful to identify the dialysate volume that is tolerated best.

C. Sleep Apnea Syndrome in Dialysis Patients

Sleep apnea is a common disorder in end-stage renal disease and chronic renal failure. It occurs in at least 60% of ESRD patients, but the diagnosis may be difficult to establish because of the similarity of uremic symptoms to those of the sleep apnea syndrome (72–79). After excluding anatomic and metabolic disorders associated with excessive sleepiness and disordered breathing in sleep and after ensuring that the patient is receiving adequate dialysis, the sleep disorder should be diagnosed using polysomnography (75). The incidence and severity of sleep apnea is similar in patients receiving chronic peritoneal dialysis and hemodialysis (80).

The causes of the increased prevalence of sleep apnea in ESRD patients are unknown and likely differ from those in the general population. Abnormalities in respiratory controller mechanisms from chronic hypocarbia, metabolic acidosis, and uremic toxins have been blamed for the occurrence of apnea in this setting (81).

The known complications of sleep apnea include arrhythmias and pulmonary hypertension. Both acute (with each apnea) and chronic daytime blood pressure elevations are frequently observed in sleep apnea patients, and occult sleep apnea is postulated as one possible cause of "primary" hypertension in middle-aged men. In addition, sleep apnea has been implicated in coronary artery disease and strokes. The contribution of sleep apnea to the high mortality from cardiac disease and stroke in peritoneal dialysis and hemodialysis patients is unknown (74).

The treatment of sleep apnea in uremic patients is similar to the treatment of the disorder in the general population, e.g., continuous positive pressure airway breathing (82). Langevin et al. reported two hemodialysis patients with sleep apnea syndrome whose symptoms and polysomnigraphy improved dramatically after succesful renal transplantation (83).

VII. DIALYSIS-ASSOCIATED HYPOXIA

Hypoxemia occurs in nearly 90% of patients during hemodialysis. Although the fall in arterial pO_2 is typically 85% of the predialysis value, this minor degree of hypoxemia may cause significant morbidity in patients with previously compromised cardiopulmonary status and may contribute to intradialytic hypotension, nausea, and muscle cramps in others (84). The hemodialysis patient slowly accumulates H^+ ions during the 44-hour interdialytic period and is in a respiratory-compensated (hyperventilation) metabolic acidosis at the start of dialysis. Indeed, a HCO_3^- level between 17 and 23 mEq/L and a rather low $Paco_2$ of 33–36 mmHg is observed. Four hours later the patient ends up with a slight degree of metabolic alkalosis, mild to moderate hypoventilation, with or without breathing irregularities (Fig. 1). Defined in another way, the dialysis patient is an acid accumulator for 44 hours followed by a 4-hour efficient period of retitration, which can be accompanied by a variable degree of hypoxemia.

Dialysis-associated hypoxemia is a topic of ongoing research. The pathophysiology of this hypoxemia depends highly on the dialysate composition and, to some extent, on the alkalinization of body fluids and the type of membrane used (Fig. 2). Two mechanisms seem to be very important: CO_2 unloading and the complement activation–hypoxemia cascade (85,86). Both mechanisms may occur separately or simultaneously depending on the dialysis technology used (biocompatibility of the membranes and type of dialysate)(85,87). Intrapulmonary leukostasis with mediator release and inflammation at the level of the pulmonary microcirculation is an early event depending upon the biocompatibility of the dialyzer membrane used and has a measurable but rather limited effect upon the Pao_2. Alveolar hypoventilation depends upon the CO_2-unloading capacity of the hemodialysis set-up, is independent of the dialyzer membrane, and can have an important effect on Pao_2. This hypoventilation can be due to extracorporeal losses of CO_2 or (and) to changes in the endogenous production of carbon dioxide (Vco_2), and consumption of oxygen (Vo_2), secondary to the metabolism of acetate.

The clinical implication of this dialysis-induced hypoxemia is of immediate importance to dialysis patients with an already compromised cardiopulmonary function. They represent 10–15% of an average dialysis population with predialysis Pao_2 values below 80 mmHg. The additional 25% decrease of Pao_2 after the start of dialysis using a bioincompatible membrane and acetate in the dialysis solution results in desaturation (88). The following measures can be undertaken to minimize the risk of hypoxemia in dialysis patients:

The use of (more expensive) biocompatible membranes
The use of a bicarbonate dialysate bath at 37 mEQ/L
Uutilization of supplemental oxygen (FiO_2 of 28%)
Optimizing the hematocrit
Sequential ultrafiltration and dialysis

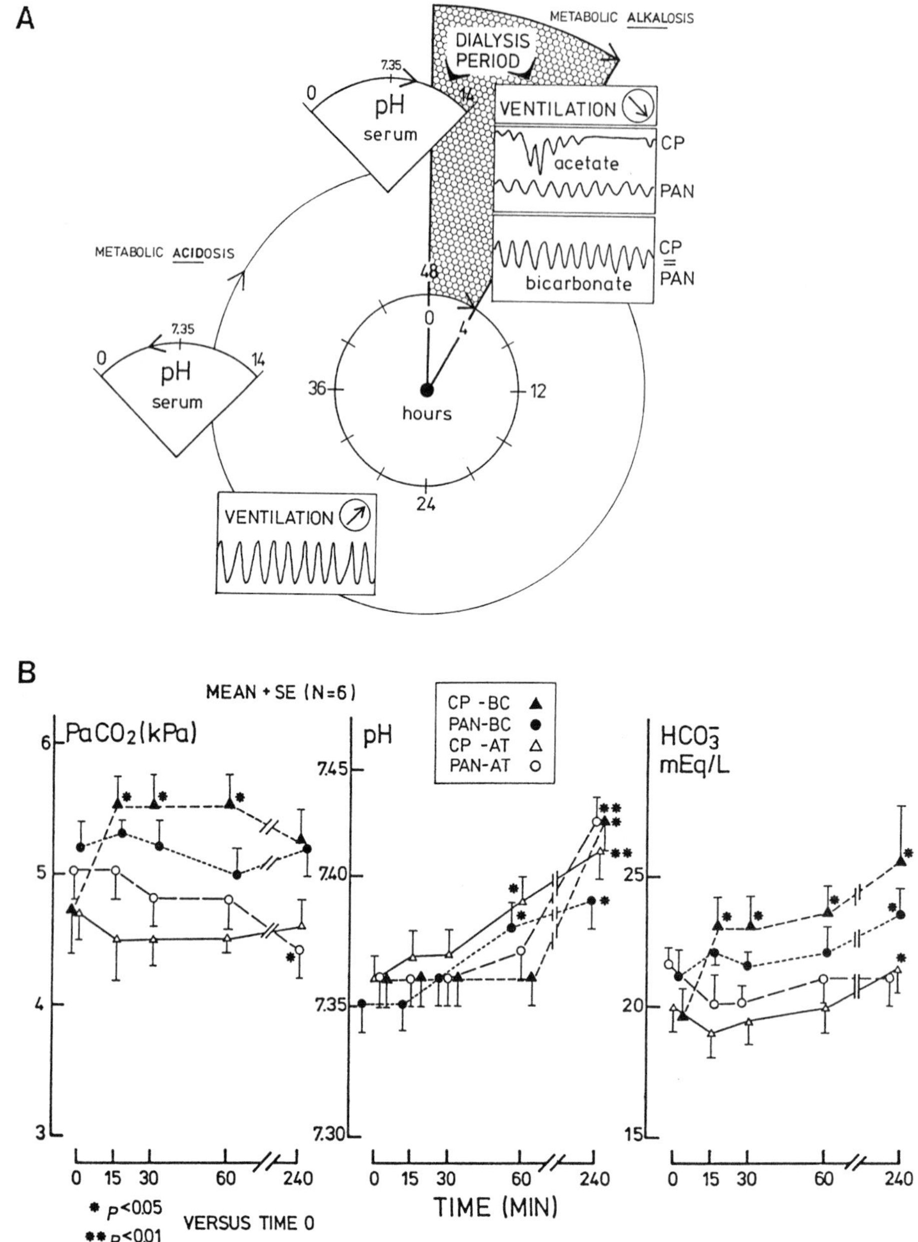

Fig. 1 (a) Acid-base and ventilation during hemodialysis. (B) $PaCo_2$, systemic pH, and arterial HCO_3^- during hemodialysis (69). CP, Cuprophane membrane; PAN, polyacrylonitrile membrane; AT, acetate-containing dialysate; BC, bicarbonate-containing dialysate; $PaCO_2$, arterial carbon dioxide tension. = regular, = irregular breathing pattern.

Some authors claim that cuprophane dialyzers can be rendered biocompatible by reuse, presumably due to coating by serum proteins (89). One study using cuprophane dialyzers rendered more biocompatible after reuse has shown an improvement in peak expiratory flow rate when compared to new cuprophane dialyzers (90). However, a task force from the National Kidney Foundation states there is no conclusive evidence to substantiate the notion that either morbidity or mortality associated with single use or reuse is different (91)

The exact role of a thrice weekly complement activation or alternative mechanisms (92,93) using bioincompatible membranes in the long-term clinical status of dialysis patients remains to be determined.

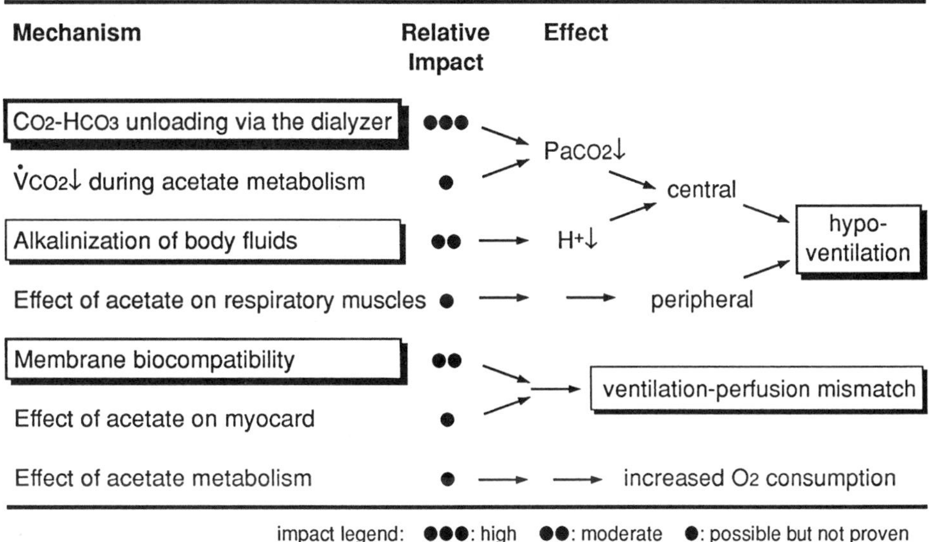

Fig. 2 Mechanisms of dialysis-associated hypoxemia: their effects and their relative impact in dialysis-related hypoxemia.

VIII. CONCLUSION

The lung is a target organ predisposed to suffer from the important disturbances in the water and electrolyte balance characteristic for the patient with end-stage renal failure.

The long term effect of thrice weekly complement activation on pulmonary function is not known. It is striking to note that the literature does not contain a prospective study of the lung function during chronic hemo- or peritoneal dialysis. Based on present knowledge, it is recommended that elderly patients, those with compromised cardiopulmonary function, patients who have experienced hypersensitivity to cellulose-based membranes, and those with acute renal failure should be dialyzed with a biocompatible membrane and bicarbonate-containing dialysate.

REFERENCES

1. Bush A, Gabriel R. Pulmonary function in chronic renal failure: effects of dialysis and transplantation. Thorax 1991; 46:424–428.
2. Grassi V, Malerba M, Boni E, Tantucci C, Sorbini C.A. Uremic lung. Contrib Nephrol 1994; 106:36–42.
3. Gavelli G, Zompatori M. Thoracic complications in uremic patients and in patients undergoing dialytic treatment: state of the art. Eur Radiol 1997; 7:708–717.
4. Guyton A, Linsey A. Effect of elevated left atrial pressure and decreased plasma protein concentration on the development of pulmonary edema. Circ Res 1959; 7: 649–657.
5. Eiser AR, Lieber JJ, Neff MS. Phlebotomy for pulmonary edema in dialysis patients. Clin Nephrol 1997; 47: 47–49.
6. Bright R. Tabular view of the morbid appearance in 100 cases connected with albuminous urine, with observations. Guys Hosp Rep 1836; 1:380–400.
7. Maher JF. Uremic pleuritis. Am J Kidney Dis 1987; 10: 19–22.
8. Berger HW, Rammohan G, Neff MS, Buhain WJ. Uremic pleural effusion. A study in 14 patients on chronic dialysis. Ann Intern Med 1975; 82:362–364.
9. Galen MA, Steinberg SM, Lowrie FG, Lazarus JM, Hampers CL, Merrill JP. Hemorrhagic pleural effusion in patients undergoing chronic hemodialysis. Ann Intern Med 1975; 82:359–361.
10. Rodelas R, Rakowski TA, Argy WP, Schreiner GE. Fibrosing uremic pleuritis during hemodialysis. JAMA 1980; 243:2424–2425.
11. Brown CM, Sloan DF, Berns AS, Kanter A. Fibrosing uremic pleuritis during hemodialysis. JAMA 1981; 245: 705.
12. Don C, Burns KD, Levine DZ. Body fluid volume status in hemodialysis patients: the value of the chest radiograph. Can Assoc Radiol J 1990; 41:123–126.
13. Bartter T, Santarelli R, Akers SM, Pratter MR. The evaluation of pleural effusion. Chest 1994; 106:1209–1214.
14. Gryminski J, Krakowka P, Lypacewicz G. The diagnosis of pleural effusion by ultrasonic and radiologic techniques. Chest 1976; 70:33–37.
15. Light RW, Macgregor I, Luchsinger PC, Ball WC. Pleural effusions: the diagnostic separation of transudates and exudates. Ann Intern med 1972; 77:507–513.

16. Criado A, Mena A, Figuerdo R, Reige E, Avello F. Late perforation of superior vena cava and effusion caused by central venous catheter. Anaesth Intensive Care 1981; 9:286–288.
17. Benz R, Schleifer C. Hydrothorax in CAPD. Succesful treatment with intraperitoneal tetracycline and a review of the literature. Am J Kidney Dis 1985; 2:136–140.
18. Spadaro JJ, Thakur V, Nolph KD. Technetium-99m-labelled macroaggregated albumin in demonstration of trans-diaphragmatic leakage of dialysate in peritoneal dialysis. Am J Nephrol 1982; 2:36–38.
19. Kennedy J. Procedures used to demonstrate a pleuroperitoneal communication: a review. Perit Dial Bull 1985; 5:168–170.
20. Adam WR, Arkles LB, Gill G., Meagher EJ, Thomas GW. Hydrothorax with peritoneal dialysis: radionuclide detection of a pleuroperitoneal connection. Aust NZ J Med 1980; 10:330–332.
21. Gibbons G, Baumert J. Unilateral hydrothorax complicating peritoneal dialysis. Use of radionuclide imaging. Clin Nucl Med 1983; 3:83–84.
22. Otsuka N, Kawai S, Fukunaga M, Ono S, Morita K, Nagai K, Tomomitsu T, Yanagimoto S, Mimura H, Ohsawa G. Confirmation of dialysate leakage by intraperitoneal administration of radioactive colloid. Radiat Med. 1992; 10:253–255.
23. Lepage S, Bisson G, Verreault J, Plante GE. Massive hydrothorax complicating peritoneal dialysis. Isotopic investigation (peritoneopleural scintigraphy). Clin Nucl Med. 1993; 18:498–501.
24. Walker F, McAllister C, McKee P, McNulty J. Intraperitoneal iopamidol, a new radiocontrast agent in the diagnosis of a pleuroperitoneal communication. Perit Dial Bull 1986; 6:108–109.
25. Scanziani R, Dozio B, Caimi F, De Rossi N, Magri F, Surian M. Peritoneography and peritoneal computerized tomography: a new approach to non-infectious complications of CAPD. Nephrol Dial Transplant 1992; 7:1035–1038.
26. Renzo S, Beatrice D, Giuliano R, Francesco C. Peritoneal x-ray and computerized tomography in evaluating abdominal complications in CAPD. Adv Perit Dial. 1990; 6:62–63.
27. Jagasia MH, Cole FH, Stegman MH, Deaton P, Kennedy L. Video-assisted talc pleurodesis in the management of pleural effusion secondary to continuous ambulatory peritoneal dialysis: a report of three cases. Am J Kidney Dis 1996; 28:772–774.
28. Anderson S, Kennefick TM, Brenner BM. Renal and systemic manifestations of glomerular disease. In: Brenner BM, ed. The Kidney. 5th ed. Philadelphia: WB Saunders, 1996:1981–2010.
29. Guntupalli K, Soffer O, Baciewicz P. Pulmonary embolism in end stage renal disease. Intensive Care Med 1990; 16:405–407.
30. Hombrouckx R, D'Halluin F, Bogaert AM, Leroy F, De Vos JY, Larno L. Fibrin sheet covering subclavian or femoral dialysis catheters. Artif Organs 1994; 18:322–324.
31. Winn MP, McDermott VG, Schwab SJ, Conlon PJ. Dialysis catheter 'fibrin-sheath stripping': a cautionary tale! Nephrol Dial Transplant 1997; 12:1048–1050.
32. Smits HFM, VanRijk PP, VanIsselt JW, Mali WPTM, Koomans HA, Blankestijn PJ. Pulmonary embolism after thrombolysis of hemodialysis grafts. J Am Soc Nephrol 1997; 8:1458–1461.
33. Zuckerman DA, Sterling KM, Oser RF. Safety of pulmonary angiography in the 1990s. J Vasc Interv Radiol 1996; 7:199–205.
34. Nilsson T, Carlsson A, Mare K. Pulmonary angiography: a safe procedure with modern contrast media and technique. Eur Radiol 1998; 8:86–89.
35. Dalen JE, Alpert JS, Hirsh J. Thrombolytic therapy for pulmonary embolism. Is it effective? Is it safe? When is it indicated? Arch Intern Med 1997; 157:2550–2556.
36. Lee HY, Stretton TB, Barnes AM. The lungs in renal failure. Thorax 1975; 30:46–53.
37. Bush A, Gabriel R. Pulmonary function in chronic renal failure: effects of dialysis and transplantation. Thorax 1991; 46:424–428.
38. Conger JD, Hammond WS, Alfrey AC, Contiguglia SR, Stanford RE, Huffer WE. Pulmonary calcification in chronic dialysis patients. Ann Intern Med 1975; 83:330–336.
39. Kuzela DC, Huffer WE, Conger JD, Winter SD, Hammond WS. Soft tissue calcification in chronic dialysis patients. Am J Pathol 1977; 86:403–424.
40. Milliner DS, Zinsmeister AR, Lieberman E, Landing B. Soft tissue calcification in pediatric patients with end-stage renal failure. Kidney Int 1990; 38:931–936.
41. Zouboulis CC, Blume-Peytavi U, Lennert T, Stavropoulos PG, Schwarz A, Runkel N, Trautmann C, Orfanos CE. Fulminant metastatic calcinosis with cutaneous necrosis in a child with end-stage renal disease and tertiary hyperparathyroidism. Br J Dermatol 1996; 135:617–622.
42. Uchida M, Sakemi T, Ikeda Y, Maeda T. Acute progressive and extensive metastatic calcifications in a nephrotic patient following chronic hemodialysis. Am J Nephrol 1995; 15:427–430.
43. Jarava C, Marti V, Gurpegui ML, Merello JI; Rdez-Quesada B, Palma A. Pulmonary calcification in chronic dialysis patients. Nephrol Dial Transplant 1993; 8:673–674.
44. Taguchi Y, Fuyuno G, Shioya S, Yanagimachi N, Katoh H, Matsuyama S, Ohta Y. MR appearance of pulmonary metastatic calcification. J Comput Assist Tomogr 1996; 20:38–41.
45. Jarava C, Marti V, Gurpegui ML, Merello JI, Rdez-Quesada B, Palma A. Pulmonary calcification in chronic dialysis patients. Nephrol Dial Transplant 1993; 8:673–674.
46. Avram MM: The Long Island College Hospital experience with the decade or longer hemodialysis patient.

In: Avram MM, ed. Prevention of Kidney Disease and Long-Term Survival. New York: Plenum, 1982:165.
47. Zidulka A, Despas PJ, Millic-Emili J, Anthonisen NR. Pulmonary function with acute loss of excess lung water by hemodialysis in patients with chronic uremia. Am J Med 1973; 55:134–141.
48. Craig DB, Wahba WM, Don HF, Couture JG, Becklake MB. Closing volume and its relationship to gas exchange in seated and supine positions. J Appl Physiol 1971; 31:717–721.
49. Robson M, Levin A, Ravid M. Serial measurement of vital capacity in patients on chronic hemodialysis. Nephron 1977; 19:60–64.
50. Brigham KL, Bernard G. Pulmonary complications of chronic renal failure. Semin Nephrol 1981; 1:188–197.
51. Wallin CJ, Jacobson SH, Leksell LG. Subclinical pulmonary oedema and intermittent hemodialysis. Nephrol Dial Transplant 1996; 11:2269–2275.
52. Metry G, Wegenius G, Hedenstrom H, Wikstrom B, Danielson BG. Computed tomographic measurement of lung density changes in lung water with hemodialysis. Nephron 1997; 75:394–401.
53. Vonk-Noordegraaf A, van der Meer BJ, de Vries JP, de Vries PM. Determination of the relation between alterations of total body water and thoracic fluid content during ultrafiltration by bioelectrical impedance analysis. Nephrol Dial Transplant 1995; 10:382–385.
54. Jones JG, Bembridge JL, Sapsford DJ, Turney JH. Continuous measurements of oxygen saturation during hemodialysis. Nephrol Dial Transplant 1992; 7:110–116.
55. Bazzi C, Amaducci S, Arrigo G, Colombo B, Moreni E, D'Amico G. Bronchial responsiveness in patients on regular hemodialysis treatment of very long duration. Am J Kidney Dis 1994; 24:802–805.
56. Berlyne GM, Lee HA, Ralston AJ, Woodlock JA. Pulmonary complications of peritoneal dialysis. Lancet 1966; 2:75–78.
57. Goggin MJ, Joekes AM. Pulmonary gas exchange during peritoneal dialysis. Br Med J 1971; 2:247–248.
58. Ahluwalia M, Ishikawa S, Gellman M, Shah T, Sekar T, MacDonnel KF. Pulmonary functions during peritoneal dialysis. Clin Nephrol 1982; 18:251–256.
59. Prezant DJ. Effect of uremia and its treatment on pulmonary function. Lung 1990; 168:1–14.
60. Khanna R, Oreopoulos DG. Complications of peritoneal dialysis other than peritonitis. In: Nolph KD, ed. Peritoneal Dialysis. The Hague: Martinus Nijhoff, 1985:441.
61. Scheldewaert R, Bogaerts Y, Pauwels R, Van der Straeten M, Ringoir S, Lameire N. Management of a massive hydrothorax in a CAPD patient: a case report and a review of the literature. Peritoneal Dial Bull 1982; 2: 69–72.
62. Freedman S, Maberly DJ. Pulmonary gas exchange during dialysis. Br Med J 1971; 3:48.
63. Prezant DJ, Aldrich TK, Karpel JP, Lynn RI. Adaptations in the diaphragm's in vitro force-length relationship in patients on continuous ambulatory peritoneal dialysis. Am Rev Respir Dis 1990; 141:1342–1349.
64. O'Brien AA, Power J, O'Brien L, Clancy L, Keogh JA. The effect of peritoneal dialysate on pulmonary function and blood gasses in CAPD patients. Irish J Med Sci 1990; 159:215–216.
65. Taveira Da Silva AM, Davis WB, Winchester JF, Coleman DE, Wei CW. Peritonitis, dialysate infusion and lung function in continuous ambulatory peritoneal (CAPD). Clin Nephrol 1985; 24:79–83.
66. Wanke T, Auinger M, Lahrmann H, Merkle M, Formanek D, Irsigler K, Zwick H. Diaphragmatic function in patients on continuous ambulatory peritoneal dialysis. Lung 1994; 172:231–240.
67. Siafakas NM, Argyrakopoulos T, Andreopoulos K, Tsoukalas G, Tzanakis N, Bouros D. Respiratory muscle strength during continuous ambulatory peritoneal dialysis (CAPD). Eur Respir J 1995; 8:109–113.
68. Cohn J, Balk RA, Bone RC. Dialysis-induced respiratory acidosis. Chest 1990; 98:1285–1288.
69. Bhatla B, Satalowich R, Khanna R. Low-volume supine peritoneal dialysis in a chronic obstructive airway disease patient. Adv Perit Dial 1994; 10:120–123.
70. Singh S, Dale A, Morgan B, Sahebjami H. Serial studies of pulmonary function in continuous ambulatory peritoneal dialysis. Chest 1984; 86:874–877.
71. Leblanc M, Ouimet D, Tremblay C, Nolin L. Peritoneal instillation test before CAPD in a case of severe pulmonary disease. Perit Dial Int 1995; 15:384–387.
72. Holley JL, Nespor S, Rault R. A comparison of reported sleep disorders in patients on chronic hemodialysis and continuous peritoneal dialysis. AM J Kidney Dis 1992; 19:156–161.
73. Wadhwa NK, Seliger M, Greenberg HE, Bergofsky E, Mendelson WB. Sleep related respiratory disorders in end-stage renal disease patients on peritoneal dialysis. Perit Dial Int 1992; 12:51–56.
74. Kraus MA, Hamburger RJ. Sleep apnea in renal failure. Adv Perit Dial 1997; 13:88–92.
75. Kimmel PL, Gavin C, Miller G, Mendelson WB, Wernli I, Neugarten J. Disordered sleep and noncompliance in a patient with end-stage renal disease. Adv Ren Replac Ther 1997; 4:55–67.
76. Hallett M, Burden S, Stewart D, Mahony J, Farrell P. Sleep apnea in end-stage renal disease patients on hemodialysis and continuous ambulatory peritoneal dialysis. ASAIO J 1995; 41:M435–441.
77. Rodriguez A, Stewart D, Hotchkiss M, Farrell P, Kliger A, Finkelstein F. Sleep apnea in CAPD. Adv Perit Dial 1995; 11:123–126.
78. Walker S, Fine A, Kryger MH. Sleep complaints are common in a dialysis unit. Am J Kidney Dis 1995; 26: 751–756.
79. Stepanski E, Faber M, Zorick F, Basner R, Roth T. Sleep disorders in patients on continuous ambulatory peritoneal dialysis. J Am Soc Nephrol. 1995; 6:192–197.

80. Wadhwa NK, Mendelson WB. A comparison of sleep-disordered respiration in ESRD patients receiving hemodialysis and peritoneal dialysis. Adv Perit Dial 1992; 8:195–198.
81. Fletcher EC. Obstructive sleep apnea and the kidney. J Am Soc Nephrol 1993; 4:1111–1121.
82. Pressman MR, Benz RL, Schleifer CR, Peterson DD. Sleep disordered breathing in ESRD: acute beneficial effects of treatment with nasal continuous positive airway pressure. Kidney Int 1993; 43:1134–1139.
83. Langevin B, Fouque D, Leger P, Robert D. Sleep apnea syndrome and end-stage renal disease. Cure after renal transplantation. Chest 1993; 103:1330–1335.
84. Ross EA, Nissenson AR. Dialysis hypoxemia. In: Dialysis Therapy. 2d ed. Philadelphia: Hanley & Belfus, 1993:130–131.
85. De Backer WA, Verpooten GA, Borgonjon DJ, Vermeire PA, Lins RR, De Broe ME. Hypoxemia during hemodialysis: effects of different membranes and dialysate compositions. Kidney Int 1983; 23:738–743.
86. Eiser AA. Pulmonary gas exchange during hemodialysis and peritoneal dialysis: interaction between respiration and metabolism. Am J Kidney Dis 1985; 6:131–142.
87. Vasiri ND, Wilson A, Mukai D, Darwish R, Rutz A, Hyatt J, Moreno C. Dialysis hypoxemia. Role of dialyzer membrane and dialysate delivery system. Am J Med 1984; 77:828–833.
88. Peces-Serrano A, Fernandez-Vega F, Alvarez-Grande J: Hypoxemia during hemodialysis in patients with impairment in pulmonary function. Nephron 1986; 42: 14–18.
89. Craddock PR, Fehr J, Dalmasso AP, Brighan KL, Jacobs HS. Hemodialysis leukopenia. Pulmonary vascular leukostasis resulting from complement activation by dialyzer cellophane membranes. J Clin Invest 1977; 59: 879–888.
90. Davenport A, Williams AJ. The effect of dialyzer reuse on peak expiratory flow rate. Respir Med 1990; 84: 17–21.
91. Task Force on Reuse of Dialyzers, Council on Dialysis, National Kidney Foundation. National Kidney Foundation report on dialyzer reuse. Am J Kidney Dis 1997; 30:859–871.
92. Camussi G, Segolini G, Rotunno M, Vercellone A. Mechanism involved in acute granulocytopenia in hemodialysis:cell-membrane direct interactions. Int J Artif Organs 1978; 1:123–127.
93. Danielson BG, Hallgren R, Benge P. Neutrophil and eosinophil degranulation by hemodialysis membranes. Contrib Nephrol 1984; 37:83–88.

28

Quality of Life and Functional Status in Chronic Hemodialysis and Peritoneal Dialysis

Maruschka Patricia Merkus and Raymond T. Krediet
Academic Medical Center, Amsterdam, The Netherlands

I. INTRODUCTION

Patients with end-stage renal disease (ESRD) cannot be cured of their underlying conditions. Because the dialysis itself has an important impact on the patient's lifestyle in terms of personal time involved and compliance required, the patient's own perception of health or quality of life (QL) is highly relevant for clinical practice. Therefore, it is necessary to define, measure, and act on assessments of the patient's health that are more broadly defined than life versus death.

The objectives of the present chapter are (a) to describe the QL concept as it is applied in health care, (b) to outline the main methodological problems in assessing QL, (c) to review existing QL measures applied in dialysis patients, (d) to identify the bottlenecks in QL research in dialysis patients, and (e) to propose directions for future QL assessment in dialysis patients, both in research and clinical practice.

II. THE CONCEPT OF QUALITY OF LIFE

The QL concept has been approached from many perspectives. These include physical well-being, the spiritual and psychological approaches, as well as social, economic, and political aspects (1). However, QL in the context of disease and treatment is generally limited to health-related quality of life. Health, according to The World Health Organization (WHO), can be defined as "a state of complete physical, psychological and social well-being and not merely the absence of disease or infirmity" (2). Consistent with this definition, there is general consensus that a comprehensive description of QL should at least cover the patient's functioning and well-being in the physical, psychological, and social domains. The physical domain comprises self-care, mobility, physical activity level, pain, and other physical symptoms experienced as a result of either the disease or treatment. Psychological status includes cognitive functioning, emotional status (e.g., anxiety, depression, and happiness), as well as general perceptions of health, well-being, and life satisfaction. The social domain refers to the ability to get along with others at the level of family, close friends, work and the general community, sexuality, and satisfaction with social contacts (1,3–5).

III. ASSESSMENT OF QUALITY OF LIFE

Because of its multidimensional nature, the patient's assessment of QL is often complex. Nevertheless, many measurement tools or instruments have been developed in an attempt to assess this outcome parameter in clinical research, patient care, and policy making. Most of the available QL instruments are structured questionnaires that depend on the patient's self-report.

A. Basic Properties of Quality-of-Life Instruments

The basic properties of an instrument to consider are its feasibility and its psychometric soundness (i.e., reliability, validity, and responsiveness).

1. Feasibility

Measures for use in routine clinical practice need to be short, simple, easy to administer and score, and low in cost, whereas longer and more complex instruments might be acceptable in the research setting (6,7). Self-administered questionnaires, particularly those that are mailed to respondents, are less expensive but have a greater likelihood of nonresponse, errors of misunderstanding, and missing items. This is especially a risk in more severely ill and elderly respondents (8,9). This creates the problem of inadequate evaluation of QL in a subgroup of patients in which this is highly relevant (4). The use of an interviewer avoids these problems to some extent and generally allows collection of a larger amount of information and more complex data. However, the use of interviewers and their training to minimize interviewer effects is more time-consuming and expensive. A compromise between the two modes may be to have the questionnaire completed under supervision or to interview by telephone. In subjects where self-reports are difficult to obtain (e.g., patients with dementia or other communication disorders), a health-care provider or a significant other (e.g. partner, child, or other close companion) can be asked to respond on behalf of the patient, the so-called proxy approach (8). However, evidence regarding the validity of caregiver information is mixed. In general, there seems to be a tendency for caregivers, both formal and informal, to underestimate QL, especially in the psychosocial area (10–12). In addition, lower patient-proxy agreement can be expected among those patients for whom the need of proxies is most salient (13).

2. Reliability

Reliability can be evaluated in terms of homogeneity or internal consistency and stability. Statistically, internal consistency is commonly measured by Cronbach's alpha, a measure of the weighted average correlation among all the items in a given instrument or scale (14). Cronbach's alpha can range between 0 (no correlation) and 1 (perfect correlation). It is generally accepted that Cronbach's alpha should be in excess of 0.70 (15). The stability of a self-report measure can be assessed by test-retest reliability, which is based on the concordance between measurements in the same subject on two occasions with the same instrument (16–18). In case of observer-rated instruments, stability can also be assessed by intra- and interrater reliability.

3. Validity

Validity refers to the degree to which a measure reflects what it is supposed to measure (15). Validity can be classified into content, criterion, construct, and clinical validity. Content validity refers to a subjective review of the extent to which a measure covers the health concept (3). For criterion validity the relationship between the measure of interest and some superior criterion or gold standard has to be examined. Since no gold-standard measure for QL is present, this type of data does not exist. More common are studies of construct validity. Construct validity can be obtained by examining the relationships between the measure of interest and measures that are intended to assess similar or dissimilar health concepts (convergent respectively discriminant validity) (15,17). Finally, clinical validity can be assessed by examining the extent to which a given measure is able to distinguish between patients with different disease states (within and between diagnoses) and between patient groups and general population samples (4,7).

4. Responsiveness

Evaluation of therapeutic or other health-care interventions is mostly performed with repeated assessments of QL over time. For this purpose, a QL measure needs to be able to detect small but clinically meaningful intrapatient health changes over time. This property is called responsiveness or sensitivity to change (17,19). Due to the absence of a gold standard for a relevant change in health status, information about the responsiveness of QL measures is scarce. Furthermore, methodological and statistical approaches to assess responsiveness are still under debate (20). Some variants are based on comparison of score changes obtained with a given QL measure to the patient's or physician's overall impression of change (17,18,21,22). An alternatively proposed strategy is to examine whether scores on a measure change in a certain direction and magnitude in parallel with changes in more objective parameters of disease severity, such as physical examination and laboratory investigations (23,24).

B. Types of QL Instruments

According to their scope and applicability, QL instruments can be classified into multidimensional or unidimensional instruments and generic or disease-specific instruments (25). The majority of QL instruments use a multidimensional approach. This has the advantage of allowing determination of the effects of a disease or treatment on different aspects of QL. Single instruments that attempt to measure all important domains of QL are called health profiles (8). A battery of scales for measuring particular dimensions or aspects of health can also be used, such as instruments to assess cognitive functioning, depression, activities of daily living, or social functioning. The use of such a series of specific and often unidimensional measures allows one to assess each relevant life domain in depth. This approach has the disadvantage that results may not be comparable across studies and that patient burden with completing such a battery may be unacceptably high (4).

Generic instruments are intended to be applicable in a wide variety of conditions, patient groups, and demographic populations. Therefore, they allow comparisons of the impact of disease across groups with different health problems. However, because they may not adequately focus on particular concerns and problems of a specific patient group, they may not be able to detect relevant and specific health changes over time or changes as a result of an intervention. In contrast, since disease-specific instruments focus on problems and concerns associated with specific diseases, patient groups, or areas of function, they are more likely to be sensitive for the detection of clinically important health changes. However, inherent to their specific nature they do not allow cross-disease comparisons (25,26).

Utility measures are an alternative approach to descriptive QL measures. The utility approach is derived from economic and decision-making theory and is aimed at the valuation of specific levels of health. Utility measures provide a single number (utility) between 0 and 1 indicating the patient's description for his or her current health state relative to death (0) and perfect health (1). As such, the technique combines the patient's overall assessment of health status with its value to him or her (27). A major advantage of the utility measurement is its amenability to cost-utility analysis. A disadvantage of the utility approach is that it does not allow examination of effect on different life domains (25). Moreover, important methodological issues concerning the methods for generating utilities and their convergence with classic QL measures still need to be resolved (4).

C. QL Instruments Used in ESRD

A wide variety of QL measures has been used in ESRD patients. In this section only published, established, multidimensional QL measures will be discussed in more detail. Table 1 provides a summary of the most important characteristics of these instruments. They include the QL dimensions assessed, mode of administration, time to complete, number of items, reference period, perspective, scoring, measurement properties, and language versions. In the following sections these characteristics will be discussed in more detail.

1. Generic Multidimensional Instruments—Descriptive

Three established generic multidimensional instruments have frequently been used in dialysis patients: the Sickness Impact Profile, The Nottingham Health Profile, and The Medical Outcomes Study 36-Item Short-Form Health Survey.

a. The Sickness Impact Profile

The Sickness Impact Profile (SIP) was designed as an outcome measure to be applicable in various patient groups as well as in populations with different cultural backgrounds. The SIP measures perceived changes in behavior judged by a patient as the consequence of being sick (28). The questionnaire contains 136 items grouped into 12 categories of activities: sleep and rest, feeding, work, home management, recreation and pastimes, body care and movement, mobility, ambulation, emotional behavior, alertness/intellectual behavior, communication, and social interaction. Endorsed statements are summed up using item weights reflecting the degree of dysfunction. Apart from category scores, scores from three categories can be combined into a physical dimension, and four category scores can be combined into a psychosocial dimension. Finally, a total SIP score can be calculated. Patients are asked to consider their current state that day and to determine which statements describe themselves and are related to their state of health. Examples of SIP items are: "I walk shorter distances or stop to rest often," "I act irritable and impatient with myself, for example, talk badly about myself, swear at myself, blame myself for things that happen," and "I isolate myself as much as I can from the rest of the family."

The SIP has been found reliable and valid in various patient and general populations (28–30). Information on its responsiveness to changes in health status is mixed (31–34). A drawback of the SIP is its relative insensitivity in populations with mild disease impact (35).

The SIP has been used extensively in dialysis patients to assess QL (36–51). Internal consistency of the SIP appeared to be acceptable (42). Construct validity was supported by correlations in the hypothesized di-

Table 1 Summary of Characteristics of Multidimensional Descriptive QL Instruments Used in ESRD Populations

Instrument (Ref.)	Dimensions/scales	Administration mode/time to complete	No. items/ reference period/ perspective	Scoring	Measurement characteristics	Languages
SIP (28–52)	Ambulation, mobility, body care, social, emotional, communication, alertness, sleep, eating, home management, recreation, employment	Self- or interviewer administered/ 20–30 min	136/today/patient	Dichotomous item response options; 12 summated category scores; 2 summated dimension (physical and psychosocial) scores; 1 summated total score (item weights)	Feasibility: ±; Reliability: + aggregated; ± item level Validity: +; Responsiveness: ±	Original: English (USA), Translations: Danish, Dutch, English (UK-FLP), Finnish, Flemish, French, German, Italian, Norwegian, Spanish, Swedish
NHP (42,53–66)	Part 1: Physical, emotional, social, pain, energy, sleep Part 2: effect on 7 life areas: home, family, social life, sex life, hobbies, holidays, employment	Self-administered/ 10 min	Part 1: 38 items; Part 2: 7 items/no specific period/ patient	Dichotomous item response options; 6 summated scale scores (item weights)	Feasibility: +; Reliability: +; Validity: +; Responsiveness: ±	Original: English (UK) Translations: Danish, Dutch, Finnish, Flemish, French, German, Italian, Norwegian, Spanish, Swedish
SF-36 (10,32,59, 63,67–85)	Physical, emotional, social, role limitations (physical and emotional), vitality, pain, general health perceptions, health change	Self- or interviewer administered/ 5–10 min	36/4 weeks (standard version) or 1 week (acute version)/ patient	Variable ordinal item response options; 8 summated scale scores; 2 aggregated physical and mental component scores	Feasibility; +; Reliability; +; Validity; +; Responsiveness: ±	Original: English (USA) Translations: Danish, Dutch, English (Australian), English (Canadian), English (UK), Flemish, French, German, Italian, Japanese, Norwegian, Spanish, Swedish
Parfrey's Instrument (92,95,96)	Symptoms, emotions, mental well-being, life satisfaction and well-being, overall physical and mental independence, functional impairment; activity, daily living, health, support and outlook	Interviewer administered/ 20 min	51/previous few weeks/patient and clinician	Variable ordinal item response options; 8 summated scale scores	Feasibility: ±; Reliability: +; Validity; +; Responsiveness: ±	Original: English (Can) Translations: none
KDQ (37,46, 47,100)	Physical symptoms (patient-specific), fatique, depression, relationship with others, frustration	Self- or interviewer administered/ 10–15 min	26/2 weeks/ patient	7 point rating scale; 5 scale scores, representing the average for all items in the scale	Feasibility: +; Reliability: +; Validity: +; Responsiveness: ±	Original: English (USA) Translations: none
KDQOL Long Form (LF), Short Form (SF) (77,102)	SF-36 dimensions, symptoms/problems, effects of ESRD on daily life, burden of ESRD, cognitive function, work status, sexual function, quality of social interaction, sleep, social support, dialysis staff support, satisfaction with care	Self- or interviewer administered/ LF: 30 min; SF: 16 min	LF:134; SF:80/ varies between 4 weeks and no specific period/patient	Variable ordinal item response options; scale scores represent the average for all items in the scale	Feasibility: LF: ±; SF: +; Reliability: LF & SF: ± (no stability data); Validity: LF & SF: +; Responsiveness LF & SF: ?	Original: English (USA) Translations: SF: Dutch, French, German, Italian, Japanese, Spanish

+: Well supported; ±: moderately supported: some aspects/some clinical areas supported/additional evidence necessary; −: not well supported; ?: not yet been assessed/not known to us.

rection between SIP scales and other instruments measuring similar or dissimilar health aspects (41,42). In addition, the SIP has been shown to be able to discriminate between dialysis patients and general population samples (36) and between patient groups with regard to age, comorbidity, and the degree of anemia (43,45,51). The responsiveness of the SIP is illustrated by the improvements that were found for several SIP subscale scores before and after transplantation (38). Total SIP scores improved after successful treatment of anemia with erythropoietin (EPO), but the separate (sub)scale scores showed inconsistent patterns (37,46,47,49,50). Due to its length the SIP is most suitable for cross-sectional studies. Recently a short version of the SIP, containing 68 items divided over six categories, has proven reliable (52).

b. Nottingham Health Profile

The Nottingham Health Profile (NHP) has been developed as a measure of perceived health for use in population surveys. The first part of the questionnaire consists of 38 items, scored yes/no, grouped into six scales: physical mobility, energy, pain, sleep, social isolation, and emotional reaction. Weighted sum scores are calculated for each scale. The second part comprises seven yes/no items that are not summed but considered separately. It assesses the impact of health on seven life areas: jobs around the house, home life, social life, sex life, hobbies, holidays, and employment. No reference period is specified. Because some of the items of part 2 seldom apply to all respondents, application of part 2 has been discouraged by The European Group for Quality of Life and Health Measurement (53). Examples of items of part 1 are: "I have trouble getting up and down stairs and steps," "The days seem to drag," and "I feel I am a burden to people."

Reliability and validity have been reported (54–56), but responsiveness studies are inconsistent (57,58). Like the SIP, the NHP lacks sensitivity in respondents with less severe health problems (59,60).

The NHP has been used in a small number of renal failure studies (42,61–66). Satisfactory reliability has been shown (42,62). Validity was shown by correlations of the physical and psychological scales in the expected direction with other measures of physical and psychological functioning (42). Furthermore, improvement in energy, physical mobility, and emotional well-being and reduced limitation in looking after home, social life, sex life, and hobbies have been found with EPO therapy (61,63,64). Compared to the SIP, the NHP was found to be somewhat more reliable and feasible, i.e., shorter and less difficult, in a sample of dialysis patients (42). In line with the intentions of the constructors, the NHP was found to be a measure of perceived health, while the SIP is more a functional measure.

c. The MOS Short Form 36

The MOS Short Form 36 (SF-36), also known as the RAND-36 Item Health Survey, was developed to meet a need for short and yet comprehensive measures that can be used in clinical settings and in studies that are unable to afford the use of longer measures (67–69). The SF-36 consists of eight multi-item scales: physical functioning, role limitations caused by physical problems, bodily pain, general health perceptions, mental well-being, role limitations caused by emotional problems, social functioning, and vitality (energy/fatigue). The first four may be combined as a physical component score and the last four as a mental component score (70). Item response options vary between 2 and 6. Patients are asked to rate the effect of their health on their lives during the previous 4 weeks (standard version) or during the previous week (acute version). Scores are summed for each scale. Examples of items are "Does your health now limit you in climbing several flights of stairs?," "How much time during the past 4 weeks have you felt downhearted and blue?," and "During the past 4 weeks, to what extent has your physical health or emotional problems interfered with your normal social activities with family, friends, neighbors or groups?"

The SF-36 has been proven to be both reliable and valid in general and patient populations (59,69,71–73). The SF-36 was capable of detecting improvement in health status after heart valve and hip replacement (32,74) and in surgical clinical trials (75). It was also responsive to changes in perceived health status over time in common clinical conditions such as menorrhagia, peptic ulcer, low back pain, and varicose veins (76).

In the dialysis context the SF-36 has been used both for investigational purposes and for individual patient monitoring (10,63,77–85). Internal consistency of the SF-36 in dialysis patients has been reported (77,80,84). The SF-36 discriminates between dialysis patients and general population samples (63,77,79,83,84), between dialysis and transplanted patients, between patients with varying degrees of comorbidity (79), and between known-group classifications such as length of hospital stay and number of medications used (77). In addition, the SF-36 has been able to detect improvements in health status with correction of anemia by EPO therapy

(63,81). The questionnaire is short and easy to administer and has a high patient acceptance (80). Teams from dialysis programs in the United States have reported promising experience in using SF-36 responses as a tool in individual patient monitoring (80,84).

2. Disease-Specific Multidimensional Instruments—Descriptive

A number of attempts, some more structured than others, have been made to construct instruments that are specifically focused on the QL impact of ESRD and its treatment (47,77,86–94). Three selected, well-documented, multidimensional ESRD-specific instruments will be discussed here in depth.

a. *Parfrey's Instrument*

The intention of Parfrey and coworkers was to develop an ESRD-specific instrument for use in the evaluation of various ESRD therapies (92,95,96). This instrument, a battery of eight scales, includes an ESRD-specific symptom and affect scale and six generic scales addressing mental well-being [Campbell's indices of general affect, life satisfaction, and well-being (97)], overall physical and mental independence [the Spitzer Subjective Quality of Life Index (98)], activity, daily living, health, support, and outlook [the Spitzer Concise Quality of Life Index (98)], and functional impairment [Karnofsky Performance Scale (99)]. The latter two scales are clinician-rated, while the other scales are self-rated. The symptom scale includes one individual-specific symptom and 11 preselected symptoms (e.g., tiredness, cramps, itching), identified by interview of 226 ESRD patients. The affect scale consists of 12 emotions, which the researchers considered to influence ESRD patients' well-being (e.g., faith, helpless, fed up). Patients are asked to rate each symptom and affect on a scale of 1 (very severe) to 5 (absent). Patients are asked to refer to the previous few weeks. Sum scores are calculated for each scale. A well-trained interviewer is necessary to administer the questionnaire, which takes about 20 minutes (92).

Intra- and interrater reproducibility was established and the instrument was found to be able to discriminate between dialysis and transplant patients with respect to physical aspects of QL. Responsiveness was supported by improvement in scores in dialysis patients after successful transplantation and unchanged scores in maintenance dialysis and transplant patients (92,96). An advantage of Parfrey's Instrument is the inclusion of generic instruments. This allows comparison with other (patient) populations. A limitation is its need for well-trained interviewers. So far, this instrument has not been used by other research groups.

b. *The Kidney Disease Questionnaire*

The Kidney Disease Questionnaire (KDQ) was developed for use in clinical trials in hemodialysis patients (37,46,47,100). Potential relevant items were identified by interviewing patients and health-care workers and review of existing QL measures. Next, 50 hemodialysis patients were asked to rank the importance of each item using a 5-point scale. The items that were found to be most important to them were retained in the final questionnaire. This questionnaire contains 26 items in five dimensions: physical symptoms, fatigue, relationships with others, depression, and frustration. The physical symptoms scale comprises six individual-specific symptoms. Patients are asked to consider the previous 2 weeks. An example of an item of the fatigue dimension is: "How often during the past 2 weeks have you felt low in energy?" All items are scored on a 7-point rating scale. Each dimension score represents the average of all items in the concerning dimension.

Performance characteristics of the KDQ were assessed in a clinical trial of EPO treatment. The KDQ scores were found to be reproducible and to display construct validity when compared with scores on the SIP, the Time Trade-Off instrument (see below) and an exercise stress test. Moreover, the KDQ appeared to be more sensitive to change in patients receiving EPO treatment than the other outcome measures used (37,46,47). The KDQ was reported to be well accepted by patients. Its administration time ranged between 10 and 15 minutes (47). The KDQ is only applicable in hemodialysis patients. A similar transplant version, the Kidney Transplant Questionnaire, has been developed by the same authors (91). Allowing patients to select the symptoms of greatest concern to them enhances the responsiveness and patient acceptance but limits the possibility of aggregating data across patients and studies (101). Like Parfrey's Instrument, the KDQ has not yet been used by other research groups.

c. *The Kidney Disease Quality of Life Instrument*

The original 134-item Kidney Disease Quality of Life Instrument (KDQOL) is a self-report instrument that includes the SF-36/RAND-36 as a generic core, supplemented with multi-item scales targeted at particular problems of individuals with kidney disease and on dialysis: symptoms/problems, effects of kidney disease on daily life, burden of kidney disease, cognitive function, work status, sexual function, quality of social interaction, and sleep. Also included were multi-item measures of social support, dialysis staff encouragement, patient satisfaction, and a single-item overall rating of health. The selection of the disease-targeted items was based on discussion groups with patients, dialysis staff, and review of the literature (77). For most items patients are asked to refer to the previous 4 weeks. For some items no specific reference period is stated. Items in the same scale are averaged together to create the scale scores. Examples of items are: "During the past 4 weeks, to what extent were you bothered by cramps?," "How much does kidney disease bother you in your ability to travel?," and "I feel frustrated dealing with my kidney disease."

Internal consistency and validity of the KDQOL were supported in a population of 165 dialysis patients in the United States (77). Because the length of the KDQOL was expected to be a drawback for practical use, the KDQOL-Short Form (KDQOL-SF) was developed. The KDQOL-SF includes the SF-36/RAND-36, supplemented with 43 items covering the same disease-targeted aspects as the original form. The KDQOL-SF has been found to be well accepted and quick to complete (16 min) (102). Support for internal consistency and validity has been provided in a sample of 165 dialysis patients. Evaluation of its responsiveness is currently ongoing (103). Like Parfrey's Instrument, the inclusion of a generic core allows comparison with other disease states and general population samples. Compared to the KDQ and Parfrey's Instrument, the KDQOL is more comprehensive in scope. Moreover, the KDQOL-SF has been translated into several languages and is currently included as an outcome measure in large-scale (multi-)national trials.

3. Utility Measures

Unlike the descriptive approaches, utility measurements in dialysis patients are rather limited. This may be explained by the fact that empirical work in utility measurement has not yet reached the same stage of development as descriptive QL measurement (104). Because the Time Trade-Off (TTO) technique has been applied in a number of QL studies in ESRD patients (37,44,46,48,87,105–107), it will be discussed here in somewhat more detail.

In the TTO approach, the respondent is asked how many years of perfect health he or she would be willing to trade for their current health (46). The choices are presented in a standardized manner by a trained interviewer using visual aids. The expected choice is a lifetime in full health. By reducing the time of perfect health and leaving the time in the suboptimal health state fixed, a point can be determined in which the patient no longer can make a preference choice (103). This indifference point is called the utility. For example, an ESRD patient may rate being in his or her current health state for 10 years as equivalent to perfect health for 5 years. This would result in a utility of patient's current health state of 0.5 on a 0-to-1 utility scale, where 0 denotes death and 1 perfect health (103).

The TTO approach has been described as a reliable and valid method in ESRD patients (105,106). The TTO appeared sensitive to changes in QL after successful transplantation (48,107) but insensitive to improvement in Kt/V dose (87) and EPO therapy (37,46). The fact that various methodological problems in utility measurements still have to be resolved, together with the relatively high patient burden and the need for well-trained interviewers, limit the use of the TTO.

D. Choosing the Appropriate QL Instrument

The choice of the appropriate QL instrument is dependent on the objective of measurement and the clinical context. In addition, the dimensions of health that are considered most relevant, the measurement properties of the instrument, and available resources are important.

As discussed earlier, instruments for use in patient care need to be short and easy to administer, simple to score and interpret, and low in cost. Lengthier and more complex questionnaires may be applied in the research setting. Regarding measurement properties, reliability and validity are always important. The importance of responsiveness to change will depend on the purpose of assessing QL. For example, in longitudinal studies and clinical trials with repeated measurements, responsiveness is an additional essential feature.

Health profiles carry the risk that, simply by chance, a significant effect is found in one or more dimensions, because many variables are tested. A single aggregate score avoids this statistical problem of multiple testing and is therefore preferred in clinical trials. However, as the same overall score can be arrived at in different ways, they may obscure important variability in treatment dimension interactions (6).

Another consideration is whether to use a generic or a disease-specific measure. Generic instruments may not be adequately sensitive to the specific QL concerns of the dialysis patient. In contrast, disease-specific measures, using dialysis patient experience in their development, are likely to be more relevant and more responsive to clinically relevant disease activity. This makes them more appropriate when the objective is to identify effects that dialysis patients experience when a new therapy is introduced. However, disease-specific instruments give limited opportunity for the establishment of the relative burden of different diseases and the relative merit of different interventions in various diseases. Therefore, generic instruments are likely to be of greatest interest to third-party payers and policy makers, while disease-specific instruments may be most suitable in clinical trials and patient care.

Utility measures are particularly relevant if the economical implications of an intervention are a major focus of investigation (8). However, various methodological problems in utility measurements have yet to be resolved (4).

From the preceding discussion it can be concluded that no single best instrument exists. In line with others (6,26,108), we consider the combination of a validated multidimensional generic and disease-specific instrument the preferable approach in most situations.

IV. RESULTS OF QL STUDIES IN ESRD

From the early days of dialysis an abundance of papers have addressed the QL of ESRD patients. Despite all these research efforts, the answer to the question as to which treatment should be recommended to which patients is still lacking. Recent reviews have summarized the results of the majority of studies (109–115).

The aim of the present review, therefore, was not to repeat the work already done by others, but to tabulate in a systematic way the methodological properties of former studies such as the design, sample size, dimensions of QL assessed, and allowance for case mix differences. The term case mix is used to describe those factors that vary in groups being compared that might affect the types of treatment outcome (116). This approach was chosen to identify the bottlenecks in the interpretation of the various studies. We focused only on studies from the last decade. The older studies were excluded because they were conducted before the era of important technological advances, including improved hemodialysis, establishment of peritoneal dialysis on a large scale, introduction of the immunosuppressant cyclosporine, and last but not least erythropoietin. Studies not published in the English language and not published in medical journals or journals of the psychosocial sciences were also excluded. Finally, interim analyses and studies designed for the sole purpose of assessing measurement properties of new QL tools were excluded too. As a comprehensive review is impossible in this limited space, representative examples of the various QL studies in ESRD patients are presented.

The results of the selected studies are summarized in Tables 2 and 3. Overall, the picture emerges that QL of successfully transplanted patients is superior to that of patients on dialysis treatment. Among dialysis patients, approximately half of the comparative studies of home hemodialysis (HHD), in-center hemodialysis (CHD), and peritoneal dialysis (PD) favored HHD over CHD and PD, while the other studies suggested QL of these modalities to be similar. No differences in QL were found in the great majority of comparisons of patients treated by CHD or PD. The other studies suggested that either CHD or PD patients attained a higher QL. With the exception of one study (117), all comparisons of QL between dialysis patients and general population samples reported that QL of dialysis patients was substantially impaired, especially regarding the physical dimension.

The impact of adequacy of dialysis on QL has only recently received attention. No association has been found between Kt/V and QL (51,78,83,85,118). A small positive association has been observed between the normalized protein catabolic rate (nPCR) and physical functioning (78,83) and bodily pain (83). However, Moreno et al. (51) found no association between PCR and QL. Additionally, univariate analysis of a small sample of CAPD patients (78) showed that patients with a total creatinine clearance (Ccr) of 65 L/week/1.73 m^2 or higher reported greater vitality than patients with a Ccr of less than 65 L/week/1.73 m^2.

With the exception of only one randomized, placebo-controlled clinical trial (37), information on the effect of EPO on QL is derived from nonrandomized studies including a large, controlled, phase IV study (63), a large-scale phase III study (64) without a concurrent control group, and numerous small-scale studies with no or improper control groups (49,50,61,119,120). Except for one small study (61), all studies were done in hemodialysis patients. A beneficial effect of EPO was observed on physical aspects of QL, especially energy level. The effect on the social and psychological aspects of QL appears less dramatic and less consistent (Table 3). Proper evaluation of the optimal dosage of EPO to provide a maximum enhancement of QL with minimal risk of adverse events of EPO therapy, such as hypertension or vascular access clotting, is indicated.

The lack of agreement between the comparative studies of QL of the various treatment modalities may partially be explained by differences in definition of QL and tools to assess QL. Though it cannot be directly inferred from Table 2, definition of QL in the late 1980s and early 1990s was heavily weighted on psychosocial well-being and life satisfaction, while less attention was paid to functional aspects. In addition, a wide array of measures, validated or not, was used In more recent years a trend is present towards a more multifaceted assessment of QL in functional, well-being, and satisfaction terms, with the application of established multidimensional instruments, such as the SIP and SF-36.

Another possible critical issue contributing to the lack of conclusive evidence is the fact that all comparative studies of QL of ESRD patients in different modalities were observational, cross-sectional, nonrandomized comparisons. Inherently, the various groups were probably heterogeneous with respect to case mix. Because ESRD is the terminal condition of very different diseases and disease processes and the choice of treatment modality depends on both medical and nonmedical factors, (112,121), case mix is an important issue in comparative studies in ESRD patients (112). The fact that patients sometimes change their modality of treatment for both medical and nonmedical reasons further complicates this issue. Therefore, not only the cross-sectional nature but also the timing of studies may be a critical issue in itself. Assessment early in the course of treatment may include patients who are unsatisfied and likely to switch modality (113). On the other hand, assessment later in the course of treatment may overestimate QL because patients who do less well may have died or switched from modality. Furthermore, patients who have experienced a prior therapy have more points of reference available: the period prior to ESRD, the period with their former treatment, the time their transplant failed, or the period after a successful transplant. Moreover, the option of changing modality will be less available to patients who have already experienced another treatment and found it unsatisfactory (122).

The importance of allowing for case mix is illustrated by the fact that significant differences in QL between different dialysis modalities disappeared once adjustment for case mix was made (43,45,51,83,122–125). In one study the rank order of dialysis modalities in terms of QL even changed after allowing for case mix (45). Table 2 shows that case mix adjustment differed between studies. Some included the full range of sociodemographic, primary kidney disease, comorbidity, anemia, and therapy history (51,83), whereas others only assessed a few variables (43,45,82,85,88,122–127). About one third of the studies did not take case mix differences into account (36,78,79,117,118,128–130). Age (43,45,51,123,125), the presence of diabetes mellitus (43,45,51), as well as other co-existent conditions (43,45,51,83,117,123,125) are the most consistently mentioned explanatory factors of impaired QL. Gender (51,117) and education (43,51) are other case mix variables that have been reported to influence QL independently. Recently, lower residual renal function was observed to be independently associated with worse QL (83). However, because to our knowledge this factor has only been studied once, further data on the effect of residual renal function on QL are necessary. Furthermore, results of intervention studies, presented in Table 3, showed that improvement of anemia with EPO significantly improved QL, especially regarding the energy level. This evidence underscores the need to adjust for the level of anemia in comparisons of QL of treatment modalities. So far, only two comparisons of treatment modalities reported adjustment for the level of anemia (51,83). Studies that did not consider level of anemia may reflect the adverse effects of anemia rather than uremia or its treatment (111).

Not only the type but also the definition of case mix variables considered differed among studies. Mostly, comorbid status was assessed by the presence of preselected types of co-existent diseases (43,85,117), and/or summing the number of co-existent conditions, each condition equally weighted (45,83,123,125). Only a few studies focused on the severity of co-existent diseases (51,130). As the number and type of co-existent diseases assessed varied, comorbid status cannot simply be compared across studies. Adjustment for therapy history varied between length of time since ESRD onset (43), length of time on ESRD treatment (88,123), length of time on dialysis (51,85,126,127), length of time on current treatment modality (43,123), and history of a failed transplant (43,51,122–124). The effect of switching dialysis modality has only been studied once (122,124). In a small sample of CAPD patients, patients who had experienced only CAPD reported somewhat higher QL than patients with previous hemodialysis treatment. Experience of a failed transplant had a detrimental effect on QL in one study (123), but no such influence was observed in another one (43). In the study of Simmons et al. (122,124), an effect of a previous failed transplant was only suggested in CAPD. Length of time on current treatment was not associated with QL in patients who were stabilized on current treatment modality for a year or longer (43). In contrast, others observed that length of time on dialysis was associated with higher psychological distress (126). The remaining studies presented in Table 2 adjusted for time on dialysis or failed transplant but did

Table 2 Results of Observational Studies in ESRD

Study (Ref.)	Aim	Design	Study populations HHD	CHD	PD	Tx	GP	QL outcome Phys	Psych	Soc	Case mix adjustment SoDe	PKi	Comb	He	THis	Main results
Hart and Evans, 1987 (43)	M	C	287	347	81	144		+	+	+	+	+	+		+	QL CHD = CAPD = HHD < Tx Age, education, diabetic renal condition, comorbidity strongest independent associations with lower QL
Oldenburg, 1988 (126)	M	C		52	50			?	+	+	+				+	PD poorer adjustment to illness; CHD more social distress Increasing psychological distress with time on dialysis
Wolcott and Nissenson, 1988 (127)	M	C		33	33			+	+	+	+		+		+	Psychosocial QL CAPD likely superior to CHD
Bremer et al., 1989 (123)	M	C	47	146	79	187	+	?	+	+	+	+	+		+	QL failed transplants < CAPD = CHD < HHD = TX Emotional well-being and life satisfaction CHD = CAPD < HHD = Tx = GP Age and comorbid status only case mix variables consistently related to QL
Björvell and Hylander, 1989 (36)	M	C		53			+	+	+	+						Physical functioning CHD < GP
Julius et al., 1989 (45)	M	C		171	125	163	+	+			+	+	+			Physical dysfunctioning CAPD > CHD > Tx; Age (older), primary kidney disease (diabetes) and higher number of comorbid conditions are by far strongest explanatory factors of higher physical dysfunction
Auer et al., 1990 (117)	M	C		78 (+12) extended study	81 (+18),		+		+	+						Overall life satisfaction CHD = CAPD = GP; Male patients, <60 yr., with additional medical and social risks, were least satisfied with life on several different assessment scales
Devins et al., 1990 (88)	M	C	39	11	15	34		+	+	+	+		?		?	Illness intrusiveness HHD = CHD = CAPD > Tx; Non-consistent modality differences in life satisfaction, happiness and pessimism/illness-related concerns
Simmons et al., 1990 (122,124)	M	C		83	510	173	+	+	+	+	+		?		+	QL CAPD = CHD < Tx Psychological QL CAPD = CHD < Tx = GP No consistent evidence of detrimental impact of failed transplant on QL
Tucker et al., 1990 (128)	M	C		29	22				+	+						QL CHD = CAPD;

Fox et al., 1991 (129)	M	C	58	13	37			+	+	+						QL CAPD = CHD < HHD
Russell et al., 1992 (107)	M	L	9	10	8				Utility measure				N/A (within subject comparison)			QL significantly improved following successful transplantation
Griffin et al., 1994 (130)	M	C		35	63			+	+	+						Functional status CHD = PD Psychological adjustment CHD > PD
Gudex, 1995 (125)	M	C	59	95	93	367	+	+	+	+	+		+			QL HHD = CHD = CAPD < Tx < GP Age, comorbidity significant influence on functional status
Kahn et al., 1995 (79)	M	C		43	27	102	+	+	+	+						QL CHD and PD combined < Tx; QL CHD and PD combined < Tx; Physical QL Tx < GP
Laupacis et al., 1996 (48)	M	L		168				+	+	+			N/A (within subject comparison)			By 6 months after transplantation QL improved in all domains and stayed improved throughout 2 years of follow-up
Meers et al., 1996 (82)	A	L		34				+	+	+	+		+			Psychosocial QL self-care CHD > full-care CHD; No change in QL before and after transfer to satellite unit in self-care CHD;
Moreno et al., 1996 (51)	M/A	C	7	963 CHD includes hemodiafiltration(71)	41			+	+	+	+	+	+	+	+	Dialysis technique (modality, total Kt/V, PCR, dialyzer membrane and dialysis solution) not related to QL; Age and comorbidity most important correlates of QL and to a lesser degree gender, education, socioeconomic status, hemoglobin
Morton et al., 1996 (85)	A	C		55	60			+	+	+	+		+		+	Total Kt/V and PCR not related to QL in either CHD or PD patients
Steele et al., 1996 (118)	A	C			49			+	?	+						Psychological symptoms much stronger determinants of overall QL than total Kt/V
Goller et al., 1997 (78)	A	C			57			+	+	+						QL CAPD < GP Impaired physical functioning related to lower nPCR Patients with a Ccr ≥ 65 L/week/1.73 m^2 higher vitality than patients with Ccr < 65 L/week/1.73 m^2 Total Kt/V not related to QL
Merkus et al., 1997 (83)	M/A	C		120	106		+	+	+	+	+	+	+	+	N/A baseline assessment of cohort study	QL CHD = CAPD < GP; Dialysis Kt/V not related to QL; Hemoglobin, comobidity and residual renal function most important correlates of QL and to a lesser degree age, renal vascular disease, employment and the nPCR

M: Impact of treatment modality on QL was (one of) the objective(s); A: impact of adequacy of dialysis on QL was (one of) the objective(s); C: cross-sectional; L: longitudinal; HHD: home hemodialysis; CHD: in-center hemodialysis; C(A)PD: continuous (ambulatory) peritoneal dialysis; Tx: successful transplantation; GP: general population; Phys: physical; Psych: psychological; Soc: social; SoDe: sociodemographic; PKi: primary kidney disease; Comb: comorbid diseases; He: hemoglobin/hematocrit; THis: therapy history (e.g., failed transplants, time since dialysis onset); Ccr: creatinine clearance; (n)PCR: (normalized) protein catabolic rate; +: assessed; ?:doubtful; N/A: not applicable.

Table 3 Results of Intervention Studies in ESRD

Study	Design		Interventions	Patients		Control group	Follow-up (Fup)				QL outcome			Main results
	Ran	Bli		HD	CAPD		Fup1	Fup2	Fup3	Fup4	Phys	Psych	Soc	
Wolcott et al., 1989 (120)			EPO, no dosage indications, no target Ht	15			1 mo after correction of Ht	10–12 mo after EPO onset			+	+	+	Improved energy levels and psychological adaptation from baseline to Fup; No improvement in social adaptation and cognitive function from baseline to Fup
Canadian Erythropoietin Study Group, 1990 (37)	+	+	Placebo EPO, target Hb 95–110 g/L EPO, target Hb 110–130 g/L	118		Placebo	6 mo				+	+	+	Marked improvement in physical aspects and non-consistent improvements in psychosocial aspects of QL from baseline to Fup with EPO; Similar QL in both EPO-groups
Co-operative Multicenter EPO Clinical Trail Group, 1990 (64)			EPO, target Ht of 0.32–0.38	329		Historical: National Kidney Dialysis and Kidney Transplantation Study	6 mo	10 mo			+	+	+	Improvement in physical and psychosocial QL, from baseline to Fup2 to level of successful transplanted historical controls; No effect of EPO on vocational status
Auer et al., 1992 (61)			EPO, no dosage indications, no target Hb/Ht		22		3–5 mo	≥6 mo after Fup1			+	+	+	Significant improvement in energy, social life from baseline to follow-up

McMahon et al., 1992 (49)	cross-over trial	+	EPO, target Hb 9 g/dL EPO, target Hb 12 g/dL	12		Target Hb of 9 g/dL	4 mo after stabilization of target Hb				+	+	+	Improvement in physical and psychosocial QL from baseline to Fup1 in both Hb target groups; Similar QL in both Hb target groups
Bárány et al., 1993 (119)			EPO, target Hb 10 g/dL	24		8 HD patients Historical: nationwide dialysis group	after correction of anemia	12–18 mo			+	+	+	Improvement in physical and emotional well-being from baseline to Fup1 to level of control group; Improvement persisted after 1 year of EPO treatment
Moreno et al., 1996 (50)			EPO no dosage indications, no target Hb/Ht	57 elderly patients		29 HD patients, age matched, not requiring EPO	3 mo	6 mo			+	+	+	Improvement in physical and psychosocial QL from baseline to Fup1 with EPO, that persisted at Fup2; No change in QL in control patients
National Co-operative rHu Erythropoietin Study, 1996 (63,81)			EPO, no dosage indications, no target Hb/Ht	469 (4 other)	11	520 old-to EPO patients (511 HD, 7 CAPD, 2 other)	within 40–180 days				+	+	+	Improvement in physical and psychosocial QL from baseline to Fup in new-to-EPO patients to level of old-to-EPO patients; No change in QL in old-to-EPO patients from baseline to Fup.
Muirhead et al., 1992 (100)	+	+	Placebo run-in period Intravenous EPO 50 U/kg Subcutaneous EPO 50 U/kg	128		Intravenous EPO	after Hb stabilization	8 wk	16 wk	24 wk	+	+	+	Similar improvement in QL in both EPO administration groups; Only improvement in physical QL with EPO
Churchill et al., 1992 (39)	+ cross-over trial	+	Conventional HD High flux HD	22		Conventional HD	4 mo				+	+	+	No difference in QL between high flux and conventional HD (mean Kt/V 1.42 vs. 1.27)

Ran: Randomized; Bli: (double) blinded; mo: months; wk: weeks; Phys: physical; Psych: psychological; Soc: social; +: done/assessed; ?: doubtful; N/A: not applicable.

not report the specific effect of therapy history on QL. Therefore, supplementary data on effect of therapy, especially regarding switching of dialysis modalities, are required.

Apart from the various definitions and assessment tools of QL and the cross-sectional study designs, the small sample size of many studies may have attributed to the absence of firm conclusions on the QL of ESRD patients, except for its being worse than the general population.

V. CONCLUSIONS AND FUTURE DIRECTIONS

Uncertainty with regard to the clinical significance of differences in QL will remain until multicenter randomized trials comparing the different dialysis modalities are completed. The same holds true with respect to the effect of adequacy of dialysis. However, randomized allocation to dialysis modality is hard to achieve. In the absence of randomized trials, longitudinal multicenter cohort studies starting at or near the date of the initiation of treatment and following patients for a considerable amount of time are the best alternative. Suitable adjustment for case mix differences should be made to provide comparison of prognostically similar groups. The case mix variables that should at least be considered are age, gender, education, socioeconomic status, level of anemia, residual renal function, therapy history, primary kidney disease, as well as the presence and severity of co-existent conditions. Regarding severity of illness, the assessment is still not well established, either in the general hospital setting or in ESRD-specific settings (101). Encouraging results have been reported on medical record based indices, such as The Index of Co-Existent Disease (ICED) (101,116,131) and The DUKE Severity of Illness Checklist (DUSOI) (101,132). Recently, a patient self-report measure, originally developed to assess severity of diabetes and comorbidity in diabetes patients, has been suggested suitable for use in ESRD patients (133). However, further evaluation is necessary. In addition, more insight is needed into both the physician and patient preferences for dialysis modalities to minimize the effect of selection bias in the evaluation of different treatment alternatives.

In our review we have focused only on published, validated instruments. To our knowledge, results of currently ongoing evaluation of other instruments for use in the dialysis setting, such as The Dartmouth COOP Charts, The DUKE Health Profile, the CHOICE Health Experience Questionnaire, and the Renal-Dependent Quality of Life Questionnaire, seem to be promising (101,134).

We conclude that QL assessment should regularly be performed in the clinical monitoring of ESRD patients. This assessment should preferably consist of the combination of a generic and a disease-specific instrument. Since the disease-specific KDQOL-SF incorporates a well-established generic core (SF-36/RAND-36) is well accepted by patients, short to complete, and translated into several languages, we consider this instrument as a clinical suitable and promising QL measure.

REFERENCES

1. Schipper H, Clinch JJ, Olweny CLM. Quality of life studies: Definitions and conceptual issues. In: Spilker B, ed. Quality of Life and Pharmacoeconomics in Clinical Trials. 2d ed. Philadelphia: Lippincott-Raven Publishers, 1996:11–23.
2. World Health Organization. The First Ten Years of the World Health Organization. Geneva: World Health Organization, 1958.
3. Fitzpatrick R, Fletcher A, Jones D, Spiegelhalter D, Cox D. Quality of life measures in health care. I: Applications and issues in assessment. Br Med J 1992; 305:1074–1077.
4. de Haan RJ, Aaronson N, Limburg M, Langton Hewer R, van Crevel H. Measuring quality of life in stroke. Stroke 1993; 24:320–327.
5. Nissenson AR. Quality of life in elderly and diabetic patients on peritoneal dialysis. Perit Dial Int 1996; 16(suppl 1):S407–S409.
6. Fletcher A, Gore S, Jones D, Fitzpatrick R, Spiegelhalter D, Cox D. Quality of life measures in health care. II: design, analysis, and interpretation. Br Med J 1992; 305:1145–1148.
7. McColl E, Christiansen T, König-Zahn C. Making the right choice of outcome measure. In: Hutchinson A, Bentzen N, König-Zahn C, eds. Cross-Cultural Health Outcome Assessment: A User's Guide. Groningen, The Netherlands: European Research Group on Health Outcomes (ERGHO), 1997:12–26.
8. Guyatt GH, Jaeschke R, Feeny DH, Patrick DL. Measurement in clinical trials: choosing the right approach. In: Spilker B, ed. Quality of Life and Pharmacoeconomics in Clinical Trials. 2d ed. Philadelphia: Lippincott-Raven Publishers, 1996:41–48.
9. Kidder LH, Judd CM, Smith ER. Questionnaires and interviews: overview of strategies. In: Kidder LH, Judd CM, eds. Research Methods in Social Relations. 5th ed. Tokyo: CBS Publishing Japan Ltd., 1986:219–235.
10. Meers C, Hopman W, Singer MA, MacKenzie TA, Morton AR, McMurray M. A comparison of patient,

nurse, and physician assessment of health-related quality of life in end-stage renal disease. Dial Transplant 1995; 24:120–124,139.
11. Sneeuw CA, Aaronson NK, Sprangers MAG, Detmar SB, Wever LDV, Schornagel JH. Value of caregiver ratings in evaluating the quality of life of patients with cancer. J Clin Oncol 1997; 15:1206–1217.
12. Sprangers MAG, Aaronson NK. The role of health care providers and significant others in evaluating the quality of life of patients with chronic disease: a review. J Clin Epidemiol 1992; 45:743–760.
13. Sneeuw CA, Aaronson, NK, Osoba D, Muller MJ, Hsu MA, Jung WK, Brada M, Newlands ES. The use of significant others as proxy raters of the quality of life of patients with brain cancer. Med Care 1997; 35:490–506.
14. Cronbach LJ. Coefficient alpha and the internal structure of tests. Psychometrika 1951; 16:297–334.
15. Hays RD, Anderson R, Revicki D. Psychometric considerations in evaluating health-related quality of life measures. Qual Life Res 1993; 2:441–449.
16. Juniper EF, Guyatt GH, Jaeschke R. How to develop and validate a new health-related quality of life instrument. In: Spilker B, ed. Quality of Life and Pharmacoeconomics in Clinical Trials. 2d ed. Philadelphia: Lippincott-Raven Publishers, 1996:49–56.
17. Guyatt G, Walter S, Norman G. Measuring change over time: assessing the usefulness of evaluative instruments. J Chron Dis 1987; 40:171–178.
18. Deyo RA, Diehr P, Patrick DL. Reproducibility and responsiveness of health status measures. Controlled Clin Trials 1991; 12(suppl):142S–158S.
19. Kirshner B, Guyatt G. A methodologic framework for assessing health indices. J Chron Dis 1985; 38:27–36.
20. Wright JG, Young NL. A comparison of different indices of responsiveness. J Clin Epidemiol 1997; 50: 239–246.
21. Deyo RA, Centor RM. Assessing the responsiveness of functional scales to clinical change: an analogy to diagnostic test performance. J Chron Dis 1986; 39: 897–906.
22. Jaeschke R, Singer J, Guyatt GH. Measurement of health status: ascertaining the minimal clinically important difference. Controlled Clin Trials 1989; 10: 407–415.
23. Meenan RF, Anderson JJ, Kazis LE, Egger MJ, Altz-Smith M, Samuelson Jr CO, Willkens RF, Solsky MA, Hayes SP, Blocka KL, Weinstein A, Guttadauria M, Kaplan SB, Klippel J. Outcome assessment in clinical trials: evidence for the sensitivity of a health status measure. Arthritis Rheum 1984; 27:1344–1352.
24. Kazis LE, Anderson JJ, Meenan RF. Effect sizes for interpreting changes in health status. Med Care 1989; 27(suppl):S178–S189.
25. Guyatt GH, Feeny D, Patrick DL. Issues in quality of life measurement in clinical trials. Controlled Clin Trials 1991; 12(suppl):81S–90S.
26. Patrick DL, Deyo RA. Generic and disease-specific measures in assessing health status and quality of life. Med Care 1989; 27(suppl):S217–S232.
27. Bennett K, Torrance G, Tugwell P. Methodological challenges in the development of utility measures of health-related quality of life in rheumatoid arthritis. Controlled Clin Trials 1991; 12(suppl):118S–128S.
28. Bergner M, Bobbitt RA, Carter WB, Gilson BS. The Sickness Impact Profile: development and final revision of a health status measure. Med Care 1981; 19: 787–805.
29. de Bruin AF, de Witte LP, Stevens, F, Diederiks JP. Sickness Impact Profile: the state of the art of a generic functional status measure. Soc Sci Med 1992; 35:1003–1014.
30. de Haan R, Limburg M, van der Meulen J, Jacobs H, Aaronson N. Quality of life after stroke: impact of stroke type and lesion location. Stroke 1995; 3:402–408.
31. Deyo RA, Inui TA. Toward clinical applications of health status measures: sensitivity of scales to clinically important changes. Health Serv Res 1984; 19: 277–289.
32. Katz JN, Larson MG, Phillips CB, Fossel AH, Liang MH. Comparative measurement sensitivity of short and longer health status instruments. Med Care 1992; 30:917–925.
33. MacKenzie CR, Charlson ME, DiGioia D, Kelley K. Can The Sickness Impact Profile measure change? An example of scale assessment. J Chron Dis 1986; 39: 429–438.
34. Tandon PK, Stander H, Schwarz Jr RP. Analysis of quality of life data from a randomized, placebo-controlled heart failure trial. J Clin Epidemiol 1989; 42: 955–962.
35. Hall J, Hall N, Fisher E, Killer D. Measurement of outcomes of general practice: comparison of three health status measures. Fam Pract 1987; 4:117–122.
36. Björvell H, Hylander B. Functional status and personality in patients on chronic dialysis. J Intern Med 1989; 226:319–324.
37. Canadian Erythropoietin Study Group. Association between recombinant human erythropoietin and quality of life and exercise capacity of patients receiving haemodialysis. Brit Med J 1990; 300:573–578.
38. Christensen AJ, Holman Jr JM, Turner CW, Smith TW, Grant MK, DeVault Jr GA. A prospective study of quality of life in end-stage renal disease: Effects of cadaveric renal transplantation. Clin Transplant 1991; 5:40–47.
39. Churchill DN, Bird DR, Taylor DW, Beecroft ML, Gorman J, Wallace JE. Effect of high-flux hemodialysis on quality of life and neuropsychological function in chronic hemodialysis patients. Am J Nephrol 1992; 12:412–418.

40. Craven J, Littlefield C, Rodin G, Murray M. The End-Stage Renal Disease Severity Index (ESRD-SI). Psychol Med 1991; 21:237–243.
41. Deniston OR, Carpentier-Alting P, Kneisley J, Hawthorne VM, Port FK. Assessment of quality of life in end-stage renal disease. Health Serv Res 1989; 24: 555–578.
42. Essink-Bot ML, Krabbe PFM, Agt van HME, Bonsel GJ. NHP or SIP-A comparative study in renal insufficiency associated anemia. Qual Life Res 1996; 5:91–100.
43. Hart LG, Evans RW. The functional status of ESRD patients as measured by The Sickness Impact Profile. J Chron Dis 1987; 40(suppl 1):117S–130S.
44. Hornberger JC, Redelmeier DA, Petersen J. Variability among methods to assess patients' well-being and consequent effect on a cost-effectiveness analysis. J Clin Epidemiol 1992; 45:505–512.
45. Julius M, Hawthorne VM, Carpentier-Alting P, Kneisley J, Wolfe RA, Port FK. Independence in activities of daily living for end-stage renal disease patients: biomedical and demographic correlates. Am J Kidney Dis 1989; 13:61–69.
46. Laupacis A, Wong C, Churchill D. The use of generic and specific quality of life measures in hemodialysis patients treated with erythropoietin. Controlled Clin Trials 1991; 12(suppl):168S–179S.
47. Laupacis A, Muirhead N, Keown P, Wong C. A disease-specific questionnaire for assessing quality of life in patients on hemodialysis. Nephron 1992; 60:302–306.
48. Laupacis A, Keown P, Krueger H, Ferguson B, Wong C, Muirhead N. A study of the quality of life and cost-utility of renal transplantation. Kidney Int 1996; 50: 235–242.
49. McMahon LP, Dawborn JK. Subjective quality of life assessment in hemodialysis patients at different levels of hemoglobin following use of recombinant human erythropoietin. Am J Nephrol 1992; 12:162–169.
50. Moreno F, Aracil FJ, Pérez R, Valderrábano F. Controlled study on the improvement of quality of life in elderly hemodialysis patients after correcting end-stage renal disease related anemia with erythropoietin. Am J Kidney Dis 1996; 27:548–556.
51. Moreno F, López Gomez JM, Sanz-Guajardo D, Jofre R, Valderrábano F, Spanish Cooperative Renal Patients Quality of Life Study Group. Quality of Life in dialysis patients. A Spanish multicentre study. Nephrol Dial Transplant 1996; 11(suppl 2):125–129.
52. de Bruin AF, Buys M, de Witte LP, Diederiks JP. The Sickness Impact Profile: SIP68, a short generic version. First evaluation of the reliability and reproducibility. J Clin Epidemiol 1994; 47:863–871.
53. Hanestad BR. The NHP. In: Hutchinson A, Bentzen N, König-Zahn C, eds. Cross Cultural Health Outcome Assessment: A User's Guide. Gröningen, The Netherlands: European Research Group on Health Outcomes (ERGHO), 1997:87–93.
54. Hunt SM, McKenna SP, McEwen J, Backett EM, Williams J, Papp E. A quantative approach to perceived health status: a validation study. J Epidemiol Community Health 1980; 34:281–286.
55. Hunt SM, McKenna SP, Williams J. Reliability of a population survey tool for measuring perceived health problems: a study in patients with osteoporosis. J Epidemiol Commun Health 1981; 35:297–300.
56. Hunt SM, McEwen J, McKenna SP. Measuring health status: a new tool for clinicians and epidemiologists. J R Coll Gen Pract 1985; 35:185–188.
57. O'Brien BJ, Banner NR, Gibson S, Yacoub MH. The Nottingham Health Profile as a measure of quality of life following combined heart and lung transplantation. J Epidemiol Commun Health 1988; 42:232–234.
58. Hunt SM, McEwen J, McKenna SP, Backett EM, Pope C. Subjective health assessments and the perceived outcome of minor surgery. J Psychosom Res 1984; 28: 105–114.
59. Brazier JE, Harper R, Jones NM, O'Cathain A, Thoms KJ, Usherwood T, Westlake L. Validating the SF-36 health survey questionnaire: new outcome measure for primary care. Br Med J 1992; 305:160–164.
60. McEwen J, McKenna SP. Nottingham Health Profile. In: Spilker B, ed. Quality of Life and Pharmacoeconomics in Clinical Trials. 2d ed. Philadelphia: Lippincott-Raven Publishers, 1996:281–286.
61. Auer J, Simon G, Stevens J, Griffiths P, Howarth D, Anastassiades E, Gokal R, Oliver D. Quality of life improvements in CAPD patients treated with subcutaneously administered erythropoietin for anemia. Perit Dial Int 1992; 12:40–42.
62. Badia X, Alonso J, Brosa S, Lock P. Reliability of the Spanish version of the Nottingham Health Profile in patients with stable end-stage renal disease. Soc Sci Med 1994; 38:153–158.
63. Beusterien KM, Nissenson AR, Port FK, Kelly M, Steinwald B, Ware Jr JE. The effects of recombinant human erythropietin on functional health and well-being in chronic dialysis patients. J Am Soc Nephrol 1996: 7:763–773.
64. Evans RW, Rader B, Manninen DL, and the Cooperative Multicenter EPO Clinical Trial Group. The quality of life of hemodialysis recipients with recombinant human erythropoietin. J Am Med Assoc 1990; 263: 825–830.
65. de Groot J, de Groot W, Vos PF, Berend K, Blankestijn PJ. Quality of life of dialysis patients in Utrecht and Willemstad: little difference (in Dutch). Ned Tijdschr Geneeskd 1994; 138:862–866.
66. Schrama YC, Krediet RT, de Rooy-Roggekamp MC, Arisz L. The relation between clinical condition and quality of life in hemodialysis patients: a clinimetric study (in Dutch). Ned Tijdschr Geneeskd 1991; 135: 1182–1185.

67. Hays RD, Sherbourne CD, Mazel RM. The RAND-36-Item Health Survey 1.0. Health Econ 1993; 2:217–227.
68. Ware Jr JE, Sherbourne CD. The MOS 36-item Short Form Health Survey (SF-36): I. Conceptual framework and item selection. Med Care 1992; 30:473–483.
69. Ware Jr JE, Snow KK, Kosinski M, Gandek B. SF-36 Health Survey: Manual and Interpretation Guide. Boston: The Health Institute, 1993.
70. Ware Jr JE, Kosinski M, Bayliss MS, McHorney CA, Rogers WH, Raczek A. Comparison of methods for the scoring and statistical analysis of the SF-36 health profile and summary measures: summary of results from the Medical Outcomes Study. Med Care 1995; 33(suppl 4):AS264–AS279.
71. McHorney CA, Ware Jr JE, Raczek AE. The MOS 36-item Short Form Health Survey (SF-36): II. Psychometric and clinical tests of validity in measuring physical and mental health constructs. Med Care 1993; 31: 247–263.
72. McHorney CA, Ware Jr JE, Lu JF, Sherbourne CD. The MOS 36-item Short-Form Health Survey (SF-36): III. Tests of data quality, scaling assumptions, and reliability across diverse patient groups. Med Care 1994; 32:40–66.
73. Ruta DA, Abdalla MI, Garratt AM, Coutts A, Russell IT. SF 36 health survey questionnaire: II. Reliability in two patient based studies. Qual Health Care 1994; 3:180–185.
74. Phillips RC, Lansky D. Outcomes management in heart valve replacement surgery: early experience. J Heart Valve Dis 1992; 1:42–50.
75. Jenkinson C, Lawrence K, McWhinnie D, Gordon J. Sensitivity to change of health status measures in a randomized controlled trial: comparison of the COOP charts and the SF-36. Qual Life Res 1995; 4:47–52.
76. Garratt AM, Ruta DA, Abdalla MI, Russell IT. SF 36 health survey questionnaire: II. Responsiveness to changes in health status in four common clinical conditions. Qual Health Care 1994; 3:186–192.
77. Hays RD, Kallich JD, Mapes DL, Coons SJ, Carter WB. Development of the Kidney Disease Quality of Life (KDQOL-TM) Instrument. Qual Life Res 1994; 3:329–338.
78. Goller JL, McMahon JM, Rutledge C, Walker RG, Wood SE. Dialysis adequacy and self-reported health status in a group of CAPD patients. Adv Perit Dial 1997; 13:128–133.
79. Kahn IH, Garrett AM, Kumar A, Cody DJ, Catto GRD, Edward N, MacLeod AM. Patients' perception of health on renal replacement therapy: evaluation using a new instrument. Nephrol Dial Transplant 1995; 10:684–689.
80. Kurtin PS, Davies AR, Meyer KB, DeGiacomo JM, Kantz ME. Patient-based health status measures in outpatient dialysis: early experiences in developing an outcomes assessment program. Med Care 1992; 30: MS136–MS149.
81. Levin NW, Lazarus M, Nissenson AR, for the National Cooperative rHU Erythropoietin Study Group. National Cooperative rHu Erythropoietin study in patients with chronic renal failure—an interim report. Am J Kidney Dis 1993; 22(suppl 1):3–12.
82. Meers C, Singer MA, Toffelmire EB, Hopman W, McMurray M, Morton AR, MacKenzie TA. Self-delivery of hemodialysis care: a therapy in itself. Am J Kidney Dis 1996; 27:844–847.
83. Merkus MP, Jager KJ, Dekker FW, Boeschoten EW, Stevens P, Krediet RT, and The Necosad Study Group. Quality of life in patients on chronic dialysis: self-assessment 3 months after the start of treatment. Am J Kidney Dis 1997; 29:584–592.
84. Meyer KB, Espindle DM, DeGiacomo JM, Jenuleson CS, Kurtin PS, Ross Davies A. Monitoring dialysis patients' health status. Am J Kidney Dis 1994; 24: 267–279.
85. Morton AR, Meers C, Singer MA, Toffelmire EB, Hopman W, McComb J, MacKenzie TA. Quantity of dialysis: quality of life—What is the relationship? ASAIO J 1996; 42:M713–M717.
86. Burton HJ, Kline SA, Lindsay RM, Heidenheim, P. The role of support in influencing outcome of end-stage renal disease. Gen Hosp Psychiatry 1988; 10: 260–266.
87. Churchill DN, Wallace JE, Ludwin D, Beecroft ML, Taylor DW. A comparison of evaluative indices of quality of life and cognitive function in hemodialysis patients. Controlled Clin Trials 1991: 12(suppl):159S–167S.
88. Devins GM, Mandin H, Hons RB, Burgess ED, Klassen J, Taub K, Schorr S, Letourneau PK, Buckle S. Illness intrusiveness and quality of life in end-stage renal disease: comparison and stability across treatment modalities. Health Psychol 1990; 9:117–142.
89. Ferrans CE, Powers MJ. Quality of life index: development and psychometric properties. Adv Nurse Science 1985; 8:15–24.
90. Ferrans CE, Powers MJ. Psychometric assessment of the Quality of Life Index. Res Nurs Health 1992; 15: 29–38.
91. Laupacis A, Pus N, Muirhead N, Wong C, Ferguson B, Keown P. Disease-specific questionnaire for patients with a renal transplant. Nephron 1993; 64:226–231.
92. Parfrey PS, Vavasour H, Bullock M, Henry S, Harnett JD, Gault MH. Development of a health questionnaire specific for end-stage renal disease. Nephron 1989; 52:20–28.
93. Park H, Bang WR, Kim SJ, Kim ST, Lee JS, Kim S, Han SJ. Quality of life of ESRD patients: development of a tool and comparison between transplant and dialysis patients. Transplant Proc 1992; 24:1435–1437.

94. Peters VJ, Hazel LA, Finkel P, Colls J. Rehabilitation experiences of patients receiving dialysis. ANNA J 1994; 21:419–426,457.
95. Parfrey PS, Vavasour H, Henry S, Bullock M, Gault MH. Clinical features and severity of nonspecific symptoms in dialysis patients. Nephron 1988; 50:121–128.
96. Parfrey PS, Vavasour H, Gault MH. A prospective study of health status in dialysis and transplant patients. Transplant Proc 1988; 20:1231–1232.
97. Campbell A, Converse PE, Rodgers WL. The Quality of American Life. New York: Russell Sage Foundation, 1976.
98. Spitzer WO, Dobson AJ, Hall J, Chesterman E, Levi J. Measuring the quality of life of cancer patients. A concise QL-index for use by physicians. J Chron Dis 1981; 34:585–597.
99. Karnofsky DA, Burchenal JH. The clinical evaluation of chemotherapeutic agents in cancer. In: MacLeod CM, ed. Evaluation of Chemotherapeutic Agents. New York: Columbia University Press, 1949:191–205.
100. Muirhead N, Churchill DN, Goldstein M, Nadler SP, Posen G, Wong C, Slaughter D, Laplante P. Comparison of subcutaneous and intravenous recombinant human erythropoietin for anemia in hemodialysis patients with significant comorbid disease. Am J Nephrol 1992; 12:303–310.
101. Rettig RA, Sadler JH, Meyer KB, Wasson JH, Parkerson Jr GR, Kantz B, Hays RD, Patrick DL. Assessing health and quality of life outcomes in dialysis: a report on an Institute of Medicine workshop. Am J Kidney Dis 1997; 30:140–155.
102. Hays RD, Kallich JD, Mapes DL, Coons SJ, Amin N, Carter WB. Kidney Disease Quality of Life Short Form (KDQOL-SFtm), Version 1.2: A Manual for Use and Scoring. Santa Monica, CA: RAND, 1995.
103. Edgell ET, Coons SJ, Carter WB, Kallich JD, Mapes D, Damush TM, Hays RD. A review of health-related quality of life measures used in end-stage renal disease. Clin Ther 1996; 18:887–938.
104. Essink-Bot ML. Health status as a measure of outcome of disease and treatment. Ph.D. dissertation, Erasmus University, Rotterdam, The Netherlands, 1995.
105. Churchill DN, Torrance GW, Taylor DW, Barnes CC, Ludwin D, Shimizu A, Smith KM. Measurement of quality of life in end-stage renal disease: The Time Trade-Off approach. Clin Invest Med 1987; 10:14–20.
106. Molzahn AE, Northcott HC, Hayduk L. Quality of life of patients with end stage renal disease: a structural equation model. Qual Life Res 1996; 5:426–432.
107. Russell JD, Beecroft ML, Ludwin D, Churchill DN. The quality of life in renal transplantation—prospective study. Transplant Proc 1992; 54:656–660.
108. Kutner NG. Assessing end-stage renal disease patients' functioning and well-being: measurement approaches and implications for clinical practice. Am J Kidney Dis 1994; 24:321–333.
109. Ahlmén J. Quality of life of the dialysis patient. In: Jacobs C, Kjellstrand CM, Koch KM, Winchester JF, eds. Replacement of renal function by dialysis. 4th ed. Dordrecht, The Netherlands: Kluwer Academic Publishers, 1996: 1466–1479.
110. Gokal R. Quality of life in patients undergoing renal replacement therapy. Kidney Int 1993; 43(suppl 40): S23–S27.
111. Gokal R. Quality of life. In: Gokal R, Nolph KD, eds. The Textbook of Peritoneal Dialysis. Dordrecht, The Netherlands: Kluwer Academic Publishers, 1994:679–698.
112. Kaplan De-Nour A, Brickman AL. Determining quality of life in the renal replacement therapies. In: Spilker B, ed. Quality of Life and Pharmacoeconomics in Clinical Trials. 2d ed. Philadephia: Lippincott-Raven Publishers, 1996:953–960.
113. Kurtin P, Nissenson AR. Variation in end-stage renal disease patient outcomes: what we know, what should we know, and how do we find it out? J Am Soc Nephrol 1993; 3:1738–1747.
114. Nissenson AR. Measuring, managing, and improving quality in the end-stage renal disease treatment setting: peritoneal dialysis. Am J Kidney Dis 1994; 24:368–375.
115. Sensky T. Psychosomatic aspects of end-stage renal failure. Psychother Psychosom 1993; 59:56–68.
116. Greenfield S, Sullivan L, Silliman RA, Dukes K, Kaplan SH. Principles and practice of case mix adjustment: applications to end-stage renal disease. Am J Kidney Dis 1994; 24:298–307.
117. Auer J, Gokal R, Stout JP, Hillier VF, Kincey J, Simon LG, Oliver DO. The Oxford-Manchester Study of Dialysis Patients: age, risk factors and treatment method in relation to quality of life. Scand J Urol Nephrol 1990; 131(suppl):31–37.
118. Steele TE, Baltimore D, Finkelstein SH, Juergensen P, Kliger AS, Finkelstein FO. Quality of life in peritoneal dialysis patients. J Nerv Ment Dis 1996; 184:368–374.
119. Bárány P, Pettersson E, Konarski-Svensson. Long-term effects on quality of life in hemodialysis patients of correction of anemia with erythropoietin. Nephrol Dial Transplant 1993; 8:426–432.
120. Wolcott DL, Marsh JT, La Rue A, Carr C, Nissenson AR. Recombinant human erythropoietin treatment may improve quality of life and cognitive function in chronic hemodialysis patients. Am J Kidney Dis 1989; 14:478–485.
121. Nissenson AR, Prichard SS, Cheng IKP, Gokal R, Kubot M, Maiorca R, Riella MC, Rottembourg J, Steward JH. Non-medical factors that impact on ESRD modality selection. Kidney Int 1993; 43(suppl 40):S120–S127.
122. Simmons RG, Anderson CR, Abress LK. Quality of life and rehabilitation differences among four end-

stage renal disease therapy groups. Scand J Urol Nephrol 1990; 131(suppl):7–22.
123. Bremer BA, McCauley CR, Wrona RM, Johnson JP. Quality of life in end-stage renal disease: a reexamination. Am J Kidney Dis 1989; 13:200–209.
124. Simmons RG, Abress L. Quality of life issues for end-stage renal patients. Am J Kidney Dis 1990; 15:201–208.
125. Gudex CM. Health-related quality of life in endstage renal failure. Qual Life Res 1995; 4:359–366.
126. Oldenburg O, MacDonald GJ, Perkins RJ. Prediction of quality of life in a cohort of end-stage renal disease patients. J Clin Epidemiol 1988; 41:555–564.
127. Wolcott DL, Nissenson AR. Quality of life in chronic dialysis patients: a critical comparison of continuous ambulatory peritoneal dialysis (CAPD) and hemodialysis. Am J Kidney Dis 1988; 11:402–412.
128. Tucker CM, Ziller RC, Smith WR, Mars DR, Coons MP. Quality of life of patients on in-center hemodialysis versus continuous ambulatory peritoneal dialysis. Perit Dial Int 1990; 11:341–346.
129. Fox E, Peace K, Neale TJ, Morrison RBI, Hatfield PJ, Mellsop G. Quality of life for patients with end-stage renal failure. Renal Failure 1991; 13:31–35.
130. Griffin KW, Wadhwa NK, Friend R, Suh H, Howell N, Cabralda T, Jao E, Hatchett L, Eitel PE. Comparison of quality of life in hemodialysis and peritoneal dialysis patients. Adv Perit Dial 1994; 10:104–108.
131. Niccolucci A, Cubasso D, Labbrozzi D, Mari E, Impicciatore P, Procaccini DA, Forcella M, Stella I, Querques M, Pappani A, Passione A, Strippoli P. Effect of co-existent diseases on survival of patients undergoing dialysis. ASAIO J 1992; 38:M291–M295.
132. Parkerson Jr GR, Broadhead WE, Tse CKJ. The DUKE Severity of Illness Checklist (DUSOI) for measurement of severity and comorbidity. J Clin Epidemiol 1993; 46:379–393.
133. Greenfield S, Sullivan L, Dukes KA, Silliman RA, D'Agostino R, Kaplan SH. Development and testing of a new measure of case mix for use in office practice. Med Care 1995; 33:AS47–AS55.
134. Bradley C. Design of a renal-dependent individualized quality of life questionnaire. Adv Perit Dial 1997; 13: 116–120.

29

Dyslipoproteinemia Associated with Chronic Renal Failure

C. H. Barton and N. D. Vaziri
University of California, Irvine, Irvine, California

I. LIPID AND LIPOPROTEIN DISORDERS IN END-STAGE RENAL DISEASE

Chronic renal failure (CRF) is an important cause of secondary dyslipoproteinemia, with abnormalities generally occurring in individuals with renal insufficiency ranging from moderate to severe (1–3). In addition, the superimposed effects of dialysis, nutrition, medications, nephrotic syndrome, and/or the coexistence of an underlying disease may further modulate the lipoprotein profile in this setting. To better understand the abnormalities in lipoprotein metabolism associated with CRF, a brief review of lipids, lipoproteins, and their normal metabolism is discussed. However, for a more comprehensive discussion of lipoprotein metabolism the reader is referred to recent reviews (4–10).

II. PLASMA LIPIDS AND LIPOPROTEINS

The three major classes of complex plasma lipids are triglycerides, cholesterol, and phospholipids. Triglycerides (TG) are formed by the esterification of glycerol with fatty acids and are mainly stored in adipose tissue, where they function as an important energy reserve as well as a reservoir for essential fatty acids. Through the process of lipolysis, free fatty acids are released into the circulation, where they are bound to albumin and carried to tissues such as muscle, liver, and heart. Depending on need, fatty acids maybe stored in adipose tissue or oxidized for energy. Cholesterol and phospholipids serve as essential components of all membranes, while cholesterol is also a necessary precursor for the synthesis of vitamin D, bile acids, and steroid hormones. Although cholesterol is made in most tissue, it is mainly synthesized by intestinal mucosa and liver from acetate through a series of some 20 reactions. The rate-limiting step in this sequence involves the conversion of 3-hydroxy-3-methyl glutaryl coenzyme A (HMG-CoA) to mevalonate, which is catalyzed by HMG-CoA reductase (6).

Because lipids are insoluble in aqueous plasma, they must circulate as component parts of larger macromolecules (lipoproteins) that are composed of a central hydrophobic lipid core of esterified cholesterol and triglycerides surrounded by a polar hydrophilic surface composed of proteins, unesterified cholesterol, and phospholipids (Fig. 1). The protein components of lipoproteins are termed apolipoproteins or apoproteins, and each apoprotein may have one or more specific functions. In addition to their critical role in solubilizing and transporting lipids in plasma, apoproteins can function as cofactors for specific enzymes or as ligands for specific receptors. Furthermore, apoproteins have important functions involving the structural formation and secretion of certain lipoproteins and in the transfer and exchange of lipids between various lipoproteins.

Plasma lipoproteins can be separated into six major classes on the basis of hydrated density or electrophoretic migration. From the least to the most dense, these include chylomicrons, very low-density lipoproteins (VLDL), intermediate-density lipoproteins (IDL), low-density lipoproteins (LDL), and high-density lipoproteins (HDL). A sixth class of lipoproteins, lipoprotein (a) [Lp(a)] has a density between LDL and HDL and migrates in the pre-β position on electrophoresis

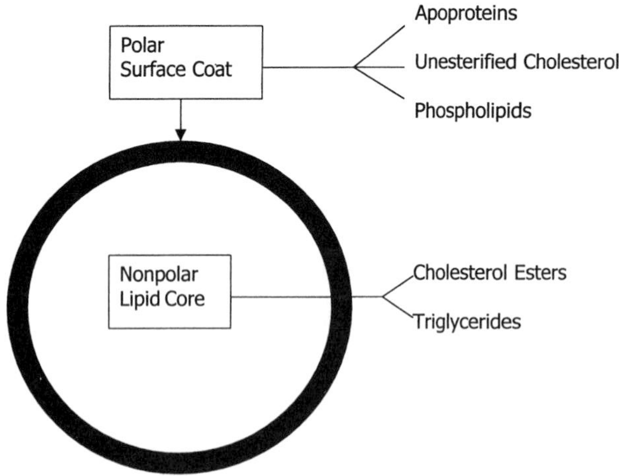

Fig. 1 Lipoprotein structure.

(11). The major characteristics of these lipoproteins are shown in Table 1.

Chylomicrons are large TG-rich lipoproteins that are synthesized and secreted by epithelial cells in the small intestine. Their formation, secretion, and subsequent catabolism serve to transport dietary lipids from the gut to various tissues such as liver, muscle, and adipose. Chylomicrons are catabolized by lipoprotein lipase (LPL), an enzyme located on the endothelial surface of capillaries.

VLDLs are large TG-rich particles that are synthesized and secreted by hepatocytes. In the fasting state virtually all plasma TGs are contained in VLDLs. IDLs and LDLs are generated from the catabolism of VLDL, which undergoes lipolysis through interaction with both LPL and hepatic triglyceride lipase (HTGL). This latter enzyme is located on the surface of hepatic endothelial cells and is also important in the lipolysis of IDL. LDLs are thus formed from the catabolism of VLDL and IDL. The resulting LDL particles are depleted in both TG and surface apoproteins (retaining only apo B-100). However, being greatly enriched with cholesterol, LDLs are the major cholesterol-transporting lipoprotein in the plasma.

The components of HDL originate from lipoprotein material secreted by both the liver and intestine. In particular, the formation of HDL is dependent on the release of specific lipids and apoproteins from circulating chylomicrons and VLDL in the course of normal lipolytic processing. The major importance of HDL is in the acquisition and transport of cholesterol (from peripheral locations) back to the liver for metabolism and excretion (12,13).

III. APOPROTEINS

The major apoproteins include A-I, A-II, B-100, B-48, C-II, C-III, E, and apo (a). With the exception of the apo B lipoproteins, most apoproteins have appreciable water solubility and can be readily exchanged between various lipoprotein particles (i.e., VLDL and HDL) (10). Apo A-I and apo A-II are the principal apoproteins in HDL. In addition to its structural role, apo A-I activates lecithin-cholesterol acyltransferase (LCAT), which catalyzes the esterification of lipoprotein choles-

Table 1 Classification and Characteristics of Lipoproteins

Lipoprotein	Origin	Density (g/mL)	Electrophoretic mobility	Major lipids	Major apoproteins
Chylomicrons	Small intestine	<0.95	Remains at origin	Triglyceride (80–90%)	A-I, A-II, A-IV, B-48, C-II, C-III, E
VLDL	Liver	<1.006	Pre-β	Triglyceride (50–70%) Cholesterol (10–20%)	B-100, C-II, C-III, E
IDL	VLDL	1.006–1.019	Slow pre-β	Triglyceride (40%) Cholesterol (30–40%)	B, E
LDL	IDL	1.019–1.063	β	Triglyceride (5–10%) Cholesterol (45–50%)	B-100
HDL	Liver Intestine Other lipoproteins	1.063–1.210	α	Triglyceride (3–5%) Cholesterol (15–25%)	A-I, A-II (C, E are variable)
Lp(a)	Apo (a) from liver binds with LDL	1.04–1.120	Slow pre-β	Cholesterol	B-100, apo (a)

terol. Other than its apparent structural role, the function of apo A-II is unknown. In plasma, apo B exists as two isoforms (B-100 and B-48) that are synthesized by a single gene. Apo B-100 is synthesized in the liver, has 4536 amino acids, and is the translation product of the full-length apo B mRNA. In contrast, apo B-48 is synthesized in the intestine, has 2152 amino acids, and is the product of a unique apo B mRNA-editing mechanism (14). Apo B-100 is an important structural protein for LDL, IDL, and VLDL and functions as a ligand for the LDL receptor. In addition, apo B-100 performs a necessary role in the intracellular assembly and secretion of VLDL. The inability of the apo B lipoproteins to transfer between lipoprotein particles is thought to be a function of the large number of nonpolar amino acid side chains that penetrate the surface monolayer (10). Apo B-48 is the major B apoprotein present on chylomicrons and plays an essential role in their assembly and secretion. The other major apoprotein that functions as a ligand for the LDL receptor is apo E, which is the putative mediator of hepatic uptake of chylomicron remnants as well as certain VLDL remnants (9). In addition, apo E appears to act as a cofactor that enhances activity of hepatic triglyceride lipase (HTGL) (15). This enzyme facilitates lipolysis of VLDL and IDL as well as hydrolysis of triglycerides and phospholipids in HDL. Apo C-II, which is present on the surface of chylomicrons and VLDL, enhances activity of LPL, an enzyme that plays an essential role in metabolism of chylomicrons and most VLDL particles (8). Conversely, apo C-III appears to inhibit or downregulate the activity of LPL (17,18). In addition, apo C-III inhibits hepatic uptake of apo E containing particles. (8) Apo (a) is a large hydrophilic glycoprotein that is present only on lipoprotein (a), a more recently isolated lipoprotein considered to be an independent risk factor for cardiovascular disease (11,19–22). The important characteristics and functions of the major apoproteins are shown in Table 2.

IV. NORMAL LIPOPROTEIN METABOLISM

The metabolism and transport of lipids can essentially be divided into three pathways (6–8, 23):

1. The exogenous pathway, which involves the absorption, processing, and transport of dietary lipids
2. The endogenous pathway, which involves hepatic synthesis and secretion of lipoproteins
3. The so-called "reverse cholesterol transport" system, which is involved in the transfer of cholesterol back to the liver from extrahepatic sites

Schematic representations of these pathways are shown in Figures 2, 3, and 4.

Table 2 Characteristics of the Major Plasma Apoproteins

Apoprotein	Molecular mass (daltons)	Source	Lipoprotein distribution	Function
Apo A-I	28,016	Liver and intestine	HDL, cylomicrons	LCAT activation Structural component of HDL
Apo A-II	17,414	Liver and intestine	HDL, chylomicrons	Structural component of HDL
Apo A-IV	44,465	Liver and intestine	HDL, chylomicrons	Possible activation of LCAT
Apo B-48	264,000	Intestine	Chylomicrons	Formation and secretion of chylomicrons
Apo B-100	540,000	Liver	VLDL, IDL, LDL	Ligand for LDL receptor; formation and secretion of VLDL
Apo C-I	6,630	Liver	VLDL, IDL, HDL Chylomicrons	LCAT activation; may inhibit hepatic remnant uptake (chylomicron and VLDL)
Apo C-II	8,900	Liver	VLDL, IDL, HDL Chylomicrons	LPL activation
Apo C-III	8,800	Liver	VLDL, IDL, HDL Chylomicrons	LPL inhibitor; may inhibit hepatic remnant uptake
Apo E	34,145	Liver	VLDL, IDL, HDL Chylomicrons	Ligand for LDL and apo E receptors

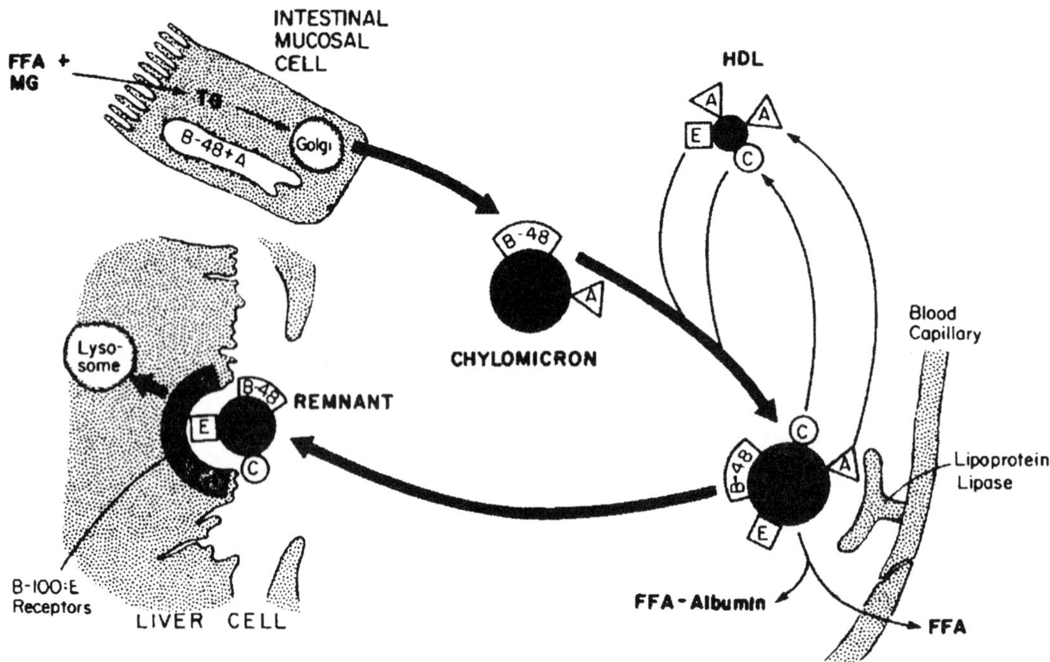

Fig. 2 The pathways for transport of dietary fat in chylomicrons, depicted here, have been deduced mainly from studies in rats, but appear, on less direct evidence, to be similar in humans. Dietary cholesterol, like fatty acids and monoglycerides, is esterified in the mucosal cells and is transported in the nonpolar core of chylomicron particles (black area) with triglycerides (dark gray area). Whereas most of the triglycerides are removed in extrahepatic tissues, almost all of the cholesteryl esters are taken up by the parencymal cells of the liver during endocytosis of chylomicron remnants. As remnants are formed, not only are certain proteins, as shown, transferred to HDL, but also a substantial fraction of the surface lipids, mainly phosphatidylcholine (lecithin). Uptake of chylomicron remnants by the liver appears to be mediated primarily by a receptor that recognizes only the E apoprotein. (Courtesy of R. J. Havel, *Medical Clinics of North America*, W.B. Saunders Company, Philadelphia, PA.)

A. Exogenous Pathway

In the exogenous pathway, dietary cholesterol and fatty acids are absorbed by intestinal cells, reesterified in the endoplasmic reticulum, and packaged into chylomicrons incorporating a surface coat of apoproteins that include B-48, A-I, A-II, and A-IV (15,23,25). The triglyceride-rich chylomicrons are then secreted by exocytosis into lacteals and transported through lymphatics to the blood stream, where additional apoproteins (C-II, C-III, and E) and cholesterol esters are acquired from HDL. Apo C-II, located on the chylomicron surface, activates vascular endothelial cell LPL, which catalyzes hydrolysis of the chylomicron core triglycerides. This causes the release of monoglycerides and free fatty acids, the latter being taken up primarily by adipose and muscle cells. During this process, apo A-I, A-II, A-IV, C-II, and C-III are transferred to HDL. The resulting chylomicron remnant particles are considerably smaller, being relatively depleted in triglycerides but enriched in cholesterol and still retaining apoproteins B-48 and E. These remnants are subsequently taken up by the liver and degraded by lysosomal enzymes, the liberated cholesterol being reesterified and utilized in the synthesis of lipoproteins and bile. Hepatic uptake of chylomicron remnants is thought to be mediated through apo E binding to LDL receptors and perhaps through binding to a putative chylomicron remnant receptor that also recognizes apo E (15).

B. Endogenous Pathway

The endogenous pathway involves the hepatic synthesis and secretion of VLDLs that are large, triglyceride-rich particles that also contain cholesterol, phospholipids, and apoproteins B-100, C-I, C-II, C-III, and E (5,8,10,23,26). There is only one molecule of apo B-100 per VLDL particle, which functions as a secretory aid. Following secretion, VLDL is hydrolyzed by LPL in a similar manner to that of chylomicrons but at a slower rate with apo C-II again acting as cofactor. This results in the progressive removal of triglyceride from

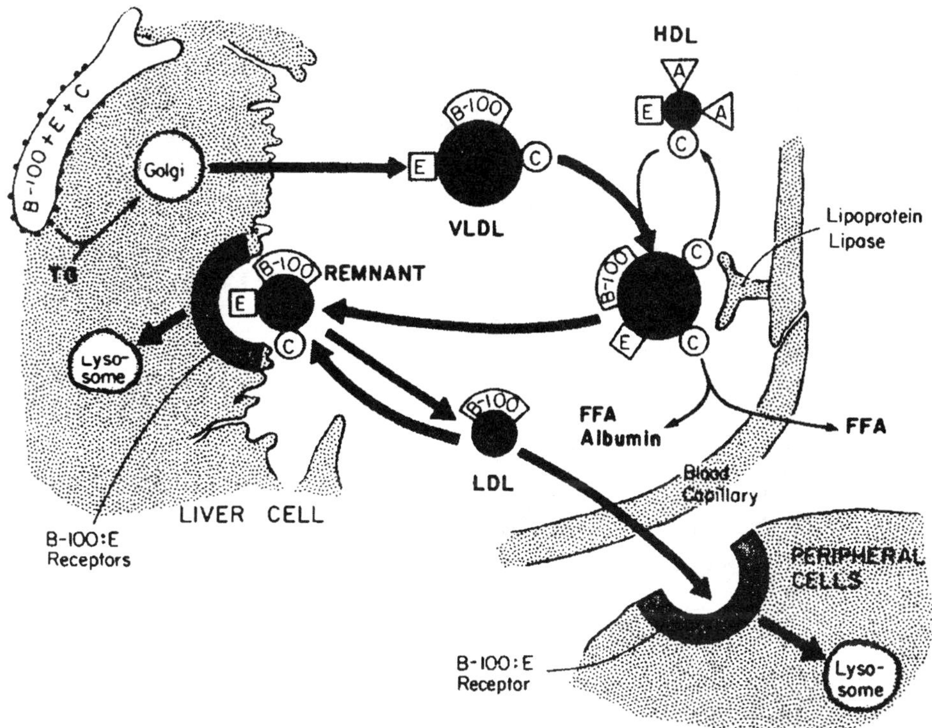

Fig. 3 The pathway of VLDL transport from the liver, shown here, resembles in several respects that of chylomicrons, but note that the protein components of newly secreted VLDL differ from those of chylomicrons. After remnants are formed in extrahepatic tissues, both VLDL and chylomicrons contain C and E apoproteins, but different B apoproteins. The B-100 protein, secreted by the liver, unlike B-48 of chylomicrons, is recognized by an hepatic lipoprotein receptor, which also recognizes apoprotein E. However, most VLDL remnants are not normally taken up by endocytosis and catabolized in the liver; rather, they are mainly catabolized further with loss of all proteins except B-100 to yield LDL. LDL is metabolized slowly by interaction with B-100, E receptors in extrahepatic tissues and liver, and also by less well-defined mechanisms. Whereas chylomicron cholesterol esters are derived mainly from the diet, the cholesterol esters of VLDL, as well as those of LDL and HDL (black areas in core of particles), are derived from the action of lecithin-cholesterol acyltransferase (see also Fig. 4). (Courtesy of R. J. Havel, *Medical Clinics of North America*, W.B. Saunders Company, Philadelphia, PA.)

VLDL and formation of VLDL remnants. Compared to chylomicrons, the slower rate of VLDL hydrolysis is perhaps a function of its smaller average particle size and diminished LPL binding. The liver takes up approximately 50–60% of VLDL remnant particles via LDL receptors that recognize apo E (10). VLDL particles vary in size with the larger particles yielding larger remnants containing more molecules of apo E as compared to the smaller particles. As a consequence, the smaller VLDL remnants have a lower affinity for hepatic LDL receptors and remain in circulation longer. These potentially more atherogenic particles (VLDL remnants and IDL) may undergo further hydrolysis, catalyzed by HTGL with apo E acting as a cofactor. The resulting LDL is a smaller, denser, cholesterol ester–rich particle that is usually devoid of all apoproteins with the exception of apo B-100. LDL particles contain about 75% of plasma cholesterol, are potentially quite atherogenic, and are normally cleared from the circulation via LDL receptors. Although LDL receptors are present in most tissue, the liver accomplishes approximately 70–80% of plasma LDL clearance. The long residence time in circulation for LDL (several days) versus VLDL (minutes to hours) is explained by the seemingly paradoxical lower affinity of LDL for the LDL receptor as compared to VLDL (10). The uptake of LDL is initiated by the monovalent binding of the LDL receptor to apo B-100, located on the surface of LDL particles. The process of endocytosis then internalizes the LDL-receptor complex. This results in the degradation of LDL by lysosomes and the release of free cholesterol. The liberated intracellular cholesterol in turn downregulates cholesterol synthesis by suppressing the activity of HMG-CoA reductase, the

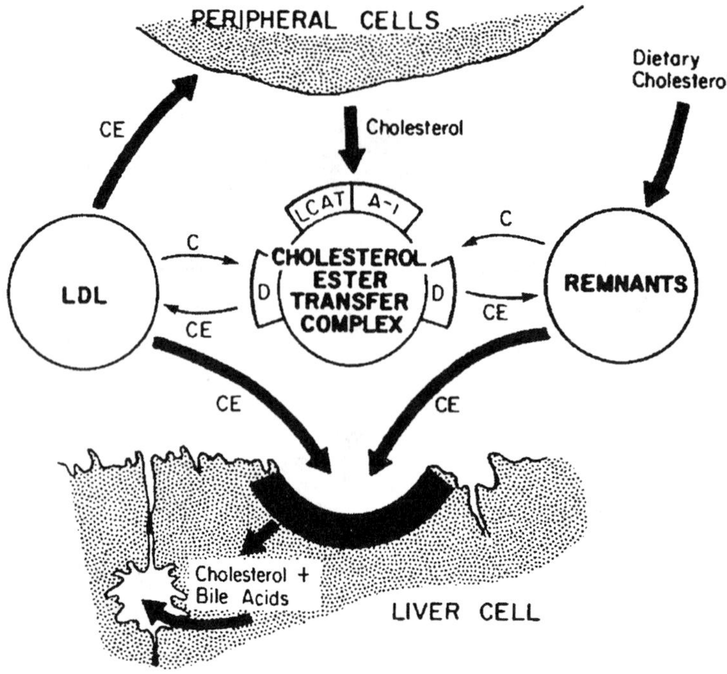

Fig. 4 This diagram depicts the current concept of the major pathway by which cholesterol in the surface coat of plasma lipoproteins and in cells is transported to the liver for excretion in the bile. The enzyme, LCAT, exists in blood plasma and probably in extravascular spaces as part of a subtraction of HDL, the cholesterol ester transfer complex, which also contains the cofactor protein for the enzyme (apoprotein A-I) and apoprotein D. The cholesterol ester-product of the transferase reaction is rapidly transferred by apoprotein D to other lipoproteins. The conversion of polar cholesterol to nonpolar cholesteryl esters creates a gradient, which permits cholesterol to be transferred continually to the complex from cells and other lipoproteins, resulting in the movement of cholesterol to cells that have active lipoprotein receptors. (Courtesy of R. J. Havel, *Medical Clinics of North America*, W.B. Saunders Company, Philadelphia, PA.)

rate-limiting enzyme in cholesterol synthesis. A second regulatory effect of intracellular cholesterol accumulation is stimulation of acyl-CoA: cholesterol acyltransferase, an enzyme that catalyzes re-esterification of cholesterol for storage purposes. A third effect is the downregulation of LDL receptor expression. Therefore, the accumulation of intracellular cholesterol inhibits both synthesis and uptake of cholesterol. This negative-feedback mechanism tightly regulates intracellular cholesterol concentration and modulates total body cholesterol metabolism through its effect on hepatocytes.

The primary mechanism for the removal of circulating lipoproteins is generally through receptor-mediated endocytosis. The most extensively studied and defined lipoprotein receptor is the LDL receptor that binds to lipoproteins containing apo B-100 (i.e., LDL) and/or apo E (i.e., VLDL, IDL, and β-migrating VLDL) (7,10,27). Recently another VLDL receptor (VLDL-R) has been described and so named based on its specific affinity for VLDL (28,29). The primary structural difference between the VLDL-R and LDL receptor is that the ligand-binding domain of the former consists of eight tandem copies of 40 cysteine-rich amino acid repeats as opposed to just 7 repeats in the latter. From a functional point, VLDL-R binds apo E-containing lipoproteins and not LDL (28,30–33). In addition to their different ligand-binding properties, the two receptors also have distinctly different tissue distributions. Thus, in contrast to the LDL receptor, which is primarily expressed in the liver, adrenal cortex, testes, and ovaries, VLDL-R is mainly expressed in skeletal muscle, heart, brain, and adipose tissue (28,33). In this regard, the tissue distribution of VLDL-R is remarkably similar to that of LPL (34). Therefore, it appears that, like LPL, VLDL-R may play an important role in the regulation of plasma VLDL and energy metabolism.

C. Reverse Cholesterol Transport

Although cholesterol may accumulate in tissue as a result of such processes as LDL cholesterol uptake and de novo synthesis, cholesterol can only be degraded and excreted by the liver. The mechanism for removal of cholesterol from cells is largely dependent on HDL, which acts as a vehicle for cholesterol transport from peripheral sites to the liver. This "reverse cholesterol transport system" appears to involve several pathways (10,23,36,37). For example, cholesterol that is taken up by HDL and esterified may be transferred to VLDL or LDL prior to its removal by the liver in a process mediated by cholesterol ester transfer protein (CETP). Alternatively, cholesterol in HDL particles may be delivered directly to the liver, where uptake may be receptor mediated (perhaps in the case of HDL particles with surface apo E), or its entry into hepatocytes may occur by some other less well-defined mechanism.

Although the origin and metabolism of HDL remain incompletely understood, it appears that its major components (apo A-I and apo A-II) are synthesized by both the liver and small intestine and are secreted into the plasma with phospholipids. This results in the formation of nascent HDL, which has a disk-like configuration. It should be noted, however, that many of the various phospholipids and apoproteins that will eventually comprise HDL are initially incorporated on the surface of chylomicrons and VLDL, only to be liberated during lipolysis and subsequently transferred to the developing nascent HDL (38,39). Free cholesterol is also initially taken up on the surface of these developing HDL particles. With the acquisition of apo A-I, nascent HDL is transformed into an ideal substrate for LCAT, an enzyme that catalyzes the esterification of cholesterol. The newly formed cholesterol esters are subsequently relocated into the HDL core, a process that transforms the particle disk like shape into a more spherical configuration. These spherical HDLs are relatively small and dense, having a low ratio of free cholesterol to phospholipid. However, after attracting and accumulating free cholesterol from cell membranes and other lipoproteins in a process catalyzed by LCAT, larger, less dense HDL_2 particles are formed. The average HDL cholesterol (HDL-C) lipid content is 32% cholesterol ester, 5% free cholesterol, 55% phospholipid, and 8% triglyceride, wherein the major apoproteins are apo A-I (70%) and apo A-II (20%) (39). However, by analytical ultracentrifugation HDL-C particles are classified into two major subtypes: the smaller, denser, cholesterol-poor HDL_3 fraction and the larger, less dense, cholesterol ester-rich HDL_2 fraction. There are also differences in apoprotein distribution between HDL subtypes, with HDL_2 generally containing only apo A-I (four apo A-I molecules per particle) and HDL_3 containing both apo A-I and A-II (two molecules of each per particle). Additionally, a third apo E–rich HDL subtype is described with a density distribution lighter than HDL_2. Although apo E–rich HDLs are thought to be important metabolically, their measurement is usually not included in HDL-C assays. HDL_2 can also be transformed to HDL_3 in a process involving the transfer of cholesterol esters to TG-rich lipoproteins such as VLDL and IDL in exchange for triglycerides (a transaction facilitated by CEPT). In a second reaction involving the hydrolysis of accumulated triglycerides (catalyzed by HTGL), HDL_2 is transformed back to HDL_3. Although plasma levels of HDL_3 and HDL_2 are in dynamic balance, normally about 60% of HDL-C are composed of HDL_3 while approximately 40% are in the HDL_2 fraction. Numerous studies have demonstrated an association between low plasma HDL-C levels and increased cardiovascular risk (40–42), with the HDL_2 fraction shown to be the better discriminator of risk (43,44). The apparent antiatherogenic properties of HDL are thought to be mediated through promotion of reverse cholesterol transport. Other proposed mechanisms include inhibition of lipoprotein peroxidation as well as inhibition of vascular smooth muscle cell proliferation (45–47). It may also be the association of low HDL-C with increased plasma levels of atherogenic TG-rich lipoprotein remnants (i.e., chylomicron remnants, VLDL remnants, and IDL) as well as small dense LDLs that confer cardiovascular risk (39,47).

In summary, the normal transport and metabolism of lipids are essential not only in providing energy for tissue such as heart and muscle but also in providing substrates necessary for the biosynthesis of cell membranes, vitamin D, steroid hormones, and bile. On the one hand, the body must be able to deliver fatty acids to tissue, such as muscle and adipose, for energy and storage purposes, and on the other hand, a mechanism must be provided where excess cholesterol can be cleared from tissue and plasma. The normal operation of the exogenous and endogenous pathways with the secretion of triglyceride-rich lipoproteins assures an ample supply of fatty acids. In addition, the secretion of VLDL provides the liver a mechanism for ridding itself of surplus triglycerides derived from lipogenesis as well as from the uptake of free fatty acids and triglyceride-rich lipoproteins. Because extrahepatic tissue cannot metabolize and excrete cholesterol, a mechanism must be provided to take up and transport excess cholesterol from these sites. A similar mechanism must also be present to take up and remove cholesterol that is released into plasma by processes such as cell membrane turnover. This is accomplished by the reverse cholesterol transport system that utilizes HDL as its principal component.

V. DISORDERS OF LIPOPROTEIN METABOLISM IN CHRONIC RENAL FAILURE

Disturbances in lipoprotein metabolism can be broadly divided into conditions that are genetic in origin versus those that are acquired (i.e., related to an underlying disease, medication, or diet). It is important, however, to consider that the clinical expression of any disease is determined by the complex interaction of environmental factors and genetic predisposition, and dyslipoproteinemia is certainly no exception to this maxim. Moreover, there now exists a large body of compelling evidence linking abnormalities in lipoprotein metabolism with atherosclerotic cardiovascular disease. For example, increased plasma concentrations of LDL, IDL, chylomicron remnants, and Lp(a) are shown to be highly atherogenic, as opposed to increased levels of HDL cholesterol, which are shown to reduce atherosclerotic risk (40,48–51).

The typical lipoprotein abnormalities associated with chronic renal failure (CRF) are shown in Table 3 (1–4). These include hypertriglyceridemia with associated elevations in VLDL, IDL, and chylomicron remnants. Both the prevalence and severity of hypertriglyceridemia directly correlate with the severity of CRF (2,17,18,52). Mild hypertriglyceridemia may be present in approximately 30% of patients with glomerular filtration rates (GFR) between 15 and 30 mL/min, whereas up to 60–80% of patients with advanced renal insufficiency demonstrate moderate HTG. Increased plasma levels of remnants of large TG-rich lipoproteins also occurs in CRF as evidenced by the frequent presence of fasting chylomicronemia as well as by the presence of slow-migrating VLDL particles (termed β-VLDL), which closely resemble particles observed in type III hyperlipidemia or broad beta disease (53–56). Furthermore, recent studies using sophisticated methodologies designed to detect remnant lipoproteins have demonstrated 2- to 10-fold increases in plasma IDL levels (57). Additionally, the magnitude of IDL elevation was shown to be proportional to elevations in plasma TG. Using plasma vitamin A ester levels as a marker, significant elevations in plasma chylomicron remnants have also been recently reported in CRF patients (54).

In CRF, total plasma cholesterol levels are generally normal but may be mildly elevated in up to 25% of patients (2). Similar to total cholesterol, LDL-C levels are also typically normal but may be elevated in a small percentage of patients, whereas HDL-C levels are usually decreased (2,17,18,56–59). In general, elevations in plasma cholesterol are directly correlated with elevations in LDL-C, VLDL-C, TG, and apoproteins B, C-II, and C-III (2,3,18,56). Elevated TG levels in CRF patients are also shown to positively correlate with plasma levels of VLDL-C and apoproteins B, C-II, and C-III but not with LDL-C. Furthermore, TG levels negatively correlate with plasma levels of HDL and apo A-I (2,3,4,18,56–60). In addition, significantly increased plasma Lp(a) levels are described in patients with end-stage renal disease (ESRD) (61–65).

Substantial changes in plasma levels of apoproteins as well as significant alterations in their distribution between the major plasma lipoprotein classes occur in CRF (Table 4) (1–4,66–69). The most predominant abnormality is an increase in apo C-III, which occurs relatively early in CRF (in both hypertriglyceridemic and

Table 3 Characteristic Changes in Plasma Lipid and Lipoprotein Values in CRF

Triglycerides usually increased
Total cholesterol usually normal
Free fatty acids usually normal
Fasting chylomicronemia often present
VLDL-C usually increased
VLDL remnants and IDL-C usually increased
LDL-C usually normal
Small dense LDL particles usually increased
HDL-C cholesterol usually decreased
Lp(a) usually increased

Table 4 Characteristic Changes in Plasma Apoprotein Values in CRF

Apo A-I usually decreased
Apo A-II usually decreased
Apo A-IV increased
Apo B may be normal or increased[a]
Apo C-I may be normal or increased[a]
Apo C-II may be normal or increased[a]
Apo C-III increased
Apo E usually normal
Apo A-I/Apo C-III reduced
Apo C-II/Apo C-III reduced
Apo C-III/Apo E increased

[a]Increased values are reported in hypertriglyceridemic subgroups.

normotriglyceridemic patients). Significant reductions in plasma apo A-I and apo A-II levels are also described in CRF (18,56,66,67). Furthermore, the magnitude of increase in apo C-III as well as the decreases in apo A-I and A-II directly correlate with the severity of renal insufficiency, while the decreases in apo A-I and A-II also parallel reductions in HDL. Abnormalities involving plasma apoproteins C-I, C-II, B, and E are less certain in CRF as some studies report moderate increases in apoproteins B, C-I, and C-II (18,56), whereas others have failed to demonstrate significant changes in these apoproteins (64,69). The presence or absence of hypertriglyceridemia may be important as significant increases in apoproteins B, C-I, and C-II have been recently reported in hypertriglyceridemic patients as opposed to normotriglyceridemic patients with CRF (56). With regard to Apo-E, most studies have not shown significant changes in plasma levels with CRF (56,66,68,69). However, apo-E levels are generally considered to be inappropriately low for the degree of plasma TG increase in CRF.

Abnormalities involving apoprotein distribution and concentration in the major plasma lipoprotein classes (VLDL, IDL, LDL and HDL) also occur in CRF (1–4,56,66,70). In VLDL, increases in apoproteins B, C-I, C-II, C-III, and E are reported, however, these increases are shown to be much greater in hypertriglyceridemic patients as opposed to normotriglyceridemic patients (56). In IDL, significant increases in apoproteins B, C-I, C-II, C-III, and E are reported, and in LDL, increases in apoproteins C-I, C-II, and C-III are reported. Finally, in HDL, significant decreases in apoproteins A-I, A-II, C-I, and C-II are reported along with an increase in apo B.

The compositional abnormalities in lipoproteins associated with CRF affect all plasma lipoprotein classes (Table 5) (1–4,17,18,56,57,66–73). The major lipoproteins (VLDL, IDL, LDL, and HDL) are substantially enriched in TG. Cholesterol content is also increased in VLDL and IDL, essentially unchanged in LDL, and decreased in HDL. Furthermore, there is an associated shift in the distribution of apoproteins B, C, and E between HDL and other major lipoproteins (VLDL, IDL, and LDL); where VLDL is enriched in apo C-III, IDL is especially enriched in apoproteins B, C, and E, LDL is enriched in apo C-peptides, and HDL is deplete in apo C-peptides and apo E. The increased total apo C-III plasma level in CRF is, therefore, mainly reflective of increased apo C-III in VLDL, IDL, and LDL. Moreover, the disproportionately greater increases of apo C-III compared to apoproteins B, C-II, and E account for the reduced apo C-II:apo C-III and increased apo C-III:apo E ratios characteristic of CRF. In addition, the combination of increased apo C-III in B-lipoproteins (VLDL, IDL, and LDL) and decreased apo A-I in non-B lipoproteins (HDL_2 and HDL_3) account for the reduced apo A-I:apo C-III ratio that is considered to be an early and perhaps the most reliable marker for dyslipoproteinemia in CRF.

Table 5 Changes in Apoprotein Content of Plasma Lipoproteins in CRF Prior to the Institution of Dialysis

	VLDL	IDL	LDL	HDL
TG	↑*	↑*	↑*	↑
Cholesterol	↑*	↑**	↔	↓**
Apo A-I	↔	↑	↓	↓**
Apo A-II	↓	↑	↓**	↓**
Apo B	↑*	↑**	↑	↑**
Apo C-I	↑*	↑**	↑*	↓**
Apo C-II	↑*	↑**	↑**	↓**
Apo C-III	↑*	↑**	↑**	↓
Apo E	↑*	↑**	↔	↓*

(↔), Essentially no change as compared to healthy controls; (↑), increased value not statistically significant; (↑*) statistically significant only in hypertriglyceridemic CRF patients compared to controls; (↑**) statistically significant in both normotriglyceridemic and hypertriglyceridemic CRF patients compared to controls.

VI. TRIGLYCERIDE METABOLISM IN CRF

In the pathogenesis of dyslipoproteinemia, the plasma concentration of a given lipoprotein is a function of both its synthesis and catabolism. With regard to hypertriglyceridemia, most reports have shown that the metabolism and plasma clearance of TG-rich lipoproteins (i.e.,VLDL, IDL, and chylomicron remnants) are reduced in CRF (Table 6) (1–4,17,18,52–60,66–75). There is also considerable evidence that the activities of both lipoprotein lipase (LPL) and hepatic triglyceride lipase (HTGL) are substantially reduced in CRF (76–88). This appears to be the major mechanism for hypertriglyceridemia in ESRD, because the hydrolysis of TG-rich lipoproteins depends on the normal function of these enzymes.

A. Decreased Activity of Lipoprotein Lipase

With regard to LPL, there appear to be a number of factors associated with CRF that impair its activity. First of all, insulin resistance that is characteristically present in CRF may play a role because insulin is

Table 6 Summary of Abnormalities involving the Metabolism of TG-Rich Lipoproteins in CRF

Decreased Triglyceride Catabolism
↓LPL activity
Insulin resistance
Heparin-related
Related to alterations in lipoprotein composition
Circulating inhibitors
Hyperparathyroidism/Increased cytosolic calcium/ abnormal gene expression
↓HTGL activity
Hyperparathyroidism/Increased cytosolic calcium/ abnormal gene expression
↓LCAT activity
apo A-I deficiency
Decreased Uptake of TG-Rich Lipoproteins
Abnormal lipid content (TG enrichment)
Abnormal apoprotein content (especially increases in apo C-III)
Modifications related to oxidation, glycation, and carbamalation
Diminished receptor function
Increased TG Production
Hyperinsulinemia
Increased carbohydrate ingestion or uptake from dialysate in PD

known to enhance LPL activity (1,2,80,89). In addition, in uremic animal models insulin administration has been shown to increase LPL activity (89). A second putative mechanism involves heparin, which is known to stimulate both LPL and HTGL (77,78). It is postulated that these enzymes are depleted as the result of chronic heparin administration during hemodialysis. Support for this concept comes from studies that have shown significant reductions in serum lipids (both triglycerides and cholesterol) in hemodialysis patients, where low molecular weight heparin (which has little effect on LPL and HTGL) was substituted for conventional heparin (90,91). A third potential mechanism for LPL dysfunction in CRF involves alterations in lipoprotein composition. With regard to VLDL and IDL, apo C-III content is increased disproportionately to that of apo C-II. Because apo C-III inhibits LPL-catalyzed lipolysis, its increased content in VLDL and IDL may contribute to impaired metabolism of these lipoproteins in CRF (18,69,73,92). In addition, increased sialylation of apo C-III is described in CRF, and this alteration is also reported to render TG-rich lipoproteins resistant to LPL-mediated catabolism (93). A fourth area of consideration involves the presence of one or more circulating inhibitors of LPL activity that are not effectively removed by dialysis. Recently, investigators have described a specific plasma inhibitor of LPL: an apo A-I–containing particle of pre-β-electrophoretic mobility residing in the lipoprotein-free fraction of plasma (86). This pre-β-HDL particle (containing free apo A-I and 3% phospholipid) appears to be an important inhibitor of LPL in both uremic and nonuremic subjects. Although plasma concentrations of total apo A-I are reduced in CRF, free apo A-I is increased compared to normal controls (94,95). Furthermore, the increase in free apo A-I appears to be a direct result of renal insufficiency because catabolism of pre-β-HDL (free apo A-I) takes place predominantly in the kidneys (96).

A final area of consideration involves abnormalities in LPL gene expression. Studies in uremic animals have shown reductions in LPL activity, as well as downregulation in LPL mRNA in association with secondary hyperparathyroidism (97,98). Moreover, these abnormalities in LPL gene expression and activity were corrected by parathyroidectomy. In humans with ESRD a positive correlation is also demonstrated between secondary hyperparathyroidism and hypertriglyceridemia (82). Furthermore, parathyroidectomy is shown to reduce plasma TG levels in experimental animals as well as humans (98–102). Although the putative mechanism by which PTH inhibits LPL activity is thought to involve PTH-mediated insulin resistance (82,88), there is other evidence indicating that excess PTH downregulates LPL gene expression. In support of this latter concept, our laboratory has shown significant reductions in LPL activity in heart, skeletal muscle and adipose tissue in rats with CRF. This was also accompanied by parallel reductions in LPL mRNA and LPL protein mass (97,98). Furthermore, the downregulation of LPL gene expression, protein mass, and activity was reversed by parathyroid ablation. This effect of PTH on LPL expression may be mediated through increases in cytosolic calcium. In summary, the reduced LPL activity observed in CRF may be the result of a combination of abnormalities including insulin resistance, heparin-related LPL depletion, altered lipoprotein composition, the presence of circulating inhibitors, as well as downregulation of LPL expression.

B. Decreased Activity of Hepatic Triglyceride Lipase

Although our understanding of the relationship between CRF and imparied HTGL activity is far from complete, decreased activity of HTGL along with downregulation of HTGL gene expression are also described in patients with CRF in association with secondary hyperparathyroidism. Moreover, these abnormalities are either ameliorated or corrected following parathyroidectomy. In addition there is evidence indicating that impaired HTGL activity in CRF may also be mediated by PTH-induced increases in cytosolic calcium (87,102). However, the fact that restoration of normal tissue expression of both LPL and HTGL (by parathyroid ablation) is accompanied by only partial correction of HTG in CRF indicates the existence of additional mechanisms (87,98).

C. Additional Abnormalities in TG Metabolism

In addition to the impairments in LPL and HGTL activity, other abnormalities involving TG metabolism are described in CRF. These include decreased activity of lecithin cholesterol acyltransferase (LCAT) (75,103,104), alterations in lipoprotein composition that may impair receptor uptake (54,56,58,105–108), and possible downregulation in VLDL receptor expression (109). There is also evidence that increased TG production may contribute to hypertriglyceridemia in a subset of patients with ESRD (74). LCAT is closely associated with HDL and is activated by apo A-I. Because LCAT catalyzes esterification of free cholesterol released during catabolism of TG-rich lipoproteins, impairment of LCAT activity could impede both TG catabolism and HDL anabolism and, moreover, cause alterations in HDL composition. A number of studies demonstrate decreased LCAT activity in CRF, which may be related to reduced levels of apo A-I in HDL (7,103,104).

Abnormalities in lipoprotein composition that may impair catabolism, uptake, and plasma clearance in CRF include an increase in apo C-III relative to apo C-II and apo E as well as a disproportional increase in TG content relative to cholesterol. In addition to functioning as an inhibitor of LPL activity, a high apo C-III content may impair catabolism and receptor uptake, while a relative decrease in apo C-II content (relative to C-III) would also function to inhibit LPL. Also, a high apo C-III content relative to E may diminish receptor affinity and, therefore, decrease or delay clearance of TG-rich remnants. Furthermore, the high TG content of VLDL, IDL, and LDL is reported to impair catabolism and clearance of these particles in CRF (54,56,58).

Our laboratory has provided evidence that VLDL-R expression may be reduced in CRF (109,110). Using a rat model, we were able to demonstrate a fourfold reduction in heart and skeletal muscle VLDL-R mRNA and protein mass following 5/6 nephrectomy. This was associated with a fivefold increase in plasma TG concentration. Moreover, the VLDL-R mRNA levels were directly related to creatinine clearance and inversely related to serum TG and VLDL concentrations. It remains to be determined whether downregulation of VLDL-R also contributes to hypertriglyceridemia in humans with ESRD. Recently, a severe defect in chylomicron remnant uptake has also been described in dialysis patients (54). Whether or not this defect involves receptor dysfunction as opposed to an abnormality in lipoprotein composition remains unknown.

To what extent increased TG production contributes to hypertriglyceridemia in CRF remains controversial. Categorically, patients with ESRD have been shown to have defective TG catabolism irrespective of TG plasma levels. However, subsets of ESRD patients with hypertriglyceridemia are shown to have higher rates of TG production than CRF patients with normal plasma TG levels (74). Certainly in the presence of impaired TG catabolism, even a modest increase in production could result in substantial elevations in plasma levels. Some investigators have shown a correlation between insulin resistance, hyperinsulinemia, and increased hepatic TG production in ESRD (111,112). Other factors that may stimulate TG production in CRF include increased fatty acid availability due to altered protein binding, carnitine deficiency, hyperglucagonemia, high glucose or acetate loads related to dialysis, as well as diets high in refined sugars.

VIII. CHOLESTEROL METABOLISM IN CRF

The typical plasma cholesterol profile observed in CRF shows normal to slightly elevated levels in LDL and total cholesterol, whereas HDL is generally decreased with greater reductions in HDL_2 compared to HDL_3 (1–4,70). More important, however, are qualitative changes in HDL that to a large extent are the consequence of impaired VLDL and chylomicron metabolism along with defective transfer of lipids and apoproteins between the large TG-rich particles undergoing breakdown and nascent HDL undergoing formation. This results in both quantitative and qualitative alterations in HDL, which in turn adversely affects overall cholesterol metabolism. In this respect abnormalities in

TG and cholesterol metabolism in CRF are closely linked. Furthermore, as a consequence of diminished LCAT activity, the rate of cholesterol esterification is substantially reduced. This, coupled with the accompanying defect in CETP, is the apparent mechanism responsible for the observed defects in cholesterol ester and apoprotein transfer between HDL and other lipoproteins (i.e., VLDL and IDL). These abnormalities may explain certain observed lipoprotein compositional changes in CRF, including the increased TG content of VLDL, IDL, LDL, and HDL, the abnormal shift in distribution of apoproteins C and E from HDL to VLDL and IDL, and the reduction of apo A-I and A-II content in HDL (18,56,59,66,71). Furthermore, the low apo A-I content in HDL is thought to contribute to impaired conversion of HDL_3 to HDL_2. Thus the combination of impaired synthesis of HDL_3 (the precursor of HDL_2) coupled with reduced conversion (HDL_3 to HDL_2) are the putative mechanisms responsible for the disproportionately low plasma HDL_2 levels described in CRF. Moreover, the resulting reduction in plasma HDL concentration (in particular HDL_2) in combination with the noted compositional changes in HDL (i.e., decreased apo A-I and increased TG content) may cause substantial impairment in reverse cholesterol transport and further predispose CRF patients to atherosclerosis.

A reduction in the plasma clearance of LDL has been reported in CRF that appears to be proportional to the severity of the renal insufficiency (56–58,60,69,75). This may be related to alterations in LDL composition, including an increased content in apo C-III, apo E, and TG that interfere with receptor uptake. There is also evidence that LDL receptor uptake may be impaired through the process of uremic-related carbamalation that chemically alters apo B-100 (105,113). An additional consideration involves alterations in the LDL apo B/E receptor per se, as a recent study has demonstrated decreased LDL-receptor function and mRNA expression in lymphocytes isolated from uremic patients (114). It is therefore possible that a decrease in LDL receptor expression (related to either a transcriptional defect or a defect in LDL receptor mRNA stability) may also contribute to reduce LDL clearance in CRF.

A. Lp(a) Metabolism in CRF

Over the past decade there have been numerous studies showing significant elevations in plasma Lp(a) levels in ESRD patients compared to controls (62–64,115). In general, Lp(a) plasma levels are shown to be controlled by the apoprotein (a) [apo(a)] gene locus on chromosome 6q2.6-q2.7 (61,116). This gene is highly polymorphic, with over 30 known alleles, and there is an inverse relationship between the molecular weight of the corresponding apo(a) isoform and Lp(a) plasma levels. That is, patients with genetically determined low molecular weight (LMW) isoforms of apo(a) have high average Lp(a) plasma levels, whereas patients with high molecular weight (HMW) apo(a) isoforms have low plasma levels of Lp(a). In CRF, however, Lp(a) levels are shown to be elevated regardless of apo(a) phenotype. Therefore, in ESRD the elevated plasma Lp(a) levels appear to be a function of renal insufficiency per se, rather than genetic factors. The fact that Lp(a) levels normalize following successful kidney transplantation in patients having HMW apo(a) phenotypes further substantiates this conclusion (117–121). By what mechanism renal failure causes the observed elevations in plasma Lp(a) remains uncertain. It has been proposed that uremic toxins might either promote increased hepatic synthesis of Lp(a) or impair its catabolism and removal from the circulation (61,63). Furthermore, Lp(a) can act as an acute phase reactant, and its levels may increase in response to proinflammatory cytokine stimulation (122). It is also possible that diseased kidneys produce a factor that directly or indirectly promotes hepatic Lp(a) synthesis. This latter concept is supported by one study demonstrating lower Lp(a) levels in nephrectomized dialysis patients (118). Conversely, other data have provided evidence suggesting direct renal involvement in the uptake and catabolism of Lp(a) in that definite reductions in its plasma concentration have been observed between the arteria and vena renalis in humans (61). Furthermore, various renal cell types express the LDL receptor–related protein, which is thought to be involved in the uptake and catabolism of Lp(a) (123,124). However, careful turnover studies will be required to determine more conclusively the relative roles of increased synthesis verses impaired catabolism of Lp(a) in the CRF setting.

Lp(a) has been shown to be an independent risk factor for atherosclerotic cardiovascular disease in both the general population and in patients with ESRD (125–133). Even though the elevated plasma Lp(a) levels in CRF patients may be nongenetic in origin, the genetically determined apo(a) phenotype is shown to be an even better predictor of atherosclerotic severity than Lp(a) plasma levels per se (61). That is, cohorts of ESRD patients with LMW apo(a) isoforms are shown to have more severe atherosclerotic disease compared to cohorts with HMW apo(a) phenotypes.

This is explained on the basis of the duration of Lp(a) elevation, in that patients with LMW apo(a) isoforms presumably have had high Lp(a) levels their entire life, whereas patients with HMW apo(a) isoforms have had elevated Lp(a) levels for only the duration of their renal failure.

IX. MECHANISMS FOR DYSLIPOPROTEINEMIA IN CRF

There are potentially a multiplicity of factors in CRF that may act either independently or in combination with other conditions to adversely affect lipoprotein metabolism. These include hormonal alterations, retained substances/toxins, altered gene expression, altered lipoprotein composition and structure, enzyme and cofactor dysfunction or deficiency, receptor dysfunction, and iatrogenic effects.

A. Hormonal

The hormonal abnormalities associated with CRF that most likely play a causal role with regard to dyslipoproteinemia are secondary hyperparathyroidism and insulin resistance. There is considerable evidence that parathyroid hormone (PTH) excess contributes to hypertriglyceridemia through its putative inhibitory effect on LPL and HTGT activity (82,87,88,97,98,102). Insulin resistance associated with CRF may also be a mechanism for decreased LPL activity (74,79,80). It is further suggested that the inhibitory effect of PTH on LPL may be mediated through a mechanism involving PTH-induced insulin resistance. In addition, there is evidence that the inhibitory effect of PTH on LPL and HTGL may be mediated through downregulation of their gene expression (97,98). Elevated levels of growth hormone are described in CRF and may also contribute to insulin resistance and hypertriglyceridemia (134). A final area of consideration with respect to hormonal abnormalities relates to the low estrogen levels in women reported in CRF (135–138). In postmenopausal women, lack of estrogen is associated with increased cardiovascular risk while estrogen replacement is shown to reduce the risk (51,139). Furthermore, the reduced cardiovascular risk of estrogen replacement is largely attributed to favorable changes in plasma lipoproteins, including reductions in LDL-C, Lp(a), and small, dense LDL, along with increases in HDL-C. It is, therefore, possible that estrogen depletion contributes to dyslipoproteinemia and cardiovascular risk in women with CRF.

B. Retained Substances of Toxins

A causal role for retained poorly dialyzable substances in the pathogenesis of hyperlipidemia needs to be better defined. To date there is good evidence for only one such substance—the recently described pre-β-HDL particle containing apo A-I and phospholipid, which appears to be an important inhibitor of LPL activity (86). It is also possible that renal insufficiency per se contributes to dyslipoproteinemia through a reduction in the metabolism of specific lipoproteins. Such a mechanism could be responsible for Lp(a) accumulation in ESRD.

C. Altered Gene Expression

An area of considerable interest involves the effect of renal failure on gene expression. There is currently a growing body of evidence that gene expression of a number of proteins may be downregulated in association with renal insufficiency. Specifically, the downregulation of LPL mRNA, HTGL mRNA, LDL-R mRNA, and VLDL-R mRNA has been described in various models of ESRD (experimental and clinical), which may have relevance in the pathogenesis of dyslipoproteinemia (87,88,97,98,114,140).

D. Compositional and Structural Abnormalities

Another area of importance involves various alterations in lipoprotein composition and structure that occur in association with CRF. Such modifications may impair not only specific lipoprotein functions, but also their catabolism, uptake, and plasma clearance (56–60). Examples of this include the increased apo C-III content in VLDL and IDL as well as the increased apo C-III, Apo E, and TG content in LDL. Furthermore, increased TG content in certain lipoproteins (e.g., LDL) may increase susceptibility to oxidation (141). Moreover, compositional changes in HDL (i.e., reduction in apo A-I) could severely impair its function and thereby impede the peripheral mobilization and transport of cholesterol (18,56,59).

Increased rates of certain specific chemical reactions occur in CRF such as carbamalation, (105,113), glycation (142), and oxidation (143–148), which may further alter lipoprotein structure. Carbamalation is a process by which isocyanic acid, derived from urea, reacts with an amino or sulfahydryl group of a macromolecule (i.e., lipoprotein), whereas glycation involves the formation of advanced glycated end products from covalent nonenzymatic interactions between aldose sugars and proteins or lipoproteins such as LDL. Both carbamalated and glycated LDLs are readily taken up by macrophages via the scavenger receptor pathway, a process linked to the formation of lipid-laden foam cells and progressive atherosclerosis (105,142,149–151). Chemical modifications, therefore, may greatly augment the atherogenic properties of lipoproteins; the best example of this is peroxidation, which will be subsequently discussed in more detail.

E. Abnormalities in Carnitine Metabolism

There is some evidence supporting a relationship between carnitine anomalies and dyslipoproteinemia in CRF (152–156). L-Carnitine is a quaternary amine that plays an important role in fatty acid metabolism and is required for the transport of long-chain fatty acids from the cytoplasm into the mitochondria, the site of oxidation. Patients on hemodialysis may become deficient in free carnitine due to dialytic losses, and it is proposed that such a deficiency could result in an increase in TG synthesis arising from the increased availability of free fatty acids. Furthermore, impaired fatty acid oxidation could result in production of large amounts of incompletely metabolized acyl moieties that are normally conjugated with free carnitine, forming acyl-carnitine. Most studies, however, have shown that total plasma carnitine levels are elevated in CRF patients not receiving dialysis (157,158). In hemodialysis patients, free carnitine levels are typically low, whereas acyl carnitine levels are generally elevated (158–160). Conversely, patients receiving peritoneal dialysis have normal total and free carnitine levels in conjunction with elevated acyl carnitine levels (161,162). To what extent these abnormalities in carnitine metabolism contribute to or affect dyslipoproteinemia in ESRD remains to be determined. To date, studies evaluating the effects of carnitine supplementation on lipid metabolism in CRF have shown inconsistent results.

F. Iatrogenic Causes

Iatrogenic causes of dyslipoproteinemia in the setting of ESRD also need consideration. The use of medications such as thiazide diuretics and beta-blockers can increase TG. The administration of heparin during hemodialysis has also been associated with abnormalities in TG metabolism (81,90). The dialysis procedure, particularly hemodialysis, may further modify lipoproteins through the stimulation of cytokines and reactive oxygen metabolites (163–170). There is considerable evidence that exposure of blood to artificial membranes of low biocompatibility (i.e., cellulosic membranes) may trigger the production of reactive oxygen species through complement activation and/or by a direct phagocyte–artificial membrane interaction. It is also possible that dialysate solution contaminants such as bacterial lipopolysaccharides (which are small enough to pass through artificial membranes and enter the circulation) further stimulate cytokine production and phagocyte oxidative metabolism (165–167). The subsequent release of reactive oxygen species (ROS) may cause lipid peroxidation resulting in lipoprotein damage. Furthermore, generated lipid peroxides can function like hydroxyl radicals causing a vicious cycle of oxidative injury and ROS production (168). In a recent study using a monoclonal antibody assay, oxidatively modified LDL was increased more than eightfold in chronic hemodialysis patients compared to normal controls (146). In addition, chronic hemodialysis patients have been shown to develop autoantibodies against oxidized LDL (ox-LDL), a process that may further contribute to vascular injury and atherosclerosis (147).

X. LIPOPROTEINS AND OXIDATIVE STRESS IN CRF

CRF, irrespective of dialysis, may also represent a state of increased oxidative stress or redox imbalance. This is evidenced by an increase (in plasma) in a number of products of lipid peroxidation that include malondialdehyde (MDA), conjugated dienes, oxidatively modified VLDL (ox-VLDL), and ox-LDL (168–170). Also, the demonstration of elevated levels of oxidized proteins such as albumin as well as the presence of increased amounts of oxidized ascorbic acid and glutathione provide additional evidence that uremia represents a condition of increased oxidative stress (171–175). Endogenous oxidant activity may be increased in uremia as a consequence of the altered metabolism and metabolic acidosis inherent in this condition. Furthermore, recent studies have reported an increased susceptibility of LDL to oxidation (141,143–147). This may be related to a reduction in vitamin E antioxidant activity in LDL and/or to its increased triglyceride content. Another lipoprotein very susceptible to oxidation is Lp(a) (65). Because the oxidation of lipoproteins generate additional ROS that begets more oxidation, this type of process may substantially contribute to the oxidative stress associated with CRF.

Two additional factors in CRF that may potentiate vascular injury and contribute to oxidative stress are the accelerated accumulation of advanced glycated end products (AGEs) and the presence of hyperhomocysteinemia (142,150,151,177–181). An accelerated accumulation of AGEs has been shown to occur in CRF, possibly as a consequence of increased oxidative stress (150,178). Furthermore, these products are not effectively removed by conventional hemodialysis and they rapidly reaccumulate in plasma even following high-flux dialysis (142). AGEs in turn may cause or contribute to vascular injury and atherosclerosis largely through their interaction with AGE-specific receptors on endothelial cells and macrophages (151,182). This interaction induces the synthesis and release of various cytokines and growth factors, which in turn may cause vascular injury through the initiation of a series of deleterious effects including increased vascular permeability, thrombogenesis, cellular proliferation, and matrix production.

Homocysteine, an atherothrombotic sulfur-containing amino acid, is shown to be an independent risk factor for cardiovascular disease (183–187). The high prevalence of hyperhomocysteinemia reported in ESRD is attributed to a marked reduction in renal uptake and clearance of total homocysteine (180,181). Hyperhomocysteinemia-induced vascular injury may be related to the ability of this amino acid to enhance LDL auto-oxidation (188). Another potential mechanism for vascular injury involves the ability of homocysteine to enhance binding of Lp(a) to fibrin, which increases the antifibrinolytic activity of Lp(a) and promotes thrombosis (189). Furthermore, either oxidative stress or other factors associated with CRF may enhance oxidation of homocysteine further increasing its atherogenic potential (148,190).

Compounding the problem of increased oxidative stress is the growing body of evidence that various endogenous antioxidant protective mechanisms are diminished in CRF (143,176,178). These include decreased activity of glutathione-dependent enzymes (i.e., glutathione 5-transferase, glutathione reductase and glutathione peroxidase) (174,175), decreased activity of superoxide dismutase (SOD) (192), as well as reduced levels and/or impaired function of vitamin E (143,193). The reduction in cytoplasmic SOD activity has been correlated with zinc deficiency, whereas the diminished activity of glutathione peroxidase may be related to selenium deficiency (194). ESRD, therefore, is a condition of increased oxidative stress resulting from the combination of increased generation of ROS coupled with defective and/or deficient antioxidant mechanisms. It is also possible that dialysis per se contributes to this dysequilibrium through previously discussed mechanisms.

XI. CONSEQUENCES OF DYSLIPOPROTEINEMIA IN CRF: CARDIOVASCULAR RISKS

Cardiovascular disease is the single greatest cause of mortality in both the general population and in ESRD, but both its prevalence and related mortality are significantly higher in ESRD patients (195–198). The most recent data (published by the USRDS and the EDTA) have shown that over the past several decades, death from myocardial infarction, congestive heart failure, and stroke accounted for over 50% of all mortality in ESRD. Furthermore, the incidence of cardiac death in dialysis patients was increased by a factor of 5–20 over the general population.

It is assumed that risk factors for cardiovascular disease in the general population are equally applicable in CRF patients. These include demographic factors such as age, gender, and race; clinical factors such as hypertension, left ventricular hypertrophy, diabetes mellitus, and smoking; biochemical determinants such as plasma lipoprotein levels, homocysteine levels, and fibrinogen levels; as well as a family history for premature cardiovascular disease (40,48,49,51,199). The lipoprotein abnormalities associated with CRF that may increase cardiovascular risk include hypertriglyceridemia decreased levels of HDL and apo A-1 levels, as well as increased levels of Lp(a), IDL, LDL, and chylomicron remnants (3,65,71,148,202). Furthermore, alterations in lipoprotein composition (i.e., increased apo C-III and TG content in VLDL, IDL, and chylomicron remnants, as well as decreased apo A-I content in HDL) may also increase risk for cardiovascular disease in CRF. In fact, there is a large body of literature suggesting that the increased frequency of atherosclerotic cardiovascular disease in CRF is primarily a consequence of the associated high prevalence of dyslipoproteinemia and hypertension (4,65,111,203–218). It should, however, be noted that additional proatherogenic factors associated with CRF may also contribute to cardiovascular risk. These include hyperhomocysteinemia, insulin resistance, the effects of proinflammatory cytokines, as well as the effects of carbamalation, glycation, and especially oxidation on circulating macromolecules and vascular tissue (148,202).

Lipid is a fundamental component of atherosclerotic plaques, and abnormalities in lipoprotein metabolism appear to play an important role in the pathogenesis of atherosclerosis. Moreover, the leading theory regarding the pathogenesis of atherosclerosis involves lipoprotein oxidative modification and the response-to-injury-hypothesis (208–210). Accordingly, circulating lipoproteins such as LDL enter the vascular subendothelial space and are taken up by macrophages. This process may result in the formation of lipid-laden foam cells, especially if uptake is accelerated. Moreover, the subsequent trapping of foam cells in the vascular intima results in formation of fatty streaks, which represent early lesions of atherosclerosis. There is now substantial evidence that oxidation also plays a critical role in the pathogenesis and acceleration of atherosclerotic disease (148,208–211). Lipoproteins such as LDL appear to undergo oxidative modification in the process of being transported from the circulation into the subendothelial space through interaction with endothelial cells. Further oxidative modification may occur through contact with resident macrophages and/or smooth muscle cells. According to the oxidative modification hypothesis, LDL is only minimally oxidized by endothelial cell contact (148,207–214). This minimally oxidized or modified LDL (mm-LDL) then acts as a direct chemoattractant for circulating monocytes and also induces vascular endothelial cells to produce monocyte chemotactic protein 1 (MCP-1) as well as granulocyte and macrophage colony-stimulating factors (215,216–222). This further stimulates monocyte recruitment and differentiation, and the ensuing accumulation of macrophages causes more extensive peroxidation of LDL (218,220). The more extensively oxidized LDLs are readily taken up by macrophages via scavenger receptors, whereas mm-LDLs are taken up by (apo) B/E–dependent LDL receptors (149,221,223). This is very significant, because in contrast to LDL receptor uptake, the uptake of ox-LDL by the scavenger-receptor pathway occurs at a more rapid rate and is not subject to negative-feedback control. Scavenger uptake of ox-LDL, therefore, is much more likely to result in massive accumulation of ox-lipoproteins with subsequent formation of foam cells. It is noteworthy that macrophages in tissue culture cannot be converted to foam cells by incubation with even very high concentrations of unoxidized LDL (224). Furthermore, cell-induced oxidative modification of LDL (in vitro) is inhibited by the addition of plasma (149). This indicates not only that normal plasma has antioxidant properties but also that oxidation in vitro for the most part must take place in a microenvironment, such as the vascular intima that is relatively shielded from naturally occurring antioxidants. In CRF, the possibility that plasma is diminished in antioxidant capability is further suggested by the increased levels of oxidatively modified lipoproteins (143,147,225).

In addition to its chemotactic properties, ox-LDL also inhibits macrophage motility, which functions to trap these developing foam cells in the arterial wall (217). Moderately oxidized lipoproteins can also stimulate the synthesis and secretion of various cytokines, (IL-1 and TNF-α), as well as growth factors (PDGF, FGF, and TGFβ) (226–228). In addition they can induce the expression of adhesion molecules such as VCAM-1 and ICAM-1 (229,230). In contrast, more extensively oxidized lipoproteins can be cytotoxic to macrophages and resident vascular cells (231–233). As a consequence of exposure to oxidized lipoproteins, activated cells (macrophages) may release a number of growth factors as well as various toxic substances such as peroxides and superoxide anions that can injure vascular tissue. In addition, cytolysis of lipid-laden cells (macrophages and vascular smooth muscle cells) causes the release of various proteolytic enzymes, oxidized lipids, as well as other reactive oxidants into the vascular wall. This results in further injury with denudation of endothelium, exposure of collagen, and platelet adherence/aggregation, which brings into play a host of additional mitogenic, vasoactive, thrombogenic, and inflammatory factors that greatly accelerate atherosclerotic injury through repeated cycles of inflammation, injury, and fibrosis (148,209,212).

It is also important to consider that oxidative modification may alter the antigenicity of macromolecules (lipoproteins), rendering them immunogenic. This is evidenced by the identification of autoantibodies against various epitopes of oxidatively modified LDL in the serum as well as in the atherosclerotic lesions per se (234–237). Furthermore, the titer of autoantibodies to MDA-LDL (an oxidized epitope of LDL) is shown to be a risk factor for progression of atheroscelosis (235). There is now a large body of evidence indicating that ESRD is a condition of increased oxidative stress (169–172). There is also evidence demonstrating increased plasma values for various lipid peroxidation products in CRF (172–177,225). This is particularly illustrated by the detection of high anti-LDL-ox titers in dialysis patients (147). Moreover, the presence of autoantibodies against oxidatively modified lipoproteins suggests another pathogenic mechanism for atherosclerosis in that anti-ox-LDL complexes may be taken up by macrophages via Fc receptors and thereby contribute to foam cell formation (149). It is also possible that oxidatively modified lipoproteins generate immune responses directed against epitopes within atherosclerotic lesions that may evoke additional vascular injury. The combination of dyslipoproteinemia, oxidative stress, and increased lipid peroxidation, therefore, may play an important role in the pathogenesis of vascular injury and accelerated atherosclerosis in CRF.

To establish whether or not a given risk factor is truly causal in the pathogenesis of cardiovascular disease, not only must its presence significantly correlate with coronary heart disease (CHD) risk, but also its elimination should significantly reduce CHD risk. These rigid criteria have only recently been established for hypercholesterolemia and hypertension in the general population. Studies specifically evaluating cardiovascular risk factors in ESRD patients, however, are relatively sparse and for the most part inconclusive. With regard to the lipoprotein abnormalities associated with CRF, there is evidence demonstrating a significant positive correlation between elevated plasma Lp(a) levels and cardiovascular mortality (65). In addition, dialysis patients with LMW apo(a) phenotypes and/or a low apo A-I: C-III ratio are also shown to be at increased risk for cardiovascular disease and related mortality (61,67). A positive correlation between plasma LDL-C, total cholesterol and TG levels, and cardiovascular risk, however, has not been clearly established in CRF patients. In fact, several recent studies have provided data suggesting an apparent paradoxical inverse relationship between cholesterol levels and cardiovascular risk in dialysis patients (238,239). Specifically, those patients with low plasma cholesterol were shown to have increased cardiovascular mortality. Furthermore, in hemodialysis patients, very low plasma cholesterol levels (<100 mg/dL) were associated with a 4.2-fold increased mortality risk as opposed to very high cholesterol levels (>350 mg/dL), which were associated with only a 1.3-fold increased mortality risk. A similar situation has also been noted with hypertension in CRF (197,238,240). That is, ESRD patients with low systolic blood pressure were found to have a higher relative risk for cardiovascular mortality. These findings, however, should not be interpreted as an indication that hypertension and hypercholesterolemia are negative risk factors for cardiovascular disease in CRF patients. Indeed, there is no credible evidence that the underlying pathophysiology or risk for cardiovascular disease is fundamentally different in CRF. It is, therefore, reasonable to assume that risk factors for CHD in the general population (hypertension and hypercholesterolemia) also convey CHD risk in ESRD.

There are a several plausible explanations for this apparent paradoxical relationship in CRF between hypertension, cholesterol, and CHD risk. In the first place, the presence of low blood pressure may simply reflect underlying severe target organ damage (e.g., cardiomyopathy) or be a manifestation of the J-curve phenomenon related to over aggressive ultrafiltration and/or treatment with antihypertensive agents. It is also possible that an unrecognized comorbid condition such as pericarditis (complicated by tamponade), chronic constrictive pericarditis, or the presence of occult infection maybe responsible for low blood pressure in a CRF patient. With regard to plasma lipids, it is important to consider the superimposed effects of protein-energy malnutrition, a condition often present in ESRD, which is strongly linked to increased mortality in dialysis patients (241,242). Important biochemical markers of malnutrition include reduced plasma levels of secretory proteins such as albumin and lipoproteins (i.e., cholesterol and apoprotein B), as well as a reduction in serum creatinine, which is a marker of somatic protein content. Therefore, one explanation for the apparent inverse relationship between cholesterol and cardiovascular risk in CRF is that protein-energy malnutrition constitutes a greater risk for mortality compared to moderately increased cholesterol levels in better nourished patients. It is important to consider that the most frequent causes of death in malnourished dialysis patients are cardiovascular disease and infection. In fact, there are a number of studies demonstrating an association between malnutrition and increased cardiovascular mortality in ESRD although the reason for this has not been fully explained (242–245). Low serum albumin, a marker for malnutrition and a strong predictor of mortality in dialysis patients, has also been associated with elevated Lp(a) levels (a known independent risk factor for cardiovascular disease) (246). Therefore, increased plasma Lp(a) levels may also be a factor in the increased cardiovascular mortality associated with hypoalbuminemia in dialysis patients.

In CRF, there is also a relationship between plasma proteins, lipoproteins, and underlying chronic inflammation. In dialysis patients, increased plasma levels of various positive acute phase reactants have been described including fibrinogen, C-reactive protein, serum amyloid A, ferritin, α_2-macroglobulin, α_1-acid glycoprotein, ceruloplasmin, and haptoglobin (247–250). In contrast, plasma levels of negative acute phase reactants (prealbumin, albumin, and transferrin) are often decreased (250). It is further noted that in conditions associated with tissue inflammation or injury including acute myocardial infarction, some lipoproteins such as Lp(a) and TG act as positive acute phase reactants, whereas other lipoproteins such as cholesterol behave as negative acute phase reactants. The most compelling evidence, however, linking CRF and inflammation is the demonstration of elevated plasma levels of proinflammatory cytokines including TNF-α, IL-1β and IL-6 in hemodialysis patients (162,251–253). The process of hemodialysis may stimulate cytokine production in circulating mononuclear cells (i.e., monocytes, T lymphocytes, and natural killer cells) (252–254). This occurs via a combination of mechanisms including the interaction of mononuclear cells with dialysis polymer materials, dialyzer-mediated complement activation, and/or contamination of blood with small molecular weight microbial products present in the dialysate (163–166,254–257). The release of proinflammatory cytokines such as TNF and IL-1 may in turn cause febrile reactions, hypotension, and anorexia. Proinflammatory cytokines may also trigger release of various neuropeptides (i.e., ACTH, corticotropin-releasing factor, and somatostatin) as well as stimulate hepatic synthesis of acute phase reactants while suppressing albumin synthesis (163). Other important actions of TNF and IL-1 include stimulation of eicosanoid synthesis, the enhancement of endothelial coagulant activity, and the expression of leukocyte adhesion molecules, as well as the stimulation of a plasminogen activator inhibitor (163,252,253,258–260). TNF and IL-1 can simultaneously upregulate cellular metabolism and increase expression of a number of genes coding for biologically active molecules while they suppress the expression of genes responsible for synthesis of albumin and lipoprotein lipase (163,258,259). Therefore, increased production and release of proinflammatory cytokines represents another potential mechanism for hypoalbuminemia and dyslipoproteinemia in hemodialysis patients. Furthermore, the typical plasma biochemical profile in ESRD, showing increased levels of positive acute phase reactants such as fibrinogen, C-reactive protein, Lp(a), and TG coupled with reduced levels of negative acute phase reactants, such as prealbumin and albumin, also appears to be cytokine-mediated. It is also noteworthy that some acute phase reactants such as Lp(a), fibrinogen, and C-reactive protein are predictive of cardiovascular risk (65,260–262). As a result of this growing body of data linking chronic inflammation with cardiovascular disease, it is postulated that proinflammatory cytokines may be important in the pathogenesis of atherosclerosis (209,250,262). Supporting this concept is a recent study showing that aspirin, an agent with anti-inflammatory properties, was most effective in reducing the risk of myocardial infarction in those patients with the highest levels of C-reactive protein (263). In hemodialysis patients, an elevated C-reactive protein level has been shown to be a strong predictor of both increased mortality and low serum albumin (247). In addition, a significant negative correlation has been demonstrated between levels of proinflammatory cytokines and levels of cholesterol and albumin, that is, hemodialysis patients with the lowest plasma cholesterol and albumin levels have been shown to have the highest cytokine levels (264). Furthermore, patients with high TNF and IL-6 levels had increased mortality compared to patients with low cytokine levels. Chronic stimulation of proinflammatory cytokines, therefore, provides another plausible explanation in hemodialysis patients for the inverse relationship between plasma albumin and Lp(a) levels and for the apparent paradoxical association of low plasma cholesterol with increased cardiovascular risk. In summary, there is considerable evidence that many CRF patients have underlying malnutrition and/or chronic inflammation. Moreover, both conditions are correlated with increased mortality and both conditions cause perturbations in plasma proteins and lipids. Therefore, any interpretation of lipoprotein abnormalities and related cardiovascular risk in CRF must also consider superimposed effects of malnutrition and chronic inflammation. Furthermore, underlying chronic inflammation (most evident in hemodialysis patients) may be involved in the pathogenesis of vascular injury and atherosclerosis.

XII. DYSLIPOPROTEINEMIA: THE EFFECTS OF DIALYSIS

The characteristic changes in lipid, lipoprotein, and apoprotein values in CRF are summarized in Table 3, while the typical changes in apoprotein content of plasma lipoproteins are summarized in Table 4. In general, the same plasma lipoprotein abnormalities that typify CRF, such as hypertriglyceridemia with TG enrichment of all major lipoprotein classes (VLDL, IDL, LDL, and HDL), decreased HDL, and increased Lp(a) values, are also characteristically present in patients treated with dialysis. Dialysis treatment, therefore, does not appear to fundamentally correct any underlying pathophysiological mechanism responsible for dyslipoproteinemia, however, treatment with either peritoneal (PD) or hemodialysis (HD) may modulate plasma lipoprotein values (17,18,52–62,68–77).

A. Hemodialysis

The most common effects of HD on plasma lipids and lipoproteins include reductions in plasma TG, total cholesterol, and LDL cholesterol levels. However, small increases in TG levels are reported in some studies, possibly as a consequence of acetate used in place of bicarbonate as a dialysate buffer (1–4,18,52,60,74,75). Moreover, when reductions in plasma cholesterol are caused by malnutrition and/or are related to an underlying inflammatory state, cardiovascular mortality is greatly increased (241–243,264). Increases in plasma saturated fatty acid levels along with decreases in monounsaturated and polyunsaturated fatty acids are also described in HD patients (265). Furthermore, elevated plasma mevalonic acid levels associated with CRF are significantly reduced with HD (266). With regard to plasma apoproteins, mild to moderate increases in apo A-I, apo A-II, apo C-III, and apo E are reported, whereas mild decreases in apo B are reported following the institution of HD. In contrast, significant decreases in apo E are reported (both in plasma and in apo B–containing lipoproteins) in anephric patients on hemodialysis, suggesting a possible role in apo E synthesis by the remnant kidneys. Overall, the effect of HD on lipid/lipoprotein abnormalities in CRF appear to be relatively minor despite theoretical concerns with regard to dialysate-related acetate loads (reported to increase hepatic TG synthesis), the use of heparin (reported to deplete LPL and HTGL as well as inhibit LCAT activity), and increased cytokine release (reported to inhibit LPL activity) (1–4,17,18,71–75,258).

B. Peritoneal Dialysis

In contrast to HD, treatment with PD may aggravate dyslipoproteinemia, causing increases in plasma TG, total cholesterol, LDL-C, VLDL-C, and Lp(a) (59,67,72,74,75,267–270). Moderate increases in total cholesterol, VLDL-C, and LDL-C occur in approximately 15–30% of patients treated with PD in contrast to HD where cholesterol levels are typically normal or low. Reductions in HDL-C are generally less severe in PD patients (compared to HD), with one study actually reporting an increase in HDL-C (270). Moderate hypertriglyceridemia is reported in 60–80% of patients receiving long-term PD, the highest TG levels usually occurring in those patients with high predialysis TG values (268,269). The increases in plasma lipoproteins observed with PD appear to some extent to be related to the amount of glucose absorbed from the peritoneal cavity (268,269). Plasma lipoprotein levels, however, often stabilize or even decline after 6–12 months of dialysis (irrespective of changes in dialysate glucose concentration), suggesting that a form of adaptation to peritoneal glucose loads may occur (267). The adverse effects of PD on plasma lipids, lipoproteins, and apolipoproteins are summarized in Table 7.

Abnormalities involving plasma apoproteins in dialysis patients are also similar to those described in predialysis CRF patients (66,67,71,72,267,268,271,272). However, when compared to HD, patients receiving PD usually demonstrate higher plasma apo A-I and apo B values but lower apo A-I:apo B ratios, indicating disproportionate increases in apo B. Elevated levels of apo A-IV are reported in predialysis CRF patients as well as in patients receiving dialysis (with slightly higher levels reported in PD vs. HD) (271). Elevated apo A-IV levels in CRF are thought to result from impaired chylomicron metabolism as increases in apo IV levels are shown to correlate with chylomicronemia (53). There is also evidence that apo A-IV may play a functional role in reverse cholesterol transport (through the stimulation of LCAT activity), and this has led to speculation that elevated apo A-IV may actually be beneficial in reducing cardiovascular risk (271,272). Increased CETP activity is described in patients receiving PD, which may be related to peritoneal protein loss (272). It is also proposed that increased CETP synthesis may be induced by elevated plasma levels of apo B–containing lipoproteins in PD patients (271). Moreover, a positive association between CETP and either LDL-C or the LDL-C:HDL-C ratio in PD patients suggests that increased in CETP activity may increase atherogenic risk (71,272).

Table 7 Adverse Effects of Peritoneal Dialysis on Plasma Lipids, Lipoproteins, and Apolipoproteins

Plasma Lipids	Effects of peritoneal dialysis
Triglyceride	Moderate increase[a]
Total cholesterol	Moderate increase[a]
Plasma Lipoproteins	
VLDL-C	Moderate increase[a]
LDL-C	Moderate increase[a]
Small dense LDL	Moderate increase[a]
Lipoprotein(a)	Moderate increase[a]
HDL-C	Mild increase
Apolipoproteins	
Apo A-I	Mild increase
Apo B	Moderate increase[a]
Apo A-I/B	Decreased[a]

[a]Statistically significant.

In addition to having increased plasma levels of atherogenic remnants of large TG-rich lipoproteins (i.e., chylomicron remnants and VLDL remnants), CRF patients are also shown to have elevated levels of highly atherogenic TG-enriched, small dense LDL particles as well as significant elevations in plasma Lp(a) values compared to controls (55,61–64,274). More specifically, the highest frequency of small TG-enriched LDL particles is described in PD patients (48%) compared to HD patients (23%) and healthy controls (7%) (274). There are also numerous studies demonstrating significantly elevated Lp(a) levels in dialysis patients compared to controls (61–65). Furthermore, Lp(a) values are generally are significantly higher in PD patients compared to HD patients.

Factors associated with PD that may adversely affect lipoprotein metabolism include excessive peritoneal glucose absorption (200–250 g/d with frequent use of hypertonic high-glucose dialysate) and/or protein losses from the peritoneal cavity (269,270). While moderate protein losses appear to be common with PD, losses can exceed 10–15 g/d (275). In addition, passive losses of virtually all plasma proteins occur via a molecular sieving effect of the peritoneal membrane (275–277). Therefore, for most proteins, losses are directly related to the plasma concentration of the respective protein and inversely related to molecular size. In accordance with this, the peritoneal clearance of HDL is greater than LDL, which is greater than VLDL. However, in contrast to what is described with most proteins, the peritoneal mass transfer and clearance of both HDL and albumin are inversely correlated with their respective plasma concentrations (275). As a result, peritoneal losses play a much greater role in lowering plasma HDL and albumin compared to other plasma proteins. Furthermore, relatively large peritoneal losses of apoproteins A-I and A-IV are reported at rates exceeding 250 and 220 mg/d, respectively, while moderate losses are reported for apo B, and comparatively small losses are reported for apoproteins A-II, C-III, C-II, and E (271,278,279). Despite the increased losses of apo A-I and apo A-IV, plasma levels of these apoproteins are generally not reduced in PD patients.

In addition to dyslipoproteinemia, abnormalities involving hemostatic factors are described in dialysis patients that may be related to abnormal lipoprotein metabolism (249,280). Elevated plasma levels of fibrinogen and coagulation factor VII were recently reported in PD patients, and significant positive correlations were found between plasma fibrinogen or factor VII levels and plasma lipid levels, including cholesterol and TG. Furthermore, elevated levels of fibrinogen and factor VII levels are also associated with increased cardiovascular risk (261,281,282). Additionally, in the general population a number of studies have reported a positive correlation between factor VII levels and plasma levels of TG and cholesterol (283,284). It is therefore possible that PD may increase cardiovascular risk by worsening both dyslipoproteinemia and related hemostatic abnormalities.

XIII. MANAGEMENT OF DYSLIPOPROTEINEMIA IN CRF

It is well established that the risk for atherosclerotic cardiovascular disease is significantly increased in CRF (195–198). Furthermore, it is acknowledged that dyslipoproteinemia may substantially contribute to this risk. Treatment of dyslipoproteinemia in CRF, however, is controversial, and consensus guidelines regarding evaluation and management have yet to be established for a number of reasons. First, the rationality for currently recommended lipid screening and treatment protocols is based on data from patient populations with normal renal function, and the appropriateness of utilizing information extrapolated from this experience in the management of dyslipemia in CRF is a debatable issue that will be subsequently discussed. Second, although patients with CRF are known to be at high risk for cardiovascular disease with many manifesting multiple risk factors (e.g., hypertension, diabetes mellitus, male gender, and advanced age) and/or exhibiting evidence for overt atherosclerotic cardiovascular disease, the relative importance of dyslipoproteinemia remains to be established. Moreover, there are no clinical trail data (in dyslipoproteinemic CRF patients) demonstrating beneficial effects of lipid-lowering therapy in terms of risk reduction. Third, the superimposed effects of malnutrition as well as that of chronic inflammation need consideration in view of their apparent high prevalence in CRF, their affect on mortality and morbidity, as well as their affect on lipoprotein metabolism.

In the general population a strong positive correlation has been established between elevated plasma cholesterol levels (especially LDL-C) and cardiovascular risk (40–42,47,51). Moreover, there are numerous studies demonstrating the value of cholesterol-lowering therapy in reducing cardiovascular mortality in high-risk asymptomatic patients (primary prevention) as well as in patients with established coronary heart disease (secondary prevention) (47,50,198,285–288). Therefore, a great deal of importance is placed on cholesterol (total cholesterol and LDL-C) in both screening

Table 8 Treatment Based on LDL-C

Patient characteristics	LDL level (mg/dL)	LDL goal (mg/dL)
Dietary Therapy		
Without CHD and <2 risks	≥160	<160
Without CHD and ≥2 risks	≥130	<130
With CHD	>100	≤100
Drug Therapy		
Without CHD and <2 risks	≥190	<160
Without CHD and ≥2 risks	≥160	<130
With CHD	≥130	<100

protocols and treatment goals, with less emphasis on other lipoprotein abnormalities particularly those involving TG metabolism. However, when currently recommended NCEP guidelines (Tables 8 and 9) are applied, the vast majority of CRF patients do not meet minimum treatment criteria because from a quantitative standpoint the lipoprotein abnormalities are typically only mild to moderate in severity (289). For example, plasma cholesterol levels in CRF are usually normal, especially in patients receiving HD. Even hypertriglyceridemia, the most predominant abnormality detectable by routine screening in CRF, would probably not be of sufficient magnitude to be targeted for treatment.

It is also important to consider that the role of triglycerides in atherosclerotic disease in the general population remains controversial. Hypertriglyceridemia per se has not been established as an independent risk factor, even though high fasting TG levels have been positively correlated with coronary heart disease (CHD) risk by univariate analysis in most case-control and prospective studies (51,290,291). This association, however, is weakened when the strong inverse relationship between HDL-C and CHD risk is taken into account, which raises an important consideration, namely, the frequent clustering of hypertriglyceridemia, low plasma HDL-C, and the increased presence of small dense LDL particles, a combination known to be highly atherogenic (292–294). This combination, however, is not surprising considering the close relationship between the catabolism of TG-rich lipoproteins (chylomicrons and VLDL) and the formation of HDL-C and LDL-C. Thus, impaired TG catabolism affects not only the plasma clearance of chylomicrons and VLDL, but also the formation and development of LDL-C and HDL-C.

There is increasing evidence supporting the concept that impaired TG catabolism with associated hypertriglyceridemia and reduced HDL is atherogenic. First of all, a number of familial and metabolic disorders expressing this dyslipemic phenotype are associated with accelerated atherosclerosis. The metabolic disorder "syndrome X" is characterized not only by this constellation of lipoprotein abnormalities (hypertriglyceridemia, decreased HDL, and small dense LDL particles) but by additional abnormalities, two of which are also typically seen in CRF—insulin resistance and hypertension (295,296). In addition, data from two recently conducted clinical studies illustrate the importance of TG values in assessing CHD risk and in predicting the outcome of lipid-lowering therapy when interpreted in combination with HDL-C and LDL-C values (297,298). In the Helsinki Heart Study, subjects with LDL-C/HDL-C ratios of >5 and TG levels of >200 mg/dL had significantly higher CHD risk compared to subjects with LDL-C/HDL-C ratios of ≤5 and TG levels of ≤200 mg/dL (297). Moreover, the high-risk group had a 71% lower incidence of CHD events with lipid-lowering therapy (gemfibrizol) than the corresponding placebo group. Moreover, CHD risk could not be predicted on the basis of LDL-C levels alone (298). Additionally, there are data from the Stockholm Ischaemic Heart Disease study indicating that TG reduction (in hypertriglyceridemic patients) is also beneficial in secondary prevention (299). Although we still lack conclusive data (from large-scale clinical trials) demonstrating cardiovascular risk reduction in association with TG-lowering treatment (in hypertriglyceridemic patients), there is nonetheless credible evidence to suggest such an outcome. In fact, the 1992 NIH Consensus Development Conference has recommended that TG-reduction therapy may be considered when TG levels are only borderline high (200–400 mg/dL) under the following circumstances: (1) established CHD, (2) family history of premature CHD, (3) concomitant high total cholesterol (>240 mg/dL) and low HDL-C, and (4) genetic forms of hypertriglyceridemia associated with increased CHD risk (e.g., familial dysbetalipoproteinemia and familial combined hyperlipidemia) (291). In summary, we have a good deal of evidence linking the combination of hypertriglyceridemia, low HDL-C, and small dense LDL with increased cardiovascular

Table 9 Definitions of Hypertriglyceridemia

Borderline-high triglycerides	<200–400 mg/dL
High triglycerides	400–1000 mg/dL
Very high triglycerides	>1000 mg/dL

Note: Treatment is generally recommended when triglyceride levels are >500 mg/dL.

risk. Moreover, several recent studies have shown beneficial effects of TG-reduction therapy in improving LDL-C:HDL-C ratios and reducing CHD risk. In view of these findings, coupled with the knowledge that CRF causes a form of dyslipoproteinemia characterized by moderate hypertriglyceridemia with increased chylomicron remnants and IDL, along with decreased HDL-C, increased small dense LDL and increased Lp(a), a good argument for aggressive TG-lowering measures can be made. Further supporting this contention is the knowledge that many CRF patients manifest multiple risk factors and/or have underlying cardiovascular disease. However, the rationale for early aggressive treatment must also be tempered by the knowledge that conclusive data (from clinical trail studies) proving efficacy and safety of lipid-lowering therapy in CRF is still lacking. Furthermore, the issue of risk is particularly germane in CRF in view of the increased potential for drug toxicity as well as concerns related to protein-energy nutrition with respect to dietary modifications. Nevertheless, based on our current understanding of lipoprotein pathophysiology, its consequences and management, along with the inference that some of the increased cardiovascular risk in CRF is dyslipoproteinemic related, a number of qualified recommendations can be made regarding the evaluation and management of this problem until more conclusive data become available.

A. Screening for Dyslipoproteinemia in CRF

First, with regard to screening, a thorough clinical and laboratory assessment should be conducted to identify lipoprotein abnormalities and other risk factors as well as the presence of underlying cardiovascular disease. The major atherogenic and antiatherogenic lipoproteins are listed in Table 10. Plasma lipid profiles should include measured total cholesterol, HDL-C, and triglyceride values with LDL-C being calculated by the Friedewald formula: LDL-C = total cholesterol − HDL-C − TG/5 (under most circumstances VLDL-C can be estimated as 1/5 × TG) (300). In contadistinction to some other forms of secondary dyslipoproteinemia, the Friedwald formula is reported to reliably estimate LDL-C in most CRF patients. However, increased plasma Lp(a) and/or compositional abnormalities in VLDL may compromise its accuracy (301). Furthermore, if TG levels exceed 400 mg/dL, VLDL-C and LDL-C cannot be accurately calculated and must be measured following centrifugation. For TG levels to be meaningful, samples must be collected after a 12-hour fast and prior to heparin administration in HD patients. The clinical utility of assessing other lipoprotein components such as Lp(a), IDL, chylomicron remnants, small dense LDL, HDL subclasses (HDL_2 and HDL_3), apo B, apo A-I, and apo III is less certain at this time because laboratories capable of performing accurate measurements are not widely available, standardization of normal ranges is often lacking, and there is no overall consensus regarding either predictive or treatment values.

Table 10 Lipoproteins and Cardiovascular Risk

Atherogenic Lipoproteins
Chylomicron remnants
VLDL remnants
IDL
LDL
Lp(a)
Antiatherogenic Lipoproteins
HDL

B. Treatment Values for Lipoproteins in CRF

Treatment values for plasma lipids (total cholesterol, LDL-C, and TG) in CRF must be extrapolated from NCEP guidelines (Tables 8 and 9) (289). It is reasonable, therefore, to treat LDL-C levels of ≥160 mg/dL in patients without CHD and only one risk factor. In addition, treatment is recommended for LDL-C levels of ≥130 mg/dL in patients with two or more risk factors, while LDL-C levels of ≥100 mg/dL should be treated in patients with known CHD as part of secondary risk prevention. It is also recommended that patients with LDL-C of >130 mg/dL be considered for treatment in the presence of a concomitant increase in Lp(a) (>30 mg/dL) and decrease in HDL (<35 mg/dL) (302). Although data supporting this strategy are limited, the risk for CHD in patients with elevated Lp(a) is further increased by elevated LDL-C levels. Moreover, there is recent evidence that Lp(a) may cease to be a risk if LDL-C levels are sufficiently reduced (303). Patients with very high LDL-C values (>190 mg/dL) should be suspected of having an underlying primary hyperlipoproteinemia or an additional secondary disorder. It should also be kept in mind that low cholesterol levels might indicate malnutrition or underlying inflammation.

In general, treatment is not recommended for mild hypertriglyceridemia (250–500 mg/dL). However, based on NCEP guidelines, borderline-high triglycerides (200–400 mg/dL) may be treated in patients with concomitant high total cholesterol levels (>240 mg/dL) and low HDL-C (<35 mg/dL) and/or in patients with established CHD (289). There are also sufficient data to consider treatment in patients with elevated triglycerides (>200 mg/dL) and an LDL-C/HDL-C ratio > 5 (297). We would further recommend that treatment of borderline-high triglycerides be considered in CRF patients with low HDL-C (<35 mg/dL), as this combination is highly indicative of severely impaired TG catabolism with associated small dense LDL and TG remnants. If available, measurements of small dense LDL, IDL, and chylomicron remnants should be monitored in patients with hypertriglyceridemia and low HDL-C.

Table 12 Additional Factors Implicated in the Pathogenesis of Cardiovascular Disease in CRF

Secondary hyperparathyroidism
Left ventricular hypertrophy
Insulin resistance
Anemia
Poor nutrition (hypoalbuminemia)
Proinflammatory cytokines and acute phase reactants
Homocysteine
Oxidative stress (lipid peroxidation)
Modified proteins (oxidation, glycosylation, carbamylation)
Thrombogenic factors
Complement activation
Inhibition of NO-synthase

XIV. MANAGEMENT OF DYSLIPOPROTEINEMIA IN CRF

Management of dyslipoproteinemia should begin with risk factor assessment (Table 11). Modifiable risks (smoking, hypertension, obesity, physical inactivity, and diabetes mellitus) should be eliminated or treated whenever possible. Additional factors in CRF implicated in the pathogenesis and progression of cardiovascular disease such as anemia, hyperhomocysteinemia, LVH, hyperparathyroidism, and poor nutrition also require appropriate management (Table 12). Furthermore, it is important to assess factors and conditions that may influence lipoprotein metabolism. These include diet and nutritional status (obesity is more common in PD patients), alcohol consumption, physical activity, type and adequacy of dialysis, and medication (beta-blockers, diuretics, glucocorticoids, and androgens may adversely affect lipids).

Table 11 Nonlipid Risk Factors

Modifiable Factors
Cigarettes
Hypertension
Obesity
Physical activity
Diabetes mellitus
Nonmodifiable Factors
Age
Male gender
Family history of premature CHD

A. Diet, Exercise, and Lifestyle Modification

Lifestyle changes shown to be beneficial in dyslipoproteinemia management include dietary modification, weight reduction in obese patients, and the employment of moderate aerobic exercise (304–307). A number of studies have demonstrated the effectiveness of dietary modification in the management of dyslipemia in CRF (303–305). In hypertriglyceridemic patients, carbohydrates should be reduced to 30–35% of total daily caloric intake, with complex carbohydrates substituted for refined sugars. This strategy may be effective in reducing hepatic VLDL synthesis. In addition, a reduction in dietary saturated fat to achieve a polyunsaturated:saturated ratio of between 1:1 and 2:1 is shown to be effective in lowering TG and raising HDL in CRF patients. Elimination of alcohol may also result in reduction of plasma TG. Protein intake of high biological value should be maintained at approximately 1.2 g/kg/d in HD patients and 1.2–1.5 g/kg/d in PD patients. Total caloric intake should also be maintained at 30–35 kcal/kg/d unless weight reduction is indicated.

In hypercholesterolemic patients, a low-cholesterol diet (<300 mg/d) is shown to reduce total plasma cholesterol as well as LDL-C levels (304). Although diets low in refined sugar, cholesterol, and saturated fat are shown to be effective in lowering VLDL and LDL-C as well as raising HDL-C levels in CRF, most studies have been short term. Moreover, there are a number of problems and concerns regarding dietary modifications. First, carbohydrate restriction is difficult to achieve in CRF, especially in PD patients where 15–30% of total caloric intake may come from glucose absorbed through the peritoneum. However, strict compliance regarding sodium intake can minimize volume-related weight gain and, therefore, the need for high-osmotic (high-glucose) dialysis solutions. Second are nutritional concerns, because many cholesterol-rich foods (meat and eggs) are excellent sources of high biological value protein, therefore, nutritional parameters must be closely monitored. Third, as the putative mechanism by which carbohydrate restriction lowers plasma triglycerides is through reduced hepatic synthesis, the rationality for this approach can be criticized on the basis that the underlying pathophysiology (defective TG catabolism) remains unaffected. In spite of these concerns, dietary therapy may be useful in the treatment of dyslipoproteinemia in CRF and is, therefore, recommended along with other appropriate lifestyle modifications in initial management.

Fish oil supplements containing omega-3 polyunsaturated fatty acids (PUFA) are also effective in lowering plasma TG levels in CRF apparently through inhibition of hepatic TG synthesis (308–311). In addition, increases in HDL-C (especially HDL_2) have been reported, whereas the effect of fish oil on LDL-C has been inconsistent. Other potentially favorable effects of omega-3 fatty acids include diminished thromboxane A_2 production (resulting in reduced platelet aggregation) and mild blood pressure reduction (311–312). The use of omega-3 PUFA (starting with dosages of 3 g/d) may be considered in hypertriglyceridemic CRF patients with the following caveats: (a) long-term compliance is often poor, (b) plasma LDL-C levels may increase, and (c) overall beneficial effects remain unproven. Furthermore, because there are concerns regarding the potential for PUFA oxidation in CRF, the co-administration (400–600 U/d) of vitamin E is recommended.

In hemodialysis patients, regular aerobic exercise (cycling, walking, and jogging) is shown to reduce plasma triglycerides and raise HDL-C (307). Aerobic exercise appears to promote VLDL catabolism by increasing LPL activity, which may be related to improved insulin sensitivity (313). Thus, at least on a theoretical basis, exercise may function to correct an underlying mechanism for dyslipemia in CRF. Furthermore, aerobic exercise has been shown to improve blood pressure control, anemia, and relieve symptoms of depression in dialysis patients (307). Therefore, every effort should be made to encourage regular exercise programs in CRF patients.

B. Additional Factors That May Affect Lipoproteins

Additional factors or measures reported to affect lipoprotein metabolism in CRF include treatment with erythropoietin, L-carnitine supplementation, vitamin D administration, use of LMW heparin, and high-flux dialysis. Erythropoietin (EPO) is reported to reduce plasma triglycerides, apo B, and total cholesterol in dialysis patients (314,315). An increase in apo A-I is also reported with EPO therapy. It is thought that EPO favorably affects lipoprotein metabolism by improving carbohydrate tolerance. Some studies, however, have failed to demonstrate any modulating effects of EPO on plasma lipids (316,317). It is also possible that the beneficial effects of EPO are related to improved exercise tolerance and increased physical activity. For sure, the widespread availability and efficacy of EPO allows virtually all CRF patients to maintain hematocrits within a range more conducive to exercise.

Administration of L-carnitine (500–1000 mg/d or 10–20 mg/kg post-HD) is reported to lower TG levels in hypertriglyceridemic patients, but a consistent TG-lowering effect has not been demonstrated (152,156,318). Treatment with $1,25(OH)_2D_3$ is also reported to lower TG levels in CRF (318). This effect may be mediated through PTH suppression because treatment of hyperparathyroidism has been shown to reduce plasma triglycerides (110,111). The long-term use of LMW heparin has also been shown to significantly lower triglycerides, apo B and cholesterol in HD patients (90,91,320). The beneficial effect of LMW heparin on plasma lipids may be attributable to its weaker lipolytic action, which results in reduced fatty acid release and less depletion of LPL.

High-flux dialysis using polysulfone membranes is reported to significantly lower total plasma triglycerides, VLDL triglycerides, VLDL cholesterol, apo B, and apo C-III compared to controls receiving low-flux dialysis using cellulose-based membranes (321–323). Significant increases in HDL-C are also reported with high-flux dialysis (321). These findings may be related to improved membrane biocompatibility because there is evidence suggesting a link between cytokine release (triggered by cellulostic membranes) and suppression of LPL activity (258,259).

Removal of a circulating inhibitor of LPL is another proposed mechanism to explain the apparent modulating effects of high-flux dialysis on lipoprotein metabolism. Other proposed beneficial effects of high-flux dialysis include increased removal of AGEs and reduced oxidative stress. There are also preliminary data indicating that antioxidant modification of dialysis membranes with vitamin E may effectively reduce oxidative stress and lipoperoxidation (324).

XV. USE OF LIPID-LOWERING DRUGS IN CRF

When conservative measures fail to achieve the desired lipid-lowering effect (including a 3- to 6-month trial of appropriate dietary and lifestyle modifications), pharmacological therapy may be considered. The salient features of the five major classes of lipid-lowering agents are shown in Table 13.

Fibric acid derivatives (gemfibrozil, clofibrate, clinofibrate, and benzafibrate) have been used in CRF to treat hypertriglyceridemia (325–329). Not only are triglycerides significantly reduced (30–70%), but increases in HDL-C are also reported. Furthermore, these agents are shown to lower apo E and apo C-III levels, but their effect on LDL-C has been variable. Currently, the only fibrate widely used in the United States is gemfibrozil. Fibrates act to increase the activity of LPL, possibly thereby increasing the catabolism and clearance of TG-rich lipoproteins (23,47). Thus, there appears to be a rational basis for using fibrates in the management of the hypertriglyceridemia/low-HDL dyslipemia typical of CRF. In addition, fibrates may also have an inhibitory effect on HMG-CoA reductase (329). Since excretion of fibrates is primarily renal, their dosage must be reduced by 50–75% in CRF to minimize toxicity. Patients should be closely monitored for signs and symptoms of myopathy/rhabodomyolysis (the most common toxic manifestation of fibrates). In addition, creatine phosphokinase levels should be closely monitored, with weekly measurements for the first several weeks and monthly measurements thereafter.

HMG-CoA reductase inhibitors (lovastatin, pravastatin, simvastatin, fluvastatin, and atorvastatin) are the drugs of choice in the management of hypercholesterolemia (330–332). Statins inhibit 3-hydroxy-3-methylglutaryl coenzyme A (the rate-limiting step in cholesterol biosynthesis) and as a consequence of reduced synthesis, hepatocellular cholesterol levels fall. This in turn causes an increase in LDL receptor synthesis, which lowers plasma cholesterol by increasing hepatocellular uptake. HMG-CoA reductase inhibitors (statins) lower total cholesterol and LDL-C levels by 20–40% in dialysis patients with minimal side effects and complications. Additionally, significant increases in HDL-C are reported as well as significant reductions in apoproteins A-II, B, C-II, C-III, and E with lowering of the B:A-I ratio. Furthermore, in a recent study, enhancing LDL receptor-mediated uptake showed pravastatin to lower IDL by 31% in dialysis patients (333). A significant reduction in VLDL cholesterol was also demonstrated, whereas VLDL triglycerides were not significantly affected. These findings are consistent with enhanced VLDL receptor uptake, which demonstrates a high affinity for the smaller VLDL-C particles while showing a low affinity for the large VLDL-TG-rich particles. In addition, much of the TG reduction associated with HMG-CoA reductase inhibition may be the result of enhanced uptake of IDL and LDL-C, which is TG-enriched in CRF. There is also evidence that compositional abnormalities may be corrected or improved through a reduction in the cholesterol content of VLDL and normalization of the TG:cholesterol ratio in VLDL (332,333). Moreover, the enhanced removal of atherogenic remnants (i.e., VLDL-C and IDL) may prove particularly beneficial in CRF and should be the focus of future studies. Because statins are primarily metabolized by the liver, they generally do not require dose modification in CRF. However, in the presence of liver disease or with the simultaneous use of fibrates or nicotinic acid, the risk for myopathy is greatly increased. In either event, patients treated with statins require periodic monitoring of muscle and liver enzymes. Atorvastatin, the latest generation HMG-CoA inhibitor, not only has powerful cholesterol-lowering effects, but is also quite effective in lowering triglycerides. However, the experience with this agent in CRF is very limited.

Nicotinic acid derivatives (niacin) effectively lower plasma triglycerides and LDL-C as well as increase HDL-C (328). These agents may modulate lipoprotein metabolism by several mechanisms, including inhibition of hepatic VLDL synthesis, inhibition of fatty acid release from adipose tissue, and stimulation of LPL activity. Increases in HDL-C are attributable to facilitated catabolism of TG-rich lipoproteins. In one study, nicotinic acid was also shown to significantly lower Lp(a) levels, however, there was a strong negative relationship between the percentage reduction of Lp(a) and pretreatment TG levels (334). However, we are unaware of any studies evaluating the efficacy of nicotinic acid in lowering Lp(a) in CRF patients. Although nicotinic acid and its derivatives may decrease both cholesterol and triglycerides and increase HDL-C in dyslipoproteinemic CRF patients, frequent side effects

Table 13 Classes of Lipid-Lowering Drugs

Class	Dose in CRF	Mechanism of action	Lipid-lowering effect	Major side effects/complications
HMG-CoA Reductase Inhibitors				
Lovastatin	10–40 mg/d	↓Cholesterol synthesis	↓Total cholesterol (20–30%)	Abnormal liver
Pravastatin	10–40 mg/d	↑LDL receptors	↓LDL-C (20–40%)	Function tests
Simvastatin	5–40 mg/d		↓VLDL-C	Myopathy/Myositis
Fluvastatin	20–40 mg/d		↓IDL	
Atorvastatin	10–40 mg/d		↓TG (10%) ↑HDL-C (10%)	
Fibric Acids				
Gemfibrozil	300–600 mg/d	↑LPL activity ↑LDL catabolism ↓VLDL synthesis	↓TG (20–60%) ↑ or ↓ LDL-C ↑HDL-C	
Nicotinic Acid				
Niacin	50–100 mg TID with gradual increases to 1–2 g TID	↓VLDL synthesis ↓LDL-C synthesis ↑LPL activity	↓TG (25–85%) ↓VLDL-C (25–35%) ↓LDL-C (15–25%) ↑HDL-C	Flushing, tachycardia, pruritis, nausea, diarrhea, abnormal liver function tests, hyperuricemia (may aggrevate gout), glucose intolerance, peptic ulcer disease, myositis
Bile Acid Resin				
Cholestyramine	8–12 g BID to TID	Interruption of enterohepatic circulation with stimulation of bile synthesis, depletion of hepatocellular cholesterol and increased synthesis of LDL receptors	↓LDL-C (15–30%) ↑HDL-C ↑TG (20%)	Constipation, nausea, abdominal discomfort, interference with absorption of other drugs
Cholestipol	10–15 g BID to TID			

(flushing, skin rashes, nausea, and abdominal pain) have limited their use (335,336). Associated complications such as increased glucose intolerance, hyperuricemia with exacerbation of gout, and/or aggravation of peptic ulcer disease further restrict the use of nicotinic acid in CRF.

Probucol is shown to have only moderate LDL-C-lowering effects, apparently mediated by increased catabolism and non–receptor LDL-C plasma clearance (23,47). Unfortunately, probucol may also cause reductions in HDL-C. Apart from its effect on lipoprotein metabolism, probucol has antioxidant properties and has been shown to inhibit LDL-C oxidation (337). Probucol appears to have relatively few side effects, however, prolongation of the QT interval may occur. Although probucol is not recommended for lipid reduction in CRF, it may prove useful as an antioxidant.

The final category of lipid-lowering drugs, the bile acid sequestrants (cholestyramine and colestipol) are shown to effectively lower LDL-C (15–30%) with modest increases in HDL-C also reported (23,47). These agents bind cholesterol-containing bile acids in the intestine, preventing their reabsorption. The interruption in enterohepatic circulation stimulates bile synthesis, which depletes hepatocellular cholesterol stores. This in turn stimulates LDL receptor production, which increases hepatocellular cholesterol uptake and causes a reduction in plasma levels. Bile acid sequestrants are often recommended as initial drug therapy in hypercholesterolemic patients. However, because these agents also increase plasma triglycerides through stimulation of hepatic VLDL synthesis, they are generally not recommended in CRF.

XVI. SUMMARY AND CONCLUSIONS

The approach to management of dyslipemia in CRF is summarized in Tables 14 and 15. Due to the complex interrelationship between many of the cardiovascular risk factors as well as the prognostic significance of multiple risks, dyslipoproteinemia needs to be evaluated in the context of overall risk. Therefore, other risk factors must be identified and every effort made to either eliminate or treat risks that are modifiable. Lifestyle changes involving diet, exercise, reduction in

Table 14 The Approach to Management of Dyslipoproteinemia in CRF

Identify and eliminate or treat modifiable risks (see Table 11)
Recommend appropriate lifestyle changes (diet, exercise, reduce alcohol, eliminate smoking, and reduce weight if appropriate)
Eliminate medications that can worsen dyslipoproteinemia
Identify and treat other conditions or factors that may adversely affect dyslipoproteinemia and/or cardiovascular risk
Secondary hyperparathyroidism
Anemia
Homocysteinemia
Consider dialysis-related modifications
Change to a more biocompatible membrane
Use high-flux dialysis
Use low molecular weight heparin
Reduction in use of hypertonic glucose solutions in PD
Use of lipid-lowering drugs (see Table 13)

alcohol intake, and appropriate weight loss are recommended as initial steps in management. In diabetic patients, better glycemic control may also improve dyslipidemia. Dialysis-related modifications shown to ameliorate dyslipoproteinemia include the use of low molecular weight heparin and high-flux dialysis with polysulfone membranes, while less frequent use of high-glucose dialysate may improve dyslipoproteinemia in patients receiving peritoneal dialysis. If conservative measures are ineffective in controlling dyslipidemia, the use of pharmacological agents may be considered. Fibrates such as gemfibrozil are effective in lowering triglycerides and raising HDL-C in CRF, however, there are concerns regarding toxicity. HMG-CoA reductase inhibitors are shown to be both safe and effective in lowering cholesterol and LDL-C. Statins may also effectively lower triglycerides and IDL as well as increase HDL-C in CRF patients. The only lipid-lowering drug shown to reduce Lp(a) is nicotinic acid, however, this effect has not been studied in CRF. Exercise as well as the administration of either estrogens or androgens are also reported to lower Lp(a) in the general population. Furthermore, in postmenopausal women estrogen replacement is shown to decrease LDL-C, increase HDL-C, and reduce cardiovascular risk. As we are not aware of any studies on the effects of estrogens on lipids or CHD risk in CRF, we are unable to make recommendations with regard to their use in dyslipoproteinemia management. However, when estrogens are used in CRF for treatment of dysfunctional uterine bleeding, in bleeding time correction or estrogen deficiency, plasma triglycerides need to be monitored because such therapy may exacerbate hypertriglyceridemia. Unfortunately, androgens cannot be recommended in Lp(a) reduction due to their adverse affect on other plasma lipoproteins, which include concomitant increases in LDL-C and decreases in HDL-C.

Table 15 Additional Strategies That May be Useful in the Management of Dyslipoproteinemia and/or Cardiovascular Risk in CRF

L-Carnitine (TG-lowering effect has been inconsistent)
Fish oil supplements (effective in lowering TG, but LDL-C may increase)
Aspirin (whether the benefits of low-dose aspirin [81–325 mg/d] in stroke and CHD risk reduction demonstrated in the general population extend to CRF patients is unknown)
Antioxidants (vitamins C and E, beta-carotene, and Probucol) are of uncertain benefit

Other conditions commonly associated with CRF that may be relevant in the management of both dyslipoproteinemia and cardiovascular risk are hyperparathyroidism, anemia, and homocysteinemia. Secondary hyperparathyroidism may not only contribute to dyslipoproteinemia but may also promote cardiovascular fibrosis and calcification, therefore, early diagnosis and aggressive management of this condition is imperative. In addition, treatment of anemia with erythropoietin may improve exercise tolerance and dyslipoproteinemia. Correction of anemia will also reduce cardiac workload and left ventricular contractility, resulting in better tolerance of myocardial ischemia in patients with CHD. Homocysteinemia (plasma levels > 16 nmol/mL) is often present in CRF and may significantly add to cardiovascular risk. We recommend routinely screening patients for this condition because homocysteinemia can be safely and effectively treated with folic acid and vitamins B_6 and/or B_{12}. Although definitive data are unavailable on optimal dosage, folic acid (1–5 mg/d), B_6 (10 mg/d), and the RDA of B_{12} are effective in lowering homocysteine levels in CRF.

Additional factors that may be involved in the pathogenesis of vascular injury and atherosclerosis in CRF include increased oxidative stress, accelerated glycation, endothelial dysfunction, hemostatic abnormalities, and inflammation. Although there is considerable evidence linking oxidative stress and lipoprotein peroxidation in the pathogenesis of atherosclerosis, there are few data at this time demonstrating efficacy of antioxidant therapy in risk reduction. While oxidative stress may be important in lipid peroxidation and vascular injury in CRF, its relative role in CHD risk needs to be clearly defined. Furthermore, to employ effective preventative measures we must acquire a better understanding of the factors involved in the pathogenesis of oxidative stress in CRF. Moreover, safe and effective antioxidant regimens can only be established from interventional clinical trail data involving CRF patients. Related areas worthy of study include (a) the possible role of trace element deficiency (zinc and/or selenium) in oxidant stress in dialysis patients, (b) the role of F_2-isoprostanes (potentially harmful byproducts of lipid peroxidation) in vascular injury (elevated levels of these prostaglandin-like compounds are reported in hemodialysis patients) (148), and (c) the relative importance of AGEs in CRF, particularly with respect to their proposed role as interactants in oxidative stress and vascular injury.

The relationship between dyslipoproteinemia, hemostatic abnormalities, and endothelial dysfunction in CRF also needs clarification with respect to the following questions:

1. What is the relative role of dyslipoproteinemia in causing endothelial dysfunction in CRF patients?
2. How important is oxidative stress in the pathogenesis of endothelial dysfunction and injury?
3. Will effective dyslipoproteinemia management and/or antioxidant therapy improve endothelial function and ameliorate the related hemostatic abnormalities and, moreover, will such treatment reduce CHD risk?

A final area of both concern and interest involves proinflammatory cytokines—the mechanisms for their induction in CRF, their potential role in vascular injury, as well as their modulating effects on lipoprotein metabolism, albumin synthesis, and acute phase reactants. The complex relationship between inflammation, coagulation, and cardiovascular risk is exemplified by fibrinogen. Hepatic synthesis and secretion of fibrinogen (an acute phase reactant and procoagulant) is enhanced by proinflammatory cytokines, while increases in plasma fibrinogen may in turn adversely affect hemostasis, blood rheology, platelet aggregation, and endothelial function, creating a hypercoagulable state associated with increased cardiovascular risk. As cytokine induction may be a function of several identifiable factors such as dialysis membrane biocompatability, contamination of dialysate water with microbial products, and/or complement activation, the potential for effective prevention appears to be good. Furthermore, with the development of cytokine-blocking agents or inhibitors such as IL-1 receptor antagonists and soluble TNF receptors, cytokine-mediated diseases may become specifically treatable. However, to better understand the complex relationships between oxidation endothelial dysfunction, hemostatic abnormalities and inflammation, their modulating influence on lipoprotein metabolism as well as their involvement in the pathogenesis of vascular injury will require additional investigative work. Moreover, without the benefit of data from prospective, randomized clinical trails in CRF patients the management of dyslipoproteinemia will continue to be based on extrapolation and inference.

REFERENCES

1. Appel G. Lipid abnormalities in renal disease. Kidney Int 1991; 39:169–183.
2. Attman P-O, Alaupovic P. Lipid abnormalities in chronic renal insufficiency. Kidney Int 1991; 39(suppl):S16–S23.
3. Attman P-O, Samuelsson O, Alaupovic P. Lipoprotein metabolism and renal failure. Amer J Kidney Dis 1993; 21(6):573–592.
4. Attman P-O, Samuelsson O, Alapovic P. Lipid Abnormalities in Progressive Renal Insufficiency. Contrib Nephrol 1997; 120:1–10.
5. Mahley RW. Biochemistry and physiology of lipid and lipoprotein metabolism. In: Becker KL, ed. Principles and Practice of Endocrinology and Metabolism. Philadelphia: JB Lippincott, 1995:1369–1378.
6. Grundy SM. Disorders of lipids and lipoproteins. In: Stein JH, ed. Internal Medicine. St. Louis: Mosby, 1994:1436–1456.
7. Brewer HB, Santamarina-Fojo S, Hoeg JM. Disorders of lipoprotein metabolism. In: De Groot LJ, ed. Endocrinology. Philadelphia: Saunders, 1995:2731–2752.
8. Scanu AM. Physiopathology of plasma lipoprotein metabolism. Kidney Int 1991; 31:S3–S7.
9. Llingworth DR. Lipoprotein metabolism. Am J Kidney Dis 1993; 22(1):90–97.
10. Havel RJ, Kane JP. Introduction: structure and metabolism of plasma lipoproteins. In Scriver CR, Beaudet AL, Sly WS, Valle D, eds. The Metabolic and Molecular Basis of Inherited Disease. New York: McGraw-Hill, 1995:1841–1851.
11. Utermann G. The mysteries of lipoprotein(a). Science 1989; 246:904–910.
12. Mahley RW. Atherogenic lipoproteins and coronary artery disease: concepts derived from recent advances in cellular and molecular biology. Circ 1985; 72:943–948.

13. Glomset JA, Norum KR. The metabolic role of lecithin cholesterol acyltransferase: perspectives from pathology. Adv Lipid Res 1973; 11:1–65.
14. Powell LM, Wallis SC, Pease RJ, Edwards YH, Knott TJ, Scott J. A novel form of tissue-specific RNA processing produces apoprotein B-48 in intestine. Cell 1987; 50:831–840.
15. Mahley RW, Hussain MM. Chylomicron and chylomicron-remnant catabolism. Curr Opinion Lipidol 1991; 2:170–175.
16. Brown BG, Zhao XQ, Sacco DE, Albers JJ. Lipid lowering and plaque regression. New insights into prevention of plaque disruption and clinical events in coronary disease. Circulation 1993; 87:1781–1791.
17. Grutzmacher P, Marz W, Peschke B, Gross W, Schoeppe W. Lipoproteins and apolipoproteins during the progression of chronic renal disease. Nephron 1988; 50:103–111.
18. Attman P-O, Alaupovic P. Lipid and apolipoprotein profiles of uremic dyslipoproteinemia: relation to renal function and dialysis. Nephron 1991; 57(4):401–410.
19. Utermann G. Lipoprotein(a). In: Scriver CR, Beaudet AL, Sly WS, Valle D, eds. The Metabolic and Molecular Bases of Inherited Disease. New York: McGraw-Hill, 1995:1887–1912.
20. Scanu AM, Lawn RM, Berg K. Lipoprotein(a) and atherosclerosis. Ann Intern Med 1991; 115:209–218.
21. Scanu AM, Fless GM. Lipoprotein(a): heterogeneity and biological relevance. J Clin Invest 1990;85:1709–1715.
22. Scanu AM. Lipoprotein(a): a genetic risk factor for premature coronary heart disease. JAMA 1992; 267: 3326–3329.
23. Disorders of lipid metabolism. In: Dale DC, Federman DD eds. Scientific American Medicine. New York: Scientific American, 1997:1–24.
24. Mahley RW, Hussain MM. Chylomicron and chylomicron remnant catabolism. Curr Opin Lipidol 1991; 2:170–176.
25. Young SG. Recent progress in understanding apolipoprotein B. Circulation 1990; 82:1574–1594.
26. Kowal RC, Herz J, Goldstein JL, Esser V, Brown MS. Low density lipoprotein receptor-related protein mediates uptake of cholesterol esters derived from apoprotein E-enriched lipoproteins. Proc Natl Acad Sci USA 1989; 86:5810–5814.
27. Brown MS, Goldstein JL. A receptor-mediated pathway for cholesterol homeostasis. Science 1986; 232: 34–37.
28. Takahasi S, Kawarabayasi Y, Nakai T, Sakai J, Yamamoto T. Rabbit very low density lipoprotein receptor: a low density lipoprotein receptor-like protein with distinct ligand specificity. Proc Natl Acad Sci USA 1992; 89:9252–9256.
29. Sakai J, Hoshino A, Takahashi S, Miura Y, Ishii H, Susuki H, Kawarabayahi Y, Yamamoto T. Structure, chromosome location, and expression of the human very low density lipoprotein receptor gene. J Bio Chem 1994; 269:2173–2182.
30. Sudhof TC, Goldstein JL, Brown MS, Russell DW. The LDL receptor gene: a mosaic of exons shared with different proteins. Science 1985; 228:815–822.
31. Goldstein JL, Brown MS. The low-density lipoprotein pathway and its relation to atherosclerosis. Annu Rev Biochem 1977; 46:897–930.
32. Oka K, Tzung KW, Sullivan M, Lindsay E, Baldini A, Chan L. Human very-low-density lipoprotein receptor complementary DNA and deduced amino acid sequence and localization of its gene (VLDLR) to chromosome band 9p24 by fluorescence in situ hybridization. Genomics 1994; 20:298–300.
33. Webb JC, Patel DD, Jones MD, Knight BL, Soutar AK. Characterization and tissue-specific expression of the human 'very low density lipoprotein (VLDL) receptor' mRNA. Hum Mol Gen 1994; 3:531–537.
34. Gafvels ME, Caird M, Britt D, Jackson CL, Patterson D, Strauss JF III: Cloning of a cDNA encoding a putative human very low density lipoprotein/apolipoprotein E receptor and assignment of the gene to chromosome 9pter-p23. Somatic Cell Mol Genet 1993; 19: 557–569.
35. Auwerz J, Leroy P, Schoonjans K. Lipoprotein lipase: recent contributions from molecular biology. Crit Rev Clin Lab Sci 1992; 29:243–268.
36. Tall AR. Plasma high density lipoproteins. Metabolism and relationship to atherogenesis. J Clin Invest 1990; 86:379–384.
37. Gwynne JT. HDL and atherosclerosis: an update. Clin Cardiol 1991; 4(2 suppl 1):117–124.
38. Kane JP, Havel RJ. Disorders of biogenesis and secretion of lipoproteins containing the B apolipoproteins. Scriver CR, Beaudet AL, Sly WS, Valle D, eds. The Metabolic and Molecular Bases of Inherited Disease. New York: McGraw-Hill, 1995:1887–1912.
39. Breslow JL. Familial disorders of high-density lipoprotein metabolism. In: Scriver CR, Beaudet AL, Sly WS, Valle D, eds. The Metabolic and Molecular Bases of Inherited Disease. New York: McGraw-Hill, 1995: 2031–2052.
40. Castelli WP, Garrison RJ, Wilson PW, Abbott RF, Kalousdian S, Kannel WB. Incidence of coronary heart disease and lipoprotein cholesterol levels. The Framingham Study. JAMA 1986; 256:2835–2838.
41. Rifkind BM. High-density lipoprotein cholesterol and coronary artery disease: survey of the evidence. Am J Cardiol 1990; 66:3A-6A.
42. Gordon DJ, Knoke J, Probstfield JL, Superko R, Tryoler HA. High-density lipoprotein cholesterol and coronary heart disease in hypercholesterolemic men: the Lipid Research Clinics Coronary Primary Prevention Trial. Circ 1986; 74:217–225.
43. Wood PD, Williams PT, Haskell WL. Physical activity and high-density lipoproteins. In: Miller NE, Miller

GJ, eds. Clinical and Metabolic Aspects of High Density Lipoproteins. Amsterdam: Elsevier, 1984:133–152.
44. Pietinen P, Huttunen JK. Dietary determinants of plasma high-density lipoprotein cholesterol. Am Heart J 1987; 133(2 Pt 2):620–625.
45. Parthasarathy S, Barnett J, Fong LG. High-density lipoproteins inhibits the oxidative modification of low-density lipoprotein. Biochim Biophys Acta 1990; 1044:275–283.
46. Khoo JC, Miller E, McLoughlin P, Steinberg D. Prevention of low density lipoprotein aggregation by high density lipoprotein of apolipoprotein A-I. J Lipid Res 1990; 31:645–652.
47. Jones PH, Grundy SM, Gotto AM Jr. Assessment and management of lipid abnormalities. In: Alexander RW, Schlant RC, Fuster V, eds. Hurst's The Heart Arteries and Veins. New York: McGraw-Hill, 1998:1553–1581.
48. Stamler J, Wentworth D, Neaton JD. Is the relationship between serum cholesterol and risk of premature death from coronary disease continuous and graded ? findings in 356,222 primary screenees of the Multiple Risk Factor Intervention Trial (MRFIT). JAMA 1986; 256:2823–2828.
49. The Expert Panel. Report of the National Cholesterol Education Program Expert Panel on Detection, Evaluation, and Treatment of High Blood Cholesterol in Adults. Arch Intern Med 1988; 148:36–69.
50. The Expert Panel. Second Report of the Expert Panel on Detection, Evaluation and Treatment of High Blood Cholesterol in Adults. NIH publication No a3–3095. Bethesda, MD: U.S. Department of Health and Human Services, 1993.
51. Maron DJ, Ridker PM, Pearson TA. Risk factors and the prevention of coronary heart disease. In: Alexander RW, Schlant RC, Fuster V eds. Hurst's The Heart Arteries and Veins. New York: McGraw-Hill, 1998: 1175–1195.
52. Chan MK, Varghese Z, Moorhead JF. Lipid abnormalities in uremia, dialysis and transplantation. Kidney Int 1981; 19:625–637.
53. Nestel PJ, Fidge NH, Tan MH. Increased lipoprotein-remnant formation in chronic renal failure. N Engl J Med 1982; 307:329–333.
54. Weintraub M, Burstein A, Rassin T, Liron M, Ringel Y, Cabili S, Blum M, Peer G, Iaina A. Severe defect in clearing postprandial chylomicron remnants in dialysis patients. Kidney Int 1992; 42:1247–1252.
55. Oda H, Yorioka N, Okushin S, Nishida Y, Kushihata S, Ito T, Yamakido M. Remnant-like particle cholesterol may indicate atherogenic risk in patients on chronic hemodialysis. Nephron 1997; 76: 7–14.
56. Attman P-O, Alaupovic P, Travella M, Knight-Gibson C. Abnormal lipid and apolipoprotein composition of major lipoprotein density classes in patients with chronic renal failure. Nephrol Dial Transplant 1996; 11:63–69.
57. Joven J, Vilella E, Ahmad S, Cheung MC, Brunzell JD. Lipoprotein heterogeneity in end-stage renal disease. Kidney Int 1993; 43: 410–418.
58. Horkko S, Huttunen K, Korhonen T, Kesaniemi Y. Decreased clearance of low-density lipoprotein in patients with chronic renal failure. Kidney Int 1994; 45: 561–570.
59. Shoji T, Nishizawa Y, Nishitani H, Yamakawa M, Morii H. Impaired metabolism of high density lipoprotein in uremic patients. Kidney Int 1992; 41:1653–1661.
60. Senti M, Romero R, Pedro-Botet J, Pelegri A, Nogues X, Rubies-Prat J. Lipoprotein abnormalities in hyperlipidemic and normolipidemic men on hemodialysis with chronic renal failure. Kidney Int 1992; 41:1394–1399.
61. Kronenberg F, Utermann G, Dieplinger H. Lipoprotein(a) in renal disease. Am J Kidney Dis 1996; 27(1): 1–25.
62. Levine DM, Gordon BR. Lipoprotein(a) levels in patients receiving renal replacement therapy: methodologic issues and clinical implications. Am J Kidney Dis 1995; 26(1):162–169.
63. Webb AT, Reavely DA, O'Donnell M, O'Connor B, Seed M, Brown EA. Lipids and lipoprotein(a) as risk factors for vascular disease in patients on renal replacement therapy. Neph Dial Transplant 1995; 10: 354–357.
64. Shoji T, Nishizawa Y, Nishitani H, Yamakawa M, Morii H. High serum lipoprotein(a) concentraions in uremic patients treated with continuous ambulatory peritoneal dialysis. Clin Nephrol 1992; 38(5):271–276.
65. Cressman MD, Heyka RJ, Paganini EP, O'Neil J, Skibinski CI, Hoff HF. Lipoprotein(a) is an independent risk factor for cardiovascular disease in hemodialysis patients. Circ 1992; 86(2):475–482.
66. Attman P-O, Alanpovic P, Gustafson A. Serum apolipoprotein profile of patients with chronic renal failure. Kidney Int 1987; 32:368–375.
67. Ohta T, Hattori S, Nishiyama S, Higashi A, Matsuda I. Quantitative and qualitative changes of apolipoprotein A I-containing lipoproteins in patients on continuous ambulatory peritoneal dialysis. Metabolism 1989; 38(9):843–849.
68. Robert D, Jeanmonod R, Favre H, Fruchart JC, Sturzenegger E, Riesen W. Changes in lipoproteins induced by the remnant kidney tissue or binephrectomy in chronic uremic patients treated by hemodialysis. Metabolism 1989; 38(6):514–521.
69. Alsayed N, Rebourcet R. Abnormal concentrations of CII, CIII, and E apolipoproteins among apolipoprotein B-containing, B-free and A-I-containing lipoprotein particles in hemodialysis patients. Clin Chem 1991; 37(3):387–393.

70. Avram MM, Goldwasser P, Burrell DE, Antignani A, Fein PA, Mittman N. The uremic dyslipidemia: a cross-sectional and longitudinal study. Am J Kidney Dis 1992; 20(4):324–335.
71. Oda H, Keane WF. Lipid abnormalities in end stage renal disease. Nephrol Dial Transplant 1998; 13(suppl 1):45–49.
72. Cassadev M, Ruiu G, Tagliaferro V, Triolo G, Pagano G. Lipoprotein and apoprotein levels in different types of dialysis. Int J Artif Organs 1989; 12:433–438.
73. Atger V, Beyne P, Frommherz K, Roullet JB, Drueke T. Presence of apo B-48 and relative apo C-II deficiency and apo C-III enrichment in uremic very-low density lipoproteins. Ann Biol Clin 1989; 47:497–501.
74. Chan MK, Varghese Z, Persaud JW, Baillod RA, Moorhead JF. Hyperlipidemia in patients on maintenance hemo-and peritoneal dialysis: the relative pathogenetic roles of triglyceride production and triglyceride removal. Clin Nephrol 1982; 17(4):183–190.
75. Dieplinger H, Schoenfeld PY, Fielding CJ. Plasma cholesterol metabolism in end-stage renal disease Difference between treatment by hemodialysis or peritoneal dialysis. J Clin Invest 1986; 77:1071–1083.
76. Bagdade J, Casaretto A, Albers J. Effects of chronic uremia, hemodialysis, and renal transplantation on plasma lipids and lipoproteins in man. J Lab Clin Med 1976; 87(1):38–48.
77. Huttunen JK, Pasternack A, Vanttinen T, Ehnholm C, Nikkila EA. Lipoprotein metabolism in patients with chronic uremia. Effect of hemodialysis on serum lipoproteins and postheparin plasma triglyceride lipases. Act Med Scand 1978; 204:211–218.
78. Chan MK, Persaud J, Varghese Z, Moorhead JF. Pathogenic roles of post-heparin lipases in lipid abnormalities in hemodialysis patients. Kidney Int 1984; 25: 812–818.
79. Savdie E, Gibson JC, Crawford GA, Simons LA, Mahony JF. Impaired plasma triglyceride clearance as a feature of both uremic and posttransplant triglyceridemia. Kidney Int 1980; 18:774–782.
80. Roullet JB, Lacour B, Yvert JP, Prat JJ, Drueke T. Factors that increase serum triglyceride-rich lipoproteins in uremic rats. Kidney Int 1985; 27:420–425.
81. Applebaum-Bowden D, Goldberg AP, Hazzard WR, Sherrard DJ, Brunzell JD, Huttunen JK, Nikkila EA, Ehnholm C. Postheparin plasma triglyceride lipases in chronic hemodialysis: evidence for a role for hepatic lipase in lipoprotein metabolism. Metabolism 1979; 28:917–924.
82. Akmal M, Kasim SE, Soliman AR, Massry SG. Excess parathyroid hormone adversely affects lipid metabolism in chronic renal failure. Kidney Int 1990; 37: 854–858.
83. McCosh EJ, Solangi K, Rivers JM, Goodman A. Hypertriglyceridemia in patients with chronic renal insufficiency. Am J Clin Nutr 1975; 28:1036–1043.
84. Mordasini R, Frey F, Flury W, Klose G, Greten H. Selective deficiency of hepatic triglyceride lipase in uremic patients. N Engl J Med 1977; 297:1362–1366.
85. Sakurai T, Oka T, Hasegawa H, Igaki N, Miki S, Goto T. Comparison of lipids, apoproteins and associated enzyme activities between diabetic and nondiabetic end-stage renal disease. Nephron 1992; 61:409–414.
86. Cheung AK, Parker CJ, Ren K, Iverius PH. Increased lipase inhibition in uremia: identification of pre-beta-HDL as a major inhibitor in normal and uremic plasma. Kidney Int 1996; 49:1360–1371.
87. Klin M, Smogorzewski M, Ni Z, Zhang G, Massry SG. Abnormalities in hepatic lipase in chronic renal failure: role of excess parathyroid hormone. J Clin Invest 1996; 97:2167–2173.
88. Akmal MS, Perkins S, Kasim SE, Oh H-Y, Smogorzewski M, Massry SG. Verapamil prevents chronic renal failure-induced abnormalities in lipid metabolism. Am J Kidney Dis 1993; 22:158–163.
89. Roullet JB, Lacour B, Yvert J-P, Drueke T. Correction by insulin of disturbed TG-rich LP metabolism in rats with chronic renal failure. Am J Physiol 1986; 250(4 Pt 1):E373–E376.
90. Schrader J, Stibbe W, Armstrong VW, Kandt M, Muche R, Kostering H, Seidel D, Scheler F. Comparison of low molecular weight heparin to standard heparin in hemodialysis/hemofiltration. Kidney Int 1988; 33: 890–896.
91. Deuber HJ, Schulz W. Reduced lipid concentrations during four years of dialysis with low molecular weight heparin. Kidney Int 1991; 40:496–500.
92. Bergesio F, Monzani G, Ciuti R, Serruto A, Benucci A, Frizzi V, Salvadori M. Lipids and apolipoproteins change during the progression of chronic renal failure. Clin Nephrol 1992; 38:264–270.
93. Holdsworth G, Stocks J, Dodson P, Galton DJ. An abnormal triglyceride-rich lipoprotein containing excess sialylated apolipoprotein C-III. J Clin Invest 1982; 69:932–939.
94. Glass CK, Pittman RC, Keller GA, Steinberg D. Tissue sites of degradation of apolipoprotein A-I in the rat. J Biol Chem 1983; 258:7161–7167.
95. Horowitz BS, Goldberg IJ, Merab J, Vanni TM, Ramakrishnan R, Ginsberg HN. Increased plasma and renal clearance of an exchangeable pool of apolipoprotein A-I in subjects with low levels of high density lipoprotein cholesterol. J Clin Invest 1993; 91:1743–1752.
96. Neary RH, Gowland E. The effect of renal failure and haemodialysis on the concentration of free apolipoprotein A-1 in serum and the implications for the catabolism of high-density lipoproteins. Clin Chem Acta 1988; 171:239–245.
97. Vaziri ND, Liang K. Down-regulation of tissue lipoprotein lipase expression in experimental chronic renal failure. Kidney Int 1996; 50:1928–1935.

98. Vaziri, ND, Wang XQ, Liang K. Secondary hyperparathyroidism downregulates lipoprotein lipase expression in chronic renal failure. Am J Physiol 1997; 273: F925–F930.
99. Henck CC, Liersch M, Ritz E, Stegmeier K, Wirth A, Mehls O. Hyperlipoproteinemia in experimental chronic renal insufficiency in the rat. Kidney Int 1978; 14:142–150.
100. Ljunghall S, Lithell H, Vessby B, Wide L. Glucose and lipoprotein metabolism in primary hyperparathyroidism: effects of parathyroidectomy. Acta Endocrinol 1978; 89:580–589.
101. Lacour B, Roullet JB, Liagre AM, Jorgetti V, Beyne P, Dubost C, Drueke T. Serum lipoprotein disturbances in primary and secondary hyperparathyroidism and effects of parathyroidectomy. Am J Kidney Dis 1986; 8: 422–429.
102. Klin M, Smogorzewski M, Khilnani M, Michnowska M, Massry SG. Mechanism of PTH-induced rise in cytosolic calcium in adult rat hepatocytes. Am J Physiol 1994; 267:G754–G763.
103. Guarnieri GF, Moracchiello M, Campanacci L, Ursini F, Ferri L, Valente M, Gregolin C. Lecithin-cholesterol acyl transferase (LCAT) activity in chronic uremia. Kidney Int 1978; 13(suppl):S26–S30.
104. McLeod R, Reeve CE, Frohlich J. Plasma lipoproteins and lecithin: cholesterol acyltransferase distribution in patients on dialysis. Kidney Int 1984; 25:683–688.
105. Horkko S, Huttunen K, Kervinenk K, Kesaniemi YA. Decreased clearance of uraemic and mildly carbamylated low-density lipoprotein. Eur J Clin Invest 1994; 24:105–113.
106. Attman P-O, Alaupovic P, Knight-Gibson C, Tavella M. The compositional abnormalities in lipoprotein density classes of patients with chronic renal failure (CRF) (abstr). Am J Kidney Dis 1989; 14:432.
107. Windler E, Havel RJ. Inhibitory effects of C apolipoproteins from rats and humans on the uptake of triglyceride-rich lipoproteins and their remnants by the perfused rat liver. J Lipid Res 1985; 26:556–565.
108. Gonen B, Goldberg AP, Harter HR, Schonfeld G. Abnormal cell-interactive properties of low-density lipoproteins isolated from patients with chronic renal failure. Metabolism 1985; 34:10–14.
109. Vaziri ND, Liang K. Down regulation of VLDL receptor expression in chronic experimental renal failure. Kidney Int 1997; 51:913–919.
110. Liang K, Oveisi F, Vaziri ND. Role of secondary hyperparathyroidism in the genesis of hypertriglyceridemia and VLDL receptor deficiency in chronic renal failure. Kidney Int 1998; 53:626–630.
111. Bagdade JD, Porte D Jr, Bierman EL. Hypertriglyceridemia. A metabolic consequence of chronic renal failure. N Engl J Med 1968; 279:181–185.
112. Attman P-O, Gustafson A. Lipid and carbohydrate metabolism in uraemia. Eur J Clin Invest 1979; 9:285–291.
113. Horkko S, Savolainen MJ, Kervinen K, Kesaniemi YA. Carbamylation-induced alterations in low-density lipoprotein metabolism. Kidney Int 1992; 41:1175–1181.
114. Portman J, Scott RC III, Rogers DD, Loose-Mitchell DS, Lemire JM, Weinberg RB. Decreased low-density lipoprotein receptor function and mRNA levels in lymphocytes from uremic patients. Kidney Int 1992; 42:1238–1246.
115. Kronenberg F, Konig P, Neyer U, Auinger M, Pribasnig A, Lang U, Reitinger J, Pinter G, Utermann G, Dieplinger H. Multicenter study of lipoprotein(a) and apolipoprotein(a) phenotypes in patients with end-stage renal disease treated by hemodialysis or continuous ambulatory peritoneal dialysis. J Am Soc Nephrol 1995; 6:110–120.
116. Murray JC, Buetow KH, Donovan M, Hornung S, Motulsky AG, Disteche C, Dyer K, Swisshelm K, Anderson J, Giblett E, Sadler E, Eddy R, Shows TB. Linkage disequilibrim of plasminogen polymorphisms and assignment of the gene to human chromosome 6q26-6q27. Am J Hum Gent 1987; 40:338–350.
117. Kronenberg F, Konig P, Lhotta K, Ofner D, Sandholzer C, Margreiter R, Dosch E, Utermann G, Dieplinger H. Apolipoprotein(a) phenotype associated decrease in lipoprotein(a) plasma concentrations after renal transplantation. Arterioscler Thromb 1994; 14:1399–1404.
118. Azrolan N, Brown CD, Thomas L, Hayek T, Zhao ZH, Roberts KG, Scheiner C, Friedman EA. Cyclosporin A has divergent effects on plasma LDL cholesterol (LDL-C) and lipoprotein(a) [Lp(a)] levels in renal transplant recipients. Evidence for renal involvement in the maintenance of LDL-C and the elevation of Lp(a) concentrations in hemodialysis patients. Arterioscler Thromb 1994; 14:1393–1398.
119. Black IW, Wilcken DEL. Decreases in apoplipoprotein(a) after renal transplantation: implications for lipoprotein(a) metabolism. Clin Chem 1992; 38:353–357.
120. Murphy BG, McNamee PT. Apolipoprotein(a) concentration decreases following renal transplantation. Nephrol Dial Transplant 1992; 7:174–175.
121. Kronenberg F, Konig P, Lhotta K, Konigsrainer A, Sandholzer C, Utermann G, Dieplinger H. Cycloporin and serum lipids in renal transplant recipients. Lancet 1993; 341:765.
122. Kario K, Matsuo T, Kobayashi H, Matsuo M, Asada R, Koide M. High lipoprotein(a) levels in chronic hemodialysis patients are closely related to the acute phase reaction. Throm Haemostasis 1995; 74:1020–1024.
123. Zheng G, Bachinsky DR, Stamenkovic I, Strickland DK, Brown D, Andres G, McCluskey RT. Organ distribution in rats of two members of the low-density lipoprotein receptor gene family, gp330 and LRP/alpha 2MR, and the receptor-associated protein (RAP). J Histochem Cytochem 1994; 42:531–542.

124. Marz W. Beckmann A, Scharnagl H, Siekmeier R, Mondorf U, Held I, Schneider W, Preissner KT, Curtiss LK, Gross W, Huttinger M. Heterogeneous lipoprotein(a) size isoforms differ by their interaction with the low density lipoprotein receptor and the low density lipoprotein receptor-related protein/a_2-macroglobulin receptor. FEBS Lett 1993; 325:271–275.
125. Sigurdsson G, Baldursdottir A, Sigvaldason H, Agnarsson U, Thorgeirsson G, Sigfussson N. Predictive value of apolipoproteins in a prospective survey of coronary artery disease in men. Am J Cardiol 1992; 69:1251–1254.
126. Wald NJ, Law M, Watt HC, Wu TS, Bailey A, Johnson AM, Craig WY, Ledue TB, Haddow JE. Apolipoproteins and ischaemic heart disease: implications for screening. Lancet 1994; 343:75–79.
127. Schaefer EJ, Lamon-Fava S, Jenner JL, McNamara JR, Ordovas JM, Davis CE, Abolafia JM, Lippel K, Levy RI. Lipoprotein(a) levels and risk of coronary heart disease in men. The Lipid Research Clinics Coronary Primary Prevention Trail. JAMA 1994; 271: 999–1003.
128. Dahlen G. The pre-beta lipoprotein phenomenon in relation to serum cholesterol and triglyceride levels, the Lp(a) lipoprotein and coronary heart disease. Acta Med Scand 1974; 570(suppl):1–45.
129. Kostner GM, Avogaro P, Cazzolato G, Marth E, Bittolo-Bon G, Qunici GB. Lipoprotein Lp(a) and the risk for myocardial infarction. Atherosclerosis 1981; 38:51–61.
130. Sandkamp M, Funke H, Schulte H, Kohler E, Assmann G. Lipoprotein(a) is an independent risk factor for myocardial infarction at a young age. Clin Chem 1990; 36:20–23.
131. Dahlen GH, Guyton JR, Attar M, Farmer JA, Kautz JA, Gotto AM Jr. Association of levels of lipoprotein Lp(a), plasma lipids, and other lipoproteins with coronary artery disease documented by angiography. Circulation 1986; 74:758–765.
132. Armstrong VW, Cremer P, Eberle E, Manke A, Schulze F, Wieland H, Kreuzer H, Seidel D. The association between serum Lp(a) concentrations and angiographically assessed coronary atherosclerosis. Dependence on serum LDL levels. Atherosclerosis 1986; 62:249–257.
133. Genest J Jr, Jenner JL, McNamara JR, Ordovas JM, Silberman SR, Wilson PWF, Schaefer EJ. Prevalence of lipoprotein(a) [Lp(a)] excess in coronary artery disease. Am J Cardiol 1991; 67:1039–1045.
134. Orskov H, Christensen NJ. Growth hormone in uremia: I. Plasma growth hormone, insulin and glucagon after oral and intravenous glucose in uremic subjects. Scand J Clin Lab Invest 1971; 27:51–60.
135. Bonomini V, Orsoni G, Sorrentino MA, Todeschini P. Hormonal changes in hemodialysis. Blood Purif 1990; 8:54–57.
136. Ferraris JR, Domene HM, Escobar ME, et al. Hormonal profile in pubertal females with chronic renal failure: before and under haemodialysis and after renal transplantation. Acta Endocrinol 1987; 115:289–291.
137. Gomez F, De La Cueva R, Wauters JP, Lemarchand-Beraud T. Endocrine abnormalities in patients undergoing long-term hemodialysis: the role of prolactin. Am J Med 1980; 68:522–525.
138. Nagel TC, Freinkel N, Bell RH. Gynecomastia, prolactin and other peptide hormones in patients undergoing chronic hemodialysis. J Clin Endocrinol Metab 1973; 36:428–431.
139. Belchetz PE. Hormonal treatment of postmenopausal women. N Engl J Med 1994; 330:1962–1971.
140. Liang K, Vaziri ND. Gene expression of LDL receptor, HMG-CoA reductase and cholesterol-7-(-hydroxylase in chronic renal failure. Nephrol Dial Transplant 1997; 12:1381–1386.
141. Alaupovic P, Tavella M, Bard JM, Wang CS, Attman PO, Koren E, Croder C, Knight-Gibson C, Downs D. Lipoprotein particles in hypertriglyceridemic states. Adv Exp Med Biol 1988; 243:289–297.
142. Vlassara H. Serum advanced glycosylation end produts: a new class of uremic toxins? Blood Purif 1994; 12:54–59.
143. Maggi E, Bellazzi R, Falaschi F, Frattoni A, Perani G, Finardi G, Gazo A, Nai M, Romanini D, Bellomo G. Enhanced LDL oxidation in uremic patients: an additional mechanism for accelerated atherosclerosis? Kidney Int 1994; 45:876–883.
144. Jackson P, Loughrey CM, Lightbody JH, McNamee PT, Young IS. Effect of hemodialysis on total antioxidant capacity and serum antioxidants in patients with chronic renal failure. Clin Chem 1995; 41:1135–1138.
145. Jain SK, Abreo K, Duett J, Sella ML. Lipofuscin products, lipid peroxides and aluminum accumulation in red blood cells of hemodialyzed patients. Am J Nephrol 1995; 15:306–311.
146. Itabe H, Yamamoto H, Imanaka T, Shimamura K, Uchiyama H, Kimura J, Sanaka T, Hata Y, Takano T. Sensitive detection of oxidatively modified low density lipoprotein using a monoclonal antibody. J Lipid Res 1996; 37:45–53.
147. Maggi E, Bellazzi R, Gazo A, Seccia M, Bellomo G. Autoantibodies against oxidatively-modified LDL in uremic patients undergoing dialysis. Kidney Int 1994; 46:869–876.
148. Becker BN, Himmelfarb J, Henrich W, Hakim RM. Reassessing the cardiac risk profile in chronic hemodialysis patients: a hypothesis on the role of oxidant stress and other non-traditional cardiac risk factors. J Am Soc Nephrol 1997; 8:475–486.
149. Steinberg D, Parthasarathy S, Carew TE, Khoo JC, Witztum JL. Beyond cholesterol. Modifications of low-density lipoprotein that increase its atherogenicity. N Engl J Med 1989; 320:915–924.

150. Hogan M, Cerami A, Bucala R. Advanced glycosylation end products block the antiproliferative effect of nitric oxide. Role in the vascular and renal complications of diabetes mellitus. J Clin Invest 1992; 90: 1110–1115.
151. Palinski W, Koschinsky T, Butler SW, Miller E, Vlassara H, Cerami A, Witzum JL. Immunological evidence for the presence of advanced glycosylation end products in atherosclerotic lesions of euglycemic rabbits. Arterioscler Thromb Vasc Biol 1995; 15:571–582.
152. Vacha GM, Giorcelli G, Siliprandi N, Corsi M. Favorable effects of L-carnitine treatment on hypertriglyceridemia in hemodialysis patients: decisive role of low levels of high-density lipoprotein-cholesterol. Am J Clin Nutrition 1983; 38:532–540.
153. Wanner C, Wieland H, Wackerle B, Boeckle H, Schollmeyer P, Horl WH. Ketogenic and antiketogenic effects of L-carnitine in hemodialysis patients. Kidney Int 1989; 36:264–268.
154. Ahmad S, Dasgupta A, Kenny MA. Fatty acid abnormalities in hemodialysis patients: effects of L-carnitine administration. Kidney Int 1989; 36:243–246.
155. Maeda K, Shinzato T, Kobayakawa H. Effects of L-carnitine administration on short-chain fatty acid (acetic acid) and long-chain fatty acid metabolism during hemodialysis. Nephron 1989; 51:355–361.
156. Golper TA, Ahmad S. L-carnitine administration to hemodialysis patients: has its time come? Seminars in Dialysis 1992; 5(2):94–98.
157. Wanner C, Forstner-Wanner S, Rossle C, Furst P, Schollmeyer P, Horl WH. Carnitine metabolism in patients with chronic renal failure: effect of L-carnitine supplementation. Kidney Int 1987; 32:132–135.
158. Bartel LL, Hussey JL, Shrago E. Pertubation of serum carnitine levels in human adults by chronic renal disease and dialysis therapy. Am J Clin Nutr 1981; 34: 1314–1320.
159. Leschke M, Rumpf KW, Eisenhauer T, Fuchs C, Becker K, Kothe U, Scheler F. Quantitative assessment of carnitine loss during hemodialysis and hemofiltration. Kidney Int 1983; 24:143–146.
160. Golper TA, Wolfson M, Ahmad S, Hirschberg R, Kurtin P, Katz LA, Nicora R, Ashbrook DW, Kopple JD. Multicenter trial of L-carnitine in maintenance hemodialysis patients. I. Carnitine concentrations and lipid effects. Kidney Int 1990; 38:904–911.
161. Moorthy AV, Rosenblum M, Rajaram R, Shug AL. A comparison of plasma and muscle carnitine levels in patients on peritoneal or hemodialysis for chronic renal failure. Am J Nephrol 1983; 3:205–208.
162. Wanner C, Forstner-Wanner S, Schaeffer G, Schollmeyer P, Horl WH. Serum free carnitine, carnitine esters and lipids in patients on peritoneal dialysis and hemodialysis. Am J Nephrol 1986; 6:206–211.
163. Dinarello CA. Cytokines: Agents provocateurs in hemodialysis? Kidney Int 1992; 41:683–694.
164. van Ypersele de Strihou C. Are biocompatible membranes superior for hemodialysis therapy? Kidney Int 1997; 62:S-101–S-104.
165. Bingel M, Lonnemann G, Shaldon S, Koch KM, Dinarello CA. Human interleukin-1 production during hemodialysis. Nephron 1986; 43:161–163.
166. Lonnemann G, Bingel M, Floege J, Koch KM, Shaldon S, Cinarello CA. Detection of endotoxin-like interleukin-1-inducing activity during in vitro dialysis. Kidney Int 1988; 33:29–35.
167. Loppnow H, Brade H, Durrbaum I, Dinarello CA, Kusumoto S, Rietschel ET, Flad HD. IL-1 induction-capacity of defined lipopolysaccharide partial structures. J Immunol 1989; 142:3229–3238.
168. Grone HJ, Walli AK, Grone EF. The role of oxidatively modified lipoproteins in lipid nephropathy. Contrib Nephrol 1997; 120:160–175.
169. Roselaar SE, Nazhat NB, Winyard PG, Jones P, Cunningham J, Blake DR. Detection of oxidants in uremic plasma by electron spin resonance spectroscopy. Kidney Int 1995; 48:199–206.
170. Witko-Sarat V, Friedlander M, Capeillere-Blandin C, Nguyen-Khoa AT, Nguyen A, Zingraff J, Jungers P, Descamps-Latscha B. Advanced oxidation protein products as a novel marker of oxidative stress in uremia. Kidney Int 1996; 49:1304–1313.
171. Price SR, Mitch WE. Metabolic acidosis and uremic toxicity: protein and amino acid metabolism. Semin Nephrol 1994; 14:232–237.
172. Galle J, Wanner C. Oxidative stress and vascular injury-relevant for atherogenesis in uraemic patients? Nephrol Dial Transplant 1997; 12:2480–2483.
173. Kumano K, Yokota S, Go M, Suyama K, Sakai T, Era S, Sogami M. Quantitative and qualitative changes of serum albumin in CAPD patients. Adv Perit Dial 1992; 8:127–130.
174. Canestrari F, Galli F, Giorgini A, Albertini MC, Galiotta P, Pascucci M, Bossu M. Erthrocyte redox state in uremic anemia: effects of hemodialysis and relevance of glutathione metabolism. Acta Haematol 1994; 91:187–193.
175. Yeung JH. Effects of glycerol-induced acute renal failure on tissue glutathione and glutathione-dependent enzymes in the rat. Meth Find Exp Clin Pharmacol 1991; 13:23–28.
176. Miyata T, Wada Y, Cai Z, Iida Y, Horie K, Yasuda Y, Maeda K, Kurokawa K, van Ypersele de Strihou C. Implication of an increased oxidative stress in the formation of advanced glycation end products in patients with end-stage renal failure. Kidney Int 1997; 51: 1170–1181.
177. Miyata T, Udea Y, Shinzato T, Iida Y, Tanaka S, Kurokawa K, van Ypersele de Strihou C, Maeda K. Accumulation of albumin-linked and free-form pentosidine in the circulation of uremic patients with end-stage renal failure: renal implications in the path-

ophysiology of pentosidine. J Am Soc Nephrol 1996; 7:1198–1206.

178. Miyata T, Maeda K, Kurokawa K, van Ypersele de Strihou C. Oxidation conspires with glycation to generate noxious advanced glycation end products in renal failure. Nephrol Dial Transplant 1997; 12:255–258.

179. Bostom AG, Shemin D, Lapane KL, Sutherland P, Nadeau MR, Wilson PW, Yoburn D, Bausserman L, Tofler G, Jacques PF, Selhub J, Rosenberg IH. Hyperhomocysteinemia, hyperfibrinogenemia, and lipoprotein(a) excess in maintenance dialysis patients: a matched case-control study. Atherosclerosis 1996; 125:91–101.

180. Bostom AG, Lathrop L. Hyperhomocysteinemia in end-stage renal disease: prevalence, etiology, and potential relationship to arteriosclerotic outcomes. Kidney Int 1997; 52:10–20.

181. Guttormsen AB, Ueland PM, Svarstad E, Refsum H. Kinetic basis of hyperhomocysteinemia in patients with chronic renal failure. Kidney Int 1997; 52:495–502.

182. Schmidt AM, Hori O, Brett J,Yan SD, Wautier J-L, Stern D. Cellular receptors for advanced glycation end products. Arteriocler Thromb 1994; 14:1521–1528.

183. McCully KS. Vascular pathology of homocysteinemia: implications for pathogenesis of arteriosclerosis. Am J Pathol 1969; 56:111–128.

184. Boushey CJ, Beresford SA, Omenn GS, Motulsky AG. A quantitative assessment of plasma homocysteine as a risk factor for vascular disease. Probable benefits of increasing folic acid intake. JAMA 1995; 274:1049–1057.

185. Arnesen E, Refsum H, Bonaa KH, Ueland PM, Forde OH, Nordrehaug JE. Serum total homocysteine and coronary artery disease. Int J Epidemiol 1995; 24P: 704–709.

186. Perry IJ, Refsum H, Morris RW, Ebrahim SB, Ueland PM, Shaper AG. Serum total homocysteine and coronary heart disease in middle-aged British men. Heart 1996; 75(suppl 1):P53.

187. Perry IJ, Refsum H, Morris RW, Ebrahim SB, Ueland PM, Shaper AG. Prospective study of serum total homocysteine concentration and risk of stroke in middle-aged British men. Lancet 1995; 346:1395–1398.

188. Blom HJ, Klevinveld HA, Boers GH, Demacker PN, Hak-Lemmers HL, TePoele-Pothoff MT, Trijbels JM. Lipid peroxidation and susceptibility of low-density lipoprotein to in vitro oxidation in hyperhomocysteinaemia. Eur J Clin Invest 1995; 25:149–154.

189. Harpel PC, Chang VT, Borth W. Homocysteine and other sulfhydryl compounds enhance the binding of lipoprotein(a) to fibrin: a potential biochemical link between thrombosis, atherogenesis, and sulfhydryl compound metabolism. Proc Natl Acad Sci USA 1992; 89:10193–10197.

190. Hultberg B, Andersson A, Arnadottir M. Reduced, free and total fractions of homocysteine and other thiol compounds in plasma from patients with renal failure. Nephron 1995; 70:62–67.

191. Dasgupta A, Hussain S, Ahmad S. Increased lipid peroxidation in patients on maintenance hemodialysis. Nephron 1992; 60:56–59.

192. Paul JL, Sall ND, Soni T, Poignet JL, Lindenbaum A, Man NK, Moatti N, Raichvarg D. Lipid peroxidation abnormalities in hemodialyzed patients. Nephron 1993; 64:106–109.

193. Cohen JD, Viljoen M, Clifford D, DeOliveria AA, Veriava Y, Milne FJ. Plasma vitamin E levels in a chronically hemolyzing group of dialysis patients. Clin Nephrol 1986; 25:42–47.

194. Richard MJ, Arnaud J, Jurkovitz C, Hachache T, Meftahi H, Laporte F, Foret M, Favier A, Cordonnier D. Trace elements and lipid peroxidation abnormalities in patients with chronic renal failure. Nephron 1991; 57: 10–15.

195. American Heart Association. Heart and Stroke Facts: 1995 Statistical Supplement. Dallas: American Heart Association, 1994.

196. Held P, Levin N, Port F: Cardiac disease in chronic uremia: an overview. In: Parfrey PS, Harnett JD, eds. Cardiac Dysfunction in Chronic Uremia. Boston: Kluwer Academic Publishers, 1992:3–17.

197. Rostand SG, Brunzell JD, Cannon RO III, Victor RG. Cardiovascular complications in renal failure. J Am Soc Nephrol 1991; 2:1053–1062.

198. United States Renal Data System. 1993 Annual Data Report, Bethesda, MD: National Institutes of Health, National Institutes of Diabetes and Digestive and Kidney Disease, 1993.

199. Farmer JA, Gotto AM Jr. Dyslipidemia and other risk factors for coronary artery disease. In: Braunwald E, ed. Heart Disease: A Textbook of Cardiovascular Medicine. Philadelphia: W. B. Saunders, 1997:1126–1160.

200. Raine AEG, Margreiter R, Brunner FP, Ehrich JH, Geerlings W, Landais P, Loirat C, Mallick NP, Selwood NH, Tufveson, et al. Report on management of renal failure in Europe, XXII. Nephrol Dial Transplant 1992; 7(suppl 2):7–35.

201. Brunner FP, Selwood NH. Profile of patients on RRT in Europe and death rates due to major causes of death groups. The EDTA Registration Committee. Kidney Int 1992; 38(suppl):S4–S15.

202. Raine AE. Can cardiovascular complications be prevented in dialysis patients? Adv Neph 1996; 25:317–339.

203. Haas LB, Wahl PW, Sherrard DJ. A longitudinal study of lipid abnormalities in renal failure. Nephron 1983; 33:145–149.

204. Cheung AK, Wu LL, Kablitz C, Leypoldt JK. Atherogenic lipids and lipoproteins in hemodialysis patients. Am J Kidney Dis 1993; 22:271–276.

205. Parfrey PS, Harnett JD, Barre PE. The natural history of myocardial disease in dialysis patients. J Am Soc Nephrol 1991; 2:2–12.
206. Lazarus JM, Lowrie EG, Hampers CL, Merrill JP. Cardiovascular disease in uremic patients on hemodialysis. Kidney Int 1975; 7(suppl):167–175.
207. Kasiske BL, O'Donnell MP, Cowardin W, Keane WF. Lipids and the kidney. Hypertension 1990; 15(5) 443–450.
208. Fuster V, Gotto AM, Libby P, Loscalzo J, McGill HC. 27th Bethesda Conference: matching the intensity of risk factor management with the hazard for coronary disease events. Task Force 1. Pathogenesis of coronary disease: the biologic role of risk factors. J Am Coll Cardiol 1996; 27:964–976.
209. Ross R. The pathogenesis of atherosclerosis: a perspective for the 1990s (review). Nature 1993; 362: 801–809.
210. Fuster V, Badimon L, Badimon JJ, Chesebro JH. The pathogenesis of coronary artery disease and the acute coronary syndromes (parts 1 and 2) (review). N Engl J Med 1992; 326:242–250, 310–318.
211. Halliwell B. The role of oxygen radicals in human disease, with particular reference to the vascular system. Haemostasis 1993; 23(suppl 1):118–126.
212. Ross R. The pathogenesis of atherosclerosis. In: Braunwald E, ed. Heart Disease: A Textbook of Cardiovascular Medicine. Philadelphia: W. B. Saunders, 1997:1105–1125.
213. Steinberg D. Role of oxidized LDL and antioxidants in atherosclerosis. Adv Exp Med Biol 1995; 369: 39–48.
214. Parthasarathy S, Wieland E, Steinberg D. A role for endothelial cell lipoxygenase in the oxidative modification of low density lipoprotein. Proc Natl Acad Sci USA 1989; 86:1046–1050.
215. Diaz MN, Frei B, Vita J, Keaney JF Jr. Antioxidants and atherosclerotic heart disease. N Engl J Med 1997; 337(6):408–416.
216. Navab M, Berliner JA, Watson AD, Hama SY, Territo MC, Lusis AJ, Shih DM, Van Lenten BJ, Frank JS, Demer LL, et al. The yin and yang of oxidation in the development of the fatty streak: a review based on the 1994 George Lyman Duff Memorial Lecture. Arterioscler Thromb Vasc Biol 1996; 16:831–842.
217. Quinn MT, Parthasarathy S, Fong LG, Steinberg D. Oxidatively modified low density lipoproteins: a potential role in recruitment and retention of monocyte/macrophages during atherogenesis. Proc Natl Acad Sci USA 1987; 84:2995–2998.
218. Parhami F, Fang ZT, Fogelman AM, Andalibi A, Territo MC, Berliner JA. Minimally modified low density lipoprotein-induced inflammatory responses in endothelial cells are mediated by cyclic adenosine monophosphate. J Clin Invest 1993; 92:471–478.
219. Rajavashisth TB, Andalibi A, Territo MC, Berliner JA, Navab M, Fogelman AM, Lusis AJ. Induction of endothelial cell expression of granulocyte and macrophage colony-stimulating factors by modified low-density lipoproteins. Nature 1990; 344:254–257.
220. Quinn MT, Parthasarathy S, Steinberg D. Lysophosphatidycholine: a chemotatic factor for human monocytes and its potential role in atherogenesis. Proc Natl Acad Sci USA 1988; 85:2805–2809.
221. Cushing SD, Berliner JA, Valente AJ, Territo MC, Navab M, Parhami F, Gerrity R, Schwartz CJ, Fogelman AM. Minimally modified low density lipoprotein induces monocyte chemotactic protein 1 in human endothelial cells and smooth muscle cells. Proc Natl Acad Sci USA 1990, 87:5134–5138.
222. Kamanna VS, Bassa BV, Kirschenbaum MA. Atherogenic lipoproteins and human disease: extending concepts beyond the heart to the kidney. Curr Opin Nephrol Hypertension 1997; 6(3):205–211.
223. Goldstein JL, Ho YK, Basu SK, Brown MS. Binding site on macrophages that mediates uptake and degradation of acetylated low density lipoprotein, producing massive cholesterol deposition. Proc Natl Acad Sci USA 1979; 76:333–337.
224. Brown MS, Goldstein JL. Lipoprotein metabolism in the macrophage: implications for cholesterol deposition in atherosclerosis. Annu Rev Biochem 1983; 52: 223–261.
225. Daerr WH, Windler ETE, Greten H. Peroxidative modification of very-low-density lipoproteins in chronic hemodialysis patients. Nephron 1993; 63: 230–231.
226. Heery JM, Kozak M, Stafforini DM, Jones DA, Zimmerman GA, McIntyre TM, Prescott SM. Oxidatively modified LDL contains phospholipids with platelet-activating factor-like activity and stimulates the growth of smooth muscle cells. J Clin Invest 1995; 96:2322–2330.
227. Stiko-Rahm A, Hultgardh-Nilsson A, Regnstrom J, Hamsten A, Nilsson J. Native and oxidized LDL enhances production of PDGF AA and the surface expression of PDGF receptors in cultured human smooth muscle cells. Arterioscler Thromb 1992; 12:1099–1199.
228. Thomas CE, Jackson RL, Ohlweiler DF, Ku G. Multiple lipid oxidation products in low density lipoproteins induce interleukin-l beta release from human blood mononuclear cells. J Lipid Res 1994; 35:417–427.
229. Frostegard J, Wu R, Haegerstrand A, Patarroyo M, Lefvert AK, Nilsson J. Mononuclear leukocytes exposed to oxidized low density lipoprotein secrete a factor that stimulates endothelial cells to express adhesion molecules. Atherosclerosis 1993; 103:213–219.
230. Marui N, Offermann MK, Swerlick R, Kunsch C, Rosen CA, Ahmad M, Alexander RW, Medford RM. Vascular cell adhesion molecule-l (VCAM-l) gene tran-

scription and expression are regulated through an antioxidant-sensitive mechanism in human vascular endothelial cells. J Clin Invest 1993; 92:1866–1874.
231. Grone H-J, Walli AK, Grone EF. The role of oxidatively modified lipoproteins in lipid nephropathy. In: Keane WF, Horl WH, Kasiske BL, eds. Lipids and the Kidney. Basel: Karger, 1997:160–175.
232. Guyton JR, Black BL, Seidel CL. Focal toxicity of oxysterols in vascular smooth muscle cell culture. A model of the atherosclerotic core region. Am J Pathol 1990; 137:425–434.
233. Smith LL, Johnson BH. Biological activities of oxysterols. Free Radic Biol Med 1989; 7:285–332.
234. Palinski W, Yla-Herttuala S, Rosenfeld ME, Butler SW, Socher SA, Parthasarathy S, Curtiss LK, Witzum JL. Antisera and monoclonal antibodies specific for epitopes generated during oxidative modification of low density lipoproteins. Arteriosclerosis 1990; 10: 325–335.
235. Salonen JT, Yla-Herttuala S, Yamamoto R, Butler S, Korpela H, Salonen R, Nyyssonen K, Palinski W, Witzum JL. Autoantibody against oxidized LDL and progression of carotid atherosclerosis. Lanet 1992; 339: 883–887.
236. Bergmark C, Wu R, de Faire U, Lefvert AK, Swedenborg J. Patients with early-onset peripheral vascular disease have increased levels of autoantibodies against oxidized LDL. Arterioscler Thromb Vasc Biol 1995; 15:441–445.
237. Kacharava AG, Tertov VV, Orekhov AN. Autoantibodies against low-density lipoprotein and atherogenic potential of blood. Ann Med 1993; 25:551–555.
238. Lowrie EG, Lew NL. Death risk in hemodialysis patients: the predictive value of commonly measured variables and an evaluation of death rate differences between facilities. Am J Kidney Dis 1990; 15:458–482.
239. Goldwasser P, Mittman N, Antignani A, Burrell D, Michel MA, Collier J, Avram MM. Predictors of mortality in hemodialysis patients. J Am Soc Nephrol 1993; 3:1613–1622.
240. Foley RN, Parfrey PS, Harnett JD, Kent GM, Murray DC, Barre PE. Hypertension, cardiomyopathy, cardiac morbidity, and mortality in ESRD (abstr). J Am Soc Nephrol 1995; 6:529.
241. Avram MM, Mittman N, Bonomini L, Chattopadhyay J, Fein P. Markers for survival in dialysis. Am J Kidney Dis 1995; 26(1):209–219.
242. Iseki K, Kawazoe N, Fukiyama K. Serum albumin is a strong predictor of death in chronic dialysis patients. Kidney Int 1993; 44:115–119.
243. Hakim RM, Levin N. Malnutrition in hemodialysis patients. Am J Kidney Dis 1993; 21(2):125–137.
244. Churchill DN, Taylor DW, Cook RJ, LaPlante P, Barre P, Cartier P, Fay WP, Goldstein MB, Jindal K, Mandin H, McKenzie JK, Muirhead N, Parfrey PS, Posen GA, Slaughter D, Ulan RA, Werb R. Canadian hemodialysis morbidity study. Am J Kidney Dis 1992; 19:214–234.
245. Ritz E, Vallance P, Nowicki M. The effect of malnutrition on cardiovascular mortality in dialysis patients: is L-arginine the answer? Nephrol Dial Transplant 1994; 9:129–130.
246. Yang WS, Kim SB, Min WK, Park S, Lee MS, Park JS. Atherogenic lipid profile and lipoprotein(a) in relation to serum albumin in haemodialysis patients. Nephrol Dial Transplant 1995; 10:1668–1671.
247. Bergstrom J, Heimburger O, Lindholm B, Quereshi AR. Elevated serum C-reactive protein is a strong predictor of increased mortality and low serum albumin in hemodialysis (HD) patients (abstr). J Am Soc Nephrol 1995; 6:573.
248. Docci D, Bilancioni R, Baldrati L, Capponcini C, Turci F, Feletti C. Elevated acute phase reactants in hemodialysis patients. Clin Nephrol 1990; 34:88–91.
249. Tomura S, Nakamura Y, Doi M, Ando R, Ida T, Chida Y, Ootsuka S, Shinoda T, Yanagi H, Tsuchiya S, Marumo F. Fibrinogen, coagulation factor VII, tissue plasminogen activator, plasminogen activator inhibitor-l, and lipid as cardiovascular risk factors in chronic hemodialysis and continuous ambulatory peritoneal dialysis patients. Am J Kidney Dis 1996; 27:848–854.
250. Wanner C, Zimmermann, Quaschning T, Galle J. Inflammation, dyslipidemia and vascular risk factors in hemodialysis patients. Kidney Int 1997; 52:S-53–S-55.
251. Ward RA, McLeish KR. Polymorphonuclear leukocyte oxidative burst is enhanced in patients with chronic renal insufficiency. J Am Soc Nephrol 1995; 5(9):1697–1702.
252. Herbelin A, Nguyen AT, Zingraff J, Urena P, Descamps-Latscha B. Influence of uremia and hemodialysis on circulating interleukin-l and tumor necrosis factor (. Kidney Int 1990; 37:116–125.
253. Herbelin A, Urena P, Nguyen AT, Zingraff J, Descamps-Latscha B. Elevated circulating levels of interleukin-6 in patients with chronic renal failure. Kidney Int 1991; 39:954–960.
254. Lonnemann G, Bingel M, Koch KM, Shaldon S, Dinarello CA. Plasma interleukin-l activity in humans undergoing hemodialysis with regenerated cellulosic membranes. Lymphokine Res 1987; 6:63–70.
255. Laude-Sharp M, Caroff M, Simard L, Pusineri C, Kazatchkine MD, Haeffner-Cavaillon N. Induction of IL-l during hemodialysis: transmembrane passage of intact endotoxins (LPS). Kidney Int 1990; 38:1089–1094.
256. Urena P, Herbelin A, Zingraff J, Lair M, Man NK, Descamps-Latscha B, Drueeke T. Permeability of cellulosic and non-cellulosic membranes to endotoxins and cytokine production during in vitro hemodialysis. Kidney Int. In press.

257. Lonnemann G, Koch KM, Shaldon S, Dinarello CA. Studies on the ability of hemodialysis membranes to induce, bind, and clear human interleukin-l. J Lab Clin Med 1988; 112:76–86.
258. Feingold KR, Soued M, Serio MK, Moser AH, Dinarello CA, Grunfeld C. Multiple cytokines stimulate hepatic lipid synthesis in vivo. Endocrinology 1989; 125:267–274.
259. Grunfeld C, Soued M, Adi S, Moser AH, Dinarello CA, Feingold KR. Evidence for two classes of cytokines that stimulate hepatic lipogenesis: relationships among tumor necrosis factor, interleukin-l and interferon-alpha. Endocrinology 1990; 127:46–54.
260. Ernst E. Fibrinogen: its emerging role as a cardiovascular risk factor. Angiology 1994; 45:87–93.
261. Ernst E. Plasma fibrinogen-an independent cardiovascular risk factor. J Intern Med 1990; 227:365–372.
262. Liuzza G, Biasucci LM, Gallimore JR, Grillo R, Rebuzzi AG, Pepys MB, Maseri A. The prognostic value of C-reactive protein and serum amyloid A protein in severe unstable angina. N Engl J Med 1997; 331:417–424.
263. Ridker PM, Cushman M, Stampfer MJ, Tracy RP, Hennekens CH. Inflammation, aspirin, and the risk of cardiovascular disease in apparently healthy men. N Engl J Med 1997; 336:973–979.
264. Bologa RM, Levine DM, Parker TS, Serur D, Stenzel KH, Rubin A, Cheigh JS. High cytokine levels may mediate the high mortality of hemodialysis (HD) patients with low albumin and/or cholesterol (TC) (abstr). J Am Soc Nephrol 1995; 6:573.
265. Varga Z, Karpati I, Paragh G, Buris L, Kakuk G. Relative abundance of some free fatty acids in plasma of uremic patients: relationship between fatty acids, lipid parameters, and diseases. Nephron 1997; 77:417–421.
266. Scoppola A, De Paolis P, Menzinger G, Lala A, DiGuilio S. Plasma mevalonate concentrations in uremic patients. Kidney Int 1997; 51:908–912.
267. Ramos JM, Heaton A, McGurk JG, Ward MK, Kerr DN. Sequential changes in serum lipids and their subfractions in patients receiving continuous ambulatory peritoneal dialysis. Nephron 1983; 35:20–23.
268. Lameire N, Matthys D, Matthys E, Beheydt R. Effects of long-term CAPD on carbohydrate and lipid metabolism. Clin Nephrol 1988 30(suppl 1):S53–S58.
269. Lindholm B, Norbeck HE. Serum lipids and lipoproteins during continuous ambulatory peritoneal dialysis. Acta Med Scand 1986; 220:143–151.
270. Breckenridge WC, Roncari DAK, Khanna R, Oreopoulos DG. The influence of continuous ambulatory peritoneal dialysis on plasma lipoproteins. Atherosclerosis 1982; 45:249–258.
271. Kandoussi C, Cachera C, Reade R, Pagniez D, Fruchart JC, Tacquet A. Apo AIV in plasma and dialysate fluid of CAPD patients: comparison with other apolipoproteins. Nephrol Dial Transplant 1992; 7:1026–1029.
272. Asayama K, Hayashibe H, Mishiku Y, Honda M, Ito H, Nakazawa S. Increased activity of plasma cholesterol ester transfer protein in children with end-stage renal disease receiving continuous ambulatory peritoneal dialysis. Nephron 1996; 72:231–236.
273. Steinmetz A, Utermann G. Activation of lecithin: cholesterol acyltransferase by human apolipoprotein A-IV. J Biol Chem 1985; 260:2258–2264.
274. O'Neal D, Lee P, Murphy B, Best J. Low density lipoprotein particle size distribution in end-stage renal disease treated with hemodialysis or peritoneal dialysis. Am J Kidney Dis 1996; 27(1):84–91.
275. Kagan A, Bar-Khayim Y, Schafer Z, Fainaru M. Kinetics of peritoneal protein loss during CAPD: II. Lipoprotein leakage and its impact on plasma lipid levels. Kidney Int 1990; 37:980–990.
276. Sniderman A, Cianflone K, Kwiterovich PO Jr, Hutchinson T, Barre P, Prichard S. Hyperapobetalipoproteinemia: the major dyslipoproteinemia in patients with chronic renal failure treated with chronic ambulatory peritoneal dialysis. Atherosclerosis 1987; 65: 257–264.
277. Kagan A, Bar-Khayim Y, Schafer Z, Fainaru M. Kinetics of peritoneal protein loss during CAPD: I. Different characteristics for low and high molecular weight proteins. Kidney Int 1990; 37:971–979.
278. Dulaney JT, Hatch FE Jr. Peritoneal dialysis and loss of proteins: a review. Kidney Int 1984; 26:253–262.
279. Saku K, Sasaki J, Naito S, Arkawa K. Lipoprotein and apolipoprotein losses during continuous ambulatory peritoneal dialysis. Nephron 1989; 51:220–224.
280. Kobayashi M, Yorioka N, Yamakido M. Hypercoagulability and secondary hyperfibrinolysis may be related to abnormal lipid metabolism in patients treated with continuous ambulatory peritoneal dialysis. Nephron 1997; 76:56–61.
281. Kannel WB, Wolf PA, Castelli WP, D'Agostino RB. Fibrinogen and risk of cardiovascular disease: The Framingham Study. JAMA 1987; 258:1183–1186.
282. Kelleher CC. Plasma fibrinogen and factor VII as risk factors for cardiovascular disease. Eur J Epidemiol 1992; 8(suppl 1):79–82.
283. Hoffman CJ, Miller RH, Hultin MB. Correlation of factor VII activity and antigen with cholesterol and triglycerides in healthy young adults. Arterioscler Thromb 1992; 12:267–270.
284. Bruckert E, Carvalho de Sousa J, Giral P, Soria C, Chapman MJ, Caen J, de Gennes J. Interrelationship of plasma triglyceride and coagulant factor VII levels in normotriglyceridemic hypercholesterolemia. Atherosclerosis 1989; 75(2–3):129–134.
285. Rossouw JE. Secondary prevention of coronary heart disease. In: Rifkind BM, ed. Lowering Cholesterol in High-Risk Individuals and Populations. New York: Marcel Dekker, 1995:46–67.
286. Shepherd J, Cobbe SM, Ford I, Isles CG, Lorimer AR, MacFarlane PW, McKillop JH, Packard CJ. Preven-

tion of coronary heart disease with pravastatin in men with hypercholesterolemia. West of Scotland Coronary Prevention Study Group. N Engl J Med 1995; 333: 1301–1307.

287. Scandinavian Simvastatin Survival Study Group. Randomized trail of cholesterol lowering in 4444 patients with coronary heart disease: the Scandinavian Simvastatin Survival Study (4S). Lancet 1994; 344:1383–1389.

288. Sacks FM, Pfeffer MA, Moye LA, Rouleau JL, Rutherford JD, Cole TG, Brown L, Warnica JW, Arnold JM, Wun CC, et al. The effect of pravastatin on coronary events after myocardial infarction in patients with average cholesterol levels. N Engl J Med 1996; 335:1001–1009.

289. National Cholesterol Education Program. Second Report of the Expert Panel on Detection, Evaluation, and Treatment of High Blood Cholesterol in Adults (Adult Treatment Panel II). Circulation 1994; 89:1333–1445.

290. Austin MA. Plasma triglyceride and coronary heart disease. Aterioscler Thromb 1991; 11(review):2–14.

291. NIH Consensus Conference. Triglyceride, high-density lipoprotein and coronary heart disease. NIH Consensus Development Panel on Triglyceride, High-Density Lipoprotein, and Coronary Heart Disease. JAMA 1993; 269:505–510.

292. Patsch W, Gotto AM Jr. High-density lipoprotein cholesterol, plasma triglyceride, and coronary heart disease: pathophysiology and management. Adv Pharmacol 1995; 32:375–426.

293. Ebenbichler CF, Kirchmair R, Egger C, Patsch JR. Postprandial state and atherosclerosis. Curr Opin Lipidol 1995; 6:286–290.

294. Genest J Jr, Cohn JS. Clustering of cardiovascular risk factors: targeting high-risk individuals. Am J Cardiol 1995; 76:8A–20A.

295. DeFronzo RA, Ferrannini E. Insulin resistance. A multifaceted syndrome responsible for NIDDM, obesity, hypertension, dyslipidemia, and atherosclerotic cardiovascular disease. Diabetes Care 1991; 14:173–194.

296. Reaven GM. Role of insulin resistance in human disease (syndrome X): an expanded definition. Annu Rev Med 1993; 44:121–131.

297. Manninen V, Tenkanen L, Koskinen P, Huttunen JK, Manttari M, Heinonen OP, Frick MH. Joint effects of serum triglyceride and LDL cholesterol and HDL cholesterol on coronary heart disease risk in the Helsinki Heart Study. Implications for treatment. Circulation 1992; 85:37–45.

298. Assmann G, Schulte H. Relation of high-density lipoprotein cholesterol and triglycerides to incidence of atherosclerotic coronary artery disease (the PROCAM experience). Prospective Cardiovascular Munster Study. Am J Cardiol 1992; 70:733–737.

299. Carlson LA, Rosenhamer G. Reduction of mortality in the Stockholm Ischaemic Heart Disease Secondary Prevention Study by combined treatment with clofibrate and nicotinic acid. Acta Med Scand 1988; 223: 405–418.

300. Friedewald WT, Levy RI, Fredrickson DS. Estimation of the concentration of low density lipoprotein cholesterol in plasma, without use of the preparative ultracentrifuge. Clin Chem 1972; 18:499–502.

301. Nauck M, Kramer-Guth A, Bartens W, Marz W, Wieland H, Wanner C. Is the determination of LDL cholesterol according to Friedewald accurate in CAPD and HD patients? Clin Nephrol 1996; 46(5):319–325.

302. Wanner C, Bartens W. Lipoprotein(a) in renal patients: is it a key factor in the high cardiovascular mortality? Nephrol Dial Transpl 1994; 9:1066–1068.

303. Maher VMG, Brown BG, Marcovina SM, Hillger LA, Zhao XQ, Albers JJ. Effects of lowering elevated LDL cholesterol on the cardiovascular risk of lipoprotein(a). JAMA 1995; 274:1771–1774.

304. D'Amico G, Gentile MG. Influence of diet on lipid abnormalities in human renal disease. Am J Kidney Dis 1993; 22(1):151–157.

305. Sanfelippo ML, Swenson RS, Reaven GM. Response of plasma triglycerides to dietary change in patients on hemodialysis. Kidney Int 1978; 14:180–186.

306. Cattran DC, Steiner G, Fenton SS, Ampil M. Dialysis hyperlipidemia: response to dietary manipulations. Clin Nephrol 1980; 13:177–182.

307. Goldberg AP, Geltman EM, Gavin JR III, Carney RM, Hagberg JM, Delmez JA, Naumovich A, Oldfield MH, Harter HR. Exercise training reduces coronary risk and effectively rehabilitates hemodialysis patients. Nephron 1986; 42:311–316.

308. Hamazaki T, Nakazawa R, Tateno S, Shishido H, Isoda K, Hattori V, Yoshida T, Fujita T, Yanos, Kumagai A. Effects of fish oil rich in eicosapentaenoic acid on serum lipid in hyperlipidemic hemodialysis patients. Kidney Int. 1984; 26:81–84.

309. Rolf N, Tenschert W, Lison AE. Results of a long-term administration of omega 3 fatty acids in haemodialysis patients with dyslipoproteinaemia. Nephrol Dial Transplant 1990; 5:797–801.

310. Fracasso A, Toffoletto P, Landini S, Morachiello P, Righetto F, Scanferla F, Genchi R, Roncali D, Bazzato G. Effect of hypertriglyceridemia correction by omega-3 fatty acids on peritoneal transport in continuous ambulatory peritoneal dialysis patients. Perit Dial Int 1993; 13(suppl 2):S437–S439.

311. Bilo HJ, Homan van der Heide JJ, Gans RO, Donker AJ. Omega-3 polyunsaturated fatty acids in chronic renal insufficiency. Nephron 1991; 57:385–393.

312. Rylance PB, Gordge MP, Sayner R, Parsons V, Weston MJ. Fish oil modifies and reduces platelet aggregability in haemodialysis patients. Nephron 1986; 43:196–202.

313. Gavin JR III, Goldberg AP, Hagberg JM, Delmez JA, Geltman E, Harter HR. Endurance exercise improves

insulin sensitivity in uremia. Clin Res 1982; 30:393–397.

314. Pollock CA, Wyndham R, Collett PV, Elder G, Field MJ, Kalowski S, Lawrence JR, Waugh DA, George CR. Effects of erythropoietin therapy on the lipid profile in end-stage renal failure. Kidney Int 1994; 45: 897–902.
315. Viron B, Donsimoni R, Michel C, al Khayat R, Mignon F. Effect of recombinant human erythropoietin on nutritional status and plasma lipids in uremic patients. Nephron 1992; 60:249.
316. Mat O, Stolear JC, Georges B. Blood lipid profile in hemodialysis patients treated with human erythropoietin. Nephron 1992; 60:236–237.
317. Prata MM, Sousa FT, Barbas JM, Rodrigues MC. Blood lipids in haemodialysis patients treated with erythropoietin (abstr). Nephrol Dial Transplant 1990; 5:474.
318. Guarnieri GM, Ranieri F, Toigo G, Vasile A, Ciman M, Rizzoli V, Moracchiell M, Campanacci L. Lipid lowering effect of carnitine in chronically uremic patients treated with maintenance hemodialysis. Am J Clin Nutr 1980; 33:1489–1492.
319. Yeksan M, Turk S, Polat M, Cigli A, Erdogan Y. Effects of 1,25 $(OH)_2D_3$ treatment on lipid levels in uremic hemodialysis patients. Int J Artif Organs 1992; 15(12):704–707.
320. Elisaf MS, Germanos NP, Bairaktari HT, Pappas MB, Koulouridis EI, Siamopoulos KC. Effects of conventional vs. low-molecular-weight heparin on lipid profile in hemodialysis patients. Am J Nephrol 1997; 17: 153–157.
321. Josephson MA, Fellner SK, Dasgupta A. Improved lipid profiles in patients undergoing high-flux hemodialysis. Am J Kidney Dis 1992; 20(4):361–366.
322. Blankestijn PJ, Vos PF, Rabelink TJ, van Rijn HJM, Jansen H, Koomans HA. High-flux dialysis membranes improve lipid profile in chronic hemodialysis patients. J Am Soc Nephrol 1995; 5:1703–1708.
323. Fishbane S, Bucala R, Koschinsky T, Giordano D, Founds H, Vlassara H. Significant reduction of plasma LDL-apo B and glycated apo B follows chronic high-flux hemodialysis in diabetic uremic patients.
324. Buoncristiani U, Galli F, Rovidati S, Albertini MC, Campus G, Canestrari F. Oxidative damage during hemodialysis using a vitamin-E-modified dialysis membrane: a preliminary characterization. Nephron 1997; 77:57–61.
325. Pasternack A, Vanttinen T, Solakivi T, Kuusi T, Korte T. Normalization of lipoprotein lipase and hepatic lipase by gemfibrozil results in correction of lipoprotein abnormalities in chronic renal failure. Clin Nephrol 1987; 27:163–168.
326. Nishizawa Y, Shoji T, Nishitani H, Yamakawa M, Konishi T, Kawasaki K, Morii H. Hypertriglyceridemia and lowered apolipoprotein C-II/C-III ratio in uremia: effect of a fibric acid, clinofibrate. Kidney Int 1993; 44:1352–1359.
327. Kijima Y, Sasaoka T, Xanayama M, Kubota S. Untoward effects of clofibrate in hemodialyzed patients. N Engl J Med 1977; 296:515.
328. Grundy SM. Management of hyperlipidemia of kidney disease. Kidney Int 1990; 37:847–853.
329. Berndt J, Gaumert R, Still J. Mode of action of the lipid-lowering agents, clofibrate and BM 15075, on cholesterol biosynthesis in rat liver. Atherosclerosis 1978; 30:147–152.
330. Wanner C, Horl W, Luley CH, Wieland H. Effects of HMG-CoA reductase inhibitors in hypercholesterolemic patients on hemodialysis. Kidney Int 1991; 39: 754–760.
331. Fiorini F, Patrone E, Ardu F, Castelluccio A. Efficacy and safety of simvastatin in the treatment of hyperlipidemia in uremic patients undergoing hemodialysis. Minerva Urol Nephrol 1992; 44:165–168.
332. Wanner C, Lubrich-Birkner I, Summ O, Wieland H, Schollmeyer P. Effect of simvastatin on qualitative and quantitative changes of lipoprotein metabolism in CAPD patients. Nephron 1992; 62:40–46.
333. Nishizawa Y, Shoji T, Emoto M, Kawasaki K, Konishi T, Tabata T, Inoue T, Morii H. Reduction of intermediate density lipoprotein by pravastatin in hemo- and peritoneal dialysis patients. Clin Nephrol 1995; 43: 268–277.
334. Carlson LA, Hamsten A, Asplund A. Pronounced lowering of serum levels of lipoprotein Lp(a) in hyperlipidemic subjects treated with nicotinic acid. J Intern Med 1989; 226:271–276.
335. Chan MK. Lipoprotein metabolism in dialysis patients. In: Nissenson AR, Fine RN, Gentile DE, eds. Clinical Dialysis. Norwalk: 1995:669–714.
336. De Vecchi A, Pini C, Castelnovo C, Rovellini A, Colombini M, Scalamogna A. Low-dose acipimox in type IIb dyslipidemia in CAPD patients. In: Ota K, et al., eds. Current Concepts in Peritoneal Dialysis. New York: Elsevier, 1992:555–571.
337. Parthasarathy S, Young SG, Witztum JL, Pittman RC, Steinberg D. Probucol enhances oxidative modification of low density lipoprotein. J Clin Invest 1986; 77: 641–644.

30

Disturbances in Carbohydrate, Protein, and Trace Metal Metabolism in Uremia and Dialysis Patients

Norbert Lameire
University Hospital of Gent and University of Gent, Gent, Belgium
Raymond Vanholder
University Hospital of Gent, Gent, Belgium
Bernadette Faller
Hospital Louis Pasteur, Colmar, France

In this chapter, disturbances in carbohydrate and insulin metabolism and protein and amino acid metabolism in chronic renal failure patients and the effects of maintenance hemodialysis and chronic peritoneal dialysis on these metabolic disturbances will be discussed. Also some selected aspects of trace metal metabolism in hemodialysis and peritoneal dialysis patients will be reviewed.

Alterations in lipoprotein metabolism are discussed in Chapter 29. Some of these metabolic disturbances have implications on the nutritional status of the dialysis patients, a subject discussed in Chapter 22.

I. CARBOHYDRATE AND INSULIN METABOLISM IN CHRONIC RENAL FAILURE AND DIALYSIS

Uremia is typically associated with impaired glucose metabolism. The most important characteristics of glucose and insulin metabolism in uremia are summarized in Table 1.

Some patients manifest fasting hyperglycemia in response to oral and intravenous glucose loads, while others are able to maintain normoglycemia by raising plasma insulin levels. As summarized in Table 1, tissue insensitivity to insulin (i.e., impaired ability of insulin to stimulate glucose uptake in peripheral tissues) is of primary importance, but augmented hepatic glucose output and alterations in insulin degradation and insulin secretion may also contribute (2–4). The variable severity of these changes in individual patients explains the variable plasma levels of insulin and glucose that may be seen, both fasting and following a glucose load.

A. Insulin Resistance

Peripheral resistance to the action of insulin occurs in almost all uremic subjects and is largely responsible for the abnormal glucose metabolism seen in this setting (2–4). Impaired tissue sensitivity to insulin has already been demonstrated in patients with only mild to moderate reductions in renal function (5). Both experimental and clinical studies suggest that skeletal muscle is the primary site of insulin resistance (2,3), presumably due to a postreceptor defect (6,7).

Normal insulin receptor binding, β-subunit phosphorylation, and kinase activation in uremic subjects have been found (8,9). In addition, the expression of GLUT-4, the major glucose transporter in striated muscle, has been found to be normal in uremic muscle (7).

Abnormalities in both oxidative as well as nonoxidative glucose metabolism contribute to the impaired insulin sensitivity in renal failure (7,10). A role for elevated endothelin-1 levels in the insulin resistance in chronic renal failure has recently been suggested (4). Accumulation of a uremic toxin or toxins may play a role in the insulin resistance.

Table 1 Characteristics of Glucose and Insulin Metabolism in Uremia

Normal fasting blood glucose
Spontaneous hypoglycemia
Fasting hyperinsulinemia
Normal, elevated, or decreased blood insulin levels in response to hyperglycemia induced by oral or intravenous glucose administration
Elevated blood levels of proinsulin and C-peptide
Elevated blood levels of immunoreactive glucagon
Impaired insulin secretion by pancreatic islets (observed only in the presence of established secondary hyperparathyroidism)
Multiple derangements in metabolism and function of pancreatic islets
Impaired glycolytic pathways
Reduced basal and glucose-stimulated ATP content
Elevated basal levels of cytosolic calcium
Decreased V_{max} of Ca^{2+}-ATPase and $Na^{+}K^{+}$-ATPase
Reduced calcium signal and response to glucose and potassium
Normal hepatic glucose production
Normal suppression of hepatic glucose production by insulin
Decreased peripheral sensitivity to insulin action
Impaired glucose tolerance (present only when insulin secretion is impaired in the presence of commonly encountered resistance to the peripheral action of insulin)
Decreased requirement for insulin by diabetic patients with diabetic nephropathy and uremia

Source: Ref. 1.

McCaleb et al. (11) reported that the sera of uremic patients contain a compound with a molecular weight of 1000–2000 daltons, which inhibits glucose metabolism by normal rat adipocytes. This compound is specific for uremia, since it is absent in the blood of patients with insulin resistance but without uremia. Other investigators proposed that hippurate and pseudouridine, which accumulate in the blood of patients with uremia, contribute to insulin resistance. It appears that both hippurate and pseudouridine inhibit glucose utilization by rat diaphragm, brain, kidney cortex, erthrocytes, or soleus muscle (12,13).

Hörl and colleagues (14,15) have isolated two proteins from uremic serum, which inhibited deoxyglucose uptake and oxidative metabolism and phorbol ester–stimulated glucose uptake in polymorphonuclear leukocytes. The observation that tissue sensitivity to insulin can be substantially improved by a low-protein diet, supplemented with an amino acid–keto acid preparation, and dialysis, is consistent with a role for uremic toxins (4,10,16). Excess parathyroid hormone (PTH) resulting from abnormalities in phosphate and vitamin D metabolism is also thought to be responsible for insulin resistance (17,18). Mak (17) showed that the acute intravenous administration of calcitriol (1,25-dihydroxyvitamin D) to hemodialysis patients enhanced insulin release and improved glucose tolerance. This effect was independent of changes in the plasma concentrations of calcium or PTH. Two longer trials demonstrated that intravenous calcitriol essentially normalized insulin sensitivity (18,19). Plasma PTH levels also fell, so that it was not possible to determine whether the improvement was due to calcitriol per se and/or to reversal of hyperparathyroidism.

Metabolic acidosis appears to be another factor that contributes to insulin resistance in uremia (4) and correction of acidosis by sodium bicarbonate treatment results in a significant, albeit moderate, increase in insulin-mediated glucose uptake in non-dialyzed uremic patients (20). Sedentary life-style contributes to the resistance to insulin action (21).

The degree of tissue insensitivity directly correlates with maximal aerobic work capacity, indicating that physical training may ameliorate insulin resistance in patients with renal failure Support for this hypothesis was provided by a study which noted that long term exercise training in a group of patients on maintenance hemodialysis was associated with significantly reduced blood glucose levels, improved glucose disappearance rates, and reduced fasting serum insulin levels (22). This explains also why at least in some studies, correction of renal anemia with erythropoietin was associated with increased insulin secretion and decreased blood glucose levels following a test meal (23) and with increased insulin-stimulated glucose disposal by about 50%. The improvement in tissue oxygen supply leads to increased exercise tolerance (24,25). In another study, however, no change in insulin secretion was seen after an oral glucose load (26).

B. Insulin Secretion

The expected response to impaired tissue sensitivity would be an augmentation in insulin secretion in an attempt to normalize glucose metabolism. In many cases, however, insulin secretion tends to be blunted; these patients tend to have the greatest impairment in glucose tolerance. It appears that the failure to secrete insulin is a generalized phenomenon since it occurs to a variety of stimuli present in uremia, such as potassium (27) and L-leucine (28)

A PTH-induced elevation in the intracellular calcium concentration may be responsible for the impairment in insulin release by decreasing both the cellular content of ATP and Na-K-ATPase pump activity in the pancreatic beta cells (29). In experimental animals, these changes can be prevented by prior parathyroidectomy or by the administration of the calcium channel blocker verapamil (28,30,31). In addition, excess PTH may interfere with the ability of the beta cells to augment insulin secretion in response to hyperglycemia or amino acids (28,32,33). Another factor that can suppress insulin release in chronic renal failure is the associated metabolic acidosis (3). The frequent deficiency of calcitriol (1,25-dihydroxyvitamin D) in chronic renal failure also may contribute to the impairment in insulin secretion. In animals, the pancreatic islets possess receptor proteins for 1,25$(OH)_2$ D_3 and for vitamin D–dependent calcium-binding protein, both of which are localized in the beta cells of the islets (34–39).

As mentioned above, acute administration of calcitriol (1,25-dihydroxyvitamin D) to hemodialysis patients has been shown to enhance insulin release and improve glucose tolerance (17). This effect was independent of changes in the plasma concentrations of calcium or PTH. The importance of the inhibiting effect of PTH and the stimulating effect of calcitriol was also suggested in a case report of a patient who developed hypoglycemia with high insulin levels after the combination of parathyroidectomy and large doses of calcitriol (40).

Leptin, a 16 kDa peptide that is encoded for by the *ob* gene and is secreted by adipocytes, has recently been shown to inhibit glucose-stimulated insulin secretion in perfused rat pancreas isolated islets (41).This finding is of potential interest in relation to insulin secretion in chronic renal failure patients, since plasma leptin concentrations are significantly elevated in undialyzed patients with a GFR of <20 mL/min (42) and in both hemodialysis (43,44) and peritoneal dialysis patients (45).

Serum leptin concentrations correlate to plasma insulin concentrations independent of body fat content in chronic renal failure (46). Recently, marked decreases of circulating leptin in diabetic rats were reversed by insulin treatment. It was hypothesized that decreased glucose transport into adipose tissue may contribute to decreased leptin production in insulin-deficient diabetes (47).

C. Insulin Degradation

The kidney plays a central role in the metabolism of insulin in normal subjects (2–4). Approximately 60% of total renal insulin clearance occurs by glomerular filtration and 40% by extraction from the peritubular vessels. The renal clearance of insulin is 200 mL/min, significantly exceeding the normal glomerular filtration rate of 120 mL/min due to the contribution of tubular secretion. This clearance corresponds with a degradation of six to eight units of insulin by the kidney each day, which accounts for approximately 25% of the daily production of insulin by the pancreas.

There is little change in the metabolic clearance rate of insulin in renal disease until there has been a substantial reduction in GFR (2). Increased peritubular insulin uptake is able to compensate for reduced filtration until the GFR has fallen to less than 15–20 mL/min (48). At this point, there is a dramatic reduction in insulin clearance (2).

The kidney also catabolizes proinsulin and C-peptide, and the renal extraction appears to be proportional to their arterial concentrations. Ligation of the renal pedicle of experimental animals results in a 75% rise in the levels of plasma insulin and a 300% increase in the levels of proinsulin and C-peptide. The kidney accounts for most of the catabolism of the insulin precursor proinsulin. It is therefore useful to remember that in patients with renal failure, high plasma levels of immunoreactive insulin represent a greater contribution of proinsulin and C-peptide than of active insulin. There may thus be a dissociation between the radioimmunoassay and the biologically active insulin when renal function decreases.

D. Hepatic Glucose Metabolism

The role of alterations in hepatic glucose metabolism is unclear. Some studies (49) found results supporting an increased hepatic production of glucose in uremia, and it was suggested that there existed an exaggerated hepatic glucagon sensitivity that contributed to the increased neoglucogenesis (50). Others, in contrast, found a normal hepatic glucose production and suggested a decreased rather than an increased sensitivity to glucagon in uremia (51,52).

The kidney accounts for approximately one third of the metabolic clearance of glucagon, the major route of glucagon removal being glomerular filtration. Plasma glucagon levels are increased in chronic renal failure, and glucagon secretion in response to stimulants is increased, but the elevated glucagon levels in uremia are apparently due to decreased metabolic clearance rather than to hypersecretion of the hormone. Both biologically active and inactive forms of glucagon accumulate in uremic patients. These patients also demonstrate a three- to fourfold increase in the hypergly-cemic response to glucagon.

E. Clinical Implications

While sophisticated tests disclose resistance to the hy-poglycemic activity of insulin in virtually all uremic subjects, most nondiabetic patients do not develop per-sistent hyperglycemia unless they have a genetic pre-disposition to diabetes (2–4). In this setting, inadequate insulin secretion may combine with uremic insulin re-sistance to produce overt diabetes.

The hyperinsulinemia normally induced by insulin resistance may also contribute to the common devel-opment of hypertriglyceridemia in chronic renal failure. Insulin enhances hepatic very low-density lipoprotein (VLDL) triglyceride synthesis and may indirectly (via decreased sensitivity of lipoprotein lipase to insulin) reduce the rate of metabolism of VLDL. Hyperinsuli-nemia can also affect fibrinolysis by stimulating the production of plasminogen activator inhibitor-1. It may therefore play a role in the decreased systemic fibri-nolytic activity characteristic of chronic renal failure (53).

F. Hypoglycemia

An unusual manifestation of disturbed glucose metab-olism in chronic renal failure is the development of spontaneous hypoglycemia (3,54,55). This complica-tion can be seen in both diabetic and nondiabetic sub-jects, and multiple factors may play a contributory role. These include decreased caloric intake, reduced renal gluconeogenesis due to the reduction in functioning re-nal mass, impaired release of the counterregulatory hormone epinephrine due to the autonomic neuropathy of renal failure, concurrent hepatic disease, and de-creased metabolism of drugs, such as alcohol, propran-olol and other nonselective β-blockers, and disopyr-amide, which might promote a reduction in the plasma glucose concentration (3). Angiotensin-converting en-zyme (ACE) inhibitors may induce hypoglycemia by increasin insulin sensitivity (56) and/or by decreasing hepatic glucose production (57).

Oral hypoglycemic drugs, particularly the first-gen-eration sulfonylureas (chlorpropamide, tolbutamide), may provoke severe hypoglycemia because of their re-duced clearance in renal failure, the presence of re-duced hepatic clearance and decreased albumin con-centration, reduced caloric intake, malnutrition, hepatic failure, alcoholism, or an associated endocrine condi-tion. The use of chlorpropamide in renal failure patients is not recommended because of its marked prolonged half-life due to its exclusive renal excretion. Other oral hypoglycemic agents should also be used with extreme caution in patients with serious renal impairment.

G. Carbohydrate Metabolism in CAPD

The absorption of glucose from the traditional dialysate in nondiabetic peritoneal dialysis patients depends on the glucose concentration used in the dialysate. It has been caculated that CAPD patients derive about 20% of their total daily energy intake from this source. This corresponds with a daily peritoneal energy intake be-tween 4 and 13 kcal/kg body weight (58).

Another concern related to high daily glucose ab-sorption is the possible development of de novo dia-betes mellitus, reported in 3 cases out of 40 and 5 cases out of 95 nondiabetic CAPD patients (59,60). In our unit, 5 cases of de novo diabetes mellitus were ob-served in 310 nondiabetic CAPD patients treated be-tween 1979 and 1996. (61).

In the case of overt or impending diabetes mellitus, this extra glucose may be responsible for the appear-ance (or worsening) of the disease, necessitating the institution (or an increase in dose) of insulin. Ex-changes with a 1.5% glucose dialysate have only mar-ginal effects on blood glucose and insulin levels (62,63); however, with the use of hypertonic glucose solutions the tendency towards the development of hy-perglycemia and hyperinsulinemia is more pronounced.

Wideröe et al. (64) reported increased plasma C-peptide levels along with an increased ratio between C-peptide and insulin levels in CAPD patients. Many other studies have shown that basal glucose and insulin levels were either normal or increased in CAPD pa-tients (65–68).

Among 9 patients followed over 6 years, we found no major alterations in the blood glucose profiles dur-ing a once-daily 4.25% glucose exchange. In addition, neither the peak plasma insulin concentrations nor the insulin concentrations at the end of a 4-hour dwell were significantly different between the start of CAPD and after 6 years (61). Peripheral insulin action, as mea-sured by the euglycemic insulin clamp technique, im-proved after 3 months of CAPD; hepatic glucose output remained unchanged (69). In diabetic patients, the in-sulin requirements may double or even quadruple if insulin is administered intraperitoneally because of en-hanced insulin degradation, adherence of insulin to the peritoneum and mesentery where it is locally degraded, adherence to the plastic dialysate bags, and extraction of about 50% of insulin by the liver, to which the insulin is delivered via the portal vein.

H. Carbohydrate Metabolism in Hemodialysis

Many studies have indicated that hemodialysis is capable of improving the carbohydrate metabolism in uremia, by amelioration of the glucose tolerance in association with an increase in tissue sensitivity to insulin (70–72). More recent studies (73) have shown that hemodialysis improved the muscle cell utilization of glucose through the pathway of nonoxidative metabolism, the latter corresponding mainly to storage as glycogen. As with the tissue sensitivity to insulin, hemodialysis has been shown to improve the insulin secretory response to glucose (74).

The exact mechanism(s) of the amelioration in carbohydrate metabolism is (are) not known, but from the previous discussion of the different factors that may play a role in the disturbed metabolism, it is clear that several of these factors are corrected or at least ameliorated by dialysis. Besides the removal of diabetogenic circulating toxins, correction of the acidosis, improvement of the hyperparathyroidism, administration of calcitriol, and correction of the anemia with erythropoietin, may all play a role. Recently, beneficial effects on glucose tolerance in hemodialysis patients were described with the administration of large dose of intravenous biotin (75). Biotin belongs to the prosthetic group of carboxylases, and the only protein proven to be specifically induced by biotin is glucokinase. A biotin-deficient state in uremia is possible due to protein restriction and losses of this low molecular weight substance into the dialysate.

I. Insulin Requirements in Diabetes Mellitus

Insulin requirements show a biphasic course in diabetic patients with renal disease. It is not uncommon for glucose control to deteriorate as renal function deteriorates, because increasing insulin resistance can affect both insulin-dependent and non–insulin-dependent diabetics. Thus, insulin requirements may increase in the former, while the institution of insulin therapy may be necessary in the latter. In comparison, the marked fall in insulin clearance in advanced renal failure often leads to an improvement in glucose tolerance. This may allow a lower dose of insulin to be given or even the cessation of insulin therapy (76,77). Decreased caloric intake, due to uremia-induced anorexia, also may contribute to the decrease in insulin requirements (3).

The institution of hemodialysis in diabetic patients may significantly influence the insulin requirements. This will in any given patient depend upon the net balance between improving tissue sensitivity and restoring normal hepatic insulin metabolism. As a result, one cannot readily predict insulin requirements in this setting, and careful observation of the patient is essential.

II. ALBUMIN METABOLISM IN CHRONIC RENAL FAILURE AND DIALYSIS PATIENTS

As emphasized in Chapter 22 of this volume, hypoalbuminemia is a strong independent risk factor for death in both hemodialysis and peritoneal dialysis patients (78,79). A change in the concentration of any plasma protein can be a consequence of a change in its rate of synthesis, a change in its rate of catabolism, the development of external losses, and/or a change in the distribution volume of the protein. Table 2 summarizes the current mechanisms of hypoalbuminemia and the determinants of the preservation of the albumin pool in patients with renal disease and dialysis.

It has recently been suggested that inflammation and not malnutrition is the primary cause of the reduced albumin synthesis in hypoalbuminemic hemodialysis patients. Recent evidence has come from the preliminary report by Bergström et al. (81) that plasma C-reactive protein (CRP) concentration was the most powerful predictor of serum albumin and was a better predictor of death at 1 year than the serum albumin concentration. Also, Kaysen et al. (82) found using multiple regression analysis that both CRP and other acute-phase proteins, such as serum amyloid A, predicted albumin concentration in a group of hemodialysis patients.

A. Disturbances in Amino Acid Metabolism in Dialysis Patients

The kidney plays a major role in the regulation of many body pools of amino acids (AA) through synthesis, degradation, and/or urinary excretion. In chronic renal failure, a specific pattern with high concentrations of several nonessential amino acids (NEAA) and low concentrations of essential amino acids (EAA), including branched-chain amino acids (BCAA), has been reported in both plasma and in muscle (83,84). It is now well accepted that the historical classification of AA as essential and nonessential is not satisfactory in chronic

Table 2 Albumin Turnover in Renal Disease and Dialysis

Hypoalbuminemic patient group	Albumin synthesis	Fractional albumin catabolic rate	External losses	Albumin distribution
Hemodialysis	Reduced	Reduced (protects albumin pool)	Minor but can be important with reuse; amino acid losses may contribute	Normal
CAPD	Variable; synthesis may increase in response to losses, but may be suppressed by malnutrition or inflammation	Reduced (protects albumin pool)	External loss is important	Normal

Source: Adapted from Ref. 80.

renal failure because hisitidine has been shown to be an essential AA, and other AA, such as glycine, tyrosine, cystine, proline, arginine, glutamine, and taurine, are generally considered as indispensable components of the normal diet.

A recent report (85) presented data on AA concentration obtained simultaneously from three different compartments [plasma, muscle, and red blood cells (RBC)] in patients with ESRD. The findings showed that RBC and plasma play independent and opposing roles in AA interorgan transport and that several AA abnormalities in all three compartments exist in uremia. The authors recommend that AA in RBC should be considered when metabolic and clinical studies of AA disturbances in uremia are undertaken. Tables 3 and 4 summarize some of the data obtained in three groups of patients (predialysis, hemodialysis, and peritoneal dialysis, compared to normal controls) taken from this study. It is clear that low values of plasma and intracellular BCAA are found in chronic renal failure patients; the mechanism for this abnormality involves accelerated BCCA decarboxylation.

This mechanism represents the reversal of the metabolic adaptation to a low-protein diet where the major response is to reduce EAA oxidation. As long as there is absence of metabolic acidosis, the adaptive responses to a low-protein diet remain intact (86). However, metabolic acidosis stimulates BCAA degradation, and correction of the acidosis also improves the protein degradation in both experimental animals as in humans (87).

Also recently, many abnormalities have been observed in plasma sulfur amino acid (sAA) concentrations in nondialyzed patients with chronic renal failure and during treatment with both hemodialysis and peritoneal dialysis (88). The major findings were significantly decreased methionine and taurine concentrations in both hemodialysis and peritoneal dialysis, while cysteine sulfinic acid and total, free, and protein-bound homocysteine and cysteine were significantly increased

Table 3 Plasma and Muscle Essential Free Amino Acid Concentration in Healthy Controls and Uremic Patients

	Concentration (μmol/L)							
	Controls		Predialysis		Peritoneal dialysis		Hemodialysis	
Amino acid	Plasma	Muscle	Plasma	Muscle	Plasma	Muscle	Plasma	Muscle
Histidine	87	592	78	515	68	523	76	540
Isoleucine	63	68	53	96	56	91	50	90
Leucine	120	133	82	151	82	146	85	178
Lysine	195	994	159	966	162	1,370	163	1,371
Phenylalanine	53	62	50	115	53	87	54	88
Threonine	128	571	108	626	106	805	114	67
Tyrosine	60	87	36	75	41	89	36	8
Valine	220	253	168	285	161	233	174	28

Table 4 Plasma and Muscle Nonessential Free Amino Acid Concentrations in Healthy Controls and Uremic Patients

	Concentration (μmol/L)							
	Controls		Predialysis		Peritoneal dialysis		Hemodialysis	
Amino acid	Plasma	Muscle	Plasma	Muscle	Plasma	Muscle	Plasma	Muscle
Alanine	316	2,249	321	2,824	395	3,318	324	3,224
Arginine	86	633	93	686	92	822	97	918
Asparagine	47	266	49	397	49	439	51	458
Citrulline	34	170	85	118	92	181	92	197
Glutamic acid	32	4,015	53	6,165	51	6,208	45	4,668
Glutamine	655	20,050	633	19,963	596	20,374	567	21,906
Glycine	248	1,304	280	1,706	258	1,981	289	2,119
Ornithine	66	493	63	364	61	434	52	372
Serine	114	584	93	796	85	770	82	706
Taurine	49	19,194	53	18,890	42	15,477	33	12,711

in all patient groups. Taurine deficiency has been considered a potential cause of dilated cardiomyopathy (89), and although the exact physiological function of taurine is not known, a role in modulating calcium fluxes, cardiac contractility, and congestive heart failure has been suspected (90). As described in the chapter on cardiovascular problems, homocysteine has recently attracted interest because of its probable association with cardiovascular disease in non-uremic as well as in uremic patients (see Chapter 15).

B. Protein Degradation and Metabolic Acidosis

The cellular mechanisms of protein degradation in acidosis include lysosomal, (calcium)-activated proteases and energy-requiring and energy-independent proteolytic pathways. Studies by Mitch et al. (91) have shown that acidosis activates the ubiquitin-proteasome–dependent pathway. Evidence for acidosis-induced activation of this pathway includes increased mRNAs for ubiquitin and subunits of the proteasome in muscle of acidotic compared with pair-fed control rats (91). Acidosis is now considered to be an important independent cause of malnutrition in uremic patients, and correction of the acidosis in both hemodialysis and peritoneal dialysis patients is mandatory.

III. TRACE ELEMENT METABOLISM IN UREMIA AND DIALYSIS

The term *trace element* dates back to the initial stage of the development of analytical methods in the nineteenth century. It described all elements in body fluids and tissues occurring in such extremely small amounts that they could not be measured accurately. This nomenclature remained, although most trace elements can now be measured very precisely.

Trace elements are divided into two categories: essential and nonessential. A trace element is essential if (a) the element should be present in healthy tissues, (b) deficiency of the element consistently produces functional impairment, (c) the abnormalities induced by the deficiency are always followed by specific biochemical changes, and (d) addition of the element prevents or corrects these changes (92). It is generally accepted that the term trace element applies to elements that occur in the body at concentrations of less than 50 ng/kg under normal conditions (92).

A. Methodology for Measurement of Trace Elements

Accurate determination of trace element concentration is essential to allow a correct interpretation of the pathophysiological events related to their accumulation or loss in chronic renal failure. Various analytical techniques can be used to measure trace elements in body fluids and tissues (93). Analytical methods for these measurements have improved substantially during the last decades with the introduction of flame/flameless atomic absorption, electron microprobe analysis, inductively coupled plasma emission spectroscopy, inductively coupled mass spectrometry, neutron activation analysis, and x-ray fluorescence.

For many elements occurring at the ng/L or ng/kg level, major difficulties arise at the stage of sample collecting and handling. Because of the very low concentration of the elements, contamination is a major problem. Utmost care should be taken to collect samples in trace element–free recipients and tubes.

The next consideration concerns the adequacy of specificity and sensitivity of the analytical methods. In addition, the possibility for the analysis of the trace element in small tissue samples should be considered.

For some studies, it may be interesting to use a multielement method that allows the estimation of several trace elements at the same time. Drawbacks of certain methods may be that they need an important infrastructure and that they are very labor intensive. The management of large numbers of samples in a relatively limited study period then becomes impossible. Radiochemical neutron activation analysis is a good illustration of such a method. Its value lies in being the pioneer in producing accurate data, and it continues to serve as a very reliable reference method for certification purposes.

For single-element analysis, the most commonly available system is flameless atomic absorption spectrometry. For multiple-element analyses, inductively coupled plasma mass spectrometry, recently introduced in the field, supersedes all other methods. There is, however, no single method that allows the measurement of all possible trace elements in body fluids and tissues.

An important source of misunderstanding and discrepancy is the lack of uniformity in reporting results. Depending on the element and the study, sometimes whole blood values are reported, while at other times concentrations in blood constituents such as serum or plasma, packed red cells, platelets, or leukocytes are reported. Concentrations in various tissues obtained on biopsy and autopsy samples are in almost all cases markedly different from blood concentrations. Certain tissues, such as the kidneys and the skin, are known for sequestering trace elements (e.g., arsenicum or cadmium).

In this section, some aspects of trace element metabolism in relation with uremia and dialysis modalities will be discussed. This discussion will not include aluminum or iron metabolism; these two elements are discussed in other chapters.

B. Trace Element Concentrations in Uremia

The extent of abnormality of trace element concentrations in body fluids and tissues in case of uremia is dependent on many factors, the most important one being the degree of renal failure. Changes in trace element concentration may also be induced by the use of one or another form of renal replacement therapy. Padovese et al. (94) demonstrated that dialysis fluids used for continuous ambulatory peritoneal dialysis (CAPD), hemodialysis, and hemofiltration may contain trace metals in various concentrations depending on the chemical composition of the salts used to prepare the final dialysis fluid. For a series of trace elements, including gold, barium, gallium, thallium, vanadium, nickel, and chromium, the weekly exposure via the dialysis fluids appeared to be 50- to 12000-fold greater than the estimated amount absorbed via the diet. In addition, some end-stage renal disease (ESRD) patients may have developed their kidney disease following an intoxication with one of these trace elements (e.g., lead). This will result in much higher values than in end-stage renal failure due to other causes.

In Table 5 the range of normal serum concentrations of various trace elements observed in several studies and the comparative values in uremia, hemodialysis, and CAPD are given, together with an indication of whether these are increased or decreased versus the reference value. Values reported in the literature during accidental intoxications with one or another trace element are not included in this table. Some of the most clinically important acute intoxications occurred with aluminum and have been reviewed by D'Haese and De Broe (116).

It is clear from Table 5 that some elements tend to rise (e.g., arsenicum, cobalt, cesium, chromium, mercury, molybdenum) with renal failure, whereas others show an overt tendency to decrease (e.g., bromine, rubidium, selenium, zinc). Furthermore, the stage of renal failure and the type of renal replacement therapy may influence trace element concentration (e.g., bromine is decreased in hemodialysis and CAPD patients but is elevated in non-ESRD patients). Similarly, differences may be present from organ to organ (117) and/or depending on the living area of the patients under study (118,119).

A detailed description of the potential toxic/depletory side effects of some trace elements is beyond the scope of this chapter and can be found in some recent reviews (95,120). Trace elements are thought to be involved in impairment of renal function (lead, germanium, cadmium, copper, mercury), enhanced susceptibility to cancer (arsenic, cadmium, selenium), cardiovascular disease (selenium, mercury, lead, cadmium, vanadate, copper and iron excess, and cobalt), glucose intolerance, bone disease/osteomalacia (both aluminum intoxication and iron overload), anemia (arsenic, aluminum accumulation, copper deficiency, va-

Table 5 Reported Serum/Plasma Concentrations of the Most Important Trace Elements in Renal Failure and Dialysis

Element	Normal values	ESRD	Hemodialysis	CAPD	
Arsenic (μg/L)	0.09–5.49	0.5–24.8 (↑)	1.6–17.5 (↑)	4.67–5.41 (↑)	96–99
Bromine (mg/L)	2.19–5	6.9 (=/↑)	1.1–1.9 (↓)	1.0 (↓)	100–102
Cadmium (μg/L)	<0.10–0.20	—	1.2 (↑)	—	103
Cesium (μg/L)	0.45–1.50	—	0.6–1.5 (↑)	1.1 (=)	101,103,104
Chromium (μg/L)	0.04–0.35	0.28		4.3 ± 1.92 (↑)	101
			6.2 ± 2.1 (↑)	7.5 ± 1.7 (↑)	105
			8.31 ± 10.91 (↑)	8.32 ± 2.86 (↑)	106
Cobalt (μg/L)	0.11 ± 0.06	0.35 (↑)	0.45 ± 0.1 (↑)	0.3 (↑)	94,101
Copper					
(mg/L)	0.98–1.07	0.8–1.3 (=/↑)	0.8–1.5 (=/↑)	1.1–1.2 (=)	101,102,103,106
(μmol/L)	18.3 ± 5		11.9 ± 2.4 (↓)	15.2 ± 3.4 (↓)	107
Fluoride (μM/L)	0.55–1.9	—	0.8–5.2 (↑)	1.7–5.2 (↑)	108
Gold (ng/L)	9–12	—	40.9 (=/↑)	—	103
Manganese (μg/L)	0.57 ± 0.13	—	—	0.58 ± 0.11 (=)	101
Mercury (μg/L)	0.55–2.1	—	2.5 (↑)	—	103
Molybdenum (μg/L)	0.28–1.17	—	2.3 (↑)		103
Rubidium (mg/L)	0.095–0.272	—	0.1 (↓)	0.17 (=)	100,101,103
Selenium					
(mg/L)	0.13 ± 0.02	0.2 (=)	0.1 (=/↓)	0.1 (↓)	100–103
(μg/L)	64.7 ± 13	44.5 ± 13.3 (↓)	52.5 ± 14.8 (↓)		109
Silicon (μg/L)	110–880	480–1300 (↑)	620–4600 (↑)		110
Strontium (μmol/L)	0.22 ± 0.06	—	0.62 ± 0.24 (↑)	—	113,114
Vanadium (μg/L)	0.01–1	—	18.4 (↑)		115
Zinc (mg/L)	0.69–1.21	0.7–0.9 (↓)	0.7–0.9 (↓)	0.85 (↓)	101,102,104,106

Source: Adapted from Ref. 95.

nadium, and high blood lead levels), enzyme dysfunction (selenium, copper and zinc, mercury, lead, vanadate and cadmium), encephalopathy/coma (acute aluminum intoxication), and immune deficiency (iron overload and selenium and zinc deficiency).

C. Specific Examples

1. Selenium

Serum selenium levels appear to be lower than normal in dialysis patients. Selenium is an essential trace element for humans (121) because it is necessary for the biological activity of glutathione peroxidase (122) and is known to neutralize harmful peroxidation taking place during metabolic processes. Recently, correlations were established between creatinine clearance and plasma levels of glutathione peroxidase, selenium, and total glutathione in undialyzed patients and patients on either peritoneal dialysis or hemodialysis. Alterations in antioxidant systems gradually increased with the degree of renal failure, rose further in patients on peritoneal dialysis, and culminated in hemodialysis patients (123).

The clinical significance of the low levels of selenium in dialysis patients is not clear but has been invoked as contributing factor in cardiovascular disease, skeletal myopathy, altered immune functions, and increased risk for cancer. Low serum selenium may be related to low selenium mineral contents in soil and food, e.g., grain (124,125).

The observation that selenium can be found in the peritoneal dialysate indicates a potential source of selenium losses through the peritoneal membrane. This selenium may cross the peritoneal membrane bound to proteins.

2. Zinc

Low serum and increased packed cell zinc levels have been observed in nondialyzed and dialyzed uremic patients (101,104). The zinc levels in the peritoneal dialysate are very low and are reduced by more than half after one dwell. Zinc is not lost into the dialysate effluent; on the contrary, significant zinc absorption from the dialysate has been observed (126,127).

After supplementation with zinc, taste acuity markedly improved in 95% of hemodialysis patients with poor appetite and zinc concentrations in hair increased in 85% of patients (128). The patients' appetites were improved, the average caloric intake increased by 675 kcal/day, and intolerance to protein diminished.

In peritoneal dialysis patients, zinc supplementation had a beneficial effect on the reduced TSH, T_4, and T_3 serum levels (129), suggesting that zinc deficiency plays a role in the disturbed biosynthesis or release of these hormones.

Interestingly, recent research (130) has found a zinc concentration–dependent increase in stimulated IL-1α and IL-1β and TNF-α release in both peripheral mononuclear cells and peritoneal macrophages from CAPD patients. A zinc concentration–dependent increase in peritoneal macrophage calcitriol release was also observed. It is known that calcitriol plays an important role in granulocyte and immune cell fuction (131).

Low serum zinc may be related to removal by hemodialysis (97)) and inefficient caloric intake (132). Although serum zinc tends to rise at the end of dialysis, this must be attributed entirely to the rise in concentration of vector proteins due to ultrafiltration (133).

3. Chromium

Chromium concentrations in both serum and red blood cells rise with chronic dialysis treatment. Extra addition to the blood was demonstrated in CAPD and hemodialysis from the impurities present in dialysate (101). In CAPD patients, the mean serum chromium levels are about 26 times higher than the normal mean values (101). The concentration of chromium in the fresh peritoneal dialysate is about 8 times the normal serum value and is absorbed for about 50% per dwell. After absorption, chromium is directly transferred to the general circulation, where it is mainly bound to transferrin (134).

Using a functional model of chromium kinetics and metabolism, long-term (10 years) treatment with CAPD should result in an accumulation of chromium with a factor of 100 in those organs, especially liver and spleen, known to have a slow exchange of chromium with the central plasma compartment (135).

The essentiality versus toxicity of chromium in humans is somewhat ambiguous. While Cr(III) is an essential element involved in glucose metabolism, Cr(VI) is a potent carcinogen (136).

4. Bromium

Bromium levels in both serum and packed blood cells fall far below the normal values in both hemodialysis (100,137) and peritoneal dialysis patients (101). The increase of bromium in the peritoneal dialysate indicates that some bromium leaves the body across the peritoneum with a half-life of about 24 hours. It is interesting to note that subnormal blood levels of bromium have been hypothesized as a cause for the insomnia of dialysis patients (137).

5. Silicon

Silicon levels in dialysis patients are markedly increased (for review, see Refs. 110–112). Elevated silicon levels may be the result of excess silicon concentrations in the dialysate, as well as of consumption of drinking water containing excess silicon (111,112,138). The clinical significance of the increased silicon levels is not yet fully understood, but recently a presumed silicon-related syndrome consisting of a perforating folliculitis of the skin and aberrant hair growth has been described in two dialysis patients (110).

D. Therapeutic Aspects

Excess trace element ingestion can be avoided by reducing intake via food and other sources and by reducing contact with environmentally contaminated material. If excess load can be attributed to presence in dialysate, water purification should be improved preferably by using reversed osmosis and ion exchange systems.

Further excess present in the toxic range can be removed by chelation (e.g., desferrioxamine for aluminum and iron or EDTA for lead). It should, however, be taken into account that an overzealous chelation may induce enhanced toxicity by itself: removal of lead from the bone compartment, where it resides in a relatively dormant form, may accelerate progress of renal failure; chelation of aluminum may temporarily induce symptoms of dementia. It is interesting to note that chelation therapy with desferrioxamine, in contrast with the effects on aluminum and iron removal, has virtually no influence on the removal of copper, zinc, or lead in CAPD patients (139). In renal failure, chelation must be combined with dialysis strategies (139,140).

It should be stressed that chelators per se may exert toxicity: desferrioxamine has been associated with immune suppression and development of opportunistic infections such as mycormycosis (140). Elements that are below the reference levels can more easily be replaced, either perorally or after addition to the dialysate. The latter solution may, however, be too expensive and labor intensive in view of the large dialysate volumes that cross the dialyzer at the occasion of each dialysis.

REFERENCES

1. Massry SG, Smogorzewski M. Carbohydrate metabolism in renal failure. In: Kopple JD, Massry SG, eds. Nutritional Management of Renal Disease. Baltimore: Williams & Wilkins, 1997:63–76.
2. Mak RM, De Fronzo RA. Glucose and insulin metabolism in uremia. Nephron 1992; 61:377–382.
3. Adrogué HJ. Glucose homeostasis and the kidney. Kidney Int 1992; 42:1266–1282.
4. Alvestrand A. Carbohydrate and insulin metabolism in renal failure. Kidney Int 1997; 52(suppl 62):S48–S52.
5. Eidemak I, Felt-Rasmussen B, Kanstrup I-L, Nielsen SL, Schmitz O, Strandgaard S. Insulin resistance and hyperinsulinemia in mild to moderate progressive chronic renal failure and its association with aerobic work capacity. Diabetologia 1995; 38:565–572.
6. Smith D, DeFronzo RA. Insulin resistance in uremia mediated by postbinding defects. Kidney Int 1982; 22: 54–62.
7. Castellino P, Solino A, Luzi L, Barr JG, Smith DJ, Petrides A, Giordano M, Carroll C, DeFronzo RA. Glucose and amino acid metabolism in chronic renal failure: effects of insulin and amino acids. Am J Physiol 1992; 262:F168–F176.
8. Friedman JE, Dohm GL, Elton CHW, Rovira A, Chen JJ, Leggett-Frazier N, Atkinson SM, Thomas FT, Long SD, Caro JF. Muscle insulin resistance in uremic humans: glucose transport, glucose transporters, and insulin receptors. Am J Physiol 1991; 261:E87–E94.
9. Bak JF, Schmitz O, Sorensen SS. Activity of insulin receptor kinase and glycogen synthase in skeletal muscle from patients with chronic renal failure. Acta Endocrinol (Copenh) 1989; 121:744–750.
10. Riggalleau V, Combe C, Blanchtier V, Aubertin J, Apacicio M, Gin H. Low protein diet diet in uremia: effects of glucose metabolism and energy production rate. Kidney Int 1997; 51:1222–1227.
11. McCaleb ML, Wish JB, Lockwood DH. Insulin resistance in chronic renal failure. Endocrine Res 1985; 11: 113–125.
12. Dzurik R, Hupkova V, Cernacek P. The isolation of an inhibitor of glucose utilization from the serum of uraemic subjects. Clin Chim Acta 1983; 46:77–83.
13. Dzùrik R, Spustovà V, Lajdovà I. Inhibition of glucose utilization in isolated rat soleus muscle by pseudouridine: implications for renal failure. Nephron 1993; 65:108–110.
14. Hörl WH, Haag-Weber M, Georgopoulos A, Block LH. The physicochemical characterization of a novel polypeptide present in uremic serum that inhibits the biological activity of polymorphonuclear leukocytes. Proc Natl Acad Sci USA 1990; 87:6353–6357.
15. Haag-Weber M, Mai B, Hörl WH. Isolation of a granulocyte inhibitory protein from uremic patients with homology to ($_2$ microglobulin. Nephrol Dial Transplant 1994; 9:382–388.
16. Mak RHK, Turner C, Thompson T, Haycock GB, Chantler C. The effects of low protein diet with amino acid/ keto acid supplements on glucose metabolism in children with uremia. J Clin Endocrin Metab 1986; 63:985–989.
17. Mak RH. Intravenous 1,25-dihydroxycholecalciferol corrects glucose intolerance in hemodialysis patients. Kidney Int 1992; 41:1049–1054.
18. Kautzsky-Willer A, Pacini G, Barnas U, Ludvik B, Strell C, Graf H, Prager R. Intravenous calcitriol normalizes insulin sensitivity in uremic patients. Kidney Int 1995; 47:200–206.
19. Lin S, Lin Y, Lu K, Diang LK, Chyr SH, Liao WK, Shieh SD. Effects of intravenous calcitriol on lipid profiles and glucose tolerance in uraemic patients with secondary hyperparathyroidism. Clin Sci 1994; 87: 533–538.
20. Reaich D, Channon SM, Scrimgeour CM, Daley SE, Wilkinson R, Goodship THJ. Correction of acidosis in humans with CRF decreases protein degradation and amino acid oxidation. Am J Physiol 1993; 265:E230–E235.
21. Stuart CA, Shangraw RE, Prince MJ, Peters EJ, Wolfe RR. Bed-rest induced insulin resistance occurs primarily in muscle. Metabolism 1988; 37:802–806.
22. Goldberg A, Hagberg J, Delmez J, Haynes ME, Harter HR. The metabolic effects of exercise training in hemodialysis patients. Kidney Int 1989; 18:754–761.
23. Kokot F, Wiecek A, Grzeszczak W, Klin M, Zukowska-Szczechowska F. Influence of erythropoietin treatment on glucose tolerance, insulin, glucagon, gastrin, and pancreatic polypeptide secretion in hemodialyzed patients with end stage renal disease. Contrib Nephrol 1990; 87:42–50.
24. Borissova AM, Djambazova A, Todorov K, Dakovska L, Tankova T, Kirilov G. Effect of erythropoietin on the metabolic state and peripheral insulin sensitivity in diabetic patients on hemodialysis. Nephrol Dial Transplant 1993; 8:93–95.
25. Mak RHK. Effect of recombinant human erythropoietin on insulin, amino acid, and lipid metabolism in uremia. J Pediatr 1996; 129:97–104.
26. Chagnac A, Weinstein T, Zevin D, Korzets A, Hirsh J, Gafter U, Levi J. Effects of erythropoieten on glucose tolerance in hemodialysis patients. Clin Nephrol 1994; 42:398–400.
27. Fadda GZ, Thanakitcharu P, Communale R, Lipson LG, Massry SG. Impaired potasium-induced insulin secretion in chronic renal failure. Kidney Int 1991; 40: 413–417.

28. Oh H, Fadda G, Smogorzewski M, Liou HH, Massry SG. Abnormal leucine-induced insulin secretion in chronic renal failure. Am J Physiol 1994; 267:F853–F860.
29. Hajjar SM, Fadda GZ, Thanakitsaru P, Smogorzewski M, Massry SG. Reduced activity of Na^+-K^+-ATPase of pancreatic islets in chronic renal failure: role of secondary hyperparathyroidism. J Am Soc Nephrol 1992; 2:1355–1363.
30. Thanakitsaru P, Fadda ZG, Hajjar SM, Levi E, Stojceva-Taneva O, Massry SG. Verapamil reverses glucose intolerance preexisting chronic renal failure: studies on mechanisms. Am J Nephrol 1992; 12:179–187.
31. Hörl WH, Haag-Weber M, Mai B, Massry SG. Verapamil reverses abnormal $[Ca^3+]$ i and carbohydrate metabolism of PMNL of dialysis patients. Kidney Int 1995; 47:1741–1745.
32. Fadda GZ, Hajjar SM, Perna AF, Zhou X-J, Lipson LG, Massry SG. On the mechanism of impaired insulin secretion in chronic renal failure. J Clin Invest 1991; 87:255–261.
33. Perna AF, Fadda GZ, Zhou XJ, Massry SG. Mechanisms of impaired insulin secretion after chronic excess of parathyroid hormone. Am J Physiol 1990; 259: F210–F216.
34. Christakos S, Norman AW. Studies of the mode of action of calciferol XXXIX. Biochemical characterization of $1,25(OH)_2$ D_3 receptors in chick pancreas and kidney cytosol. Endocrinol 1981; 108:140–149.
35. Pike JW. Receptors for 1,25 dihydroxyvitamin D3 in chick pancreas: a partial physical and functional characterization. J Steroid Biochem 1981; 16:385–395.
36. Roth J, Bonner-Weir S, Norman AW, Orci L. Immunocytochemistry of vitamin D-dependent calcium-binding protein in chick pancreas: exclusive localization in cells. Endocrinology 1982; 110:2216–2218.
37. Morrisey RL, Bucci TJ, Empson RN, Lufkin EG. Calcium-binding proteins: its cellular localization in jejunum, kidney and pancreas. Proc Soc Exp Biol Med 1975; 148:56–60.
38. Pochet R, Pipeleers DG, Malaisse WJ. Calbindin D-27 Kda preferential localization in non-β islet cells of the rat pancreas. J Biol Cell 1987; 61:155–161.
39. Narbaitz R, Stumpf WE, Sar M. The role of autoradiographic and immunocytochemical techniques in the clarification of sites of metabolism and action of vitamin D. J Histochem Cytochem 1981; 29:91–100.
40. Nadkarni M, Berns JS, Rudnick MR, Cohen RM. Hypoglycemia with hyperinsulinemia in a chronic hemodialysis patient following parathyroidectomy. Nephron 1992; 60:100–103.
41. Emilsson V, Liu Y-L, Cowthorne MA, Morton NM, Davenport M. Expression of the functional leptin receptor mRNA in pancreatic islets and direct inhibitory action of leptin on insulin secretion. Diabetes 1997; 46:313–316.
42. Heimbürger O, Lönnqvist F, Danielsson A, Nordenström J, StenvinkelP. Serum immunoreactive leptin concentration and its relation to the body fat content in chronic renal failure. J Am Soc Nephrol 1997; 8: 1423–1430.
43. Nishizawa Y, Shoji T, Tanaka S, Yamashita M, Morita A, Emoto M, Tabata T, Inoue T, Morii H. Plasma leptin level and its relationship with body composition in hemodialysis patients. Am J Kidney Dis 1998; 31: 655–661.
44. Sharma K, Considine RV, Michael B, Dunn SR, Weisberg LS, Kurnik BR, Kurnik PB, O'Connor J, Sinha M, Caro JF. Plasma leptin is partly cleared by the kidney and is elevated in hemodialysis patients. Kidney Int 1997; 51:1980–1985.
45. Dagogo-Jack S, Ovalle F, Landt M, Gearing B, Coyne DW. Hyperleptinemia in patients with end-stage renal disease undergoing continuous ambulatory peritoneal dialysis. Perit Dial Int 1998; 18:34–40.
46. Stenvinkel P, Heimbürger O, Lonnqvist F. Serum leptin concentrations correlate to plasma insulin concentrations independent of body fat content in chronic renal failure. Nephrol Dial Transplant 1997; 12:1321–1325.
47. Havel PJ, Uriu-Hare JY, Stanhope KL, Stern JS, Keen CL, Ahren B. Marked and rapid decreases of circulating leptin in streptozotocin diabetic rats: reversal by insulin. Am J Physiol 1998; 274:R1482–R1491.
48. Rabkin R, Simon NM, Steiner S, Colwell JA. Effects of renal disease on renal uptake and excretion of insulin in man. N Engl J Med 1970; 282:182–187.
49. Rubenfeld S, Garber AJ. Abnormal carbohydrate metabolism in chronic renal failure: the potential of accelerated glucose production, increased gluconeogenesis, and impaired glucose disposal. J Clin Invest 1978; 62:20–28.
50. Sherwin RS, Bastl C, Finkelstein FO, Fisher M, Black H, Hendler R, Felig P. Influence of uremia and hemodialysis on the turnover and metabolic effects of glucagon. J Clin Invest 1976; 57:722–731.
51. DeFronzo RA, Alvestrand A, Smith D, Hendler R, Hendler E, Wahren J. Insulin resistance in uremia. J Clin Invest 1981; 67:563–568.
52. Schmitz O. Peripheral and hepatic resistance to glucagon in uremic subjects. Acta Endocrinol (Copenh) 1988; 118:125–134.
53. Hong S, Yang D. Insulin levels and fibrinolytic activity in patients with end-stage renal disease. Nephron 1994; 68:329–333.
54. Peitzman SJ, Agarwal BN. Spontaneous hypoglycemia in end stage renal failure. Nephron 1977; 19:131–140.
55. Arem R. Hypoglycemia associated with renal failure. Endocrinol Metab Clin North Am 1989; 18:103–121.
56. Arauz-Pacheco C, Ramirez LC, Rios JM, Raskin P. Hypoglycemia induced by angiotensin converting enzyme inhibitors in patients with non-insulin dependent

diabetes receiving sulfonylurea therapy. Am J Med 1990; 89:811–813.

57. Pollare T, Lithell H, Berne C. A comparison of the effects of hydrochlorothiazide and captopril on glucose and lipid metabolism in patients with hypertension. N Engl J Med 1989; 321:868–873.
58. Bergström J, Fürst P, Alvestrand A, Lindholm B. Protein and energy intake, nitrogen balance and nitrogen losses in patients treated with continuous ambulatory peritoneal dialysis. Kidney Int 1993; 44:1048–1057.
59. Kurtz SB, Wong VH, Anderson CF, Vogel JP, McCarthy JT, Mitchell C. Continuous ambulatory peritoneal dialysis. Three years' experience at the Mayo Clinic. Mayo Clin Proc 1983; 58:633–639.
60. Lindholm B, Bergström J. Nutritional aspects of CAPD. In: Gokal R, ed. Continuous Ambulatory Peritoneal Dialysis. Edinburgh: Churchill Livingstone, 1986:228–237.
61. Lameire N, Matthys D, Matthys E, Beheyt R. Effects of long-term CAPD on carbohydrate and lipid metabolism. Clin Nephrol 1988; 30(suppl 1):S53–S58.
62. Armstrong VW, Buschman U, Ebert R, Fichs C, Rieger J, Scheler F. Biochemical investigations of CAPD: plasma levels of trace elements and amino acids and impaired glucose tolerance during the course of treatment. Int J Artif Organs 1980; 3:237–241.
63. Heaton A, Ramos M, Johnston D, Gokal R, Ward MK, Kerr DNS. Glucose and lipid metabolism in continuous ambulatory peritoneal dialysis. Kidney Int 1982; 22:220–221.
64. Wideröe TE, Smeby LC, Myking OL. Plasma concentrations and transperitoneal transport of native insulin and C-peptide in patients on continuous ambulatory peritoneal dialysis. Kidney Int 1984; 25:82–87.
65. Heaton A, et al. Carbohydrate and lipid metabolism during continuous ambulatory peritoneal dialysis (CAPD): the effect of a single dialysis dwell. Science 1983; 65:539–545.
66. Armstrong V, Creutzfeldt W, Ebert R, Fuchs C, Hilgers R, et al. Effect of dialysate glucose load on plasma glucose and hormones in CAPD patients. Nephron 1985; 39:141–145.
67. Lindholm B, Karlander S. Glucose tolerance in patients undergoing continuous ambulatory peritoneal dialysis. Acta Med Scand 1986; 220:477–483.
68. Smith W, Hanning I, Johnston D, Brown C. Pancreatic beta cell function in CAPD. Nephrol Dial Transplant 1988; 3:448–453.
69. Heaton A, Taylor R, Johnston D, Ward M, Wilkinson R. Hepatic and peripheral insulin action in chronic renal failure and during continuous ambulatory peritoneal dialysis. Clin Sci 1989; 77:383–388.
70. Hampers C, Soelder JS, Doak PB, Merrill JP. Effect of chronic renal failure and hemodialysis on carbohydrate metabolism. J Clin Invest 1966; 45:1719–1731.
71. Graf H, Prager R Koverik J, Luger A, Schernthaner G, Pinggera WF. Glucose metabolism and insulin sensitivity in patients on chronic hemodialysis. Metabolism 1985; 34:974–977.
72. Oshida Y, Sato Y, Shiraishi S, Sakamoto N. studies on glucose tolerance in chronic renal failure: estimation of insulin sensitivity before and after initiation of hemodialysis. Clin Nephrol 1987; 28:35–38.
73. Foss MC, Gouveia LMFB, Neto MM, Paccola GMGF, Piccinato CE. Effect of hemodialysis on peripheral glucose metabolism of patients with chronic renal failure. Nephron 1996; 73:48–53.
74. DeFronzo, RA, Tobin JD, Rowe JW, Andres R. Glucose intolerance in uremia. Quantification of pancreatic beta cell sensitivity to insulin and tissue sensitivity to insulin. J Clin Invest 1978; 62:425–435.
75. Koutsikos D, Foutounas C, Kapetanaki A, Agroyannis B, Tzanatos H, Rammos G, Kopelias I, Bosiolis B, Bovoleti O, Darema, M, Sallum G. Oral glucose tolerance test after high-dose i.v. biotin administration in normoglycemic hemodialysis patients. Ren Fail 1996; 18:131–137.
76. Runyan JW, Hurwitz D, Robbins SL. Effect of Kimmelstiel-Wilson syndrome on insulin requirements in diabetes. N Engl J Med 1955; 252:388–391.
77. Weinrauch LA, Healy RW, Leland OS Jr, Goldstein HH, Libertino JA, Takacs FJ, Bradley RF, Gleason RE, D'Elia JA. Decreased insulin requirements in acute renal failure in diabetic nephropathy. Arch Intern Med 1978; 138:399–402.
78. Lowrie EG, Lew NL. Death risk in hemodialysis patients: the predictive value of commonly measured variables and an evaluation of death rates differences between facilities. Am J Kidney Dis 1990; 15:458–482.
79. Avram MM, Goldwasser P, Erroa M, Fein PA. Predictors of survival in continuous ambulatory peritoneal dialaysis patients: the importance of prealbumin and other nutritional and metabolic markers. Am J Kidney Dis 1994; 32:91–98.
80. Kaysen GA. Albumin turnover in renal diasease. Miner Electrolyte Metab 1998; 24:55–63.
81. Bergström J, Heimbürger O, Lindholm B, Qureshi AR. Elevated serum CRP is a strong predictor of increased mortality and low serum albumin in hemodialysis patients (abstr). J Am Soc Nephrol 1995; 6:573.
82. Kaysen GA, Rathore V, Depner TA. C reactive protein (CRP) and serum amyloid A (SAA) levels predict serum albumin levels in hemodialysis patients (abstr). J Am Soc Nephrol 1996; 7:1486.
83. Klahr S. Effects of renal insufficiency on nutrient metabolism and endocrine function. In: Mitch WE, Klahr S, eds. Handbook of Nutrition and the Kidney. 3rd ed. Philadelphia: Lippincott-Raven, 1998:25–44.
84. Reaich D, Maroni BJ. Protein and amino acid metabolism in renal disease and renal failure. In: Kopple

JD, Massry SG, eds. Nutritional Management of Renal Disease. Baltimore: Williams and Wilkins, 1997:1–33.

85. Divino Filho JC, Bàràny P, Stehle P, Fürst P, Bergström J. Free amino-acid levels simultaneously collected in plasma, muscle, and erthrocytes of uaemic patients. Nephrol Dial Transplant 1997; 12:2339–2348.

86. Mitch WE. Uremic acidosis and protein metabolism. Curr Opin Nephrol Hypert 1995; 4:488–492.

87. Reaich D, Graham KA, Channon SM, Hetherington C, Scrimgeour CM, Wilkinson R, Goodship THJ. Insulin mediated changes in protein degradation and glucose utilization following correction of acidosis in humans with CRF. Am J Physiol 1995, 268:E121–E126.

88. Suliman, ME, Anderstam B, Lindholm B, Bergström J. Total, free, and protein-bound sulphur amino acids in uraemic patients. Nephrol Dial Transplant 1997; 12: 2332–2338.

89. Moise SN, Pacioretty LM, Kallfelz FA, et al. Dietary taurine deficiency and dilated cardiomyopathy in the fox. Am Heart J 1996; 121:541–547.

90. Huxtable RJ. Physiological actions of taurine. Physiol Rev 1992; 72:101–163.

91. Mitch WE, Medina R, Greiber S, May RC, England BK, Price SR, Bailey JL, Goldberg AL. Metabolic acidosis stimulates muscle protein degradation by activating the ATP-dependent pathway involving ubiquitin and proteasomes. J Clin Invest 1994; 93:2127–2133.

92. Mertz W. Trace element nutrition in health and disease: contributions and problems of analysis. Clin Chem 1975; 21:468–475.

93. Alfrey AC. Trace elements and regular dialysis. In: Maher JF, ed. Replacement of renal function by dialysis. Dordrecht: Kluwer Academic, 1989:996–1003.

94. Padovese P, Galleini M, Brancaccio D, Petra R, Fortaner S, Sabbioni E, Minoia C, Markakis K, Berlin A. Trace elements in dialysis fluids and assessment of the exposure of patients on regular hemodialysis, hemofiltration, and continuous ambulatory peritoneal dialysis. Nephron 1992; 61:442–448.

95. Vanholder R, Cornelis R, Dhondt A, Ringoir S. Trace element metabolism in renal disease and renal failure. In: Kopple JD, Massry SG, eds. Nutritional Management of Renal Disease. Baltimore: Williams and Wilkins, 1997:395–414.

96. De Kimpe J, Cornelis R, Mees L, Van Lierde S, Vanholder R. More than tenfold increase of arsenic in serum and packed cells of chronic hemodialysis patients. Am J Nephrol 1993; 13:429–434.

97. Van Renterghem D, Cornelis R, Vanholder R. Behaviour of 12 trace elements in serum of uremic patients on hemodiafiltration. J Trace Elem Electrolytes Health Dis 1992; 6:169–174.

98. Zhang X, Cornelis R, De Kimpe J, Mees L, Vanderbiesen V, De Cubber A, Vanholder R. Accumulation of arsenic species in serum of patients with chronic renal disease. Clin Chem 1996; 42:1231–1237.

99. Zhang X, Cornelis R, De Kimpe J, Mees L, Lameire N. Study of arsenic-protein binding in serum of patients in continuous ambulatory peritoneal dialysis. Clin Chem 1998; 44:141–147.

100. Cornelis R, Ringoir S, Lameire N, Mees L, Hoste J. Blood bromine in uremic patients. Mineral Electrolyte Metab 1979; 2:186–192.

101. Wallaeys B, Cornelis R, Mees L, Lameire N. Trace elements in serum, packed cells, and dialysate of CAPD patients. Kidney Int 1986; 30:599–604.

102. Tsukamoto Y, Iwanami S, Marumo F. Disturbances of trace element concentrations in plasma of patients with chronic renal failure. Nephron 1980; 26:174–179.

103. Van Renterghem D, Cornelis R, Vanholder R. Behaviour of 12 trace elements in serum of uremic patients on hemodiafiltration. J Trace Elem Electrolytes Health Dis 1992; 6:169–174.

104. Cornelis R, Mees L, Ringoir S, Hoste J. Serum and red blood cell Zn, Se, Cs and Rb in dialysis patients. Mineral Electrolyte Metab 1979; 2:88–93.

105. Halls DJ, Leung ACT, Henderson IS, Fell GS, Dobbie JW, Kennedy AC. Serum chromium concentrations in patients with renal failure. In: Mills CF, Bremmer I, Chesters JK, eds. Trace Element metabolism in Man and Animals (TEMA-5). Commenwealth Agricultural Bureaux, 1984:819–822.

106. Thomson NM, Stevens BJ, Humpherey TJ, Atkins RC. Comparison of trace elements in peritoneal dialysis, hemodialysis and uremia. Kidney Int 1983; 23:9–14.

107. Emenaker NJ, DiSilvestro RA, Nahman NS, Percival S. Copper-related blood indexes in kidney dialysis patients. Am J Clin Nutr 1996; 64:757–760.

108. Al-Walkeer JS, Mitwalli AH, Huraib S, Al-Mohaya S, Abu-Aisha H, Chaudhary SA, Al-Majed SA, Memon N. Serum ionic fluoride levels in haemodialysis and continuous ambulatory peritoneal dialysis patients. Nephrol Dial Transplant 1997; 12:1420–1424.

109. Bonomini M, Forster S, Manfrini V, De Risio F, Steiner M, Vidovich MI, Klinkmann H, Ivanovich P, Albertazzi A. Geographic factors and plasma selenium in uremia and dialysis. Nephron 1996; 72:197–204.

110. Saldanha LF, Gonick HC, Rodriguez HJ, Marmelzat JA, Repique EV, Marcis CL. Silicon-related syndrome in dialysis patients. Nephron 1997; 77:48–56.

111. Gitelman HJ, Alderman FR, Perry SJ. Silicon accumulation in dialysis patients. Am J Kidney Dis 1992; 19:140–143.

112. Gitelman HJ, Alderman F, Perry SJ. Renal handling of silicon in normals and patients with renal insufficiency. Kidney Int 1992; 42:957–959.

113. Mauras Y, Ang KS, Simon P, Tessier B, Cartier F, Allain P. Increase in blood plasma levels of boron and strontium in hemodialyzed patients. Clin Chim Acta 1986; 156:315–320.

114. Smythe WR, Alfrey AC, Craswell PW, Crouch CA, Ibels LS, Kubo H, Nunnelley LL, Rudolph H. Trace element abnormalities in chronic uremia. Ann Int Med 1982; 96:302–310.
115. Hosokawa S, Yoshida O. Serum vanadium levels in chronic hemodialysis patients. Nephron 1993; 64: 388–394.
116. D'Haese PC, De Broe ME. Adequacy of dialysis: trace elements in dialysis fluids. Nephrol Dial Transplant 1996; 11(suppl 2):92–97.
117. Zevin D, Weinstein T, Levi J, Djaldetti M. X-ray microanalysis of the fingernails of uremic patients treated by hemodialysis. Clin Nephrol 1991; 36:302–304.
118. Smythe WR, Alfrey AC, Craswell PW, Crouch CA, Ibels LS, Kubo H, Nunnelley LL, Rudolph H. Trace element abnormalities in chronic uremia. Ann Intern Med 1982; 96:302–310.
119. Bonomini M, Forster S, Manfrini V, De Risio F, Steiner M, Vidovich MI, Klinkmann H, Ivanovich P, Albertazzi A. Geographic factors and plasma selenium in uremia and dialysis. Nephron 1996; 72:197–204.
120. Gilmour ER, Hartley GH, Goodship THJ. Trace elements and vitamins in renal disease. In: Mitch WE, Klahr S, eds. Nutrition and the Kidney. 2nd ed. Little, Brown and Company, 1993:114–131.
121. Young VR. Selenium: a case for its essentiality in man. N Engl J Med 1981; 304:1228–1230.
122. Rotruck JT, Pope AL, Ganther HE, Swanson AB, Hafemen DG, Hoekstra WG. Selenium: biochemical role as component of gluthathione peroxidase protein. Science 1973; 179:588–590.
123. Ceballos-Picot I, Witko-Sarsat V, Merad-Boudia M, Nguyen AT, Jaudon MC, Zingraff J, Verger C, Jungers P, Descamps-Latscha B. Glutathione antioxidant system as a marker of oxidative stress in chronic renal failure. Free Radid Biol Med 1996; 21:845–853.
124. Maksimovic ZJ. Selenium deficiency and Balkan endemic nephropathy. Kidney Int 1991; 40:S12–S14.
125. Dworkin B, Weseley S, Rosenthal W, Schwartz E, Weiss L. Diminished blood selenium levels in renal failure patients on dialysis: correlations with nutritional status. Am J Med Sci 1987; 293:6–11.
126. Tamura T, Cornwell PE, Vaughn WH, Waldo FB, Kohaut EC. Zinc levels in peritoneal dialysate (abstr). Am J Clin Nutr 1985; 41:865.
127. Zlotkin SH, Rundle MA, Hanning RM, Buchanan BE, Balfe JW. Zinc absorption from glucose and amino acid dialysis solutions in children on continuous ambulatory peritoneal dialysis (CAPD). J Am Coll Nutr 1987; 6:345–350.
128. Atkin-Thor E, Goddard BW, O'Nion J, Stephen RL, Kolff WJ. Am J Clin Nutr 1978; 10:1948–1951.
129. Arreola F, Paniagua R, Pérez A, Diaz-Bensussen S, Junco E, Villalpando S, Exaire E. Effect of Zinc treatment on serum thyroid hormones in uremic patients under peritoneal dialysis. Horm Metab Res 1993; 25: 539–542.
130. Kimmel PL, Phillips TM, Lew SQ, Langman CB. Zinc modulates mononuclear cellular calcitriol metabolism in peritoneal dialysis patients. Kidney Int 1996; 49: 1407–1412.
131. Rice JC, Haverty TP. Vitamin D and immune function in uremia. Sem Nephrol 1990; 3:237–239.
132. Hosokawa S, Kohira S, Imai T, Tomoyoshi T, Nishio T, Sawanishi K. Zinc transfer during hemodialysis in chronic renal failure patients. Blood Purif 1983; 1: 225–230.
133. Hachache T, Meftahi H, Foret M, Kuentz F, Milongo R, Christollet M, Cordonnier DJ, Arnaud J, Favier A. Evolution du taux sérique du zinc à court (1 séance) et moyen terme (6 mois) chez 33 hémodialysés. Néphrologie 1989; 10:87–90.
134. Borguet F, Cornelis R, Delanghe J, Lambert MC, Lameire N. Study of the chromium binding in plasma of patients on continuous ambulatory peritoneal dialysis. Clin Chim Acta 1995; 283:71–84.
135. Borguet F, Wallaeys B, Cornelis R, Lameire N. Transperitoneal absorption and kinetics of chromium in the continuous ambulatory peritoneal dialysis patient. Nephron 1996; 72:163–170.
136. IARC Monographs on the Evaluation of the Carcinogenic Risk of Chemicals to Humans. Lyon: International Agency for Research on Cancer, 1987 (suppl 7):165–168.
137. Oe DL, Vis RD, Meijer JM, Van Langevelde F, Allon W, Van De Meer C, Verheul H. Bromine deficiency and insomnia in patients on dialysis. In: Howell MJCC, Gawthorne JM, White CL, eds. Trace Element Metabolism in Man and Animals. Australian Academy of Science, 1981:516.
138. D'Haese PC, Shaheen FA, Huraib SO, Djukanovic L, Polenakovic MH, Spasovski G, Shikole A, Schurgers ML, Daneels RF, Lamberts LV, Van Landeghem GF, De Broe ME. Increased silicon levels in dialysis patients due to high silicon content in the drinking water, inadequate water treatment procedures, and concentrate contamination: a multicentre study. Nephrol Dial Transplant 1995; 10:1838–1844.
139. Navarro JA, Granaldillo VA, Rodriguez-Iturbe B, Garcia R, Salgado O, Romero RA. Removal of trace metals by continuous ambulatory peritoneal dialysis after desferrioxamine B chelation therapy. Clin Nephrol 1991; 35:213–217.
140. Boelaert JR, de Locht M, Van Cutsem J, Kerrels V, Cantinieaux B, Verdonck A, Van Landuyt HW, Schneider YJ. Mucormycosis during deferoxamine therapy as a siderophore-mediated infection—in vitro and in vivo animal studies. J Clin Invest 1993; 91: 1979–1986.

31

Neurological Complications of Dialysis

Stefano Biasioli
Legnago Hospital, Legnago, Italy

Neurological complications in dialysis populations are common but frequently misunderstood. Some of them relate to the persistence of uremia, some relate to the dialytic treatment "per se," while others are independent of both uremia and dialysis (1–9). This chapter provides an overview of the most common neurological problems seen in the hemodialysis (HD) and peritoneal dialysis (PD) patient.

I. PERSISTING UREMIC ENCEPHALOPATHY

In presence of adequate efficiency of dialytic therapy, the clinical pattern of overt uremic encephalopathy (UE) is rarely seen in a regular dialysis patient. Patients with chronic renal failure may or may not develop symptoms of UE (ranging from mild sensorial clouding to tremors followed by delirium and coma) if they are constantly followed by physicians so that adequate water and electrolyte balance is achieved, blood pressure is controlled, the nutritional status is normal, and iatrogenic intoxication is avoided.

Even after the institution of an "adequate" dialytic program, some patients may continue to show some subtle nervous system abnormalities such as a decrease in alertness and attention span, a reduced ability to concentrate, an impaired mentation, a generalized weakness, and signs of peripheral neuropathy. Although the weakness may be caused by several nonneurological factors (mainly linked to anemia and to the well-known protein-calorie malnutrition), the other symptoms are all due to a mild form of UE. Tremors and asterixis are two typical motor abnormalities of a mild, stable UE, while myoclonus is usually associated with a clouded sensorium and with stupor.

As shown in Table 1, uremia is only one of the several causes of metabolic encephalopathy (ME), but many (at least seven) of the conditions listed can be present in the uremic status. Metabolic and toxic disorders all produce similar effects on the central nervous system (CNS), including disturbances of mental function (also called sensorial clouding), neurological disturbances (dysarthria, tremors, asterixis), motor abnormalities (asthenia, clumsiness) and hormonal changes. In uremic individuals, UE may remain subclinical for a long period, but it sometimes becomes evident in the early stages of renal failure. Therefore, the clinical features of UE can be divided into early and late disturbances (Table 2).

A. Pathophysiology of CNS Alterations in Uremia

CNS alterations in uremia (10–57) can be mainly functional. Malnutrition or amino acid (AA) imbalance can alter the levels of putative neurotransmitters [e.g., glutamine, γ-aminobutyric acid (GABA), or glycine], of some derived substances [e.g., glycine branched-chain AA (BCAA) ratios], of monoamines (mainly dopamine and serotonin), and possibly also of neuropeptides. This AA imbalance can be directly responsible for many of the clinical features of UE. The early phase of UE could be attributed to AA derangements such as increased levels of glycine or organic acids (from phenylalanine), to elevations in free-tryptophan, to de-

Table 1 Causes of Metabolic Encephalopathy

Anemia
Body temperature changes
Decreased psychosocial adaptation
Endocrinopathies
Fluid, electrolyte, and acid-base changes
Impaired glucose metabolism
Infections
Intoxications (drugs, etc.)
Liver diseases (necrosis, portal-systemic shunts)
Respiratory diseases
Uremia

creased glutamine-GABA values, and to altered dopamine metabolism. Sensorial clouding, dyskinesias, asthenia, humoral changes, and reduced sexual activity can be explained by AA derangements. On the other hand, the persistence of very low GABA values and of very high glycine levels and 5-HT:DO ratios could induce the late phase of UE. Subcortical dementia, uremic twitching, seizures, and significant endocrine abnormalities may appear at this stage.

Table 2 Clinical Features of Uremic Encephalopathy

Early changes	Late changes
Disturbances of Mental Function	
Malaise	Defective cognition
Anxiety	Obtundation
Loss of recent memory	Errors of perception
Impaired concentration	Illusion
Insomnia	Visual hallucinations
Fatigue	Agitation
Apathy	Delirium
Stupor	
Coma	
Neurological Disturbances	
Dysarthria (slow, slurred, thickened speech)	Myoclonus Tetany
Tremors	
Asterixis	
Motor Abnormalities	
Clumsiness	Limb muscle tone alteration
Unsteadiness	Stretch-reflex asymmetry
Increase of grasp reflexes	Hemiparesis Convulsions
Asthenia	
Hormonal Changes	
Altered prolactin secretion	Hyperprolactinemia Increased PTH
Increased PTH(?)	Increased free radicals

In general, the unified theory of UE is based on AA derangements and on the subsequent imbalance of neurotransmitters. The altered "balance" between stimulating and depressing neurotransmitters causes disturbances in mental, neurological, motor, and hormonal functions. If this hypothesis is correct, only a minor role is attributable to the "classic uremic factors," such as parathyroid hormone (PTH), aluminum, and idiogenic osmoles (41–50).

It is now evident that a single mechanism cannot explain UE. A number of neurotoxic substances are retained in chronic renal failure (CRF), among them blood urea nitrogen (BUN) (>200 mg%), ammonia, cyanide, phenol-like compounds, and middle molecules (MMs). All of these may contribute to UE. There is no evidence supporting a dominant role of MMs in the pathogenesis of UE, even though some studies have found an inverse association between EEG abnormalities and middle molecular (B_{12}) clearance (51–53).

It is well known that in uremia PTH can directly increase the calcium content of the brain, which may play an indirect role in the wasting syndrome and in the AA imbalance (9,54) contributing to altered prolactin secretion. UE is not associated with aluminum toxicity; intestinal absorption of aluminum per se is unable to cause encephalopathy in patients who have not undergone dialysis (55).

If the hypothesis proposed for the genesis of UE is correct, some well-known small molecules (i.e., certain AAs and their derivatives) could replace many unknown middle molecules, which have been sought since the early 1970s but not yet been found. Small molecules could at least be implicated in many uremic symptoms, including gastrointestinal (urea), hematological (guanidines), and hormonal and neurological (AAs) abnormalities.

Many points need further clarification before a unified hypothesis on UE can be accepted. For example, is there a relationship between uremic encephalopathy and uremic malnutrition? What is the role of nitric oxide and free radicals in UE? It is well known that glutathione peroxidase (GPx) is decreased in uremia (56), but there are no data concerning the relationships between glutathione (GSH), GPx, superoxide dismutase (SOD), and related enzymes in CRF patients.

Finally, recent evidence suggests that the anemia of chronic renal failure may have a direct effect on brain function (43–50). Abnormalities of cognitive function tests, as well as electrophysiological measurements of brain function, significantly improve with correction of the anemia with recombinant erythropoietin. There are at least three possible explanations for the better CNS function accompanying the rise in hematocrit level; all are probably based on improvement in brain metabolism. First, increased hematocrit will lead to enhanced brain oxygen delivery with a beneficial effect on brain metabolism. Second, when the hematocrit rises, cerebral blood flow falls, thus correcting localized "brain uremia" because of the decreased delivery to the brain of uremic toxins. Finally, the decrease in cerebral blood flow may decrease intracranial pressure and diminish subtle cerebral edema. CNS function in dialysis patients improves but does not normalize after improvement of anemia with EPO, suggesting that anemia is only one of several factors important in the pathogenesis of UE (57). Table 3 lists the distinctive features of UE.

B. Evaluation of Uremic Encephalopathy

Many methods of evaluation can be used, such as electroencephalogram (EEG), evoked potentials (EPs), psychological testing, cerebrospinal fluid (CSF) analysis, brain density on CT, and hormonal or amino acid studies.

In 87 patients with CRF early auditory evoked potentials (BAERs) demonstrated changes in wave morphology and abnormal prolongations of all wave latencies and interpeak intervals. The direct positive effect of HD was reflected in shortening all wave latencies. Recording of the intraindividual course of a BAER allowed documentation of worsened cerebral function even in patients with constant uremic conditions (10).

Detailed information on the different tests is beyond the scope of this chapter. (For further information, see Refs. 11–40.)

Table 3 Distinctive Features of Uremic Encephalopathy

Features	Ref.
No specific morphological brain change	16, 17
No correlation between the degree of UE and CSF or plasma abnormalities of commonly measured solutes	5
No cerebral edema or cellular volume changes	11, 16, 17, 19
Normal CSF concentrations of electrolytes	5, 42
Normal CSF pH	5, 8, 9, 42
Increase in brain osmolality (urea + idiogenic somoles)	25, 32
Increase in the calcium content in cortical gray matter and hypothalamus	9
In dogs, a relationship between EEG abnormalities and increased brain calcium content	4
Altered AA ratios both in CSF and in plasma	18, 31, 42
Increased serum levels of 5-HT, PTH, PRL, FSH, and LH	37, 38, 40
Malnutrition	
Free radicals and nitric oxide	
Anemia	43–50

C. Effect of Dialysis and Transplantation on UE

Little has been defined about the physiopathology of dialysis-associated encephalopathy: several hypotheses have been proposed during the last 30 years (58–73). Many of them have been rejected, and some are still being evaluated.

Whatever the genesis, the "functional" lesions can be rapidly reversed. When a patient, even showing severe clinical neurological manifestations, is transplanted, the whole UE syndrome clears up within days, in parallel with the improvement in renal function. On the other hand, when a patient with severe uremic complications starts dialysis, the major neurological signs rapidly disappear within days or weeks, but mild signs of encephalopathy may persist, or even appear later on, despite dialysis.

II. DIALYSIS-ASSOCIATED ENCEPHALOPATHIES

Dialytic treatment has been associated with the appearance of some peculiar both acute and chronic disorders of the CNS (Table 4). These disorders include dialysis disequilibrium, dialysis dementia, subdural hematoma, typical electrolyte disorders, hydrosoluble vitamin deficiency, acute intoxication with trace elements, hypertensive encephalopathy, and the effects of drugs.

III. ACUTE NEUROLOGICAL COMPLICATIONS ASSOCIATED WITH DIALYSIS

A. Dialysis Disequilibrium Syndrome

Symptoms suggesting an acute metabolic encephalopathy may develop either during the hemodialysis session or as long as 24 hours after dialysis has been completed (58–73). They range from mild symptoms

Table 4 Neurological Complications in Dialysis

Acute complications
Epidural and subdural hematomas
Subarachnoid bleeding
Cerebral embolus and infarcts
Transient ischemic attacks
Altered body fluid osmolality
Hypo-hypernatremia
Intradialytic hypotension
Epidural abscess
Hypertensive encephalopathy
Hypoglycemia
Hypercalcemia
Cranial nerve paralysis or convulsions of unknown origin
Chronic complications
Dialysis encephalopathy
Dialysis dementia
Depletion syndrome
Wernicke-like syndrome
Autonomic system dysfunction
Cranial nerve disorders
Peripheral neuropathy

(distress, headache, tremors, muscle cramps, anorexia, dizziness) to more severe manifestations (restlessness, blurring of vision, emesis, hypertension, confusion, stupor), which may progress to convulsions and coma (74–86). Such episodes, rarely fatal, tend to resolve themselves within a few days and usually occur when dialysis therapy is being initiated (i.e., during the first sessions) rather than during chronic treatment, assuming that abrupt changes of dialytic strategies are avoided.

Dialysis disequilibrium syndrome (DDS) is more common in younger patients. It is well known that muscle cramps may also be caused by too rapid fluid loss or to an error in the estimated dry weight. The other symptoms are peculiar to DDS; they usually are of relatively short duration, but in case of major symptoms, recovery may take 2 to 3 days. To avoid mistakes, it is important to stress the fact that the diagnosis of DDS should be a diagnosis of exclusion (Table 5).

DDS was originally attributed to a plasma-brain urea imbalance, followed by an osmotic gradient, causing a shift of water inducing cerebral edema and brain swelling. Results of studies in animals and humans (87–89) did not support either this view or another theory, which was based on electrolyte imbalance. Later, the focus was placed on the generation of osmotically active agents, lowering the pH of both cerebrospinal fluid (CSF) and brain cell water (15–18, 90–93). It was suggested that organic acids accumulating during HD could be the cause of the decline in pH and of the consequent brain swelling. A gradual reduction of elevated blood urea, together with the addition of osmotically active solutes (glucose, glycerol, fructose, NaCl, mannitol) in the dialysate was suggested as prevention (90–93).

Table 5 Differential Diagnosis of Dialysis Disequilibrium Syndrome

Acute cerebrovascular accident
Cardiac arrhythmia
Cerebral embolus secondary to shunt clotting
Copper intoxication
Depletion syndrome
Dialysis dementia
Excessive ultrafiltration
Hyperparathyroidism with hypercalcemia (serum Ca >14)
Hyponatremia (serum Na^+ <125 mEq/L)
Hypoglycemia
Malignant hypertension
Nickel intoxication
Nonketotic hyperosmolar coma with hyperglycemia
Subdural hematoma
Uremia, per se
Wernicke's encephalopathy
Malfunction of fluid-proportioning system

Whatever the cause of DDS, the following must be taken into account:

1. Since the introduction of bicarbonate HD instead of acetate HD, the frequency of DDS has been greatly reduced.
2. Any technique leading to pure ultrafiltration (without dialysis) avoids the appearance of DDS.
3. DDS can be prevented by decreasing dialysis length and reducing dialysis efficiency.
4. At the initiation of HD treatment, it is advisable to perform "soft sessions" (5), i.e., sessions of brief duration, with a low blood flow and a minimal weight loss.
5. In PD patients, DDS has been observed only in intermittent peritoneal dialysis (IPD) patients treated with hyperosmolar solutions which are at present in disuse.
6. In CAPD patients treated with standard PD solutions, DDS has not yet been reported.
7. A DDS-induced coma in a HD patient is normally reversed several hours after the HD session, even though no pharmacological intervention, except bedrest, has been utilized.

B. Dialytic Changes in Water Content in CNS: Details

As outlined before, according to the old pathogenetic hypothesis, dialysis disequilibrium is associated with cerebral edema. Urea removal from the blood would occur more rapidly than from the CSF and brain tissue, and a urea osmotic gradient could be generated, causing a movement of water into brain cells (reverse urea effect). At the same time, HD generates a CO_2 gradient between plasma and CSF, lowering the pH both in the CSF and in brain tissue. These changes will be followed by an increase in brain intracellular osmolality because of the rise of H^+ concentration and the in situ generation of idiogenic osmoles. These osmoles are primarily acid radicals derived from protein metabolism. This osmotic imbalance causes tissue swelling and cerebral edema. This hypothesis was based on studies performed by Arieff et al. (5) on animals and by Port et al. (68) on humans. More recently, other pathogenetic theories have been proposed based on studies with computerized axial tomography in HD patients (88,89). Morphological and densitometric analysis of the brain (before and after the HD session) revealed a reduction of parenchymal density after the session, which was interpreted as cerebral edema. In the early 1980s, La Greca et al. (16,17), measuring the brain density on CT scan of HD and CAPD populations, found that uremic subjects showed a consistent reduction in density during dialysis without change in brain volume.

Using the bioimpedance technique we have shown that during the last phase of the hemodialysis session there is an increase of the water cellular content in the body, while in the first half, it decreases (94). It is thus possible that in DDS a major role could be attributed to the water shifts between intra- and extracellular volumes. Too-rapid volume changes could induce the symptoms of DDS.

Subsequent studies performed on a large population (controls, ESRF, HD, IPD, and CAPD patients) and using more sophisticated techniques suggested the following (16,17):

1. No morphological modifications of cerebral tracts, cysternal-ventricular systems, and subarachnoid spaces were noted. Rare cases of atrophy did not change after dialysis.
2. Cerebral density values in normal subjects range from 35 to 50 Houndsfield units (HU) in the gray matter and from 20 to 30 HU in the white matter. The variability range is about 8%.
3. In HD and IPD patients, cerebral density values before dialysis were higher than normal and ranged from 45 to 55 HU in the gray matter and from 30 to 40 HU in the white matter.
4. In HD and IPD patients, cerebral density in both gray and white matter decreased significantly after dialysis, reaching values similar to those recorded in the normal population. In the interdialytic period, cerebral density progressively increases and reaches high values before the subsequent dialysis session.
5. In contrast, in nondialyzed uremic subjects and patients undergoing CAPD, density values are similar to those seen in controls (88,89).

Since cerebral density is inversely correlated to brain water content, it was concluded that, in the postdialytic period, cerebral edema does not occur and brain water content returns to normal values from a predialytic dry status. Since these variations in cerebral density do not occur in continuous dialysis treatment, it appears that a nonphysiological treatment, such as the intermittent ones, causes the observed modifications of the brain water content. These alterations could be induced by water transport following electrolyte, acid-base, and osmotic changes, but are not consistent with the hypothesis of postdialytic edema as a primary cause of DDS. In addition, pressure analyses performed before and after the dialysis session did not confirm the presence of CSF hypertension generated by dialysis. Finally, the continuous and periodic modifications of brain water content—and, therefore, of the metabolic and electrophysiological activities of the brain cells—could play an important long-term role in the pathogenesis of chronic encephalopathy in dialyzed patients (89).

The effects of rapid HD in rats were recently investigated (90). It was shown that in HD animals (compared with nondialyzed uremic controls) there was an increase (during the session) in brain water and in the brain-to-plasma urea ratio. The retention of brain urea was able to account for the increase in brain water observed in the rapidly dialyzed animals. Major organic osmolytes in the brain (including glutamine, glutamate, taurine, and myoinositol) did not decrease significantly after rapid dialysis. According to this paper (90), the "cerebral edema" in this model of DDS was primarily due to a large brain-to-plasma urea gradient and not to the formation of organic osmolytes. However, this work does not focus on the point that the brain water content of HD rats (before the session) is similar to that of nondialyzed uremic controls.

IV. OTHER ACUTE NEUROLOGICAL COMPLICATIONS

A. Hemorrhagic Complications

Hypertension and anticoagulant therapy are the two main nontraumatic causes of intracranial hemorrhage. Many HD patients have a long history of hypertension in the predialytic phase, which often persists during the dialytic life. Heparin and antiplatelet agents are routinely used in these patients.

This explains the high potential risk of cerebral hemorrhage. Subdural hematoma is not an exceptional cause of death in HD patient. The early symptoms such as headache, nausea, and vomiting are not uncommon, but if they are followed by signs of increased intracranial pressure, such as loss of consciousness and coma, a diagnosis of cerebral bleeding should be excluded. Subacute and chronic subdural hematoma may cause pseudodementia, drowsiness, confusion, and mild hemiparesis. The diagnosis can usually be made by CT scan or, when available, by magnetic resonance imaging (MRI). Subarachnoidal bleeding or a subdural hematoma can be identified in this way. Such episodes in uremic patients may be fatal unless early surgery is performed. When waiting for a CT scan examination, if the patient's symptoms worsen and signs of localized neurological disease or signs of meningeal irritation appear, a subdural hematoma should be suspected (96,98).

Subarachnoidal bleeding can be considered as an important cause of death in HD and is often related to excessive anticoagulant therapy or to congenital defects of the cerebrovascular bed. Any *intracranial hemorrhage* may first appear as convulsions and subsequently evolve to coma. *Epidural hematoma* is exceptional but may occur in patients under anticoagulation and cause spinal cord compression and bilateral loss of sensibility in the lower limbs.

On CT scan intracerebral blood leakage forms a roughly circular mass, displacing and compressing the adjacent brain structures. Large hemorrhagic lesions may displace midline structures, damaging the vital nuclei. The ventricular system may become hemorrhagic. The clinical symptoms have a sudden onset, followed by a gradual or rapid evolution phase. A CT scan may help in the diagnosis in showing hemorrhages of ≥ 1.5 cm wide. Puncture of CSF should be avoided in the presence of signs of intracranial hypertension.

The therapeutic possibilities are few, but surgical drainage is mandatory in the case of a large (>3 cm) cerebellar hematoma with mild dysfunction of brainstem. The prognosis is poor when large hematomas are present. Small hematomas may be associated with a better recovery of brain function than ischemic brain infarcts because the brain tissue is often displaced rather than destroyed.

Cerebral embolus must be suspected when a sudden neurological complication appears after a maneuver of shunt declotting (once) or of declotting of a central venous catheter. Such a complication is very rare, considering the thousands of catheters placed in HD patients all over the world. The heart is the main source of cerebral emboli, with atrial fibrillation being the most common cause. Anticoagulants are effective in preventing such embolisms, but anticoagulation must be delayed for several days if the infarct is hemorrhagic. Emboli could cause unilateral visual disturbances with visual transient loss (cotton effect) or blurring of half of one visual field (amaurosis fugax).

B. Cerebral Infarcts

A thrombotic stroke may be the consequence of a progressive process, lasting hours or days. The main event happens during sleep or in the period shortly after awakening.

Size and localization of infarcts will condition the clinical neurological pattern. Cerebral infarcts may be shown by magnetic resonance within hours and by CT scan within days. On CT scan, minor hypodensity and an enhanced contrast appear; a spontaneous hyperdensity on the contrary means intracranial bleeding.

C. Transient Ischemic Attacks

Transient ischemic attacks (TIA) are temporary focal cerebral deficits mainly due to ischemia. They are transient or temporary because they last less than 24 hours, ranging from a few seconds to several hours. They are focal when the damaged zone is very small.

TIAs are often associated with stenosis of several arteries and are predictors of both cerebral infarcts and extracerebral, mainly myocardial, infarcts. Up to 50–70% of carotid strokes (due to extracranial carotid occlusion) are preannounced by TIAs, strokes occurring a few days after a TIA episode.

The main cause of TIA is the embolization of fibrin platelet material related from atherosclerotic sites. Differential diagnosis must exclude focal epilepsy, migraine, vertigo, syncope, and Stokes-Adam attacks. Obviously, the clinical manifestations depend on the type of artery involved and on the entity of the lesion (Table 6).

Table 6 Transient Ischemic Attacks

Area of damage	Symptoms
Carotid territory	Controlateral weakness
	Controlateral paraesthesiae
	Ipsilateral visual disturbances
Vertebrobasilar system	Hemianopia
	Diplopia
	Dysarthria
	Weakness (one or both sides)
Middle cerebral artery	Single attack

D. Osmolality Changes

Altered body fluid osmolality can be caused by an improper proportioning of dialysate (not followed by alarms to stop the treatment) with consequent hypo- or hypernatremia. In both cases acute neurological complications (seizures and coma) appear, but the clinical picture is different.

In acute hypernatremia, the pattern is characterized by thirst, spasticity, muscle rigidity followed by irritability, seizures, and coma. In acute hyponatremia (serum Na^+ <125 mEq/L), the clinical pattern is characterized by weakness, fatigue, dulled sensorium progressing to seizures, coma, and respiratory arrest. In both cases death may occur if the problem is not properly identified, the treatment is not stopped, and the dialysis monitor is not changed.

E. Intradialytic Hypotension

This complication has been extensively discussed in other chapters. It is sufficient to stress that the rare appearance of seizures during episodes of hypotension (as a consequence of cerebrovascular insufficiency) may be mistaken for DDS, especially in cases of diabetes mellitus or in the presence of serious vascular alterations (99–106).

F. Infections

Infections of vascular access, mycotic aneurysms, pulmonary infections, toxoplasmosis, and systemic infections may all involve the CNS causing the appearance of meningitis, acute encephalopathy, and/or hemorrhage. Although a common sign in HD patients, headache should always be carefully evaluated, especially when it appears at the end of dialysis and when it is associated with a fast decline of neurological status.

Meningitis (cervical rigidity and positive Kernig's sign) should be excluded. The presence of sources for a direct spread of the infection to the meninges (mastoiditis, sinusitis) should be looked for. A CT scan may help when brain abscesses are suspected.

Of 10 HD patients who developed an epidural abscess, 8 had dual-lumen intravenous catheters for HD access and 5 had received parenteral antibiotics for catheter salvage. Severe, debilitating back pain was the only consistent initial complaint. It was concluded (107) that attempts at catheter salvage with parenteral antibiotics carry significant risks for neurological complications. Severe and debilitating back pain, with or without neurological signs, in HD patients with recently treated or ongoing bacteremia should raise the suspicion of an occult epidural abscess.

V. HYPERTENSIVE ENCEPHALOPATHY

Hypertensive encephalopathy is caused by a sharp rise in blood pressure to very high levels (250–240/140–150 mmHg). As in eclampsia or in nonuremic patients, acute and severe neurological and ophthalmological changes appear. Nausea, vomiting, drowsiness, confusion, agitation, convulsions, and—sometimes—neck stiffness may appear. A raised CSF pressure, a brain swelling of the white matter on CT scan, irregular vascular changes (vasospasms mixed with segmental vascular dilatation), and permeability changes of penetrating arterioles all rapidly appear after the onset of the acute blood pressure elevation. The rapid increase in blood pressure is counterbalanced by a sharp rise in cerebrovascular resistance, mainly at the intracerebral small arteries situated at the level of the second and third cortical cell layers. A breakdown of this physiological biofeedback causes a segmental dilatation of those small vessels where the muscular contractility is unable to counter the dangerous, sudden rise in pressure at the cortical level.

Malignant hypertension is a well-known cause of acute encephalopathy in both normal subjects and HD patients. This complication, occurring frequently in the early days of dialysis when less was known about sodium and water balance during a dialytic session, is actually very rare. The main reasons for this improvement are (a) a better interdialytic pressure control, thanks to the effectiveness of several antihypertensive drugs, (b) a better definition of the "ideal dry weight" in each patient thanks to strict clinical evaluation and the use of bioimpedance and weight formulas (94), (c) the tailoring of treatment to individual clinical needs, and (d) automatic strict ultrafiltration control according to the preset program. In our experience malignant hypertension can also be avoided in obese patients (weighing more than 100 kg) with dramatic interdialytic increases in body weight (more than 10 kilos!) and a sustained ultrafiltration (i.e., 7–8 kg in 5 hours!).

Malignant hypertension is in fact relatively more frequent in patients with very high diastolic blood pressure values for a long period before institution of dialysis. In many of such subjects hypertension is never definitely overcome, and from time to time it reappears, becoming worse as the session progresses. Clinical symptoms appear—headache, cramps (mainly abdominal, possibly due to ischemia of the mesenterial bed), nausea, vomiting, and muscular spasticity—as signs of central nervous involvement.

VI. BIOCHEMICAL CHANGES

A. Hypoglycemia

Hypoglycemia is a rare dialysis complication, first, because many dialysate solutions contain glucose at a concentration equal to the blood glucose level and, second, because even in absence of glucose in dialysate, neurological complications linked to moderate hypoglycemia can usually be avoided if short sessions are used and if a snack is given to patients during or (preferably) after the session.

B. Hypercalcemia

Hypercalcemia has been reported in HD patients receiving dialysis with inappropriately high dialysis fluid calcium concentrations and/or large doses of vitamin D and/or calcium-based chelating agents. Whatever the cause, these patients show evidence of a severe encephalopathy, ranging from impaired intellectual functioning to delirium, stupor, and coma. The handling includes hemo- or peritoneal dialysis with calcium-free solutions, i.v. calcitonin (4 U/kg/12 h), and prednisone (1 mg/kg/d).

VII. MISCELLANEOUS

Several recent observations have drawn attention to neurological problems related to some peculiar causes.

A. Malnutrition

Folate, water-soluble vitamins, and vitamin C are removed during dialysis. Folate deficiency, leading to axonal degeneration, demyelination, and neuronal death, and thiamine (B_1) and B_{12} deficiencies may all induce the classical signs of metabolic encephalopathies.

These deficiencies may be associated with high homocysteine blood levels, which carry an elevated risk for atherosclerosis (108). In some patients (even those treated by regular bicarbonate dialysis with a Kt/v >1.2), plasma homocysteine levels may be 10 times normal: supplementation with folic acid and water-soluble vitamins is mandatory in such cases (109).

Low-dose megestrol (20 mg orally, twice daily) may increase serum albumin levels of malnourished HD patients (increase of albumin >0.3 g/dL) (110).

B. Role of Erythropoietin

Delanty et al. (111) have recently shown that human recombinant erythropoietin (EPO) may cause hypertensive encephalopathy. In six of their patients EPO induced hypertension, headache, and seizures. Four of six patients had showed changes in the posterior white matter on CT scan. This so-called hypertensive posterior leukoencephalopathy can be managed by prompt antihypertensive and anticonvulsant treatment and by discontinuation of EPO.

C. Aluminum Encephalopathy

Recently Wang et al. (112) showed that treatment with improperly processed dialysis water and administration of aluminum compounds were the major causes of aluminum toxicity in uremic patients. Anemia, encephalopathy, and bone disease may occur. Due to the close correlation between the DFO test and bone aluminum level, this test may be useful for the diagnosis of aluminum toxicity, and DFO therapy (20–40 mg/kg twice a week i.v.) may decrease aluminum body content when patients have a serum aluminum concentration higher than 200 μg/L or a bone aluminum concentration 10 times greater than controls.

D. Neurocognitive Function in HD Patients

Well-dialyzed HD patients do not show neuropsychological deficit when compared with age- and education-matched medical controls. Pliskin et al. (113) applied a comprehensive neuropsychological test battery, including measures of intelligence, immediate and delayed memory, attention and speed of mental processing, language abilities, complex problem solving, motor skills, and depression, to 16 well-dialyzed ($Kt/V_{urea} = 1.46 \pm 0.24$) patients and 12 controls. The lack of clear neuropsychological deficits in these ESRD patients of low average intelligence led to the hypothesis that previously observed apparent deficits resulted from very low dialysis delivery or from comparison with poorly matched historical controls. There were significant deficits in language ability and intelligence in ESRD patients with higher-than-median scores on the Beck Depression Inventory compared with less depressed ESRD patients. However, this effect of depression did not result in differences between dialysis and non-ESRD patient groups.

VIII. THE PROBLEM OF DIALYSIS DEMENTIA

Dialysis dementia (DD) is related to UE and to some acute neurological changes (114–156). Dialysis dementia or dialysis encephalopathy is a slowly progressive but fatal neurological pathology. First described in the early 1970s (114–125), it is now considered as being part of a multisystemic disease involving the brain (encephalopathy), bone osteomalacia, muscle (proximal myopathy), and bone marrow. Twenty-eight years after its initial description, the etiology of this strange syndrome remains controversial. Starting from the original view of Arieff et al. (5) implicating an aluminum intoxication of the uremic brain through intermediate steps, we are now convinced that DD probably represents the endpoint of several etiologies.

As shown in Table 7, DD can be divided into three major forms: (a) a *childhood form*, in which DD is associated with congenital or postpartum uremia and in which the young brain, exposed to uremic toxins, may develop several neurological disorders, (b) an adult sporadic-endemic form, in which aluminum does not play any role, and (c) an adult *epidemic type* in which a relationship between aluminum-contaminated dialysate and the syndrome has been suggested.

The first reports concerned the endemic form in patients who dialyzed for more than 2 years before the onset of the neurological signs. Only later did it become clear that these symptoms were similar to those typical of UE: slurring and stuttering of the speech (due to dysarthria), personality changes (mainly depression), decreased memory and loss of attention, difficulty of concentration, slowing of comprehension, and more severe signs—myoclonus, seizures, dementia, apathy, and lethargy. Symptoms initially appear intermittently and worsen during session. After a few months they become constant, and death follows after 6–18 months. The patient vegetates and becomes completely apathic:

Table 7 Features of Dialysis Dementia

Groups
Infants-childhood: (a) uremic toxins on immature brain, (b) Al-independent
Adult sporadic-endemic: (a) worldwide distribution, (b) Al-independent, (c) no therapy
Adult epidemic: (a) geography dependent, (b) Al-dependent (Al in dialysis water), (c) epidemic, (d) trace elements in water
Differential diagnosis
In dialysis dementia, Al accumulates in brain structures (cortical gray matter, glial cells, choroid epithelia) different from those (nucleus, neurofibrillary tangles) found in Alzheimer's disease.
Possible causes
Al intoxication, in the adult epidemic form
Trace elements intoxication
Neurotransmitter imbalance
Malnutrition
Aging
Normal pressure hydrocephalus
Slow virus infection
Cerebral blood flow alterations

a severe protein-calorie malnutrition often ensues and constitutes the main cause of inevitable death. Despite the typical clinical signs (speech alterations, 90%; motor disturbances, 75%; convulsions, 70–90%), brain histology is nonspecific. The EEG pattern is similar to that found in several metabolic encephalopathies, with multifocal bursts of steep delta waves altering the normal background pattern in the early phase.

In 1976, Alfrey et al. (125) showed that, in DD patients, the aluminum content of the brain gray matter was significantly elevated when compared to normal HD patients and normal subjects (11 vs. 3 vs. 1, respectively). The same was true for soft tissues and bone, and hence aluminum-containing phosphate binders were implicated in the disease. The intriguing question remained why DD strikes only a small minority of dialysis patients, if at that time all of them took aluminum phosphate binders.

Finally, Prior (133) showed a strong association between the aluminum content in dialysate water, the epidemic form of DD, and severe dialysis osteodystrophy. From this observation the use of de-ionized water or osmotically treated water to prepare the dialysis solution was derived. For reasons of safety, the dialysate aluminum must be lower than 20 μg/L, and aluminum pipes must be avoided in the dialysis water system.

In general, modern water treatment could prevent CNS toxicity by removing a number of trace elements, especially cadmium, manganese, lead, mercury, copper, and nickel. An increased manganese content was found in the cortical white matter of eight patients with UE and elevated aluminum levels in the gray matter. Even though properly deionized water for dialysate (with very low aluminum levels) is used, DD appeared (134) in HD patients who showed serum aluminum levels four times higher than other dialysis patients using the same dose of aluminum binders. Again, a greater individual aluminum absorption could play a role. Thus, the true role of aluminum in the genesis of DD remains to be clarified. It is fairly certain that aluminum does not play any role in the childhood and the adult-sporadic forms of DD. In the third form (adult epidemic) it could make some contribution by itself or in combination with other agents such as other trace elements, amino acid imbalance, or aging.

According to several authors (135–138) DD shows some similarities with Alzheimer disease. However, several differences exist.

In 1987, Altmann (153) showed that low levels of erythrocyte DPRA (dihydropteridine reductase activity) inversely correlated with plasma aluminum levels, doubling after a desferrioxamine treatment. He suggested (but it was not proven) that high aluminum levels could cause a decrease of brain DPRA. This could result in a reduced synthesis of two major neurotransmitters such as tyrosine and acetylcholine. According to Altmann, it is possible that patients developing DD have a lower blood transferrin-binding capacity or a greater quantity of brain transferrin receptors.

In 1996 Reusche et al. (154) correlated drug-related aluminum intake and HD treatment with the deposition of argyrophilic aluminum containing inclusions in CNS of patients with dialysis-associated encephalopathy. CNS tissue and peripheral organs of 50 autopsy cases with chronic renal failure (CRF) and dialysis treatment were evaluated for aluminum-containing argyrophilic inclusions using the Howell and Black method as modified by Reusche. Morphological alterations were correlated with the duration of HD and with the amount of prescribed aluminum-containing drugs for better control of hyperphosphatemia. Significant correlations were found between the degree of morphological alterations and aluminum intake up to 2.5 kg, as well as between morphology and duration of long-term HD. The most sensitive structure for CNS deposits were the choroid epithelia, followed by glial cells and neurons. Autonomic ganglia, heart, ovary/testis, parathyroids, adrenals, and pituitary demonstrated reliably peripheral deposits. Aluminum-containing drugs, preferentially administered during HD, explain the additional significance of aluminum uptake and the correlation with the duration of dialysis. The deposition of aluminum-containing proteinaceous inclusions is apparently irreversible. After successful renal transplantation, the aluminum-induced argyrophilic degradation products remain unchanged in the cellular cytoplasm for up to 10 years.

Some papers (141,142) have shown that with alteration of the blood-brain barrier (BBB), an increased brain aluminum content appears. This involves not only UE but all metabolic encephalopathies (e.g., hepatic), metastatic cancer, and aging.

After 30 years, many questions about DD remain unsolved. The best water treatment, the use of new phosphate binders, and attention to the dialytic adequacy and the nutritional status have reduced but not eliminated DD.

In our opinion, DD is a syndrome frequently associated with some basic risk factors, such as a biological aging greater than the natural aging and evident malnutrition. Age, homocysteine levels, and nutritional status could be at least as important as aluminum levels (108,109). Only six cases of normal pressure hydrocephalus have been described (142), but controls were lacking. It is well known that a slight ventricular dilatation with cerebral atrophy can be found in ESRD patients without DD. Only one slow virus has been isolated from the brain of patients who died of DD.

Briefly, DD can be seen as the final stage of a metabolic encephalopathy caused by several factors and possibly by different mechanisms. The role of aluminum is evident only in the adult epidemic type. No satisfactory treatment exists. There is a 6- to 18-month interval between diagnosis and death. Several approaches have been tested: increase in dialysis frequency (4–5 times/week) with soft dialysis, administration of parenteral nutrition during the dialysis sessions, the use of keto-analogs of branched-chain amino acids, bromocriptine (to lower both PRL and PTH), and deferoxamine.

The use of deferoxamine (143–148) has not changed the natural history of DD patients in the last 15 years. None of the other approaches have been successful except kidney transplantation (149–152). The latter may reverse both dialysis-associated encephalopathy syndrome and DD (149–151).

IX. DEPLETION SYNDROME

Several factors may enhance the risk of abnormal vitamin levels in renal diseases such as decreased vitamin intake, increased degradation, losses into dialysate, and interference of drugs with the kinetics of vitamins (155). While vitamin A, E, and riboflavin deficiencies have been rarely observed in uremic patients, thiamine deficiency may induce mental changes. Vitamin B_6 deficiency is not uncommon in chronic renal failure, causing anorexia, increased plasma and tissue oxalate levels, high plasma homocysteine levels, and increased risk for vascular disease.

Even though consistent findings suggest that renal failure patients should be routinely prescribed folic acid (5–10 mg/d), vitamin B_6 (100 mg/d), and B_{12} (1 mg/d) to decrease plasma homocysteine levels, further studies are necessary to justify these suggestions (108–109,155). Experimental biotin (B_8) deficiency induces mild depression, muscle pains, hyperesthesia, anorexia and, later on, maculosquamous dermatitis. In general, effects of vitamin status of patients treated for decades have not yet been studied, but it is evident that several vitamin deficiencies may induce significant changes in the metabolism and vascular status of such patients.

Decreased selenium and zinc levels induce peroxidative damage to cells (56) and decrease taste and small acuity. Changes of mental function and neurological complications could appear, since the plasma amino acid pattern is abnormal in CRF and tends to become more pronounced in malnutrition (28,30–33,123,141).

X. WERNICKE SYNDROME

This syndrome is characterized by ataxia and changes in ocular motility: nystagmus, abducens palsy, or palsy of conjugate gaze. When associated with a Korsakoff psychosis, patients show also a defective recent memory, confusion, and confabulation. High doses of thiamine reduce the ataxia and the ocular disturbances, while they show no effect on the mental symptoms. Vomiting, restricted food intake, and neurotoxic drugs may play a role.

XI. AUTONOMIC SYSTEM DYSFUNCTION

Uremic neuropathy is not limited to impairment of motor function. Autonomic dysfunction is common, being more extensive in predialysis patients. The efferent sympathetic pathway is intact, but the efferent parasympathetic pathway is significantly abnormal and the baroreceptor sensitivity is depressed (42,77–79,101–106). In fact, while the cold pressure test and the response to sudden loud noise are usually normal, the expiration:inspiration ratio, the lying:standing ratio, the Valsalva ratio, and the baroreceptor sensitivity slope were found to be significantly abnormal in nondialyzed patients. The lower baroreflex sensitivity could contribute to volume-depletion hypotension during dialysis (77,78).

The development of bradycardia and hypotension during hemodialysis appears to be related to a sudden parasympathetic vagal overactivity and could be attributed to the Bezold-Jarisch reflex (79,99–101). Other signs of ASD are postural hypotension (not due to a wrong dry-weight!), impaired sweating, low heart rate response to standing, and a significant reduction of day/night blood pressure variations.

XII. CRANIAL NERVE DISORDERS

Cranial nerves can be affected in uremic subjects. Facial asymmetry, miosis, transient nystagmus, and heterophoria are sometimes observed (4,6–9).

When the eighth cranial nerve is affected, both auditory and vestibular divisions are involved. Varying degrees of nystagmus, hearing loss, and sixth nerve palsy are well described (14).

XIII. PERIPHERAL NEUROPATHY

Polyneuropathy (PN) is one of the most frequent complications of uremia, with an incidence ranging from 10 to 83% (1–4,6–9). Nearly all HD patients show some alterations of nerve function, while a symptomatic neuropathy affects about 10% of the dialysis population, males being more affected than females (11).

Severity and progression of dialysis PN are extremely different; the changes are usually slow, but in the case of severe superimposed clinical illness, lower motor neurones (LMN) or primary sensory neurones (PSN) can be affected. Muscle cramps and the restless legs syndrome are early manifestations of LMN involvement: they usually disappear when clinical signs of neuropathy appear (14,42,57,70).

The first sign of sensorial neuropathy is the perception of light touch over distal lower limbs. When the neuropathy progresses further, other sensorial signs become apparent: diffuse paraesthesia, pain, and burning feet. Only a minority of patients show clinical signs of neuropathy in the upper limbs, although alterations of conduction velocity are present in all limbs (74).

The neurophysiological investigations of HD patients have demonstrated a slowing of conduction in all the peripheral nerves: motor and sensory nerve fibers are equally affected in the four limbs. Measurement of nerve conduction velocity (NCV) is less suitable than that of light touch and of vibratory perception thresholds, expressing the clinical functions of large myelinated fibers. The study of the amplitude of nerve action potentials is very important, since the finding of an important decrease of this sensory potential means that a significant loss of large myelinated fibers has occurred in the studied nerve.

Adequate HD prevents deterioration of neuropathy and may even show a slow improvement, even though NCV shows only minor changes. Again, serial determinations of the clinical functions of large myelinated fibers are more suitable in detecting changes in nerve function than NCV studies (74,77–78).

In uremic neuropathy, the degeneration of nerve fibers is characterized by a structural impairment of axons and myelin sheathes. The axonal disorder is the primary one, while the demyelination is secondary to the primary axonal lesion. Besides morphological changes, functional lesions (partially reversed by a single HD session) are also present, being responsible for some functional disturbances and probably caused by some removal of circulating toxins.

The etiology of PN is unclear. Some major pathogenetic mechanisms have been proposed: deficiency, uremic toxins, and hormonal imbalance. There is no doubt that the uremic population shows several deficiencies involving either vitamins (mainly water-soluble ones) or other neurological nutrients.

The "depletion syndrome" (see above) may possibly play a role. B_1 deficiency is usually associated with a PN but B_1 deficiency has yet to be demonstrated in the HD population, and the administration of B_1 neither prevents nor cures PN.

As far as toxins are concerned, PN could be caused by some toxins inducing the inhibition of several enzymes (153). Many toxins have been looked for in the last 30 years (middle molecules, methylguanidine, myoinositol, etc.), but a correlation between the plasma levels of any of these compounds and the severity of PN has not been found.

Toxins inhibiting transketolase (an enzyme present in the CNS) and glutamic oxalacetic transaminase could induce a polyneuropathy. Some dialyzable substances could also block onabain-sensitive, potassium-dependent ATPase, thus decreasing sodium transport across cell membranes and slowing the conduction along nervous membranes.

The role of PTH is a subject of debate (137–148). Raised PTH levels could increase the calcium concentration in the peripheral nerves, but several arguments against the role of PTH in the genesis of PN exist. It is now clear that no correlation exists between the different forms of PTH and NCV, that high PTH levels do not mean PN, and that motor NCV is not improved by parathyroidectomy (156). The influence of several other hormones on PN is still unclear.

XIV. CONCLUSIONS

When the several effects induced by dialysis on uremic brain are considered, it is evident that many concomitant factors may play a role. In the long dialysis exposure, each repeated acute change (at least 156 times a year) becomes an important part of a complex system determining the onset and the worsening of the chronic encephalopathy. The unphysiology of dialytic treatment has a detrimental effect on CNS, but malnutrition, anemia, hypertension, atherosclerosis, free radicals, amino acid imbalance, hormonal disorders, trace elements, and drugs all play a role, even in different ways.

Why then do many patients (even though dialyzed for more than 20 years) show no clear signs of dialytic encephalopathy but only mild signs of UE? In the last 10 years, new information in this field has been relatively scarce. Many aspects of UE and of DE still need clarification. New techniques (NMR, bioimpedance, computer-aided imaging, new laboratory tests, biosensors) and possibly better clinical cooperation between nephrologists and neurologists should enable us to write a more adequate chapter on this topic in the next 5–10 years!

REFERENCES

1. Addison T. On the disorders of the brain connected with diseased kidneys. Guy's Hosp Rep 1839; 4:1–7.
2. Hun H. Nervous symptoms associated with Bright's Disease. Alb Med Ann 1895; 16:139–151.
3. Tyler HR. Neurologic disorders in renal failure. Am Med 1968; 44:734–748.
4. Tyler HR. Neurologic complications of uremia. In: Strauss MB, Welt LG, eds. Diseases of the Kidney. 2d ed. Boston: Little, Brown, 1971:334–342.
5. Arieff AI, Massry SG, Barrientos A, Kleeman GR. Brain water and electrolyte metabolism in uremia: effects of slow and rapid HD. Kidney Int 1973; 4:177–187.
6. Nissenson AR, Levin ML, Klawans HL, Nausieda PL. Neurological sequelae of end stage renal disease (ESRD). J Chron Dis 1977; 30:705–733.

7. Bolton CF, Johnson WJ, Dick PJ. Neurologic manifestations of renal failure. In: Earley LE, Gottschalk CW, eds. Strauss and Welt's Diseases of the Kidney. 3d ed. Boston: Little, Brown, 1979:371–392.
8. Arieff AI. Neurological complications of uremia. In: Brenner BM, Rector FC, eds. The Kidney. 2d ed. Philadelphia: WB Saunders, 1981:2306–2343.
9. Mahoney CA, Arieff AI, Leach WJ, Lazarowitz VC. Central and peripheral nervous systems effects of chronic renal failure. Kidney Int 1983; 24:170–177.
10. Balzer S, Kuttner K. Early auditory evoked potential. A diagnostic parameter in uremic encephalopathy. HNO 1996; 44:559–566.
11. Blagg CR: Brain abnormalities. In: Massry SG, Glassock RJ, eds. Textbook of Nephrology. 2d ed. Baltimore: Williams & Wilkins, 1983:7.15–7.19.
12. Kiley JE, Pratt KL, Gisser DG, Schaffer CA. Techniques of EEG frequency analysis for evaluation of uremic encephalopathy. Clin Nephrol 1976; 5:279–285.
13. Kiley JE, Woodruff MW, Pratt KL. Evaluation of encephalopathy by EEG frequency analysis in chronic dialysis patients. Clin Nephrol 1976; 5:245.
14. Teschan PE, Ginn HE, Bourne JR. Quantitative indices of clinical uremia. Kidney Int 1979; 15:676–697.
15. Arieff AI, Lazarowitz VC, Guisardo R. Experimental dialysis disequilibrium syndrome; prevention with glycerol. Kidney Int 1978; 14:270–278.
16. La Greca G, Dettori P, Biasioli S. Studies on morphological and densitometrical changes in brain after hemo and peritoneal dialysis. ASAIO Trans 1981; 27: 40–44.
17. La Greca G, Biasioli S, Chiaramonte S. Studies on brain density in hemo and peritoneal dialysis. Nephron 1982; 31:146–150.
18. Biasioli S, Chiaramonte S, Fabris A. Neurotransmitter imbalance in plasma and cerebrospinal fluid during dialytic treatment. ASAIO Trans 1983; 29:44–49.
19. Olsen S. The brain in uremia. Acta Psychiatr Scand 1961; 36(suppl 156):1–10.
20. Savazzi GM, Cusmano F, Degasperi T. Cerebral atrophy in patients on long-term regular hemodialysis treatment. Clin Nephrol 1985; 23:89–95.
21. Gulyassy PF, Peters JH, Lin SC, Ryan PM. Hemodialysis and plasma amino acid composition in chronic renal failure. Am J Clin Nutr 1968; 21:565–570.
22. Giordano C, De Pascale C, De Santo NG, Esposito R, Cirilli C, Stangerlin P. Disorder in the metabolism of some amino acids in uremia. In: Proceedings of the 4th International Congress of Nephrol. Basel: Karger, 1970:196–205.
23. Alvestrand A, Fürst P, Bergstrom J. Plasma and muscle free amino acids in uremia: influence of nutrition with amino acids. Clin Nephrol 1982; 18:297–305.
24. Letendre CH, Nagaiah K, Guroff G. Brain amino acids. In: Biochemistry of Brain. Oxford, England: Pergamon Press, 1980; 343–382.
25. McGale EHF, Pye IF, Stonier C, Hutchinson EC, Aber GM. Studies of the interrelationship between cerebrospinal fluid and plasma amino acid concentration in normal individuals. J Neurochem 1977; 29:291–297.
26. Pardridge WM, Oldendorf WH. Transport of metabolic substrates through the blood brain barrier. J Neurochem 1977; 5:28–35.
27. Pye IF, McGale EHF, Stonier C, Hutchinson EC, Aber GM. Studies of cerebrospinal fluid and plasma amino acid in patients with steady state chronic renal failure. Clin Chim Acta 1979; 9:65–72.
28. Deferrari G, Garibotto G, Robaudo C, Ghiggeri GM, Tizianello A. Brain metabolism of amino acids and ammonia in patients with chronic renal insufficiency. Kidney Int 1981; 20:505–510.
29. Pauli HG, Vorburger C, Reubi F. Chronic derangement of cerebrospinal fluid acid-base components in man. J Appl Physiol 1962; 17:993–996.
30. Biasioli S, D'Andrea G, Chiaramonte S. The role of neurotransmitters in the genesis of uremic encephalopathy. Int J Artif Organs 1984; 7:101–106.
31. Sullivan PA, Murnaghan D, Callaghan N. Katmaneni BD, Curzon G. Cerebral transmitter precursors and metabolites in advanced renal disease. J Neurol Neurosurg Psychiatry 1978; 41:581–588.
32. Biasioli S, D'Andrea G, Fabris A. The pathogenesis of uremic encaphalopathy. Int J Artif Organs 1985; 8: 20–22.
33. Howard JJ, Jeppson, Ziparov V, Fischer JE. Hyperammonaemia, plasma amino acid imbalance and BBB amino acid transport: a unified theory of portal systemic encephalopathy. Lancet 1979; 2:772–775.
34. Tyler HR, Leavitt S. Asterixis. J Chron Dis 1965; 18: 409–415.
35. Young SN, Lal S, Sourkes TL, Feldmuller F, Aronoff A, Martin JB. Relationship between tryptophan in serum and CSF and 5-HIAA in CSF of man: effect of cirrhosis of liver and probenecid administration. J Neurol Neurosurg Psychiatry 1975; 38:322–330.
36. Jellinger K, Irsigler K, Kothbauer P, Riederer P. Brain monoamines in metabolic coma. Int Congress Series 1977; 427:169–175.
37. Biasioli S, Feriani M, Chiaramonte S. The serotoninergic system in uremia: relationship to hormonal status. In: Friedman E, Beyer M, De Santo, eds. Prevention of Progressive Uremia. New York: Field & Wood, 1989:79–82.
38. Biasioli S, D'Andrea G, Micieli G, Feriani M, Borin D, Chiaramonte S. Hyperprolactemia as a marker of neurotransmitter imbalance in uremic population. Int J Artif Organs 1987; 10:245–257.
39. Biasioli S, D'Andrea G, Feriani M. Uremic encephalopathy: an updating. Clin Nephrol 1986; 25:57–63.
40. Biasioli S, Mazzali A, Foroni R, D'Andrea G, Feriani M, Chiaramonte S. Chronobiological variations of prolactin (PRL) in chronic renal failure (CRF). Clin Nephrol 1988; 30:86–92.

41. Lowrie EG, Steinberg SM, Galen MA. Factors in the dialysis regimen which contribute to alternations in the abnormalities of uremia. Kidney Int 1976; 10:409–422.
42. Ronco C, Biasioli S, Borin D, Brendolan A, Chiaramonte S, Fabris A. Patologia neurologica in dialisi. Min Nefrol 1982; 4:185–193.
43. Nissenson AR, Marsh JT, Brown WS, Wolcott DL. Central nervous system function in dialysis patients: a practical approach. Semin Dial 1991; 4(2):115–123.
44. Nissenson AR. Recombinant human erythropoietin: impact on brain and cognitive function, exercise tolerance, sexual potency, and quality of life. Semin Nephrol 1989; 9(suppl 2):25–31.
45. Marsh JT, Wolcott DL, Harper R, Nissenson AR. Impairment of brain function by anemia: ameliorative effects on brain and cognitive function of rHuEPO in dialysis patients. Kidney Int 1991; 29:155–163.
46. Matthew RJ, Rabin P, Stone WJ, Wilson WH. Regional cerebral blood flow in dialysis encephalopathy and primary degenerative dementia. Kidney Int 1985; 28:64–68.
47. Grotta JC, Manner C, Pettigrew LC. Yatsu FM. Red blood cell disorders and stroke. Stroke 1986; 17:811–817.
48. Sagales T, Gimeno V, Planella MJ, Raguer N, Bartolome J. Effects of rHuEPO on Q-EEG and event-related potentials in chronic renal failure, Kidney Int 1993; 44:1109–1115.
49. Grimm G, Stockenhuber F, Schneeweiss B, Madl C, Zeithlhofer J, Schneider B. Improvement of brain function in hemodialysis patients treated with erythropoietin. Kidney Int 1990; 38:480–486.
50. Brown WS, Marsh JT, Wolcott D. Cognitive function, mood and P3 latency: effects of the amelioration of anemia in dialysis patients. Neuropsychologia 1991; 29:34–45.
51. Mahoney CA, Sarnacki P, Arieff AI. Uremic encephalopathy: role of brain energy metabolism. Am J Physiol 1984; 247(Renal Fluid Electrolyte Physiol 16): F527–F532.
52. Fraser CL, Sarnacki P, Arieff AI. Altered Na transport in brain of uremic rats: Relation to neurotransmission in uremia? Clin Res 1984; 32:532A.
53. Kiley JE. Residual renal and dialyzer clearance, EEG slowing, and nerve conduction velocity. ASAIO J 1981; 4:1–8.
54. Massry SG, Procci WR, Goldstein DA, Kletzky OA. Sexual dysfunction. In: Textbook of Nephrology. Baltimore: Williams & Wilkins, 1983:7.89–7.92.
55. Gilli P, Fagioli F, Malacarne F. Serum aluminum levels and peritoneal dialysis. Int J Artif Organs 1984; 7: 107–110.
56. Schiavon R, Biasioli S, De Fanti E. The plasma glutathione peroxidase enzyme in hemodialyzed subjects. ASAIO J 1994; 40:968–971.
57. McGonigle RJS, Bewick M, Weston MJ, Parsons V. Progressive, predominantly motor, uremic neuropathy. Acta Neurol Scand 1985; 71:379–384.
58. Kennedy AC, Linton AL, Eaton JC. Urea levels in cerebrospinal fluid after hemodialysis. Lancet 1962; 1: 410–411.
59. Arieff AI. Dialysis disequilibrium syndrome: current concepts on pathogenesis. In: Schreiner GE, Winchester JR, eds. Controversies in Nephrology. Washington, DC: George Washington University Press, 1982:367–376.
60. Pagel MD. Acetate and bicarbonate fluctuations and acetate intolerance during dialysis. Kidney Int 1982; 21:513–515.
61. Rodrigo F, Shideman J, McHugh R, Buselmeier T, Kjellstrand C. Osmolality changes during hemodialysis: natural history, clinical correlations, and influence of dialysate glucose and intravenous mannitol. Ann Intern Med 1977; 86:554–557.
62. Van Stone JC, Carey J, Meyer R, Murrin C. Hemodialysis with glycerol containing dialysate. ASAIO J 1979; 2:119–121.
63. Arieff AI. Dialysis disequilibrium syndrome: current concepts on pathogenesis and prevention. Kidney Int 1994; 45:629–631.
64. Grushkin CM, Korsch B, Fine RN. Hemodialysis in small children. JAMA 1972; 221:869–871.
65. de Peterson H, Swanson AG. Acute encephalopathy occurring during hemodialysis. Arch Intern Med 1964; 113:877–891.
66. Fukusige M. Hemodialysis with kill-type artificial kidney: clinical study on disequilibrium syndrome. Acta Urol Jpn 1971; 17:89–92.
67. Mawdsley C. Neurological complications of hemodialysis. Proc R Soc Med 1972; 65:871–874.
68. Port FK, Johnson WJ, Klass DW. Prevention of dialysis disequilibrium syndrome by use of high sodium concentration in the dialysate. Kidney Int 1973; 3: 327–333.
69. Arieff AI, Leach W, Park R, Lazarowitz VC. Systemic effects of NaHCO3 in experimental lactic acidosis in dogs. Am J Physiol 1982; 242:586–588.
70. Fraser CL, Arieff AI. Nervous system complications in uremia. Ann Intern Med 1988; 109:143–144.
71. Rouby JJ, Rottenbourg J, Durande JP. Hemodynamic changes induced by regular hemodialysis and sequential ultrafiltration hemodialysis: a comparative study. Kidney Int 1980; 17:801–804.
72. Rosa AA, Shideman J, McHugh R, Duncan D, Kjellstrand CM. The importance of osmolality fall and ultrafiltration rate on hemodialysis side effects. Nephron 1981; 27:134–136.
73. Gutman RA. Controlled comparison of hemodialysis and peritoneal dialysis: Veterans Administration multicenter study. Kidney Int 1984; 26:459–463.
74. Dyck PJ, Johnson WJ, Lambert EH. Detection and

evaluation of uremic peripheral neuropathy in patients on hemodialysis. Kidney Int 1975; 7:S201–S205.
75. Di Giulio S, Chkoff N, Lhoste F. Parathormone as a nerve poison in uremia. N Engl J Med 1978; 299: 1134–1135.
76. Brismar T, Tegner R. Excitability changes reveal decreased sodium permeability in neuropathy. Exp Neurol 1985; 87:177–180.
77. Mallamaci F, Zoccali C, Ciccarelli M, Briggs JD. Autonomic function in uremic patients treated by hemodialysis or CAPD and in transplant patients. Clin Nephrol 1986; 25:175–180.
78. Zoccali C, Ciccarelli M, Mallamaci F, Maggiore Q. Parasympathetic function in hemodialysis patients. Nephron 1986; 42:285–289.
79. Naik RB, Mathias CJ, Wilson CA. Cardiovascular and autonomic reflexes in hemodialysis patients. Clin Sci 1981; 60:165–170.
80. Marsden CD. Basal ganglia disease. Lancet 1982; 1: 1141–1147.
81. Raju SF, White AR, Barnes TT. Improvement in disequilibrium symptoms during dialysis with low glucose dialysate. Clin Nephrol 1982; 181:126–129.
82. Platts MM, Anastassiades E. Dialysis encephalopathy: precipitating factors and improvement in prognosis. Clin Nephrol 1981; 15:228–233.
83. Smith EC, Mahurkar SD, Mamdani BH, Dunea G. Diagnosing dialysis dementia. Dial Transplant 1978; 7: 1264–1274.
84. Alfrey AC, Mishell JM, Burks J. Syndrome of dyspraxia and multifocal seizure associated with chronic hemodialysis. ASAIO Trans 1972; 18:257–261.
85. Mahurkar SD, Salta P, Smith EC. Dialysis dementia. Lancet 1973; 1:1412–1415.
86. Alfrey AC. Dialysis encephalopathy. Kidney Int 1986; 18:S53–S57.
87. La Greca G, Biasioli S, Chiaramonte S, Dettori P, Fabris A, Feriani M. Brain density studies during hemodialysis. Lancet 1980; 2:582.
88. Dettori P, La Greca G, Biasioli S, Chiaramonte S, Fabris A, Feriani M. Changes of cerebral density in dialyzed patients. Neuroradiology 1982; 23:95–99.
89. Ronco C, Biasioli S, Chiaramonte S, Feriani M, Fabris A, Pisani E. Modifiche ematoliquorali indotte dalla dialisi extracorporea e peritoneale. In: d'Amico G, ed. Nefrologia, Dialisis e Trapianto. Milan: Witchtig, 1982: 311–325.
90. Silver SM. Cerebral edema after rapid dialysis is not caused by an increase in brain organic osmoles. J Am Soc Nephrol 1995; 6:1600–1606.
91. Arieff AI, Massry SG, Barientos A, Kleeman CR. Brain water and electrolyte metabolism in uremia: effects of slow and rapid hemodialysis. Kidney Int 1973; 4:177–182.
92. Mann H, Stiller S. Elimination of sodium chloride as the cause of dialysis disequilibrium syndrome (abstr). Kidney Int 1980; 17:401.
93. Arieff AI, Guisado R, Massry SG, Lazarowitz VC. Central nervous system pH in uremia and the effect of hemodialysis. J Clin Invest 1976; 58:306–310.
94. Biasioli S, Talluri T. La Bioimpedenza in Nefrologia. Vicenza: Egida, 1996.
95. Arieff AI, Cooper JD, Armstrong D, Lazarowitz VC. Dementia, renal failure and brain aluminum. Ann Intern Med 1979; 90:741–744.
96. Snyder M, Renaudin J. Intracranial hemorrhage associated with anticoagulation therapy. Surg Neurol 1977; 7:31–33.
97. Bechar M, Lakke JPW, Van der Hem GK, Beks JFW, Penning L. Subdural hematoma during long term hemodialysis. Arch Neurol 1972; 26:513–515.
98. Leonard A, Shapiro FL. Subdural hematoma in regularly hemodialyzed patients. Ann Intern Med 1975; 82:650–654.
99. Orofino L, Marcen R, Quereda C, Villafruela J, Sabater J, Matesanz R, Pascual J, Ortuño J. Epidemiology of symptomatic hypotension in hemodialysis: Is cool dialysate beneficial for all patients? Am J Nephrol 1990; 10:177–181.
100. Capuano A, Sepe V, Cianfrone P, Castellano T, Andreucci VE. Cardiovascular impairment, dialysis strategy and tolerance in elderly and young patients on maintenance haemodialysis. Nephrol Dial Transplant 1990; 5:1023–1026.
101. Jost CM, Agarwal R, Khair P, Grayburn PA, Victor RG, Henrich WL. Effects of cooler temperature dialysate on hemodynamic stability in 'problem' dialysis patients. Kidney Int 1993; 44:606–610.
102. Acute intradialytic well-being: results of a clinical trial comparing polysulfone with cuprophan. Bergamo Collaborative Dialysis Study Group. Kidney Int 1991; 40: 714–720.
103. Hakim RM, Pontzer MA, Tilton D, Lazarus JM, Gottlieb MN. Effects of acetate and bicarbonate dialysate in stable chronic dialysis patients. Kidney Int 1985; 28:535–538.
104. Diamond SM, Henrich WL. Acetate dialysate versus bicarbonate dialysate: a continuing controversy (review). Am J Kidney Dis 1987; 9:3–7.
105. Malberti F, Surian M, Colussi G, Minetti L. The influence of dialysis fluid composition on dialysis tolerance. Nephrol Dial Transplant 1987; 2:93–99.
106. DiBello V, Bianchi AM, Caputo MT. Fractional shortening/end-systolic stress correlation in the evaluation of left ventricular contractility in patients treated by acetate dialysis and lactate haemofiltration. Nephrol Dial Transplant 1990; 3(suppl 1):115–120.
107. Kovalik EC, Raymond JR, Albers F. A clustering of epidural abscesses in chronic HD patients. J Am Soc Nephrol 1996; 7:2264–2267.
108. Welch GN, Loscalzo J. Homocysteine and atherothrombosis. N Engl J Med 1998; 338:1042–1050.
109. Zideck W. Homocysteine. A new atherosclerotic risk

factor in end stage renal failure. Nephron 1997; 75: 249–250.
110. Lien YH, Ruffenach SJ. Low dose megestrol increases serum albumin in malnourished dialysis patients. Int J Artif Organs 1996; 19:147–150.
111. Delanty N, Vaughan C, Frucht S, Stubgen P. Erythropoietin-associated hypertensive posterior leukoencephalopathy. Neurology 1997; 49:686–689.
112. Wang G, Zhu P, Wang S. The causes, diagnosis and treatment of Al toxicity in patients with CRF undergoing dialysis. Chung Hua Nei Ko Tsa Chin 1996; 35: 36–40.
113. Pliskin HN, Yurk HM, Umans JG. Neurocognitive function in chronic HD patients. Kidney Int 1996; 49: 1435–1440.
114. Mahurkar, SD. Dialysis dementia. Lancet 1973; 1: 1412–1413.
115. Alfrey AC. Syndrome of dysphaxia and multifocal seizures associated with chronic hemodialysis. Trans Amer Soc Artif Intern Organs 1972; 18:257–260.
116. Barratt LJ, Lawrence JR. Dialysis-associated dementia. Aust NZJ Med 1975; 5:62–64.
117. Chokroverty S, Bruetman ME, Berger V, Reyes MG. Progressive dialytic encephalopathy. J Neurol Neurosurg Psychiatry 1976; 39:411–413.
118. Mahurkar SD, Myers L, Cohen J, Kamath RV, Dunea G. Electroencephalographic and radionucleotide studies in dialysis dementia. Kidney Int 1978; 13:306–311.
119. Nadel AM, Wilson WP. Dialysis encephalopathy: a possible seizure disorder. Neurology 1976; 26:1130–1133.
120. Noriega-Sanchez A, Martinez-Maldonado M, Haiffe RM. Clinical and electroencephalographic changes in progressive uremic encephalopathy. Neurology 1978; 28:667–672.
121. Flendrig JA. Aluminum and dialysis dementia. Lancet 1976; 1:235–236.
122. La Greca G, Biasioli S, Borin D, Brendolan A, Chiaramonte S, Fabris A. Dialytic encephalopathy. Contrib Nephrol 1985; 3:14–28.
123. Iversen LL. Neurotransmitter and CNS disease. Lancet 1982; 2:914–918.
124. Sorenson JRJ, Campbell IR, Tepper LB, Lingg RD. Aluminum in the environment and human health. Environ Health Perspect 1974; 8:3–95.
125. Alfrey AC, Le Gendre GR, Kaenhy WD. The dialysis encephalopathy syndrome: possible aluminum intoxication. N Engl J Med 1976; 294:184–188.
126. Alfrey AC, Smithe WR. Trace element abnormalities in chronic uremia. Proc 11th Contractr Conf Artif Kidney Chron Uremia Prog NIAMDD 1978; 11:137–139.
127. Arieff AI, Cooper JD, Armstrong D, Lazarowitz VC. Dementia, renal failure, and brain aluminum. Ann Intern Med 1979; 90:741–747.
128. McDermott JR, Smith AI, Ward MK. Brain aluminum concentration in dialysis encephalopathy. Lancet 1978; 1:901–904.
129. Pascoe MD, Gregory MC. Dialysis encephalopathy: aluminum concentration in dailysate and brain. Kidney Int 1979; 16:90.
130. Dunea G, Mahurkar SD, Mamdami B, Smith EC. Role of aluminum in dialysis dementia. Ann Intern Med 1978; 88:502–504.
131. Nathan E, Pedersen SE. Dialysis encephalopathy in a nondialyzed uremic boy with aluminum hydroxide orally. Acta Paediatr Scand 1980; 69(6):793–796.
132. Griswald WR, Reznik V, Mendoza SA. Accumulation of aluminum in a nondialyzed uremic child receiving aluminum hydroxide. Pediatrics 1983; 71:56–58.
133. Prior JC. Dialysis encephalopathy and osteomalacic bone disease. Am J Med 1982; 72:33–37.
134. Ward MK. Osteomalacia dialysis osteodystrophy: evidence for a water-borne aetiological agent, probably aluminum. Lancet 1978; 1:841–844.
135. Katzman R. Alzheimer's disease. N Engl J Med 1986; 314:964–965.
136. Brun A, Dictor M. Senile plaques and tangles in dialysis dementia. Acta Path Microbiol Scand 1981; 89: 193–195.
137. Good PF, Perl DP. A laser microprobe mass analysis study of aluminum distribution in the cerebral cortex of dialysis encephalopathy. J Neuropathol Exp Neurol 1988; 47:321–325.
138. Farrar G. Defective gallium-transferrin binding in Alzheimer disease and Down syndrome: possible mechanism for accumulation of aluminum in brain. Lancet 1990; 335:747–749.
139. Farrar G., Morton AP, Blair JA. The Intestinal Spectiation of Gallium: Possible Models to Describe the Bioavailability of Aluminum. In: Bratter P, Schramel P, eds. Trace Element Analytical Chemistry in Medicine and Biology. Berlin: Walter de Gruyter, 1988: 343–347.
140. Perl DP, Good PF. Microprobe studies of aluminum accumulation in association with human central nervous system disease. Environ Geochem Health 1990; 12:97–99.
141. Banks WA, Kastin AJ. Aluminum increases permeability of the blood-brain barrier to labelled DSIP and b-endorphin: possible implications for senile and dialysis dementia. Lancet 1983; ii:1227–1228.
142. Matthew RJ, Rabin P, Stone WJ. Regional cerebral blood low in dialysis encephalopathy and primary degenerative dementia. Kidney Int 1985; 28:64–67.
143. Malluche HH, Smith AJ, Abreo K. The use of deferoxamine in the management of aluminum accumulation in bone in patients with renal failure. N Engl J Med 1984; 311:140–146.
144. Ackrill P, Raltson AJ, Day JP. Role of desferrioxamine in the treatment of dialysis encephalopathy. Kidney Int 1986; 18:S104–S107.

145. Sprague SM, Corwin HL, Wilson R. Encephalopathy in chronic renal failure responsive to desferrioxamine therapy; another manifestation of aluminum neurotoxicity. Arch Intern Med 1986; 146:2063–2064.
146. Hood SA, Clark WF, Hodsman AB. Successful treatment of dialysis osteomalacia and dementia using desferrioxamine infusions and oral 1α hydroxy-cholecalciferol. Am J Nephrol 1984; 4:369–374.
147. Milne FJ, Sharp B, Bell P, Meyers AM. The effect of low aluminum water and desferrioxamine on the outcome of dialysis encephalopathy. Clin Nephrol 1983; 20:202–207.
148. Payton CD, Junor BJ, Fell GS. Successful treatment of aluminum encephalopathy by intraperitoneal desferrioxamine. Lancet 1984; 1:1132–1133.
149. Sullivan D, Murnaghan DJ, Callaghan N. Dialysis dementia, recovery after transplantation. Br Med J 1977; 2:740.
150. Davison AM, Giles GR. The effect of transplantation on dialysis dementia. Proc Eur Dial Transplant Assoc 1979; 16:407–412.
151. Mattern WD, Krigman MR, Blythe NB. Failure of successful renal transplantation to reverse the dialysis-associated encephalopathy syndrome. Clin Nephrol 1977; 7(6):275–278.
152. O'Hare JA, Callaghan NM, Murnaghan DJ. Dialysis encephalopathy: clinical, electroencephalographic, and interventional aspects. Medicine 1983; 62:129–141.
153. Altmann P. Serum Al levels and erythrocyte dihydropteridine reductase activity in patients on HD. N Engl J Med 1987; 317:80–83.
154. Reusche E, Koch V, Friedrich HJ. Correlation of drug related Al intake and dialysis treatment with deposition of argyrophilic-Al-containing inclusions in CNS of patients with dialysis associated encephalopathy. Clin Neuropathol 1996; 15:342–347.
155. Chazot C, Kopple JD. Vitamin metabolism and requirements in renal disease and renal failure. In: Kopple JD, Massry SG, eds. Nutritional Management of Renal Disease. Baltimore: Williams & Wilkins, 1997: 415–477.
156. Said G. Neurological aspects of dialysis patients. In: Jacobs C, Kjellstrand CM, Koch KM, Winchester JF, eds. Replacement of Renal Function by Dialysis. Boston: Kluwer Academic Publisher, 1996:1243–1260.

32

Psychiatric and Psychosocial Complications in Chronic Dialysis

Bum-Hee Yu
Samsung Medical Center, Sungkyunkwan University, Seoul, Korea

Joel E. Dimsdale
University of California, San Diego, San Diego, California

I. INTRODUCTION

Patients with end-stage renal disease (ESRD) have complications in virtually every organ system. Psychiatric difficulties with depression, coping problems, delirium with disturbed behaviors, noncompliance, and marital/family problems are commonly encountered (1). Such patients often show profound quality-of-life complications of chronic dialysis. There are also ethical issues regarding stopping dialysis treatment in ESRD patients. Psychotropic medications need special attention in this medically fragile population. Children and adolescents receiving dialysis can have additional serious problems in both physical and psychological development. Nephrologists need to consider all of these aspects of maintaining dialysis treatment in ESRD patients.

II. QUALITY OF LIFE AND BEHAVIORAL COMPLIANCE PROBLEMS

A. Quality of Life During Dialysis

ESRD patients experience a lower quality of life compared to the general population, and restoration of optimal quality of life should be one of the major goals of ESRD treatment program. As many as 50–70% of chronic dialysis patients report moderate to severe levels of stress related to health status, social relationships and function, and vocational function (2). Low quality of life in dialysis patients may eventually lead to noncompliance and treatment failure. Medical, social, and psychological difficulties in chronic dialysis patients can be obvious contributors to their poor quality of life (3). There are numerous sources of severe psychological stress, including chronic fatigue, other physical symptoms of ESRD, excessive dependence on other people, loss of previous social functioning, and difficulties in maintaining hope in the face of an uncertain future (4).

Psychosocial adaptation in chronic dialysis patients is independent of medical adaptation. Therefore, adequate psychosocial interventions might improve chronic dialysis patients' psychosocial adaptation even though their medical condition remains stable or deteriorates (5). To increase the quality of life in chronic dialysis patients, physicians should assess what is the patients' most important psychosocial stress as well as their medical problems during dialysis. Psychosocial interventions to resolve their most pressing problems are helpful, and psychiatric referrals should be made in the case of patients with severe adaptation problems. Renal transplantation can help many patients because transplant recipients usually report better quality of life than dialysis patients (6). However, physicians should remember that diminished quality of life and depression might be particularly pronounced in people who have had failed transplants and require resumption of dialysis.

B. Noncompliance and Disruptive Behavior of Dialysis Patients

Noncompliance is a commonly seen problem in the treatment of dialysis patients. Because of the regimen's complexity, many people have difficulty adhering to the necessary diet, medication, and schedule of appointments. Adherence is likely to be influenced in a complex manner by multiple factors, including age, gender, locus of control, social adjustment, and past psychiatric history (7). Compliant patients appear to have fewer family problems, receive more assistance from their spouses, and have better family communications (8). In general, younger patients are more likely to skip treatments than older patients, and behavioral compliance styles are greatly influenced by social support and by the severity of medical illness (9,10). The most pervasive problem is fluid noncompliance as measured by excessive weight gains between dialysis sessions (11). Serum urea, potassium, phosphorus, and interdialytic weight gain are commonly used as objective data in estimating noncompliance (12).

Many dialysis patients are unhappy and resentful about being ill. A small error on the part of medical staff may evoke an exaggerated anger response on the part of a patient. Similarly, frustration with life's disappointment may be displaced onto the treatment regimen (13). Anger and noncompliance may also be manifestations of a patient's perception of loss of independence. In that case, appropriate medical advice should be given, and anxiety can be managed with behavioral techniques or minor tranquilizers.

The following guidelines are suggested for physicians to deal with noncompliance of dialysis patients. First, physicians need to be alert to conflicts between dialysis patients and their caretakers—both family members and the dialysis staff. Sometimes patients express their anger or aggression indirectly by noncompliant behavior. Second, it is important to recall that patients cannot comply with instructions they don't understand. The dialysis regimen with its nutritional limitation is indeed complex to grasp, even for highly intelligent, motivated patients. It is very important for physicians to communicate medical information about dialysis repeatedly to their patients. Use of mixed media education can be helpful (individual meeting with staff, group meeting, pamphlet, videotape). Third, imputing moral failure to noncompliant patients should be avoided, because it could result in further deterioration of the rapport between patients and medical staffs. Patients have the right to make choices, even bad choices; our task is to ensure that they are informed about the consequences. Fourth, to the extent that the regimen is less intrusive (e.g., frequency of medication), patients comply better with treatment. Finally, physicians should keep in mind that noncompliant behavior can also result from depression or other neuropsychiatric disturbances accompanied by cognitive impairment.

In many cases, supportive psychotherapy in conjunction with an educational approach by physicians helps to solve noncompliance problems of dialysis patients. A formal psychiatric consultation is advisable when psychiatric diagnosis is questionable, when physicians are at an impasse with patients, or when physicians experience extreme frustration in dealing with difficult noncompliance problems. Frequently the noncompliance problem relates to multiple complicated life situations of the patients outside of the dialysis setting. Cognitive behavioral approaches can be useful in dealing with compliance problems. Because adherence to prescription is important for patient survival, strategies to address different behavioral compliance styles will be necessary to ensure adequate delivery of dialysis (9). Noncompliance during dialysis can be the best predictor of noncompliance following transplantation (14), so transplantation in patients with a history of noncompliance should be considered only after resolving these problems.

Dialysis staffs occasionally deal with disruptive patients who threaten to interrupt their own care and sometimes threaten the safety of medical staff or other patients receiving dialysis. It is important to provide appropriate medical care for the ESRD patients, but the needs and the rights of the other patients and the health care providers must also be respected. Any ESRD program is a joint endeavor entailing shared responsibilities between all the participants, i.e., each patient and his or her family, the medical staffs, the other patients of the dialysis facility, and the facility itself (15).

Skills in handling disruptive patients in the dialysis unit require the same attention to detail as some of the technical factor related to dialysis. Consistent guidelines in managing disruptive patients are frequently helpful, although each problem should be approached on an individual basis. Education and training to cope with disruptive dialysis patients is required, especially for direct patient-care staffs. They are at the highest risk for receiving abuse from patients, yet they are unlikely to have had any skilled training in dealing with these problems (16).

Disruptive patients should be dealt with by a team approach. The effort should include the patient's physician, administrator, renal staff nurses and social worker, and, if possible, a psychiatrist or psychologist. Early conferences with patients should be recommended when disruptive behavior is first noticed. It is also helpful to have a meeting with the disruptive patient, his or her family, and the dialysis team to discuss options available in terms of "quality-of-life" issues and decisions that are in the best interest of the patient (15). Sometimes it may be necessary to make a relatively formal contract between the dialysis unit and the patient with very specific wording that conveys what is expected of both parties. The contract should be simple, plain, direct, and concise and can be changed flexibly as the situation dictates (16). Mediation, a process in which a professional, neutral third party helps disputing parties reach a mutually acceptable agreement, can also be helpful in managing disruptive patients (17).

It should be remembered that the disruptive patient is also sick. The patient may not understand what is expected of him, and the irrational behavior may well be a manifestation of the patient's anxiety or fear. Some patients may have a personality disorder, poor impulse control, or other undiagnosed psychiatric disease (16). To stop caring for the patient and refer to another facility should be a last option after all other efforts have been proved to be ineffective.

III. SOME ETHICAL ISSUES IN CHRONIC DIALYSIS PATIENTS

After cardiovascular diseases, dialysis termination is the second leading cause of death in ESRD patients, accounting for 17% of all deaths. These patients are usually older and have multiple medical problems with a recent deterioration (18). The life expectancy of a 65-year-old patient who initiates treatment with chronic dialysis is only 3.5 years; nonetheless, about 50% of patients who begin dialysis in the United States are age 60 years or older (19). Because of the increasing age of patients on dialysis, withdrawal of treatment will probably become more common in the future.

What are the indications to stop dialysis? There has been much debate about this issue. To a certain extent, the careful guidelines for stopping dialysis in demented patients may be broadly useful (20). Five considerations have been listed in such circumstances:

1. Obtain patients' views about how they would want to be treated if they became incompetent, specifically asking if and when they would want dialysis stopped.
2. When the patient has permanently deteriorated, establish and maintain good communication with the family to discuss the state of the patient and their view on the treatment plan.
3. If the condition should be irreversible and progressive and the patient can no longer communicate with family and treatment team, it is appropriate to stop dialysis.
4. If the hardship and suffering induced by the dialysis procedure itself is in excess of any benefit, again it is appropriate to stop dialysis.
5. It is recommended that decisions of this type be made not by the physician in isolation, but in communication with other professionals such as nurses and social workers.

Advance directives in ESRD may simplify issues such as cardiopulmonary resuscitation and dialysis discontinuation and they may assist ESRD patients, families, and staff with end-of-life decisions (21). Even though the actual number of ESRD patients who have completed formal advance directives is small, patients can react to them by feeling empowered and secure, and may experience an increased control at the end of life (22). One study reported that patients usually died less than a week after stopping dialysis, did not experience substantial pain or mental confusion, had an opportunity to communicate meaningfully with a supportive family and staff, and died in the presence of loved ones (23).

IV. COMMON NEUROPSYCHIATRIC SYNDROMES IN CHRONIC DIALYSIS PATIENTS

A. Depression

Depression is the most prevalent psychiatric problem in patients with ESRD treated with dialysis. Although there are varying estimates of its prevalence, it should be apparent that a high frequency of moderate, debilitating levels of depression exists among patients with renal disease. The prevalence rate ranges from 6.5% for major depression and 17.7% for minor depression to 43% including both moderate and severe depression (24–28) (Table 1). Depression may affect hemodialysis patients in immunological function, nutrition, and compliance (29) and can increase risk of early death in dialysis patients (30).

Table 1 Prevalence of Major Depressive Disorder in ESRD Patients

Prevalence (%)	Sample size	Ref.
25	20	24
43	23	25
18	83	26
8.1	99	27
6.5	124	28

There are several possible explanations for the occurrence of depression in ESRD patients. Psychological loss and/or actual loss in renal condition, role of workplace and family, and sexual function can contribute to the depression. Uremic toxins, especially if inadequately treated, may also aggravate depression (31).

It is not easy to diagnose depression accurately in dialysis patients because of lack of standardized diagnostic criteria in patients with severe medical problems. Depression has both physical and psychological symptoms. Many typical symptoms of major depression may actually be sequelae or clinical manifestations of uremia, thus making diagnosis much more difficult. Classification according to the *Diagnostic and Statistical Manual of Mental Disorders IV* (32) requires at least a 2-week period of either depressed mood or loss of interest or pleasure. In addition, five of nine depressive symptoms (Table 2) that cannot be explained by the results of physical examination and laboratory studies must be present (33). If physicians detect such symptoms, psychiatric consultation should be obtained to assess the psychiatric condition more accurately. It is more helpful to consult a psychiatrist who is familiar with the complexities of dialysis and who routinely treats medically ill patients. After the diagnosis is established, it is prudent to start antidepressant medications.

As a diagnosis of depression is established in patients receiving dialysis, effective treatment strategies should be considered, including cognitive-behavioral interventions and antidepressant medications. Pharmacotherapy in depressive patients with dialysis treatment includes tricyclic antidepressants, serotonin-selective reuptake inhibitors, nefazodone, psychostimulants such as methylphenidate, neuroleptics, and lithium. Tricyclic antidepressants such as nortriptyline, desipramine, and imipramine, which are potentially sedating with relatively moderate anticholinergic side effects, can be used as first-line antidepressants, especially when the depressive symptom of insomnia, agitation, or irritability is prominent. However, because patients maintained with dialysis seem to be frequently more sensitive to side effects associated with these medications (34), serotonin-selective reuptake inhibitors (e.g., fluoxetine, sertraline, paroxetine, and fluvoxamine) and nefazodone can be also prescribed; these newer agents on the whole have fewer side effects and lower suicide patients. Despite constant advertisements testifying to the increased rapidity of onset of antidepressants, physicians should wait 2–4 weeks to assess response. Sometimes it is hard for physicians to wait for more than 2 weeks when the patients cannot tolerate the side effects of these antidepressant medications or their depression is too severe for physicians to wait for the delayed effect of the medications. In that case, use of psychostimulants or electroconvulsive therapy can be considered as an alternative treatment of depression. The pharmacotherapy of depression will be discussed in the latter part of this chapter.

Table 2 Signs and Symptoms of Depression Syndromes

Depressed mood
Loss of interest or pleasure
Significant weight loss or gain
Insomnia or hypersomnia
Psychomotor agitation or retardation
Fatigue or loss of energy
Feelings of worthlessness
Diminished ability to think or concentrate; indecisiveness
Recurrent thoughts of death, suicidal ideation, suicide attempt, or specific plan for suicide

Source: Adapted from Ref. 33.

Physicians may use various brief self-rating scales to diagnose depression (35–37) (Table 3). ESRD patients' perception of their illness, rather than the objective medical severity or extent of role disruption, can determine the level of depression experienced (38). It is necessary to differentiate depressive symptoms from uremic symptoms because many symptoms of uremia such as fatigue, anorexia, and sleep disorders are also prominent features of depression. In addition, sleep apnea, anemia, and medical therapy may produce symptoms similar to the somatic ones of depression, and alternative explanations for the symptoms should also be considered (e.g., inadequate dialysis, hypothyroidism, hypercalcemia, hyponatremia, vitamin B_{12} deficiency).

B. Delirium and Cognitive Dysfunctions

Cognitive dysfunctions are common among ESRD patients and are frequently noted as deficits in attention

Table 3 Diagnostic Self-Rating Scales for Depression

Instrument	Rater	Ref.
Center for Epidemiological Studies Depression Scale (CES-D)	Self	35
Beck Depression Inventory	Self	36
Primary Care Evaluation of Mental Disorder (Prime-MD), Mood Module	Self and clinician	37

and memory, reduced mental alertness, fatigability, and decreased concentration. Patients who have cognitive dysfunctions are frequently referred to psychiatrists because adequate cognition is central to regimen compliance and for maximizing quality of life. In addition, these cognitive dysfunctions may result from depression, which is common in ESRD patients. Some patients manifest subclinical symptoms such as restlessness, anxiety, irritability, distractibility, or sleep-wake disruption immediately before an overt delirium begins. Clinical features of delirium include diffuse cognitive impairment, disorganized thought, language disturbances ranging from mild dysarthria to dysphasia or muteness, illusions or hallucinations, psychomotor retardation or agitation, paranoid delusions, and labile affect. Slowing with triphasic delta waves can be seen in EEG. DSM-IV diagnostic criteria for delirium are listed in Table 4 (32).

Numerous factors can provoke delirium in medically ill patients, and the differential diagnosis of delirium may be extensive. Therefore, a careful assessment is required in ESRD patients with delirium. Laboratory and radiological evaluation of patients with delirium has two levels: basic and additional tests (33) (Table 5).

Table 4 Diagnostic Criteria for Delirium

Disturbance of consciousness (i.e., reduced clarity of awareness of the environment) with reduced ability to focus, sustain, or shift attention
A change in cognition (such as memory deficit, disorientation, language disturbance) or the development of a perceptual disturbance that is not better accounted for by a preexisting, established, or evolving dementia
Disturbance developing over a short period of time (usually hours to days) and tending to fluctuate during the course of the day
Evidence from the history, physical examination, or laboratory findings of a medical condition or substance intoxication or withdrawal judged to be etiologically related to the disturbance

Source: Adapted from Ref. 32.

Despite adequate dialysis, uremic patients often present with subjectively reported memory-concentration complaints (39). The reason for a general decline in cognitive function in chronic renal failure patients is not clear, but an ill-defined impairment in processing information without gross learning disabilities is currently recognized (40). In brain-imaging studies, cerebral damage is frequently seen in MRI findings of chronic hemodialysis patients (41). There is a disturbed pattern of cerebral blood flow in hemodialysis patients, although regional single photon emission tomography abnormalities did not correspond to the severity of cognitive dysfunction (42).

Toxic metabolic conditions associated with dementia in chronic renal failure are uremic encephalopathy and dialysis dementia. When GFR falls to about 10% of normal, uremic encephalopathy occurs. Uremic patients demonstrate mild to moderate impairment on tests that evaluate cognitive flexibility, sustained concentration/attention, perceptual motor speed, learning/memory, and constructional ability. Deficits in verbal intellectual ability tend to be less severe than those in the nonverbal visual-spatial sphere (43). Thus the severity of deficits may be missed on casual examination. Affect and personality factors may also be associated with memory-concentration complaints in hemodialysis patients (39).

Dialysis itself is associated with at least three distinct disorders of the central nervous system: dialysis disequilibrium syndrome, dialysis dementia, and progressive intellectual dysfunction (44). Dialysis disequilibrium is a transient condition usually seen within the first several treatments and is correlated with a rapid reduction in circulating blood urea nitrogen levels. Dialysis dementia is a distinct form of cognitive decline found among patients who have been on dialysis for at least 2 years, and death typically occurs within 6 months after dementia appears. Some authors report that significant amounts of aluminum can be found in the cytoplasm of choroidal epithelium, glia, and neurons in patients with dialysis-associated encephalopathy (45). Aluminum can contribute to the pathogenesis of dialysis dementia, and physicians should keep in mind that aluminum salt in dialysate fluid may provoke or aggravate the dementia progress of patients during chronic dialysis. Progressive intellectual dysfunction is a general decline in cognitive capacity among some patients with chronic renal failure undergoing dialysis.

Table 5 Assessment of the Patient with Delirium

Physical status
History
Physical and neurological examination
Review of vital signs and anesthesia record if postoperative
Review of medical records, medications, and correlation with behavioral changes
Mental status
Interview and cognitive tests
Basic laboratory tests (consider in every patient with delirium)
Blood chemistries (electrolytes, glucose, calcium, albumin, BUN, creatinine, serum SGOT, bilirubin, alkaline phosphatase, magnesium, PO_4^-, VDRL)
Complete blood count
Serum drug levels (e.g., digoxin, theophylline, phenobarbital, cyclosporine)
Arterial blood gases or oxygen saturation
Urinalysis and connection for culture and sensitivity
Urine drug screen
Electrocardiogram and chest x-ray
Additional laboratory tests (order as indicated by clinical condition)
Electroencephalogram
Lumbar puncture
Brain computed tomography (CT) or magnetic resonance imaging (MRI)
Blood chemistries [e.g., heavy metal screen, B_{12} and folate levels, lupus erythematosus (LE) Prep, antinuclear antibody (ANA), urinary prophyrins, human immunodeficiency virus]

Source: Adapted from Ref. 33.

A deterioration in total intelligence as measured by the Wechsler Adult Intelligence Scale–Revised has been found. Verbal skills are typically maintained at the original levels, but performance IQ deteriorates. Memory function, particularly working memory, is frequently affected (46).

C. Sleep Disturbances

Sleep disturbances are common among renal dialysis patients. They lead to daytime sleepiness and decreased mental acuity, which contribute to suboptimal daily functioning. Insomnia, restless leg syndrome, and sleep apnea are commonly reported sleep disorders in dialysis patients (47).

The most common type of insomnia in dialysis patients is mild, transient insomnia related to psychosocial stressors. Insomnia secondary to anxiety or depression is also commonly seen because depression is so common in dialysis patients. Some drugs such as antihypertensives, diuretics, clonidine, cimetidine, thyroxine, and steroids can cause insomnia. Behavioral management techniques, such as progressive muscular relaxation, biofeedback, hypnosis, and improvement of sleep hygiene can help dialysis patients with insomnia. Often a few simple alterations in a patient's habits or sleep environment can be effective (48) (Table 6).

Benzodiazepines including clonazepam, lorazepam, nitrazepam, oxazepam, and temazepam can be used for the treatment of insomnia. Zolpidem, an imidazopyridine sedative, also can be used as a hypnotic in patients with ESRD, although dosage reduction is usually recommended (49).

In recent years, it has been recognized that more than 50% of ESRD and dialyzed patients suffer from sleep apnea (50), and most of the hemodialysis patients who complain of daytime fatigue or sleepiness reveal significant sleep apnea in polysomnographic studies (51). Obstructive sleep apnea syndrome is thought to be related to metabolic factors. During metabolic acidosis, compensatory hyperventilation leads to hypocapnia, generating periodic respiration and destabilization of respiratory control. In addition, uremic toxins or other metabolic abnormalities can influence respiratory control (51). Therefore screening for obstructive sleep apnea might well become a routine part of the management of hemodialysis patients in the future (52). However, the effect of dialysis on sleep apnea is still controversial.

Restless leg syndrome is one of the more distressing concomitants of ESRD, and 20% of ESRD patients report moderate to severe restless leg syndrome symptomatology (53). Patients with this illness complain of an achy or crawling paresthesia, usually in the lower

Table 6 Tips for Promoting Sleep Hygiene

Keep regular wake and sleep onset times.
Ensure that an appropriate length of time is spent in bed—neither too short nor too excessive.
Eat meals regularly and eat a light snack before going to bed, if hungry.
Get more exercise every day, but avoid stimulating exercise before bedtime.
Avoid daytime naps.
Encourage evening activities, either outside or in the home but avoid emotionally upsetting activities or conversations immediately before bedtime.
Bathing in warm water or drinking a cup of warm milk may help sleep induction.
Avoid intake of stimulants such as caffeine (coffee, tea, cocoa, colas), nicotine, and alcohol, especially immediately before bedtime.
Avoid activities associated with wakefulness in bed (e.g., watching TV or listening to the radio).
Learn relaxation techniques to relieve tension or worries that may keep you awake, and avoid dwelling on mental problems in bed.
Make a pleasant sleep environment, which includes sleeping on a comfortable mattress with adequate bed covers and insulating the bedroom against excessive noise, light, cold, and heat.

Source: Adapted from Ref. 48.

extremities, which disturbs sleep maintenance. Roughly 80% of restless leg syndrome patients may also manifest periodic limb movement disorder, in which involuntary movements of the affected limbs occur roughly every 20–40 seconds during sleep (54). Levodopa produced significant clinical effects on this illness compared to ordinary hypnotics, and 100–200 mg/day of levodopa proved to be effective without noticeable side effects (55). Carbamazepine may also produce favorable clinical effects (56).

Nocturnal muscle cramp is not an infrequent complaint among hemodialysis (HD) patients, and 300 mg/day of quinine sulfate may be effective in preventing nocturnal cramps if blood levels are periodically obtained and dosage is adjusted accordingly (57).

D. Suicide

Patients undergoing dialysis are more prone to suicide than the general population (58). Roughly 1 or 2 out of 1000 dialysis patients commit suicide, but the rate of attempting suicide is much higher than this (13). One study reported that the suicide rate is estimated to be 10–25 times more frequent in dialysis patients than in the general population. The assumed reasons for the high rate are as follows (59):

1. Impaired quality of life on maintenance dialysis may lead to depression, multiple somatic symptoms during hemodialysis, sexual problems, and anxiety.
2. Hemodialysis patients have easy ways of ending their life that other people do not have.
3. Dialysis patients are older than the general population, and suicide rate is known to rise with increasing age.

To prevent suicide in dialysis patients, careful evaluations of patients, including comprehensive social and psychological assessment, should be obtained. Patients should be adequately informed concerning the medical and psychological problems that they may face prior to starting dialysis. Psychotropic medications may be needed. Motivated individuals with psychological problems should be considered for psychotherapy.

E. Sexual Dysfunctions

Patients with chronic renal failure frequently show reduced sexual potency after the onset of kidney disease. The cause of sexual dysfunction in ESRD patients is not completely understood. In addition to the multiple psychosocial difficulties, zinc deficiency, autonomic neuropathy, abnormalities in penile blood supply, hormonal disturbances due to hypothalamic-pituitary-gonadal axis dysfunction, secondary hyperparathyroidism, and antihypertensive medications may contribute to the sexual dysfunction. Not infrequently, physicians prescribe antidepressants for patients with ESRD because depression is so common. Tricyclic antidepressants can occasionally decrease erectile and ejaculatory function in men and delay orgasm in women. Serotonin-selective reuptake inhibitors also occasionally decrease libido somewhat and can reduce sexual excitement. They can decrease ability to achieve erection and delay ejaculation in men and inhibit orgasm in women. Monoamine oxidase inhibitors may diminish orgasmic function in both men and women, reducing the firmness of erections and the ability to ejaculate in men without altering libido in men or women (60). Though these drug side effects are usually dose-dependent, physicians should be alert to these effects of antidepressants.

Chronic sexual dysfunction in ESRD patients can lead to multiple emotional problems and marital conflicts and may aggravate depression and noncompliance problems with patients receiving renal replacement therapy. On the other hand, some authors report that

35% of ESRD patients with sexual dysfunction have a subsequent increase in sexual potency after beginning dialysis (61), but the effect of dialysis in these patients is still controversial.

V. PSYCHOTROPIC MEDICATIONS IN DIALYSIS PATIENTS

A. Antidepressants

1. *Tricyclic Antidepressants*

Depression is the most common psychiatric problem in patients during dialysis. Tricyclic antidepressants (TCAs) are largely eliminated via the liver and are not subject to being dialyzed out. For this reason, dose reduction is generally not necessary. However, it is prudent to start dialysis patients on lower doses since such patients appear to be somewhat more sensitive to the side effects of TCAs (34). Increased concentrations of conjugated drug forms and an abnormal distribution or delayed elimination of unconjugated and conjugated metabolites may contribute to the apparent hypersensitivity of TCAs in chronic renal failure patients, particularly because glucuronides may exert peripheral pharmacological effects (62). Therefore, the initial dose should be low and slowly increased on the basis of clinical response and side effects. TCAs can be very helpful to patients with severe depression.

Nortriptyline, desipramine, and imipramine are usually the drugs of choice in the group of TCA medications. The usual adult dose is 75–100 mg/day in nortriptyline, and 150–250 mg/day in desipramine and imipramine. Amitriptyline, although effective, often cannot be tolerated because of its high anticholinergic side effects. Common side effects of TCA medications include postural hypotension, sexual dysfunction, and anticholinergic side effects such as dry mouth, blurred vision and constipation. These side effects are usually more prominent in the elderly.

2. *Serotonin-Selective Reuptake Inhibitors, Monoamine Oxidase Inhibitors, and Nefazodone*

Serotonin-selective reuptake inhibitors (SSRIs); have few anticholinergic side effects, but nausea, headache, nervousness, and insomnia can be common adverse effects. Because their metabolism is largely hepatic, doses are generally not changed for dialysis patients (63). The usual doses of fluoxetine and sertraline are 20–40 mg/day and 50–100 mg/day, respectively. Physicians should be alert to drug interactions of SSRIs. SSRIs are highly bound to plasma protein, and administration of another highly protein-bound drug may cause increased free concentrations of the drug, potentially resulting in adverse effects. In addition, many SSRIs are potent inhibitors of cytochrome P450 IID_6, which governs the oxidative metabolism of many drugs, thereby increasing the blood level of many therapeutic agents. Table 7 shows possible drug interactions of fluoxetine (60,64).

Monoamine oxidase inhibitors (MAOIs) are also protein bound, and protein-binding inhibition in ESRD can produce higher blood levels at the same dosage (65). Postural hypotension, light-headedness, dizziness, coldness, and headache are common side effects of MAOIs. Therapeutic serum levels of MAOIs have not been established. Therefore, decision as to adequate dose of these drugs should be based on remission of clinical symptoms. MAOIs can produce serious hypertensive reactions when they are used simultaneously with tyramine-rich foods (e.g., cheese, other fermented foods, beer, wine) or with medications such as cold remedics, nasal decongestants, cough syrup, and any prescription or over-the-counter remedy containing vasoconstrictor or stimulant-type drugs. In addition, meperidine, hydralazine, methyldopa, ephedrine, epinephrine, or other bronchodilators may also produce hypertensive reactions in MAOI-treated patients. It is necessary to warn patients against the use of cocaine while taking MAOIs because cocaine abuse can produce moderate hypertension in these patients. Although the incidence of hypertensive crisis during treatment of MAOIs is actually very low, careful instruction about

Table 7 Drug Interactions of Fluoxetine

Blood levels and adverse effects of the following drugs are increased:
- Antidepressant—tricyclics and trazodone
- Barbiturate
- Benzodiazepines—except lorazepam and oxazepam
- Carbamazepine
- Narcotics—particularly pentazocine, dextromethorphan, and meperidine
- Neuroleptics
- Phenytoin
- Valproate
- Calcium channel blockers—verapamil, nifedipine
- Insulin or related compounds
- Highly protein-bound medications—anticoagulants, digitalis, digitoxin

Source: Adapted from Refs. 60, 64.

restrictions of diet and medications should be given by physicians before starting treatment (60).

Nefazodone is a new antidepressant that inhibits neuronal uptake of serotonin and norepinephrine. Renal function impairment has no effect on steady-state nefazodone plasma concentration. The recommended initial dose in dialysis patients is 100 mg/day on a twice-daily schedule, and the effective dosage range is generally 300–600 mg/day. It is recommended that nefazodone not be used in combination with a MAOI or within 14 days of discontinuing treatment with a MAOI. Nefazodone is an inhibitor of cytochrome P450 III_A and is highly bound to plasma protein. Thus, it can increase the plasma concentrations of drugs such as nonsedating antihistamines, benzodiazepines, and digoxin (66).

3. *Stimulants*

The above antidepressants generally require 2–4 weeks before effectively treating the depression. Stimulants such as dextroamphetamine, pemoline, and methylphenidate are often useful, particularly in hospitalized medical patients with depression, in whom it is desirable to achieve an initial mood improvement in a short period of time (67). There are extensive studies of the safety of such drugs even in medically unstable patients who are in intensive care unit settings. Methylphenidate has been reported to be useful in elderly depressed patients with renal failure in some studies (68). Methylphenidate, which is metabolized in the liver and eliminated by the kidney, has metabolites with only minimal clinical activity. Doses of 5–10 mg may be administered one to three times daily safely in patients with ESRD. This drug should be prescribed with care because it is Class II controlled substance, although limited dosage for brief interventions presents little risk of dependency (60).

4. *Lithium and Carbamazepine*

Lithium can be useful in the treatment of treatment-resistant depression and bipolar disorder. Patients with ESRD have potential problems with lithium since it is largely excreted by the kidney. Excessive doses may be nephrotoxic, especially in ESRD patients. Lithium is readily dialyzable and should be replaced after each dialysis. To determine appropriate dosage, a lithium level should be checked just prior to dialysis. A single dose, usually 600 mg, is given after the dialysis run (65). Hyperlithemia can be toxic, but its rapid correction can be more toxic because of hyponatremia. Gradual rather than abrupt correction of hyperlithemia might decrease the risk of neurotoxicity (69).

Carbamazepine has been found to be useful in the treatment and prophylaxis of recurrent depression, and 200–600 mg/day may improve depressed mood when used alone or in combination with a tricyclic or MAOI antidepressant (70). It is largely metabolized in the liver, but physicians should keep in mind that several cases of carbamazepine-induced acute renal failure have been reported (71). Neurotoxicity with dizziness, diplopia, headache, and nausea may occur when carbamazepine is combined with calcium channel blockers or angiotensin-converting enzyme inhibitors (60).

B. Sedatives and Anxiolytics

Benzodiazepines are widely prescribed for anxiety and sleep disorders in medically ill patients. Benzodiazepines that are not converted to active metabolites can be used (e.g., clonazepam, lorazepam, nitrazepam, oxazepam, temazepam). Initial dosage of these drugs should be about two thirds of what would be given to a patient with normal kidney function. Diazepam, flurazepam, and chordiazepoxide have active polar metabolites that may accumulate in patients with chronic renal failure and cause prolonged sedation. For this reason, long-term use of these agents should be avoided (65). Elderly patients are particularly sensitive to cognitive side effects produced by benzodiazepines, and physicians should be aware that benzodiazepines can aggravate cognitive dysfunction in elderly patients receiving dialysis. Zolpidem appears to have little daytime hangover effect. The major metabolic route includes oxidation and hydroxylation in the liver, and it may be used as a hypnotic in ESRD patients even though dosage reduction is recommended in such patients (49). The use of barbiturates is not recommended because of their slow elimination and potential side effects in patients with ESRD.

C. Antipsychotics

Antipsychotic agents are not subject to being dialyzed out, and the metabolism and excretion of these drugs occurs via liver. As a group, they tend to be highly bound to serum protein, making their tissue levels variable and potentially higher in renal failure patients than in those with normal kidney function. Therefore, these drugs should be used with adequate caution in a two thirds of normal dosage (65). Haloperidol is the drug of first choice to treat a patient with delirium. The initial recommended dosage for medically ill or elderly patients with delirium is 1.0–5.0 mg two to three times a day. Occasionally much higher doses are necessary for severe agitation. Haloperidol may produce acute dystonia or extrapyramidal syndromes such as facial immobility, muscular rigidity, reduction and slowing of voluntary movement, tremor, stooped posture, festinating gait, and akathisia. However, these side effects are not common when lower dosages are used in delirious patients. After the confusion has cleared, haloperidol administration should be continued and tapered off over 1–5 days (33).

VI. SPECIAL ISSUES OF CHRONIC DIALYSIS IN CHILDREN AND ADOLESCENTS

Children and adolescents with ESRD are usually not long-term dialysis candidates because the ultimate goal is kidney transplantation. Continuous ambulatory peritoneal dialysis has become a good alternative to hemodialysis in the treatment of school-age children with ESRD because it can return children to school and help them to restore a normal life more effectively than in-center hemodialysis (72). However, ESRD children may have serious problems in growth and physical appearance and undergo greater psychological stress when continuous ambulatory peritoneal dialysis therapy is prolonged. Low self-esteem, school maladjustment, depression, and separation anxiety have been found (73). These problems can also affect other family members. Parental relationship problems, high levels of anxiety, depression, and psychosomatic problems in parents have all been noted (74). In addition, healthy siblings may suffer from reduced attention within the family.

Adolescents on hemodialysis tend to be more angry, have more body image problems, be more isolated from peers, and be more noncompliant when compared with adult patients. These differences reflect the fact that the stresses of chronic dialysis for adolescents lie in areas that are already problematic because they involve crucial developmental tasks of adolescence (75).

Noncompliance is a major problem in children and adolescents receiving dialysis. Behavior modification regimens such as token reward systems can be used successfully to improve dietary compliance and control disruptive behavior while on hemodialysis. However, the effect of these regimens tends to be transient unless a maintenance reinforcement schedule is provided (76). To encourage the psychological adjustment of children and/or parents, counseling, psychotherapy or family therapy can be crucially effective.

Children with ESRD may be especially vulnerable to the neuropsychological effects of uremia. Visual motor coordination, attention, and memory can be impaired, and these cognitive deficits, together with the psychological disturbances, may interfere markedly with learning, scholastic performance, and social interactions (77). Early dialysis and proper nutritional intervention will positively affect neuropsychological development in infants and children with ESRD (78,79). Dialysis therapy can also improve neuropsychological performance in older children and adolescents. However, physicians should keep in mind that some neuropsychological deficits may become permanent, especially after long periods of chronic renal failure (80).

The chronic metabolic insult of renal failure can interfere with normal neural development during the critical period of rapid growth of the brain. In previous studies, significant developmental delays, seizures, hypotonia, microencephaly, dyskinesia, EEG abnormalities, and signs of severe osteodystrophy and hyperparathyroidism were reported in some children with ESRD (81,82). Poor nutrition and the use of aluminum salts in dialysate fluid may play a role in the etiology of the developmental delay. Therefore it is prudent to limit aluminum salts, especially in younger children with ESRD (83).

For pediatric patients with ESRD, adequate educational opportunities and vocational training are important prerequisites for achieving independence in adult life (84). Factors such as home dialysis, a successful transplant, and the absence of medical complications promote rehabilitation and help to determine whether the young adult patients complete their education, get a job, become independent of parents, and establish long-term relationships outside the family. The ultimate goal of any therapy for ESRD in children and adolescents is to allow them to become as self-sufficient as possible (83).

From childhood to old age, there are major psychiatric issues confronted by ESRD patients. Successful treatment must address these problems with the same meticulous attention that is given to alteration in electrolytes.

REFERENCES

1. House A. Psychiatric referrals from a renal unit: a study of clinical practice in a British hospital. J Psychosom Res 1989; 33:363–372.

2. Kaplan DA. Psychological adjustment to illness scale (PAIS): a study of chronic hemodialysis patients. J Psychosom Res 1982; 26:11–22.
3. Steele TE, Baltimore D, Finkelstein SH, Juergensen P, Kliger AS, Finkelstein FO. Quality of life in peritoneal dialysis patients. J Nerv Ment Dis 1996; 184:368–374.
4. Farmer CJ, Bewick M, Parsons V, Snowden SA. Survival on home hemodialysis: its relationship with physical symptomatology, psychosocial background and psychiatric morbidity. Psychological Med 1979; 9:515–523.
5. Wolkott DL, Nissenson AR, Landsverk J. Quality of life in chronic dialysis patients: factors unrelated to dialysis modality. Gen Hosp Psychiatry 1988; 10:267–277.
6. Gudex CM. Health-related quality of life in end stage renal failure. Qual Life Res 1995; 4(4):359–366.
7. Sensky T, Leger C, Gilmour S. Psychosocial and cognitive factors associated with adherence to dietary and fluid restriction regimens by people on chronic hemodialysis. Psychoth Psychosomatics 1996; 65(1):36–42.
8. Hartman P, Becker M. Non-compliance with prescribed regimen among chronic hemodialysis patients: a method of prediction and educational diagnosis. Dial Transplant 1978; 9:978–987.
9. 9. Kimmel PL, Peterson RA, Weihs KL, Simmens SJ, Boyle DH, Verme D, Umana WO, Veis JH, Alleyne S, Cruz I. Behavioral compliance with dialysis prescription in hemodialysis patients. J Am Soc Nephrol 1995; 5:1826–1834.
10. Kimmel PL, Peterson RA, Weihs KL, Simmens SJ, Boyle DH, Umana WO, Kovac JA, Alleyne S, Cruz I, Veis JH. Psychologic functioning, quality of life, and behavioral compliance in patients beginning hemodialysis. J Am Soc Nephrol 1996; 7:2152–2159.
11. Streltzer J, Hassell LH. Noncompliant hemodialysis patients: a biopsychosocial approach. Gen Hosp Psychiatry 1988; 10:255–259.
12. Lamping DL, Campbell KA. Hemodialysis compliance: assessment, prediction, and intervention, Part I. Semin Dial 1990; 3:52–56.
13. Levy NB. Central and peripheral nervous systems in uremia. In: Massry SG, Glassock RJ, eds. Textbook of Nephrology. 3rd ed. Baltimore: Williams & Wilkins, 1995:1325–1338.
14. Rodriguez A, Diaz M, Colon A, Santiago-Delpin EA. Psychosocial profile of noncompliant transplant patients. Transplant Proc 1991; 23(2):1807–1809.
15. Baskin S. Ethical issues in dialysis: guidelines for treating the disruptive dialysis patient. Nephrol News Issues 1994; 8(3):43, 50.
16. Burns GC. Empowering dialysis professionals in the management of the aggressive and disruptive patient. Dial Transplant 1995; 24(4):184–186.
17. Johnstone S, Seamon VJ, Halshaw D, Molinari J, Longknife K. The use of mediation to manage patient-staff conflict in the dialysis clinic. Adv Renal Replacement Ther 1997; 4:359–371.
18. Catalano C, Goodship TH, Graham KA, Marino C, Brown AL, Tapson JS, Ward MK, Wilkinson R. Withdrawal of renal replacement therapy in Newcastle upon Tyne: 1964–1993. Nephrol Dial Transplant 1996; 11: 133–139.
19. Nissenson AR. Dialysis therapy in the elderly patient. Kidney Int 1993; 40(suppl):S51–57.
20. Kaye M, Lella JW. Discontinuation of dialysis therapy in the demented patient. Am J Nephrol 1986; 6:75–79.
21. Rutecki GW, Rodriguez L, Cugino A, Jarjoura D, Hastings F, Whittier FC. End of life issues in ESRD: a study of three decision variables that affect patient attitudes. ASAIO J 1994; 40(3):M798–802.
22. Cohen LM, McCue JD, Germain M, Woods A. Denying the dying: advance directives and dialysis discontinuation. Psychosomatics 1997; 38:27–34.
23. Cohen LM, McCue JD, Germain M, Kjellstrand CM. Dialysis discontinuation. Arch Intern Med 1995; 155: 42–47.
24. Cramond WA, Knight PR, Lawrence JR. The psychiatric contribution to a renal unit undertaking chronic hemodialysis and renal hemo-transplantation. Br J Psychiatry 1967; 113:1201–1212.
25. Holcomb JL, MacDonald RW. Social functioning of artificial kidney patients. Soc Sci Med 1973; 7:109–119.
26. Lowry MR, Atcherson E. A short-term follow-up of patients with depressive disorder on entry into home dialysis training. J Affective Disorder 1980; 2:219–227.
27. Craven JL, Rodin GM, Johnson L, Kennedy SH. The diagnosis of major depression in renal dialysis patients. Psychosom Med 1987; 49:482–492.
28. Hinrichsen GA, Lieberman JA, Pollack S, Steinberg H. Depression in hemodialysis patients. Psychosomatics 1989; 30:284–289.
29. Kimmel PL, Weihs K, Peterson RA. The role of depression. J Am Soc Nephrol 1993; 3:12–27.
30. Soucie JM, McClellan WM. Early death in dialysis patients: risk factors and impact on incidence and mortality rates. J Am Soc Nephrol 1996; 7(10):2169–2175.
31. Israel M. Depression in dialysis patients: a review of psychological factors. Can J Psychiatry 1986; 31:445–451.
32. American Psychiatric Association. Diagnostic and Statistical Manual of Mental Disorders. 4th ed. Washington, DC: American Psychiatric Press, Inc., 1994.
33. Rundell JR, Wise MG. Textbook of Consultation-Liaison Psychiatry. Washington, DC: American Psychiatric Press, Inc., 1996.
34. Stoudemire A, Moran MG, Fogel BS. Psychotropic drug use in the medically ill, Part I. Psychosomatics 1990; 31:377–391.
35. Radoff LS. The CES-D scale: a new self report depression scale for research in the general population. Appl Psychol Meas 1977; 1:385–401.

36. Beck AT, Steer RA, Garbin MG. Psychometric properties of the Beck Depression Inventory: twenty five years of evaluation. Clin Psychol Rev 1988; 8:77–100.
37. Spitzer RL, Williams JBW, Kroenke K, Linzer M, deGruy FV 3rd, Hahn SR, Brody D, Johnson JG. Utility of a new procedure for diagnosing mental disorders in primary care: the Prime-MD 1000 study. JAMA 1994; 272:1749–1756.
38. Sacks CR, Peterson RA, Kimmel PL. Perception of illness and depression in chronic renal failure. Am J Kidney Dis 1990; 15:31–39.
39. Brickman AL, Yount SE, Blaney NT, Rothberg S, De-Nour AK. Pathogenesis of cognitive complaints in patients on hemodialysis. Gen Hosp Psychiatry 1996; 18: 36–43.
40. Brown TM, Brown RLS. Neuropsychiatric consequences of renal failure. Psychosomatics 1995; 36:244–253.
41. Fazekas G, Fazekas F, Schmidt R, Kapeller P, Offenbacher H, Krejs GJ. Brain MRI findings and cognitive impairment in patients undergoing chronic hemodialysis treatment. J Neurol Sci 1995; 134:83–88.
42. Fazekas G, Fazekas F, Schmidt R, Flooh E, Valetitsch H, Kapeller P, Krejs GJ. Pattern of cerebral blood flow and cognition in patients undergoing chronic hemodialysis treatment. Nucl Med Commun 1996; 17:603–608.
43. Nissenson AR, Fine RN, Gentile DE. Clinical Dialysis. 3rd ed. East Norwalk, CT: Appleton & Lange, 1995.
44. Fraser CL, Arieff AI. Metabolic encephalopathy as a complication of renal failure: mechanisms and mediators. New Horizons 1994; 2:518–526.
45. Reusche E, Seydel U. Dialysis-associated encephalopathy: light and electron microscopic morphology and topography with evidence of aluminum by laser microprobe mass analysis. Acta Neuropathol 1993; 86(3): 249–258.
46. Cohen LM. Renal Disease. In: Rundell JR, Wise MG, eds. American Psychiatric Press Textbook of Consultation-Liaison Psychiatry. Washington, DC: American Psychiatric Press, Inc., 1996:573–578.
47. Walker SL, Fine A, Kryger MH. Sleep complaints are common in a dialysis unit. Am J Kidney Dis 1995; 26: 751–756.
48. Kaplan HI, Sadock BJ. Comprehensive Textbook of Psychiatry. 6th ed. Baltimore: Williams & Wilkins, 1995:1407.
49. Salva P, Costa J. Clinical pharmacokinetics and pharmacodynamics of zolpidem: therapeutic implications. Clin Pharmacokinetics 1995; 29(3):142–153.
50. Jean G, Piperno D, Francois B, Charra B. Sleep apnea incidence in maintenance hemodialysis patients: influence of dialysate buffer. Nephron 1995; 71:138–142.
51. Fletcher EC. Obstructive sleep apnea and the kidney. J Am Soc Nephrol 1993; 4(5):1111–1121.
52. Hallett MD, Burden S, Stewart D, Mahony J, Farrell PC. Sleep apnea in end-stage renal disease patients on hemodialysis and continuous ambulatory peritoneal dialysis. ASAIO J 1995; 41:M435-M441.
53. Winkelman JW, Chertow GM, Lazarus M. Restless legs syndrome in end-stage renal disease. Am J Kidney Dis 1996; 28:372–378.
54. Walters AS. Towards a better definition of the restless legs syndrome. Movement Disord 1995; 10:634–642.
55. Trenkwalder C, Stiasny K, Pollmacher Th, Wetter Th, Schwaez J, Kohnen R, Kazenwadel J, Kruger HP, Ramm S, Kunzel M, Oertel WH. L-dopa therapy of uremic and idiopathic restless legs syndrome: a double-blind, crossover trial. Sleep 1995; 18:681–688.
56. Yoshioka M, Ishii T, Fukunishi I. Sleep disturbance of end-stage renal disease. Japanese J Psychiatry Neurol 1993; 47:847–851.
57. Mandal AK, Abernathy T, Nelluri SN, Stitzel V. Is quinine effective and safe in leg cramps? J Clin Pharmacol 1995; 35:588–593.
58. Abram HS, Moore GL, Westervelt FB. Suicidal behavior in chronic dialysis patients. Am J Psychiatry 1971; 127:119–120.
59. Haenel Th, Brunner F, Battegay R. Renal dialysis and suicide: occurrence in Switzerland and in Europe. Compr Psychiatry 1980; 21:140–145.
60. Bernstein JG. Handbook of Drug Therapy in Psychiatry. 3rd ed. St. Louis: Mosby-Year Book, Inc., 1995.
61. Abram HS, Hester LR, Sheridan WF, Epstein GM. Sexual functioning in patients with chronic renal failure. J Ner Ment Dis 1975; 160:220–226.
62. Liberman JA, Cooper TB, Suckow RF, Steinberg H, Borenstein M, Brenner R, Kane JM. Tricyclic antidepressant and metabolite levels in chronic renal failure. Clin Pharmacol Ther 1985; 37:301–307.
63. Levy NB, Blumenfield M, Beasley CM, Dubey AK, Solomon RJ, Todd R, Goodman A, Bergstrom RR. Fluoxetine in depressed patients with renal failure and in depressed patients with normal kidney function. Gen Hosp Psychiatry 1996; 18:8–13.
64. USP DI. Drug Information for the Health Care Professional. 18th ed. Rockville, MD: The United States Pharmacopeial Convention, Inc., 1998:1472–1475.
65. Levy NB. Use of psychotropics in patients with kidney failure. Psychosomatics 1985; 26:699–709.
66. Drug Facts and Comparisons. St. Louis, MO: Facts and Comparisons, 1998:1635–1653.
67. Chiarello RJ, Cole JO. The use of psychostimulants in general psychiatry. Arch Gen Psychiatry 1987; 44:286–295.
68. Stiebel VG. Methylphenidate plasma levels in depressed patients with renal failure. Psychosomatics 1994; 35:498–500.
69. Swartz CM, Jones P. Hyperlithemia correction and persistent delirium. J Clin Pharmacology 1994; 34:865–870.
70. Folks DG. Carbamazepine treatment of selected affectively disordered inpatients. Am J Psychiatry 1982; 139: 115–117.

71. Lambert M, Fournier A. Acute renal failure complicating carbamazepine hypersensitivity. Rev Neurol 1992; 148:574–576.
72. Baum M, Powell D, Calvin S, McDaid T, McHenry K, Mar H, Potter D. Continuous ambulatory peritoneal dialysis in children: comparison with hemodialysis. N Engl J Med 1982; 307(25):1537–1542.
73. Fukunishi I, Kudo H. Psychiatric problems of pediatric end-stage renal failure. Gen Hosp Psychiatry 1995; 17(1):32–36.
74. Brownbridge G, Fielding DM. Psychosocial adjustment and adherence to dialysis treatment regimes. Pediatr Nephrol 1994; 8:744–749.
75. De-Nour AK. Adolescents' adjustment to chronic hemodialysis. Am J Psychiatry 1979; 136:430–434.
76. Fennell RS, Foulkes LM, Boggs SR. Family-based program to promote medication compliance in renal transplant children. Transplant Proc 1994; 26(1):102–103.
77. Weiss RA, Edelmann CM, Jr. Children on dialysis. N Engl J Med 1982; 307:1574–1575.
78. Osberg JW, Meares GJ, McKee DC, Burnett GB. Intellectual functioning in renal failure and chronic dialysis. J Chron Dis 1982; 35:445–457.
79. Warady BA, Kriley M, Lovell H, Farrell SE, Hellerstein S. Growth and development of infants with end-stage renal disease receiving long-term peritoneal dialysis. J Pediatr 1988; 112:714–719.
80. Fennell RS, Fennel EB, Carter RL, Mings EL, Klausner AB, Hurst JR. Association between renal function and cognition in childhood chronic renal failure. Pediatr Nephrol 1990; 4(1):16–20.
81. Rotundo A, Nevins TE, Lipton M, Lockman LA, Mauer SM, Michael AF. Progressive encephalopathy in children with chronic renal insufficiency in infancy. Kidney Int 1982; 21:486–491.
82. McGraw ME, Haka-Ikse K. Neurologic-developmental sequalae of chronic renal failure. J Pediatr 1985; 106: 579–583.
83. Fennell RS. Psychosocial problems related to dialysis in pediatric patients. In: Nissenson AR, Fine RN, Gentile DE, eds. Clinical Dialysis. 3rd ed. East Norwalk, CT: Appleton & Lange, 1995:839–847.
84. Rosenkranz J, Bonzel KE, Bulla M, Michalk D, Offner G, Reichwald-Klugger E, Scharer K. Psychosocial adaptation of children and adolescents with chronic renal failure. Pediatr Nephrol 1992; 6:459–463.

33

Gastrointestinal Complications in the Dialysis Patient

Pradeep Ramamirtham and Thomas J. Savides
University of California, San Diego, San Diego, California

Before the advent of hemodialysis, gastrointestinal (GI) involvement was a common complication of uremia. Despite the universal application of hemodialysis, GI problems are still frequent in patients with end-stage renal disease (ESRD). This verifies the role of the kidney beyond that of only a metabolic filter. Some GI complications are inherent to renal disease and others to hemodialysis. This chapter will focus on those GI issues that will be most frequently encountered by the nephrologists and primary care physicians managing dialysis patients (Table 1).

I. GASTROINTESTINAL BLEEDING

GI bleeding is a common clinical problem requiring more than 300,000 hospitalizations annually in the United States. Among the general population, it has been estimated that 150 patients per 100,000 are hospitalized annually for upper GI hemorrhage. Accurate figures are unavailable for lower GI hemorrhage, but it is much less common (1). Although the exact incidence is not known, there is a higher frequency of upper GI bleeding in uremic patients on maintenance hemodialysis compared to controls (2). Heparinization may play a role in this regard because mucosal lesions are more likely to bleed with the interruption of the normal clotting cascade.

Common causes of upper GI bleeding in the United States include peptic ulceration (duodenal and gastric ulcers), erosive gastritis, varices, and gastroesophageal junction mucosal tears (Mallory-Weiss tears). The etiology of bleeding in patients with chronic renal failure appears similar to that of control patients (3). There appears to be no difference in the incidence of peptic ulcers in uremic subjects compared to the general population (4). However, approximately half of patients on chronic hemodialysis have endoscopic findings of gastroduodenal inflammation, a much higher proportion than found in patients not on hemodialysis (5,6). There are conflicting reports on whether peptic ulcers or inflammation account for the greater proportion of upper GI bleeding in patients on hemodialysis (7–9).

A. *Helicobacter pylori* Infection and Peptic Ulcer Disease

Over the past several years it has become increasingly clear that the bacterium *Helicobacter pylori* contributes to peptic ulcer formation. Virtually all *H. pylori*–positive patients display antral gastritis, which resolves with treatment of the bacteria. Nearly all patients with duodenal ulcers have *H. pylori* gastritis. Thus, infection of the stomach with this organism appears to be a prerequisite for the development of duodenal ulcers in the absence of other precipitating factors such as nonsteroidal anti-inflammatory drugs (NSAIDs) or Zollinger-Ellison syndrome. The association with gastric ulcers is slightly less strong, with 80% of gastric ulcer patients also having *H. pylori* infection. The majority of individuals infected with *H. pylori* do not develop ulcers, which indicates that host characteristics, strain variability, or other factors play a role in the pathogenesis.

H. pylori infection can cause microscopic changes of chronic gastritis, intestinal metaplasia, or atrophic gastritis. There may be an association between *H. py-*

Table 1 GI Complications in the Dialysis Patient

Gastrointestinal bleeding
Helicobacter pylori infection and peptic ulcer disease
Angiodyplasia
Lower GI bleeding
Occult GI blood loss
Treatment of GI bleeding
Pancreatitis
Acute pancreatitis
Chronic pancreatitis
Treatment of pancreatitis
Viral hepatitis
Hepatitis C
Hepatitis B
Hepatitis G
Gastric emptying
Gastroesophageal reflux disease
Amyloidosis

lori and gastric adenocarcinoma and gastric lymphoma. The association of *H. pylori* in the pathogenesis of nonulcer dyspepsia or functional upper abdominal pain remains to be clearly defined (10).

There is no difference between the incidence of *H. pylori* infection in hemodialysis patients and in the general population. Further, there is no correlation between the incidence of dyspeptic symptoms in dialysis patients and the finding of *H. pylori* infection (12).

Patients generally should only be treated with antibiotics to eradicate *H. pylori* infection if there is documented peptic ulceration (13). Numerous antibiotic regimens have been studied in the treatment of *H. pylori* infection. A 2-week combination of H_2 blockers with bismuth subsalicylate, tetracycline, and metronidazole can yield eradication rates of over 90%. Other two- and three-drug combinations including the use of amoxicillin, clarithromycin, metronidazole, and proton pump inhibitors can achieve similar efficacy (10). The only combination specifically evaluated in dialysis patients is from Japan using a combination of lanzoperazole, amoxicillin, and plaunotol, which achieved a 78% eradication rate (11).

B. Angiodysplasia

Angiodysplasia, or vascular ectasia, is frequently associated with chronic renal failure and is more likely to bleed in these patients than in those with normal renal function. There is no proven cause for angiodysplasia, nor is it known why there is an association with renal disease. Studies by Boley and colleagues (14) suggest that colonic angiodysplasias are acquired lesions of aging, which develop as a result of increased intraluminal pressure leading to dilatation and tortuosity of the submucosal veins. This dilatation progresses to the mucosal veins and venules and eventually to the capillary rings. As the capillary rings dilate, incompetence of the precapillary sphincter ensues, with eventual development of a small arteriovenous communication or angiodysplasia.

Angiodysplasia in dialysis patients may be as common as in the general population, but lesions may bleed more frequently in uremic patients with impaired coagulation. Although angiomas are most often found in the right colon, they can occur anywhere in the GI tract and account for a major portion of upper GI hemorrhages in dialysis patients (7). In one series, they were more common than peptic lesions as the cause for upper intestinal bleeding in renal failure patients, accounting for 53% of episodes compared with 40% for non–renal failure patients (9).

C. Lower GI Bleeding

Causes of lower gastrointestinal hemorrhages in uremic patients are not different from those with normal renal function. These include hemorrhoids, diverticular disease, inflammatory bowel disease, polyps and neoplasms, and angiodysplasia. There is an increased detection of colonic angiodysplastic lesions bleeding in hemodialysis patients. Polycystic kidney disease is associated with a greater frequency of diverticular disease than age-matched controls (15).

D. Occult GI Blood Loss

Occult blood loss is a common finding in chronic renal failure, with patients frequently exhibiting guaiac-positive stools without a drop in hematocrit (16,17). One study of asymptomatic hemodialysis patients with hemoccult-positive stools found that the most common cause was gastroduodenal inflammation (17).

Hemoccult testing was developed for the screening of colon cancer, for which the American population carries a 5% risk. If a stool specimen obtained from an asymptomatic person is positive, evaluation of the entire large bowel is necessary, usually with colonoscopy. Despite the high false-positive rate of hemoccult testing in the general population, it has been deemed cost-effective for detecting early colon cancer, with an average cost of $40,000 per life saved. This compares favorably with other screening programs, such as mammography. Patients with renal failure have a higher false-positive rate of fecal occult blood testing than non–renal failure patients, which may result in hemoccult testing for renal failure patients being less cost-effective for colon cancer screening than in the general population (16,17). In the United States it is recommended that some form of colorectal cancer screening be performed in all patients over 50 years of age, regardless of renal function, with either screening flexible sigmoidoscopy, barium enema, colonoscopy, or fecal occult blood testing.

Chronic gastrointestinal blood loss with decreased hematocrit and iron deficiency is frequently encountered in uremic patients. Upper endoscopy and/or colonoscopy should be performed starting with whichever is likely to have a higher yield based on patient history. If no lesions are found, a small bowel x-ray series can be obtained to exclude small bowel tumors or inflammatory bowel disease, although the yield of such evaluation is often low in patients who have iron deficiency without symptoms (18).

E. Treatment of GI Bleeding

Management of gastrointestinal bleeding is no different in patients with or without renal failure. However, there is an increased need for transfusion, emergency surgery, and mortality rate in patients with renal compromise (19). Patients with acute upper gastrointestinal hemorrhage should undergo urgent endoscopic evaluation and treatment after hemodynamic stabilization. Patients with lower gastrointestinal hemorrhages should have an urgent bowel preparation over 4–6 hours using 4 L of a balanced electrolyte solution (e.g., polyethylene glycol, Colyte). Oral sodium phosphate solutions (e.g., Fleets Phospha-Soda) bowel prep should be avoided in patients with renal failure because of the large amounts of sodium and phosphate that may be absorbed.

Angiodysplasias can be treated with simple iron supplementation to keep up with chronic losses. If this proves to be insufficient, endoscopic cauterization of detectable lesions may decrease transfusion requirement. Failing this, uncontrolled trials have suggested that conjugated estrogens may help decrease blood loss from these lesions (20,21). Sloand and Schiff (22) studied four patients with chronic GI bleeding from angiodysplasia and applied transdermal estrodiol 50–100 g in 24 hours every 3.5 days for 2 months. They noted decreased transfusion requirements in all four patients, with improved bleeding times and no adverse reactions (22). In one case report, the use of a somatostatin analog given at a dose of 100 μg subcutaneously twice daily for 26 months was efficacious in stopping recurrent anemia in a 37-year-old woman with angiodysplasia (23).

II. PANCREATITIS

Acute pancreatitis is a clinical syndrome characterized by abdominal pain and increased serum pancreatic enzyme levels. More than 80% of cases in the United States are attributed to gallstones or alcohol. Other causes for acute pancreatitis include medications, infections, hyperlipidemia, vascular disease, and microlithiasis. The incidence of pancreatitis in the general population ranges from 1 to 5 per 10,000 per year.

A. Acute Pancreatitis

The diagnosis of acute pancreatitis can be difficult in patients with chronic renal failure. Symptoms consistent with acute pancreatitis, abdominal pain, retching, and vomiting are not uncommon in these patients. Further, the usual diagnostic laboratory assays, such as amylase and lipase, are frequently elevated in these patients due to decreased renal clearance of these enzymes (24). CT scanning, which shows pancreatic edema, can help confirm the diagnosis.

The incidence of acute pancreatitis in chronic renal failure is approximately 1 per 100 per patient-year, which is higher than in the general population. Alcohol and biliary tract disease only account for 50% of these cases, while there is a larger proportion of idiopathic cases compared to the general population (25). This argues that renal failure in and of itself, through as-yet-unclear mechanisms, may be associated with, or even cause, acute pancreatitis (25).

Grading the severity of acute pancreatitis and establishing a prognosis can provide valuable information to the clinician by guiding interventions and allowing evaluation of the success or failure of therapeutic measures. Currently, the most commonly used clinical assessments of acute pancreatitis are Ranson's criteria (Table 2) and the Acute Physiology and Chronic Health Evaluation (APACHE) II criteria.

Using Ranson's criteria, patients with fewer than two signs have very low rates of morbidity (<5%) and mortality (<1%). With greater than six signs the rates are greatly increased to 90% and 20%. These figures are only applicable to patients with previously normal renal function because those on maintenance hemodialysis who develop acute pancreatitis have a more severe course of disease. With greater than three of Ran-

Table 2 Ranson's Criteria for Severe Acute Pancreatitis

On admission	Within 48 hours
Age > 55 years	Hematocrit decrease > 10%
WBC > 16,000	Urea nitrogen increase > 5 mg/dL
LDH > 350 IU/L	Serum calcium < 8 mg/dL
Glucose > 200 mg/dL	Arterial pO_2 < 60 mmHg
AST > 250 IU/L	Base deficit > 4 mEq/L
	Estimated fluid sequestration > 6 L

son's criteria the observed mortality in dialysis patients is near 70% compared with 11% for non–chronic renal failure patients.

Severe pancreatitis is more common in renal failure patients with mild disease (0–2 Ranson's criteria) occurring in 79% compared with 52% of controls, and severe disease (>3 criteria) occurring in 48% versus 21% of controls (25). This suggests that when acute pancreatitis occurs in dialysis patients, it is more likely to be severe and have a worse prognosis than in those without renal failure.

Local complications of acute pancreatitis are no more common in renal failure patients, with equal occurrence of abscesses, pseudocysts, ascites, and splenic vein thromboses. However, systemic complications are more frequently encountered in dialysis patients. In one study, 66% of dialysis patients had one or more of pulmonary, cardiovascular, hematological, or septic complications compared to 27% of those with initially normal renal function (25).

B. Chronic Pancreatitis

Chronic pancreatitis is rare in most settings other than those accounted for by alcohol. However, in autopsy studies in patients who were on long-term hemodialysis, changes of chronic pancreatitis are more frequent than those of acute pancreatitis. These changes include pancreatic fibrosis, calcification, cystic changes, hemosiderin deposition, and abscess formation. In one study, histological pancreatitis (acute and chronic) was found in 50% of patients with end-stage renal failure compared with 15% of controls (27). Most of these patients did not present with clinical pancreatitis during their lifetime.

C. Treatment of Pancreatitis

The treatment of acute pancreatitis in patients with end-stage renal disease is not different from that of the general population. Conservative measures are generally used including restricting oral intake, narcotic analgesia, replacing electrolytes as necessary, and monitoring for complications. Should complications such as an infected pseudocyst, pancreatic abscess, or necrosis arise, invasive management and drainage may be necessary. This can be pursued with surgical, radiological, or advanced endoscopic techniques. When invasive therapy is required, it may be prudent to discontinue peritoneal dialysis in favor of hemodialysis until the pancreatitis has fully healed. There are varying results when peritoneal dialysis is discontinued with transfer to hemodialysis in uncomplicated pancreatitis, and therefore it cannot be recommended routinely (28).

Chronic pancreatitis can present with either pain or pancreatic insufficiency manifest as diabetes or malabsorption. Management of pain from chronic pancreatitis can be very difficult, and it is often advisable to involve a pain specialist because narcotics are the usual mainstay of therapy. There is some evidence for the use of acid suppression via proton-pump inhibitors (omeprazole, lanzoprazole), non–enteric-coated pancreatic enzyme supplementation (Viokase), and low-dose tricyclic antidepressants (amitriptyline 10 mg) to reduce the pain from chronic pancreatis. Celiac plexus blocks with alcohol injections have produced mixed results with occasional benefits, which usually do not last more than a few months. In the setting of pancreatic obstruction demonstrated by dilated pancreatic ducts, endoscopic therapy with stricture dilation and pancreatic duct stenting has been successful in reducing pain. If medical therapy fails, surgical treatment can then be considered. The type of surgery depends on the ductal morphology. When ductal obstruction is thought to be the mechanism of pain, a partial pancreatic resection with pancreatojejunostomy or a lateral pancreaticojejunostomy (modified Peustow's procedure) can be performed. When no ductal obstruction is evident and the mechanism of pain is thought to be diffuse parenchymal disease, a partial pancreatic resection may be considered.

Exocrine pancreatic insufficiency, manifested by malabsorption, steatorrhea, and weight loss, can be managed with pancreatic enzyme replacements with each meal. Because gastric acid can denature the pancreatic enzymes, patients receiving pancretic enzymes should also receive either daily histamine receptor antagonists or proton pump inhibitors.

III. VIRAL HEPATITIS

Elevations in transaminases occur in 10–44% of chronic hemodialysis patients. In a necropsy study of

78 patients who had undergone dialysis, 90% displayed some hepatic abnormality. In addition to hepatomegaly and chronic passive congestion from cardiac disease, these changes included periportal fibrosis, fatty metamorphosis, triaditis, and hemosiderosis, which are likely due to viral hepatitis (29). In the past, approximately half of the hepatic abnormalities were attributed to non-A, non-B hepatitis, with the remaining cases implicating hepatitis B, Epstein-Barr virus (EBV), cytomegalovirus (CMV), and drugs such as alcohol and cyclosporine. However, since 1989, when hepatitis C virus (HCV) was cloned, it has been identified as the cause for over 90% of posttransfusion non-A, non-B hepatitis in the United States. Twenty-five percent of hemodialyzed patients carry anti-HCV antibodies. These antibodies are associated with detectable viremia in 85% and chronic hepatitis in 90% despite normal transaminases in over half of them (30). (Both hepatitis C and B are covered extensively in Chapter 38 of this volume.)

IV. GASTRIC EMPTYING

Symptoms of nausea and vomiting, extremely common in the general population and common side effects of many prescribed drugs, are particularly common among renal failure patients. The underlying etiology may be difficult to determine in the dialysis patient. They may be the only presenting symptoms of uremia, gastroesophageal reflux, gastroparesis, poor gastric emptying, infection, side effects of medication, or a mechanical obstruction. Because diabetes mellitus is a common cause of chronic renal failure, many of the symptoms overlap with those of dialysis patients. Many diabetics with chronic renal failure demonstrate poor gastric emptying, especially those with both sympathetic and parasympathetic autonomic neuropathy, the majority of whom will remain relatively asymptomatic (31,32). Dialysis in and of itself does little to delay solid and liquid emptying times as determined by radioisotope markers (33). In CAPD patients, the physical presence of peritoneal dialysate in the abdomen can retard solid food gastric emptying, which is resolved when the dialysate is drained (34). Evaluation of these symptoms in this patient population again begins with a history and physical. If any alarm symptoms of GI bleeding, weight loss, dysphagia, or abdominal pain are illicted, examination via endoscopic or radiographic measures is appropriate. Otherwise, it may be prudent to offer a trial of a promotility agent such as metaclopramide or cisapride before searching for an organic cause. If 8 weeks of therapy with full-dose pro-motility agents (metaclopramide 10 mg qid, cisapride 10 mg qid) does not relieve symptoms, emperic therapy can be considered a failure. Further evaluation with solid phase gastric emptying study may then be pursued to document disease. Macrolide antibiotics and oral antifungals (e.g., fluconazole, ketoconazole) can have interactions with cisapride, leading to prolonged QT intervals predisposing to lethal arrythmias. Therefore, these medications are contraindicated when using cisapride.

V. GASTROESOPHAGEAL REFLUX DISEASE

Gastroesophageal reflux, the movement of gastric contents from the stomach to esophagus, is a normal physiological process occurring in virtually everyone several times a day without producing symptoms. When it does produce symptoms of tissue injury in the esophagus, oropharynx, or respiratory tract, it is a pathological process referred to as gastroesophageal reflux disease (GERD). The most common symptoms are heartburn, chest pain, and regurgitation. Conditions predisposing to GERD are incompetency of the internal lower esophageal sphincter, loss of support from the crural diaphragm (as may occur in hiatal hernias), and delayed gastric emptying. As the latter condition is common in diabetics, this may be a frequent disease in the dialysis patient.

Dialysis and renal failure in and of themselves do not predispose to GERD. Management begins with lifestyle modification. These include raising the head of the bed, smoking cessation, reducing alcohol consumption, reducing dietary fat, reducing meal size and bedtime snacks, and weight reduction. Foods that precipitate symptoms include chocolates, spearmints and peppermints, coffee, tea, carbonated beverages, and tomato and citrus juices. Prescription medications such as anticholinergics, theophylline, benzodiazepines, narcotics, calcium channel blockers, and progesterone have been noted to worsen symptoms.

Should lifestyle modification alone fail to alleviate symptoms, than it is appropriate to use concurrent medical treatment. Oral antacids may be contraindicated in the dialysis patient because they contain aluminum, phosphorus, and magnesium. Oral H_2 blockers (cimetidine, ranitidine, famotidine, nizatidine) or cisapride are good first-line agents. Failing these, the use of proton pump inhibitors, either alone or in combination with a promotility agent, is usually efficacious. When medical therapy fails or when indicated by lifestyle (avoidance of medication), laparoscopic surgery is increasingly used to treat GERD. A gastric fundoplication (Nissen procedure) wraps the fundus of the stomach around the terminal esophagus to form an effective barrier to acid reflux, with symptoms recurring in about 10% of patients.

Complications of GERD include strictures and Barrett's esophagus (columnar intestinal metaplasia). Strictures can be dilated endoscopically with biopsies to exclude malignancy followed by maintenance proton pump inhibitors. Barrett's esophagus carries a risk for esophageal adenocarcinoma. The 30- to 40-fold increased risk in Barrett's translates into an overall risk of about 3%. These patients should undergo surveillance endoscopy with biopsy every 1–2 years.

VI. AMYLOIDOSIS

Amyloidosis is not a single disease but rather a term for diseases that share the common feature of deposition of pathological insoluble fibrillar proteins in organs and tissue. Patients undergoing dialysis are prone to develop secondary amyloidosis Carpal tunnel syndrome, known to develop in dialysis patients, is related to the duration of treatment and is almost inevitable after 8 years. In approximately half of such cases, amyloid is demonstrable in the synovial tissue as well as the rectal mucosa (35). Amyloidosis has also been observed as deposits throughout the gastrointestinal tract, liver, and pancreas. Although it has yet to be implicated in clinical hepatic or pancreatic dysfunction, when it involves the gastrointestinal tract it can present as bleeding, perforation, or pseudo-obstruction. Neural involvement may also cause an autonomic neuropathy and lead to diarrhea (3,36,37). Unlike primary amyloidosis, which contains fragments of light chain immunoglobulins, secondary amyloidosis due to dialysis is associated with chains of β_2-microglobulin. No effective treatment as yet exists for this form of amyloidosis, and symptom relief governs the course of therapy.

VII. SUMMARY

Gastrointestinal complications are common in the dialysis patient. Lesions accounting for gastrointestinal bleeding is similar to that of the general population, but when they occur they are more usually more severe in the renal failure patient. Renal failure through as-yet-unidentified mechanisms probably predisposes to acute pancreatitis, which also takes a more severe course in the dialysis patient. Treatment of acute and chronic pancreatitis does not vary according to degree of preexisting renal impairment. Viral hepatitis, especially hepatitis C, is commonly encountered in dialysis centers, and ongoing studies will help determine the optimal course of therapy for these patients. Gastric emptying problems and GERD are common consequences of motility disturbances in the diabetic dialysis patient for which there are effective medical, endoscopic, and surgical therapies. Amyloid deposits in renal failure can have a myriad of presentations, for which no effective therapy exists except those offering symptom relief.

REFERENCES

1. Elta G. Approach to the patient with gross gastrointestinal bleeding. In: Yamada et al., eds. Textbook of Gastroenterology. Vol. 1. 2d ed. Philadelphia: Lippincott, 1995:671–698.
2. Posner, et al. Endoscopic findings in chronic hemodialysis patients with upper gastrointestinal bleeding. Am J Gastroenterol 1983; 78:720.
3. Alvarez L, Puleo, J, Balint JA, et al. Investigation of gastrointestinal bleeding in patients with end stage renal disease. Am J Gastroenterol 1993; 88:30–33.
4. Kang J. The gastrointestinal tract in uremia. Dig Dis Sci 1993; 38(2):257.
5. Wee A, Kang JY, Ho MS, Choong HL, Wu AYT, Sutherland IH. Gastroduodenal mucosa in uraemia: endoscopic and histological correlation and the prevalence of Helicobacter-like organisms. Gut 1990; 31:1093–1096.
6. Kang JY, Wu AYT, Sutherland IH, Vathsala A. Prevalence of peptic ulcer in patients undergoing maintenance hemodialysis. Dig Dis Sci 1988; 33:774.
7. Chalasani N, Cotsonis G, Wilcox CM. Upper gastrointestinal bleeding in patients with chronic renal failure: role of vascular ectasia. Am J Gastroenterol 1988; 91(11):2329–2332.
8. Tsai C-J, Hwang J-C. Investigation of upper gastrointestinal hemorrhage in chronic renal failure. J Clin Gastroenterol 1996; 22(1):2–5.
9. Zuckerman GR, Corbette GL, Clause RE, Harter HR. Upper gastrointestinal bleeding in patients with chronic renal failure. Ann Int Med 1985; 102:588.
10. NIH Consensus Conference. Helicobacter pylori in peptic ulcer disease. JAMA 1994; 272:65–69.
11. Tamura H, Tokushima H, Murakawa M, Matsumura O, Itoyama S, Sekine S, et al. Eradication of Helicobacter in patients with end-stage renal disease under dialysis treatment. Am J Kidney Dis 1997; 29:86–90.
12. Luzza F, Imeneo M, Maletta M, Mantelli I, Tancre D, Merando G, et al. Helicobacter pylori-specific IgG in

chronic haemodialysis patients: relationship of hypergastrinaemia to positive serology. Nephrol Dial Transpl 1996; 11:120–124.
13. Moustafa, et al. Helicobacter pylori and uremic gastritis: a histopathologic study and correlation with endoscopic and bacteriologic findings. Am J Nephrol 1997; 17:165–171.
14. Boley SJ, Sammarantano R, Adams A, DiBiase A, Kleinhaus S, Sprayregen S. On the nature and etiology of vascular ectasisas of the colon: degenerative lesions of aging. Gastro 1977; 72:650–660.
15. Scheff RT, Zuckerman G, Harter H, Delmez J, Kopehler R. Diverticular disease in patients with chronic renal failure due to polycystic kidney disease. Ann Intern Med 1980; 92:202.
16. Rosenblatt et al. Gastrointestinal blood loss in patients with chronic renal failure. Am J Kidney Dis 1982; 1: 232.
17. Akmal M, Sawelson S, Karubian F, Gadallah M. The prevalence and significance of occult blood loss in patients with predialysis advanced chronic renal failure (CRF), or receiving dialytic therapy. Clin Nephrol 1994; 42(3):198–202.
18. Rockey DC, Cello JP. Evaluation of the gastrointestinal tract in patients with iron-deficiency anemia. N Engl J Med 1993; 329(23):1691–1695.
19. Silverstein, et al. The National ASGE survey on upper gastrointestinal bleeding. ii. Clinical prognostic factors. Gastrointest Endosc 1981; 27:30–93.
20. Bronner MH, Pate MB, Cunningham JT, Marsh WH. Estrogen-progesterone therapy for bleeding gastrointestinal telangiectasias in chronic renal failure. Ann Int Med 1986; 105:371–374.
21. Van Cutsem E, Rutgeerts P, Vantrappen G. Treatment of bleeding gastrointestinal vascular malformations with oestrogen-progesterone. Lancet 1990; 335:953–955.
22. Sloand JA, Schiff MJ. Beneficial effect of low-dose transdermal estrogen on bleeding time and clinical bleeding in uremia. Am J Kidney Dis 1995; 26:22–26.
23. Andersen MR, Aaseby J. Somatostatin in the treatment of gastrointestinal bleeding caused by angiodysplasia. Scand J Gastroenterol 1996; 31:1037–1039.
24. Vaziri, et al. Pancreatic enzymes in patients with end-stage renal disease maintained on hemodialysis. Am J Gastroenterol 1988; 83:410–412.
25. Pitchumoni CS, Arguello P, Agarwal N, Yoo J. Acute pancreatitis in chronic renal failure. Am J Gastroenterol 1996; 91(12):2477–2482.
26. Lee SP, Nicholls JH, Park HZ. Biliary sludge as a cause of acute pancreatitis. N Engl J Med 1992; 326:589–593.
27. Vaziri ND, Chang D, Malekpour A, Radaht S. Pancreatic pathology in chronic dialysis patients: an autopsy study of 78 cases. Nephron 1987; 46:347–349.
28. Joglar FM, Saade M. Outcome of pancreatitis in CAPD and HD patients. Peritoneal Dial Int 1995; 15:264–266.
29. Pahl MV, Vaziri MD, Dure-Smith B, Miller R, Mirahmadi MK. Hepatobiliary pathology in hemodialysis patients: an autopsy study of 78 cases. Am J Gastroenterol 1986; 81:783.
30. Pol S, Thiers V, Carnot F, Zins B, Romeo R, bethelot P and Brechot C. Effectiveness and tolerance of interferon-alpha 2b in the treatment of chronic hepatitis C in haemodialysis patients. Nephrol Dial Transpl 11(suppl 4):58–61.
31. Kao, et al. Delayed gastric emptying in patients with chronic renal failure. Nuclear Med Commun 1996; 17: 164–167.
32. Dumitrascu DL, Barnert J, Kischner T, Weinbeck M. Antral emptying of semisolid meal measured by real-time ultrasonography in chronic renal failure. Dig Dis Sci 1995; 40:636–644.
33. Soffer, et al. Gastric emptying in chronic renal failure patients on haemodialysis. J Clin Gastroenterol 1987; 9:651–653.
34. Brown-Cartwright, et al. Gastric emptying of an indigestible solid in patients with end-stage renal disease on continuous ambulatory peritoneal dialysis. Gastro 1988; 95:46–51.
35. Schwartz A, Keller F, Seyfert S, Poll W, Molzahn M, Distler A. Carpal tunnel syndrome: a major complication in long term hemodialysis patients. Clin Nephrol 1984; 22:133–137.
36. Araki H, Muramaoto H, Oda K, Koni I, Mabuchi H, Mizukami Y, et al. Severe gastrointestinal complications of dialysis-related amyloidosis in two patients on long-term hemodialysis. Am J Nephrol 1996; 16:149–153.
37. Ikegaya N, Kobayashi S, Hishida A, Kaneko E, Furushashi M, Murayama Y. Colonic dilatation due to dialysis-related amyloidosis. Am J Kidney Dis 1995; 25: 807–809.

34

Ocular Complications in Dialysis Patients

Jean-Jacques De Laey and Bart Lafaut
University Hospital of Gent, Gent, Belgium

Anita Leys
University Hospital St.-Rafaël, Leuven, Belgium

A number of ocular problems associated with renal failure may persist in patients under hemodialysis. It is thus difficult to discuss complications related to hemodialysis independently from those caused by the underlying renal problem. Most of these complications will also be found in patients who underwent renal transplantation, although in this group specific ocular problems may result from iatrogenic immunosuppression.

I. CONJUNCTIVA AND CORNEA

Hemodialysis patients may present with an inflamed pingueculum. A pingueculum is an elastic degeneration of interpalpebral connective tissue and is considered in patients with chronic renal failure as an accelerated age-related change associated with exposure (1). Such a pingueculitis is not to be distinguished clinically from pinguecular inflammation unassociated with renal failure.

The "red eye" of renal failure is relatively rare but characteristic. It presents as a diffuse waxy red episcleral and conjunctival hyperemia, which extends beyond the palpebral fissure and is not associated with exudates. The inflammatory reaction causes mild to moderate pain and irritation. It appears to be related to a high serum calcium concentration and subsides once the calcium concentration normalizes (2).

Corneal calcifications and, even more frequently, conjunctival calcifications are common complications in patients with chronic renal failure. Most patients on regular dialysis show limboconjunctival calcification, which is due to raised serum calcium and phosphate levels. Limbal calcification in renal failure may resemble or even be undistinguishable from Vogt's white limbus girdle, a relatively common, supposedly age-related change (Fig. 1). The severity of the calcification correlates with the duration of renal failure (3). The corneal calcification may spread towards the center of the cornea. It is typically situated in the middle third, corresponding to the palpebral fissure, and may eventually interfere with vision (band-shaped keratopathy) (Figs. 2 and 3). The corneal calcification may flake off, causing extremely painful corneal erosions. If the band-shaped keratopathy interferes with vision or is painful, it can be removed with application of ethylene diamine tetraacetic acid (EDTA) on the desepithelialized cornea.

Painful cornea erosions, not necessarily associated with band keratopathy, occur more frequently in patients with Alport's disease or with diabetes mellitus, two conditions known to be associated with a fragile corneal epithelium.

II. INTRAOCULAR PRESSURE

Earlier reports mention an average transient intraocular pressure rise of 5.9 (4) to 8.1 mmHg (5) during hemodialysis. Urea has been extensively used as an oc-

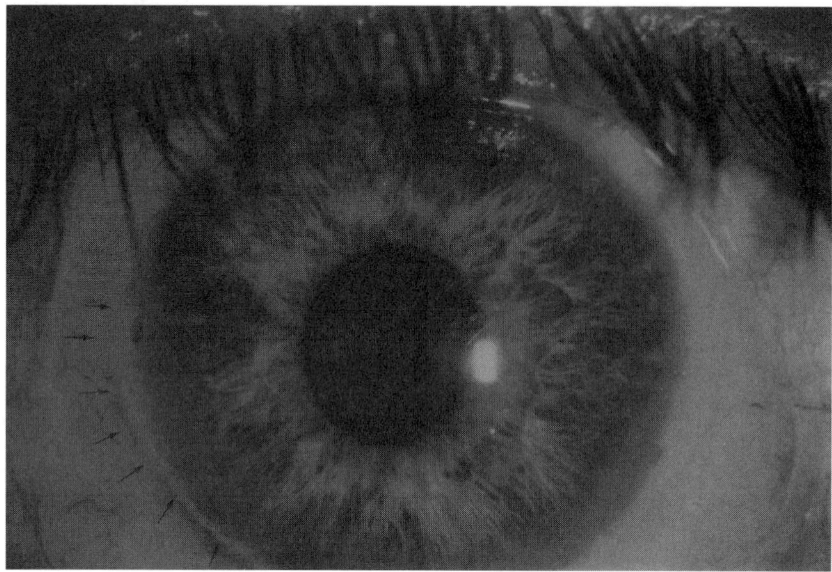

Fig. 1 Corneal calcification at the lumbus (Vogt's white limbus girdle).

ular hypotensive agent in the acute treatment of closed angle glaucoma, because of its established osmotic ocular gradient (6). A delayed transport of urea across the blood-aqueous barrier has been demonstrated (7). Rapid removal of urea from the plasma by hemodialysis will thus not significantly lower the concentration of urea in the aqueous. A rise in intraocular pressure could thus result from the osmotic movement of water from the plasma into the aqueous (4). This effect of a decrease in blood urea on the intraocular pressure as a result of a change in osmolarity can be counteracted by adding glucose to the dialysate or by combining hemodialysis with ultrafiltration (8).

Acute glaucoma is a rare complication of hemodialysis (8). Prevention of glaucoma includes control of intraocular pressure of patients who start long-term hemodialysis. Patients at risk should be closely followed with repeated visual field testing and optic disc evalu-

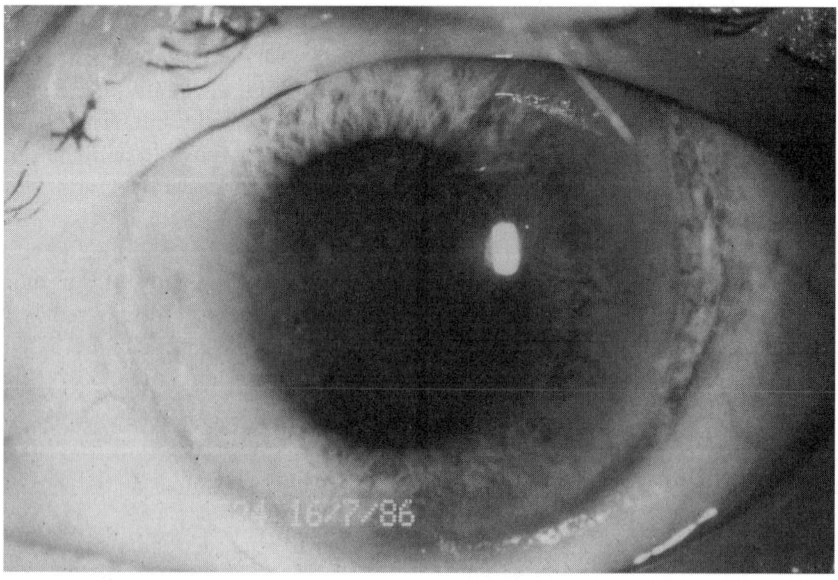

Fig. 2 Corneal and perilimbal corneal calcification in renal failure.

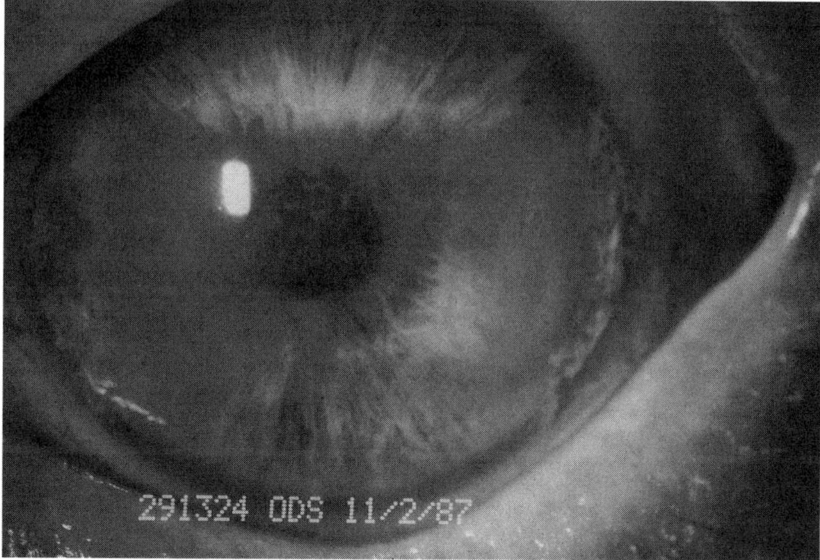

Fig. 3 Band-shaped keratopathy. (Same eye as Fig. 2, 7 months later.)

ation as well as tonometry and receive, if necessary, a medical treatment if the eye pressure fluctuates too much.

III. LENS

In her monograph on the ocular complications of hemodialysis and kidney transplantation, Polak (8) mentions the observation by Avello in 1963 of a reversible cataract in a 17-year-old dialysis patient and the occurrence of an irreversible cataract during dialysis reported by Abrams in 1966. In 37 dialysis patients, Polak noted only three patients with coronary cataract unrelated to the treatment and three with incipient cataract presumably caused by the corticosteroid treatment. However, other authors suspect a possible causal relationship between rapidly progressive cataracts and hemodialysis (9–11).

IV. RETINA AND OPTIC PATHWAYS

There are a number of oculorenal syndromes leading to renal failure and presenting with fundus lesions, such as familial nephronophthisis (Senior-Loken syndrome), cystinosis, primary hyperoxaluria, Zellweger syndrome, Alport's syndrome, or membranoproliferative glomerulonephritis. The fundus lesions will progress independently of the renal condition.

The microangiopathy of diabetes mellitus mainly affects retina and kidney. In patients with diabetic nephropathy, retinopathy is always present and proliferative retinopathy is common. Retinopathy tends to deteriorate as renal failure develops, particularly in patients with poorly controlled blood pressure and in patients in whom no retinal treatment has been given before the renal failure. Treatment of the hypertension and of end-stage renal failure, on the other hand, may have a favorable influence on diabetic retinopathy, particularly on macular edema (12).

Hemodialysis patients with proliferative diabetic retinopathy present an increased risk of bleeding because of the intermittent heparinization needed for hemodialysis. This may be, for some nephrologists, an additional argument to opt for peritoneal dialysis. In the presence of proliferative diabetic retinopathy, panretinal photocoagulation is mandatory. Once the new vessels have regressed, the risk of bleeding is reduced. If, however, because of persisting vitreous hemorrhage panretinal photocoagulation can only be partially performed or is even not possible, vitrectomy associated with endophotocoagulation during the surgery has to be considered. The results are usually favorable if the diabetic retinopathy is not complicated by a traction retinal detachment and an extinction of the retinopathy can be obtained. The choice of peritoneal dialysis or hemodialysis should thus not so much be influenced by the condition of the eye, but be decided by the nephrologist taking into account the respective advantages or disadvantages of the two dialysis modalities.

Renal failure and dialysis preferably affect the vascular system of the patient (13). Patients under main-

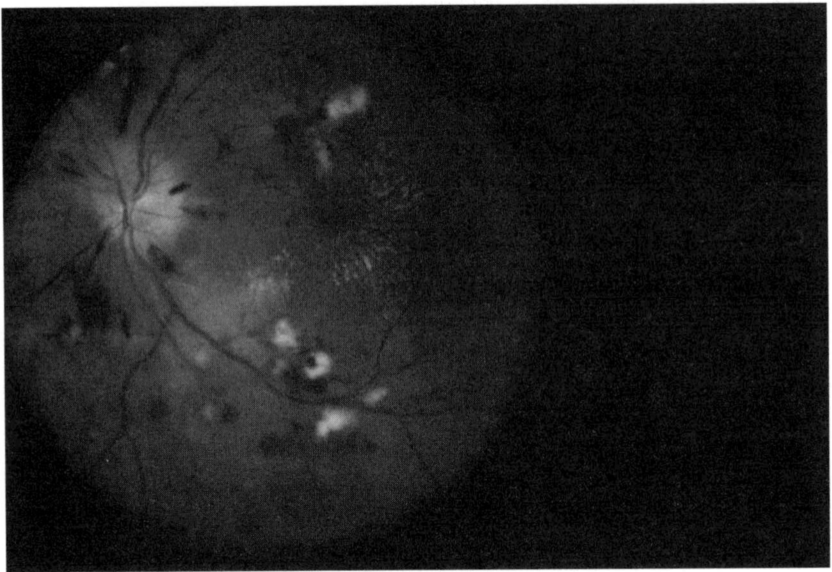

Fig. 4 Hypertensive retinopathy with flame-shaped hemorrhages, cotton-wool exudates, and a macular star of lipoid exudates.

tenance hemodialysis have an increased mortality rate as a consequence of hyperlipidemia and hypertension. In general it is thought that lipid abnormalities of patients with chronic renal failure are insufficiently influenced by dialysis.

The retinal signs of malignant arterial hypertension are retinal edema, hard exudates, cotton wool spots, flame-shaped hemorrhages, and papil edema (Fig. 4). The manifestations of hypertensive retinopathy regress when the arterial hypertension is controlled. Careful ophthalmoscopy or fluorescein angiography may, however, reveal permanent scarring of the retinal vasculature with areas of capillary dropout and vascular remodeling (14).

Accelerated hypertension may provoke localized serous detachment of the retina (15,16) (Fig. 5). This is a possible complication of toxemia of pregnancy and is due to hypertensive choroidopathy. Fluorescein angiography shows a considerable reduction in choroidal flow. This in turn causes retinal pigment dysfunction.

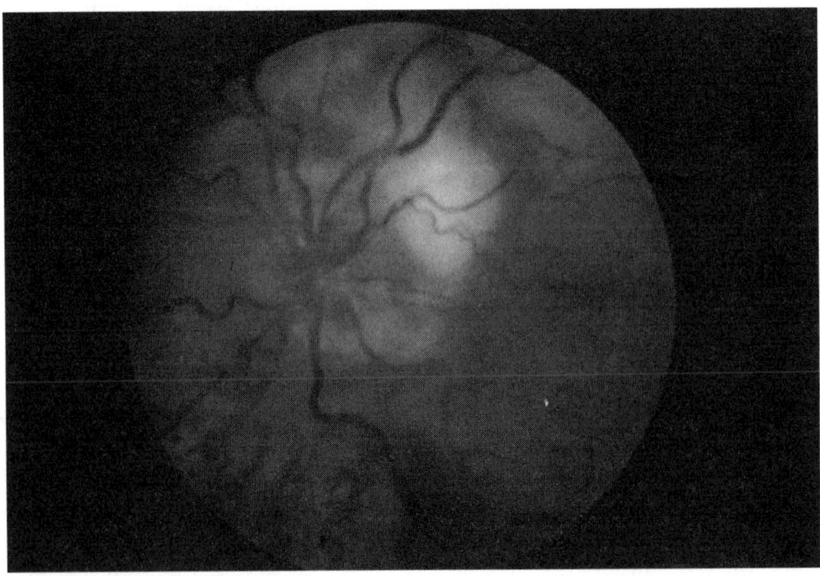

Fig. 5 Hypertensive chorioretinopathy with localized serous detachment of the retina and subretinal hemorrhages.

The normalization of the arterial tension will result in a reperfusion of the choriocapillaris, followed by resolution of the detachment. The involvement of the retinal pigment epithelium eventually leads to localized or more diffuse pigment changes (16). This sometimes takes the form of a small area of hyperpigmentation surrounded by depigmentation (Elschnig's spot), choroidal vascular opacification (Siegrist's line), or more widespread pigmentary changes.

Gass described two female patients with bullous retinal detachment and multiple retinal pigment epithelial detachments while under hemodialysis (18). Neither patient presented evidence of uncontrolled hypertension or disorders associated with disseminated intravascular coagulopathy, which are also known causes of choroidal ischemia and exudative retinal detachment. Fluorescein angiography showed multiple detachments of the retinal pigment epithelium. The detachment in the left eye of the first patient was considered to be rhegmatogenous, although no retinal hole was found. It underwent an unsuccessful scleral buckling procedure. The left, blind eye of the second patient was enucleated for suspicion of malignant melanoma. Histopathology revealed a funnel-shaped retinal detachment, proteinaceous subretinal fluid, and a necrotizing granulomatous anterior scleritis and cyclitis consistent with the diagnosis of uveal effusion. The findings in these two patients resemble those found in healthy, middle-aged men with severe idiopathic central serous chorioretinopathy. A similar condition was also observed following renal or cardiac transplantation, and psychological stress could play a key role as a precipitating factor (19). Such cases may respond to laser treatment of the areas of pigment epithelial detachment.

The majority of hemodialysis patients, if not all, present obvious retinal signs of arteriosclerosis, such as abnormal arteriovenous crossings with venous compression, copper wire, and silver wire appearance of the arterioles (8). They thus present an increased risk of retinal arterial or venous occlusions leading to visual loss. Pratt and de Venecia observed a unilateral central retinal vein occlusion, which occurred within 72 hours of peritoneal dialysis, followed by the administration of one unit packed cells and one unit of whole blood. They suggest that the hemoconcentration due to blood transfusion and rapid weight loss in a patient with preexisting arteriosclerotic changes in the central retinal vessels may have precipitated the vascular occlusion (20). A sudden arterial hypotension related to the reduction of intravascular volume may precipitate retinal arterial occlusions, acute ischemic optic neuropathy, or cerebrovascular accidents associated with visual field loss. Such events are illustrated in the following case history.

Case 1

A 63-year-old man had a sudden decrease of vision in his left eye. His medical history showed arterial hypertension, end-stage renal disease, and cardiopathy. His renal problems included chronic interstitial nephritis due to abuse of analgesics and an invasive papilloma. Hemodialysis was started at age 61, and in the same period a pacemaker was inserted. Several surgical interventions were required for the papilloma (nephroureterectomy and cysto-prostato-urethrectomy). Two months before his ocular problems were noticed, a cerebrovascular accident occurred, with aphasia and paresis of the right arm. Initial eye examination revealed in his left eye a branch retinal vein occlusion with dense hemorrhages and several cotton-wool spots in the superotemporal field of the posterior pole (Fig. 6). In the noninvolved area of the left fundus and in the right fundus, retinal arteries were narrow and sclerotic. During further follow-up, intraretinal hemorrhages and cotton-wool spots slowly resorbed in the area of branch occlusion and visual acuity returned to 0.2. However, neovascularization developed on the optic nerve head and a vitreous hemorrhage occurred (Fig. 7), which required laser treatment.

Retinal hemorrhages are frequently found (20) but are mostly asymptomatic. They are usually scattered, small, and found at the posterior pole or in the midperiphery (21). They may be an expression of associated diabetic retinopathy or of a uremic toxic of heparin-conditioned tendency to bleeding (22).

Purtscher's retinopathy is a vaso-occlusive process affecting the retinal arterioles in the posterior pole, characterized by scattered infarctions of the retinal nerve fiber layers, superficial flame-shaped hemorrhages, and edema, resulting in sudden visual loss. This condition is classically associated with a severe head or chest trauma. A similar fundus aspect, sometimes referred to as Purtscher's-like retinopathy, has been reported in acute pancreatitis, auto-immune disorders, amniotic fluid embolism, or even retrobulbar anesthesia. A Purtscher's-like retinopathy was also observed in three young women with chronic retinal failure, one of whom was undergoing dialysis (23). The condition was bilateral in two and unilateral in one patient. Based on the fluoroangiographic characteristics, an embolization is most likely, although its cause is still unclear.

Uremic optic neuropathy refers to visual loss, possibly up to no light perception, in a matter of weeks,

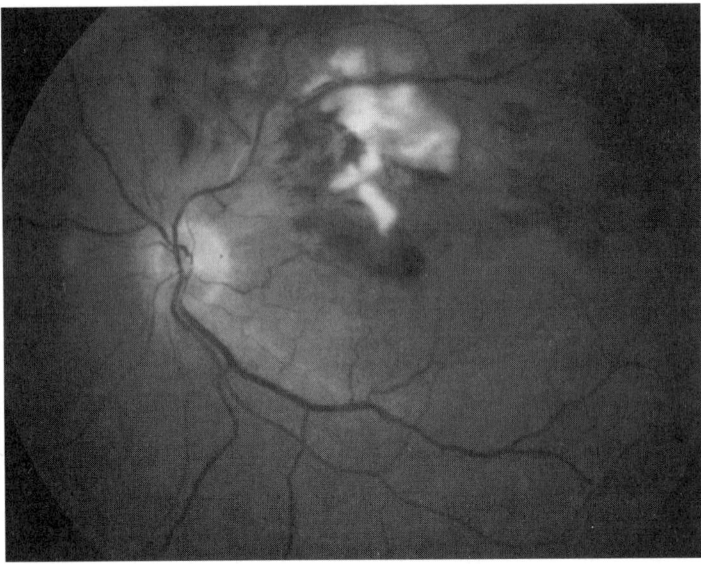

Fig. 6 Branch retinal vein occlusion in a 63-year-old patient with arterial hypertension, renal disease, and cardiopathy.

with sluggish or absent pupil reactions, optic disc swelling, and visual field loss. Hypertension alone cannot explain the findings. Anemia and especially uremia (blood urea nitrogen levels >35.7 mmol/L or 100 mg/dL) may be important in its etiology (24). Uremic encephalopathy with brain edema may cause cortical blindness (uremic amaurosis) (25).

One patient described by Hilton et al. (21) required placement of a shunt to treat hydrocephalus of undetermined cause. This resulted in regression of papil edema. The pathogenesis of intracranial hypertension in uremia is unknown, but it could be related to alterations of the blood-brain barrier. Knox et al. recommend prompt dialysis and periocular steroid treatment to reverse the visual loss from uremic optic neuropathy (24).

Hamed et al. (26) examined three patients who developed optic neuropathy while undergoing chronic hemodialysis. The first patient recovered completely after

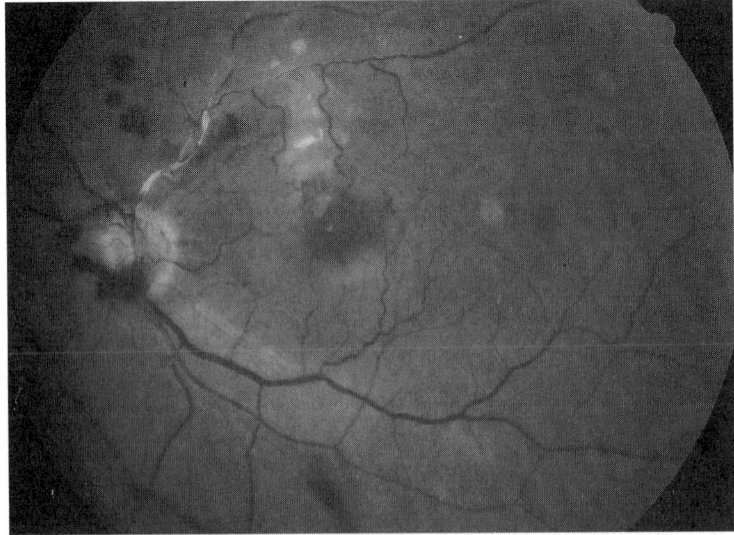

Fig. 7 Branch retinal vein occlusion with neovascularization at the optic disc (same patient as Fig. 6).

discontinuing desferroxamine chelation therapy, which had been started 2 months earlier to reduce increased serum aluminum levels (2 g after each hemodialysis session). In the second patient bilateral visual loss was associated with chronic papil edema due to an atypically severe anterior ischemic optic neuropathy. The latter two patients showed little improvement with high-dose intravenous methylprednisolone therapy combined with more vigorous hemodialysis, better blood pressure control, and blood transfusions.

Long-term desferroxamine treatment for iron or aluminum overload may cause an acute retrobulbar optic neuropathy evidenced by sudden visual loss, color vision disturbances, and visual field defects (27). In the majority of the reported cases, the visual loss is reversible. The drug is also toxic for the retinal pigment epithelium.

Rahi et al. (28) documented light and electron microscopic changes in the retinal pigment epithelium following treatment with high-dose desferroxamine for systemic iron overload. Iron deposits were found in the nonpigmented ciliary epithelium, the ciliary muscle, stromal cells of the choroid, the sclera, and the peripheral retina and occasionally in the photoreceptor layer or in the retinal pigment epithelium. The latter showed patchy depigmentation and degeneration. Clinically the presumed desferroxamine retinal pigment epitheliopathy is characterized by pigment mottling in the posterior pole and in the periphery, progressing to geographic macular atrophy, with abnormal electroretinography (ERG) and electro-oculography (EOG) (27,29) (Fig. 8). However, Mathys et al. (30), who followed 14 dialysis patients under desferroxamine treatment, noted only two patients with subnormal ERG and three with a subnormal EOG. In contrast, with desferroxamine optic neuropathy, which is usually reversible, the retinopathy may progress despite the discontinuation of the drug. Desferroxamine is not necessarily always responsible for the retinal degeneration in dialysis patients, and the direct role of chronic iron overload may not be disregarded.

De Doncker et al. (31) followed a 30-year-old patient with renal failure due to glomerulonephritis and treated with chronic hemodialysis. This patient already presented peripheral and macular pigmentary changes, progressing to choriocapillaris atrophy before desferroxamine was given. They also examined 10 pediatric cases with secondary hemosiderosis. Nine of them were under dialysis and only 5 were treated with desferroxamine. Eight patients (four with desferroxamine, four not treated with desferroxamine) showed pigmentary changes.

The difficulty of diagnosing desferroxamine toxicity is illustrated by the following case histories.

Case 2

A 48-year-old man complained of blurred vision and night blindness. He had been diagnosed with acute glomerulonephritis at the age of 12 years. His medical history revealed chronic glomerulonephritis and arterial hypertension, end-stage renal disease at age 28, repeated rejection of kidney transplants, chronic hemodialysis for nearly 20 years, renal osteodystrophy, and chronic iron overload, treated for several months with desferroxamine. An ophthalmic examination showed slightly decreased visual acuity and keratopathy with prominent limbal degeneration and calcium precipitates nasally and temporally in the interpalpebral area of both eyes. There were also a few opacities located centrally in the cornea. Bilateral fundus changes were noted with pale optic discs, narrow retinal arteries, and pronounced changes of the retinal pigment epithelium with drusen and atrophic changes (Fig. 9). Study of the record revealed that the macular and peripheral drusen and pigmentary changes existed several years before the short-term treatment with desferroxamine was started. A presumed diagnosis of membranoproliferative glomerulonephritis type 2–associated ocular changes was made, although no biopsy was available to prove the underlying renal disease. During the following months a decrease of vision and increase of keratopathy were noted, with multiple small whitish opacities and mild band-shaped keratopathy, which further progressed to dense calcified plaques and blindness. Several treatments of the keratopathy with calcium-chelating agents resulted in only short-term improvement of his vision. In addition, both eyes were painful, with signs of dry eye and with several particularly painful events of cornea erosion.

Case 3

A 62-year-old female hemodialysis patient with chronic renal failure due to phenacetin abuse complained of progressive visual loss. She was seen for the first time in April 1991. Her vision was 8/10 in the right eye and 6/10 in the left eye. She presented discrete subcapsularis posterior lens opacities, probably related to chronic corticosteroid treatment. Fundus examination revealed perifoveal pigmentary changes in both eyes, associated with some choriocapillaris atrophy in the left eye (Fig. 10a). Desferroxamine treatment was started in November 1991. In December 1991, the vision in

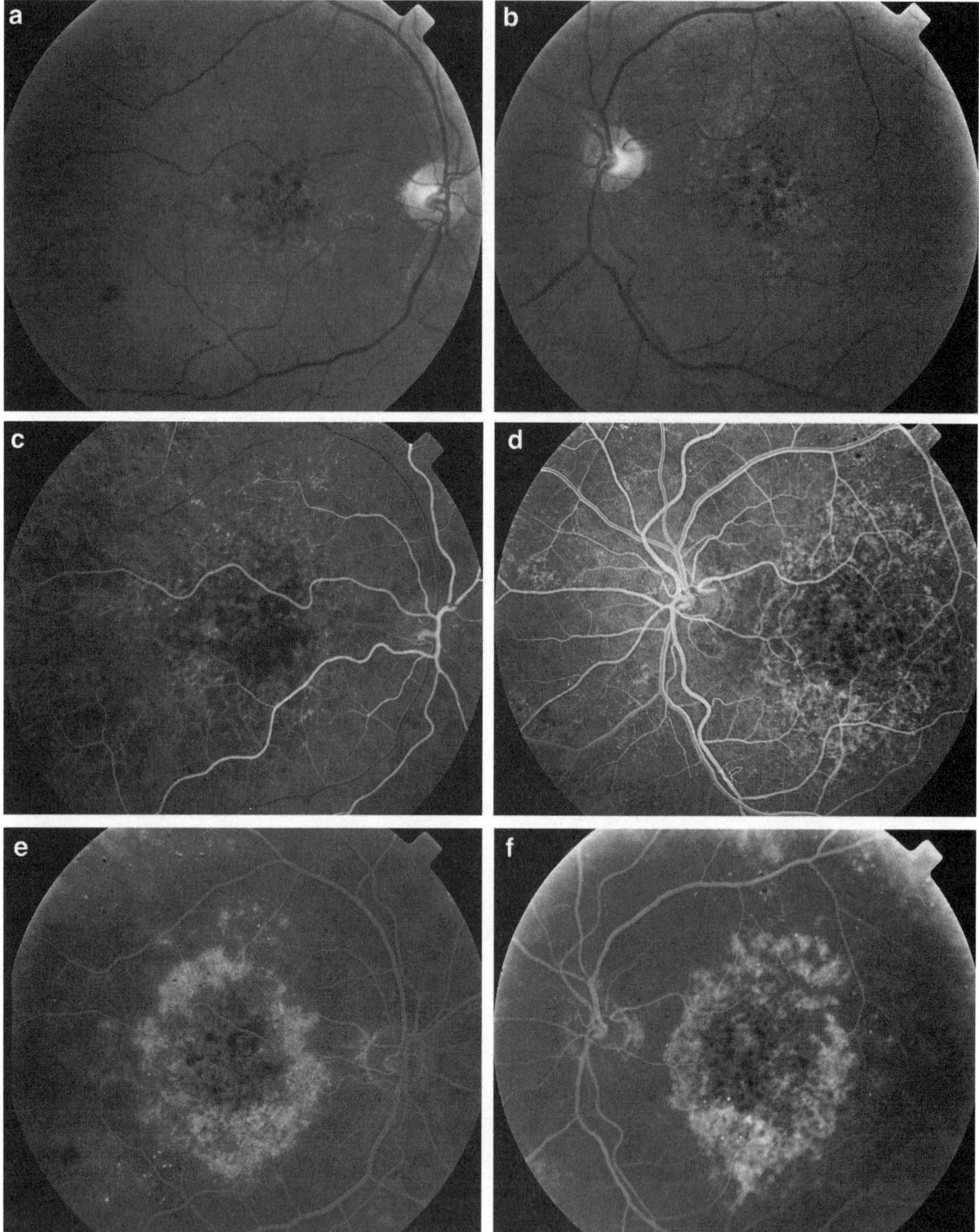

Fig. 8 Red free (a and b) and fluorescein angiographic (c, d, e, and f) aspects of desferroxamine retinal pigment epitheliopathy. Marked pigment epithelial changes. The photopic ERG was subnormal. The EOG was pathological with a light-to-dark ratio of 133% in the right eye and 128% in the left eye.

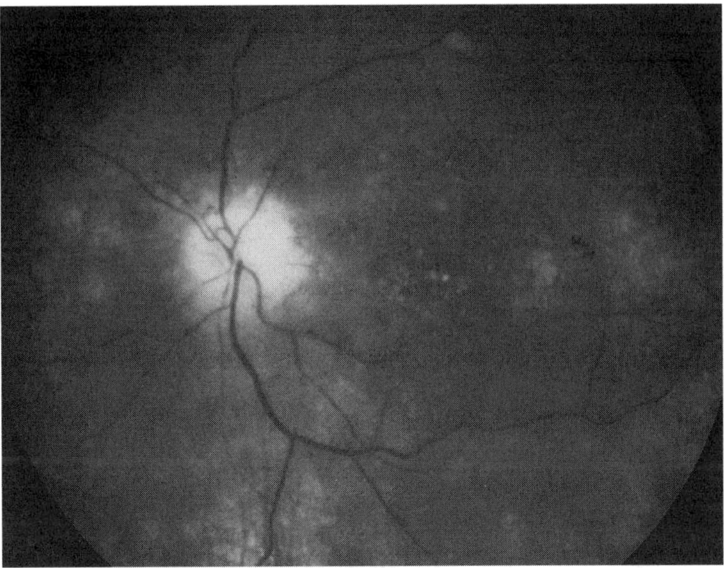

Fig. 9 Macular pigment epithelial atrophy, drusen of Bruch's membrane, and pole optic disc in a 48-year-old patient with end-stage renal disease—presumed diagnosis of membrane proliferative glomerulonephritis type 2.

the right eye was still 8/10 but was decreased to 1/10 in the left eye. The lesion in the left eye has progressed to a one-disc-diameter large area of well-delineated choroidal atrophy (Fig. 10b). In January 1992, the vision of the right eye had diminished to 2/10. The ERG was normal but the EOG was slightly subnormal with a light:dark ratio of 159% in the right eye and 163% in the left eye. Desferroxamine treatment was discontinued in May 1992. Two years later, the vision was 1/10 in both eyes and both macular regions presented a 1.5 disc diameter large area of choriocapillaris atrophy (Fig. 10c).

These two cases showed pigmentary fundus lesions and vision loss before desferroxamine treatment was initiated. They could be considered as related to membranoproliferative glomerulonephritis in the first and to age-related changes in the second patient. Desferroxamine may have precipitated macular changes in an already compromised fundus. Also the direct deleterious role of iron overload should not be overlooked.

As long as the exact effect of desferroxamine on the retinal pigment epithelium is not known, this chelating drug should be used with caution, especially in patients already presenting pigmentary changes in the fundus. Patients under desferroxamine should be screened regularly with fluorescein angiography to permit the detection of early pigmentary changes.

V. ORBIT

Two orbital problems have been associated with renal failure and dialysis: brown tumors of the orbit and mucormycosis. Brown tumors are focal bony lesions due to hyperparathyroidism resulting from the direct effects of parathyroid hormone on bone. They are not uncommon in primary hyperparathyroidism. They are less frequent in secondary hyperparathyroidism, associated with chronic renal failure, and rarely involve orbital bones. Brown tumors of the orbit present as fibrous and giant-cell proliferation in a hemorrhagic stroma with osseous metaplasia and may cause visual loss, proptosis, diplopia, ocular motility problems, and nasal obstruction (32).

Mycormycosis is an infection caused by fungi of the class Zygomycetes order Mucorales. Several cases of mucormycosis of orbit or of nasal and paranasal cavities have been reported in dialysis patients treated with desferroxamine for either iron or aluminum overload (33). This is an acute and life-threatening infection. The orbital disease not only causes intraocular complications such as retinal ischemia and panophthalmitis, but may invade posteriorly into the intracranial cavity (34).

Boelaert et al. (35) have suggested that mucormycosis in desferroxamine-treated patients is mediated by the siderophore activity of the drug. Mainly hemodi-

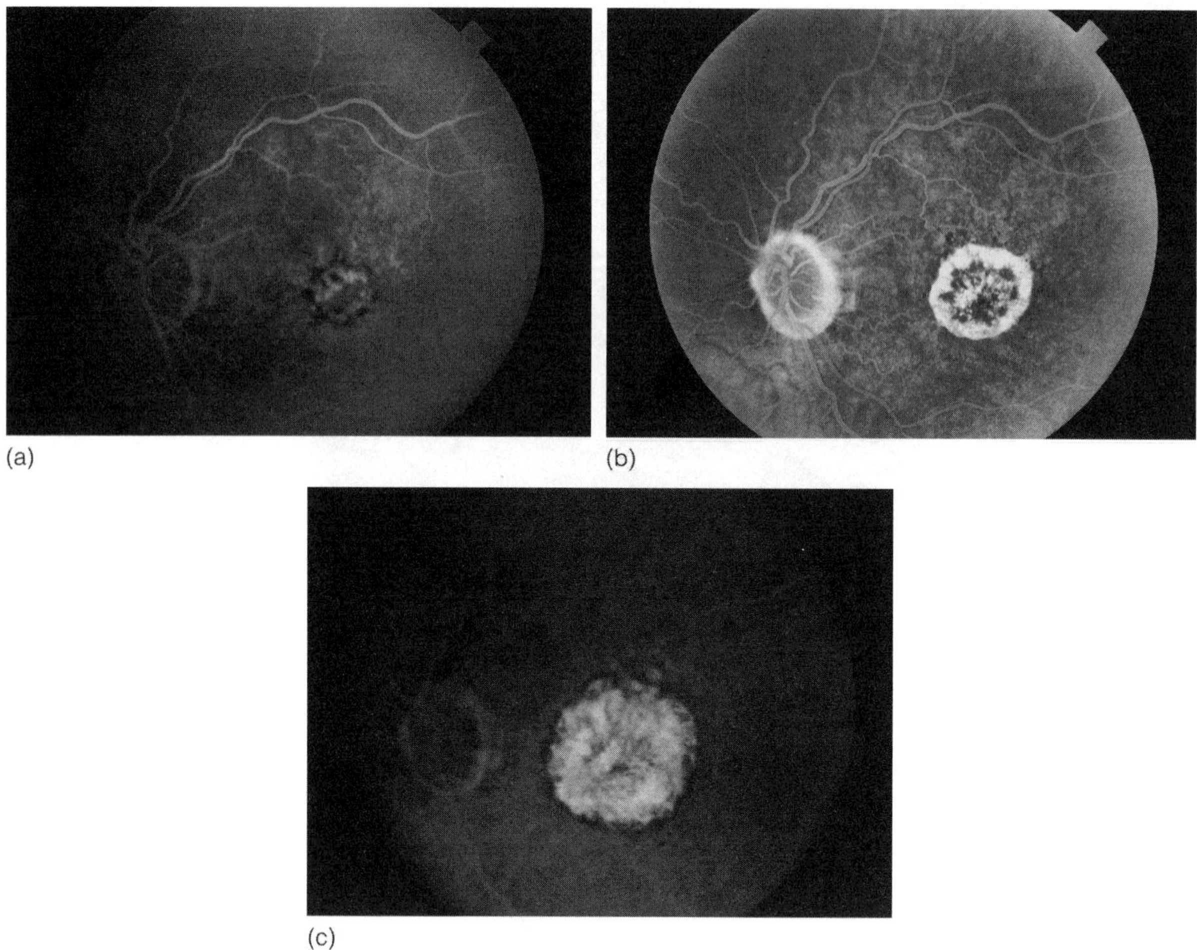

Fig. 10 Fluorescein angiography of the macular region of the left eye of a 62-year-old hemodialysis patient: (1) April 1991, (b) December 1991, (c) May 1992.

alysis patients treated with desferroxamine have been reported to develop mucormycosis. It is only exceptionally seen in patients with normal renal function. Other risk factors are diabetic or metabolic ketoacidosis and immunosuppression.

VI. CONCLUSION

Hemodialysis may be associated with a number of ocular problems, some of which are related to the preexisting cause of renal failure, others to the associated vascular lesions. In order to evaluate the actual importance and frequency of ocular complications in dialysis patients, the records of two large hemodialysis centers (Algemeen Ziekenhuis Sint-Jozef, Leuven, and Universitair Ziekenhuis Leuven, Belgium) were retrospectively studied.

The most frequent ocular complications were pain, subconjunctival hemorrhages, and visual loss due to vascular accidents or diabetic retinopathy. Mild pain and irritation were usually caused by dry eyes with markedly decreased tear flow. Dialysis patients with a typical "red eye" complained of more pronounced pain. The most severe pain was experienced with cornea erosions due either to a fragile corneal epithelium (more frequently in patients with Alport's disease or diabetes mellitus) or to severe band-shaped keratopathy.

Spontaneous subconjunctival hemorrhages or even larger hematomas after minor trauma spontaneously regressed and were usually not associated with visual loss. Visual loss usually occurred in patients with vascular lesions of the retina, the optic nerve head, or the visual pathways. Several types of vascular lesions were observed:

1. Cerebrovascular accidents, frequently associated with a homonymous visual field loss or with central scotomas due to occipital lesions
2. Ischemic eye due to carotid artery occlusion
3. Anterior ischemic optic neuropathy resulting from an infarction of the optic nerve head
4. Central retinal vascular occlusions either arterial of venous
5. Diabetic retinopathy

Less frequent complications are, however, not less sight-threatening. This is the case for choroidal ischemia, serous retinal detachment, or optic neuropathy either related to uremia or desferroxamine treatment. The potential retinal toxicity of desferroxamine means that nephrologists must use this substance with caution, especially in patients already presenting pigmentary changes, although the causal relationship between desferroxamine and retinal pigmentary changes is not absolutely clear. Finally, mucormycosis is a potentially life-threatening condition that can occur in hemodialysis patients, and it should be rapidly recognized by the ophthalmologist.

In general, we recommend that a dialysis patient without particular ocular symptoms be evaluated twice a year by an experienced ophtalmologist.

ACKNOWLEDGMENTS

Dr. D. van Caesbrouck, Algemeen Ziekenhuis, Sint-Joseph Instituut, Turnhout, Belgium, was extremely helpful in the retrospective analysis of the ocular complications in the dialysis patients under his care. Dr. A. de Wachter, Department of Ophthalmology, Algemeen Ziekenhuis Sint-Jan, Brugge, Belgium, provided Fig. 8.

REFERENCES

1. Ehlers N, Krusehansen F, Hansen ME, Jensen OA. Corneoconjunctival changes in uremia; influence of renal allotransplantation. Acta Ophthalmol 1972; 50:83–94.
2. Klaassen-Broekema N, van Bijsterveld OP. Red eyes in renal failure. Br J Ophthalmol 1992; 76:268–271.
3. Porter R, Crombie AL. Corneal and conjunctival calcification in chronic renal failure. Br J Ophthalmol 1973; 57:339–343.
4. Sitprija V, Holmes JH, Ellis PP. Intraocular pressure changes during artificial kidney therapy. Arch Ophthalmol 1964; 72:626–631.
5. Watson AG, Greenwood WR. Studies on the intraocular pressure during hemodialysis. Can J Ophthalmol 1966; 1:301–307.
6. Galin MA, Davidson R, Pasmanik S. An osmotic comparison of urea and mannitol. Am J Ophthalmol 1963; 55:244–247.
7. Galin MA, Davidson R, Pasmanik S. Aqueous and blood urea nitrogen levels after intravenous urea administration. Arch Ophthalmol 1961; 65:805–807.
8. Polak BCP. Ophthalmological complications of haemodialysis and kidney transplantation. Doc Ophthalmol 1980; 49:1–96.
9. Straub W, Freund J. Katarakt nach extrakorporaler Dialysebehandlung? Klin Mbl Augenheilk 1970; 157:51–52.
10. Laqua H. Katarakt bei chronischer Nierinsuffizienz und Dialysebehandlung. Klin Mbl Augenheilk 1972; 160: 346–350.
11. Koch JR, Siedek M, Weikenmeier P, Metzler U. Katarakt bei intermittierender Hämodialyse. Klin Mbl Augenheilk 1976; 168:346–353. Leys AM. The eye and renal disease. In: Tasman W, Jaeger EA, eds. Duane's clinical ophthalmology, Philadelphia, Publisher Lippincott-Raven, 1997, Vol. 5, Ch. 37.
12. Bell DSH. Diabetic nephropathy: changing concepts of pathogenesis and treatment. Am J Med Sci 1991; 301: 195–200.
13. Lazarus JM, Denker BM, Owen WF. Organ system abnormalities in hemodialysis. In: Brenner BM, ed. The Kidney. Philadelphia: W.B. Saunders, 1991:2451–2472.
14. Lafaut BA, De Vriese ASP, Stulting AA. Fundus fluorescein angiography of patients with severe hypertensive nephropathy. Graefe's Arch Clin Exp Ophthalmol 1997; 235:749–754.
15. de Venecia G, Jampol LM. The eye in accelerated hypertension. Localized serous detachments of the retina in patients. Arch Ophthalmol 1984; 102:68–73.
16. Gaudric A, Coscas G, Bird AC. Choroidal ischemia. Am J Ophthalmol 1982; 94:489–498.
17. De Laey JJ. Fluorescein angiography of the choroid in health and disease. Int Ophthalmol 1983; 6:125–138.
18. Gass JDM. Bullous retinal detachment and multiple retinal pigment epithelial detachments in patients receiving hemodialysis. Graefe's Arch Clin Exp Ophthalmol 1992; 230:454–458.
19. Friberg TR, Eller AW. Serous detachment resembling central serous chorioretinopathy following organ transplantation. Graefe's Arch Clin Exp Ophthalmol 1990; 228:305–309.
20. Pratt MV, de Venecia G. Central retinal vein occlusion following peritoneal dialysis. Am J Ophthalmol 1970; 70:337–340.
21. Hilton AF, Harrison JD, Lamb AM, Petrie JJB, Hardie I. Ocular complications in haemodialysis and renal transplant patients. Am J Ophthalmol 1976; 2:114–116.
22. Pambor R, Pap I. Netzhautveränderungen unter der Hämodialysis. Folia Ophthalmol 1976; 2:114–116.
23. Stoumbos VD, Klein ML, Goodman S. Purtscher's-like

retinopathy in chronic renal failure. Ophthalmology 1992; 99:1833–1839.

24. Knox DL, Hanneken AM, Hollows FC, Miller NR, Schick HL, Gonzales WL. Uremic optic neuropathy. Arch Ophthalmol 1988; 106:50–54.
25. Walsh FB, Brown AB. Bilateral blindness of sudden onset. Trans Ophthalmol Soc Austr 1963; 23:13–27.
26. Hamed LM, Winward KE, Glaser JS, Schatz NJ. Optic neuropathy in uremia. Am J Ophthalmol 1989; 1098: 30–35.
27. Lakhanpal V, Schocket SS, Jiji R. Desferroxamine (Desferral) induced toxic retinal pigmentary degeneration and presumed optic neuropathy. Ophthalmology 1984; 91:443–451.
28. Rahi AHS, Hungerford JL, Ahmed AI. Ocular toxicity of desferroxamine: light microscopic histochemical and ultrastructural findings. Br J Ophthalmol 1986; 70:373–381.
29. Arden GB, Wonke B, Kennedy C, Muehms ER. Ocular changes in patients undergoing long-term desferroxamine treatment. Br J Ophthalmol 1984; 68:873–877.
30. Mathys B, Baeck A, Verougstraete C, Verstappen A, Dhaene M, Zanen A. Altération pigmentaire de la rétine chez des patients dialysés traités par la desferroxamine. Bull Soc Belge Ophtalmol 1988; 224:49–60.
31. De Doncker R, Casteels I, Leys A, Missotten L. Desferroxamine and ocular toxicity, causal or concomitant relationship. Bull Soc Belge Ophtalmol 1987; 220:61–67.
32. Parrish CM, O'Day DM. Brown tumor of the orbit. Case report and review of the literature. Arch Ophthalmol 1986; 104:1199–1202.
33. Boelaert JR, Fenves AZ, Coburn JA. Desferroxamine therapy and mucormycosis in dialysis patients: report of an international registry. Am J Kidney Dis 1991; 18: 660–667.
34. Naumann GOH, Apple DJ. Pathology of the Eye. New York: Springer Verlag, 1986:131–132.
35. Boelaert JR, de Locht M, van Cutsem J, Kerrels V, Cantinieaux B, Verdonck A, van Landuyt HW, Scheider YJ. Mucormycosis during desferroxamine therapy is a siderophore-mediated infection. In vitro and in vivo animal studies. J Clin Invest 1993; 91:1979–1986.

35

Complications of Renal Replacement Therapy in the ICU

Claudio Ronco
St. Bortolo Hospital, Vicenza, Italy

Aldo Fabris and Mariavalentina Pellanda
Nephrology and Dialysis Service, City Hospital, Bassano del Grappa, Italy

I. INTRODUCTION

Some patients admitted to intensive care units (ICUs) may require dialytic therapy. In most cases the pathological condition is acute renal failure, although it is not infrequent to treat patients with chronic renal failure and acute illness of different origin.

The choice of renal replacement therapy (RRT) (continuous or intermittent hemodialysis or peritoneal dialysis) depends on logistics and the patient's clinical conditions. The presence of multiple organ failure, the presence of well-trained personnel, the availability of dialysis machines, and the degree of cooperation between intensivists and nephrologists are all factors affecting the final choice of the technique. Each of the aforementioned treatments has advantages, disadvantages, and possible complications.

Continuous renal replacement therapies (CRRT) are generally characterized by a good clinical tolerance and hemodynamic stability. This is at least in part related to the use of biocompatible membranes and the slow continuous fluid removal with a consequent plasma refilling. The possibility of manipulating the extracellular fluid composition with different substitution fluids that may also act as a source of calories, the absence of rebound in plasma solute concentration, and the stability of the targeted patient's hydration all make continuous treatments particularly indicated in critically ill patients. However, due to their invasive nature, these extracorporeal therapies are not free of complications, and treatment should be carefully monitored at any given moment.

Despite its many advantages, including high efficiency, shortness of the session, low heparinization, possibility of rapid correction of water, electrolyte, and acid-base derangements, intermittent hemodialysis is frequently complicated by cardiovascular instability, hypoxemia, postdialytic plasma solute rebound, and fluid and solute shifts among body compartments. All these complications make its utilization possible only in a select population. The choice of intermittent hemodialysis may also be hampered by the impact that this therapy has on the prognosis of and recovery from acute renal failure (ARF), particularly if bioincompatible membranes, such as Cuprophan, are used (1–3).

Peritoneal dialysis does not provoke hemodynamic instability, significant disequilibrium, or hypoxemia and does not require anticoagulation; therefore, it is well suited for patients with head trauma, cardiovascular instability, and high risk of bleeding. Due to the slow removal of low molecular weight solutes, such as urea and creatinine, this technique is not suitable for highly catabolic patients.

This chapter will describe the complications of different techniques and provide possible measures to prevent and manage problems associated with RRT in the ICU.

II. COMPLICATIONS OF CRRT

CRRT are widely used as treatment of ARF in critically ill patients. Due to the severe illness of these patients, it is sometimes difficult to distinguish between complications related to the therapy and those related to the illness. The rapid evolution in technology and the newer indications for continuous therapies have led to a parallel change in the frequency and severity of various complications. For example, while disconnection of the lines in 1985 represented about 8% of all complications, this event seldom occurred in 1995 and represented only 0.5% of overall complications (4).

Continuous therapies are generally well tolerated with a low rate of complications. The potential complications are summarized in Table 1.

Because CRRT involves invasive techniques, certain typical risks have to be considered. We can schematically distinguish between technical and clinical complications, even though these two categories are always merging together in clinical practice.

A. Technical Complications

Technical complications have a variable frequency depending on the technique employed. When continuous arteriovenous hemofiltration (CAVH) is used, the utilization of the arterial access introduces a series of possible complications that are not seen when a venovenous approach is utilized. In CAVH, the most severe complications are mainly associated with arterial access (5). The venovenous access reduces the complication rate considerably (6).

Table 1 Complications of Continuous Renal Replacement Therapies

Technical complications
Vascular access malfunction
Blood flow reduction and circuit clotting
Line disconnection
Air embolism
Fluid and electrolyte balance errors
Loss of filter efficiency
Clinical complications
Bleeding
Thrombosis
Infection and sepsis
Bioincompatibility and allergic reactions
Hypothermia
Nutrient losses
Inadequate blood purification

1. Vascular Access Malfunction and Circuit Clotting

Vascular access malfunction is a serious complication because it causes a reduction of the blood flow available in the extracorporeal circuit. In CAVH, the arterial access is critical in ensuring sufficient blood flow. A reduction of the inner diameter of the catheter even by a simple kinking causes a significant reduction of the blood flow and sometimes blocking of the circuit (7). In CVVH these complications are not common, since a blood pump provides a stable blood flow and double lumen catheters are placed in a central vein. The use of blood pump and double lumen catheters may in turn lead to other potential complications. First, the circuit has a negative pressure in the line segment before the blood pump. This leads to the risk of vessel damage and suction of air into the circuit with a consequent risk of air embolism. Both situations are potentially dangerous and require accurate pressure- and air-monitoring devices in the circuit. Recirculation is a dangerous situation in which the viscosity of the blood in the extracorporeal circuit increases progressively until a point at which ultrafiltration ceases and the filter is blocked. Accurate monitoring of pressures in the circuit makes it possible to overcome this problem and to employ measures for restoring a normal access function.

2. Line Disconnection

At the high perfusion rate of the extracorporeal circuit (especially in the absence of alarms and monitoring), any accidental disconnection of blood lines is acutely life-threatening. Therefore, it must always be assured that all connections are well locked and that the whole circuit is visible (e.g., not covered by blankets). Continuous surveillance by a competent nurse must always be ensured. It is generally accepted that the occurrence of technical complications clearly correlates with competence and intensity of nursing care. In the presence of a blood pump, the correct function of alarms and pressure monitors should be periodically checked. If there is an alarm failure, dangerous variations in pressures could occur inside the circuit and occasionally the circuit may even explode.

3. Air Embolism

Air embolism in modern, pump-driven systems is prevented by the presence of special monitoring and alarm systems, which immediately stop perfusion when air is detected in the system. Except for technical defects, this safety system excludes any possibility of air embolism. Air embolism is prevented in CAVH by the positive pressure in all sections of the circuit. Despite this, air embolism could occur when a disconnection happens at the venous access and negative inspiratory pressure sucks air into the venous system.

4. Fluid and Electrolyte Balance Errors

Accidental fluid overload is a constant danger of continuous hemofiltration techniques, especially when a high fluid turnover is maintained. Meticulous monitoring and recording of fluid intake and output are mandatory. Everybody must be aware of the danger of possible errors. Furthermore, the clinical status of the patient must carefully and critically be taken into account. Machines with fluid-balancing systems are used to prevent mistakes resulting from the manual handling of the balance (8). However, the possibility of a failure of the system must always be considered, and careful monitoring should be part of the standard protocol. Mistakes in the preparation of the replacement solutions may occur, especially when high fluid turnover is scheduled. It is a good practice to keep record of any bottle or bag utilized for reinfusion and to keep the empty containers until the end of the nurse and doctor shifts (9,10).

When high fluid turnover is scheduled, the possibility of a negative thermal balance should be considered and adequate fluid warming should then be provided.

5. Loss of Filter Efficiency

It has been demonstrated that CAVH filters operate in conditions of low blood flow and filtration pressure equilibrium. This depends on the characteristics of the filters and their blood path resistance. As a consequence, high rates of filter clotting and low efficiency in terms of ultrafiltration are generally observed in CAVH. In CVVH, the blood pump has solved the problem of maintaining adequate blood flows, and the resistance of the hemofilter is no longer an issue. However, in CVVH, a significant reduction in membrane permeability to water and solutes may occur over time. The sieving coefficients of solutes tend to decrease, thus reducing the efficiency of the system. Therefore, even though high filtration rates are mechanically maintained, the effective solute removal may be less than expected due to this phenomenon (11).

At the same time, the protein layer deposition at the blood membrane interface tends to reduce the hydraulic permeability of the membrane, and lower filtration rates may be observed over time. All of these factors may result in a significant decrease in the effective delivery of treatment.

B. Clinical Complications

Clinical complications may be related to the unstable clinical condition of the patient and/or to the complex nature of different renal replacement techniques and their impact on the patient's physiology.

1. Bleeding

In arteriovenous treatment, percutaneous vessel puncture and introduction of large cannulas by modified Seldinger technique may lead to bleeding and unwanted vessel perforation or damage. With careful technique and experience, this happens only exceptionally. However, in case of local arteriosclerosis, serious bleeding may occur due to injury of the arterial wall and plaques detachment. Therefore, when severe local arteriosclerosis is anticipated, another access (preferably venovenous) should definitely be chosen. Venous puncture may also be complicated by an accidental puncture of the artery, especially in the jugular region. On the other hand, the cannulation of the subclavian vein may also be complicated by accidental damage of the pleural membrane with effusion or pneumothorax. In recent years, the use of ultrasonic guidance has resulted in a dramatic reduction in accidents during vessel cannulation.

During the course of hemofiltration, careful control of the anticoagulation (low-dose heparinization) reduces the risk of bleeding. However, at the end of the procedure bleeding may result from the removal of the catheter. Careful and persistent compression is mandatory, especially if arterial vessels are involved. If bleeding continues, the decision for surgical repair of the arterial wall should be made without further delay. The infection of a large persistent hematoma may cause an abscess that is difficult to treat, especially in the femoral region.

The anticoagulation achieved by heparin infusion should be directed toward a maximal effect in the extracorporeal circuit but minimal or absent effects in the systemic circulation. Alternative procedures in the critically ill patient with bleeding tendency can be undertaken. Local heparinization, prostacyclin, low molecular weight heparin, citrate, predilution, and other alternative techniques have been tried to improve the bleeding diathesis of the patient while maintaining an efficient antithrombogenesis in the extracorporeal circuit (12,13). Heparin-coated surfaces are being studied and may in the future provide a good alternative in these patients.

2. Thrombosis

Local thrombosis at the arterial site occurs rather often (~3%). This may occasionally critically impede the perfusion of the leg, in which case prompt surgical intervention is mandatory. Frequent and regular control of perfusion of the leg (e.g., by Doppler sonography) is thus highly recommended. Especially in severe arteriosclerosis, local thrombosis becomes a considerable risk. Another situation in which this complication should be considered is in the neonate. The large size of the cannula may occupy the entire lumen of the vessel, not only disturbing the perfusion of the leg or the arm but also facilitating local thrombus formation.

In venovenous hemofiltration local thrombosis may occur in the vein and may extend up to the superior or inferior vena cava. Continuous monitoring of the venous system may therefore prevent a dangerous complication.

3. Infection and Sepsis

Local infections at the site of catheter insertion (especially infected hematomas) are serious complications because they may lead to systemic infections or reduced arterial perfusion in the region. The extracorporeal circuit must be handled with extreme care: sterile handling, avoidance or drastic reduction of disconnections for blood sampling, avoidance of bleeding, and prevention of hematoma formation should be priorities. The patient in the ICU setting is highly susceptible to infections because of immune system suppression. The extracorporeal circuit can be the cause of bacterial invasion of the patient. Connections, sampling ports, and indwelling catheters may all represent a port for bacteria entry. Furthermore, once bacterial invasion has occurred, endotoxin concentrations may rise due to bacterial killing and the patient may enter the "slippery slope" of septic syndrome. Patients may also be subject to these complications because of pinholes in the membrane and back-transport of endotoxin fragments from contaminated dialysate. Transmembrane signaling and monocyte activation may also occur in the absence of the physical transfer of endotoxin from dialysate into the blood. Early signs of inflammatory response may be seen in the patient in these cases, and they are mostly reflected by an increased blood level of proinflammatory cytokines (14).

4. Bioincompatibility and Allergic Reactions

Prolonged contact with artificial membranes and plastic materials of catheters and blood lines may cause adverse reactions due to residual substances of the sterilization procedures, spallation of plastic particles, and blood-membrane chemical interactions. In a patient with a potent immunostimulation due to infections and other pathological events, maximal care should be given to trying to prevent such complications. In particular, formation of bradykinin in patients treated with ACE inhibitors and negatively charged dialysis membrane surfaces or monocyte stimulation from bioincompatible surfaces with a consequent increase of circulating cytokine levels should be carefully avoided (2,15,16). It has been demonstrated that blood contact with the extracorporeal artificial surfaces in cardiopulmonary bypass conditions is sufficient per se to evoke a systemic inflammatory response syndrome (SIRS).

5. Hypothermia

Hypothermia can occasionally occur when large amounts of ultrafiltrate are exchanged. A simple warming of substitution fluid may correct this inconvenience. On the other hand, continuous hemofiltration can be effectively used to reduce the body temperature in case of hyperthermia. At the same time, the negative thermal balance provided by the hemofilter/dialyzer (that can be considered a potent heat exchanger) must be taken into consideration when the caloric intake is scheduled and the energy balance is evaluated.

6. Nutrient Losses

The critically ill patient is often severely catabolic, and adequate protein and energy intakes should be carefully planned. Amino acids and other nutrients are lost in the ultrafiltrate and they must be replaced using adequate substitution fluids. Protein losses occur in continuous therapies, as in the case of CAPD or intermittent extracorporeal therapies. The amount of protein losses per week in continuous therapies, however, does not exceed that observed in peritoneal dialysis or in intermittent treatments. An average loss of 40–60 g of protein per week has been measured in continuous hemofiltration (3) without significant changes in total plasma protein or albumin concentrations. Such complications should be carefully considered when protein synthesis by the liver is impaired and the treatment is carried out for a prolonged period of time. Vitamin losses have been reported in continuous therapies, even though a real vitamin depletion syndrome is not commonly observed. It is of interest that attention has been recently placed on the possible oxidative stress experienced by the patient undergoing extracorporeal renal replacement. The use of glutathione solutions, vitamin E supplementation, or even vitamin E–bonded dialysis membranes has been suggested as possible means to counterbalance oxidative stress.

Hypophosphatemia has been described, and, as for other elecrolytes or nutrients and drugs, solute imbalances can easily be avoided by frequent monitoring of ultrafiltrate and plasma concentrations and adjustments of the replacement fluid composition (17).

7. Inadequate Blood Purification

The issue of treatment adequacy in acute renal failure has recently been raised by some authors (18,19). CAVH frequently provided insufficient amounts of ultrafiltrate to counterbalance the toxin production by the catabolic patient. Several new techniques are now employed to enhance solute clearances, and the adequacy of blood purification is no longer a real limitation of continuous therapies. Clearances up to 60 L per day may be obtained, and even the most catabolic patient can be maintained under adequate control.

In conclusion, complications are less common with CRRT than with intermittent treatments. The invasive nature of the technique, however, means that a series of potential adverse events must be considered. A careful monitoring of the technique, adequate nursing procedures, and a precise schedule for the therapy may help to prevent the majority of potential risks and complications.

III. COMPLICATIONS OF INTERMITTENT DIALYSIS TREATMENTS

Although several lines of evidence have demonstrated that CRRT may be better tolerated in critically ill patients, intermittent hemodialysis is still largely employed in the treatment of acute renal failure. Complications of intermittent dialysis treatments can be distinguished according to their clinical or technical nature (Table 2). A separate discussion would not permit an adequate presentation of the various interactions among different phenomena, therefore the description of hemodialysis complications will be made without distinction between technical and clinical aspects.

Clinical complications in hemodialysis are mostly related to the intermittent nature of the technique.

Table 2 Major Complications of Intermittent Hemodialysis

Clinical complications
Hypotension
Hypovolemia
Cardiovascular response to hypovolemia
Dialyzer reactions
Hypoxemia
Dialysis disequilibrium syndrome
Febrile reactions
Bleeding
Arrhythmias
Technical complications
Air embolism
Hemolysis
Inappropiate electrolyte composition of dialysate
Low or high sodium content
Low or potassium-free content
Low calcium content
Hard water syndrome

Rapid short correction of a patient's symptoms strongly affects the tolerance of treatment.

A. Hypovolemia and Hypotension

Intradialytic hypotension is one of the most frequent complications observed in hemodialysis, occurring in 20–30% of the sessions. In chronic patients it is often correlated with other symptoms such as muscle cramps, nausea, and vomiting. In the critically ill patient this is often detected by the monitors and from the signals from Swan-Ganz catheters. The exact mechanism of hypotension is not completely understood, because many factors, sometimes interrelated, may be involved in its pathogenesis. Hypovolemia with a fall in cardiac filling pressure and cardiac output is generally the most important cause of hypotension. In ICU patients, this mechanism is also related to the myocardial dysfunction that is commonly observed in sepsis and other critical illness. In the critically ill patient, a defect in the regulation of vascular tone with an inappropriate increase in vascular resistance is also frequently observed. Despite pharmacological support with norepinephrine or other vasoactive drugs, some patients are unable to recover adequate vascular tone or to maintain sufficient arterial pressure. In these conditions, the rapid fall in circulating plasma volume in rapid short sessions of ultrafiltration cannot be offset by adequate plasma refilling, and hypotension is inevitable (20), which will result in further alterations of tissue perfusion and oxygenation.

In patients with renal failure, the fluid that has accumulated in body compartments must be removed during dialysis by ultrafiltration. Since the fluid is initially drained from the intravascular compartment, blood volume rapidly declines, but its change will depend on the ratio of removal to refilling rate from the interstitial space. Under normal circumstances, the refilling depends on the Starling capillary forces, i.e., the equilibrium between oncotic and hydrostatic pressures, the latter determined by systemic arterial pressure and the pre- to postcapillary resistance ratio (21). During ultrafiltration, the removal of protein-free fluid from the intravascular compartment leads to an increase in plasma protein concentration and the oncotic pressure. This, combined with a decrease in capillary hydrostatic pressure, promotes a fluid shift from the interstitium into the intravascular space, thus counteracting the hypovolemia (22). If ultrafiltration takes place at a rate that exceeds the capacity of the interstitial fluid to migrate into the intravascular compartment, a rapid fall in plasma volume with consequent hypotension will result (22). Fluid shifts among body compartments are also modulated by plasma osmolality, since its reduction may hamper plasma refilling. The rapid extracellular reduction of osmotically active solutes, such as urea, is not accompanied by an equivalent cellular reduction; this event favors the passage of water from a hypoosmolar (extracellular) to a hyperosmolar (intracellular) compartment, so that less fluid is available to refill the vascular bed (23). These mechanisms have been supposed to play a pivotal role in the perpetuation of renal ischemia since fresh necrotic lesions have been observed in the kidney even after a long-lasting period of anuria (1). Even the electrolyte composition of dialysis fluid is important; when a dialysate with low sodium concentration is used, fluid shifts into the intracellular space due to a reduced "driving force" of plasma sodium; this may compromise vascular refilling and contribute to hypovolemia (24). Finally, plasma refilling is hampered when interstitial tissue pressure is reduced owing to underestimation of the patient's dry weight (25). Although inappropriate fluid removal is an important factor responsible for dialysis hypotension, it alone cannot account for all the hypotensive episodes.

A compensatory systemic response to hypovolemia normally activates hemodynamic mechanisms, such as reduction in capacitance of venous system and activation of cardiopulmonary and baroreceptor reflexes, which are responsible for the increase in heart rate, cardiac contractility, and systemic vascular resistances. The venous compliance, which represents 80–85% of the overall systemic compliance, determines the cardiac filling pressure and the distribution of blood volume between systemic and cardiopulmonary circulation. It also determines the distribution of the extracellular fluid volume (ECFV) between plasma and interstitial space (26). Normally, reciprocal variations of blood volume and venous compliance maintain constant cardiac filling pressures (26). This equilibrium results from the monitoring of the filling pressure by cardiopulmonary receptors. During hypovolemia, the reduced cardiopulmonary blood volume and cardiac filling pressure decrease the activity of stretch-sensitive cardiopulmonary receptors, which no longer inhibit the vasomotor centers (27). Sympathetic activation produces arteriolar and venous constriction, with consequent decrease in venous compliance and hemodynamically inactive blood volume (unstressed volume). This results in a passage of blood from systemic veins to the cardiopulmonary compartment, thus maintaining cardiac filling (28,29). The adjustments of venous capacitance, particularly in the splanchnic and the cutaneous circulations, depend on active venoconstriction and passive venous recoil. This is a consequence of arteriolar vasoconstriction, which reduces regional postcapillary flow and venuous pressure—the so-called DeJager-Krogh phenomenon (30). The precapillary arteriolar constriction also reduces the capillary hydrostatic pressure, favoring vascular refilling from the interstitium (31).

As long as the circulatory system is able to respond with these modifications to volume contraction, hypotension does not occur. A fall in arterial pressure, however, is facilitated whenever the response of cardiac output and peripheral resistances to hypovolemia are inadequate. Several factors, such as autonomic dysfunction, acetate, dialysate temperature, membrane biocompatibility, splanchnic fluid sequestration, and tissue ischemia, could be responsible for the inadequate increase in peripheral vascular resistances during hypovolemia.

Dysfunction of sympathetic activity with inadequate increase in heart rate and in peripheral resistance has been shown to be an important cause of dialysis hypotension in chronic patients (32,33). Critically ill patients are very often in shock, which would be a further reason for inadequate response to ultrafiltration.

Experimental studies demonstrated that acetate was a potent cardiodepressor (34); however, it has been demonstrated that acetate infusion has no effect on myocardial contractility (35). The cardiodepressant action of acetate has been confirmed in patients with impaired cardiac function (36). Furthermore, acetate is a direct vasodilator (37) that decreases the precapillary arterial vasoconstriction and thus increases the capillary hydrostatic pressure opposing refilling (38). For the reasons above, acetate dialysate should not be utilized in ICU patients who are prone to cardiovascular instability.

It has been suggested that an increase in body temperature could cause dialysis hypotension (39). There is a correlation between a positive thermal balance during hemodialysis and increase in heart rate, decrease in systemic vascular resistance, and diastolic blood pressure.

The use of relatively warm dialysate produces a small elevation of the central temperature, necessitating heat dissipation through the skin; blood is then sequestered in the cutaneous veins and cutaneous flow is increased at the expense of perfusion in the more vital circulatory beds. It has been demonstrated that cold dialysis with a dialysate temperature of approximately 35°C improves venous and arterial reactivity and ventricular contractility (40).

Bioincompatibility plays an important role in dialysis hypotension, which seems to be secondary to an enhanced secretion of proinflammatory cytokines (41). The production of these substances by the monocyte-macrophage system are stimulated by blood contact with bioincompatible artificial membranes, by acetate, or by endotoxin fragments coming from contaminated dialysate (42–44). It has been suggested that the vasodilating action of proinflammatory cytokines is mediated through the accumulation of nitric oxide in vascular smooth muscle cells (45).

Splanchnic fluid sequestration and tissue ischemia may also be involved in the genesis of hypotension. The former causes reduced vasoconstriction of the resistance vessels in the splanchnic area, resulting in an increased venous capacitance in this area and reduced venous return (20). Inappropriate peripheral venodilation with increased "unstressed" volume has also been proposed as an important contributor to the development of dialysis-induced hypotension (46).

Diastolic dysfunction has also been claimed as an important cause of dialysis hypotension (47). Patients prone to hypotension and with left ventricle hypertrophy display a decreased ratio of atrial waves E (early diastolic filling) to atrial waves A (atrial filling), decreasing further during hypotension as has been shown on echocardiography (47). The altered ratio could be due to the stiffness of the left ventricle, which hampers passive diastolic filling. The lower filling rate produces a smaller systolic output and hypotension, sometimes accompanied by bradycardia (48). In fact, the cardiac underfilling may induce profound inhibition of the sympathic system through the Bezold-Jarish reflex, a vagal reflex initiated by the stimulation of cardiac mechanoreceptors by vigorous contraction of an underfilled left ventricle (49).

Finally, hypoxemia correlated with the use of acetate and/or bioincompatible membranes, underlying cardiac disease, impaired miocardial contractility caused by a low calcium dialysate, and presence of arrhythmias are all frequent conditions in ICU patients. These conditions make the patients severely unstable and prone to dialysis hypotension.

On the basis of pathophysiology, many hypotensive episodes can be prevented. Because low serum albumin levels are frequently observed in critically ill patients with multiple organ failure, the use of albumin infusion during the first 15–30 minutes of dialysis helps to promote fluid mobilization from the interstitial space to the intravascular one, thus facilitating refilling (50). Pharmacological agents like the norepinephrine precursor L-DOPS (51), midodrine (52), and other vasoactive agents like lysine vasopressin (53) have been successfully utilized to prevent hypotension. Hypotensive episodes can be further prevented by decreasing blood flow and dialyzer surface area, decreasing ultrafiltration per unit of time, increasing the dialysate sodium concentration to 140–145 mEq/L, using bicarbonate-buffered dialysate, maintaining adequate calcium dialysate concentration, cooling the dialysate to 35°C, utilization of more biocompatible membranes, such as PMMA and polysulfone, and finally switching to diffusive-convective or convective techniques such as hemodiafiltration and hemofiltration. The latter are hemodynamically better tolerated than standard hemodialysis.

Acute treatment of intradialytic hypotension often requires an increase in norepinephrine dosage and infusion of normal saline. Unfortunately, fluid infusion expands extracellular volume; therefore, the patient will soon need greater ultrafiltration because of wet lung with increased possibility for further hypotension. Hypertonic saline solutions may offer a better alternative. When studying an intravenous bolus of either 10 mL of a 23% saturated hypertonic saline or 30 mL of a 7.5% hypertonic saline, each containing osmolar loads of 80 mOsm, the more concentrated solution produced a greater increase in systolic blood pressure (54).

Dextrans are useful plasma expanders to employ in the management of hypotension. Recent autopsy and biopsy studies have, however, documented extracellular deposition of dextrans in various tissues of chronically dialyzed patients (55). This report suggests some caution in the indiscriminate use of this plasma expander. Even mannitol (50 mL 20%), commonly utilized for treating dialysis hypotension, has the problem of accumulation.

Finally, continuous infusion of norepinephrine, dobutamine, and dopamine maintained, with adequate adjustments, acceptable blood pressure values during dialysis. Adjustments in the oxygen supply provided by mechanical ventilation techniques may be of further help in improving cardiac performance.

B. Hypersensitivity Reactions and Biocompatibility Issues

Dialyzer-related reactions are not completely understood, but they may be a sign of immunochemical alterations resulting from the contact of blood with a noncompatible or a poorly compatible artificial surface. Classic cellulosic membranes like Cuprophan have been claimed to present a much lower biocompatibility compared to the more recent synthetic membranes. In a prospective randomized study involving 52 critically ill patients, the group dialyzed with Cuprophan dialyzers had a lower survival rate compared to the group treated with AN-69 dialyzers. The Cuprophan group experienced a higher incidence of death from sepsis, while the survivors required a greater number of dialysis sessions and had a delayed recovery from ARF compared to patients treated with AN-69 dialyzers (2).

Recovery of renal function was significantly greater and the median number of dialysis treatments required significantly smaller in another group of patients treated with polymethylmethacrylate (PMMA) compared to patients treated with Cuprophan membranes (3). This aspect, however, is still controversial, and other studies have reported a similar mortality rate for patients treated with Cuprophan membranes and those treated with more biocompatible membranes (56). The absence of overt beneficial effects of the use of biocompatible membranes for the course and outcome in patients with ARF has been further debated (57,58), and no definite conclusions have been drawn yet on this matter.

Recently, some authors considered the biocompatibility of the entire system rather than the biocompatibility of the membrane (59). For these authors, the use of sterile dialysate and of dialytic membranes more efficient in removing high molecular weight compounds perhaps represents a better approach to minimizing the bioincompatibility of the dialysis procedure than does modification of the biocompatibility characteristics of the membrane itself.

As for the issue of biocompatibility, the treatment of patients with acute hepatic failure deserves special attention. Because cerebral edema remains a significant cause of mortality in this group of patients, the treatment of choice in ARF patients with hepatic failure should utilize a technique that causes no change or minimal change in intracranial pressure (ICP). Because Cuprophan hemodialysis has been reported to exacerbate cerebral edema in patients with ARF (60), ICP was registered during intermittent hemofiltration sessions carried out with polyamide and polyacrylonitrile hemofilters (61). The increase in ICP registered with both membranes was significantly lower than that in patients treated by hemodialysis (60). Because a greater fall in arterial oxygen tension and in total peripheral white blood cell count was observed in the polyamide patients, the increased ICP was attributed to less biocompatibility of polyamide compared to PAN. The same authors have demonstrated that in this group of critically ill patients, continuous modes of renal replacement therapies result in superior cardiac and intracranial stability compared to intermittent renal replacement techniques (62).

Among the dialyzer reactions, the first-use syndrome that occurs within minutes of the initial use of cellulosic membrane is the most frequent (63). Chest and/or back pain, nausea, malaise, pruritus, and hypotension are the most prominent symptoms. However, the clinical presentation may not be different from that associated with hypersensitivity reactions, from which it can be distinguished by the appearance of a new cellulosic membrane, the absence of specific IgE antibodies, and the absence of eosinophilia. The pathogenetic mechanism is related to the activation of complement with production of potent anaphylactoxins C3a and C5a (63). Of course, in critically ill patients these reactions may be masked by the clinical condition of the patient, who may be sedated or even in a coma. The medical therapy for this reaction involves the administration of antihistamines, antipyretics, and glucocorticoids.

C. Hypoxemia

During hemodialysis, Pao_2 tends to fall 10–20 mmHg; this drop has no clinical consequences in patients with normal oxygen tension, while in seriously ill patients with predialytic hypoxemia, the drop in Pao_2 can be catastrophic. This drop can be identified in a patient on ventilator by digital plethysmography, optic fibers, Swann-Ganz, or by hemogasanalysis.

The cause of hypoxemia is multifactorial, but it is principally related to the use of acetate dialysate and bioincompatible membranes. Acetate provokes hypoxemia by at least two mechanisms: increased oxygen consumption and decreased CO_2 production in the metabolism of acetate to bicarbonate (64) and intradialytic loss of carbon dioxide (65). Dialysis-induced hypoxemia can be attenuated by increasing the CO_2 content of the dialysate either by direct administration or by substitution of acetate with bicarbonate-buffered dialysate.

The interaction between blood and cellulosic membranes activates the alternate complement pathway, which leads to activation of neutrophils. This activation results in increased expression of neutrophil receptors specific for phagocytosis and adhesion, as well as other receptors, which cause adhesion of neutrophils to endothelium and their possible sequestration in the pulmonary circulation. Neutropenia occurs maximally at 15 minutes with new Cuprophan membranes, and it is followed by a rebound leucocytosis at 120 minutes. As an additional mechanism, the pulmonary microemboli of leukocytes might lead to an impairment of pulmonary gas diffusion and consequent hypoxia (66).

In critically ill patients, who may already have some degree of predialytic hypoxia, it is necessary to increase the ventilated volumes and/or the percentage of Fio_2.

D. Dialysis Disequilibrium Syndrome

Dialysis disequilibrium syndrome (DDS) is a neurological disorder, more common in patients starting on dialysis, especially if they have a high predialysis BUN. It is also common in elderly and pediatric patients with preexisting brain damage or severe metabolic acidosis. In the moderate form, symptoms are limited to headache and nausea. In more severe forms, restlessness, hypertension, confusion, disorientation, blurred vision, seizures, coma, and possibly death are observed. The pathophysiology of this syndrome is ascribed to brain edema caused by a different removal rate of urea from blood and cerebrospinal fluid. The blood-brain barrier acts as a membrane in which diffusion of urea is partially restricted. A rapid decrease in blood urea is accompanied by a smaller and slower fall of intracellular urea, with consequent transfer of water into brain cells (67). Additionally, a paradoxical development of cerebrospinal fluid acidosis with an increase in osmotic activity due to intracerebral accumulation of osmolytes such as inositol, glutamine and glutamic acid may play a role (68).

The simplest strategy for the prevention of DDS is to reduce the dialytic efficiency by using a smaller dialyzer, decreasing blood flow, or increasing dialysis duration. Additional strategies include prophylactic administration of osmotic agents such as mannitol, glucose, fructose, glycerol, urea, and sodium chloride, either intravenously or via the dialysate, with the aim at minimizing the decline in serum osmolality. Since modern dialysis machines can easily increase dialysate sodium levels, the use of high-sodium dialysate may be the most convenient approach. Seizures can be treated with intravenous diazepam. It should be definitely stated, however, that this syndrome is never seen in continuous renal replacement therapies and is only the result of the unphysiology of intermittent treatments.

E. Febrile Reactions

Endotoxins or their fragments are the most important determinants of pyrogenic reactions. These reactions are characterized by fever, chills, cephalea, myalgias, and hemodynamic instability.

Endotoxins are lypopolysaccharides (LPS) with high molecular weight derived from the outer membrane of gram-negative bacteria. It has been suggested that the passage through dialytic membranes is possible only when intact molecule is fragmented in products of lower molecular weight (69). The principal source of dialysate contamination may be the liquid bicarbonate concentrate. The key consequence of the action of LPS is the release of pyrogenic cytokines from monocytes and endothelial cells mediating several clinical events (69).

Another important cause of febrile reaction during dialysis may be infection of the vascular access. A typical patient with or without interdialytic fever may show during dialysis a great increase in temperature due to widespread bacterial diffusion arising from a vascular catheter. These infections are often caused by *Staphyloccus aureus*, and the best treatment is removal of the infected catheter.

F. Bleeding

Bleeding tendency is generally increased in ICU patients with acute renal failure. This tendency is mainly due to platelet dysfunction, although it may be amplified by liver dysfunction, sepsis, infection, and tissue damage.

Bleeding tendency is manifested by spontaneous mucosal bleeding, prolonged bleeding from skin puncture sites, and excessive postoperative bleeding. In these critical situations the anticoagulation of the extracorporeal circuit for intermittent therapies is a persisting challenge. Alternatives to systemic heparinization include regional heparinization with protamine, low-dose heparinization, low molecular weight heparins, saline-flush protocols with no anticoagulant, and regional citrate anticoagulation. The incidence of systemic bleeding events and extracorporeal clotting was evaluated in 57 critically ill ARF patients treated with intermittent hemodialysis (IHD) or continuous arteriovenous hemodialysis (CAVHD) using low-dose systemic heparinization, regional citrate, and saline flush with no anticoagulant (70). In the IHD with low-dose heparin, new bleeding events occurred during 26% of 35 courses and during 0% of 24 courses in the IHD with regional citrate. The saline-flush protocol for IHD (Sal IHD) did not cause bleeding, but clotting in the extracorporeal circuit occurred in 9% of procedures, so that 28% of 29 courses of Sal IHD were terminated for this reason.

Therefore, in ICU patients at high risk of bleeding, many alternatives to systemic heparinization are available, and they should be all considered to prevent any possible increase in bleeding risk. On the other hand, it should be remarked that low-dose heparin infusion as a standard procedure may be able to achieve a good antithrombogenesis in the circuit with minimal or absent systemic effect if carried out with a continuous monitoring of coagulation parameters. Among the medications utilized against bleeding tendency, the most popular are desmopressin (71), conjugated estrogens (72), and cryoprecipitates (73).

G. Cardiac Arrhythmias

Arrhythmias frequently occur in ICU patients, and particularly in those treated with hemodialysis. Patient- and treatment-related factors are involved in their onset.

Patient-related factors include age, heart and/or lung failure, the state of extracellular fluid volume, electrolyte and acid-base derangements, cardiac or major vascular surgery, digoxin therapy, and others. Treatment-related factors include potassium, calcium, and acid-base changes produced by dialysis.

Hemodialysis leads to rapid changes in serum potassium levels, mainly when a low potassium dialysate is utilized. Hypokalemia, with increased ratio between intracellular and extracellular potassium with consequent increase in negative membrane potential, facilitates the appearance of arrhythmias, particularly in patients on digoxin therapy. A reduction of arrhythmias can be obtained by substituting bicarbonate to acetate; this reduction may be explained by the more progressive correction of acidosis with the use of bicarbonate. As regarding the dialysate-calcium content, a concentration of 1.75 mmol/L, although it improves hemodynamic stability (74), may induce a higher incidence of nonsymptomatic arrhythmias (75).

Disturbances of cardiac rhythm, are extremely common in ICU patients because of many possible factors including mild or severe cardiac dysfunction. It is essential to distinguish between benign occasional arrhythmias and severe malignant and life-threatening cardiac rhythm disorders.

H. Air Embolism

Although extracorporeal systems are designed with many safeguards to avoid air embolism, the occurrence of this complication is not rare. The clinical severity depends on the quantity of the injected air, the rate of air entry, and the site of entry. During hemodialysis, the emboli are typically venous. The clinical manifestations depend on the patient's body position at the time of embolization (50). In the sitting position, air will flow along the venous system to reach the central circulation and will then back-flow into the cerebral venous system. The patient may become aware of the sound of the air in his or her vessels, lose consciousness, and develop seizures (50).

In the recumbent patient air will reach the right atrium and the right ventricle. There foam develops that flows in the pulmonary vasculature, which becomes occluded and causes pulmonary hypertension. The patient will present with chest pain, shortness of breath, cyanosis, and cough followed by cardiovascular collapse. Some air flowing through capillaries and pulmonary arterovenous shunts will reach the left heart and then systemic arterial circulation, where it may provoke coronary and cerebral embolization (50). If the patient is in the Trendelenburg position, air occludes the venous vasculature of the legs with the appearance of patchy cyanosis.

Therapeutic interventions include Trendelenburg positioning with the left side down to reduce the movement of air to the brain and trapping air bubbles in the right ventricle. This air trapping minimizes foaming, which takes place mainly in the right ventricle. If significant foaming has occurred in the right ventricle causing cardiac arrest, cardiac puncture and aspiration should be performed to remove the foam. Hyperbaric oxygen therapy is an additional aid in treating air embolism (76). Patients with cerebral air embolism may benefit from this therapy even after a prolonged delay. Even normobaric oxygen may be useful, particularly if mechanical ventilation is employed; the prompt application of mechanical ventilation with an FiO_2 of 1.0 dramatically enhances the removal of air from cerebral vessels (77).

I. Hemolysis

Clinically significant hemolysis may be observed due to the dialysis procedure. Kinked blood lines, contamination of dialysis fluid with hydrogen peroxide (because of inadequate rinsing of the water treatment system after disinfection), residual formaldehyde in reused dialyzers, accidental hypochlorite infusion, presence of copper, zinc, nitrates, or chloramines in the dialysate, and overheated or hypoosmolar dialysate may all induce hemolysis (50). Patients complain of malaise, nausea, headache, abdominal and back pain, and hypertension. Fatal hyperkalemia may occur. Dialysis must be stopped; controls of electrolytes, acid-base status, and hematocrit should be carried out, and a new treatment should be started immediately.

J. Electrolyte Derangements

Markedly low-sodium dialysate may be accidentally utilized during dialysis if the conductivity limits of the dialysis machine are not appropriately adjusted or calibrated. The consequent plasma hypoosmolality causes water intoxication, hemolysis, and cerebral edema. Patients complain of abdominal pain, leg cramps, hypertension, neurological symptoms, and hyperkalemia. Treatment consists of cessation of dialysis, initiation of another dialysis, and use of hypertonic saline infusion if hyponatremia is life-threatening.

Hypernatremia may also occur for technical problems. The consequent plasma hyperosmolality causes cellular dehydration. Clinically, patients complain of neurological symptoms, such as headache, disorientation, seizures, coma, and profound thirst. Therapy consists of the use of a new dialytic treatment with appropriate sodium concentration in the dialysate, intravenous administration of 5% glucose, and drinking of water when possible.

Hypokalemia frequently occurs when the patient is dialyzed against a very low-potassium or potassium-free dialysate. A rapid shift of potassium from the extracellular to the intracellular space as a result of metabolic alkalosis may also cause hypokalemia. Hypokalemia is more pronounced if predialytic values are moderately low or in the normal range. In these cases it may be responsible for sudden death, particularly in acutely ill patients. Adequate levels of potassium and buffer in the dialysate are mandatory to prevent this complication, and intravenous potassium can be administered during dialysis when needed.

Hyperkalemia as a complication of dialytic treatment is infrequent; the most common cause is hemolysis. A rapid start of a new treatment will normalize shortly the potassium levels. Post-dialytic hypercalcemia, partly due to increased plasma protein concentration and release of calcium from bone, is transient and does not lead to symptoms. A more important complication is the "hard-water syndrome" (78). This syndrome occurs when a fault in the purification of water (water softener or deionizer) causes an abnormally elevated concentration of calcium and magnesium in the dialysate. Patients complain of nausea, vomiting, warm skin sensation, tachycardia, hyper- or hypotension, headache, seizures. Treatment consists of the use of dialysate containing appropriate amounts of the divalent cations.

It should be noted that all these symptoms, normally observed in awake patients, may be masked in sedated patients or comatose patients. This should always be kept in mind, and accurate biochemical monitoring should be performed with adequate frequency to avoid fatal complications not anticipated by typical symptoms.

IV. COMPLICATIONS OF PERITONEAL DIALYSIS

Before the advent of continuous renal replacement therapies, peritoneal dialysis played an important role in ICU patients with ARF as a complication of medical or surgical illness or as a part of the multiorgan failure (MOF) syndrome. It is a slow continuous therapy that permits fluid removal without causing hemodynamic instability and leads to blood purification without rebound in solute concentration. With this technique there is no problem regarding biocompatibility of the membrane, because it uses peritoneal membrane, which is a natural membrane with excellent permeability to uremic toxins, ultrafiltration capacity, and easy access. This technique is more often used in children with ARF because of its relative simplicity and safety (79,80).

Access to the peritoneal cavity is obtained by the insertion of a soft and biocompatible plastic catheter (the most used is the Tenckhoff catheter) by surgical or peritoneoscopic technique. Solutions employed are slightly hyponatremic compared to plasma and contain 0–2 mmol/L of potassium and 1.25–1.75 mmol/L of calcium. The buffer most commonly used is lactate (35–40 mmol/L), while bicarbonate-containing solutions (about 34 mmol/L) are still under clinical evaluation. The most used osmotic agent is glucose. Commercially available solutions contain different concentrations (1.5–4.25 %) of glucose that have, obviously, different capacities for generating ultrafiltration. Dialysis solutions containing different osmotic agents (e.g., amino acids, glycerol, or polyglucose) are also commercially available (79).

Peritoneal dialysis techniques used in ARF patients include (79,81):

A manual technique lasting 48–72 hours with rapid exchanges (each cycle—inflow, dwell, outflow—lasting about 1 hour). Exchange volume is ≤2 L depending on the size of the patient and peritoneal cavity and the possible presence of pulmonary disease or recent abdominal surgery.

Cycler-assisted peritoneal dialysis, in which instillation and drainage of the peritoneal dialysis solution can be regulated by the use of an automatic device called a cycler. This machine, using electric clamps activated by electric timers, controls the succession of peritoneal dialysis cycles (each one comprising instillation, dwell time, and drainage). This technique is safer than manual procedures, allows very short dwell times with increased clearances of small solutes, but it is more expensive.

Continuous equilibration peritoneal dialysis (CEPD), which utilizes relatively long dwell times (2–6 hours cycle time, 1–2 L of dialysate per cycle). Exchanges can be done manually or by automated methods.

The main complications of peritoneal dialysis are summarized in Table 3.

Table 3 Complications of Peritoneal Dialysis

Technical complications
Catheter-related problems
Mechanical complications
Inflow pain
Outflow failure
Clinical complications
Complications related to increased intra-abdominal pressure:
Hernia
Genital and abdominal edema
Leakages
Hydrothorax
Alterations of respiratory function
Metabolic complications
Hyperglycemia
Hypo/Hypernatremia
Hypo/Hyperkalemia
Acidosis/Alkalosis
Protein and amino acid losses
Infectious complications
Peritonitis
Exit site infection
Tunnel infection

A. Technical Complications

1. Catheter-Related Problems

Catheter-related problems include perforation of the intestine or bladder, hemorrhage, migration of the catheter from the pelvis, occlusion by fibrin plugs, omental wrapping around the catheter, and leakage of peritoneal fluid at the insertion site (82). Leakage can occur more often in patients undergoing intra-abdominal surgery and can be an important source of infections. Leakage is also more likely to occur in patients treated with mechanical ventilation in the prone position.

2. Mechanical Complications

Mechanical complications include inflow pain, related either to adherence of the catheter tip to intra-abdominal organs or to dialysate composition (e.g., low pH, type of buffer used); other causes of inflow pain may be temperature, additives such as antibiotics, or air accidentally introduced into peritoneal cavity (82).

Outflow failure could be either associated with inflow failure, due to catheter kink or obstruction by a clot, or it may be isolated. Isolated outflow failure is due to catheter migration, omental wrapping, or adherence of intra-abdominal organs to the catheter (82).

B. Clinical Complications

1. Complications Related to Increased Intra-Abdominal Pressure

When dialysis fluid is instilled into the peritoneal cavity, intra-abdominal pressure increases linearly from normal values in an empty peritoneal cavity (0.5–2.2 cm H_2O) to 2–10 cm H_2O or more if large volumes are used (83,84). Intra-abdominal pressure may reach elevated values in case of coughing and may be influenced by weight, age, and body position (83–85). Increase of the intra-abdominal pressure may compromise lung function, reducing functional residual capacity and gas exchange efficiency with consequent decrease in PaO_2. These effects are particularly important in patients with the acute respiratory distress syndrome (ARDS), in whom this technique may not be feasible (79). Intra-abdominal pressure may significantly increase during positive pressure mechanical ventilation, and this may strongly affect the distribution of fluid in the abdominal cavity, especially in the presence of hernias.

The most common hernias in peritoneal dialysis patients are umbilical and inguinal at a previous surgical or at catheter incision site. The risk of hernia formation is greater in midline than in paramedian incisions through the rectus muscle (86,87). Another potential area of hernia formation is processus vaginalis, especially in children, when its obliteration after the migration of the testes did not occur (88). Clinical presentation of hernias varies from painless swelling, genital edema, and occasional discovery on physical examination to peritonitis due to incarcerated or perforated bowel (89).

Genital and abdominal wall edema may be due to dialysate leak through a patent processus vaginalis or through the soft tissue from a defect at the catheter-insertion site. Hernias may be associated with these complications. Leaks may also occur through surgical wound due to a peritoneo-fascial defect. If vaginal leak occurs, perforation by the catheter has to be ruled out because leak through the fallopian tubes, although possible, is rare.

Hydrothorax can be caused by the accumulation of dialysis fluid in the pleural cavity. Leak of peritoneal fluid into the pleural space can occur through tendinous defects of diaphragm or through diaphragmatic lymphatics. It can be asymptomatic and detected on routine chest x-ray examination or may be so severe as to cause respiratory failure. Hydrothorax is more common in females and located on the right side.

2. Metabolic Complications

Some metabolic complications such as hyperglycemia may occur with the use of hypertonic solutions. These solutions, by increasing ultrafiltration, may even cause hypernatremia, because sodium moves across peritoneal membrane more slowly than water. Glucose absorbed transperitoneally increases caloric intake: this can be advantageous in ICU patients but can also result in overfeeding, with increased lipogenesis and CO_2 production, which can worsen respiratory failure (79).

Hyponatremia and hyperkalemia are rare complications occurring with the use of inappropriate dialysis solutions, while hypokalemia is observed more frequently. Excessive potassium removal or cellular shift of this cation when acidosis is overcorrected are the principal causes.

In patients with lactic acidosis, lactate-containing solutions can worsen the acidosis when lactic acid cannot be rapidly metabolized. Therefore, solutions containing bicarbonate must be used. Alkalosis may occur as a consequence of overcorrection of acidosis.

Protein and amino acid losses are more important in chronic than in acute conditions, but in ARF patients protein losses in the dialysate (averaging 6–14 g/d or more in severe catabolic patients or when peritonitis is present) and amino acid losses of about 1–3.5 g per day must be taken into account (79).

3. Infectious Complications

Infectious complications of peritoneal dialysis include peritonitis, exit site, and tunnel infections. Penetration of infectious organisms into the peritoneal cavity takes place by several routes. Contamination through the catheter lumen occurs after accidental touch contamination of the connector site; other routes of infection are represented by disconnection of the dialysis tubing, accidental contamination during drug injection into the peritoneal cavity, or use of infected fluid (90).

Transmural or intestinal infections secondary to transcolonic migration of bacteria from intra-abdominal infected viscera (i.e., diverticulitis) are the major causes of gram-negative infections.

Exogenous contamination across the abdominal wall occurs as a consequence of exit site or tunnel infection. Endogenous contaminations via the blood stream may occur particularly in septic patients. Contamination through the female genital tract is also possible.

Gram-positive bacteria account for the majority of peritonitis episodes, while gram-negative bacteria and fungi, mainly *Candida* species, are less commonly involved. The most common gram-positive organism isolated in peritonitis is *Staphylococcus epidermidis*, a coagulase-negative staphylococcus that is present in normal skin flora, while some episodes of peritonitis are due to *S. aureus*, which produces toxins responsible for the severity of the infection.

In peritonitis caused by gram-negative organisms, Enterobacteriacae and *Pseudomonas* species are frequently involved. Anaerobic bacteria are responsible for a relatively low percentage of episodes. Whenever peritoneum is infected by *Bacteroides* and/or *Clostridium* species, bowel perforation and fecal leakage is almost certain; in this situation surgical repair is mandatory (91).

Positive Gram stain culture of peritoneal dialysis fluid, cloudy effluent (>100 cells/mm^3, with 50% or more neutrophils), and presence of symptoms of peritoneal inflammation are the criteria used to diagnose peritonitis. This diagnosis requires the presence of any two of these criteria (92).

Cloudy dialysate is present in 90% of cases, and abdominal pain of variable severity, ranging from mild discomfort to acute pain, is present in 80–95% of cases. Fever is not always present, and it is moderate in most cases; toxic manifestations are unusual. *S. aureus* infection is present, while nausea, vomiting, and diarrhea are present in variable percentage (90).

To treat peritoneal infections it is advisable to carry out a few rapid exchanges to remove inflammatory products. Antibiotic treatment should be started as soon as possible using vancomicin 1–2 g by intraperitoneal or intravenous route for gram-positive cover. An aminoglicoside or Ceftazidime is used in addition to cover intestinal organisms. Appropriate adjustments of therapy are necessary when organisms have been identified and antibiotic sensitivity is known; the duration of therapy varies according to the causative organism.

Catheter removal can be necessary if *Pseudomonas aeruginosa* or fungi are the causative organisms (93,94).

4. Inadequate Fluid and Solute Removal

Because of typical limitations in peritoneal clearances and ultrafiltration, peritoneal dialysis has been for the most part abandoned. It may still be used in children and newborns where vascular access represents a major problem. In adults with ARF, however, this technique does not help in achieving sufficient targets or adequate fluid balance control. This is even more evident in critically ill patients, where hypercatabolism and overhydration may be frequently present.

V. CONCLUSIONS

In conclusion, several complications may affect the efficiency and safety of various renal replacement techniques. Each technique has its own specific problems of either a technical or a clinical nature. When starting renal replacement, all pros and cons for each possible option should be considered. The final choice should be made on the basis of appropriate evaluation of the possible risks to which the patient can be exposed. Of course these are in most cases life-saving procedures, and even in the presence of high risk the procedure must be undertaken to fulfill clinical priorities. Based on our experience we see continuous renal replacement techniques as the most efficient and least risky therapies in the critically ill patient. We should not forget, however, that all procedures are safely carried out only in skilled hands and by expert and trained personnel. Adequate investment in education and training is therefore the key for a significant reduction in technical complications relative to each specific procedure.

REFERENCES

1. Conger JD. Does hemodialysis delay recovery from acute renal failure? Semin Dial 1990; 3:146–148.
2. Schiffl H, Lang SM, Koenig A, Strasser T, Haider MC, Held E. Biocompatible membranes in acute renal failure: a prospective case controlled stury. Lancet 1994; 344:570–572.
3. Hakim RM, Wingard RL, Lawrence P, Parker RA, Schulman G. Use of biocompatible membranes improves outcome and recovery from acute renal failure (abstr). J Am Soc Nephrol 1992; 3:367.
4. Bellomo R, Ronco C. Acute renal failure in the intensive care unit: which treatment is the best? In: Bellomo R, Ronco C, eds. Update in Intensive Care and Emergency Medicine. Heildeberg: Springer-Verlag, 1995: 385–407.
5. Kramer P, Wigger W, Rieger J, Matthaei D, Scheler F. Arteriovenous hemofiltration: a new and simple method for treatment of overhydrated patients resistant to diuretics. Klin Wochenschrift 1977; 55:1121–1122.
6. Ronco C. Continuous renal replacement therapies in the treatment of acute renal failure in intensive care patients. Part 1: Theoretical aspects and techniques. Nephrol Dial Transplant 1994; 9(suppl 4):191–200.
7. Lauer A, Saccaggi A, Ronco C, Belledonne M, Glabman S, Bosch JP. Continuous arterio-venous hemofiltration in the critically ill patient. Ann Intern Med 1983; 99:455–460.
8. Ronco C, Digito A, Dan M. Continuous high flux dialysis (CHFD). In: Vincent JL, ed. Yearbook of Intensive Care and Emergency Medicine. Heidelberg: Springer-Verlag, 1994: 671–677.
9. Ronco C, Fecondini L, Gavioli L, Conz P, Milan M, Dell'Aquila R, Bragantini L, Chiaramonte S, Brendolan A, Crepaldi, Farina M, La Greca G. A new blood module for continuous renal replacement therapies. Int J Art Organs 1993; 1:14–18.
10. Kierdorf H, Leue C, Heintz B, Riehl J, Melzer H, Sieberth HG. Continuous venovenous hemofiltration in acute renal failure: Is a bicarbonate- or lactate-buffered solution better? Contrib Nephrol 1995; 116:38–47.
11. Clark WR, Mueller BA, Alaka KJ, Macias WL. A comparison of metabolic control by continuous and inter-

mittent therapies in acute renal failure. J Am Soc Nephrol 1994; 4:1413–1420.

12. Stork M, Harte WH, Zimmerer E, Inthorn D. Comparison of pump-driven and spontenaous continuous hemofiltration in postoperative acute renal failure. Lancet 1991; 337:452–455.
13. Langenecker SA, Felfemig M, Werba A, Mueller CM, Chiari A, Zimpfer M. Anticoagulation with prostacyclin and heparin during continuous venovenous hemofiltration. Crit Care Med 1994; 22:1774–1781.
14. Millar AB, Armstrong L, van der Lind. Cytokine production and hemofiltration in children undergoing cardiopulmonary bypass. Ann Thorac Surg 1993; 56: 1499–1502.
15. Hakim RM, Wingard RL, Parker RA. Effect of the dialysis membrane in the treatment of patients with acute renal failure. N Engl J Med 1994; 20:1338–1342.
16. Bellomo R, Ronco C. Acute renal failure in the critically ill. In: Bellomo R, Ronco C, eds. Update in Intensive Care and Emergency Medicine. Heidelberg: Springer-Verlag, 1995.
17. Ronco C. Continuous renal replacement therapies for the treatment of acute renal failure in intensive care patients. Clin Nephrol 1993; 4:187–198.
18. Frankenfield DC, Reynolds HN, Wiles CE, Badellino MM, Siegel JN. Urea removal during continuous hemofiltration. Crit Care Med 1994; 22:407–412.
19. Bellomo R, Ronco C. Acute renal failure in the ICU: adequacy of dialysis and the case for continuous therapies. Nephrol Dial Transplant 1996; 11:424–428.
20. Daugirdas JG. Dialysis hypotension: a hemodynamic analysis. Kidney Int 1991; 39:233–246.
21. Michel CC. Fluid movement through capillary walls. In: Handbook of Physiology. Bethesda, MD: American Physiology Society, 1984:375–400.
22. Koomans HA, Geers AB, Dorhout Mees EJ. Plasma volume recovery after ultrafiltration in patients with chronic renal failure. Kidney Int 1984; 26:848–854.
23. Fleming SJ, Wilkinson JS, Greenwood RN, Aldridge C, Baker LRI, Cattle WR. Effect of dialysate composition on intercompartment fluid shift. Kidney Int 1987; 32: 267–275.
24. Daugirdas JT, Purandare VV, Ing TS, Chen WT, Popli S, Hano JE, Klok MA. Ultrafiltration hemodynamics in an animal model: effect of a decreasing plasma sodium level. Trans Am Soc Artif Intern Organs 1984; 30:603–609.
25. Stiller S, Thommes A, Konigs F, Schallenberg U, Mann H. Characteristic profiles of circulating blood volume during dialysis therapy. Trans Am Soc Artif Intern Organs 1989; 35:530–532.
26. London GM, Safar ME, Simon AC, Alexandre JM, Levenson JA, Weiss YA. Total effective compliance, cardiac output and fluid volumes in essential hypertension. Circulation 1978; 57:995–999.
27. London GM, Guerin AP, Bouthier JD, London AM, Safar ME. Cardiopulmonary blood volume and plasma renin activity in normal and hypertensive humans. Am J Physiol 1985; 249:H807–815.
28. Bennett TD, Wyss CR, Scher AM. Changes in vascular capacity in awake dogs in response to carotid sinus occlusion and administration of catecholamines. Circ Res 1984; 55:440–453.
29. Hirsch AT, Levenson DJ, Cutler SS, Dzau VJ, Creager Ma. Regional vascular response to prolonged body negative pressure in normal subjects. Am J Physiol 1989; 257:H219–225.
30. Rothe CF. Reflex control of veins and vascular capacitance. Physiol Rev 1983; 63:1281–1342.
31. London G, Marchais S, Guerin AP. Blood pressure control in chronic hemodialysis patient. In: Jacobs C, Kjellstrand CM, Koch KM, Winchester JF, eds. Replacement of Renal Function by Dialysis. Dordrecht: Kluwer Academic Publishers, 1996:966–989.
32. Zoccali C, Ciccarelli M, Maggiore Q. Defective reflex control of heart rate in dialysis patients. Evidence for an afferent autonomic lesion. Clin Sci 1982; 63:285–292.
33. Chaignon M, Chen WT, Tarazi RC, Nakamoto S, Bravo EL. Blood pressure response to hemodialysis. Hypertension 1981; 3:333–339.
34. Kirkendol PL, Robie NW, Gonzalez FM, Devia CJ. Cardiac and vascular effects of infused sodium acetate in dogs. Trans AM Soc Artif Intern Organs 1978; 24: 714–717.
35. Wizemann V, Suetanto R, Thormann J, Lubbecke F, Kramer W. Effects of acetate on left ventricular function in hemodialysis patients. Nephron 1993; 64:101–105.
36. Leunissen KML, Hoorntje SJ, Fiers HA. Acetate versus bicarbonate dialysis in critically ill patients. Nephron 1986; 42:146–151.
37. Daugirdas JT, Nawab ZM. Acetate relaxation in isolated vascular smooth muscle. Kidney Int 1987; 32:39–46.
38. Hsu CH, Swartz RD, Somermeyer MG, Raj A. Bicarbonate hemodialysis: influence on plasma refilling and hemodynamic stability. Nephron 1984; 38:202–208.
39. Maggiore Q, Pizzarelli F, Zoccali C, Sisca S, Nicolo F, Parlongo S. Effect of extracorporeal blood cooling on dialytic arterial hypotension. Proc Eur Dial Transplant Assoc 1981; 18:597–602.
40. Levy FL, Grayburn PA, Foulks CJ, Brickner ME, Henrich WL. Improved left ventricular contractility with cool temperature hemodialysis. Kidney Int 1992; 41: 961–965.
41. Henderson LW, Koch KM, Dinarello CA, Shaldon S. Hemodialysis hypotension: the interleukin hypothesis. Blood Purif 1988; 1:3–8.
42. Chenoweth DE, Cheung AK, Henderson LW. Anaphylatoxin formation during hemodialysis. Effects of different hemodialyzer membranes. Kidney Int 1983; 24: 764–769.

43. Bingel N, Lonnemann G, Koch KM, Dinarello CA, Shaldon S. Enhancement of in-vitro human interleukin-1 production by sodium acetate. Lancet 1987; 1:14–16.
44. Laude-Sharp M, Caroff M, Simard L, Pusineri C, Kazatchkine MD, Haeffner-Cavaillon N. Induction of IL-1 during hemodialysis: transmembrane passage of intact endotoxin (LPS). Kidney Int 1990; 38:1089–1094.
45. Beasley D, Brenner BM. Role of nitric oxide in hemodialysis hypotension. Kidney Int 1992; 42(suppl 38): S96–100.
46. Maeda K, Fujita Y, Shinzato T, Morita H, Kobayakawa H, Takai I. Mechanism of dialysis-induced hypotension. Trans Am Soc Artif Intern Organs 1989; 35:245–247.
47. Ritz E, Ruffmann K, Rambausek M. Dialysis hypotension. Is it related to diastolic left ventricular malfunction? Nephrol Dial Transplant 1987; 2:293–297.
48. Santoro A, Mancini E, Spongano M, Rossi M, Paolini F, Zucchelli P. A hemodynamic study of hypotension during hemodialysis using electrical bioimpedance cardiography. Nephrol Dial Transplant 1990; (suppl 1): 147–153.
49. Mark AL. The Bezold-Jarisch replex revisited: clinical implications of inhibitory reflexes originating in the heart. J Am Coll Cardiol 1983; 1:90–97.
50. Mujais SK, Ing T, Kjellstrand C. Acute complication of hemodialysis and their prevention and treatment. In: Jacobs C, Kjellstrand CM, Koch KM, Winchester JF, eds. Replacement of Renal Function by Dialysis. Dordrecht: Kluwer Academic Publishers, 1996:688–725.
51. Iida N, Tsubakihara Y, Shirai D, Imada A, Suzuki M. Treatment of dialysis-induced hypotension with L-threo-3,4-dihydroxyphenylserine. Nephrol Dial Transplant 1994; 9:1130–1135.
52. Cruz DN, Mahnensmith RL, Perazzella MA. Intradialytic hypotension: Is midodrine beneficial in symptomatic hemodialysis patients? Am J Kidney Dis 1997; 30:772–779.
53. Lindberg JS, Copley JB, Melton K, Wade CE, Abrams J, Goode D. Lysine vasopressin in the treatment of refractory hemodialysis-induced hypotension. Am J Nephrol 1990; 10:269–263.
54. Gong R, Lindberg J, Abrams J, Whitaker WR, Wade CE, Gouge S. Comparison of hypertonic saline solutions and dextran in dialysis-induced hypotension. J Am Soc Nephrol 1993; 3:1801–1812.
55. Bergonzi G, Paties C, Vassallo G, Zangrandi A, Poisetti PG, Ballocchi S, Fontana F, Scarpioni L. Dextran deposits in tissue of patients undergoing hemodialysis. Nephrol Dial Transplant 1990; 5:54–58.
56. Cosentino F, Chaff C, Piedmonte M. Risk factors influencing survival in ICU acute renal failure. Nephrol Dial Transplant 1994; 9(suppl 4):179–182.
57. Mehta R, McDonald B, Gabbai F, Pahl M, Farkas A, Pascual M, Fowler V. Effect of biocompatible membranes on outcome of acute renal failure (abstr). J Am Soc Nephrol 1996; 7:1457.
58. Jacobs C. Membrane biocompatibility in the treatment of acute renal failure: what is the evidence in 1996? Nephrol Dial Transplant 1997; 12:38–42.
59. Shaldon S, Vianken J. Biocompatibility: Is it a relevant consideration for today's hemodialysis? Int J Artif Organs 1996; 19:201–214.
60. Hanid MA, Davies M, Mellon PJ. Clinical monitoring of intracerebral pressure in fulminant hepatic failure. Gut 1980; 21:866–869.
61. Davenport A, Davison AM, Will EJ. Are changes in intracranial pressure during intermittent machine hemofiltration dependent upon membrane biocompatibility? Int J Artif Organs 1989; 12:703–707.
62. Davenport A, Will EJ, Davison AM. Effect of renal replacement therapy on patients with combined acute renal and fulminant hepatic failure. Kidney Int 1993; 43(suppl 41):245–251.
63. Hakim RM, Breillatt J, Lazarus JM, Port FK. Complement activation and hypersensitivity reactions to dialysis membranes. N Engl J Med 1984; 34:878–882.
64. Oh MS, Uribarri J, Dal Monte ML, Heneghan WE, Kee CS, Friedman EA, Carroll H. A mechanism of hypoxemia during hemodialysis: consumption of CO_2 in metabolism of acetate. Am J Nephrol 1985; 5:366–372.
65. Sherlock J, Ledwith J, Letteri J. Hypoventilation and hypoxemia during hemodialysis: reflex response to removal of CO_2 across the dialyzer. Trans Am Soc Artif Intern Organs 1977; 23:406–409.
66. Craddox PR, Fehr J, Brigham KL, Kronenberg RS, Jacob HS. Complement and leukocyte-mediated pulmonary dysfunction in hemodialysis. N Engl J Med 1977; 296:770–778.
67. Kennedy AC, Linton AL, Eaton JC. Urea levels in cerebrospinal fluid after haemodialysis. Lancet 1962; 1: 410–415.
68. Arieff AI, Guisado R, Massry SG, Lazarowitz VC. Central nervous system pH in uremia and the effects of hemodialysis. J Clin Invest 1976; 58:306–315.
69. Lemke HD, Grassmann A, Vienken J, Shaldon S. Biocompatibility: clinical aspects. In: Jacobs C, Kjellstrand CM, Koch KM, Winchester JF, eds. Replacement of Renal Function by Dialysis. Dordrecht: Kluwer Academic Publishers, 1996:734–749.
70. Ward DM, Mehta RL. Extracorporeal management of acute renal failure patients at high risk of bleeding. Kidney Int 1993; 43(suppl 41):237–244.
71. Mannucci PM, Remuzzi G, Pusineri F, Lombardi R, Valsecchi C, Mecca G, Zimmerman TS. The amino 8-D-arginine vasopressin shortens the bleeding time in uremia. N Engl J Med 1983; 308:8–12.
72. Viganò G, Gaspari F, Locatelli M, Pusini F, Bonati M, Remuzzi G. Dose-effect and pharmacokinetics of estrogens given to correct bleeding time in uremia. Kidney Int 1988; 34:853–858.
73. Jansen PA, Jubelirer SJ, Weninstein MS, Deykin D. Treatment of bleeding tendency in uremia with cryoprecipitate. N Engl J Med 1980; 303:1318–1322.

74. Van Kuijk WHM, Mulder WA, Hanff GA, Leunissen KML. Influence of changes in ionized calcium on cardiovascular reactivity during hemodialysis. Clin Nephrol 1997; 47:190–196.
75. Nishimura M, Nakanishi T, Yasui A, Tsuji Y, Kunishige H, Hirabayashi M, Takahashi H, Yoshimura M. Serum calcium increases the risk of arrhythmias during acetate hemodialysis. Am J Kidney Dis 1992; 19:149–155.
76. Weiss LD, Van MK. The applications of hyperbaric oxygen therapy in emergency medicine. Am J Emerg Med 1992; 10:558–564.
77. Dunbar EM, Fox R, Watson B, Akrill P. Successful late treatment of venous air embolism with hyperbaric oxygen. Postgrad Med J 1990; 66:469–475.
78. Freeman RM, Lawton RL, Chamberlain MA. Hard-water syndrome. N Engl J Med 1967; 276:113–118.
79. Lameire N. Principles of peritoneal dialysis and its applicaton in acute renal failure. In: Ronco C, Bellomo R, eds. Critical Care Nephrology. Dordrecht: Kluwer Academic Publishers, 1998:1357–1371.
80. Ash SR, Bever SL. Peritoneal dialysis for acute renal failure: the safe, effective and low-cost modality. Adv Renal Replacement Ther 1995; 2:160–163.
81. Steiner RW. Continuous equilibration peritoneal dialysis. Perit Dial Int 1989; 9:5–7.
82. Bargman JM. Non-infectious complications of peritoneal dialysis. In: Gokal R, Nolph KD, eds. The Textbook of Peritoneal Dialysis. Dordrecht: Kluwer Academic Publishers, 1994:555–570.
83. Gotloib L, Mines M, Garmizo L. Hemodynamic effects of increasing intra-abdominal pressure in peritoneal dialysis. Perit Dial Bull 1981; 1:41–45.
84. Twardowski ZJ, Prowant BF, Nolph KD. High volume, low frequency continuous ambulatory peritoneal dialysis. Kidney Int 1983; 23:64–69.
85. Twardowski ZJ, Khanna R, Nolph KD. Intra-abdominal pressures during natural activities in patients treated with continuous ambulatory peritoneal dialysis. Nephron 1986; 44:129–133.
86. Apostolidis NS, Tzardis PJ, Manouras AJ, Kosinidou MD, Katiztzoglou AN. The incidence of post-operative hernia as related to the site of insertion of permanent peritoneal catheter. Am Surg 1988; 54:318–322.
87. Gokal R, Ash S, Helfrich GB. Peritoneal catheter and exit-site practices: toward a optimum peritoneal access. Perit Dial Int 1993; 1-3:29–33.
88. Tank ES, Hatch DA. Hernias complicating CAPD in children. J Pediatr Surg 1986; 21:41–46.
89. Gigenis G, Khanna R, Mattews R, Oreopoulos DG. Abdominal hernias in patients undergoing CAPD. Perit Dial Bull 1982; 2:115–120.
90. Keane WF, Vas SI: Peritonitis. In: Gokal R, Nolph KD, eds. The Textbook of Peritoneal Dialysis. Dordrecht: Kluwer Academic Publishers, 1994:473–485.
91. Vas SI. Microbiological aspects of chronic ambulatory peritoneal dialysis. Kidney Int 1983; 23:83–93.
92. Pierratos A. Peritoneal dialysis glossary. Perit Dial Bull 1984; 4:2–10.
93. Keane WF, Everett ED, Golper T. Peritoneal dialysis related peritonitis—treatment recommendations 1993 update. Perit Dial Int 1993; 13:14–25.
94. Fabris A, Chiaramonte S, La Greca G, Feriani M, Ronco C, Brendolan A, Bragantini L, Conz P, Pellanda MV, Crepaldi C. Fungal peritonitis. In: La Greca G, Chiaramonte S, Fabris A, Feriani M, Ronco C, eds. Peritoneal Dialysis. Milan: Wichtig Editore, 1988:73–76.

36

Complications of Acute and Chronic Dialysis in Children

Timothy E. Bunchman
The University of Michigan, Ann Arbor, Michigan

Norma J. Maxvold
Pediatric Critical Care Medicine, The University of Michigan Health System, Ann Arbor, Michigan

This chapter is written to help troubleshoot problems arising in children with acute renal failure (ARF), end-stage renal disease (ESRD), or on dialysis. When a problem occurs, the reader needs to evaluate the different causes that could result in the clinical problem and implement a plan of action to correct it (Table 1). A typical dialysis prescription for a routine treatment is given at the beginning of the dialysis sections. The typical prescription by no means is the only way to dialyze a child using that modality but is a common prescription use for that modality.

I. PERITONEAL DIALYSIS

A. Chronic Peritoneal Dialysis

Once stable, the goal would be to attain a KT/V of ~2 for maximal benefit of dialysis. A typical prescription would be glucose concentration based upon ultrafiltration needs (remembering that many children have high urine output), volume of dialysate delivered per pass of ~40 ml/kg/pass or 1100 ml/m^2/pass, with a last fill volume of 50% of volume per pass. Often children require additional midday passes (especially if anuric) for optimal clearance and best chance for growth. Heparin use (250–500 units/L) would be used on a PRN basis based upon fibrin content of the dialysate (1).

B. Acute Peritoneal Dialysis

A typical prescription would be glucose concentration based upon ultrafiltration needs, volume per pass 10–15 ml/kg/pass, heparin 250–500 units/L of dialysate, and frequency of cycles based upon ultrafiltration and solute clearance needs but frequently every hour (2).

C. Complications of Peritoneal Dialysis

Exit site leaks occur in children for multiple reasons. The most common would be using the catheter too soon after placement of the peritoneal dialysis (PD) catheter. Each center has its own experience with break-in and the data to date do not suggest the optimal rate but clearly that final filling volumes of 30–40 ml/kg/pass or 900–1200 ml/m^2/pass should not be achieved until 3–4 weeks after the catheter has been in place. Additional reasons for exit site leak would be that of poor wound healing, which would be related to malnutrition, tissue edema, chronic use of steroids, or exit site infections. Therefore, inspection of the exit site would be necessary.

Peritonitis occurs in chronic PD at a rate of between 0.6 and 1.6 episodes per year per child. It is most commonly related to bacterial peritonitis, although other causes could be chemical peritonitis either secondary to eosinophilic reaction to the catheter (usually after

Table 1 Complications of Dialysis and Possible Causes

Complication	Possible causes
Peritoneal Dialysis—Chronic	
Leak at exit site	Early use of catheter
	Poor wound healing/nutrition
	Exit site infection
Peritonitis	Bacterial
	Fungal
	Chemical (menses, eosinophilic)
Diminished serum proteins	Protein/Immunoglobulin losses
	Inadequate protein intake
	Increase in permeability of pediatric/infant peritoneal membrane
Hyponatremia	Sodium content of dialysate 132 mEq/L
	Majority of children ≤10 years of age have urinary sodium wasting due to renal dysplasia
Inadequate dialysis	Inadequate dialysate exposure
	Impaired peritoneal transport
	Relatively large dead space of tubing in automated dialysis machines relative to small volume of dialysis delivered
Dialysate flow inhibition	Laying on the catheter
	Catheter dislodged (acute access)
	Fibrin clot inhibiting inflow or outflow
Peritoneal Dialysis—Acute	
Metabolic acidosis	Inadequate dialysis (see above)
	Lactate based solution
Ventilation problems	Hydrothorax
	Increase in intraperitoneal pressure causing ventilation resistance
Hemodialysis—Chronic/Acute	
Hypotension	Excessive ultrafiltration
	Large extracorporeal circuit relative to intravascular blood volume
	Dialysis membrane reaction
Dysequilibrium	Rapid solute clearance with a rapid decrease in BUN, rapid increase in sodium, or both
Inadequate clearance	Inadequate blood flow
	Inadequate time on dialysis
	Recirculation due to poor access
	Small of dialysis membrane or (reuse) protein layering causing lack of expose surface area of membrane
Metabolic acidosis	Inadequate dialysis (see above)
	Lactate-based solution
Bleeding	Systemic over anticoagulation
Hypothermia	Dialysate temperature improperly set—worse in infants with high body surface heat loss
Hemofiltration	
Hypotension	Excessive ultrafiltration/inaccurate ultrafiltration monitor
	Large extracorporeal circuit relative to intravascular blood volume
	Dialysis membrane reaction
Hypothermia	Heat loss in children (worse in infants with high body surface heat loss) and lack of warming device in dialysate/blood circuit
Inadequate clearance	Inadequate blood flow
	Recirculation due to poor access
	Too small of hemofilter or protein layering causing lack of expose surface area of hemofilter
Metabolic acidosis	Inadequate dialysis (see above)
	Lactate-based solution
Bleeding	Systemic overanticoagulation

Table 1 Continued

Complication	Possible causes
Low serum protein	Loss of amino acids and nutritional components across hemofilter
Hemofiltration on ECMO (in addition to what is seen with standard hemofiltration)	
Excessive clearance	Relatively high blood flow relative to small body surface area
Metabolic alkalosis	Bicarbonate-based solution in addition to carbogen added to ECMO circuit
Access Complications—External	
Inadequate blood flow from catheter	"Arterial" side up against a wall of a blood vessel
	Blood clot in access
	Low intravascular blood volume
	Extrinsic compression upon catheter/vessel (seen with femoral-based access abdominal organomegally or tense ascites)
	Catheter kinked at insertion site
	Child moving (common with femoral based catheters)
	Access too small
Inadequate blood flow back to patient	Blood clot in access
	High intrathoracic pressure (seen when patient on high-frequency ventilation)
Subclavian stenosis	Placement of large hemodialysis catheter at subclavian site instead of internal jugular
Access line sepsis	Introduction of bacteria at the time of handling access
	Exit site infection
Access Complications—Internal	
Inadequate blood flow from access	"Arterial" thrombosis or stenosis
	Low intravascular blood volume
	Extrinsic compression upon vessel
Inadequate blood flow back to patient	Blood clot in access
	Venous stenosis "downstream" from return site
Electrolyte Disturbances When Using Nonstandard Dialysis Solution (PD or HF)	
	Incorrect components of dialysate added together
Complications of Acute Renal Failure in Children	
Mortality related to cause of ARF	
Fluid and electrolyte disturbances	
Complications of End-Stage Renal Disease in Children	
Renal osteodystrophy	Multifactorial due to all components above in addition to abnormal growth hormone/insulin like growth factor axis
Metabolic acidosis	
Inadequate nutrition	
Volume depletion	
Anemia	
Growth inhibition	
Complications in Children Requiring RRT from Inborn Error of Metabolism	
Mortality related to cause of ARF	
Fluid and electrolyte disturbances	
Standard dialysis solution not optimal due to risks of hypophosphatemia, lactic acidosis	
Complications Unique to Specific Age Groups with ESRD	
Neonate/Infants:	
Higher incidence of multiple congenital anomalies with morbidity/mortality related to multiple organ dysfunction	
Children:	
Attainment of adequate dialysis to support the growing child	
Adolescence:	
Lack of compliance to medical regimen	

placement) or in adolescent females during the time of menses. Retrograde menses can occur by the fallopian tube causing intermittent bloody dialysate. Finally, fungal peritonitis can occur in children and is often related to chronic use of antibiotics or is associated timewise to placement of a gastro-feeding tube. Bacterial peritonitis is usually treated with specified antibiotics, whereas the general treatment of fungal peritonitis should be directed toward removal of the catheter with the potential use of systemic antifungal agents. The return of the peritoneum after fungal peritonitis is in the range of 30–40% (3).

Protein loss can occur in children on chronic PD. This is secondary to increased permeability of the pediatric or infant peritoneal membrane (compared to adults) with a high loss of proteins and immunoglobulins, which may increase the risk of peritonitis. These losses may be additive in children who have inadequate protein intake. Necessary protein intake could be 2–3 g/kg/day and in babies up to 4 g/kg/day in order to offset the loss of proteins across the peritoneal membrane (4).

Hyponatremia can occur in children on PD primarily related to the relatively low dialysate sodium (132 mEq/L) that is used in all standard dialysate solutions. This is usually additive in children who often have salt wasting nephropathy. Seventy percent of children less than 10 years of age have renal dysplasia or a component thereof causing sodium and water wasting. The solution for this is to increase the oral sodium intake or (rarely) add sodium to the dialysate sodium. The latter should be avoided, for an increased risk of peritonitis could occur every time a bag of dialysate is invaded (1,5).

Inadequate dialysis can occur in children for multiple reasons. In the smaller infant on automated dialysate solution, the dead space of the tubing may be 40–50 mL. Therefore, children who are on an automated system with a 40 mL dead space who receive less than 400 cc (10 times) of dialysate solution may have the equivalent of recirculation secondary to dead space of the tubing. Therefore, the dead space of the tubing must be taken into account relative to the dialysate delivered volume. Additionally, other causes of inadequate dialysis are either related to dialysis peritoneal membrane permeability defect or inadequate dialysate exposure. A simple PET test can be used to assess clearance across the membrane. At a 3–4 hour PET test, 90% of the BUN and 80% of the creatinine should have come across the membrane as a measure of dialysate adequacy. If not, peritoneal membrane failure may be occurring. Further, in the growing child, often a measured KT/V of 1.8–2.5 is required for adequate growth.

Identification of the other major cause for inadequate dialysis is based on chemistry criteria and is often related to inadequate dialysis exposure, which equates to inadequate time on dialysis. This can be adjusted be higher peritoneal volumes, potential use of tidal PD, use of extra midday passes, or longer time on dialysis on the cycler machine at night (6).

Dialysate flow inhibition can occur in children due to kinking of the catheter at the time of either inflow or outflow. This kinking is usually related to the child rolling over on it or kinking of the tubing at the inflow or outflow. Other differential causes of dialysate flow inhibition are related to fiber clot formation, which could be a sign of peritonitis, either chemical or bacterial.

D. Acute Complications

Metabolic acidosis can be related to either inadequate dialysis (see above) or metabolic acidosis and the concomitant use of a lactate-based dialysate solution. No commercially made bicarbonate solution is available for acute PD, and therefore all the solutions to date contain lactate. Often children who have hepatic dysfunction or who are septic have an underlying metabolic acidosis secondary to lactate production. The use of a lactate-based dialysate solution may exacerbate this solution. The substitution of a bicarbonate-based solution as an alternative solution (Table 2) may allow for correction of this metabolic acidosis.

Ventilation problems can occur in children with either acute or chronic dialysis. Such problems can be related to hydrothorax or to a change in intraperitoneal pressure causing ventilation resistance. The incidence

Table 2 Peritoneal Dialysis Solutions

Constituents	Standard peritoneal dialysis solution	Specialized bicarbonate solution
Dextrose (g/L)	15, 25, 42.5	15,25,42.5
Sodium (mEq/L)	132	92–100[a]
Chloride (mEq/L)	92	92–100
Lactate (mEq/L)	40	0
Sodium bicarbonate (mEq/L)	0	40[a]
Potassium (mEq/L)	0–5[b]	0–5[b]
Calcium	3.5	2–4
Magnesium (mEq/L)	0.5	0.5

[a]Total sodium needs to be physicological (130–145 mEq/L).
[b]Standard potassium bath is zero, but up to 5 mEq/L may be added.

of hydrothorax in children on acute PD is in the 7–10% range (7). This can be seen as a loss of ultrafiltration or true change in ventilation mechanics. Further, in children on PD at even small volumes, changes in peritoneal pressures may cause ventilation resistance resulting in a change in pulmonary resistance (8). Attention to this with potentially more frequent passes or less ultrafiltration or more time on dialysis may be necessary to avoid the change in ventilation.

II. HEMODIALYSIS

A. Chronic Hemodialysis

Like in PD the goal would be a KT/V of ~2 for optimal dialysis and growth. A typical prescription would be a blood circuit volume not to exceed 10% of the child's intravascular blood volume with a dialysis membrane surface area proportional to the child. The blood flow rate is 4–5 ml/kg/min, duration of treatment is 3–4 h/treatment 3–4 times per week, heparin load of 20 units/kg/dose and an infusion of 10–20 units/kg/h, with a dialysate rate of 30 L/h. The potassium bath would be 2 mEq/dL and the calcium one 3.5 mEq/dL. Ultrafiltration needs would be based upon dry weight, but an average of 0.2 ml/kg/min of ultrafiltration would occur (9).

B. Acute Hemodialysis

Procedure would be similar to chronic treatment with more attention to risk of dialysis equilibrium and excessive ultrafiltration. Heparin use is based upon risk of heparin at that time; potassium and calcium contents of the dialysate bath are dependent upon the needs of the child.

C. Complications—Acute or Chronic

Hypotension on hemodialysis (HD) may be due to different causes related to either excessive ultrafiltration, large extracorporeal circuit relative to intravascular blood volume, or potential of dialysate membrane reaction (9,10). All HD machines to date have a ultrafiltration monitor, yet variation may be ±100 mL/h. In larger patients this is insignificant, but in a small child who may only have a 800 cc intravascular blood volume, being off by 200–300 cc (100 cc variation per hour × 3 h) will result in shock. Therefore, understanding the limits of the ultrafiltration monitor and infusing back saline at a rate matching the possible ultrafiltration monitor error is necessary to avoid hypotension due to excessive ultrafiltration. Extracorporeal blood volume is important to know relative to the patient's intravascular blood volume. A child weighing less than 10 kg will have an intravascular blood volume of 80 mL/kg, while larger children will be 70 mL/kg. The rule of thumb is that no greater than 10% of the blood volume should be extracorporeal in order to avoid hypotension. Therefore, an 8 kg child with an intravascular blood volume of 640 cc should have a 64 cc circuit or less in order to avoid blood priming. If blood priming is necessary, the risk of complications relating to hyperkalemic bolus from the blood bank blood, antigen exposure with higher incidence of antibody production effecting transplant options, as well as increased infection can occur. Therefore, attention to the extracorporeal circuit and work with the local HD companies is important to minimize extracorporeal blood volume. To date, the smallest extracorporeal blood volume for chronic HD is 38 cc in order to allow for infants on chronic dialysis at 4 kg or greater to avoid blood priming each time. Finally, dialysate membrane reactions can occur causing anaphylaxis and secondary hypotension in children (10). While this incidence is rare, it can be related to some of the less biocompatible membranes. Therefore, attention to the first run for any potential risk of anaphylaxis is necessary to avoid this problem.

Dialysis dysequilibrium can occur in children but is preventable. This is often related to rapid changes in solute usually due to a rapid drop in blood urea nitrogen (BUN) or a rapid rise in sodium or a combination of both. Therefore, if a child has a high BUN (usually >100 mg/dL), an inadequate or inefficient run may be necessary in order to avoid dropping the BUN too rapidly. A "first run" protocol is used in many programs to avoid a rapid change in BUN and resultant dialysis dysequilibrium. On a standard HD run, two thirds of urea is usually cleared over a 3-hour treatment; the first-run protocol usually results in only about a 50% clearance. This inefficient run can be the result of (a) a smaller dialysis membrane than normal, (b) "current" dialysate lines as opposed to countercurrent, or (c) lower blood flow rates in the 2 mL/kg/min blood flow rate.

Inadequate clearance is usually related to inadequate blood flow, which may be dependent on the access, inadequate time on dialysis, recirculation due to poor access or too small of a dialysis membrane, or potential protein layering across the membrane (11). Assessment of blood flow is important. Standard blood flow is 4–5 mL/kg/min on chronic or acute HD. Time on dialysis relates to KT/V, which for chronic treatment should be

1.8–2.5 for optimal growth and dialysis adequacy. Recirculation due to poor access is not uncommon in patients with externalized duel lumen venous access. Therefore, if that is a concern, a formal recirculation study assessing both the "venous" into "arterial" as well as the peripheral BUN is necessary. Recirculation should be ≤5% in order to give adequate dialysis. The access placement may impact upon recirculation, for in a small vessel or in someone whose diminished cardiac output the risk of recirculation may increase due to poor blood flow. Finally, if the blood flow rate is adequate and time on dialysis is adequate, one should then consider whether one needs to go to a larger dialysis membrane. To date there is no comparison of high-efficiency versus normal-efficiency dialysis membranes, but intuitively high-efficiency dialysis membranes should give better clearance.

Metabolic acidosis is an uncommon complication but can still be seen on HD. This is usually secondary to two different causes: inadequate dialysis (see above) or use of an acetate- or lactate-based solution. Historically, acetate was used as a buffer for HD, but now bicarbonate solution is the accepted solution. Some bicarbonate adjustment can occur in most machinery with the level of roughly 30–50 mEq/L, although standard bicarbonate of 40 mEq/L is usually adequate.

Bleeding is a rare complication that can occur during either chronic or acute dialysis. It is usually related to systemic coagulation problems of the patient themselves or secondary to systemic anticoagulation. If one is using heparin for either acute of chronic HD, then the use of a bedside clotting monitor may be necessary (12). Activated clotting (ACT) can be used in order to target an ACT level of between 150–200. Heparin bolus of 10–20 units/kg/dose and then 10–20 units/kg/hour infusion may be necessary for a target ACT of 150–200. Adjustments need to be made based on those ranges if a monitor is used.

Hypothermia is a rare complication but can be seen on HD (13). This is more common in the smaller child, usually secondary to large body surface area with body surface heat loss as well as a large extracorporeal blood volume with heat loss. Therefore, with children who are at higher risk for hypothermia (usually ≤20 kg), turning the dialysate temperature up to 40°C may be necessary.

III. HEMOFILTRATION

A typical hemofiltration (HF) prescription would be a blood flow of 4–5 mL/kg/min, the use of either pre- or postfilter replacement fluid or countercurrent dialysate at 2000 mL/h/1.73 m^2 (corrected for body surface area), a hemofilter circuit volume of less then 10% of the intravascular blood volume, and a goal of 0.5–2 mL/kg/h of ultrafiltration. Anticoagulation would be either none, citrate, or heparin (load of 10–20 units/kg/dose and a infusion of 10–20 units/kg/hr) with a goal ACT of 170–200 seconds (14,15).

A. Complications on Hemofiltration

The complications of hemofiltration (HF) are similar to those seen on HD but have some specific uniqueness. To date, only very few treatment centers have ultrafiltration monitors and the goal on HF is solute clearance as well as ultrafiltration. Hemodynamic stability will relate to the accurate control of ultrafiltration as well as intravascular/extravascular volumes.

Hypotension can be related to excessive ultrafiltration, inadequate replacement infusion (on pre- or post-hemofilter infusion), or to large extracorporeal blood volume relative to intravascular blood volume or related to blood dialysis membrane reaction. The newer machines (e.g., Prisma, Cobe, Lakewood, CO; BM-25, Baxter Corp., of Deerfield, IL) do have ultrafiltration monitors on them. In addition (with pre- or postfilter replacement fluid) the infusion system (often regular intravenous pumps) may not be 100% accurate for infusion volume when not using the new machine. Therefore, an additive effect of excessive ultrafiltration as well as inadequate infusion may have a tendency to affect intravascular volume integrity. In smaller children who are more at risk for this, potential weighing of infusion and ultrafiltrate bags may be necessary. In HF machines that do not have ultrafiltration monitors, infusion pumps are often used for ultrafiltration control. Infusion pumps (IV pumps) may have inaccuracy rates of 4–30%, therefore attention to this potential complication is necessary (16).

The extracorporeal blood volume in the circuit is important to note. Often children on HF are hemodynamically less stable than those on HD. Therefore, again using the 10% rule, if one has ≥10% blood volume extracorporeal than potential blood, priming may be necessary. The complications of blood priming include hyperkalemic bolus, which is often seen with blood bank blood, as well as hyperviscosity, seen with standard blood. Therefore, dilution with 1:1 saline is often necessary to give an infusion rate on blood priming of roughly a hematocrit of 40.

Dialysis membrane reactions are a rare complication but can be seen on HF. As with all other biocompatible membranes, it is important to make sure that there is no anaphylaxis reaction to the membrane.

A final but rare complication of hypertension on HF is a blood leak. This can occur at the pump circuit or at the membrane itself; therefore, attention to any blood leaking is necessary.

Hypothermia is a common complication seen on HF of children (17). To date, there is only makeshift machinery to allow for thermal control of either dialysate or blood in children on HF. Therefore, realizing that these children often develop systemic hypothermia is important. The use of overhead warmers, warm dialysate, blood warmer, or dialysate warmer may be necessary to maintain normal thermal conditions. In a patient on HF who has hypothermia, this may mask a temperature spike that could be a sign of sepsis; therefore, attention to the hemodynamic stability is important in this setting.

Inadequate dialysis can be seen on hemofiltration. This is often secondary to inadequate blood flow, recirculation due to poor access, inadequate dialysate/infusion solution use, or, finally, a too small hemofilter or potentially protein layering across the hemofilter. To date there are no data about adequate blood flow on HF. Our standard has been 4–5 mL/kg/min, allowing for a "venous" pressure of roughly ≤200. Recirculation on HF is probably less of a problem as compared to HD because of its continuous nature. If one is trying to clear high BUN and is not getting adequate clearance, then potential recirculation evaluation may be necessary. To date there is no optimal dose of dialysate or infusion fluid to be used. Studies by this group have shown that a blood flow rate of 4–5 mL/kg/min with a surface area membrane of 0.3 m^2 using either a countercurrent dialysate solution or a prefilter infusate solution equivalent to 2 L/h adjusted to 1.7 m^2 body surface area will give an optimal BUN clearance of 30 mL/h (14). Therefore, this has become the accepted local standard of care for clearance. If inadequate clearance is seen on HF, potential adjustment of the countercurrent dialysis or the infusion flow to that level will be necessary. Further, studies to date at this institution show that at equal rates of countercurrent dialysis or infusate solution, identical BUN is identified, therefore, it is our opinion that it makes no difference in the mode of infusing solution or dialysis for BUN clearance.

Finally, a surface membrane that is too small may be responsible for inadequate clearance. This is less of a problem on HF because of the porosity seen in these filters. Ofter after these filters have been on for 2–3 days, protein layering can occur across the membrane, decreasing the surface area membrane that allows for dialysis. If one is concerned about the lack of free membrane for clearance, the simultaneous "arterial" (prehemofilter) BUN as well as an ultrafiltrate BUN can be done. If they are essentially equal, then adequate surface area is available. If the ultrafiltrate urea is markedly less than the plasma "arterial" urea, then changing the filter would be necessary.

Metabolic acidosis can be seen in children on HF. It can be related either to inadequate dialysis (see above), metabolic acidosis generated by the patient that is not being overcome due to inadequate solute clearance, or the use of a nonbicarbonate solution. To date, there is no standard bicarbonate solution used for HF, yet many programs use a bicarbonate solution to avoid using lactate-based solutions (Table 3). The alternative would be the use of a lactate-based solution and a continuous infusion of bicarbonate. Studies to date in adults have shown that lactate-based and bicarbonate-based solutions show similar clearance, yet there is a tendency to have a bit more metabolic acidosis based on a lactate solution of 40 (18). Therefore, the preference by many programs is the use of a pharmacy-made bicarbonate solution (19).

Bleeding is rare but can occur on HF. Systemic anticoagulation is not necessary in over 50% of patients on HF. Increasing the blood flow is believed to result in running "heparin free" with the idea that stagnant blood will clot. Although this practice is common, in our practice no data to date support this approach. If systemic anticoagulation is necessary, it can either be

Table 3 Bicarbonate-Based Replacement Fluid/Dialysate Solutions

Constituents	Phosphorus-based replacement fluid/dialysate	Calcium-based replacement fluid/dialysate
NaCl (mEq/L)[a]	60–100[a]	60–100[a]
$NaHCO_3$ (mEq/L)[a]	80–40[a]	80–40[a]
KCI (mEq/L)	2	2–4
K_3PO_4 (mEq/L)	2	0
$MgSO_4$ (mEq/L)	0.5–1.5	0.5–1.5
Dextrose (g/L)	0–2.0 (0.0.2%)	0–2.0 (0–0.2%)
$CaCl_2$ (mEq/L)	0	3–4[b]
Lactate (mEq/L)	0	0

The addition of 2 mEq/L of K_3PO_4 will provide potassium at 2 mEq/L and phosphorus at 4 mg/dL.

[a]Total sodium should be between 130–145 mEq/L.

[b]Calcium does not precipitate out even with 80 mEq/L of $NaHCO_3$.

based at the level of heparin or citrate. Heparin again is a commonly used drug that can be used at a bolus of 10–20 units/kg/dose and in constant infusion of 10–20 units/kg/h to maintain a target ACT of between 150–200 (12). Citrate anticoagulation has been successfully used in adults; although it has been only used to a limited extent in pediatrics, it is an acceptable approach to anticoagulation in this population (20). Studies to date have been conflicting as to whether heparinization prolongs the life of the filter, yet those studies have been used in a mixed population of children, some of whom are hypercoagulable to begin with as opposed to others who have normal coagulation factors. Therefore, no pediatric study to date has identified in the normal coagulation patient whether anticoagulation prolongs the life of the membrane.

Protein and amino acid losses across the membrane can occur on HF. The studies to date by this group have suggested that at a standard 1.5 g/kg/day of TPN nutrition, these children remain in negative protein balance (14). This is less significant than loss of amino acids and total urea nitrogen across the membrane. Therefore, optimal nutrition may exceed 2 g/kg/day to achieve adequate nutrition in these children.

B. Complications of Extracorporeal Membrane Oxygenation

Complication of HF on extracorporeal membrane oxygenation (ECMO) are similar to those related to complication of HF in general. Some unique issues related to ECMO need to be addressed.

The commonality of complications on HF versus HF and ECMO are related to hypotension, metabolic acidosis, bleeding, as well as total protein losses. Therefore the reader should refer back to the section on HF and complications of pediatrics for that area. The two unique areas related to HF and ECMO are as follows.

Excessive solute clearance can occur in patients on HF and ECMO. This is often seen in the very small child who is on ECMO. Standard ECMO flow rates are roughly 100 mL/kg/min (21). The HF circuit that is linked into the ECMO circuit can have a blood flow rate of at least 150–180 mL/min. In a 3 kg child this can result in blood flow rates of 50–60 mL/kg/min, i.e., turning over blood volume roughly once every 2 minutes as opposed to HD or HF, where blood volume replaced is every 20 minutes. This excessive blood turnover will give much more blood exposure, and therefore will result in more clearance. This is important in patients who are small, who have high blood flow rates, and who have high BUN, for it may predispose them toward dialysis dysequilibrium. As the patient gets roughly above 20 kg, the impact upon this rapid clearance is less. Alternatively, in the larger child who is 70–80 kg with a blood flow rate of roughly 150–180 mL/min, inadequate clearance may occur. Therefore, increasing the surface area of the membrane of the hemofilter or increasing the dialysate or infusate flow may be necessary for adequate clearance (22).

Metabolic alkalosis can occur in patients on ECMO with HF. This combination is usually related to the use of a bicarbonate-based solution for the dialysate or infusate solution in addition to use of carbogen, which is used by the ECMO specialist for pH buffering. Past experience has shown that patients with a pH of 7.1–7.2 who receive both a combination of carbogen from the ECMO circuit added and a bicarbonate could experience a pH rise to 7.8 which would be potentially problematic to the child. Therefore, decreasing the bicarbonate-based solution from a standard 40 to a roughly 20–25 mEq/L as well as avoiding carbogen may be necessary to avoid raising the pH (21).

IV. VASCULAR ACCESS

Chronic vascular access for HD in children remains difficult because of the diverse sizes of the children. Chronic access in children on HD is shown to be roughly 60% externally using a duel lumen "venous" access and about 35% fistula or cortex graft to date (23,24). Access complications can be divided into external use catheter versus internal use catheter.

A. Externally Utilized Access Complications

Inadequate blood flow from children on dialysis is not unusual. The causes of impaired blood flow are usually related to the "arterial" side of the catheter being pressed up against the blood vessel, a blood clot in the access, intravascular volume depletion, external compression upon that access, kinking of the catheter at the site of insertion, too little access for the needs of the prescribed blood flow, excess movement (seen as more of a problem in femoral access), or in patients who have acute femoral access with high intraabdominal pressure (due to tense acites or organomegally) compressing upon the IVC.

The "arterial" side up against the wall is not an uncommon phenomenon. The configuration of the access has the "arterial" side coming off the side with the "venous" return roughly 18–22 mm downstream. This then sets up the scenario that if someone has a large vascular access in a small vessel, the "arterial" side may suck up against the vessel wall. Other than changing the access, reversal of the flow may be necessary. Reversing the flow may give less efficient dialysis because of the higher incidence of recirculation.

A blood clot in the access of the "arterial" or "venous" side may also be problematic. Chronic vascular access is hypercoagulable, with an increased incidence of clotting. No data to date have suggested the optimal way to keep the access or the area around the access free of clot, but many programs use a combination of high-dose heparin (2500 units) in combination with urokinase (2500 units) to lock off the access between treatments.

Low intravascular blood volume can be seen children with high-output renal sufficiency predisposing toward intravascular volume depletion, which then would predispose toward inadequate blood flow. Therefore, in some patients who have inadequate blood flow, volume loading with saline may be necessary to give adequate blood flow rate.

The access size relative to the size of the patient is also important. Correlation to the size of the access to the patient is important for optimal blood flow (Table 4).

Inadequate blood flow back to the patient can be related either to a clot on the return side or high intrathoracic pressure. A clot on the return side is again related to the way the access is locked off, and use of a higher heparin or heparin/urokinase solution may be necessary to prevent clotting.

In patients on high-frequency ventilation who require HD or HF, adequate blood flow may be a problem. These patients often have a high intrathoracic pressure secondary to high-frequency ventilation, which may give a high "venous" pressure inhibiting blood flow back to the patient.

An optimal site for vascular access, if it is chronic, would be the intrajugular as opposed to the subclavian due to the fact that the incidence of subclavian stenosis may be in excess of 50% in the pediatric population.

Chronic external access for HD may be predisposed to line sepsis. Whereas data to date is limited, most programs identify an average time for infection between day 30 and day 50 after placement of the line. Often these lines can be adequately treated with systemic antibiotics without removal of the HD catheter. Common bacteria are gram-positive, with institution of vancomycin with or without rifampin for treatment. If one uses vancomycin, then vancomycin clearance needs to be kept in mind, noting that normal dialysis membranes clear less than 10% per treatment while high-flux dialysis membranes will clear 50% per treatment.

B. Internal Access Complications

Inadequate blood flow from the patient is usually related to arterial thrombosis or stenosis, low intravascular blood volume, or extrinsic compression upon the vessel. Therefore, an angiography evaluation may be necessary for further evaluation of that graft.

Table 4 Recommendations for the Selection of Insertion Site of Vascular Access Based on Patient Size

Patient Size	Catheter Size	Insertion Site	Source
Neonate	18 g, 16 g, 14 g single lumen	Femoral artery Femoral vein	Cook
	16 g single lumen	Femoral artery Femoral vein Umbilical vein	Argyle
	7.0 F dual lumen	Femoral vein	Cook Medcomp
3–6 kg	7.0 F dual lumen	Femoral vein Subclavian vein Int/Ext jugular vein	Cook Medcomp
6–30 kg	8 F dual lumen	Femoral vein Subclavian vein	Kendall Medcomp
>15–30 kg	9.0 F dual lumen	Femoral vein Subclavian vein Int/Ext jugular vein	Medcomp
	5.0 F (internal lumen) single lumen	Femoral artery Femoral vein	Medcomp
>30 kg	10.0 F dual lumen	Femoral vein Subclavian vein	Arrow, Neostar Quinton

Inadequate blood flow back to the patient includes the same differential of either "venous" clot or stenosis downstream. Therefore, if it persists an angiography for further evaluation may be necessary.

V. ELECTROLYTE DISTURBANCES USING NONSTANDARD DIALYSATE SOLUTION ON PD OR HF

Many programs use a nonstandard dialysate solution utilizing bicarbonate for either PD or HF. HD machines have an internal calibration check, which verifies the contents of the solution for safety. If one is using commercially made PD or HF solutions, a calibration check occurs at the site of manufacturing for safety. In pharmacy-made solutions, there is no check system; therefore, many programs measure an aliquot of the solution of either the PD or the HF solution to ensure its electrolyte safety. In programs that utilize citrate anticoagulation, the pharmacy also needs to make a specific replacement solution in order to avoid sodium excess. Therefore, this is one more site of potential electrolyte solution error that needs to be checked for accuracy.

VI. COMPLICATIONS OF ACUTE RENAL FAILURE IN CHILDREN

The morbidity and mortality in ARF in children are usually related to the underlying cause (25). Studies to date have suggested that the likelihood for surviving when the cause of ARF is secondary to primary renal disease is much greater than if it is from a nonrenal disease. Mortality rates to date range from 20 to 80% based on the cause of the renal failure in children (26). No prospective pediatric data to date have identified completely the outcome of this population.

VII. COMPLICATIONS OF ESRD IN CHILDREN

Common complications seen in children with ESRD include renal osteodystrophy, metabolic acidosis, inadequate nutrition, chronic volume depletion, anemia, and growth inhibition (27).

Renal osteodystrophy is not unique to children but is more significant due to the additive effect of vitamin D/phosphorus derangement of ESRD in a growing child. Therefore, attention to phosphorus control either by the use of phosphate binders (calcium carbonate, calcium acetate) and vitamin D supplementation is important. The use of aluminum-based phosphorus binders are absolutely contraindicated in children and should never be used due to the deposition of aluminum into the bone and brain (28). The optimal level of intact PTH is in the range of two to three times the normal baseline. In patients with an intact PTH that is too well under control, an adynamic bone disease can occur. Alternatively, in patients with an intact PTH that is too high, renal osteodystrophy can result (29). Therefore, many programs target intact PTH of 150–200 pg/mL for optimal level of parathyroid activity. This is often done with a combination of calcium carbonate for phosphorus binding as well as the use DHT or 1,25-dihydroxy D_3.

Metabolic acidosis secondary to uremia can impair growth. Therefore, in patients who are not on dialysis, supplementation with bicarbonate or bicitra may be necessary. Citrate-based buffers may increase the absorption of aluminum in the diet, therefore, bicarbonate would be preferable. In patients who have persistent metabolic acidosis while on dialysis, attention to the source of the buffer on dialysis or the adequacy of dialysis may be necessary.

Inadequate nutrition occurs commonly in children with ESRD. Infants have been shown to require 40% more nutrition than the nonrenal failure patient when measured by RDA to attain growth. Therefore, early use of nutritional intervention is necessary to maintain not only brain growth but somatic growth. In small infants it is often necessary to use a enteral feeding tube. In infants and small children who have polyuric renal insufficiency who are on a fluid-based formula, the use of diluted formula is optimal. A concentrated formula used in this population gives a higher osmolar (solute) load, worsening their volume depletion and affecting their nutrition and remaining relative renal function. Therefore dilute feedings with the addition of sodium may be necessary to maintain intravascular volume integrity as well as to give high-volume nutrition via formula (30). Volume depletion can occur in children, especially those with obstructive uropathy. Seventy percent of children less than 10 years of age have high-output renal insufficiency predisposing to chronic volume depletion. Therefore, when these children go on dialysis, they often require dialysis for urea and phosphorus clearance, but not volume depletion. If one maintains intravascular volume integrity with the use of extra salt and sodium water supplementation in this population, often dialysis can be avoided or postponed until a later date and potentially these children can be maintained and be preemptively transplanted.

Anemia is common to children with ESRD and can affect their school performance. Therefore, attention to the use of erythropoietin with iron supplementation is necessary. Erythropoietin can be instituted either as a subcutaneous or venous injection. Many programs continue to use the standard 100 units/kg/dose three times a week for chronic dialysis, while other programs use 300–400 units/kg/dose every 7 days to avoid extra shots. In patients who have erythropoietin nonresponse, the causes would either be related to chronic infection, secondary hyperparathyroidism that is not well controlled, or iron deficiency. Therefore, attention to those matters may be necessary in patient who do not have adequate response to erythropoietin.

Growth inhibition can occur in children with ESRD and is multifactorial, including all the issues stated above. Data to date suggest that children with ESRD would do well on growth hormone, yet studies have been very clear that growth hormone therapy should not be used in patients unless all of the above issues, including renal osteodystrophy, metabolic acidosis, nutrition, as well as anemia, are taken care of ahead of time. If not, not only will growth hormone not be as effective, but there will be an increased risk of complications, especially that of femoral head necrosis. Therefore, growth hormone should only be instituted in patients who have inadequate growth after all the factors affecting growth noted above are taken into account. In patients who are started on growth hormone, hip films at baseline as well as every 6 months or one year are in order in order to make sure there is no problem with femoral head necrosis. In patients who develop worsening secondary hyperparathyroidism, growth hormone should be stopped immediately in order to avoid complications. Other complications of growth hormone include a rare complication of pseudo tumor cerebri as well as a potential increased risk of malignancies. Studies to date have not shown the malignancy risk to be a problem in the ESRD population (27).

VIII. COMPLICATIONS IN CHILDREN UNDERGOING ACUTE DIALYSIS FOR INBORN ERROR OF METABOLISM

Often a combination of HD for acute treatment with a transition to HF for "maintenance" is ideal until the cause is identified and a medical therapy is effective (31). The difference between HD or HF for treatment of inborn error of metabolism as opposed to ARF or ESRD is that these children do not have renal failure. Therefore they have ongoing urine output (which predisposes to volume depletion) and can develop hypophosphatemia or hypokalemia if this risk is not anticipated. A typical HD prescription is identical to that for acute or chronic HD or HF with these modifications:

1. No net ultrafiltration is needed.
2. Phosphorus is added to the "B" jug of the dialysate bath to give a phosphorus bath that is physiological.
3. Potassium is added to the bath to maintain a normal physiological potassium.

The mortality in this population is usually related to the underlying need for dialysis. Examples of this would be patients with hyperammonemia, proprionic acidemia, as well as methylmalonic acidemia. It is important to realize that children who require HD or HF for inborn error of metabolism have to be thought about as unique individuals and should not be given the same prescription that one would use or ARF or ESRD. Rapid clearance of ammonia or lactate can be accomplished in children with inborn error of metabolism without risk of osmolar shifts or dialysis dysequilibrium as long as there is not accompanying acute renal failure.

IX. COMPLICATIONS UNIQUE TO SPECIFIC AGE GROUPS WITH ERSD

Neonates and infants with ESRD are a unique population. Often these children have extrarenal multiorgan dysfunction. In the neonate population with acute or chronic renal failure, excluding problems with cardiac or cerebral diseases is important. Studies have suggested that infants with ESRD are at a much higher risk if more than one organ other than kidney are affected (32).

In the pediatric and adolescent populations, the major complications seen in chronic dialysis are related to access complications, growth and development, compliance to medical regimens, as well as maintaining the goal of eventual transplantation. This is further complicated by the fact that as the child approaches adolescence and adult age, the cause or ESRD changes making the child more fluid retentive as opposed to fluid wasting. The variety of diagnosis that results in ESRD in children requires understanding each individual disease and prescribing appropriately instead of a "one-prescription-for-all" approach. Attention to the underlying cause of the renal insufficiency in ESRD is necessary in order to give adequate dialysis therapy.

Immunization complications in children with ESRD are few but important to note. Live virus vaccines can be used in patients with ESRD. Therefore, no immunization is excluded in children on chronic dialysis. Complications of immunization are usually located at the site of the injection as well as a low-grade chance of spreading live virus vaccine (OPV, MMR, VZV) to other are risk. The risk of spreading in a nonimmunized peer who is normal or immunosuppressed is extremely low, and therefore should not prohibit the use of immunizations.

X. SUMMARY

The care of the child with acute renal failure requiring renal replacement therapy is a cooperative effort between pediatric nephrologists and intensivists. Their combined expertise should allow for optimal care of the child, including RRT, good nutrition, and intensive care, if necessary, which should correlate with the best chance for survival.

Care of the child with ESRD is best done by pediatric nephrologists who have expertise in the areas of psychological, social, and sexual development along with growth and nutrition in the growing child. Care of children with ESRD by nonpediatric nephrologists may jeopardize the health of these children.

A continuing factor that inhibits optimal renal replacement therapy in children, whether acute or chronic, is a lack of pediatric-specific equipment; therefore, advancement in the areas of access, pediatric-specific equipment, ultrafiltration controllers, as well as blood warmers is necessary in the care of these children. Further research in nutritional requirements for the growing child who is maintained in a catabolic state, whether on acute or chronic renal replacement therapy, is necessary.

REFERENCES

1. Alexander SR. Peritoneal dialysis. In: Holliday MA, Barratt TM, Aver ED, eds. Pediatric Nephrology. Baltimore: Williams and Wilkens, 1994:1339–1353.
2. Reznik VM, Griswold WR, Peterson BM, Rodarte A, Ferris ME, Mendoza SA. Peritoneal dialysis for acute renal failure in children. Pediatr Nephorol 1991; 5:715.
3. Enriquez JL, Kalia A, Travis LB. Fungal peritonitis in children on peritoneal dialysis. J Pediatr 1990; 117:839.
4. Fivush BA, Case B, May MW, Lederman HM. Hypogammaglobulinemia in children undergoing continuous ambulatory peritoneal dialysis. Pediatr Nephrol 1989; 3:186–188.
5. Warady BA, Hebert D, Sullivan EK, Alexander SR, Tejani A. Renal transplantation, chronic dialysis, and chronic renal insufficiency in children and adolescents. The 1995 Annual Report of the North American Pediatric Renal Transplant Cooperative Study. Pediatr Nephrol 1997; 11:49–64.
6. Warady BA. Adequacy of peritoneal dialysis in the pediatric patient. Perit Dial Intern 1997; 17(suppl 3):S50–S52.
7. Bunchman TE, Wood EG, Lynch RE. Hydrothorax as a complication of pediatric peritoneal dialysis. Perit Dial Bull 1987; 7:237.
8. Bunchman TE, Meldrum MK, Meliones JE, Sedman AB, Kershaw DB. Pulmonary function variation in ventilator dependent critically ill infants on peritoneal dialysis. Adv Perit Dial 1992; 8:75.
9. Donckerwolke RA, Bunchman TE. Hemodialysis in infants and small children. Pediatr Nephrol 1994; 8:103.
10. Himmelfarb J, Rubin NT, Chandran P, Parker RA, Wingard RL, Hakim R. A multicenter comparison of dialysis membranes in the treatment of acute renal failure requiring dialysis. J Am Soc Nephrol 1998; 9:257–266.
11. Harmon WE, Jabs K. Hemodialysis. In: Holliday MA, Barratt TM, Aver ED, eds. Pediatric Nephrology. Baltimore: Williams and Wilkens, 1994: 1354–1372.
12. Geary DF, Gajaria M, Fryer-Keeze S, Willemsen J. Low dose and heparin free hemodialysis in children. Pediatr Nephrol 1991; 5:220.
13. Bunchman TE. Chronic dialysis in the infant less than one year of age. Pediatr Nephrol 1995; 9:S18–S22.
14. Maxvold NJ, Smoyer WE, Bunchman TE. Prospective comparison of 24 hour nitrogen balance, amino acid losses, and urea clearance between CVVH and CVVHD during pediatric continuous hemofiltration. Crit Care Med 1998; 26(1)(#300):A121.
15. Bunchman TE, Donckerwolcke R. CAVH(D), CVVH(D), modalities in infants and children. Pediatr Nephrol 1994; 8:96.
16. Jenkins R, Harrison H, Chen B, Arnold D, Funk J. Accuracy of intravenous infusion pumps in continuous renal replacement therapies. Trans Am Soc Artif Intern Organs J 1992; 38:808.
17. Bunchman TE, Maxvold NJ, Kershaw DB, Sedman AB, Custer JR. Continuous venovenous hemodiafiltration in infants and children. Am J Kid Dis 1995; 25: 17.
18. Morgera S, Heering P, Szentandrasi T, Masnassa E, Heintzen M, Willers R, Passlick-Deetjen J, Grabensee B. Comparison of a lactate versus acetate based hemofiltration replacement fluid in patients with acute renal failure. Renal Failure 1997; 19:155–164.
19. Smoyer WE, Sherbotie JR, Gardner JJ, Bunchman TE. A practical approach to continuous hemofiltration in infants and children. Dial Transpl 1995; 24:633–640.

20. Mehta RL, McDonald BR, Aguilar NM, et al. Regional citrate anticoagulation for continuous arteriovenous hemodialysis in critically ill patients. Kidney Int 1990; 36: 976–981.
21. Smoyer WE, Maxvold NJ, Remenapp R, Bunchman TE. Renal replacement therapy. In: Furhman BP, Zimmerman JJ, eds. Pediatric Critical Care. 2d ed. St. Louis: Mosby, 1998: 764–778.
22. Maxvold NJ, Bunchman TE, Bartlett RH. Dialyzer surface area effect upon solute removal ECLS, a single patient experience. Presented at the ELSO Meeting, September 1993, Dearborn, MI.
23. Bunchman TE. Pediatric hemodialysis: lessons from the past, ideas for the future. Kidney Int 1996; 49(suppl 53):S64–S67.
24. Bunchman TE, Gardner JJ, Kershaw DB, Maxvold NJ. Vascular access for hemodialysis or CVVH(D) in infants and children. Dial Transplant 1994; 23:314.
25. Parekh RS, Bunchman TE. Dialysis support in the pediatric intensive care unit. Adv Renal Replacement Ther 1996; 3:326–336.
26. Maxvold NJ, Smoyer WE, Gardner JJ, Bunchman TE. Management of acute renal failure in the pediatric patient: hemofiltration versus hemodialysis. Am J Kidney Dis 1997; 30(5)(suppl 4): 84–88.
27. Fine RN. Pathophysiology of growth retardation in children with chronic renal failure. J Pediatr Endocrinol 1994; 7:79–83.
28. Sedman A. Aluminum toxicity in childhood. Pediatr Nephr 1992; 6:383–393.
29. Goodman WG, Veldhuis JD, Belin TR, Juppner H, Salusky IB. Suppressive effect of calcium on parathyroid hormone release in adynamic renal osteodystrophy and secondary hyperparathyroidism. Kidney Int 1997; 51: 1590–1595.
30. Sedman AS, Parekh RS, DeVee JL, Flynn JT, Gregory MJ, Kershaw DB, Smoyer WE, Valentini RP, Bunchman TE. Cost-effective management of children with polyuric renal failure. J Am Soc Nephrol 1996; 7:1398.
31. Gregory MJ, Kershaw DB, Sedman AB, Valentini RP, Bunchman TB. Adaptation of standard hemodialysis for the treatment of acute hyperammonemic crisis in infants and children. J Am Soc Nephrol 1994; 5:415.
32. Ellis EN, Pearson D, Champion B, Wood EG. Outcome of infants on chronic peritoneal dialysis. Adv Perit Dial 1995; 11:266–269.

37

Dialysis in Patients with Human Immunodeficiency Virus Infection

Jorge Diego and Jacques J. Bourgoignie
University of Miami School of Medicine, Miami, Florida

The impact of the acquired immunodeficiency syndrome (AIDS) pandemic on the treatment of patients with end-stage renal disease (ESRD) is felt throughout the world, but nowhere more palpably than in the United States. Through June 30, 1997, a cumulative total of 612,078 persons with AIDS were reported to the Centers for Disease Control (CDC). Currently, nearly 240,000 people are living with AIDS in the United States, with an annual incidence of 50,000–60,000 new cases per year. It is estimated that over one million persons are infected with the human immunodeficiency virus (HIV). Worldwide, by the beginning of 1997 a cumulative total of 29.4 million people had been infected with HIV and a cumulative 8.4 million cases of AIDS had been documented (1,2). For the first time, however, the number of deaths among patients with AIDS declined in the United States from 50,700 in 1995 to 39,200 in 1996. As improvements in antiretroviral therapy and prophylaxis of opportunistic infections continue, more patients with AIDS will live longer and may be at risk for developing ESRD (3–5).

I. NATURAL HISTORY OF HIV INFECTION

The natural history of HIV infection in dialysis is best understood in the context of its behavior in the absence of renal failure. For simplicity, HIV-1 infection can be divided into the following stages: (a) viral transmission, (b) primary HIV infection, (c) seroconversion, (d) clinical latency, (e) early symptomatic HIV infection (formerly known as the aids-related complex, or ARC), (f) AIDS, and (g) advanced AIDS with a CD4 count <50 cells μL. In the absence of treatment, the usual rate of CD4 cell decline is between 30 and 90 cells/μL per year (6,7). The rate of immunological deterioration is determined by several factors, most importantly by the level of viral burden. Recent seminal observations on the pathogenesis of HIV infection have demonstrated a high and continuous steady-state level of viral replication and cell destruction on the order of 10^9 cells per day (8). Relatively steady levels of T cells and viral burden are ensured by a steady turnover of new cells to replace the dying cells daily. Immunological depletion occurs as the cell turnover rate exhausts lymphocyte reserves, heralding the eminent decline in host immunity that ushers into AIDS. The median time to the development of an AIDS-defining condition from the onset of immunological AIDS (defined as a CD4 count of <200) is 12–18 months in patients not taking antiviral therapy (9,10). The median CD4 count at the time of an AIDS-defining opportunistic infection is 67 cells/μL (11). In the absence of treatment, the mean survival of an HIV-infected patient is 10 years and the mean survival for patients with a CD4 count of <200 is 38–40 months (12). Once severe CD4 cell depletion occurs (CD4 <50 cells/μL), the median survival is only 12–18 months (9,13,14). The CD4 count and the viral burden primarily determine the rate of progression of AIDS and death. Indeed, a now famous analogy made by John Coffin (15) is that the CD4 count is like the length of a railroad track leading to an abyss; the viral load is the speed at which a train on that track is approaching. To date, the four interventions that have made a difference in survival of patients with HIV infection are antiretroviral therapy, *Pneumocystis carinii* prophylaxis, *Mycobacterium avium* prophylaxis, and care by clinicians with HIV experience (3–5,16,17). This background may help appreciate the phenomenon of HIV infection in dialysis patients.

II. HIV AND CHRONIC DIALYSIS

A. Prevalence and Incidence of HIV Infection

The prevalence of HIV infection among patients with ESRD is not well defined. Estimates based on surveys conducted jointly by the CDC and the Health Care Financing Administration (HCFA) suggest that, in 1995, approximately 1.4% of the ESRD population in the United States was HIV infected. Moreover, 39% of centers provided dialysis to HIV-positive patients (18). These figures represent significant increases in comparison to an earlier survey conducted in 1985 when the prevalence of HIV infection was 0.3% and the number of centers dialyzing HIV-positive patients was only 11% (Table 1). The prevalence of HIV is clearly influenced by temporal, geographic, and socioeconomic factors ranging from 2.8% in Baltimore, Maryland, to 23% in Miami, Florida, and 39% in Brooklyn, New York, in 1987 (19–21). At the end of 1997, the prevalence of HIV infection was 9% among 200 patients on chronic hemodialysis at the University of Miami/Jackson Memorial Medical Center in Miami, Florida. Outside the United States, HIV infection rates range from 2.2% in Brazil to between 0 and 5% in European countries (22).

Between 6 and 10% of patients with HIV infection will develop renal complications of HIV infection, and, among these, 40% may require renal replacement therapy (22,23). Incidence estimates for HIV infection and AIDS among dialysis patients are not well defined. Based on an analysis of data from the New York State ESRD network, where approximately 25% of all HIV patients on dialysis in the United States are located, Winston and Klotman (24) estimated that between 480 and 750 new cases of HIV-associated glomerulosclerosis (HIVAN) will occur nationally each year and that the increase in the observed incidence of HIVAN at 20% per year would make HIVAN the third leading cause of ESRD among African Americans between the ages of 20 and 64 by the year 2000. In San Francisco, the annual incidence of HIV patients beginning dialysis has steadily increased from 2% in 1986 to 15% between 1992 and 1994 (25). In the United States, however, through mid-1977 only 26 states had statutory requirements for confidential reporting of HIV infection. Improvements in HIV reporting and in the HCFA entering renal diagnosing form for new ESRD patients are needed to more clearly appreciate the magnitude of HIV infection as a cause and contributor to ESRD morbidity and mortality in the United States (25).

B. Survival of HIV Patients on Chronic Dialysis

1. Hemodialysis

Table 2 lists in chronological order the data available on survival of patients with HIV infection or AIDS undergoing maintenance hemodialysis. Early reports influenced the widely held perception of an abysmal outcome for AIDS patients on maintenance dialysis. In 1987, Rao et al. (42) reported that only 2 out of 73 patients with AIDS survived longer than 6 months and that none survived beyond 1 year. In 1988, Ortiz et al. (41) reported a mean survival of only 93 ± 32 days among 17 patients with AIDS. Similar outcomes were reported by others, and the status of dialysis in patients with AIDS was controversial and pessimistic (43). Nevertheless, it was appreciated that not all patients with HIV infection needing dialysis fared poorly. Indeed, Ortiz et al. (41) noted that patients with asymptomatic HIV infection fared relatively well without the benefit of optimal antiviral therapy, consistent and effective prophylaxis for opportunistic infections or reliable permanent vascular access, surviving for a mean duration of 16 ± 2 months. Schoenfeld et al. (31) performed a multivariate analysis of 55 patients dialyzed over 10 years at the San Francisco General Hospital. In their analysis they included variables such as baseline CD4 count, serum albumin, zidovudine use, dialysis modality, and cognitive motor dysfunction. Only cognitive motor dysfunction and CD4 counts correlated significantly with survival. The median survival time for the group was 16 months. When stratified by baseline CD4 count above (55%) and below (45%) 200 cells/μL, there was a significant difference in median survival at 26 ± 24 months in the higher group compared with 8.4 ± 7.1 months in the lower. The predictive power of the baseline clinical stage and CD4 cell count of patients on dialysis was confirmed by Perinbasekar et al. (30). In their study, 24 consecutive HIV-infected patients on hemodialysis were evaluated prospectively and retrospectively over 7 years (1987–1993), and clinical and laboratory baseline variables were recorded. All the patients dialyzed with a surgically constructed vascular access. The mean CD4 count in the

Table 1 Long-Term Hemodialysis Centers Reporting Patients with HIV Infection, 1985–1995, United States

Year	Centers with HIV infection No. (%)	Patients with HIV infection No. (%)	Patients with clinical AIDS No. (%)
1985	134 (11)	244 (0.3)	—
1986	238 (18)	546 (0.6)	332 (0.4)
1987	351 (24)	924 (1.0)	462 (0.5)
1988	401 (25)	1253 (1.2)	670 (0.6)
1989	456 (26)	1248 (1.0)	663 (0.5)
1990	493 (26)	1533 (1.1)	739 (0.5)
1991	601 (29)	1914 (1.2)	967 (0.6)
1992	737 (34)	2501 (1.5)	1126 (0.7)
1993	792 (34)	2780 (1.5)	1350 (0.7)
1994	914 (37)	3144 (1.5)	1593 (0.8)
1995	1022 (39)	3090 (1.4)	1606 (0.7)

Source: Ref. 18.

Table 2 Survival of Patients with HIV infection or AIDS on Maintenance Hemodialysis

Study period	N	IVDA (%)	CD4 (mean)	AIDS (%)	HIV (%)	Survival on dialysis (mean)	Ref.
1984–96	102		122 ± 169			50% 1 year, 32% 3 years	26
1997	34	59.0	140 ± 150	95	5	57 ± 50 months (4–196	27
1994–95	36					Standardized mortality ratio: 2.46	28
1986–96	36		250 ± 206			15 months (median)	29
1987–93	24	63.0	<200	58	32	11 ± 8 months	30
1985–94	55	61.0	219 ± 209	49	51	16 ± 19 months; 8.4 ± 7.1 CD4 > 200 cells mm^3 vs. 26 ± 24 CD4 < 200 cells mm^3	31
1987–94	61	45.0	<200	72	28	50% 1 year, 10% 3 years	32
1984–92	31					15 ± 9.9 months	33
1983–91	160	73.0				8 months (median)	34
1987–90	3	67.0				Anecdotal experience with 3 patients, no staging	35
1982–89	36	67.0		22	78	HIV: 96.2% 1 year, 54.5% 5 years; AIDS: 25% 6 months, 12.5% 12 months	36
1986–89	5	80.0		100		7 months (median, 2–42 months) survival after AIDS diagnosis	37
—	15	73.0		33	67	AIDS: 14.5 ± 2 months; HIV: 15.7 ± 3 months	38
1986–89	39	62.0		15	85	15 ± 2.4 months; AIDS 5/6 dead 3.6 months after diagnosis	39
1986–88	31	84.0		13	87	HIV 15.8 months, AIDS 27 months	40
1983–87	51	55.0		33	67	AIDS: 30 days median; ARC 243 days, HIV 243 days	41
1982–86	49	43.0		100	0	AIDS 1–1.4 months median; only 2/49 >6 months	42

group was 178 ± 143 cells/μL (range 1–461). In a multivariate analysis, the baseline CD4 count had the greatest correlation with survival with an overall mean survival of 11 ± 8 months (range 2–32) (Fig. 1).

More recent experience with AIDS and HIV infection in hemodialysis suggests that survival is improving. Ifudu et al. (27) reported a mean duration of survival on hemodialysis of 57 ± 50 months (4–196) in New York in an inner-city cohort of 35 HIV patients (59% with a history of intravenous drug abuse) of whom 29 (83%) had clinical AIDS. The mean CD4 count in this population was 140 ± 150 (2–500) cells/μL. In 15 patients the CD4 counts were less than 50 cells/μL. The mean duration of known HIV infection was 50 ± 34 (2–144) months. Importantly, all these patients had a permanent vascular access with a mean urea reduction rate of 65 ± 9%. Alarmingly, 12 (35%) of the patients had prior opportunistic infections, and only 6 (18%) were reported to be on antiretroviral therapy (5 zidovudine alone, 1 DDI alone), and only one patient was receiving trimethropim-sulfamethoxazole for *Pneumocystis carinii* pneumonia prophylaxis. Finally, compliance with appointments in a comprehensive HIV intervention program was poor. The reasons for the apparent improvement in survival in this study are unclear.

In 1993, the classification of AIDS was modified by the CDC to include three new indicator conditions (pulmonary tuberculosis, recurrent bacterial pneumonia, and invasive cervical cancer), in addition to including all HIV-positive patients with CD4+ T-lymphocyte count <200/μL or <14% of total lymphocytes (44). Thus, inclusion of asymptomatic HIV-positive dialysis patients among AIDS patients by current CDC criteria could have favorably improved the survival data. Factors related to the delivery of dialysis, including permanent vascular access, optimal dialysis dosage, and erythropoietin therapy, may have also contributed to this effect. Unknown yet is whether aggressive combinations of antiviral therapy, prophylaxis for opportunistic infections, and attention by experienced HIV clinicians would further improve the outcome of HIV-infected patients on dialysis as it has for individuals without chronic renal failure (3–5,16,17).

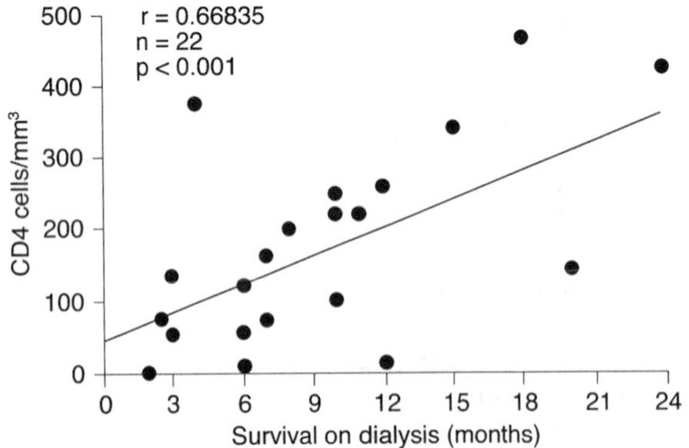

Fig. 1 Correlation between baseline CD4 lymphocyte count and survival on dialysis.

2. Peritoneal Dialysis

The reported experience with peritoneal dialysis in HIV-positive patients is small in comparison with that of hemodialysis. Theoretical concerns related to protein losses, infections, and patient physical, cognitive, and social ability to successfully perform peritoneal dialysis have tempered enthusiasm for peritoneal dialysis, particularly in patients with AIDS. Nevertheless, the reported success with this therapeutic modality has been favorable in HIV-infected patients. Tebben et al. (45) reported their experience in a well-performed and comprehensive study of 39 HIV-infected patients, predominantly intravenous drug abusers, treated with peritoneal dialysis. Once again, the authors noted a strong correlation between the clinical stage of HIV-infection and both survival and complications. The patients were divided into two groups on the basis of the stage of the HIV infection. Twelve asymptomatic patients [HIV infection stage II and III] (46) with a median CD4 count of 600 cells/μL (range 271–1540) were compared to 27 symptomatic (stage IV) patients with a median CD4 count of 31 cells/μL (range 0–310). Four patients died in the first group after a median survival of 12.1 months (death rate was 0.27/year of observation). The remaining 8 patients were alive after a median duration of follow-up of 9.8 months. In the symptomatic group, 20 deaths occurred (death rate 0.8/year of observation) after a median follow-up of only 5.2 months (range 1–30 months). The remaining 7 patients were alive after a median follow-up period of 16.7 months (range 3.6–51.4). Among the symptomatic group, 17 patients fulfilled the 1987 CDC criteria for AIDS (46). The death rate in this subset was significantly higher (1.17/year of observation).

In a contemporaneous study, Kimmel and colleagues (33) reported their experience with 392 patients entering chronic dialysis between 1984 and 1992. Thirty-one patients were HIV infected, of whom 8 (75% stage IV) were treated with peritoneal dialysis and 23 (78.3% stage IV) were treated exclusively with hemodialysis. In contrast with Tebben et al. (45), patients were predominantly homosexuals. The median survival for the

31 HIV-infected patients was 13 months in comparison to 38 months for the non–HIV-infected group. There was, however, no significant difference in median survival between the HIV-infected peritoneal dialysis group (18.5 months) and the hemodialysis group (13 months). The crude death rates in the peritoneal dialysis and hemodialysis HIV groups were 0.59 versus 0.71 per 1000 patient year. In contrast, the mortality rates in the non–HIV-infected peritoneal dialysis and hemodialysis groups were significantly lower at 0.22 and 0.23 death per patient-year, respectively.

In San Francisco, Schoenfeld et al. (31) reported their experience with nine HIV-infected patients enrolled in a chronic peritoneal dialysis program between 1985 and 1994. Eight of these patients had CD4+ cell counts of >200 cells/μL, and their median survival was correspondingly excellent (31 months) in accord with Tebben's findings of improved outcomes in patients with more intact immune systems.

C. CD4+ Lymphocytes and Viral Load

There is a paucity of biological information on the dynamics of HIV infection in patients on dialysis. Despite a variable period of clinical latency after primary HIV infection, there is no equivalent period of viral latency. Indeed, approximately 10 billion new HIV virions are produced daily with an equivalent number of CD4+ lymphocytes infected and destroyed (8). Moreover, it is now apparent that the level of plasma HIV RNA is a primary determinant of the clinical course of HIV infection (47,48). In an early study, Kimmel et al. (49) demonstrated a higher prevalence of HIV culture-positive plasma among patients with chronic renal insufficiency or ESRD than in HIV-positive patients without renal dysfunction. But the proportion of HIV-positive patients with renal insufficiency or on dialysis who were viremic was the same, prompting the authors to conclude that dialysis per se had little effect on the prevalence of plasma viremia. The authors also found that there was no correlation between CD4 cell counts or the administration of zidovudine with the prevalence of plasma viremia. Recently, Winston and Klotman (50) measured plasma HIV RNA in seropositive patients with renal disease before and after entering chronic hemodialysis. They found mean viral loads of 3.55 log (10) prior to dialysis and 5.02 log (10) in dialysis patients, suggesting that viral replication increased significantly with dialysis. In another study, these authors also reported that HIV-associated nephropathy (HIVAN) is a late complication of HIV-1 infection. In a group of patients studied since 1995 they found that all patients with biopsy-proven HIVAN had CD4 counts of <200 cells/μL, with a mean count of 77 ± 29 cells/μL in 17 patients prior to initiating dialysis. Disturbingly, 5 of 6 patients starting hemodialysis in 1995 and 5 of 11 patients starting in 1996 had died of AIDS (51). Clearly, more information on viral kinetics and response rates to complex antiretroviral regimens in dialysis patients are needed. On a relevant note, a recent study of 12 patients analyzed the effect of hemodialysis and antiretroviral therapy on plasma HIV-1 viral load (52). In six patients dialyzing with cellulose acetate dialyzers, pre- and posthemodialysis viral loads were measured by quantitative-competitive reverse transcription PCR (Amplicor, Roche). There was a consistent decrease in viral load of 45% posthemodialysis from 4.97 log (10) to 4.76 log (10). HIV-1 RNA was not found in the ultrafiltrate. Among patients receiving antiretrovirals, 6 received one and the other 6 two nuceloside reverse transcriptase inhibitors. Those receiving two drugs had lower mean viral loads [4.04 log (10) versus 5.53 log (10)] and higher CD4+ cell counts (386 ± 103 cells/μL vs. 101 ± 50 cells/μL). The authors concluded that viral load determinations should be obtained prior to hemodialysis because heparin and possibly other dialysis-related factors can interfere with the measurement of HIV-1 viral RNA. Variability in CD4 count determinations attributed to hemodialysis was reported by Elfatih et al. (53), who measured absolute and relative CD4 counts in HIV-infected patients before, during, and at the end of hemodialysis. They found that both absolute counts and percentages rose during dialysis. The message from this study was that CD4 measurements should be obtained and performed prior to dialysis.

III. COMPLICATIONS IN DIALYZED HIV PATIENTS

A. Anemia and Response to Erythropoietin

The response rate of HIV-infected patients to erythropoietin has been the subject of considerable study and obvious concern to nephrologists caring for these patients. The causes of anemia in HIV-infected patients are multiple and include marrow resistance, infiltrative diseases, malignancy, drug toxicity, and opportunistic infections. Spivak et al. (54) reported a prevalence of anemia in 18% of 22 asymptomatic HIV-infected patients, 50% of 26 patients with ARC, and 75% of 104 patients with AIDS. They also demonstrated that serum erythropoietin levels were relatively low in AIDS patients, yet production was intact but blunted. Fischl et al. (55) demonstrated that the responsiveness to exogenous erythropoietin of AIDS patients treated with zidovudine was proportional to the baseline erythropoietin level, with levels greater than 500 IU/L predictive of drug failure. In AIDS patients not receiving zidovudine, treatment with 100 U/kg of rHuEPO intravenously three times a week resulted in a decrease in transfusion requirements and a mean 5% increase in the hematocrit (56).

With this background, studies on the efficacy of erythropoietin in HIV-infected patients with ESRD on maintenance hemodialysis were conducted in New York. In the first study, 30 HIV-positive patients were compared to a group of 30 HIV-negative patients on maintenance hemodialysis. After collection of baseline data, including serum immunoreactive erythropoietin levels, each group of patients was treated with 100 IU/kg of rHuEPO thrice weekly. After 8 weeks of therapy, the mean increase in hematocrit in each group was similar (5.8% HIV group, 6.7% non-HIV groups). Remarkably, 50% of the responding HIV-positive patients had opportunistic infections and 33% were prescribed zidovudine. Finally, the authors also found that the baseline serum erythropoietin levels differed between the responding and the nonresponding HIV and non-HIV patients alike (HIV 17.7 ± 11.8 U/mL vs 416 ± 184.5 U/mL; non-HIV 13.3 ± 4.6 U/mL vs. 210.1 ± 189.1 U/mL, respectively) (57). In a subsequent study, Ifudu et al. (58) refined these observations by performing a cross-sectional study of the clinical determinants of effectiveness of erythropoietin in 33 (29 AIDS) HIV-infected patients on hemodialysis. The variables considered in the study included CD4 cell count, measures of iron storage, erythropoietin dosage, delivered dose of dialysis and serum albumin. The median CD4 count was 72 cells/μL and the median duration of known HIV infection was 48 months. In comparison with a control group of patients without HIV infection, the mean dose of rHuEPO administered thrice weekly was lower (90 ± 52 U/kg vs. 62 ± 36 U/kg). Nevertheless, the mean hematocrit in the HIV-infected group did not differ from the controls (27.4% ± 4.7 vs. 27.6% ± 3.7, respectively. A multivariate analysis showed that only the delivered dose of dialysis and transferrin saturation significantly correlated with a good response to erythropoietin. To some surprise, the degree of immunosuppression, assessed by the CD4 count and the duration of HIV infection, did not predict erythropoietin failure. Thus, it seems that for HIV-infected and noninfected patients alike, the delivery of an optimal dose of hemodialysis is the sine qua non condition for patient well-being.

B. Malnutrition

The reports that have stressed the dismal prognosis of AIDS patients on hemodialysis have noted a high incidence of failure to thrive, malnutrition, cognitive dysfunction, and opportunistic infections as preterminal events. In an early series, Rao et al. (42) noted that severe malnutrition and a failure to thrive despite aggressive nutritional support was a common problem that challenged the care of these patients. Schoenfeld et al. (31) and Perinbasekar et al. (30) noted similarly low baseline serum albumin levels (2.2 ± 1 to 2.48 ± 0.7) in their patients with AIDS starting maintenance hemodiaylsis. More recent studies in prevalent AIDS patients on hemodialysis by Lorch et al. (28) and Ifudu et al. (27) reported mean serum albumin levels of 3.28 and 3.5 g/dL, respectively. The importance of nutrition for survival of patients on chronic dialysis is well described (59) and is particularly relevant in AIDS patients who are uniquely susceptible to malnutrition as a group (60,61). Malnutrition in AIDS patients is not only prevalent but also strongly correlates with poor survival independently of CD4+ lymphocyte counts (62,63). The pathophysiology of cachexia in AIDS is complex, and associations with increased cytokine production, malabsorption, and endocrine abnormalities such as growth hormone resistance have been demonstrated (60,64). Efforts to improve nutritional parameters in AIDS patients, albeit with variable success, include pharmacotherapy with progestational agents (65,66), thalidomide (67), IGF-1 and rHu growth hormone (68,69), anabolic steroids (70,71), testosterone (72,73), and dronabinol (74). Finally, both enteral and parenteral therapy have been used with limited success as adjunctive forms of treatment (75,76).

C. Cognitive Dysfunction

Cognitive dysfunction is a frequent neurological complication of AIDS affecting up to one third of patients (77). The reported frequency of this complication in AIDS patients on dialysis ranges from 19 to 50% (31,40,41). Little is known about the effect of uremia on the clinical manifestations of HIV encephalopathy, but some clinicians report that this complication may be more prevalent among patients on chronic dialysis and certainly may impact on the initiation of renal replacement therapy (31). Some clinical success in the treatment of this condition with antiretroviral agents such as zidovudine may lessen the burden of cognitive disability in dialysis patients with AIDS (78).

D. Access-Related Issues

1. Vascular Access

There are a few but provocative reports on the subject of permanent vascular access in HIV-infected patients on hemodialysis (79–82). Obailo et al. (79) noted a mean duration of av access thrombus-free survival of 12.2 ± 6 months in 10 patients with end-stage renal disease and HIV nephropathy. Overall patency rates in these patients at 6 and at 12 months were 100% and 89%, respectively. In a recent report the same authors found a cumulative rate in synthetic arteriovenous (AV) graft-patency of 85% at one year in 13 HIV-infected hemodialysis patients. By comparison, the cumulative one-year graft patency rates in 8 patients with idiopathic focal and segmental glomerulosclerosis and in 15 patients with hypertensive nephrosclerosis were 0% and 65%, respectively (80). Similar favorable thrombosis-free rates have been reported by others. Nannery et al. (81) examined the clinical course of 22 HIV-infected patients (5 AIDS, 6 ARC, 11 asymptomatic) in whom 28 access operations were performed (24 AV grafts) over a 60-month period. In this study there were only three AV graft thromboses despite a patient population made up entirely of intravenous drug users. The principal complication in this group were 4 AV graft infections, a frequency well within the norm for non–HIV-infected patients at the time. Brock et al. (82) also examined the influence of HIV infection on complications of hemodialysis access surgery in a group of 29 HIV-infected patients (11 AIDS, 18 asymptomatic) and 79 HIV-negative patients undergoing 169 graft procedures (117 PTFE grafts, 44 AV fistulas, 8 unknown). Of note, 23% of these patients were intravenous drug users, and the majority of these were HIV positive. The overall 12-month graft patency rate in this study was 41%, and this was not affected by the patients HIV status or history of intravenous drug use. Unlike Nannery's experience, the PTFE graft infection rate in the group of patients with AIDS (48%) and asymptomatic HIV infection (36%) was significantly greater than that in the non-HIV group (15%). Confounding these findings, however, was the markedly increased PTFE graft infection rate among intravenous drug users (41%) versus the infection rate in patients who did not have a history of intravenous drug use (13%). Thus, the apparent increased susceptibility of HIV-infected patients to develop PTFE graft infections could not be separated from the practice of intravenous drug use since a separate group of non–HIV-infected intravenous drug users was not examined. Nevertheless, the authors made the influential and transcendent recommendation to avoid placing PTFE grafts in AIDS patients, preferring alternative access such as hemodialysis catheters that could be more easily removed in case of an infection. The validity of this conclusion, however, is unacceptable in view of more recent findings. Emphasizing the importance of patient characteristics in assessing the risk of graft infection, Obailo et al. (80) did not appreciate an increased rate of vascular access infection in a group of 13 HIV-infected patients, of whom 10 were not intravenous drug users.

Strategies to prevent AV access infections that have had success in other dialysis populations, such as the eradication of nasal staphylococcal colonization, which is prevalent in HIV-infected patients and contributes to bacteremia and wound infections, need to be considered as an adjunct to patient hygiene and protection of the patient's hemodialysis access from abuse (83–85).

2. Peritonitis

One of the principal concerns with peritoneal dialysis in patients with HIV infection has been the specter of an increased frequency of peritonitis. Several authors have reported both an increased rate of peritonitis and a distinct frequency and distribution of pathogens, particularly *Staphylococcus aureus* and fungal and *Pseudomonas* species (45,86–92). For example, in the study conducted by Tebben et al. (45), the overall rate of peritonitis in the HIV-infected group of 39 patients in the New Haven CAPD unit was 3.9 episodes per outpatient CAPD year. In contrast, the peritonitis rate among 435 non–HIV-infected patients was 1.5 episodes per outpatient CAPD year. The frequency of pathogens among the HIV-infected patients included gram-negative bacilli (24.4%), fungi (7.4%), and *Pseudomonas* species (8.3%). During the same period, the frequency of *Pseudomonas* and fungal peritonitis among non-HIV patients was 2% and 3%, respectively. Two key observations of this study deserve comment. One, the rate of peritonitis was increased among active intravenous drug abusers compared to non–drug users (5.8 vs. 2.9 episodes per CAPD year) emphasizing the effect of behavioral patterns on susceptibility to peritonitis. Two, the rate of peritonitis was lower in patients using Y-connectors instead of straight set systems (2.6 vs. 7.1 episodes per CAPD year). In a study by Kimmel et al. (33), there was no significant difference in peritonitis rates between primarily homosexual patients with HIV infection and non–HIV-infected CAPD patients (2.4 ± 1.6 vs. 1.7 ± 1.4 episodes per CAPD year). In agreement with these data, Wasser et al. (93)

also reported no differences in the prevalence of peritonitis between HIV-infected and uninfected patients.

E. Hospitalizations

There are few data on the rates of hospitalization in patients with HIV infection maintained on CAPD. Tebben et al. (45) reported a rate of 4.2 hospitalizations per patient-year on peritoneal dialysis (151 hospitalizations in 436 patient-months) with a mean hospitalization duration of 53.4 days per maintenance dialysis year. By comparison, Nolph (94) reported an average of 2–23 days of hospitalization per year among non–HIV-infected patients. Patients with advanced HIV infection spent twice as many days per year hospitalized than those with asymptomatic infection (67.6 days/year vs. 29.1 days/year); peritonitis and catheter-related complications, however, accounted for only 39% of the hospitalizations in the former group but 75% of hospitalizations in the latter.

IV. INFECTION CONTROL

A. Hemodiaylsis

1. Patient-to-Patient Transmission.

The specter of transmission of a deadly bloodborne pathogen in the dialysis setting where exposure to blood and body substances is commonplace raises serious concerns for patients, their families, and dialysis staff alike. The CDC addressed this issue with the publication of guidelines for the prevention of HIV transmission in the dialysis setting, stressing the role of universal precautions and disinfection of dialysis machinery (18,95,96). Their recommendations specifically note that routine testing of patients and hemodialysis staff is not necessary, nor is it advised to isolate patient and hemodialysis equipment. Fortunately, to date, the transmission of HIV between patients on hemodialysis in the United States has not been recognized and only one case of HIV transmission from an HIV-infected patient to a dialysis technician has been documented (18). Supporting these findings are the results of several single and multicenter studies in which the transmission of HIV infection could not be documented (97–99).

The catastrophic consequences of breaches in infection-control measures were dramatically illustrated by reports of HIV transmission among hemodialysis patients in Argentina, Colombia, and Egypt (100–102). In Argentina, 20 of 34 patients in a hemodialysis unit in the town of La Plata and 33 patients in a hemodialysis unit in Cordoba were found to be HIV positive. The cause of these outbreaks was attributed to inadequate infection-control policies, reuse of dialysis equipment, and the sharing of multidose heparin vials (101). In Colombia, 13 of 23 dialysis patients in one center were found to be HIV positive. By assaying sera stored for purposes of renal transplantation, it was determined that 9 of these patients had seroconverted over a period of 6 months in 1992. Most of the seroconversions occurred while patients were dialyzing at the time a new HIV-positive patient started dialysis. Genetic typing of the HIV isolates in four of the HIV seroconverters demonstrated strong sequence similarities between them and significant differences from unrelated Colombian specimens. Investigation of the practices of this unit revealed that reused hemodialysis needles were disinfected in common containers of benzalkonium chloride and at times the disinfectant solution was replaced only every 7 days (102).

2. Patient-to-Staff Transmission

The reported risk of HIV transmission after percutaneous exposure is approximately 0.32% based on unstratified pooled data from 25 prospective studies of occupational exposure and transmission of HIV-1 (103). In comparison, the average risk for transmission of hepatitis B and hepatitis C after percutaneous exposure is 2–4% and 3–10%, respectively (104). A recent case-control study conducted by the CDC (105) identified four factors that increased the risk of HIV transmission: deep injury (intramuscular), visible blood on sharp device, needle used to enter a blood vessel, and source patient with preterminal AIDS. Zidovudine prophylaxis soon after exposure was shown to reduce the risk of transmission by 79% [odds ratio 0.21 (CI 0.1–0.6)]. Dialysis staff is particularly susceptible to percutaneous injury by large-bore hollow needles that may be used for dialyzing patients with advanced stages of HIV infection and high viral loads. Gilbert and Bennett (104) estimated that in 1993 between 13 and 33 instances of HIV transmission to dialysis workers could have occurred based on the national prevalence of HIV (1.5%) in the hemodialysis population at the time and the results of a national survey of needle stick frequencies conducted among medical personnel (106). The fact that only one documented episode of HIV transmission to a dialysis health care worker has occurred may suggest that the frequency of needlestick injury among dialysis workers is overestimated, perhaps in part because of precautions learned from experience with the hepatitis viruses. On a technical note, Ortiz-Butcher et al. (107) and Ahuja et al. (52) were unable to detect HIV RNA in dialysis ultrafiltrates collected during conventional hemodialysis sessions in HIV-infected patients. This is reassuring given the potential risk of accidental mucocutaneous exposure with infectious material from splashed spent dialysate.

B. Peritoneal Dialysis

Several investigators have demonstrated the presence of HIV-1 in dialysate from HIV-infected peritoneal dialysis patients. Breyer and Harbison (108) isolated HIV-1 from the peritoneal fluid of an asymptomatic HIV-infected patient and from a patient with AIDS. Scheel et al. (109) successfully cultured HIV-1 from the peritoneal fluid of 12 of 14 patients (mean CD4 count 310 cells/μL) on maintenance peritoneal dialysis. In a series of experiments to define the survival kinetics of HIV-1, the same authors demonstrated survival of HIV-1 in peritoneal dialysate at room temperature for up to 7 days (110). Survival on dried, experimentally inoculated peritoneal dialysis tubing was demonstrated for up to 48 hours. Lastly, the authors demonstrated successful disinfection of HIV-1–containing peritoneal dialysate with a 1:512 dilution of 50% Amukin and 10% bleach solution after a 10-minute period of exposure. The National Kidney Foundation–National Institute of Health Task Force on AIDS and Kidney Disease (111) provided guidelines for disposing of peritoneal dialysis solutions in hospitals that included placing used dialysate bags in covered containers until the end of the day and disposal of dialysate into a sink or toilet using barrier precautions to prevent accidental splash contamination. Following the disposal of dialysate, it was recommended that 200 mL of 10% bleach solution be carefully poured into the sink or toilet and allowed to dwell for 30 minutes. The remaining peritoneal dialysis supplies should be discarded into properly labeled and sealed biohazard containers. Recently, Scheel and Malan (112) argued for the direct addition

Table 3 Advice About Prophylaxis After Exposure to Human Immunodeficiency Virus

	Advice per attributes of source patient		
Attributes of exposure	Asymptomatic, known low titer	AIDS symptomatic infection	Preterminal AIDS, acute infection, known high titer
Percutaneous injuries			
Superficial injury	Offer	Recommend	Strongly encourage
Visibly bloody device used in artery or vein	Recommend	Recommend	Strongly encourage
Deep intramuscular injury or actual injection	Recommend	Strongly encourage	Strongly encourage
Mucosal contacts			
Small volume and brief contact	Offer	Offer	Offer
Large volume or prolonged contact	Offer	Recommend	Recommend
Large volume and prolonged contact	Recommend	Recommend	Strongly encourage
Cutaneous contacts			
Small volume and brief contact	Offer if obvious portal of entry	Offer if obvious portal of entry	Offer if obvious portal of entry
Large volume or prolonged contact	Offer (recommend if obvious portal of entry)	Offer (recommend if obvious portal of entry)	Offer (recommend if obvious portal of entry)
Large volume and prolonged contact	Offer (recommend if obvious portal of entry)	Recommend (especially with portal of entry)	Recommend (especially with portal of entry)

Source: Ref. 103.

of a disinfectant into the patient's peritoneal dialysis bag in order to improve disinfection and facilitate the safe disposal of the fluid. Of the solutions (Amukin, bleach, and povidone iodine) with proven efficacy against HIV-1 in peritoneal dialysis fluid, only Amukin is currently formulated in a container that is modified to fit over a typical peritoneal dialysis drain bag connector (112,113).

C. Management of HIV Exposure

Every dialysis facility should have an infection-control plan in place to efficiently deal with the inevitable occurrences of high-risk exposures. The CDC and others have published recommendations for postexposure counseling and antiviral prophylaxis based on the risk category of the exposure (3,103,114). The effectiveness of postexposure prophylaxis in humans was first demonstrated by the CDC case-control study wherein zidovudine conferred a 79% decreased risk of HIV seroconversion after percutaneous exposure with HIV-1–contaminated blood (105). Taking into consideration possible antiviral resistance, current recommendations favor combination antiviral regimens including zidovudine and a protease inhibitor for all high-risk exposures. Each regimen should be modified by any information, particularly the history of antiretroviral drug usage and the clinical stage of illness in the source patient. Although the optimal timing and duration of therapy is unknown, it is recommended that therapy be initiated within the first 2 hours following exposure and carried out for a minimum of 4 weeks (Table 3).

Table 4 Antiretroviral Drugs

Nucleoside reverse transcriptase inhibitors		
Drug	**Metabolism**	**Daily dose dialysis**
Zidovudine (AZT) (3-2-3-dideoxythymidine) (115–117)	Glucuronidation to 5-O ether glucuronide; glucuronide excreted in urine (10–20% excreted unchanged in urine)	Negligible removal by hemodialysis or peritoneal dialysis; 50% daily dose (300 mg/day)
Didanosine (ddI) (2-3-dideoxyinosine) (118)	60% excreted unchanged in urine; clearance reduced >4-fold in renal failure	Reduce oral dose by 25–50%; supplemental dose after dialysis not needed
Zalcitabine (ddC) (2-3-dideoxycytidine) (119, 120)	75% excreted unchanged in urine; elimination t1/2 increased from 0.5–2.2 h to >8 h in renal failure	Reduce oral dose (0.75 mg/day)
Stavudine (D4T) (2-3-didehydro-3-deoxythymidine) (120)	Renal and nonrenal; >40% eliminated unchanged in urine	Reduce oral dose 50% (20–40 mg/day)
Laminvudine (3TC) (2-deoxy-3-thiacytidine) (120, 121)	Excreted largely unchanged in urine (68–71% of oral/IV dose)	Reduce oral dose (50–150 mg/day)
Protease inhibitors (122)		
Name	**Metabolism**	**Dosage in dialysis**
Indinavir	Hepatic (P450 3A) 20% elimination in urine	Unknown
Nelfinavir	Hepatic (P450 3A)	Unknown
Ritonavir	Hepatic (P450 CYP3A)	Unknown
Saquinavir mesylate	Hepatic (P450 3A)	Unknown
Saquinavir	Hepatic (P450 3A)	Unknown
Nonnucleoside reverse transcriptase inhibitors (121–125)		
Name	**Metabolism**	**Dosage in dialysis**
Delavirdine	Hepatic	Unknown
Nevirapine	Hepatic	Unknown

V. ANTIVIRAL THERAPY

Without targeted antiviral therapy it is not possible to provide optimal care for HIV-infected patients. Just a few years ago there was insufficient basic and clinical knowledge about the pathophysiology of HIV infection to warrant the aggressive approaches to drug therapy that are prevalent today. HIV patients on dialysis often come from medically underserved groups and may display behavior characteristics of medical nonadherence with prescribed therapies. The increasing complexity of the antiviral regimens in use today are added to the heavy medication, diet, and time burdens that dialysis patients already have. For the physician caring for these patients, the choices of medications are complicated by uncertainties over the pharmacokinetics of these regimens in ESRD. With these elements in mind, an outline of antiretroviral drugs is presented in Table 4. For guidelines on drug selection, timing, and clinical follow-up, the reader is referred to the most current International AIDS Society's updated recommendations (3). In brief, current antiretroviral therapy should use one or combine two reverse transcriptase inhibitors for all patients. Aggressive triple therapy, including a protease inhibitor, is recommended for patients (a) symptomatic of AIDS, (b) asymptomatic with CD4+ lymphocytes <500 cells/μL, and (c) asymptomatic with CD4+ lymphocytes >500 cells/μL but viral load >5,000–10,000. Because of the complexities of HIV management introduced by the new classes of antiretroviral agents, patients should be managed by clinicians experienced in their use whenever possible (122,126).

REFERENCES

1. The World Health Report 1997: Conquering Suffering, Enriching Humanity. Report of the Director-General. Geneva: World Health Organization, 1997.
2. Centers for Disease Control and Prevention. HIV/AIDS Surveillance Report 1997; 9(1):1–37.
3. Carpenter CC, Fischl MA, Hammer SM, Hirsch MS, Jacobsen DM, Katzenstein DA, Montaner JS, Richman DD, Saag MS, Schooley RT, Thompson MA, Vella S, Yeni PG, Volberding PA. Antiretroviral therapy for HIV infection in 1997. Updated recommendations of the International AIDS Society-USA panel. JAMA 1997; 277:1962–1969.
4. Fischl MA, Dickinson GM, La Voie L. Safety and efficacy of sulfamethoxazole and trimethoprim chemoprophylaxis for *Pneumocystis carinii* pneumonia in AIDS. JAMA 1988; 259:1185–1189.
5. Pierce M, Crampton S, Henry D, Heifets L, LaMarca A, Montecalvo M, Wormser GP, Jablonowski H, Jemsek J, Cyanamon M, Yangco BG, Notario G, Craft JC. A randomized trial of clarithromycin as prophylaxis against disseminated *Mycobacterium avium* complex infection in patients with advanced acquired immunodeficiency syndrome. N Engl J Med 1996; 335: 384–391.
6. Mellors JW, Rinaldo CR, Jr., Gupta P, White RM, Todd JA, Kingsley LA. prognosis in HIV-1 infection predicted by the quantity of virus in plasma. Science 1996; 272:1167–1170.
7. Stein DS, Lyles RH, Graham NM, Tassoni CJ, Margolick JB, Phair JP, Rinaldo C, Detels R, Saah A, Bilello J. Predicting clinical progression or death in subjects with early-stage human immunodeficiency virus (HIV) infection: a comparative analysis of quantification of HIV RNA, soluble tumor necrosis factor type II receptors, neopterin, and beta$_2$-microglobulin. Multicenter AIDS Cohort Study. J Infect Dis 1997; 176:1161–1167.
8. Ho DD, Neumann AU, Perelson AS, Chen W, Leonard JM, Markowitz M. Rapid turnover of plasma virions and CD4 lymphocytes in HIV-1 infection. Nature 1995; 373:123–126.
9. Easterbrook PJ, Emami J, Moyle G, Gazzard BG. Progressive CD4 cell depletion and death in zidovudine-treated patients. J AIDS 1993; 6:927–929.
10. Karon JM, Buehler JW, Byers RH, Farizo KM, Green TA, Hanson DL, Rosenblum LS, Gail MH, Rosenberg PS, Brookmeyer R. Projections of the number of persons diagnosed with AIDS and the number of immunosuppressed HIV-infected persons—United States, 1992–1994. MMWR 1992; 41:1–29.
11. Taylor JM, Sy JP, Visscher B, Giorgi JV. CD4+ T-cell number at the time of acquired immunodeficiency syndrome. Am J Epidemiol 1995; 141:645–651.
12. Osmond D, Charlesbois E, Lang W, Shiboski S, Moss A. Changes in AIDS survival time in two San Francisco cohorts of homosexual men, 1983 to 1993. JAMA 1994; 271:1083–1087.
13. Yarchoan R, Venzon DJ, Pluda JM, Lietzau J, Wyvill KM, Tsiatis AA, Steinberg SM, Broder S. CD4 count and the risk for death in patients infected with HIV receiving antiretroviral therapy. Ann Intern Med 1991; 115:184–189.
14. Mocroft AJ, Lundgren JD, d'Armino Monforte A, Ledergerber B, Barton SE, Vella S, Katlama C, Gerstoft J, Pedersen C, Phillips AN. Survival of AIDS patients according to type of AIDS-defining event. The AIDS in Europe Study Group. Int J Epidemiol 1997; 26:400–407.
15. Coffin JM. HIV viral dynamics. AIDS 1996; 10(suppl 3):S75–84.
16. Kitahata MM, Koepsell TD, Deyo RA, Maxwell CL, Dodge WT, Wagner EH. Physicians' experience with

the acquired immunodeficiency syndrome as a factor in patients' survival. N Engl J Med 1996; 334:701–706.

17. Laraque F, Greene A, Triano-Davis JW, Altman R, Lin-Greenberg A. Effect of a comprehensive intervention program on survival of patients with human immunodeficiency virus infection. Arch Intern Med 1996; 156:169–176.
18. Tokars JI, Miller ER, Alter MJ, Arduino MJ. National surveillance of dialysis associated diseases in the United States. ASAIO J 1998; 44:98–107.
19. Anonymous. Human immunodeficiency virus infection in hemodialysis patients. Baltimore-Boston Collaborative Study Group. Arch Intern Med 1988; 148:617–619.
20. Perez G, Ortiz-Interian C, Lee H, de Medina M, Cerney M, Allain JP, Schiff E, Parks E, Parks W, Bourgoignie JJ. Human immunodeficiency virus and human T-cell leukemia virus type I in patients undergoing maintenance hemodialysis in Miami. Am J Kidney Dis 1989; 14:39–43.
21. Chirgwin K, Rao TK, Landesman SH. HIV infection in a high prevalence hemodialysis unit. AIDS 1989; 3:731–735.
22. Murthy BV, Pereira BJ. A 1990s perspective of hepatitis C, human immunodeficiency virus, and tuberculosis infections in dialysis patients. Semin Nephrol 1997; 17:346–363.
23. Bourgoignie JJ, Meneses R, Ortiz C, Jaffe D, Pardo V. The clinical spectrum of renal disease associated with human immunodeficiency virus. Am J Kidney Dis 1988; 12:131–137.
24. Winston JA, Klotman PE. Are we missing an epidemic of HIV-associated nephropathy? J Am Soc Nephrol 1996; 7:1–7.
25. Schoenfeld P, Rodriguez R, Mendelson M. Patients with HIV infection and end-stage renal disease. Adv Renal Replacement Ther 1996; 3:287–292.
26. Laradi A, Mallet A, Beaufils H, Allouache M, Martinez F. HIV-associated nephropathy: outcomes and prognostic factors. J Am Soc Nephrol 1997; 8:141A.
27. Ifudu O, Mayers JD, Matthew JJ, Macey LJ, Brezsnyak W, Reydel C, McClendon E, Surgrue T, Rao TK, Friedman EA. Uremia therapy in patients with end-stage renal disease and human immunodeficiency virus infection: has the outcome changed in the 1990s? Am J Kidney Dis 1997; 29:549–552.
28. Lorch JA, Pollak VE. Outcomes in AIDS patients treated by dialysis. J Am Soc Nephrol 1996; 7:1455A.
29. Barth RH. Long survival of chronically dialyzed patients with HIV disease. J Am Soc Nephrol 1996; 7:1439A.
30. Perinbasekar S, Brod-Miller C, Pal S, Mattana J. Predictors of survival in HIV-infected patients on hemodialysis. Am J Nephrol 1996; 16:280–286.
31. Schoenfeld P, Mendelson M, Rodriguez R. Survival of ESRD patients with the HIV infection. J Am Soc Nephrol 1995; 6:561A.
32. Harrison D, Nerves R, Villalon V, Weinmann A, Sondheimer J, Cadnapaphornchai P. Outcome of HIV infected patients on hemodialysis. J Am Soc Nephrol 1995; 6:532A.
33. Kimmel PL, Umana WO, Simmens SJ, Watson J, Bosch JP. Continuous ambulatory peritoneal dialysis and survival of HIV-infected patients with end-stage renal disease. Kidney Int 1993; 44:373–378.
34. Valeri A, Neusy AJ. The impact of HIV infection in ESRD. J Am Soc Nephrol 1991; 2:72P(A).
35. Katz LA. Excellent dialysis tolerance in HIV-positive patients without AIDS. Kidney Int 1990; 37:330A.
36. Ribot S, Dean D, Goldbalt M, Saavedra M. Prognosis of HIV-positive dialysis patients. Kidney Int 1990; 37:315A.
37. Zara AC, Berlyne GM, Barth RH. Prolonged survival in AIDS with end-stage renal disease. Kidney Int 1990; 37:325A.
38. Feinfeld DA, Kaplan R. Dressler R, Lynn RI. Survival of human immunodeficiency virus-infected patients on maintenance dialysis. Clin Nephrol 1989; 32:221–224.
39. Reiser IW, Shapiro WB, Porush JG. The incidence and epidemiology of human immunodeficiency virus infection in 320 patients treated in an inner-city hemodialysis center. Am J Kidney Dis 1990; 16:26–31.
40. Gordinho JJ, Weaver M, Whaley BP, Lasker N. Survival of IVDA-HIV positive and negative patients on dialysis. Kidney Int 1989; 35:2481A.
41. Ortiz C, Meneses R, Jaffe D, Fernandez JA, Perez G, Bourgoignie JJ. Outcome of patients with human immunodeficiency virus on maintenance hemodialysis. Kidney Int 1988; 34:248–253.
42. Rao TK, Friedman EA, Nicastri AD. The types of renal disease in the acquired immunodeficiency syndrome. N Engl J Med 1987; 316:1062–1068.
43. Pennell JP, Bourgoignie JJ. Should AIDS patients be dialyzed? ASAIO Trans 1988; 34:907–911.
44. 1993 revised classification system for HIV infection and expanded surveillance case definition for AIDS among adolescents and adults. MMWR 1992; 41:1–19.
45. Tebben JA, Rigsby MO, Selwyn PA, Brennan N, Kliger A, Finkelstein FO. Outcome of HIV infected patients on continuous ambulatory peritoneal dialysis. Kidney Int 1993; 44:191–198.
46. Anonymous. Classification system for human T-lymphotrophic virus type III/lymphadenopathy-associated virus. MMWR 1986; 35:334–339.
47. Mellors JW, Kingsley LA, Rinaldo CR, Jr., Todd JA, Hoo BS, Kokka RP, Gupta P. Quantitation of HIV-1 RNA in plasma predicts outcome after seroconversion. Ann Int Med 1995; 122:573–579.

48. Mellors JW, Munoz A, Giorgi JV, Margolick JB, Tasoni CJ, Gupta P, Kingsley LA, Todd JA, Saah AJ, Detels R, Phair JP, Rinaldo CR, Jr. Plasma viral load and CD4+ lymphocytes as prognostic markers of HIV-1 infection. Ann Int Med 1997; 126:946–954.
49. Kimmel PL, VedBrat SS, Pierce PF, Umana WO, Shepherd L, Verme DA, Hirsch RP, Hellman KB. Prevalence of viremia in human immunodeficiency virus-infected patients with renal disease. Arch Int Med 1995; 155:1578–1584.
50. Winston J, Klotman P. Plasma HIV-1 in seropositive patients with renal disease. J Am Soc Nephrol 1996; 7:1345A.
51. Winston J, Fozialoff A, Klotman M, Klotman PE. HIV-associated nephropathy is a late, not early complication of HIV-1 infection. J Am Soc Nephrol 1997; 8:99A.
52. Ahuja T, Paar D, Velasco A, Watts BA. Effect of hemodialysis and antiretroviral therapy on plasma viral load in HIV-1 infected hemodialysis patients. J Am Soc Nephrol 1997; 8:226A.
53. Elfatih A, Suboth JS, Chan MM, Wasser WG. Effect of hemodialysis on the T-helper lymphocyte count in human immunodeficiency virus infected patients on chronic hemodialysis maintenance. J Am Soc Nephrol 1996; 7:1470A.
54. Spivak JL, Barnes D, Ferracioli GF. Serum immunoreactive erythropoietin and anemia in HIV-infected patients. JAMA 1989; 261:3104–3107.
55. Fischl M, Galpin JE, Groopman JE, Henry DH, Kennedy P, Miles S, Robbins W, Starrett B, Zalusky R, Abels RI, Nelson RA, Thompson D, Rudnick SA. Recombinant human erythropoietin and the treatment of anemia in patients with AIDS treated with zidovudine. N Engl J Med 1990; 322:1488–1493.
56. Henry DH, Jemsek JG, Levin AS, Levine JD, Abels RI, Nelson RA, Thompson D, Rudnick SA. Recombinant human erythropoietin and the treatment of anemia in patients with AIDS or advanced ARC not receiving ZDV. J AIDS 1992; 5:847–848.
57. Shrivastava D, Rao TK, Sinert R, Khurana E, Lundin AP, Friedman EA. The efficacy of erythropoietin in human immunodeficiency virus-infected end-stage renal disease patients treated by maintenance hemodialysis. Am J Kidney Dis 1995; 25:904–909.
58. Ifudu O, Matthew JJ, Mayers JD, Macey LJ, Brezsnyak W, Reydel C, McClendon E, Surgrue T, Rao S, Friedman EA. Severity of AIDS and the response to EPO in uremia. Am J Kidney Dis 1997; 30:28–35.
59. Lowrie EG, Lew NL. Death risk in hemodialysis patients: the predictive value of commonly measured variables and an evaluation of death rate differences between facilities. Am J Kidney Dis 1990; 15:458–482.
60. Grunfeld C, Feingold KR. Metabolic disturbances and wasting in the acquired immunodeficiency syndrome. N Engl J Med 1992; 327:329–337.
61. Babameto G, Kotler DP. Malnutrition in HIV infection. Gastroenterol Clin North Am 1997; 26:393.
62. Palenicek JP, Graham NM, He YD, Hoover DA, Oishi JS, Kingsley L, Saah AJ. Weight loss prior to clinical AIDS as a predictor of survival. Multicenter AIDS Cohort Study Investigators. J AIDS Hum Retrovirol 1995; 10:366–373.
63. Suttmann U, Ockenga J, Selberg O, Hoogestraat L, Deicher H, Muller MJ. Incidence and prognostic value of malnutrition and wasting in human immunodeficiency virus-infected outpatients. J AIDS Hum Retrovirol 1995; 8:239–246.
64. Mcnurlan MA, Garlick PJ, Steigbigel RT, Decristofaro KA, Frost RA, Lang CH, Johnson RW, Santasier AM, Cabahug CJ, Fuhrer J, Gelato MC. Responsiveness of muscle protein synthesis to growth hormone administration in HIV-infected individuals declines with severity of disease. J Clin Invest 1997; 100:2125–2132.
65. Graham KK, Mikolich DJ, Fisher AE, Posner MR, Dudley MN. Pharmacologic evaluation of megestrol acetate oral suspension in cachectic AIDS patients. J AIDS 1994; 7:580–586.
66. Von Roenn JH, Armstrong D, Kotler DP, Cohn DL, Klimas NG, Tchekmedyian NS, Cone L, Brennan PJ, Weitzman SA. Megestrol acetate in patients with AIDS-related cachexia. Ann Intern Med 1994; 121: 393–399.
67. Reyesteran G, Sierramadero JG, Delcerro VM, Arroyofigueroa H, Pasquetti A, Calva JJ, Ruizpalacios GM. Effects of thalidomide on HIV-associated wasting syndrome—a randomized, double-blind, placebo-controlled clinical trial. AIDS 1996; 10:1501–1507.
68. Waters D, Danska J, Hardy K, Koster F, Qualls C, Nickell D, Nightingale S, Gesundheit N, Watson D, Schade D. Recombinant human growth hormone, insulin-like growth factor 1, and combination therapy in AIDS-associated wasting—a randomized, double-blind, placebo-controlled trial. Ann Intern Med 1996; 125:865.
69. Frost RA, Lang CH, Gelato MC. Growth hormone insulin-like growth factor axis in human immunodeficiency virus associated disease. Endocrinologist 1997; 7:23–31.
70. Hengge UR, Baumann M, Maleba R, Brockmeyer NH, Goos M. Oxymetholone promotes weight gain in patients with advanced human immunodeficiency virus (HIV-1) infection. Br J Nutr 1996; 75:129–138.
71. Berger JR, Pall L, Hall CD, Simpson DM, Berry PS, Dudley R. Oxandrolone in AIDS-wasting myopathy. AIDS 1996; 10:1657–1662.
72. Coodley GO, Coodley MK. A trial of testosterone therapy for HIV-associated weight loss. AIDS 1997; 11:1347–1352.
73. Cofrancesco J, Whalen JJ, Dobs AS. Testosterone replacement treatment options for HIV-infected men. J AIDS Hum Retrovirol 1997; 16:254–265.

74. Beal JE, Olson R, Lefkowitz L, Larenstein L, Bellman P, Yangco B, Morales JO, Murphy R, Powderly W, Plasse TF, Mosdell KW, Shepard KV. Long-term efficacy and safety of dronabinol for acquired immunodeficiency syndrome-associated anorexia. J Pain Symptom Management 1997; 14:7–14.
75. Ockenga J, Suttmann U, Selberg O, Schlesinger A, Meier PNH, Gebel M, Schedel I, Deicher H. Percutaneous endoscopic gastrostomy in AIDS and control patients: risks and outcome. Am J Gastroenterol 1996; 91:1817–1822.
76. Melchior JC, Chastang C, Gelas P, Carbonnel F, Zazzo JF, Boulier A, Cosnes J, Bouletreau P, Messing B. Efficacy of 2-month total parenteral nutrition in AIDS patients: a controlled randomized prospective trial. The French Multicenter Total Parenteral Nutrition Cooperative Group Study. AIDS 1996; 10:379–384.
77. Lipton SA. Neuropathogenesis of acquired immunodeficiency syndrome dementia. Curr Opinion Neurol 1997; 10:247–253.
78. Melton ST, Kirkwood CK, Ghaemi SN. Pharmacotherapy of HIV dementia. Ann Pharmacother 1997; 31:457–473.
79. Obailo CI, Brathwaite M, Howard A, Cleveland W. Reduced shunt thrombosis in AIDS nephropathy. J Am Soc Nephrol 1996; 7:1416A.
80. Obailo CI, Robinson T, Brathwaite M. Variable vascular access survival in a sub population of African Americans hemodialysis patients. Am J Kidney Dis 1998; 32:250–256.
81. Nannery WM, Stoldt HS, Fares LG, 2d. Hemodialysis access operations performed upon patients with human immunodeficiency virus. Surg Gyn Obst 1991; 173:387–390.
82. Brock JS, Sussman M, Wamsley M, Mintzer R, Baumann FG, Riles TS. The influence of human immunodeficiency virus infection and intravenous drug abuse on complications of hemodialysis access surgery. J Vasc Surg 1992; 16:904–910.
83. Jacobson MA, Gellermann H, Chambers H. *Staphylococcus aureus* bacteremia and recurrent staphylococcal infection in patients with acquired immunodeficiency syndrome and AIDS-related complex. Am J Med 1988; 85:172–176.
84. Boelaert JR, Van Landuyt HW, Gordts BZ, De Baere YA, Messer SA, Herwaldt LA. Nasal and cutaneous carriage of *Staphylococcus aureus* in hemodialysis patients: the effect of nasal mupirocin. Infect Control Hosp Epidemiol 1996; 17:809–811.
85. Kluytmans J, van Belkum A, Verbrugh H. Nasal carriage of *Staphylococcus aureus*: epidemiology, underlying mechanisms, and associated risks. Clin Microbiol Rev 1997; 10:505–520.
86. Ramaswamy CR, Sreedhara R, Fein PA, Dedios A, Avram MM. Characteristics of peritonitis in HIV positive dialysis patients. J Am Soc Nephrol 1997; 8: 270A.
87. Lewis M, Gorban-Brennan NL, Kliger A, Cooper K, Finkelstein FO. Incidence and spectrum of organisms causing peritonitis in HIV positive patients on CAPD. Adv Periton Dial 1990; 6:136–138.
88. Dressler R, Peters AT, Lynn RI. Pseudomonal and candidal peritonitis as a complication of continuous ambulatory peritoneal dialysis in human immunodeficiency virus-infected patients. Am J Med 1989; 86: 787–790.
89. Perazella M, Eisen T, Brown E. Peritonitis associated with disseminated Mycobacterium avium complex in an acquired immunodeficiency syndrome patient on chronic ambulatory peritoneal dialysis. Am J Kidney Dis 1993; 21:319–321.
90. Yinnon AM, Solages A, Treanor JJ. Cryptococcal peritonitis: report of a case developing during continuous ambulatory peritoneal dialysis and review of the literature. Clin Infect Dis 1993; 17:736–741.
91. Parsonnet J. Trichosporon beigelii peritonitis. South Med J 1989; 82:1062–1063.
92. Abitbol C, Zilleruello G, Strauss J, Martin L. Dialysis treatment of pediatric patients infected with the human immunodeficiency virus. J Am Soc Nephrol 1997; 8: 215A.
93. Wasser WG, Boyle MJ, Brandon S, Gruber SJ, Winston RV, Feldman NS. HIV positivity does not predispose peritoneal dialysis patients to peritonitis. J Am Soc Nephrol 1991; 2:369A.
94. Nolph K. Comparison of continuous ambulatory peritoneal dialysis and hemodialysis. Kidney Int 1988; (suppl 24):S123–S131.
95. Anonymous. Recommendations for providing dialysis treatment to patients infected with the human T-lymphotrophic virus type III/lymphadenopathy-associated virus. MMWR 1986; 35(23):376–378.
96. Anonymous. Recommendations for prevention of HIV transmission in health-care settings. MMWR 1987; 36(suppl2):1S–18S.
97. Marcus R, Favero MS, Banerjee S, Solomon SL, Bell DM, Jarvis WR, Martone WJ, and the Cooperative Dialysis Study Group, Atlanta, Georgia. Prevalence and incidence of human immunodeficiency virus among patients undergoing long-term hemodialysis. Am J Med 1991; 90:614–619.
98. Perez GO, Ortiz C, de Medina M, Schiff E, Bourgoignie JJ. Lack of transmission of human immunodeficiency virus in chronic hemodialysis patients. Am J Nephrol 1988; 8:123–126.
99. Assogba U, Park RA, Rey MA, Barthelemy A, Rottembourg J, Gluckman JC. Prospective study of HIV I seropositive patients in hemodialysis centers. Clin Nephrol 1988; 29:312–314.
100. Hassan NF, el Ghorab NM, Abdel Rehim MS. HIV infection in renal patients. AIDS 1994; 8:853.
101. Dyer E. Argentinean doctors accused of spreading AIDS. BMJ 1993; 307:584.

102. Velandia M, Fridkin S, Cardena V, Boshell J, Ramirez G, Bland L, Iglesias A. Transmission of HIV in dialysis centre. Lancet 1995; 345:1417–1422.
103. Gerberding JL. Prophylaxis for occupational exposure to HIV. Ann Intern Med 1996; 125:497–501.
104. Gilbert DN, Bennett W. Patients with the human immunodeficiency virus infection in the hemodialysis unit. How vulnerable are the caregivers? Arch Intern Med 1995; 155:1575–1576.
105. Anonymous. Case-control study of HIV seroconversion in health care workers after percutaneous exposure to HIV-infected blood—France, United Kingdom, and United States, January 1988 to August 1994. MMWR 1995; 44:929–933.
106. Stotka JL, Wong ES, Williams DS, Stuart CB, Markowitz SM. An analysis of blood and body fluid exposures sustained by house officers, medical students, and nursing personnel on acute care general medical wards: a prospective study. Infect Contr Hosp Epidem 1991; 12:583–590.
107. Ortiz-Butcher C, Pennell JP, Walling J, Zjacic B, Fletcher M. Analysis of hemodialysis ultrafiltrate by RT-PCR for HIV after an accidental splash of a dialysis provider. J Am Soc Nephrol 1997; 8:248A.
108. Breyer AJ, Harbison MA. Isolation of human immunodeficiency virus from peritoneal dialysate. Am J Kidney Dis 1993; 21:23–25.
109. Scheel PJ, Jr., Farzadegan H, Ford D, Malan M, Watson A. Recovery of human immunodeficiency virus from peritoneal dialysis effluent. J Am Soc Nephrol 1995; 5:1926–1929.
110. Farzadegan H, Ford D, Malan M, Masters B, Scheel PJ, Jr. HIV-1 survival kinetics in peritoneal dialysis effluent. Kidney Int 1996; 50:1659–1662.
111. Schoenfeld P, Feduska NJ. Acquired immunodeficiency syndrome and renal disease: report of the National Kidney Foundation-National Institutes of Health Task Force on AIDS and Kidney Disease. Am J Kidney Dis 1990; 16:14–25.
112. Scheel PJ, Jr., Malan M. Disposal of dialysate in HIV-positive patients: an update. Adv Ren Replacement Ther 1996; 3:298–301.
113. Breyer J, Harbison MA. Isolation and quantification of human immunodeficiency virus type 1 (HIV-1) from peritoneal dialysate: implications for infection control. Perit Dialysis Int 1995; 15:179–180.
114. Anonymous. Update: provisional Public Health Service recommendations for chemoprophylaxis after occupational exposure to HIV. MMWR 1996; 45:468–480.
115. Pioger JC, Taburet AM, Colin JN, Colaneri S, Fillastre JP, Singlas E. Pharmacokinetics of zidovudine (AZT) and its metabolite (G-AZT) in healthy subjects and in patients with kidney failure. Therapie 1989; 44:401–404.
116. Kremer D, Munar MY, Kohlhepp SJ, Swan SK, Stinnett EA, Gilbert DN, Young EW, Bennett WM. Zidovudine pharmacokinetics in five HIV seronegative patients undergoing continuous ambulatory peritoneal dialysis. Pharmacotherapy 1992; 12:56–60.
117. Kimmel PL, Lew SQ, Umana WO, Li PP, Gordon AM, Straw J. Pharmacokinetics of zidovudine in HIV-infected patients with end-stage renal disease. Blood Purif 1995; 13:340–346.
118. Knupp CA, Hak LJ, Coakley DF, Falk RJ, Wagner BE, Raasch RH, van der Horst CM, Kaul S, Barbhaiya RH, Dukes GE. Disposition of didanosine in HIV-seropositive patients with normal renal function or chronic renal failure: influence of hemodialysis and continuous ambulatory peritoneal dialysis. Clin Pharm Ther 1996; 60:535–542.
119. Klecker RW, Collins JM, Yarchoan RC. Pharmacokinetics of 2′-3′ dideoxycytidine in patients with AIDS and related disorders. J Clin Pharm 1988; 28:837–842.
120. Dudley MN. Clinical pharmacokinetics of nucleoside antiretroviral agents. J Infect Dis 1995; 171:S99–112.
121. Angel JB, Hussey EK, Hall ST. Pharmacokinetics of 3TC (GR109714X) administered with and without food to HIV-infected patients. Drug Invest 1993; 6: 70–74.
122. Flexner C. HIV-protease inhibitors. N Engl J Med 1998; 338(18):1281–1292.
123. Luzuriaga K, Bryson Y, McSherry G, Robinson J, Stechenberg B, Scott G, Lamson M, Cort S, Sullivan JL. Pharmacokinetics, safety, and activity of nevirapine in human immunodeficiency virus type 1-infected children. J Infect Dis 1996; 174:713–721.
124. Chang M, Sood VK, Kloosterman DA, Hauer MJ, Fagerness PE, Sanders PE, Vrbanac JJ. Identification of the metabolites of the HIV-1 reverse transcriptase inhibitor delavirdine in monkeys. Drug Metab Dispos 1997; 25:814–827.
125. Cheng CL, Smith DE, Carver PL, Cox SR, Watkins PB, Blake DS, Kauffman CA, Meyer KM, Amidon GL, Stetson PL. Steady-state pharmacokinetics of delavirdine in HIV-positive patients: effect on erythromycin breath test. Clin Pharm Therap 1997; 61:531–543.
126. Palella FJ, Delaney KM, Moorman AC, Loveless MO, Fuhrer J, Satten GA, Aschman DJ, Holmberg SD. Declining morbidity and mortality among patients with advanced human immunodeficiency virus infection. N Engl J Med 1998; 338(13):853–860.

38

Hepatitis and Dialysis

Geert Leroux-Roels and Annemieke Dhondt
University Hospital of Gent, Gent, Belgium

Patients on maintenance hemodialysis are at increased risk for parenterally transmitted hepatitis viruses. These include hepatitis B virus (HBV), hepatitis C virus (HCV), hepatitis D virus (HDV or delta agent), and hepatitis G virus (HGV or GB virus C). HDV is a defective virus that depends on HBV as a helper virus for replication and infection. Its epidemiology, transmission prevention, and therapy therefore closely parallel that of HBV. HGV is a recently discovered parenterally transmitted virus (1,2). It has been molecularly characterized and turned out to be a member of the Flaviviridae family (for review, see Ref. 3). Since its discovery, HGV has received much attention and its occurrence has been studied in numerous conditions including hemodialysis patients. Patients on hemodialysis are at increased risk for HGV/GBV-C infection (4,5), and HGV and HCV infections frequently occur concomitantly. Recent evidence suggests that HGV is not causing hepatitis (6). The present review will focus mainly on HBV and HCV, which remain the most problematic viral hepatic infections in hemodialysis patients. HGV will be discussed briefly in the final section of this review.

I. THE HEPATITIS B VIRUS

The hepatitis B virus is a small, circular, double-stranded DNA virus, which belongs to the family of the hepadna viruses. The genome of the virus is approximately 3200 nucleotides in length and possesses 4 open reading frames. The S region codes for the three proteins of the viral envelope that share the 226 carboxy-terminal amino acids comprising the small protein, generally known as the hepatitis B surface antigen (HBsAg). The two other envelope proteins have amino-terminal extensions of 55 (preS2) and 120 (preS1) amino acids and are known as the middle (preS2+S) and large (preS1+preS2+S) envelope proteins, respectively. The C gene codes for the nucleoprotein, better known as the hepatitis B core antigen (HBcAg) and the HBeAg. The latter is a secreted protein that largely overlaps with HBcAg but has an amino-terminal extension of 10 amino acids and a carboxy-terminal truncation of varying length. The P gene codes for the multifunctional *pol* protein. Its amino-terminal part forms the terminal protein for initiating DNA-minus strand synthesis; the central part forms the reverse transcriptase and most likely also the DNA-dependent polymerase for synthesis of the DNA-plus strand; the carboxy-terminal part forms the Rnase H, which is necessary for the degradation of the RNA pregenome during the synthesis of the DNA-minus strand. The X gene encodes the X protein, the function of which is not clearly established. Since HBx activates the transcription of mRNAs and the pregenome, an enhancement of viral protein production is most likely one major function of HBx. The genome organization, transcription pattern of covalently closed HBV DNA, and physical structure of the virion are shown in Fig. 1. Detailed information on numerous structural and functional aspects of the molecular virology of HBV can be found in an excellent review article (7).

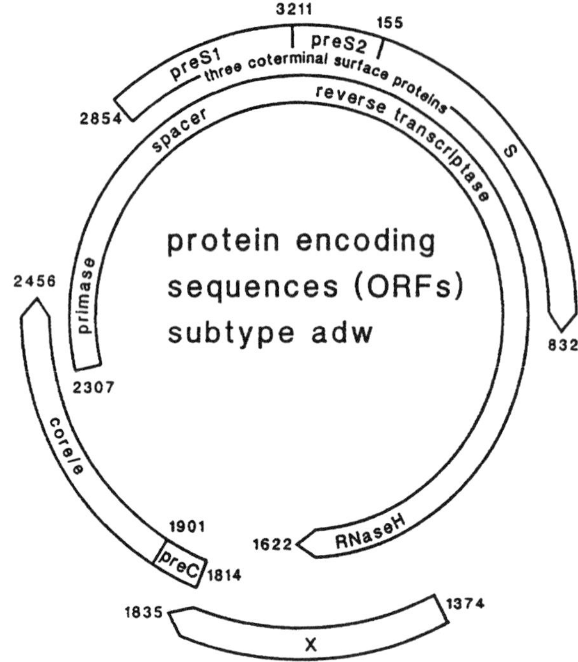

Fig. 1 Genome organization of HBV, transcription pattern of covalently closed HBV DNA, and physical structure of virion DNA.

A. Markers of HBV Infection

HBV infection can be diagnosed by the presence of viral antigens and by the host production of antibodies against these viral antigens. HBV replicates in infected hepatocytes and produces new viral particles, known as Dane particles. Apart from these infectious particles, with a diameter of 42 nm, the infected cells also produce a large excess of smaller (22 nm) empty, noninfectious viral shells. These surface particles and the Dane particles express HBsAg antigenicity that can easily be detected in every patient with acute or chronic HBV infection. Following an acute HBV infection it usually takes 8–12 weeks for the anti-HBs response (HBsAb) to become discernible. This serological evolution hallmarks a definitive resolution of the disease. Following an HBV infection, HBsAbs may persist for many years and convey a natural protection against new HBV infections that is artificially induced by hepatitis B vaccination (see further). Infected hepatocytes also secrete HBeAg. During an acute HBV infection, HBeAg and HBsAg appear almost concomitantly. HBeAg is also found in a large proportion of the patients suffering from chronic HBV infections. When an acute HBV infection is resolving, the HBeAg disappears from the circulation and the host's anti-HBe response becomes discernible. This seroconversion precedes the HBsAg-HBsAb conversion. HBeAbs often disappear years after acute infection. When an HBeAg-to-HBeAb seroconversion occurs in a patient with an established chronic HBV infection, it is usually accompanied by an arrest of the viral replication and the disappearance of the hepatic inflammation and hepatocellular damage.

Until recently, chronic HBV patients lacking HBeAg and carrying HBeAbs were considered as hardly infectious and with nonevolutive liver disease. The introduction and widespread use of HBV DNA detection assays have drastically changed this view. Indeed, a large proportion of these HBeAg^{neg}/HBeAb^{pos} patients were found to have circulating HBV DNA, and their disease patterns and infectivity rates were not as harmless as initially estimated. These patients were found to harbor an HBV carrying a mutation in the preCore region (frequently nucleotide 1869) that leads to the introduction of a stop codon in the precore sequence and the inability to produce HBeAg.

In the past few years, mutant HBV viruses have been the topic of numerous reports and some excellent review articles (8,9). The viral genome of HBV is contained within a nucleoprotein that is known as the HBcAg. With the conventional immunoassays HBcAg can never be found in the circulation of an infected person. This antigen, however, rapidly induces an anti-HBc or HBcAb response in all HBV-infected subjects irrespective of the course of the disease. Total HBcAb (IgM+IgG) is almost universally present at the onset of disease. The diagnosis of acute HBV infection is based on the detection of IgM anti-HB in serum by commercially available assays. IgM anti-HBc may also be found in the serum of chronically infected subjects, but the threshold for positivity of the commercial assays is set at a higher level to allow the discrimination of acute from chronic infections. The conventional serological approach for the diagnosis of acute or chronic HBV infections is based on the markers shown in Table 1.

These classical HBV markers have been around for two decades, and most clinicians are very skilled in their use and interpretation (10). This is not the case for the detection and/or quantification of HBV DNA. This new marker has been introduced more recently and is still not available in all diagnostic laboratories. HBV DNA is a marker of active viral replication detectable during acute hepatitis B and in patients with chronic HBV infections. HBV DNA can be detected by several methods. Because HBV is generally present in the serum in large copy numbers, it is possible to detect

Table 1 Serological Markers for Hepatitis B Virus Infection

Marker	Description
HBsAg	Hepatitis B surface antigen; earliest indicator of the presence of acute infection; also indicative of chronic infection
anti-HBs	Antibody to hepatitis B surface antigen; usually indicates clinical recovery and subsequent immunity to hepatitis B virus; may be present in the blood following active immunization with hepatitis B vaccine or passive immunization with HBIG (hepatitis B immunoglobulins; passive immunity may be acquired following blood transfusions
anti-HBc	Total antibody to hepatitis B core antigen; early indicator of acute infection; usually also a lifelong marker representing past exposure as well as active infection in the acute/chronic period
anti-HBc IgM	High levels of anti-HBc IgM detectable during the acute stage of hepatitis B; used to differentiate current from past infection
HBeAg	Hepatitis B e antigen; early indicator of acute active infection, appears shortly after HBsAg; presence of HBeAg indicates still active viral replication; HBV DNA will be found
anti-HBe	Antibody to hepatitis B e antigen; seroconversion from e antigen to e antibody during acute stage prognostic for resolution of infection; presence of anti-HBe and absence of HBeAg in presence of HBV DNA highly suggestive for the presence of a mutant HBV

and even quantify HBV DNA by direct hybridization methods such as dot and slot blot assays (11), liquid phase hybridization (Abbott Genostics), or DNA-RNA hybridization assays (Digene). The sensitivity of these assays is rather limited and allows the detection of approximately 10^6 genome equivalents per mL (±5 pg/mL). By amplifying the signal, the detection limit can be lowered to approximately 3×10^5 genome equivalents/mL (Quantiplex, Chiron Corporation). The most sensitive results are obtained by amplification of the target as is done during a polymerase chain reaction (PCR). Until recently it was extremely difficult to perform quantitative PCRs, and the method was prone to error. This has changed recently, and it is now possible to perform quantitative assays of HBV DNA in the range of 10^3–10^7 genome equivalents/mL. These assays are most useful to monitor the response of a patient to antiviral therapy (12).

B. Diagnosis of HBV in Dialysis Patients

The immune deficiency of patients with end-stage renal disease (ESRD) and of hemodialysis patients impairs the elimination of the virus (13). Nonuremic adults who are infected with HBV usually develop an acute hepatitis B that is accompanied by jaundice, fever, fatigue, and a flu-like syndrome. Overall, 5–10% of nonuremic adults with HBV infection will be unable to clear the virus and become chronically infected with HBV. Patients undergoing dialysis who are infected with HBV usually have a mild or even asymptomatic disease course (14), but more than 60% of them become chronic HBsAg carriers (15,16). The risk of a chronic evolution increases with the duration of the HBsAg positivity. When a subject has been HBsAg positive for 5 months, the chance of remaining positive is 89% (15). The diagnosis of acute or chronic HBV infections is based on the traditional serological markers described above. The measurement of HBV DNA may aid in estimating the viral load and in determining patients carrying a precore mutant virus.

A peculiar finding in hemodialysis patients, reported by several investigators (17,18), is the isolated presence of HBsAg in the absence of anti-HBc or any other marker of HBV infection of immunity. This phenomenon turned out to be due to the appearance in the circulation of HBsAg of vaccine origin. It is transient and rarely persists for more than 20 days. Therefore, it is recommended that dialysis patients are not screened for HBV markers within one month following an HBsAg vaccine administration. The reappearance of HBsAg in hemodialysis or kidney transplant patients who had seemingly eliminated the virus has been reported (19). This rather unexpected situation is not the result of a laboratory error but the consequence of a relapse of the HBV infection that is due to a drastic reduction of the patient's immune function. Recent observations in patients with normal renal function suggest that it may take years before the HBV is completely eliminated from the body; it may even be that complete clearance never occurs (20). As long as the immune system functions normally, the virus persists in the body at extremely low levels (only detectable with nested PCR) without causing any harm. Severe immunosuppression may lead to the reappearance of the virus and the clinical picture of chronic HBV infection.

C. Epidemiology of HBV in Dialysis Patients

Viral hepatitis was a serious problem in hemodialysis units during the late 1960s. Since the discovery of the "Australia antigen" by Blumberg et al. (21,22), HBV has been recognized as the responsible agent for the outbreaks of dialysis-associated hepatitis reported both in Europe and in the United States. From 1972 to 1973, HBsAg was present in 16.8% of dialysis patients and in 2.4% of medical staff, anti-HBs was detected in 34% of patients and 31% of staff members (23). In the period 1976–1993, the incidence of HBV infections decreased from 3 to 0.1% of patients and from 2.6 to 0.02% among staff members, with the largest decline occurring during 1976–1980 (24). Likewise, the prevalence of HBsAg in patients decreased from 7.8% in 1976 to 1.2% in 1993, and the prevalence in staff members declined from 0.9% in 1980 to 0.3% in 1993 (24). The former data are from U.S. centers, but a similar decrease was also observed in Europe. This positive evolution does not imply that the hepatitis B problem is solved. In 1990, 880 dialysis patients and 81 dialysis staff personnel were contaminated in European centers. The average prevalence of HBsAg in European dialysis centers in 1990 was 6.1%, but considerable regional differences were observed, ranging from 0.3% in Sweden and Finland to 25.9% in Poland (25).

D. Transmission and Preventive Measures

The most obvious form of HBV transmission is by transfusion of contaminated blood products. HBV infection in dialysis patients was correlated with the number of units of blood transfused (14). With the advent of universal blood screening for HBsAg in 1972, the most important control measure was instituted. With the introduction of recombinant human erythropoietin, fewer blood transfusions were required, and this reduced further the spread of transfusion-associated hepatitis.

It is very likely that environmental contamination played a substantial role in the spread of hepatitis B in dialysis units. Indeed, HBV infection in dialysis patients could be correlated with the time on chronic hemodialysis (14,23) and the incidence of new HBV infections could be correlated with the prevalence of hepatitis B carriers in the dialysis unit.

HBsAg was demonstrated in most body fluids including blood, saliva, semen, breast milk, tears, and ascites fluid; even sneeze samples tested positive in 35% (26). The virus can gain entry into the body through skin lesions or through intact mucous membranes, and oral transmission appears to be possible as well. HBV is an enveloped virus that resists harsh environmental conditions and that requires drastic procedures for inactivation. HBV can remain viable for up to 7 days (27), even in the absence of visible blood. Contamination of dialysis machine buttons and control surfaces with infected blood or secretions can lead to spread of HBV to staff and patients (28).

Accidental needlestick exposure from a HBsAg-positive patient is a common form of transmission. The risk of developing HBV infection after an accidental puncture with an HBsAg positive needle is estimated at 45% (29).

In the past, outbreaks of hepatitis B have also been related to cross-contamination of pressure monitors.

HBV is a spherical particle with a diameter of 42 nm. Since the cut-off of dialysis membranes never exceeds 7 nm, it would appear that hemodialysis membranes offer a safe barrier against the passage of the virus. HBV DNA or HBsAg in the dialysate or ultrafiltrate from positive patients was not demonstrated (30,31). However, despite theoretical considerations, some authors have demonstrated the passage of HBV from blood to the ultrafiltrate across the dialysis membrane (32,33). Hence, the dialysate should also be considered as a possible route of transmission.

To prevent nosocomial transmission of HBV, strict adherence to infection-control strategies is indispensable. The most important control strategies are summarized in Table 2.

HBsAg-positive patients should be segregated from other patients and separate equipment should be used. Separation of HBsAg-positive patients within a separate room using dedicated machines significantly lowered the incidence of HBV infection (24,34). It has not been demonstrated that reprocessing of hemodialyzers increases the risk of hepatitis B (34). However, we do not recommend dialyzer reuse in HBsAg-positive patients.

When handling infected patients, the use of protecting eyeglasses is warranted. Masks should always be put on to prevent bacterial infection.

Outbreaks of HBV infections have been blamed on contamination of multidose medication vials (36). Patients preparing their own medications from a common

Table 2 Infection-Control Strategies for Hepatitis B

Handwashing before and after all patient contacts
Routine use of gloves when handling patients
No sharing between patients of fistula pressing clamps, gauzes, tourniquets, thermometers, blood pressure cuffs, or other devices
Wearing protecting eyeglasses
Appropriate labeling of all specimens
No eating, drinking, or smoking in the dialysis unit
Isolation of HBsAg-positive patients within a separate room, using dedicated machines
Exclusion of HBsAg-positive patients from reuse programs
Disinfection protocol for monitors, chairs, environmental surfaces, and surroundings (e.g., hypochlorite 0.5%) and instruments (e.g., glutaraldehyde 2%)
Discarding needles directly after use into appropriate containers, without recapping

preparation area, as occur in outpatient facilities, can be a source of infection. It can be hypothesized that basic sterility rules are less respected by patients than by nurses. Therefore one should be very cautious in delegating tasks to patients. Such outbreaks justify the use of "ready-to-use" single-dose syringes rather than multidose vials, even if the latter turn out to be cheaper.

It is also important to monitor the serological status of dialysis patients at regular intervals. Patients who underwent successful vaccination should be controlled for the persistence of antibodies to HBsAg. An anti-HBs titer above 10 U/L is considered protective. It might, however, be prudent to set this safety limit at 100 U/L and administer a booster dose as soon as the patient's titer goes below this limit. In nonresponders to HB vaccination and in chronically infected patients, one should determine HBsAg, anti-HBc, HBeAg, anti-HBe, and HBV DNA (see above) to detect a new infection (unprotected vaccinees) or to monitor changes in the serostatus such as a HBeAg/anti-HBe seroconversion, the appearance of a precore mutant, or, rarely, a spontaneous clearance. It is safe to monitor patients who successfully cleared a natural HBV infection because reactivation of the disease has been documented, especially in situations where the immune system is deteriorating.

It is important to inform infected patients and their relatives in order to prevent familial spread. When spouses of infected patients are negative for HBV markers, they should be vaccinated without delay.

For known HBsAg carriers presenting with ESRD, some nephrologists prefer peritoneal dialysis to hemodialysis, especially in centers not dialyzing HBsAg-positive patients. However, this technique requires a careful approach. Indeed, spread of HBV infection through spilled peritoneal dialysate from peritoneal dialysis patients seropositive for HBV has been demonstrated (37–39).

E. Vaccination

Since the late 1970s a decline in the incidence of HBV infection in both hemodialysis patients and personnel has been observed (40). This decline was due to the implementation of infection-control strategies including separation of HBsAg-positive patients from HBsAg-negative patients, regular routine serological screening on a regular basis, and routine cleaning and disinfection procedures. In the early 1980s, plasma-derived hepatitis B vaccines became commercially available. This vaccine had initially to gain acceptance even among the groups for which it was recommended. The systematic administration of this vaccine to susceptible subjects resulted in a further decline of HBV infections in both patients and staff of hemodialysis centers (41).

In patients with ESRD in whom hemodialysis is anticipated, vaccination can be applied in the predialysis phase or as soon as dialysis is started. Based on the assumption that the immune response might be superior in the predialysis phase, some authors have advocated to start hepatitis vaccination in this phase. An analysis of cost-effectiveness revealed that immunizing patients with ESRD in the predialysis phase can prevent additional cases of HBV infection (42). However, the cost per case prevented is substantially higher for the predialysis approach, namely \$31,111 for predialysis vaccination as compared to \$25,313 for dialysis vaccination. The former strategy could become cost-saving if the price of vaccine were to decrease from \$114 to \$1.50 or if the incidence of infection were to rise from 0.6 to 38%. The issue of timing of vaccination may become less important now that many countries are implementing systematic vaccination for HBV during early childhood or adolescence in the context of the WHO Program for the eradication of HBV (43).

Over the years different vaccines (plasma-derived and recombinant yeast), different vaccine doses (mostly 20 μg/dose versus 40 μg/dose), different vaccination schedules, and different injection routes (intramuscular and intradermal) have been evaluated. Table 3 represents a selection of clinical vaccine evaluations that have been performed in the past two decades. Only studies involving intramuscular (deltoid muscle) vaccine administration to patients with ESRD or on hemodialysis were included. An immune response to HB

Table 3 Hepatitis B Vaccine Studies Performed Between 1981 and 1997

Author(s)	Year	Ref.	Subjects: Diagnosis	Subjects: Number	Type of vaccine	Vaccine (μg/dose)	Number of doses[a]	Vaccination scheme (months)	Response rate (%): >10 U/L[b]	Response rate (%): >100 U/L
Crosnier et al.	1981	44	HD	72	PlaD[2]	20	3	0, 1, 2	60	
Desmyter et al.	1983	45	HD	201	PlaD	3	4	0, 1, 2, 5	75	56
Stevens et al.	1984	46	HD	657	PlaD	40	3	0, 1, 6	50	
Benhamou et al.	1984	47	HD	70	PlaD	20	3	0, 1, 2	45.6	
			HD	69	PlaD	40	3	0, 1, 2	75	
			HD	76	PlaD	20	4	0, 1, 2, 4	69	
Jilg et al.	1986	48	HD	49	YD	40	3	0, 1, 6	65.3	
Fujiyama et al.	1987	49	HD	39	PlaD	20	3	0, 1, 6	59	
Seaworth et al.	1988	50	Predial.	21	YD	20	3	0, 1, 6	42	
			Predial.	20	YD	40	3	0, 1, 6	69	
			Predial.	20	PlaD	40	3	0, 1, 6	75	
Steketee et al.	1988	51	HD	444	PlaD				47	
Bruguera et al.	1990	52		80	YD				80	
Docci et al.	1990	53	HD	24	YD	20	4	0, 1, 2, 6	58.3	
Fujiyama et al.	1990	54	HD	22	YD	20	3	0, 1, 6	86.4	
				10	YD	40	3	0, 1, 6	90	
Smit-Leys et al.	1990	55	HD	99	PlaD ± preS2	5 or 20	4 or 6	0, 1, 2, (4), 6, (12)	71	
Albertoni et al.	1991	56	HD	236	PlaD				58.5	
Fleming et al.	1991	57	HD	83	YD	20	3	0, 1, 6	32.5	
Allegra et al.	1992	58	HD	34	YD	20	4	0, 1, 2, 6	52.9	17.6
Buti et al.	1992	59	HD	60	YD	20	4	0, 1, 2, 6	73	
Docci et al.	1992	60	HD	35	YD	20	4	0, 1, 2, 6	60	
Fanelli et al.	1992	61	HD	18	YD	40	3	0, 1, 6	61.1	
Jungers et al.	1994	62	Predial.	58	PlaD	5	4	0, 1, 2, 4	59	
			Predial.	59	YD (+preS2)	20	4	0, 1, 2, 4	71	
Marangi et al.	1994	63	HD	63	YD	40	4	0, 1, 2, 6	92	65
Rault et al.	1995	64	HD	48	YD-Recvax		3	0, 1, 6	71	
			HD	50	YD-Engerix		4	0, 1, 2, 6	74	
Fabrizi et al.	1996	65	HD	118	YD	40	3	0, 1, 2	67	57
Fernandez et al.	1996	66	HD	64	YD					
Khan et al.	1996	67	PD	47	YD	40	4	0, 1, 2, 6	53	
			HD	50	YD	40	4	0, 1, 2, 6	74	
Mitwalli	1996	68	HD	42		20	3	0, 1, 2, & 0, 1, 6	82.3 & 80	
Navarro et al.	1996	69	HD	56	YD	40	3		76.7	53.5
Cheng et al.	1997	70	HD	50	YD	40	5	0, 1, 2, 6, 12	76.1	
Peces et al.	1997	71	HD	80	YD	40	4	0, 1, 2, 12	77.5	72.5
Radovic et al.	1997	72	HD	28	YD	40	4	0, 1, 2, 6		97.5

[a]Vaccines were administered intramuscularly in the deltoid muscle.
[b]Anti-HBs response was generally measured 4 weeks after the administration of the last dose.
HD, Hemodialysis patient; predial., ESRD before dialysis, PD, peritoneal dialysis; PlaD, plasma derived; YD, recombinant, yeast derived.

vaccine is considered adequate and protective when an anti-HBs antibody titer of >10 U/L is reached one month after the third of fourth vaccine dose (depending on the schedule used). A protective immune response is reached in about 95% of healthy adult vaccine recipients. This is not the case in patients with ESRD where the immune response is often inadequate and where a protective titer is attained in 32–97% (Table 3).

Numerous factors are contributing to the poor responsiveness to HB vaccine of patients with ESRD. First, one has to consider the major impairment of both the innate and the adaptive immunity that is present in patients with ESRD, irrespective of its cause. The underlying immune defect is complex and involves monocytes, T cells, and B cells at different levels of their functioning and interplay (for review, see Ref. 73). This immune defect not only hampers the immune response to HB vaccination, it also impedes the responses to other highly recommended vaccines such as tetanus (74,75), diphtheria (76), and influenza (77) and is responsible for the frequent evolution to chronicity following HBV infection.

The immune response of healthy adult vaccinees to HB vaccine seems to be controlled by MHC-linked immune response genes. An increased incidence of poor responsiveness in subjects with HLA-DR3 and DR7 has been reported by several groups (78–84). Such an association between nonresponsiveness to HB vaccine and HLAA1, B8, DR3, DQ2 has also been observed in patients with ESRD (85–88).

Apart from uremia and genetic determinants, numerous other factors seem to contribute to the poor responsiveness to HB vaccine. Older age (44,46, 65,66,89), male gender (68,69,88), poor nutritional status (65,66), as well as obesity (67) and diabetes (65) have all been found to be associated with poorer response. In several studies the influence of a concomitant HCV infection on the anti-HBs response was examined. Navarro et al. (69,90) had the impression that HCV infection reduced the effectiveness of HB vaccination in hemodialysis patients, whereas others (70,91,92) could not observe such a reduction.

Numerous strategies have been designed and evaluated to overcome this poor responsiveness of ESRD patients. Table 3 shows a limited selection of studies that have looked at the effects on antibody responses of increased vaccine doses, altered vaccination schedules, and changes in vaccine production and content. Several studies have been performed to evaluate the safety, efficacy, and cost-reducing effects of intradermal vaccine administration for primovaccinations as well as for revaccination of poor responders. On many occasions this route turned out to be a safe, efficacious, and cost-effective alternative to intramuscular vaccination (89,94–96).

Pilot studies involving limited numbers of subjects were performed to examine the adjuvant effects of interferon-γ (91), GM-SCF (97), and thymopentin (98,99). Promising results were obtained that need to be conformed in randomized, placebo-controlled trials involving larger numbers of subjects. Subcutaneous administration of low doses of interleukin-2 (IL-2) has been reported to induce systemic immune responses in hemodialysis patients who did not respond to previous HB vaccination (100). However, this observation could not be confirmed in a randomized placebo-controlled trial (101). The effect of recombinant human erythropoietin (rHuEPO) on the immune system of hemodialysis patients has been studied by evaluating their response to HB vaccination (102). A beneficial effect was observed, the underlying mechanisms of which remain to be elucidated. Finally, several attempts have been made to improve the immunogenicity of HB vaccines by adding preS2 (103–105) or preS1+preS2 sequences (106–108) or selected regions thereof (109,110) to the S sequence that is now used as the vaccine compound. In some studies (104,105,107,109,110), addition of the preS sequences did not improve the response to the HB vaccine, whereas others suggest an improved anti-HBs response (106,108). Only one study involved hemodialysis patients (among other nonresponder groups) (108) and suggested that the preS1+preS2–containing vaccine is endowed with remarkable qualities. However, this study did not include an appropriate control group, an omission that greatly undermines the validity of the conclusions.

Vaccination is not only important for hemodialysis patients, it should also be systematically administered to all susceptible medical staff. Several studies (111,112) have demonstrated that hepatitis B vaccination of medical personnel of hemodialysis centers is a safe and efficacious way to reduce the incidence of clinical and subclinical hepatitis B among health professionals and to prevent secondary cases among their families.

When an unprotected person (patient or staff member) has a potentially HBV-infected exposure via the skin or the mucous membranes, hepatitis B immune globulin (HBIg) should be administered intramuscularly (0.06 mL/kg) within 24 hours following the exposure, and a first vaccine dose should be given within one week, to be followed by a second and third at 1 and 6 months, respectively.

F. Therapy

In the general population (nondialysis patients), approximately one third of patients treated with a 4-month course of interferon-α attain a stable remission. The markers that are associated with a good response to treatment include elevated serum aminotransferase activities, circulating HBV DNA levels not exceeding 200 pg/mL, and liver histology showing moderate or severe inflammatory activity. Patients to be treated with interferon-α should be less than 65 years of age, in otherwise good health, and without signs of decompensated cirrhosis. Standard treatment consists of 5 million units of interferon-α-2b given subcutaneously and daily or 10 million units three times a week for a period of 16 weeks (113). Nucleoside analogs such as lamivudine and famciclovir are now under study in nonuremic patients. To our knowledge, no studies are available in dialysis patients.

G. Kidney Transplantation

Some concern was raised about the outcome of HBV-infected patients after kidney transplantation (114,115). A comparative study between HBsAg-positive renal transplant patients and HBsAg-positive dialysis patients demonstrated a less favorable outcome in transplant patients as far as liver disease and overall mortality were concerned (116). HBsAg-positive patients may be considered good candidates for renal transplantation, provided that there is no chronic active hepatitis and that markers of viral replication such as HBeAg and HBV DNA are not detectable (117).

II. THE HEPATITIS C VIRUS

Hepatitis C virus (HCV) is a positive-sense, single-stranded enveloped RNA virus that belongs to the Flaviviridae family. The genome of the virus is approximately 9500 nucleotides in length and possesses a unique open reading frame, coding for a single polyprotein, flanked by untranslated regions at both the 5′ and 3′ ends. The genomic organization of the HCV RNA is illustrated schematically in Fig. 2. According to the isolate examined, the length of the polyprotein varies from 3008 to 3037 amino acids. The nascent viral polyprotein is processed by a combination of host and viral proteinases into mature viral proteins. At least 10 distinct viral proteins have so far been identified, which are arranged as shown in Fig. 2. Recent review articles (118,119) provide detailed information on numerous structural and functional aspects of the molecular virology of HCV.

A. Markers of HCV Infection

As for most viral diseases, the diagnosis of HCV infections is based on two types of test. Indirect tests detect antibodies produced by the host against viral components. These include enzyme immunoassays (EIAs), which contain HCV antigens from the core and nonstructural genes, and recombinant immunoblot assays (RIBAs), which contain the same antigens in an immunoblot format. Direct tests reveal the RNA virus itself and are based on amplification techniques such as PCR. Direct tests that are based on immunological detection techniques are in adequate to detect HCV in body fluids because the viral concentrations are too low.

The discovery and the cloning of HCV by Houghton et al. (120) quickly led to the first diagnostic test for HCV (EIA-1) (121). This assay employed a recombinant HCV antigen (C100-3) representing a portion of NS4 as capturing antigen. This assay was useful to demonstrate for the first time that most transfusion-associated non-A, non-B hepatitis was caused by HCV. However, this assay lacked sensitivity (122,123) and specificity (124,125). It was soon replaced by second-generation assays (EIA-2), which included a larger NS4 protein (C200) and antigen from core (C22-3) and NS3 regions. These multiantigenic EIA-2s were introduced in 1992 and led to a substantial improvement in sen-

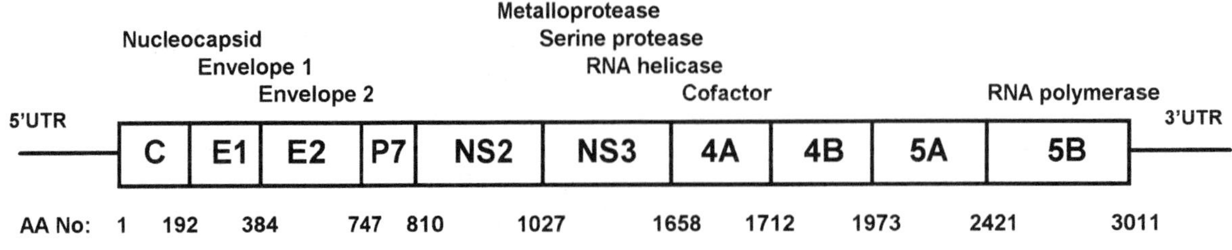

Fig. 2 Genome organization of HCV RNA.

sitivity and a slight increase in specificity (122,126). The addition of NS3 and even moreso of core antigens allowed a more rapid detection of anti-HCV antibodies and thus reduced the "window" phase. Indeed, the interval between inoculation with the virus and seroconversion shortened from average 16 weeks with EIA-1 to 10 weeks with EIA-2. Recently, third-generation anti-HCV tests (EIA-3) were introduced. These contain reconfigured core, NS3 and NS4 antigens, and an additional NS5 antigen not present in EIA-2. Several studies (127–131) have demonstrated an increased sensitivity and specificity for detecting HCV infection in blood donors and patients with hepatic disorders. The quest for better EIA goes on, and preliminary studies suggest that the addition of HCV envelope proteins E1 and/or E2 may lead to further assay improvement (132), serve as a marker of active viral replication (133,134), and be helpful in discriminating sustained responders from relapsers during interferon therapy (135,136).

Supplemental assays for anti-HCV were developed to resolve false-positive EIA results, which occurred more frequently in EIA-1 than in the superior EIA-3. The second-generation recombinant immunoblot assay (RIBA-2) which is the only supplemental assay approved by the FDA, contains the same HCV antigens as EIA-2 in an immunoblot format. A RIBA is considered positive when two or more antigens are positive, indeterminate when one antigen is positive, and negative when no reactivity is observed. Third-generation supplemental tests (RIBA-3, LIA-III) have been developed and are in use in Europe. These appear to be more specific than the RIBA-2 test. This is based on a better correlation with PCR results and a lower frequency of indeterminate results (137,138). Supplemental RIBA testing is most useful for the confirmation of positive EIA results in low-risk individuals or in a low-prevalence setting (blood banking). In these conditions 40–50% of the EIA-2–positive specimens turn out to be RIBA negative. If the RIBA result is negative, the anti-HCV EIA is likely to have been false-positive, and the patient is unlikely to have hepatitis C. If the RIBA result is positive, the patient may have or have had hepatitis C. Here the detection of HCV-RNA by PCR will demonstrate on ongoing viremia. In a high-prevalence setting such as a university referral laboratory, approximately 93% of EIA-2–positive samples are also RIBA-2 positive (139).

A direct method to detect HCV hepatitis is based on the highly sensitive reverse transcription PCR (RT-PCR). This method has become an essential tool to confirm the diagnosis of an HCV infection and to monitor the response to antiviral therapy. Although this test is undoubtedly the best confirmatory test, it is hard to standardize and is prone to errors. A survey of 31 European laboratories has shown that only 16% of laboratories scored perfectly on a standardized test panel (140). Now that PCR is increasingly applied and has shifted from the research environment to the clinical setting, the need for rigorous quality-control procedures and proficiency testing by diagnostic laboratories cannot be overemphasized. Recently Roche Molecular Diagnostics introduced the Amplicor® test kit for qualitative HCV RNA detection by the RT-PCR technique. This assay has built-in controls for assay sensitivity and specificity but does not obviate the need for rigorous training of qualified laboratory technicians and appropriate quality-control measures (139).

It is becoming increasingly apparent that the determination of the viral load may be a useful tool for the management of chronic hepatitis C (141). Two different technologies are in use to assess HCV RNA levels in body fluids of patients: a target amplification method using RT-PCR and a signal amplification method. According to the manufacturer, the Roche Amplicor HCV Monitor™ allows the detection of 500 copies/mL and has a dynamic range of 4 logs (5×10^6/mL). The major strengths of this assay are its sensitivity and convenience. The bDNA HCV RNA assay (Quantiplex™ HCV RNA, Chiron Corporation) requires no PCR amplification but relies on a series of nucleic acid hybridizations to achieve amplified signals. The linear range of the bDNA version 1.0 is between 350,000 and 58,000,000 equivalents/mL. This allows the detection of 72–86% of HCV viremic specimens as compared to RT-PCR. The most recent version, Quantiplex 2.0, has improved sensitivity and detects 93% of HCV viremic specimens (141). bDNA is easy to perform and is less prone to contamination than RT-PCR because target RNA molecules are not amplified. Its major drawback is its lack of sensitivity. Patients who are negative by bDNA must therefore be retested with RT-PCR to rule out low viremia.

In the past few years, HCV RNA has been quantified in different clinical settings, and these studies have led to the following observations:

HCV RNA levels appear to be relatively stable in most patients with chronic HCV infection (142).

Patients with advanced liver disease have higher HCV levels than asymptomatic carriers (143–145).

There seems to be no correlation between HCV levels and the histological score of patients with chronic HCV (143–145).

HCV levels are extremely high in immunosuppressed subjects such as following liver transplantation or during HIV infections (146–148).

Patients with a low level of HCV RNA have a higher likelihood of sustained response to interferon therapy; 50–70% of patients with undetectable HCV RNA by bDNA (<300.000 equivalents/mL) have sustained response to treatment compared to 10–20% of bDNA positives (149–152).

Recent studies have shown that an early disappearance of circulating virus appears to be the best indicator of a sustained response to treatment (153,154).

Studies of the viral load at the start of an interferon therapy have demonstrated a very fast half-life of HCV (mean 5 hours) and a very high production rate (2×10^{11} virions/day) (155).

The HCV genome is extremely heterogeneous. Based on their genetic relatedness, HCV can be classified in different genotypes. At present 11 major genotypes and at least 70 subtypes have been reported (156). The international scientific community now widely uses a nomenclature wherein the genotypes are represented by an Arabic numeral and extended for the subtypes, by a lowercase letter (e.g., type 1, subtype 1a). Various methods have been used for genotyping: sequencing, genotype-specific primers for PCR, restriction fragment length polymorphism, differential hybridization, and immunological techniques (serotyping). It is becoming increasingly evident that typing and subtyping for HCV is clinically important. Relevant clinical differences have emerged with respect to the efficacy of interferon-α therapy, the natural course and severity of liver disease, and the outcome of transplantation. Furthermore, different genotypes seem to follow different routes of parenteral transmission. Molecular analysis of infecting viral strains has been helpful in providing unequivocal evidence for nosocomial transmission of HCV within a hemodialysis unit (157). However, the immense heterogeneity of HCV dramatically complicates the design of prophylactic and therapeutic strategies.

B. Diagnosis of HCV in Dialysis Patients

In view of their immunocompromised state, ESRD patients respond less well to environmental and vaccine antigens. The response to HCV presents no exception to this. Numerous studies have demonstrated that screening of hemodialysis patients with EIAs does not provide accurate information and generally underscores the frequency of HCV infection among hemodialysis patients. The immunosuppressive state of hemodialysis patients not only induces false negativity of anti-HCV tests, it also weakens the intrahepatic antiviral immune response and thus masks the biochemical evidence of hepatitis. Recent studies by Pol et al. (158) using RT-PCR and Chan et al. (159) using anti-HCV to detect HCV infection showed that only one third of the infected patients had elevated transaminase levels. Based on these observations, numerous authors suggest that the direct detection of HCV RNA is required to correctly diagnose HCV infections in a hemodialysis setting. Since not all hemodialysis centers have access to this technology, alternative strategies to detect HCV infections have been explored. Caramelo et al. (160) advocate in dialysis patients decreasing the threshold for "normal values" of transaminases that are currently considered. However, our own evaluation of anti-HCV tests for the detection of HCV infections in dialysis patients is less worrisome. We recently examined sera from 213 chronic hemodialysis patients for the presence of HCV (161). Antibodies to HCV were measured using second- or third-generation EIAs. HCV-RNA was detected by a qualitative RT-PCR (Amplicor®). HCV RNA was found in seven sera, all of which were positive for HCV antibodies. This shows that these chronically HCV-infected hemodialysis patients are able to mount a detectable anti-HCV response despite their compromised immune status. In nine other patients anti-HCV antibodies were found in the absence of HCV-RNA. Whether these represent false-positive EIA results or can be considered as the serological scar of a past or self-limited HCV infection remains unsolved.

C. Morbidity of HCV in Hemodialysis Patients

The acute phase of HCV infection is infrequently associated with icterus, while the ALT levels are fluctuating with successive peaks that may eventually lead to chronicity (162). Spontaneous clearance of the virus is uncommon. HCV has an indolent progression; biopsy data reveal lesions ranging from discrete portal fibrosis or minimal changes, hemosiderosis, chronic persistent hepatitis, chronic active hepatitis to cirrhosis and hepatocellular carcinoma (163–165).

D. Epidemiology of HCV in Dialysis Patients

After the decline in incidence of HBV, non-A, non-B hepatitis became the major form of hepatitis in dialysis patients. With the introduction of the screening tests for antibodies directed against HCV, it was found that most dialysis patients suffering from hepatitis were infected with HCV (162). The European Dialysis and Transplantation Association (EDTA) survey in 1993 revealed an average HCV prevalence of 18%, with a large variation among the different countries, ranging from 1% in Finland to 44% in Egypt (166). In Table 4, the incidence of seroconversion per 1000 patients in 1994 is illustrated for the different EDTA registry countries: the highest incidence occurred in Eastern European and some Mediterranean countries (167). In the United States in 1993, the HCV prevalence was 9.7%

Table 4 Incidence of Seroconversion per 1000 Patients

Country	No. patients
Algeria	55
Austria	4
Belgium	3
Bulgaria	57
Cyprus	0
Czechoslovakia	36
Denmark	0
Egypt	23
Finland	0
France	8
Germany	5
Greece	25
Hungary	30
Iceland	0
Ireland	0
Israel	23
Italy	19
Lebanon	12
Libya	—
Luxembourg	0
Malta	0
Morocco	26
Netherlands	0
Norway	0
Poland	83
Portugal	19
Romania	27
Spain	20
Sweden	4
Switzerland	10
Syria	—
Tunesia	29
Turkey	35
United Kingdom	5
Total	29

Source: Ref. 167.

(24). Worldwide, the highest HCV prevalence in hemodialysis patients has been recorded in Saudi Arabia (168), Venezuela (169), Taiwan (170), and Indonesia (171), with values around 70%.

There is a considerably lower prevalence of anti-HCV among peritoneal dialysis patients compared with patients on chronic hemodialysis (172–176), particularly after exclusion of those patients who previously underwent hemodialysis (177–179). Likewise, home hemodialysis is also associated with a lower prevalence of HCV (175).

The prevalence of anti-HCV in hemodialysis staff workers is rather low, ranging from 0 to 6.7% (24,172,173,180–187); this is comparable with the prevalence found among other health care workers, although it is higher compared to blood donors (180).

E. Transmission and Prevention

The high prevalence of HCV infections in hemodialysis patients is due to transfusion and nosocomial transmission. Only a limited number of HCV-positive dialysis patients suffered from renal insufficiency due to HCV-associated nephropathies.

1. Transfusion

Numerous studies demonstrate a direct association between the number of blood transfusions and the prevalence of HCV among hemodialysis patients (168,188–191). In some studies HCV was found only in transfused patients (192). Since in most countries blood donors are screened for HCV, this route of transmission almost disappeared. Moreover, with the introduction of rHuEPO, transfusion requirements have markedly diminished.

2. Nosocomial Transmission

Other papers did not find any association between the number of transfusions and HCV positivity (173,193–195). HCV has even been detected in a substantial number of patients that had never been transfused (164,165,168,188,191,194,196–199). A correlation between the length of time on hemodialysis and the risk of HCV infection was demonstrated (168,173,182, 184,189,196,200). Furthermore, home hemodialysis and peritoneal dialysis (172,175) both have a lower prevalence of HCV compared to hospital hemodialysis. The difference between peritoneal and hemodialysis can, however, be at least in part attributed to the higher transfusion requirements of hemodialysis patients. Identical genomic sequences of HCV isolates were found in patients dialyzed in the same unit (157,201). Furthermore, the incidence of HCV infection is directly correlated with the HCV prevalence in the dialysis unit (202). All these findings strongly suggest that nosocomial transmission must be considered as a major source of HCV infection.

On theoretical grounds, nosocomial transmission can be considered in terms of time and space. Transmission from patient to patient dialyzed in the same shift will be called "horizontal" transmission; infection of a patient dialyzed on the same monitor after an infected patient will be called "vertical" transmission. In practice, however, these different forms are difficult to differentiate.

In a prospective study, horizontal transmission was demonstrated, finding a higher risk for HCV infection for patients dialyzed adjacent to an HCV-positive patient (188). In another study, the HCV incidence was lower in units that used separate rooms for HCV-positive patients (202); whether the latter was due to the reduction of horizontal or vertical transmission is not clear. Vertical transmission has been repeatedly described (162,203–205). HCV infection has been documented in patients being dialyzed after an HCV-positive patient on the same monitor (162); the incidence of HCV seroconversion was higher among patients sharing a dialysis machine with an HCV-positive patient (204); the incidence was lower in units where machines to HCV-positive patients were dedicated (202). In a prospective study, two patients seroconverted during the follow-up period; both patients were dialyzed in the last shift of the day, sharing the monitor with a HCV-positive patient (205). In contrast to the abovementioned studies, Gilli et al. observed in their prospective study no seroconversion when HCV-positive and HCV-negative patients shared the same dialyzer monitor (206).

Theoretically, the passage of HCV through the intact dialyzer membrane seems unlikely because the viral particle is much larger (35 nm) (207) than the membrane pores of a dialyzer. However, alterations in pore size or disruption of membrane integrity, associated with the production process, the dialysis session itself, or dialyzer reuse, can hypothetically allow the passage of the virus into the dialysate compartment. Literature data about this issue are conflicting. Three studies reported that neither low-flux cuprophane nor high-flux cellulose diacetate, polysulfone, and PAN dialyzers allow contamination of the dialysis ultrafiltrate with HCV (208–210). In contrast, two recent studies detected HCV RNA in the ultrafiltrate, albeit in only a small fraction of patients (211, 212).

Conflicting data have been published about the safety of dialyzer reuse (200,202,213). Although the HCV incidence in dialysis units that reprocessed dialyzers was not significantly different from units that did not reprocess dialyzers, the incidence of HCV infection was lowest in those units that used separate rooms for reprocessing dialyzers from HCV-positive patients or did not reprocess these dialyzers at all. Using Renalin® as sterilant was also accompanied by a lower incidence compared to formaldehyde (202). These data suggest that contamination of dialyzers in the reprocessing room may be a vector for HCV transmission. Also, Hung et al. described an increased HCV prevalence with dialyser reuse (213). Although in theory reuse is a safe procedure, in practice human errors may reduce its safety. It is also conceivable that with repeated use, membrane integrity can be lost, leading to contamination of the dialysate. Based on these observations and considerations, we would discourage the reuse of dialyzers of HCV-infected patients. The CDC, however, does not share this view and does not recommend a ban on reuse of dialyzers from these patients (214).

HCV-infected patients represent only a low risk of contamination for hemodialysis staff (215). Transmission can occur through a needlestick (216,217), although the risk of contracting HCV is smaller compared to HBV. The source of HCV outbreaks in hemodialysis units has rarely been identified or at least exceptionally published. Breakdown in standard infection-control practices, such as the sharing of a multidose heparin vial between patients and the lack of glove use or the failure to change gloves between patients, have been associated with outbreaks of HCV infection (183,218,219).

To prevent nosocomial transmission of HCV, strict adherence to infection-control strategies is essential (see before). Several groups of investigators have reported an absence or low rate of seroconversion in units where strict universal precautions were rigorously implemented (190,205,206). The question as to whether or not HCV-positive patients should be dialyzed in a separate room on a separate monitor remains unanswered. No criteria have been firmly established on the issue of isolating HCV-positive patients. This absence of consensus exists not only because of the lack of information about routes of HCV transmission among dialysis patients but also because most units does not have the infrastructure for isolating infected patients. Some authors do not feel that isolation of HCV-infected patients is warranted. Caramelo et al. concluded that sharing the same dialysis machine does not represent an additional risk, provided antiseptic measures are carefully observed (208). Others suggest that it is sufficient to consider every dialysis patient as potentially infectious, strictly adhering to the universal precautions for prevention of transmission of bloodborne antigens (219) and that segregation of HCV-positive patients may lead to faulty nursing with cross-infection of different HCV strains (220,221).

In-between solutions have been proposed, such as dialyzing HCV-positive patients in the last session of the day in order to disinfect the monitor properly without losing time and causing organizational problems (205). Blumberg et al. prevented HCV spread by limited isolation procedures, such as dedicated area and dialysis equipment (222). Others recommend reserving a separate section (197,203,204,223,224) or complete isolation (197,203,224).

We dialyze HCV-positive patients in a separate room with two separate monitors. This attitude is based on the reported possibility of horizontal and/or vertical nosocomial transmission. When HCV-positive patients are isolated, nurses are more attentive to the infectivity of the patient and extended precautions are taken. Accidental violation of infection-control measures can always occur, but by isolating infective patients its consequences can be limited. At the present time, the CDC does not recommend either dedicated machines or isolation for HCV-positive patients (214).

Before isolation of all HCV-positive patients becomes possible, serological testing is necessary. Screening chronic hemodialysis patients is generally accepted; in contrast, screening patients suffering from acute renal failure is more problematic due to the impossibility of asking for permission (intubated, seriously ill patients) and the fact that nephrologists in the ICU are in general only consultants and not the treating physicians. Screening of patients on acute hemodialysis is of importance as well, especially when risk factors are present such as drug abuse, living in endemic areas, and/or hemophilia.

Information about transmission routes of HCV must be given to HCV-infected dialysis patients and to their relatives. In an Italian study, 3 out of 52 tested family members of HCV-positive dialysis patients were found to be infected (225). A Chinese study demonstrated that, although the prevalence of HCV antibodies in family members was not significantly different from that of age-matched controls, the risk of infection was higher in spouses of infected dialysis patients in comparison to the other family members (226). In contrast, in other studies it was found that all sexual partners of HCV-positive dialysis patients were negative for HCV (183,205,227). Whether HCV is sexually transmitted remains controversial, but the transmission rate is considered to be low. The habit of sharing a toothbrush in the family has been reported as a risk factor of HCV infection (197). We instruct patients not to share utensils that might be contaminated, i.e., toothbrushes and other dental devices (tooth pick), razors, and handkerchiefs. Wounds and body fluids should be handled with care. The peritoneal effluent of HCV-infected peritoneal dialysis patients should be considered as infectious, and HCV RNA was detected in the peritoneal dialysate of seropositive patients (174,228,229), even after a storage time of up to 24 hours at room temperature (229). In contrast, Caramelo et al. did not find HCV RNA in peritoneal effluent (208).

F. Therapy of HCV-Infected Dialysis Patients

As in any liver disease, the intake of alcohol should be avoided. Moreover, with HCV infection, a synergy exists between HCV and alcohol, since viral replication increases with alcohol intake (230).

Few data are available concerning the treatment of HCV-infected dialysis patients, but the response rate seems to be better than in patients with normal renal function. Interferon-α can result in initial normalization of the transaminase levels in 67–100% and in negativation of HCV RNA in 28.5–100%. Long-term follow-up revealed a biochemical response in 29–100% and virological clearance in 14.2–92% (231). Evaluation of the therapy can be biased by the differences in pathogenicity of the HCV strains. The available studies include only a limited number of patients, and more extended and long-term studies are necessary to evaluate the efficacy and safety of interferon in dialysis patients.

Ribavirin, a nucleoside analog, has been proposed to treat hepatitis C in combination with interferon-α. However, hemolytic anemia is a major side effect, and the renal elimination and, consequently, the long half-life make this product less suitable for use in hemodialysis patients.

As in the general population, HCV-infected dialysis patients are prone to develop hepatocellular carcinoma, and, therefore, repeated hepatic ultrasound evaluation is advisable (232).

G. Renal Transplantation

Compared to HCV-negative patients, HCV-positive patients have a worse outcome after renal transplantation with an increased risk for liver disease (233,234), sepsis (233,234), kidney graft rejection (234), graft loss (233), and death (233). In contrast, other studies did not find an increased risk for graft loss and mortality (234–236). Recently, an improved survival has been observed in HCV-positive patients who were transplanted compared to those who remained on dialysis (237). Considering the large number of HCV-positive patients that has been transplanted in the past, HCV infection as such should not be considered a contraindication to renal transplantation.

III. THE HEPATITIS G VIRUS OR GB VIRUS-C

In 1995 the GB virus-C (GBV-C) and the hepatitis G virus (HGV) were isolated independently by research groups at Abbott Laboratories (1) and Genelabs Technologies (2), respectively, as novel viruses associated with acute and chronic nonA-nonE hepatitis. Detailed analyses of nucleotide and polyprotein sequences of GBV-C and HGV revealed that both viruses were separate isolates of the same virus.

HGV/GBV-C has a single-stranded genome of approximately 9000 nucleotides and has the structure of a virus in the Flaviviridae family. This single open reading frame encodes for a polyprotein that is processed into at least two structural proteins (the envelope proteins E1 and E2) and five nonstructural proteins (NS2b, NS3, NS4, NS5a, NS5b). NS2a and NS3 are endowed with protease activities and play a role in the processing of the polyprotein, NS5b is the RNA-dependent RNA polymerase of the virus. The HGV/GBV-C capsid does not seem to be coded in the same manner as in HCV. It may be completely absent, or it may be provided by an as-yet-undefined helper virus or by a cellular protein that plays the role of a capsid protein. Unlike the envelope proteins of HCV, E1 and E2 of HGV are devoid of hypervariable regions. HGV/GBV-C is transmitted parenterally by transfusion of blood or blood products, much like HCV. In patients infected with HCV, 10–25% are coinfected with HGV (238–240).

Until recently, HGV/GBV-C could only be detected by very sensitive RT-PCR assays. Most of the published epidemiological data are based on the detection of circulating HGV/GBV-C genomes in subjects with persistent viremia. Surveys performed in different parts of the world have demonstrated the ubiquitous nature of the virus and the variation in its distribution among different population groups. In healthy volunteer blood donors the prevalence of HGV/GBV-C ranges from 0.6% (6) to 1.12% (241), whereas prevalence in commercial blood donors and in injected drug users are 12.9% and 15.8%, respectively (1). The prevalence of HGV/GBV-C in chronic hemodialysis patients ranges from 3% (4) over 8.9% (241) and 16% (5) up to 58% (242).

Recently, immunoassays to detect antibodies directed towards HGV-E2 have been developed. Using these assays, much higher proportions of the examined populations were exposed to HGV/GBV-C than was suggested by HGV RNA detection alone. In healthy blood donors the seroproevalence of anti-E2 antibodies was 6% in a survey in Belgium (241) and 10% in a German population (243). In hemodialysis patients anti-E2 antibodies were found in 14.2% (241) and 30.2% (243) of patients. Anti-E2 seropositive subjects were generally negative for circulating HGV RNA, and HGV RNA positive patients seldom had anti-E2 antibodies. Anti-E2 therefore seems to be a marker of ongoing clearance of or past exposure to HGV/GBV-C.

Since its discovery HGV/GBV-C has drawn a lot of scientific attention, and a host of virological and epidemiological data has been generated. Many questions about the virus remain unanswered. The most important question is whether HGV/GBV-C is really a hepatitis virus that causes significant hepatic damage. If it is, a systematic screening of all blood and blood products for this virus becomes mandatory; if not, there is no need to introduce this costly preventive measure. Recent data show that most HGV/GBV-C infections are not associated with hepatitis. HGV does not worsen the course of concurrent HCV infection, and no causal relation between HGV infection and hepatitis has been established (6,240).

IV. CONCLUSION

It might be hypothesized that, besides the known parenterally transmitted hepatitis viruses (HBV, HCV, HDV, HGV), other yet-undefined but potentially dangerous viruses may exist. Every nephrologist has some dialysis patients with inexplicable liver disease in which no responsible virus has been identified. Therefore, it seems advisable to consider all patients as potentially infectious, especially since the level of transaminase is not always a reliable maker for the detection of liver damage in the dialysis population.

Isolation of infected patients and adherence to extended precautions when handling these patients is time consuming and labor intensive. However, actual restrictions in health care budgets lead to the reduction of staff personnel in dialysis units. Furthermore, isolation procedures are warranted not only for viral infection but also for bacterial infection such as methicillin-resistant staphylococci, vancomycin-resistant enterococci, and ceftazidime-resistant bacteria. How should the future dialysis unit then be designed? Should it consist of many separate room, rather than the classic one-room unit of today? Can dialysis then be performed safely in separate rooms with only a limited number of staff? Finally, does not spatial isolation of the patient induce social isolation? Another issue of concern is related to "holiday dialysis." Because dialysis patients are becoming increasingly mobile and are able to travel abroad, the risk for import pathologies increases. Which countries can be recommended, and which centers should be avoided? There are but a few questions and considerations nephrologist will have to confront in the years to come.

REFERENCES

1. Simons JN, Leary TP, Dawson GJ, Pilotmatias TJ, Muerhoff AS, Schlauder GG, Desai SM, Mushahawar IK. Isolation of novel virus-like sequences associated with human hepatitis. Nat Med 1995; 1:564–569.
2. Linnen J, Wages J, Zhangkeck ZY, Fry KE, Krawczynski KZ, Alter H, Koonin E. Gallagher M, Alter M, Hadziyannis S, Karayiannis P, Fung K, Nakatsuji Y, Shih JWK, Young L, Piatak M, Hoover C, Fernandez J, Chen S, Zou JC, Morris T, Hyams KC, Ismay S, Lifson JD, Hess G, Foung SKH, Thomas H, Bradley D, Margolis H, Kim JP. Molecular cloning and disease association of hepatitis G virus: a transfusion-transmissible agent. Science 1996; 271:505–508.
3. Simons JN, Desai SM, Mushahawar IK. The GB viruses: isolation, characterization, diagnosis and epidemiology. Viral Hepatitis Rev 1996; 2:229–246.
4. Masuko K, Mitsui T, Iwano K, Yamazaki C, Okuda K, Meguro T, Murayama N, Inoue T, Tsuda F, Okamoto H, Miyakawa Y, Mayumi M. Infection with hepatitis GB virus C in patients on maintenance hemodialysis. N Engl J Med 1996; 334:1485–1490.
5. Cornu C, Jadoul M, Loute G, Goubau P. Hepatitis G virus infection in haemodialysed patients: epidemiology and clinical relevance. Nephrol Dial Transplant 1997; 12:1326–1329.
6. Alter HJ, Nakatsuji Y, Melpolder J, Wages J, Wesley R, Shih WK, Kim JP. The incidence of transfusion-associated hepatitis G virus infection and its relation to liver disease. N Engl J Med 1997; 336:747–754.
7. Gerlich WH, Bruss V. Functions of hepatitis B virus proteins and molecular targets for protective immunity. In: Ellis RW, ed. Hepatitis B Vaccines in Clinical Practice. New York: Marcel Dekker, 1993:41–82.
8. Tillmann H, Trautwein C, Walker D, Michitaka K, Kubicka S, Boker K, Manns M. Clinical relevance of mutations in the precore genome of the hepatitis B virus. Gut 1995; 37:568–573.
9. Hadziyannis SJ. Hepatitis B e antigen negative chronic hepatitis B: from clinical recognition to pathogenesis and treatment. Viral Hepatitis 1995; 1:7–36.
10. Sjögren MH. Serologic diagnosis of viral hepatitis. Med Clin North Am 1996; 80:929–956.
11. Zyzik E, Gerlich WH, Uy A, Köchel H, Thomssen R. Assay of hepatitis B virus genome titers in sera of infected subjects. Eur J Microbiol 1986; 5:330–335.
12. Gerlich WH, Heermann KH, Thomssen R, Eurohep Group. Quantitative assays for hepatitis B virus DNA: standardization and quality control. Viral Hepatitis Reviews 1995; 1:53–57.
13. Lee B, Yap H, Tan M, Guan R, Quak S, Choong L, Murugasu B, Woo K, Jordan S. Cell-mediated immunity in patients on haemodialysis: relationship with hepatitis B carrier status. Am J Nephrol 1991; 11:98–101.
14. Garibaldi R, Forrest J, Bryan J, Hanson B, Dismukes W. Hemodialysis-associated hepatitis. JAMA 1973; 225:384–389.
15. London WT, Drew JS, Lustbader ED, Werner BG, Blumberg BS. Host responses to hepatitis B infection in patients in a chronic hemodialysis unit. Kidney Int 1977; 12:51–58.
16. Ribot S, Rothstein M, Goldblat M, Grasso M. Duration of hepatitis B surface antigenemia (HBsAg) in hemodialysis patients. Arch Intern Med 1979; 139: 178–180.
17. Janzen L, Minuk GY, Fast M, Bernstein KN. Vaccine-induced hepatitis B surface antigen positivity in adult hemodialysis patients: incidental and surveillance data. J Am Soc Nephrol 1996; 7:1228–1234.
18. Kear TM, Wright LS. Transient hepatitis B antigenemia in hemodialysis patients following hepatitis B vaccination. ANNA J 1996; 23:331–337.
19. Ortiz-Interian CJ, de Medina MD, Perez GO, Bourgoignie JJ, Watkins F, Velez-Robinson E, Schiff E. Recurrence and clearance of hepatitis B surface antigenemia in a dialysis patient infected with the human immunodeficiency virus. Am J Kidney Dis 1990; 16: 154–156.
20. Michalak TI, Pasquellini S, Guilhot S, Chisari FV. Hepatitis B virus persistence after recovery from acute viral hepatitis. J Clin Invest 1994; 93:230–239.
21. Blumberg B, Alter H, Visnich S. A new antigen in leukemia sera. JAMA 1965; 191:541–546.
22. Blumberg B, Sutnick A. London W. Hepatitis and leukemia their relation to australia antigen. Bull NY Acad Med 1968; 44:1566–1586.
23. Szmuness W, Prince A, Grady G, Mann M, Levine R, Friedman E, Jacobs M, Josephson A, Ribot S, Shapiro F, Stenzel K, Sudi W, Vyas G. Hepatitis B infection: a point-prevalence study in 15 US hemodialysis centers. JAMA 1974; 227:901–906.

24. Tokars J, Alter M, Favero M, Moyer L, Miller E, Bland L. National surveillance of dialysis associated diseases in the United States, 1993. ASAIO Journal 1996; 42:219–229.
25. Geerlings W, Tufveson G, Brunner F, Ehrich J, Fassbinder W, Landais P, Mallick N, Margreiter R, Raine A, Rizzoni G, Selwood N. Combined report on regular dialysis and transplantation in Europe, XXI, 1990. Nephrol Dial Transplant 1991; 6(suppl 2):5–29.
26. Villarejos V, Visona K, Gutierrez A, Rodriguez A. Role of saliva, urine and feces in the transmission of type B hepatitis. N Engl J Med 1974; 291:1375–1378.
27. Bond W, Favero M, Peterson N, Gravelle C, Ebert J, Maynard J. Survival of hepatitis B virus after drying and storage for one week. Lancet 1981; 1:550.
28. Shusterman N, Singer I. Infectious hepatitis in dialysis patients. Am J Kidney Dis 1987; 9:447–455.
29. Alter H, Seeff L, Kaplan P, McAuliffe V, Wright E, Gerin J, Purcell R, Holland P, Zimmerman H. Type B hepatitis: the infectivity of blood positive for e antigen and DNA polymerase after accidental needlestick exposure. N Engl J Med 1976; 295:909–913.
30. de Jong G, de Bruin W, Verresen L, Moshage H, Desmyter J, Yap S. High-flux membranes are not permeable to hepatitis B virus DNA. Nephron 1992; 60:368.
31. Andrew R, Hariharan S, Vaskar Saha, Jacob T, Kirubakaran M, Shastry J. Biochemical evaluation of ultrafiltrate in dialysis-dependent HBsAg-positive patients. Nephron 1988; 49:88.
32. Moynot A, Lazizi Y, Dubreuil P, Buisson C, Pillot J. Nature of Ag Hbs ultrafiltrate of haemodialyzed patients. Presence of viral DNA (abstr). Nephrol Dial Transplant 1992; 7:732.
33. Kroes A, van Bommel E, Niesters H, Weimar W. Hepatitis B viral DNA detectable in dialysate. Nephron 1994; 67:369.
34. Alter M, Favero M, Maynard J. Impact of infection control strategies on the incidence of dialysis-associated hepatitis in the United States. J Infect Dis 1986; 153:1149–1151.
35. Favero M, Deane N, Leger R, Sosin A. Effect of multiple use of dialyzers on hepatitis B incidence in patients and staff. JAMA 1981; 245:166–167.
36. Alter M, Ahtone J, Maynard J. Hepatitis B virus transmission associated with a multiple-dose vial in a hemodialysis unit. Ann Intern Med 1983; 99:330–333.
37. Goodman W, Gallagher N, Sherrard D. Peritoneal dialysis fluid as a source of hepatitis antigen. Nephron 1981; 29:107–109.
38. Spector D. Hepatitis B miniepidemic in a peritoneal dialysis unit. Arch Int Med 1977; 137:1030–1031.
39. Vas S, Oreopoulos D. Handle with care: hepatitis B antigen carriers in peritoneal dialysis units. Nephron 1981; 29:105–106.
40. Alter MJ, Favero MS, Maynard JE. Hemodialysis-associated hepatitis in the United States. In: Vyas GN, Dienstag JL, Hoofnage JH, eds. Viral Hepatitis and Liver Disease. New York: Grune & Stratton Inc., 1984:636.
41. Alter MJ, Favero MS, Moyer LA, Miller JK, Bland LA. National surveillance of dialysis-associated diseases in the United States, 1988. ASAIO Trans 1990; 36:107–118.
42. Oddone EZ, Cowper PA, Hamilton JD, Feussner JR. A cost-effective analysis of hepatitis B vaccine in predialysis patients. Health Serv Res 1993; 28:97–121.
43. Kane MA. 16 Global control of hepatitis B through universal infant immunization. In: Ellis RW, ed. Hepatitis B Vaccines in Clinical Practice. New York: Marcel Dekker, 1993; 309–322.
44. Crosnier J, Jungers P, Couroucé AM, Laplanche A, Benhamou E, Degos F, Lacour B, Prunet P, Cerisier Y, Guesry P. Randomised placebo-controlled trial of hepatitis B surface antigen vaccine in French haemodialysis units: II. Haemodialysis patients. Lancet 1981; i:797–800.
45. Desmyter J, Colaert J, De Groote G, Reynders M, Reerink-Brongers EE, Dees PJ, Ielie PN, Reesink HW and the Leuven Renal Transplantation Collaborative Group. Efficacy of heat-inactivated hepatitis B vaccine in haemodialysis patients and staff. Double-blind placebo-controlled trial. Lancet 1983; ii:1323–1328.
46. Stevens CE, Alter HJ, Taylor PE, Zang EA, Harley EJ, Szmuness W and the Dialysis Vaccine Trial Study Group. Hepatitis B vaccine in patients receiving haemodialysis. Immunogenicity and efficacy. N Engl J Med 1984; 311:496–501.
47. Benhamou E, Courouce AM, Jungers P, Laplanche A, Degos F, Brangier J, Crosnier J. Hepatitis B vaccine: randomized trial of immunogenicity in hemodialysis patients. Clin Nephrol 1984; 21:143–147.
48. Jilg W, Schmidt M, Weinel B, Kishuttler T, Brass H, Bommer J, Mishuller R, Schulte B, Schwarzbeck A, Deinhardt F. Immunogenicity of recombinant hepatitis B vaccine in dialysis patients. J Hepatol 1986; 3:190–195.
49. Fujiyama S, Yoshida K, Sagara K, Sato T, Nishimura Y, Shimada H. Efficacy and safety of hepatitis B vaccination in haemodialysis patients. J Gastroenterol Hepatol 1987; 2:167–173.
50. Seaworth B, Drucker J, Starling J, Drucker R, Stevens C, Hamilton J. Hepatitis B vaccines in patients with chronic renal failure before dialysis. J Infect Dis 1988; 157:332–337.
51. Steketee RW, Ziarnik ME, Davis JP. Seroresponse to hepatitis B vaccine in patients and staff of renal dialysis centers. Am J Epidemiol 1988; 127:772–782.
52. Bruguera M, Rodicio JL, Alcazar JM, Oliver A, Del Rio G, Esteban Mur R. Effects of different dose levels and vaccination schedules on immune response to a recombinant DNA hepatitis B vaccine in haemodialysis patients. Vaccine 1990; 8:S47–S62.

53. Docci D, Cipolloni PA, Baldrati L, Capponcini C, Turci F, Feletti C. Immune response to a recombinant hepatitis B vaccine in hemodialysis patient. Int J Artif Organs 1990; 13:451–453.
54. Fuijiyama S, Yoshida K, Sato T, Shimada H, Deguchi T. Immunogenicity and safety of recombinant yeast-derived hepatitis B vaccine in haemodialysis patients. Hepatogastroenterology 1990; 37(suppl 2):140–144.
55. Smit-Leijs MB, Kramer P, Heijtinck RA, Hop WC, Schalm SW. Hepatitis B vaccination of haemodialysis patients: randomized controlled trial comparing plasma-derived vaccine with and without pre-S2 antigen. Eur J Clin Invest 1990; 20:540–545.
56. Albertoni F, Battilomo A, Di Nardo V, Franco E, Ippolito G, Marinucci G, Perucci CA, Petrosillo N, Sommella L and The Latium Hepatitis Prevention Group. Evaluation of a region-wide hepatitis B vaccination program in dialysis patients: experience in an Italian region. Nephron 1991; 58:180–183.
57. Fleming SJ, Moran DM, Cooksley WG, Faoagali JL. Poor response to a recombinant hepatitis B vaccine in dialysis patients. J Infect 1991; 22:251–257.
58. Allegra V, Vasile A, Maschio M, Mengozzi G. Immune response after vaccination with recombinant hepatitis surface antigen in maintenance hemodialysis patients and healthy controls. Nephron 1992; 61:339–340.
59. Buti M, Viladomiu L, Jardi R, Olmos A, Rodriguez JA, Bartolome J, Esteban R, Guardia J. Long-term immunogenicity and efficacy of hepatitis B vaccine in hemodialysis patients. Am J Nephrol 1992; 12:144–147.
60. Docci D, Cipolloni PA, Mengozzi S, Baldrati L, Capponcini C, Feletti C. Immunogenicity of a recombinant hepatitis B vaccine in hemodialysis patients: a two-year follow-up. Nephron 1992; 61:352–353.
61. Fanelli V, Sanna G, Solinas A. Expectation of impaired response to recombinant hepatitis B vaccination. Nephron 1992; 61:293–295.
62. Jungers P, Chauveau P, Couroucé AM, Abbassi A, Devillier P, Marie FN, Bailleux F, Excler JL, Cerisier JE, Saliou P. Vaccin recombinant et vaccin d'extraction contre l'hépatite B chez l'insuffisant rénal: immunogénicité comparée. Presse Med 1994; 23:277–280.
63. Marangi al, Giordano R, Montanaro A, De Padova F, Schiavone MG, Dongiovanni G, Basile C. Hepatitis B virus infection in chronic uremia: long-term follow-up of a two-step integrated protocol of vaccination. Am J Kidney Dis 1994; 23:537–542.
64. Rault R, Freed B, Nespor S, Bender F. Efficacy of different hepatitis B vaccination strategies in patients receiving hemodialysis. ASAIO J 1995; 41:M717–M719.
65. Fabrizi F, Di-Filippo S, Marcelli D, Guarnori I, Raffaele L, Crepaldi M, Erba G, Locatelli F. Recombinant hepatitis B vaccine use in chronic hemodialysis patients. Long-term evaluation and cost-effectiveness analysis. Nephron 1996; 72:536–543.
66. Fernandez E, Betriu MA, Gomez R, Montoliu J. Response to the hepatitis B virus vaccine in haemodialysis patients: influence of malnutrition and its importance as a risk factor for morbidity and mortality. Nephrol Dial Transpl 1996; 11:1559–1563.
67. Khan AN, Bernardini J, Rault RM, Piraino B. Low seroconversion with hepatitis B vaccination in peritoneal dialysis patients. Perit Dial Int 1996; 16:370–373.
68. Mitwalli A. Responsiveness to hepatitis B vaccine in immunocompromised patients by doubling the dose scheduling. Nephron 1996; 73:417–420.
69. Navarro JF, Teruel JL, Mateos ML, Marcen R, Ortuno J. Antibody level after hepatitis B vaccination in hemodialysis patients: influence of hepatitis C virus infection. Am J Nephrol 1996; 16:95–97.
70. Cheng CH, Huang CC, Leu ML, Chiang CY, Wu MS, Lai PC. Hepatitis B vaccine in hemodialysis patients with hepatitis C viral infection. Vaccine 1997; 15: 1353–1357.
71. Peces R, de la Torre M, Alcazar R, Urra JM. Prospective analysis of the factors influencing the antibody response to hepatitis B vaccine in hemodialysis patients. Am J Kidney Dis 1997; 29:239–245.
72. Radovic MM, Ostric V, Djukanovic L. Complete seroconversion after vaccination against hepatitis B virus in hemodialysis patients. Clin Nephrol 1997; 47:206.
73. Descamps-Latscha B, Chatenoud L. T cells and B cells in chronic renal failure. Seminars in Nephrology 1996; 16:183–191.
74. Girndt M, Pietsch M, Kohler H. Tetanus immunization and its association to hepatitis B vaccination in patients with chronic renal failure. Am J Kidney Dis 1995; 26:454–460.
75. Guerin A, Buisson Y, Nutini MT, Saliou P, London G, Marchais S. Response to vaccination against tetanus in chronic haemodialysed patients. Nephrol Dial Transplant 1991; 7:323–326.
76. Kreft B, Klouche M, Kreft R, Kirchner H, Sack K. Low efficiency of active immunization against diphtheria in chronic hemodialysis patients. Kidney Int 1997; 52:212–216.
77. Rautenberg P, Teifke I, Schlegelberger T, Ullman U. Influenza subtype-specific IgA, IgM and IgG responses in patients on hemodialysis after influenza vaccination. Infection 1988; 16:323–328.
78. Walker M, Szmuness W, Stevens CE, Rubinstein P. Genetics of anti-HBs responsiveness: I. HLA DR7 and nonresponsiveness to hepatitis vaccination. Transfusion 1981; 21:601.
79. Usonis V, Kühnl P, Brede HD, Doerr HW. Humoral immune response after hepatitis B vaccination: kinetics of anti-HBs antibodies and demonstration of HLA antigens. Zbl Bakt Hyg 1986(A); 262:377–384.

80. Craven DE, Awdeh ZL, Kunches LM, Yunis EJ, Dienstag JL, Werner BG, Polk BF, Snydman DR. Platt R, Crumpacker CS, Grady GF, Alper CA. Nonresponsiveness to hepatitis B vaccine in health care workers. Results of revaccination and genetic typings. Ann Intern Med 1986; 105:356–360.
81. Varla-Leftherioti M, Papanicolaou M, Spyropoulou M. HLA-associated nonresponsiveness to hepatitis B vaccine. Tissue Antigens 1990; 35:60–63.
82. Weissman JY, Tsuchiyose MM, Tong MJ, Co R, Chin K, Ettinger RB. Lack of response to recombinant hepatitis B vaccine in nonresponders to the plasma vaccine. JAMA 1988; 260:1734–1738.
83. Dondi E, Finco O, Mantovani V, Mele L, Ruberto G, Cuccia M. Involvement of HLA and C4 in the nonresponsiveness to hepatitis B vaccine. Fund Clin Immunol 1996; 4:73–78.
84. Desombere I, Willems A, Leroux-Roels G. Response to hepatitis B vaccines: multiple HLA-genes are involved. Tissue Antigens 1998; 51:593–604.
85. Krämer A, Herth D, von Keyserlingk HJ, Ludwig WD, Hampl H, Sommer D, Hahn EG, Riecken EO. Non-responsiveness to hepatitis-B vaccination: revaccination and immunogenetic typing. Klin Wochenschr 1988; 66:670–674.
86. Pol S, Legendre C, Mattlinger B, Berthelot P, Kreis H. Genetic basis of nonresponse to heaptitis B vaccine in hemodialyzed patients. J Hepatol 1990; 11:385–387.
87. Caillat Zucman S, Gimenez JJ, Albouze G, Lebkiri B, Naret C. Jungers P, Bach JF. HLA genetic heterogeneity of hepatitis B vaccine response in hemodialyzed patients. Kidney Int 1993; 41:S157–S160.
88. Stachowski J, Kramer J, Füst G, Maciejewski J, Baldamus CA, Petranyi GG. Relationship between the reactivity to hepatitis B virus vaccination and the frequency of MHC class I, II and III alleles in haemodialysis patients. Scand J Immunol 1995; 42:60–65.
89. Waite NM, Thomson LG, Goldstein MB. Successful vaccination with intradermal hepatitis B vaccine in hemodialysis patients previously nonresponsive to intramuscular hepatitis B vaccine. J Am Soc Nephrol 1995; 5:1930–1934.
90. Navarro JF, Teruel JL, Mateos M, Ortuno J. Hepatitis C virus infection decreases the effective antibody response to hepatitis B vaccine in hemodialysis patients. Clin Nephrol 1994; 41:113–116.
91. Quiroga JA, Castillo I, Porres JC, Casado S, Saez F, Gracia Martinez M, Gomez M, Inglada L, Sanchez-Sicilia L, Mora A, Galiana F, Barril G, Carreno V. Recombinant gamma-interferon as adjuvant to hepatitis B vaccine in hemodialysis patients. Hepatology 1990; 12:661–663.
92. Jaiswal SB, Chitnis DS. Antibody response to hepatitis B vaccine among haemodialysis patients. Lancet 1995; 346:1363.
93. Fabrizi F, Andrulli S, Bacchini G, Corti M, Locatelli F. Intradermal versus intramuscular hepatitis B re-vaccination in non-responsive chronic dialysis patients: a prospective randomized study with cost-effectiveness evaluation. Nephrol Dial Transport 1997; 12:1204–1211.
94. Ono K, Kashiwagi S. Complete seroconversion by low-dose intradermal injection of recombinant hepatitis B vaccine in hemodialysis patients. Nephron 1991; 58:47–51.
95. Mettang T, Schenk U, Thomas S, Machleidt C, Kiefer T, Fischer FP, Kuhlmann U. Low-dose intradermal versus intramuscular hepatitis B vaccination in patients with endstage renal failure. A preliminary study, Nephron 1996; 72:192–196.
96. Quiroga JA, Castillo I, Porres JC, Casado S, Saez F, Gracia Martinez M, Gomez M, Inglada L, Sanchez-Sicilia L, Mora A, Galiana F, Barril G, Carreno V. Recombinant gamma-interferon as adjuvant to hepatitis B vaccine in hemodialysis patients. Hepatology 1990; 12:661–663.
97. Hess G, Kreiter F, Kosters W, Deusch K. The effect of granulocyte-macrophage colony-stimulating factor (GM-CSF) on hepatitis B vaccination in haemodialysis patients. J Viral Hepat 1996; 3:149–153.
98. Ervo R, Faletti P, Magni S, Cavatorta F. Evaluation of treatments for the vaccination against hepatitis B + thymopentine. Nephron 1992; 61:371–372.
99. Melappioni M, Baldassari M, Baldini S, Radicioni R, Panichi N, Saldini S. Use of immunomodulators (thymopentine) in hepatitis B vaccine in elderly patients undergoing chronic hemodialysis. Nephron 1992; 61: 358–359.
100. Meuer SC, Dumann H, Meyer zum Büschenfelde KH, Köhler H. Low-dose interleukin-2 induces systemic immune responses against HBsAg in immunodeficient non-responders to hepatitis B vaccination. Lancet 1989; 7:15–17.
101. Jungers P, Devillier P, Salomon H, Cerisier JE, Courouce AM. Randomised placebo-controlled trial of recombinant interleukin-2 in chronic uraemic patients who are non-responders to hepatitis B vaccine. Lancet 1994; 344:856–857.
102. Sennesael JJ, Van der Niepen P, Verbeelen DL. Treatment with recombinant human erythropoietin increases antibody titers after hepatitis B vaccination in dialysis patients. Kidney Int 1991; 40:121–128.
103. Kuroda S, Fujisawa Y, Iino S, Akahane Y, Suzuki H. Induction of protection level of anti-pre-S2 antibodies in humans immunized with a novel hepatitis B vaccine consisting of M (pre-S2 + S) protein particles (a third generation vaccine). Vaccine 1991; 9:163–169.
104. Pillot J, Poynard T, Elias A, Maillard J, Lazizi Y, Brancer M, Dubreuil P, Budkowska A, Chaput JC. Weak immunogenicity of the preS2 sequence and lack of circumventing effect on the unresponsiveness to the hepatitis B virus vaccine. Vaccine 1995; 13:289–294.

105. Miskovsky E, Gershman K, Clements ML, Cupps T, Calandra G, Hesley T, Ioli V, Ellis R, Kniskern P, Miller W, Gerety R, West D. Comparative safety and immunogenicity of yeast recombinant hepatitis B vaccines containing S and pre-S2 + S antigens. Vaccine 1991; 9:346–350.
106. Zuckerman JN, Sabin C, Craig FM, Williams A, Zuckerman AJ. Immune response to a new hepatitis B vaccine in healthcare workers who had not responded to standard vaccine: randomised double blind dose-response study. BMJ 1997; 314:329–333.
107. Raz R, Dagan R, Gallil A, Brill G, Kassis I, Koren R. Safety and immunogenicity of a novel mammalian cell-derived recombinant hepatitis B vaccine containing pre-S1 and pre-S2 antigens in children. Vaccine 1996; 14:207–211.
108. Hemmerling AE, Müller R, Firusian N, Grötz J, Haubitz M, Thoma HA. Clinical experience with the preS1-containing hepatitis B vaccine (HG-3) in different nonresponder groups. In: Nishioka K, Suzuki H, Mishiro S, Oda T, eds. Viral Hepatitis and Liver Disease. Tokyo: Springer, 1994:540–542.
109. Leroux-Roels G, Desombere I, Cobbaut L, Petit AM, Desmons P, Hauser P, Delem A, De Grave D, Safary A. Hepatitis V vaccine containing surface antigen and selected preS1 and preS2 sequences. 2. Immunogenicity in poor responders to hepatitis B vaccines. Vaccine 1997; 15:1732–1736.
110. Leroux-Roels G, Desombere I, De Tollenaere G, Petit AM, Desmons P, Hauser P, Delem A, De Grave D, Safary A. Hepatitis B vaccine containing surface antigen and selected preS1 and preS2 sequences. 1. Safety and immunogenicity in young, healthy adults. Vaccine 1997; 15:1724–1731.
111. Szmuness W, Stevens CE, Harley EJ, Zang EA, Oleszko WR, William DC, Sadovsky R, Morrison JM, Kellner A. Hepatitis B vaccine. Demonstration of efficacy in a controlled clinical trial in a high-risk population in the United States. N Engl J Med 1980; 303: 833–841.
112. Crosnier J, Jungers P, Couroucé AM, Laplanche A, Benhamou E, Degos F, Lacour B, Prunet P, Cersisier Y, Guesry P. Randomized, placebo-controlled trial of hepatitis B surface antigen vaccine in French haemodialysis units: I. Medical Staff. Lancet 1981: 1:455–459.
113. Lee W. Hepatitis B virus infection. N Engl J Med 1997; 337:1733–1745.
114. Pirson Y, Alexandre G, Van Ypersele de Strihou C. Long-term effect of HBs antigenemia on patients survival after renal transplantation. N Engl J Med 1977; 296:194–196.
115. Fornairon S, Pol S, Legendre C, Carnot F, Mamzer-Bruneel M, Bréchot C, Kreis H. The long-term virologic impact of renal transplantation on chronic hepatitis B virus infection. Transplantation 1996; 62:297–299.
116. Harnett J, Zeldis J, Parfrey P, Kennedy M, Sircar R, Steinmann T, Guttmann R. Hepatitis B disease in dialysis and transplant patients. Further epidemiologic and serologic studies. Transplantation 1987; 44:369–376.
117. Paparella M, Tarantino A, Ponticelli C. How to manage the dialysis patient with chronic viral hepatitis who is considered for renal transplantation? Nephrol Dial Transplant 1996; 11:2122–2124.
118. Major ME, Feinstone SM. The molecular virology of hepatitis C. Hepatology 1997; 25:1527–1538.
119. Clarke B. Molecular virology of hepatitis C virus. J Gen Virol 1997; 78:2397–2410.
120. Choo QL, Kuo G, Weiner AJ, Overby LR, Bradley DW, Houghton M. Isolation of a cDNA clone derived from a blood-borne non-A, non-B viral hepatitis genome. Science 1989; 244:359–362.
121. Kuo G, Choo QL, Alter HJ, Gitnick GL, Redeker AG, Purcell RH, Miyamura T, Dienstag JL, Alter MJ, Stevens CE, Tegtmeier GE, Bonino M, Lee WS, Kuo C, Berger K, Shuster JR, Overby LR, Brandley DW, Houghton M. An assay for circulating antibodies to a major etiologic virus of human non-A, non-B hepatitis. Science 1989; 244:362–364.
122. Kleinman S, Alter H, Busch M, Holland P, Tegtmeier G, Nelles M, Lee S, Page E, Wilber J, Palito A. Increased detection of hepatitis C virus (HCV)-infected blood donors by a multiple antigen HCV enzyme immunoassay. Transfusion 1992; 32:806–813.
123. Alter HJ, Purcell RH, Shih JW, Melpolder JC, Houghton M, Choo QL, Kuo G. Detection of antibody to hepatitis C virus in prospectively followed transfusion recipients with acute and chronic non-A, non-B hepatitis. N Engl J Med 1989; 321:1494–1500.
124. Esteban JI, Gonzalez A, Hernandez JM, Viladomiu L, Sanchez C, Lopez-Talavera JC, Lucea D, Martin-Vega C, Vidal X, Esteban R, Guardia J. Evaluation of antibodies to hepatitis C virus in a study of transfusion-associated hepatitis. N Engl J Med 1990; 323:1107–1112.
125. Esteban JI, Esteban R, Viladomiu L, Lopez-Talavera JC, Gonzalez A, Hernandez JM, Roget M, Vargas V, Genesca J, Buti M. Hepatitis C virus antibodies among risk groups in Spain. Lancet 1989; 2:294–297.
126. Aach Rd, Stevens CE, Hollinger FB, Mosley JW, Peterson DA, Taylor PE, Johnson RG, Barbosa LH, Meno GJ. Hepatitis C virus infection in post-transfusion hepatitis. An analysis with first- and second-generation assays. N Engl J Med 1991; 325:1325–1329.
127. Uyttendaele S, Claeys H, Mertens W, Verhaert H, Vermylen C. Evaluation of third generation screening and confirmatory assays for HCV antibodies. Vox Sang 1994; 66:122–129.
128. Barrera J, Prancis B, Ercilla G, Nelles M, Achord D, Darner J, Lee S. Improved detection of anti-HCV in post-transfusion hepatitis by a third-generation ELISA. Vox Sang 1995; 768:15–18.

129. Huber KR, Sebesta C, Bauer K. Detection of common hepatitis C virus subtypes with a third-generation enzyme immunoassay. Hepatology 1996; 24:471–473.
130. Kao JH, Yang PM, Lai MY, Chen PJ, Wang TH, Chen DS. Evaluation of third-generation hepatitis C antibody assay in chronic hepatitis C and chronic non-B, non-C hepatitis. Viral Immunol 1995; 8:135–139.
131. Vrielink H, Zaaijer HL, Reesink HW, van der Poel CL, Cuypers HTM, Lelie PN. Sensitivity and specificity of three third-generation anti-hepatitis C virus ELISAs. Vox Sang 1995; 69:14–17.
132. Leon P, Lopez JA, Domingo C, Echevarria JM. Evaluation of laboratory assays for screening antibody to hepatitis C virus. Transfusion 1993; 33:268–270.
133. Yuki N, Hayashi N, Kasahara A, Hagiwara H, Mita E, Kazuyoshi O, Katayama K, Fusamoto H, Kamada T. Quantitative analysis of antibody to hepatitis C virus envelope 2 glycoprotein in patients with chronic hepatitis C virus infection. Hepatology 1996; 23:947–952.
134. Lesnieuwski R, Okasinkski G, Carrick R, Van Sant C, Desai S, Johnson R, Scheffel J, Moore B, Mushahwar I. Antibody to hepatitis C virus second envelope (HCV E2) glycoprotein: a new marker of HCV infection closely associated with viremia. J Med Virol 1995; 45: 415–422.
135. Mangia A, Maertens G, Cascavilla I, Saracco G, Santantonio T, Gentile R, Annese V, Andriulli A. Circulating E1 and E2 antibodies in HCV chronic carriers. Hepatology 1997; 26:213A.
136. Depraetere S, Van Kerschaver E, Elewaut A, Brouwer J, Niesters B, Schalm S, Maertens G, Leroux-Roels G. Antibodies to E1 and E2 in patients infected with HCV 1b: evolution of antibody levels after interferon therapy. Hepatology 1997; 26:213A.
137. Pawlotsky JM, Bastie A, Pellet C, Remire J, Darthuy F, Wolfe L, Sayada C, Duval J, Dhumeaux D. Significance of indeterminate third-generation hepatitis C virus recombinant immunoblot assay. J Clin Microbiol 1996; 34:80–83.
138. Damen M, Zaaijer HL, Cuypers HTM, Vrielink H, van der Poel CL, Reesink HW, Lelie PN. Reliability of the third-generation recombinant immunoblot assay for hepatitis C virus. Transfusion 1995; 35:745–749.
139. Gretch DR. Diagnostic tests for hepatitis C. Hepatology 1997; 26(suppl 1):43S–47S.
140. Zaaijer HL, Cuypers HT, Reesink HW, Winkel IN, Gerken G, Lelie PN. Reliability of polymerase chain reaction for detection of hepatitis C virus. Lancet 1993; 34:722–724.
141. Gretch D, dela Rosa D, Corey L, Carithers R. Assessment of hepatitis C viremia using molecular amplification technologies. Viral Hepatitis Rev 1996; 2:85–96.
142. Brillanti S, Garson JA, Tuke PW. Effect of alpha-interferon therapy on hepatitis C viraemia in community-acquired chronic non-A, non-B hepatitis: a quantitative polymerase chain reaction study. J Med Virol 1991; 34:136–141.
143. Gretch D, Corey L, Wilson J, dela-Rosa C, Wilson R, Carithers R Jr, Busch M, Hart J, Sayers M, Han J. Assessment of hepatitis C virus RNA levels by quantitative competitive RNA polymerase chain reaction: high-titer viremia correlates with advanced stage of disease. J Infect Dis 1994; 169:1219–1225.
144. Hagiwara H, Hayashi N, Mita E, Naito M, Kasahara A, Fusamoto H, Kamada T. Quantitation of hepatitis C virus RNA in serum of asymptomatic blood donors and patients with type C chronic liver disease. Hepatology 1993; 17:545–550.
145. Kato N, Yokosuka O, Hosoda K, Ito Y, Ohto M, Omata M. Quantification of hepatitis C virus by competitive reverse transcription-polymerase chain reaction: increase of the virus in advanced disease. Hepatology 1993; 18:16–20.
146. Gretch DR, Bacchi CE, Corey L, dela-Rosa C, Lesniewski RR, Kowdley K, Gown A, Frank I, Perkins JD, Carithers RL. Persistent hepatitis C virus infection after liver transplantation: clinical and virological features. Hepatology 1995; 22:1–9.
147. Feray C, Gigou M, Samuel D, Paradis V, Wilber J, David MF, Urdea M, Reynes M, Brechot C, Bismuth H. The course of hepatitis C virus infection after liver transplantation. Hepatology 1994; 20:1137–1143.
148. Eyster Em, Fried MW, Di Bisceglie AM, Goedert JJ. Increasing hepatitis C virus RNA levels in hemophiliacs: relationship to human immunodeficiency virus infection and liver disease. Blood 1994; 84:1020–1023.
149. Kobayashi Y, Watanabe S, Konishi M, Yokoi M, Kakehashi R, Kaito M, Kondo M, Hayashi Y, Jomori T, Suzuki S. Quantitation and typing of serum hepatitis C virus RNA in patients with chronic hepatitis C treated with interferon-β. Hepatology 1993; 18:1319–1325.
150. Yuki N, Hayashi N, Kasahara A, Hagiwara H, Takehara T, Oshita M, Katayama K, Fusamoto H, Kamada T. Pretreatment viral load and response to prolonged interferon-α course for chronic hepatitis C. J Hepatol 1995; 22:457–463.
151. Lau JYN, Davis GL, Kniffen J, Qian KP, Urdea MS, Chan CS, Mizokami M, Neuwald PD, Wilber JC. Significance of serum hepatitis C virus RNA levels in chronic hepatitis C. Lancet 1993; 341:1501–1504.
152. Hagiwara H, Hayashi N, Mita E, Takehara T, Kasahara A, Fusamoto H, Kamada T. Quantitative analysis of hepatitis C virus RNA in serum during alpha interferon therapy. Gastroenterology 1993; 104:877–883.
153. Orito E, Mizokami M, Suzuki K, Ohba K, Ohno T, Mori M, Hayashi K, Kato K, Iino S, Lau JY. Loss of serum HCV RNA at week 4 of interferon-alpha therapy is associated with more favorable long-term re-

sponse in patients with chronic hepatitis C. J Med Virol 1995; 46:109–115.

154. Marcellin P, Pouteau M, Martinot-Peignoux M, Degos F, Duchatelle V, Boyer N, Lemonnier C, Degott C, Erlinger S, Benhamou JP. Lack of benefit of escalating dosage of interferon alfa in patients with chronic hepatitis C. Gastroenterology 1995; 109:156–165.

155. Bekkering FC, Brouwer JT, Leroux-Roles G, Van Vlierberghe H, Elewaut A, Schalm SW. Ultrarapid Hepatitis C virus clearance by daily high dose interferon in nonresponders to standard therapy. Hepatology 1997; 26:415A.

156. Maertens G, Stuyver L. Genotypes and genetic variation of hepatitis C virus. In: Harrison TJ, Zuckerman AJ, eds. The Molecular Medicine of Viral Hepatitis. London: John Wiley & Sons Ltd., 1997;183–233.

157. Stuyver L, Claeys H, Wyseur A, Van Arnhem W, De Beenhouwer H, Uytendaele S, Beckers J, Matthijs D, Leroux-Roels G, Maertens G, De Paepe M. Hepatitis C virus in a hemodialysis unit: molecular evidence for nosocomial transmission. Kidney Int 1996; 49:889–895.

158. Pol S, Romeo R, Zins B. Hepatitis C virus RNA in anti-HCV positive hemodialysis patients: Significance and therapeutic implications. Kidney Int 1993; 44:1097–1100.

159. Chan TM, Lok ASF, Cheng IKP, Chan RT. Prevalence of hepatitis C virus infection in hemodialysis patients: a longitudinal study comparing the results of RNA and antibody assays. Hepatology 1993; 17:5–8.

160. Caramelo C, Bartolomé J, Albalate M, de Sequera P. Navas S, Bermejillo T, Oliva H, Marriott E, Ortiz A, Ruiz Tunon C, Casado S, Cerreno V. Undiagnosed hepatitis C virus infection in hemodialysis patients: value of HCV RNA and liver enzyme levels. Kidney Int 1996; 50:2027–2031.

161. Roobrouck A, Depraetere S, Couvent S, Van Kerschaver E, Maertens G, Leroux-Roels G. Prevalence of GBV-C/HGV and HCV in 4 hemodialysis units in Flanders (Belgium). Hepatology 1997; 26:591A.

162. Simon N, Courroucé A, Lemarrec N, Trépo C, Ducamp S. A twelve year natural history of hepatitis C virus infection in hemodialyzed patients. Kidney Int 1994; 46:504–511.

163. Caramelo C, Ortiz A, Aguilera B, Porres J, Navas S, Marriott E, Alberola M. Alamo C, Galera A, Garron M, Gonzales-Parra E, Fernandez de Gabriel M, Oliva H, Carreno V. Liver disease patterns in hemodialysis patients with antibodies to hepatitis C virus. Am J Kidney Dis 1993; 22:822–828.

164. Dussol B, Berthezene P, Brunet P, Roubicek C, Berland Y. Hepatitis C virus infection among chronic dialysis patients in the south of France: a collaborative study. Am J Kidney Dis 1995; 25:399–404.

165. Al-Wakeel J, Malik G, Al-Mohaya S, Mitwalli A, Baroudi F, El Gamal H, Kechrid M. Liver disease in dialysis patients with antibodies to hepatitis C virus. Nephrol Dial Transplant 1996; 11:2265–2268.

166. Valderrabano F, Jones E, Mallick N. Report on management of renal failure in Europe, XXIV, 1993. Nephrol Dial Transplant 1995; 10(suppl 5):1–25.

167. Valderrabano F, Berthoux F, Jones E, Mehs O. Report on management of renal failure in Europe, XXV, 1994. Nephrol Dial Transplant 1996; 11(suppl 1):2–21.

168. Huraib S, Al-Rashed R, Aldrees A, Aljefry M, Arif M, Al-Faleh F. High prevalence of and risk factors for hepatitis C in haemodialysis patients in Saudi Arabia: a need for new dialysis strategies. Nephrol Dial Transplant 1995; 10:470–474.

169. Pujol F, Ponce J, Lema M, Capriles F, Devesa M, Sirit F, Salazar M, Vasquez G, Monsalve F, Blitz-Dorfman L. High incidence of hepatitis C virus infection in hemodialysis patients in units with high prevalence. J Clin Microb 1996; 34:1633–1636.

170. Chen K, Lo S, Lee N, Leu M, Huang C, Fang K. Superinfection with hepatitis C virus in hemodialysis patients with hepatitis B surface antigenemia: its prevalence and clinical significance in Taiwan. Nephron 1996; 73:158–164.

171. Soetjipto, Handajani R, Lusida M, Darmadi S, Adi P, Soemarto, Ishido S, Katayama Y, Hotta H. Differential prevalence of hepatitis C virus subtypes in healthy blood donors, patients on maintenance hemodialysis, and patients with hepatocellular carcinoma in Surabaya, Indonesia. J Clin Microbiol 1996; 34:2875–2880.

172. Chan T, Lok A, Cheng I. Hepatitis C infection among dialysis patients: a comparison between patients on maintenance haemodialysis and continuous ambulatory peritoneal dialysis. Nephrol Dial Transplant 1991; 6:944–947.

173. Besso L, Rovere A, Peano G, Menardi G, Fenoglio M, Fenoglio S, Ghezzi P. Prevalence of HCV antibodies in a uraemic population undergoing maintenance dialysis therapy and in the staff members of the dialysis unit. Nephron 1992; 61:304–306.

174. Gladziwa U, Schlipköter U, Lorbeer B, Cholmakow K, Roggendorf M, Sieberth H. Prevalence of antibodies to hepatitis C virus in patients on peritoneal dialysis—a multicenter study. Clin Nephrol 1993; 40:46–52.

175. Barril G, Traver J. Spanish multicentre study group. Prevalence of hepatitis C virus in dialysis patients in Spain. Nephrol Dial Transplant 1995; 10(suppl 6):78–80.

176. Golan E, Korzets Z, Cristal-Lilov A, Ben-Tovim and J Bernheim. Increased prevalence of HCV antibodies in dialyzed Ashkenazi Jews-a possible ethnic predisposition. Nephrol Dial Transplant 1996; 11:684–686.

177. Gorriz J, Miguel A, Garcia-Ramon R, Perez-Contreras J, Olivares J, Gomez-Roldan C, Alvarino J, Lanuza

M. Prevalence and risk factors for hepatitis C virus infection in continuous ambulatory peritoneal dialysis patients. Nephrol Dial Transplant 1996; 11:1109–1112.

178. Huang C, Wu M, Lin D, Liaw Y. The prevalence of hepatitis C virus antibodies in patients treated with continuous ambulatory peritoneal dialysis. Perit Dial Int 1992; 12:31–33.

179. Ng Y, Lee S, Wu S, Liu W, Chia W, Huang T. The need for second-generation antihepatitis C virus testing in uremic patients on continuous ambulatory peritoneal dialysis. Perit Dial Int 1993; 13:132–135.

180. Jadoul M, El Akrout M, Cornu C, Van Ypersele de Strihou C. Prevalence of hepatitis C antibodies in health-care workers. Lancet 1994; 344:339.

181. Jankovic N, Cala S, Nadinic B, Varlay-Knobloch V, Pavlovic D. Hepatitis C and hepatitis B virus infection in hemodialysis patients and staff: a two year follow-up. Int J Artif Organs 1994; 17:137–140.

182. Niu M, Coleman P, Alter M. Multicenter study of hepatitis C virus infection in chronic hemodialysis patients and hemodialysis center staff members. Am J Kidney Dis 1993; 22:568–573.

183. Niu M, Alter M, Kristensen C, Margolis H. Outbreak of hemodialysis-associated non-A, non-B hepatitis and correlation with antibody to hepatitis C virus. Am J Kidney Dis 1992; 19:345–352.

184. Hardy N, Sandroni S, Danielson S, Wilson W. Antibody to hepatitis C increases with time on haemodialysis. Clin Nephrol 1992; 38:44–48.

185. Mondelli M, Cristina G, Piazza V, Cerino A, Villa G, Salvadeo A. High prevalence of antibodies to hepatitis C virus in hemodialysis units using a second generation assay. Nephron 1992; 61:350–351.

186. Oguchi H, Miyasaka M, Tokunaga S, Hora K, Ichikawa S, Ochi T, Yamada K, Nagasawa M, Kanno Y, Aizawa T, Watanabe H, Yoshizawa S, Sato K, Terashima M, Yoshie T, Ogushi S, Tanaka E, Kiyosawa K, Furuta S. Hepatitis virus infection (HBV and HCV) in eleven Japanese hemodialysis units. Clin Nephrol 1992; 38:36–43.

187. Cantu P, Mangano S, Masini M, Limido A, Crovetti G, DeFilippo C. Prevalence of antibodies against hepatitis C virus in a dialysis unit. Nephron 1992; 61: 337–338.

188. Jadoul M, Cornu C, Van Ypersele de Strihou C and the UCL collaborative group. Incidence and risk factors for hepatitis C seroconversion in hemodialysis: a prospective study. Kidney Int 1993; 44:1322–1326.

189. Knudsen F, Wantzin P, Rasmussen K, Ladefoged S, Lokkegaard N, Rasmussen L, Lassen A, Krogsgaard K. Hepatitis C in dialysis patients: relationship to blood transfusion, dialysis and liver disease, Kidney Int 1993; 43:1353–1356.

190. Zeuzem S, Scheuermann E, Waschk D, Lee J, Blaser C, Franke A, Roth K. Phylogenetic analysis of hepatitis C virus isolates from hemodialysis patients. Kidney Int 1996; 49:896–902.

191. Hayashi J, Nakashima K, Kajiyama W, Noguchi A, Morofuji M, Maeda Y, Kashiwagi S. Prevalence of antibody to hepatitis C virus in hemodialysis patients. Am J Epidemiol 1991; 134:651–657.

192. Moroni G, Cori P, Marelli F, Del Prete M, Padovese P, Gallieni M, Anelli A, Brancaccio D. Indirect evidence for transfusion role in conditioning hepatitis C virus. Prevalence among dialysis patients. Nephron 1991; 57:371–372.

193. Schlipköter U, Roggendorf M, Ernst G, Rasshofer R, Deinhardt F, Weise A, Gladziwa U, Luz N. Hepatitis C virus antibodies in haemodialysis patients. Lancet 1990; 335:1409.

194. Gilli P, Moretti M, Soffritti S, Menini C. Anti-HCV positive patient in dialysis units? Lancet 1990; 336: 243–244.

195. Elisaf M, Tsianos E, Mavridis A, Dardamanis M, Pappas M, Siamopoulos K. Antibodies against hepatitis C virus (anti-HCV) in haemodialysis patients: association with hepatitis B serologic markers. Nephrol Dial Transplant 1991; 6:476–479.

196. Muller G, Zabaleta M, Arminio A, Colmenares C, Capriles F, Bianco N, Machado I. Risk factors for dialysis-associated hepatitis C in Venezuela. Kidney Int 1992; 41:1055–1058.

197. Calabrese G, Vagelli G, Guaschino R, Gonella M. Transmission of anti-HCV within the household of haemodialysis patients. Lancet 1991; 338:1466.

198. Yamaguchi K, Nishimura Y, Fukuoka N, Machida J, Ueda S, Kusumoto Y, Futami G, Ishii T, Takatsuki K. Hepatitis C virus antibodies in haemodialysis patients. Lancet 1990; 335:1409–1410.

199. Medin C, Allander T, Roll M, Jacobson S, Grillner L. Seroconversion to hepatitis C virus in dialysis patients: a retrospective and prospective study. Nephron 1993; 65:40–45.

200. Lin D, Lin H, Huang C, Liaw Y. High incidence of hepatitis C virus infection in hemodialysis patients in Taiwan. Am J Kidney Dis 1993; 21:288–291.

201. Allander T, Medin C, Jacobson S, Grillner L, Persson M. Hepatitis C transmission in a hemodialysis unit: molecular evidence for spread of virus among patients not sharing equipment. J Med Virol 1994; 43:415–419.

202. Pinto dos Santos J, Loureiro A, Cendoroglo Neto M, Pereira B. Impact of dialysis room and reuse strategies on the incidence of hepatitis C virus infection in haemodialysis units. Nephrol Dial Transplant 1996; 11: 2017–2022.

203. Pru C, Cuervo C, Ardila M, Teran M. Hepatitis C transmission through dialysis machines. ASAIO 1994; 40:M889–M891.

204. Garcia-Valdecasas J, Bernal M, Cerezo S, Garcia F, Pereira B. Strategies to reduce the transmission of

HCV infection in hemodialysis units (abstr). J Am Soc Nephrol 1993; 4:347.

205. Fabrizi F, Lunghi G, Guarnori I, Raffaele L, Crepaldi M, Pagano A, Locatelli F. Incidence of seroconversion for hepatitis C virus in chronic haemodialysis patients: a prospective study. Nephrol Dial Transplant 1994; 9: 1611–1615.
206. Gilli P, Soffritti S, De Paoli Vitali E, Bedani P. Prevention of hepatitis C in dialysis units. Nephron 1995; 70:301–306.
207. Yuasa T, Ishikawa G, Manabe S, Sekigushi S, Takeuchi K, Miyamura T. The particle size of hepatitis C virus estimated by filtration through microporous regenerated cellulose fibre. J Gen Vir 1991; 72:2021–2024.
208. Caramelo C, Navas S, Alberola M, Bermejillo T, Reyero A, Carreno V. Evidence against transmission of hepatitis C virus through hemodialysis ultrafiltrate and peritoneal fluid. Nephron 1994; 66:470–473.
209. Hubmann R, Zazgornik J, Gabriel C, Garbeis B, Blauhut B. Hepatitis C virus-does it penetrate the haemodialysis membrane? PCR analysis of haemodialysis ultrafiltrate and whole blood. Nephrol Dial Transplant. 1995; 10:541–542.
210. Manzini P, Amore A, Brunetto M, Martina G, Verme G, Bonino F, Coppo R. Is hepatitis C virus RNA detectable in dialysis ultrafiltrate? Nephron 1996; 72; 102–103.
211. Sampietro M, Graziani G, Badalamenti S, Salvadori S, Caldarelli R, Como G, Fiorelli G. Detection of hepatitis C virus (HCV) in dialysate and in blood ultrafiltrate of HCV-positive patients. Nephron 1994; 68: 140.
212. Lombardi M. Cerrai T. Dattolo P, Pizzarelli F, Michelassi S, Maggiore Q, Zignego A. Is the dialysis membrane a safe barrier against HCV infection? Nephrol Dial Transplant 1995; 10:578–579.
213. Hung K, Chen W, Yang C, Lee S, Wu D. Hepatitis B and C in hemodialysis patients. Dial Transplant 1995; 24:135–139.
214. Moyer L, Alter M. Hepatitis C virus in the hemodialysis setting: a review with recommendations for control Semin. Dial 1994; 7:124–127.
215. Kiyosawa K, Sodeyama T, Tanaka E, Nakano Y, Furuta S, Nishioka K, Purcell R, Alter H. Hepatitis C in hospital employees with needlestick injuries. Ann Intern Med 1991; 115:367–369.
216. Mitsui T, Iwano K, Masuko K, Yamazaki C, Okamoto H, Tsuda F, Tanaka T, Mishiro S. Hepatitis C virus infection in medical personnel after needlestick accident. Hepatology 1992; 16:1109–1114.
217. Zuckerman J, Clewley G, Griffiths P, Cockroft A. Prevalence of hepatitis C antibodies in clinical healthcare workers. Lancet 1994; 343:1618–1620.
218. Okuda K, Hayashi H, Kobayashi S, Irie Y. Mode of hepatitis C infection not associated with blood transfusion among chronic hemodialysis patients. J Hepatology 1995; 23:28–31.
219. Gilli P, Moretti M, Soffritti S, Marchi N, Malacarne F, Bedani P, De Paoli Vitali E, Fiocchi O, Menini C. Non-A non-B hepatitis and anti-HCV antibodies in dialysis patients. Int J Artif Organs 1990; 13:737–741.
220. Jadoul M. Transmission routes of HCV infection in dialysis. Nephrol Dial Transplant 1996; 11(suppl 4): 36–38.
221. Goessens C, Jadoul M, Walon C, Burtonboy G. Cornu C. Hepatitis C virus genotypes in hemodialyzed patients: a multicentric study. Clin Nephrol 1997; 47: 367–371.
222. Blumberg A, Zehnder C, Burckhardt J. Prevention of hepatitis C infection in haemodialysis units. A prospective study. Nephrol Dial Transplant 1995; 10: 230–233.
223. Chiaramonte S, Tagger A, Ribero M, Grossi A, Milan M, La Greca G. Prevention of viral hepatitis in dialysis units: isolation and technical management of dialysis. Nephron 1992; 61:287–289.
224. Vagelli G, Calabrese G, Guaschino R, Gonella M. Effect of HCV+ patients isolation on HCV infection incidence in a dialysis unit. Nephrol Dial Transplant 1992; 7:1070.
225. Petrarulo F, Maggi P, Sacchetti A, Pallotta G, Dagostino F, Basile C. HCV infection occupational hazard at dialysis units and virus spread, among relatives of dialyzed patients. Nephron 1992; 61:302–303.
226. Hou C, Chen W, Kao J, Chen D, Yang Y, Chen J, Lee S, Wu D, Yang S. Intrafamilial transmission of hepatitis C virus in hemodialysis patients. J Med Virol 1995; 45:381–385.
227. Ippolito E, Aterini S, Salvadori M, D'Elia G, Amato M. HCV incidence in a dialysis center: preliminary reports. Nephron 1992; 61:375–376.
228. Galdziwa U, Schlipköter U. Evidence of hepatitis C virus infection in peritoneal fluid but not in dialysate and ultrafiltrate or hemofiltrate. Nephron 1995; 71:98.
229. Krautzig S, Tillmann H, Wrenger E, Manns M, Koch K, Brunkhorst R. Hepatitis C virus in peritoneal dialysis. Clin Nephrol 1994; 41:120.
230. Oshita M, Hayashi N, Kasahara H, Hagiwara H, Mita E, Naito M, Katayama K, Fusamoto H, Kamada T. Increased serum hepatitis C virus RNA levels among alcoholic patients with chronic hepatitis C. Hepatology 1994; 20:1115–1120.
231. Diego J, Roth D. When and how should dialysis patients with anti-hepatitis C antibodies be treated? Semin Dial 1997; 10:251–258.
232. Sakai Y, Izumi N, Tazawa J, Uchihara M, Akiba T, Marumo F, Sato C. Characteristics of anti-HCV antibody-positive patients with hepatocellular carcinoma on chronic hemodialysis: recommendation of periodic ultrasonography for early detection. Nephron 1996; 74:386–389.

233. Pereira B, Wright T, Schmid C, Levey A. The impact of pretransplantation hepatitis C infection on the outcome of renal transplantation. Transplantation 1995; 60:799–805.
234. Roth D, Zucker K, Cirocco R, DeMattos A, Burke G, Nery J, Esquenazi V, Babischkin S, Miller J. The impact of hepatitis C virus infection on renal allograft recipients. Kidney Int 1994; 45:238–244.
235. Stempel C, Lake J, Kuo G, Vincenti F. Hepatitis C-Its prevalence in end-stage renal failure patients and clinical course after kidney transplantation. Transplantation 1993; 55:273–276.
236. Ponz E, Campistol J, Bruguera M, Barrera J, Gil C, Pinto J, Andreu J. Hepatitis C virus infection among kidney transplant recipients. Kidney Int 1991; 40: 748–751.
237. Knoll G, Tankersley M, Lee J, Julian B, Curtis J. The impact of renal transplantation on survival in hepatitis C-positive end-stage renal disease patients. Am J Kidney Dis 1997; 29:608–614.
238. Berg T, Naumann U, Fukumoto T, Bechstein W, Neuhaus P, Lobeck H, Höhne M, Schreier E, Hopf U. GB virus C infection in patients with chronic hepatitis Band C before and after liver transplantation. Transplantation 1996; 62:711–714.
239. Dawson G, Schlauder G, Pilot-Matias T, Thiele D, Leary T, Murphy P, Rosenblatt J, Simons J, Martinson F, Gutierrez R, Lentino J, Pachucki C, Muerhoff A, Widell A, Tegtmeier G, Desai S, Mushahwar I. Prevalence studies of GB virus-C infection using reverse transcriptase-polymerase chain reaction. J Med Virol 1996; 50:97–103.
240. Alter M, Gallagher M, Morris T, Moyer L, Meeks E, Krawczynski K, Kim J. Margolis H. Acute non-A-E hepatitis in the United States and the role of hepatitis G virus infection. N Engl J Med 1997; 336:741–746.
241. Sheng L, Widyastuti A, Kosala H, Donck J, Van Renterghem Y, Setijoso E, Soumillion A, Verslype C, Schelstraete R, Emonds M, Hess G, Yap S. High prevalence of hepatitis G virus infection compared with hepatitis C virus infection in patients undergoing chronic hemodialysis. Am J Kidney Dis 1998; 31: 218–223.
242. de Lamballerie X, Charrel R, Dussol B. Hepatitis GB virus-C in patients on hemodialysis. Lancet 1996; 334: 195–196.
243. Nubling C, Billeck H, Fursch A, Scharrer I, Schramm W, Seifreid E, Schmidt U, Staszewki S, Lower J. Frequencies of GB virus C/hepatitis G virus genomes and of the specific antibodies in German risk and non-risk populations. J Med Virol 1997; 53:218–224.

39

Complications of Dialysis in Diabetic Patients

Anne Marie Miles and Eli A. Friedman
SUNY Health Science Center at Brooklyn, Brooklyn, New York

I. INTRODUCTION

Diabetic dialysis patients comprise the largest subgroup of patients in end-stage renal disease treatment programs in developed countries and are unfortunately also subject to greater morbidity and mortality when compared to nondiabetic dialysis patients (1). Older age at the time of dialysis initiation and the presence of often advanced multisystem, micro- and macrovascular disease account for this excess rate of complications and death on dialysis. The management of diabetic dialysis patients requires an aggressive, preemptive, multidisciplinary, and patient education–oriented approach, which must often be led by the nephrologist, who has most frequent contact with the patient. Peripheral vascular, cardiovascular, and cerebrovascular disease, retinopathy, gastropathy, and dialysis-associated complications are the major contributors to co-morbidity in diabetic dialysis patients (2), and this review will address the latter group of complications (Table 1).

II. HEMODIALYSIS-RELATED COMPLICATIONS IN DIABETIC DIALYSIS PATIENTS

A. Hypotension

Intradialytic hypotension occurs with 20% greater frequency in diabetics compared to nondiabetics (3). Dialysis-associated hypotension is often heralded by nausea and vomiting and may occur despite obvious clinical volume overload and edema, hence limiting fluid removal during dialysis. Recurrent intradialytic hypotension in diabetics may also contribute to underdialysis (4) by reducing clearance through reductions in blood flow rate or early termination of dialysis. The etiology of intradialytic hypotension in diabetics is often multifactorial. Reduced left ventricular systolic ejection fraction associated with atherosclerotic coronary artery disease (5) is a major contributor and may produce hypotension soon after initiation of dialysis as the volume of blood within the extracorporeal circuit depletes intravascular volume and further compromises a marginal cardiac output. Angina pectoris and acute myocardial infarction may occur as a consequence of or be a contributory factor to hypotension in this setting. In patients with inoperable coronary artery disease and dialysis-precipitated angina, maintaining the hematocrit level above 30%, nasal oxygen during dialysis, and topical or sublingual nitroglycerin given just prior to dialysis are useful in preventing attacks of intradialytic angina.

Diastolic dysfunction related to diabetic cardiomyopathy with resultant decreased left ventricular compliance and filling (6) can also contribute to reduced cardiac output and intradialytic hypotension in diabetics.

Diabetic autonomic neuropathy may produce postural or persistent hypotension, which is exacerbated during dialysis. Autonomic neuropathy results in abolition of the reflex increase in heart rate and increased peripheral vascular resistance, which usually prevent hypotension before interstitial fluid is mobilized into the intravascular compartment.

Table 1 Dialysis-Associated Complications in Diabetic Patients

Hemodialysis-associated complications
Intradialytic hypotension
Hypertension
High interdialytic weight gain
Vascular access-related complications
Access thrombosis
Vascular steal syndrome
Ischemic monomelic neuropathy
Venous hypertension
Bone disease
Diabetic retinopathy
Malnutrition
Hyperglycemia
Peritoneal dialysis-associated complications
Peritonitis
Underdialysis
Malnutrition
Hyperglycemia

Table 2 Management Strategies for Intradialytic Hypotension in Diabetics

Bicarbonate dialysate
High-sodium (140–145 mmol/L) dialysate with linear sodium modeling
Slow rate of ultrafiltration
Sequential ultrafiltration (if grossly edematous)
Prime dialysis circuit with hypertonic albumin
Maintain hematocrit at or above 30 vol% with erythropoietin
No antihypertensive medications on morning of dialysis
Restrict meals immediately before or during hemodialysis
Leg toning exercises to improve venous return
Decrease dialysate temperature (particularly near end of dialysis)
Medications: α-agonists (e.g., midodrine, fludrocortisone)

Anemia contributes to intradialytic hypotension by reducing blood viscosity and peripheral vascular resistance and impairing the ability to maintain blood volume during ultrafiltration (7). Anemia may produce dialysis-related angina pectoris and a recent fall in hematocrit should always be sought in the diabetic patient who develops new onset or worsening angina.

Diabetics who are nephrotic or malnourished are hypoalbuminemic, and the resultant low colloid oncotic pressure reduces the plasma refilling rate and also contributes to hypotension (7).

A slight build-up of core heat during hemodialysis, in association with a reduction in heat loss caused by cutaneous vasoconstriction in response to hypovolemia early in dialysis, may result in reflex vasodilation of the cutaneous blood vessels near the end of dialysis and cause sudden hypotension. This theory of thermal amplification has been proposed by Gotch et al. (8). Reducing dialysate temperature by 2–3 degrees during the last hour of dialysis may prevent or ameliorate hypotension occurring on this basis.

Approaches to managing dialysis-related hypotension are listed in Table 2. In some cases, recurrent hypotension on hemodialysis may be severe enough to require change to peritoneal dialysis.

B. Hypertension

Hypertension is more common in diabetic than nondiabetic hemodialysis patients and is a major contributor to death from cardiovascular disease. Fifty percent of hemodialyzed diabetics require antihypertensive medications compared with 27.7% of nondiabetics (6). Although hypertension is largely volume dependent in most diabetics, improves as a hemodialysis session proceeds, and ameliorates or disappears as dry weight is attained, some patients continue to require antihypertensive medications after initiation of hemodialysis, and some may, in addition, experience progressive elevation in blood pressure during hemodialysis sessions or at the end of treatment. Exacerbated hypertension during dialysis in some hemodialysis patients may be due to acute activation of the renin-angiotensin system by reduction in intravascular volume produced by ultrafiltration (9). Use of angiotensin-converting enzyme inhibitors as part of an antihypertensive regimen or at the start of or during dialysis usually controls this problem. Calcium channel blockers and central vasodilators such as clonidine are recommended for treatment of hypertension in diabetic dialysis patients. In those with recalcitrant hypertension, it may be necessary to add minoxidil for blood pressure control. Unless indicated for cardiac reasons, β-blockers should be avoided in diabetics because they exacerbate hypertriglyceridemia, worsen glucose control, and can mask symptoms of severe hypoglycemia.

C. High Interdialytic Weight Gain

Diabetics gain 30–50% more weight in interdialytic periods than nondiabetics, and while in an early study weight gain did not correlate with glycemic control, age, duration of ESRD, continuing urine output, dry weight, or duration of diabetes (6), correlation between degree of hyperglycemia and amount of interdialytic weight gain was reported in a later study (10). In many patients, noncompliance with sodium and water restrictions contributes to large increments in weight (>5–10 lb) between dialysis sessions. High intracellular sodium content in diabetic patients, producing increased thirst, is one proposed mechanism for excessive weight gain between dialyses (11).

Volume overload worsens hypertension and contributes to cardiovascular morbidity and mortality in diabetics. The estimated dry weight of hemodialysis patients should be challenged progressively until normotension or near normotension is attained. This goal may be hindered, however, by painful muscle cramps and intradialytic hypotension. Intensive dietary counseling and improved glycemic control may help to reduce interdialytic weight gain. Intradialytic cramps are helped by intravenous boluses of hypertonic saline or sodium bicarbonate. In nondiabetic patients, 50% dextrose water may also be used to abrogate muscle cramps. Oral quinine sulfate 260 mg (Quinamm, Marion Merrell Dow Inc., Kansas City, MO) 1–2 tablets taken 30–60 minutes before dialysis and increasing dialysis time to enable slower ultrafiltration also ameliorate the problem of dialysis-related cramps.

D. Vascular Access

Problems related to vascular access are particularly prevalent and severe in diabetic patients, and an experienced vascular access surgeon is an invaluable asset in the management of diabetic hemodialysis patients. Advanced peripheral vascular disease related to medial arterial calcinosis and older age combined with destruction of veins due to previous intravenous cannulation or injections often preclude creation of an endogenous Brescia-Cimino fistula in diabetic patients or result in maturation failure of the fistula, if created. In addition, most predialytic diabetics (64%) are not told to avoid venepunctures or intravenous cannula placement in either arm in order to protect the veins for permanent dialysis access (12). Hence, most diabetic patients on hemodialysis have a synthetic, usually polytetrafluoroethylene (PTFE), graft. In a review of diabetic hemodialysis patients above 65 years of age hospitalized for failed vascular access between January 1, 1987, and December 31, 1991, at Kings County Hospital, Brooklyn, New York, only 1 of 40 (2%) diabetic patients had a fistula compared to 5 of 48 (10%) nondiabetic hemodialysis patients in the same age group hospitalized during the same time period for failed vascular access (13) Ninety-five percent of diabetics had an upper arm anteriovenous graft. Despite the risk of failure, whenever possible creation of an endogenous fistula should be first attempted in diabetic patients.

E. Access Thrombosis

Thrombosis of arteriovenous accesses is most often due to venous outflow stenosis occurring just distal to the venous anastomosis where the jet of blood shunted across the access impinges on the wall and produces intimal hyperplasia (14). Coexistent infection of the access may be present in the absence of local signs of infection and may result in overwhelming sepsis if not diagnosed early; hence, thrombectomy or revision of the graft should ideally be performed within 24–48 hours. Whether diabetic patients have an increased propensity to thrombose their vascular accesses is controversial. In vitro evidence indicates that diabetic platelets tend to aggregate more easily (15) and to produce higher levels of thromboxane B_2 (16), and in addition, increased levels of von Willebrand factor have been found in diabetic sera (11). The 1991 report of the USRDS implicated diabetes as a risk factor for arteriovenous access thrombosis: diabetic hemodialysis patients underwent 0.42 hospitalizations per years at risk for vascular access complications compared to 0.35 hospitalizations per years at risk for nondiabetics (1). National statistics in 1993 indicated that diabetic hemodialysis patients had more frequent and more prolonged hospitalizations than nondiabetics (17). Recent evidence refutes diabetes as a specific risk factor in access thrombosis, however. An analysis of 784 incident hemodialysis patients enrolled in the USRDS Case Mix Adequacy Study in 1990 (a systematic sample of patients from 523 hemodialysis units across the United States) (18) revealed that of 245 hemodialysis patients with an endogenous fistula, 71 (29%) were diabetic, while of 539 patients with a graft, 219 (41%) were diabetic. Hence three times as many grafts as fistulae were placed in diabetic patients. One-year survival rates for arteriovenous fistulae versus grafts were 70% versus 47% in this study, and although initial evaluation suggested an increased tendency for access failure in diabetics, on Cox's proportional hazard analysis, diabetes was not an independent predictor of access failure, the only such factor being peripheral vascular disease. It is likely, therefore, that the grater number of synthetic grafts placed in diabetic patients, with their associated higher failure rate, accounts for the apparent predisposition of diabetic patients to access thrombosis in earlier reports.

F. Vascular Steal Syndromes

An arteriovenous access (particularly a brachiocephalic access or a side-to-side radiocephalic fistula) creates a low-pressure run-off system, which may short-circuit blood from the palmar arch and ulnar arteries to such a degree that a steal syndrome results. With the preexisting, severe medial arterial calcinosis of the ulnar and digital arteries, which is common in diabetic dialysis patients (19), progressive ischemic pain leading to dry gangrene of one or more fingers may develop days to weeks after placement of the access. Nonhealing wounds of the fingers may also be a manifestation of vascular steal (20), and in cases of clinical uncertainty, digital pressures of <50 mmHg on noninvasive vascular studies and arteriography help to confirm the diagnosis. In severe cases of arterial steal syndromes, the onset may be more acute, within hours of creation of the access, and signs of acute arterial insufficiency such as pallor and pulselessness may be seen. Ligation of the distal limb of the radial artery in a side-to-side radiocephalic fistula or ligation or removal of a brachiocephalic access is necessary to correct the syndrome. Amputation of one or more digits and even below elbow amputation may sometimes be necessary.

G. Ischemic Monomelic Neuropathy

The term ischemic monomelic neuropathy was coined in 1983 by Wilbourn (21). It is a complication of vascular access seen almost exclusively in diabetic patients (22) and refers to the development of acute pain, weakness, and paralysis of the muscles of the forearm and hand, often with sensory loss, developing immediately after placement of an arteriovenous access, usually in the brachiocephalic or antecubital location. The condition results from diversion of the blood supply to the nerves of the forearm and hand, the ischemic insult being severe enough to damage nerve fibers but insufficient to produce necrosis of other tissues. Hence, unlike in vascular steal syndromes, the radial pulse is usually present, digital pressures normal or only mildly decreased, and necrosis, ulcers, and gangrene of the digits are absent. The propensity to development of the complication with brachiocephalic accesses relates to the fact that the brachial artery constitutes the sole arterial inflow to the forearm and hand and, in the absence of collateral vessels about the elbow, diversion of all or most brachial arterial blood through a fistula or graft results in distal ischemia. Nerve conduction studies are helpful in diagnosing the syndrome, and early access removal or ligation is necessary to prevent permanent paralysis of the hand. Unfortunately, even with prompt access closure, paralysis of the hand may be permanent.

H. Venous Hypertension

Chronic swelling of the hand, and especially of the thumb ("sore thumb" syndrome), related to the presence of the distal segment of the vein used for creation of the access, may occur in both diabetic and nondiabetic patients. Venous hypertension occurs in association with venous stenosis of the access or a more proximal stenosis at the level of the subclavian vein, which may have been previously catheterized for temporary vascular access. Ligature of the distal venous limb of the fistula or graft will usually correct the problem.

III. BONE DISEASE

Adynamic bone disease is a form of renal osteodystrophy commonly seen in diabetics, particularly those on peritoneal dialysis (23). It is characterized by low rates of bone turnover without excess unmineralized osteoid and is associated with parathyroid hormone levels below 100 pg/mL. Decreased osteoblast proliferation and defective mineralization contribute to a low rate of bone formation in diabetic rats (24), and a similar mechanism may underlie adynamic bone disease in humans. Diabetic dialysis patients also tend to experience higher rates of low-turnover bone disease associated with aluminum deposition: reduced bone formation may allow time for enhanced deposition of aluminum on the ossification front, and within 1 year of hemodialysis, aluminum deposition (usually related to use of aluminum-containing phosphate binders) is observed on bone surfaces in diabetics, and symptoms of bone pain and fractures related to aluminum bone disease may start as early as 2 years after initiation of hemodialysis (25). Aluminum bone disease may also be unmasked or accelerated after parathyroidectomy. Aluminum-containing phosphate binders should therefore be avoided in diabetics, and all diabetics with bone pain and/or fractures should have plasma aluminum levels measured before and after a single infusion of desferrioxamine. Aluminum-associated bone disease in hemodialyzed diabetics responds to a regimen of vitamin D, calcium, and desferrioxamine.

IV. DIABETIC RETINOPATHY

Visual loss in diabetic ESRD patients is most commonly related to proliferative retinopathy with associated vitreous hemorrhage and retinal detachment but may also result from macular edema, glaucoma, cataracts, and corneal disease. The presence of proliferative retinopathy is correlated with age of onset and duration of diabetes, glycemic control, and degree of blood pressure control. Heparin use during hemodialysis is no longer considered a significant contributor to progression of diabetic retinopathy or to intraocular hemorrhage. No reports definitively link heparin use on dialysis with progression of diabetic retinopathy or visual loss. Indeed, in a study of 112 diabetics followed for 20 months, progression of retinopathy was shown to be independent of dialysis modality (hemo- or peritoneal dialysis), while the significant correlation between blood pressure control and vision preservation was reinforced (26). In addition, because of the rarity (0.05%) of intraocular hemorrhage in diabetics treated with thrombolytic agents, diabetic retinopathy is not considered a contraindication to thrombolytic therapy for acute myocardial infarction (27). Focal or panretinal laser photocoagulation can reduce the incidence of serious visual loss in patients with proliferative retinopathy, and vitrectomy may restore vision in patients with vitreous hemorrhage.

V. UNDERNUTRITION

Malnutrition is frequently seen in diabetic hemodialysis patients, particularly in the presence of intercurrent illnesses. Causes of malnutrition in diabetics on hemodialysis include (a) poor glycemic control leading to gluconeogenesis and catabolism of muscle, (b) gastroparesis leading to nausea and vomiting, (c) diabetic diarrhea, and (d) underdialysis related to difficulties with vascular access or to repeated early termination of dialysis sessions caused by recurrent hypotension (28). A diet of 25–30 kcal/kg/day, with 50% of the calories coming from complex carbohydrates, and protein content of 1.3–1.5 g/kg/day is recommended for hemodialyzed diabetics. In diabetic hemodialysis patients who develop intercurrent illnesses (e.g., sepsis), early and intensive nutritional support with enteral or peripheral parenteral nutrition is necessary. Dialysate fluid should contain at least 200 mg/dL glucose because use of glucose-free dialysate results in rapid glucose loss, hypoglycemia, and production of acute starvation with acidosis and hyperkalemia (29).

VI. HYPERGLYCEMIA

Insulin requirements after beginning maintenance hemodialysis vary (30), and it is important to teach patients home glucose monitoring so as to determine changing insulin requirements. Most diabetic patients with ESRD experience reduction in insulin needs due to decreased renal excretion and catabolism of injected and endogenous insulin. Many diabetics who start dialysis will no longer need insulin, and some type 2 diabetics previously on insulin may achieve glycemic control with a small dose of a short-acting sulfonylurea drug such as glyburide or glipizide, or indeed with no hypoglycemic medications at all. The new oral hypoglycemic agent troglitazone has been approved for use in type 2 diabetics to decrease insulin requirements or for use alone or in combination with a sulfonylurea to prevent need for insulin therapy. The drug works by increasing the sensitivity of peripheral tissues to insulin and decreasing hepatic glucose production. It undergoes hepatic metabolism and hence does not require dose reduction in renal failure. It is effective in only 50% of treated patients, however, and produces mild liver injury in 1.9% of patients and sporadic cases of fulminant hepatic failure requiring liver transplantation. Liver function tests should be monitored at the start of therapy with troglitazone and at monthly intervals for the first 6 months of therapy, and then every 2 months for the remainder of the first year. Rosiglitazone appears to be a safer option with equivalent efficacy.

With control of uremia by dialysis, improved appetite and weight gain in some diabetics may result in increased insulin needs. In addition, noncompliance with hypoglycemic medications related to depression in the often stormy period surrounding dialysis initiation may contribute to hyperglycemia. Hyperosmolar coma is uncommon in diabetics on dialysis unless there is significant residual renal function. Ketoacidosis is also not frequently seen but may occur in association with sepsis or other severe intercurrent illness. Both conditions are managed by low-dose hourly regular insulin infusions for blood sugar levels above 450–500 mg/dL. It is usually possible to achieve rapid control of blood sugar, and indeed in some patients an initial single dose of 10 units of regular insulin may suffice if the patient is not seriously ill. The usual fluid replenishment regimens for nonuremic diabetics are of course not required unless the patient is in shock. Usually, fluid replacement during hemodialysis suffices.

VII. COMPLICATIONS OF PERITONEAL DIALYSIS IN DIABETIC PATIENTS

Eleven percent of diabetics entering renal replacement programs in the United States are treated with some form of peritoneal dialysis (2). In other countries such as Canada, the percentage of diabetic ESRD patients treated by peritoneal dialysis (PD) is much higher, indeed, PD is the treatment of choice for diabetics with ESRD in these countries. Physician bias, national resources, patient preference, and the presence of severe cardiovascular disease are the major factors that determine the selection of PD over hemodialysis in diabetics. The more gentle ultrafiltration afforded by CAPD will prevent or ameliorate hypotension in diabetics so prone because of left ventricular dysfunction or autonomic neuropathy.

Diabetic hemodialysis patients younger than 60 years have a similar or lower relative risk of death than diabetics of the same age on CAPD (31,32). In diabetic CAPD patients older than 60 years, there is a 19% higher relative risk of death compared with diabetic hemodialysis patients (26). The higher death rate in elderly diabetics treated with CAPD is related to advanced atherosclerotic cardiovascular and cerebrovascular disease. Diabetics are subject to a similar spectrum and rate of technique-related complications as in nondiabetics on CAPD, and a discussion of some of the most common problems of diabetics on PD follows.

A. Peritonitis

Within the first year of starting PD, 49% of patients will switch to another modality of renal replacement therapy (33), while only 37% of hemodialysis patients change treatment modality during the first year. It is more likely that a CAPD or continuous cyclic PD (CCPD) patient will switch to hemodialysis (15.6%) than that a hemodialysis patient will switch to CAPD (4.4%) (34). The high technique failure rate on CAPD is due mainly to peritonitis (35). Recurrent peritonitis, usually caused by *Staphylococcus epidermidis* or *Staphylococcus aureus*, often in association with exit site infections, is the major disadvantage of CAPD. Peritonitis in diabetic CAPD patients occurs at a rate of one episode per 11–21 patients per month (26,29,36). Diabetics on CAPD need twice the number of hospitalization days as nondiabetic CAPD patients (37), and peritonitis accounts for 30–50% of the hospitalization days (38). Fungal peritonitis is seen more commonly in diabetic than in nondiabetic CAPD patients and usually requires removal of the peritoneal catheter. There is, however, no overall increased risk of peritonitis in diabetics over nondiabetics (39), and the rates of catheter replacement are the same in both groups.

Because of delayed wound healing, dialysate leakage and exit site infections may occur in diabetics if a newly implanted Tenchoff catheter is used too early; and we recommend that, if possible, at least 2–3 weeks elapse before starting regular CAPD exchanges through a newly implanted Tenchoff catheter in a diabetic. Alternatively, starting nighttime cycling exchanges 1–2 weeks after catheter insertion and leaving the abdomen dry during the daytime to reduce intra-abdominal pressure during ambulation may reduce the risk of dialysate leakage. The Moncrief-Popovich peritoneal catheter is a recently introduced double-cuffed catheter with an external cuff, which is longer than that of the standard Tenchoff catheter, and whose external segment (external cuff and tubing) is buried subcutaneously for 4–6 weeks before being externalized and used (40). Because tissue ingrowth into the external cuff has occurred during the period of subcutaneous implantation, it is anticipated that the rates of leaks and peritonitis will be less with this catheter, and indeed we have had excellent results, with no dialysate leaks so far with this catheter.

B. Underdialysis

Patients on CAPD tend to have higher levels of blood urea nitrogen and creatinine than hemodialysis patients, and there is concern about the adequacy of CAPD as long-term uremia therapy (41). Based on peritoneal equilibration testing, a minimum clearance of 6–7 L/day is recommended for patients on peritoneal dialysis. The amount of dialysis delivered on CAPD may have to be increased with time as residual renal function is lost, and peritoneal clearance decreases owing to advanced vascular disease or recurrent episodes of peritonitis. Microangiopathy and increased vascular permeability to small and large molecules and resultant increased diffusive transport of glucose (42) may produce type I ultrafiltration failure in some diabetic patients.

C. Undernutrition

Malnutrition may occur in up to 40% of long-term CAPD patients (43,44). Malnutrition in CAPD-treated diabetics may occur because of (a) reduced appetite caused by the large glucose load in dialysate or by early satiety from increased intra-abdominal pressure or (b) large protein losses (8–10 g/day) in the dialysate effluent that may lower serum albumin and total protein levels (45). Loss of protein through the peritoneal membrane is increased during episodes of peritonitis and may worsen with time because of a generalized increase in permeability related to diabetic microangiopathy involving the peritoneal vessels or nausea and vomiting related to diabetic gastroparesis. To maintain adequate nutrition, CAPD patients should ingest at least 1.5 g protein/kg/day and between 130 and 150 g carbohydrates/day.

D. Hyperglycemia

Blood glucose control may sometimes be difficult in diabetics on CAPD because of the absorption of a mean of 182 ± 61 g glucose/day from the peritoneal cavity (46). A combination of subcutaneous and intraperitoneal insulin administration usually results in adequate glucose control, however. The total dose of intraperitoneal regular insulin required is usually two to three times the usual subcutaneous total dose. Oral antidiabetic agents (sulfonylureas with short half-lives and hepatic metabolism, e.g., glipizide, glyburide) to reduce the risk of prolonged hypoglycemia may be used in patients requiring less than 20–25 units of insulin per day.

VIII. SUMMARY

Diabetic dialysis patients require extra effort on the part of nephrologists to prevent and treat macro- and microvascular disease, to manage intradialytic complications, and to achieve the usually difficult goal of maintaining good vascular access. A multidisciplinary team approach is required, and the services of an experienced vascular access surgeon are invaluable. As the epidemic of type 2 diabetes mellitus afflicting developed countries continues and diabetics comprise an increasing percentage of incident and prevalent ESRD patients, nephrologists must target the problems peculiar to, or prevalent in the diabetic dialysis population in order to reduce morbidity and mortality in this high-risk group.

REFERENCES

1. U.S. Renal Data System, USRDS 1997 Annual Data Report. Bethesda, MD: National Institutes of Health, National Institute of Diabetes and Digestive and Kidney Diseases, 1991.
2. Miles AMV, Friedman EA. Managing co-morbid disorders in the uremic diabetic patient. Sem Dial 1997; 10:225–230.
3. Shideman JR, Buselmeier TJ, Kjellstrand CM. Hemodialysis in diabetics. Arch Intern Med 1976; 136:1126–1130.
4. Collins AL, Liao A, Umen A, Hanson G, Keshaviah P. Diabetic hemodialysis patients treated with a high Kt/V have a lower risk of death than standard Kt/V. J Am Soc Nephrol 1991; 2:318.
5. Nakamoto M. The mechanism of intradialytic hypotension in diabetic patients. Nippon Jinzo Gakkai Shi. Jap J Nephrol 1994; 36:374–381.
6. Ritz E, Strumpf C, Katz F, et al. Hypertension and cardiovascular risk factors in hemodialyzed diabetic patients. Hypertension 1985; 7(suppl II):118–124.
7. Daugirdas JT. Dialysis hypotension: A hemodynamic analysis. Kidney Int 1991; 39:223–246.
8. Gotch FA, Keen ML, Yarian SR. An analysis of thermal regulation in hemodialysis with one and three compartment models. Trans Am Soc Artif Intern Organs 1989; 35:622–624.
9. Dorhout Mees EJ. Rise in blood pressure during hemodialysis ultrafiltration: a paradoxical situation? Int J Artificial Organs 1996; 19:569–570.
10. Ifudu O, Dulin A, Lundin AP, et al. Diabetics manifest excess weight gain on maintenance hemodialysis. Am Soc Artif Intern Org 1992; 21:85.
11. Jones R, Poston R, Hinestrota A, et al. Weight gain between dialysis in diabetics. Possible significance of raised intracellular sodium content. Br Med J 1980; 1: 153–154.
12. U.S. Renal Data System. USRDS 1997 Annual Data Report. Bethesda, MD: National Institutes of Health, National Institute of Diabetes and Digestive and Kidney Diseases, 1997.
13. Miles AMV, Hong JH, Sumrani N, et al. Outcome and complications of vascular access placement in elderly diabetic patients with end stage renal disease. J Korean Am Med Assoc 1996; 2:25–28.
14. Taber TE, Maikranz PS, Haag BW, et al. Maintenance of adequate hemodialysis access. Prevention of neointimal hyperplasia. ASAIO J 1995; 41:842–846.
15. Gensini GF, Abbate R, Favilla S, Neri Serneri GC. Changes of platelet function and blood clotting in diabetes mellitus. Thromb Hemost 1979; 42:983–993.
16. Halushka PV. Increased platelet thromboxane. J Lab Clin Med 1981; 97:87–92.
17. U.S. Renal Data System. USRDS 1993 Annual Data Report. Bethesda, MD: National Institutes of Health.

National Institute of Diabetes and Digestive and Kidney Diseases, 1993.
18. Woods JD, Turenne MN, Strawderman RL, et al. Vascular access survival among incident hemodialysis patients in the United States. Am J Kidney Dis 1997; 30: 50–57.
19. Tzamaloukas AH, Murata GH, Harford AM, et al. Hand gangrene in diabetic patients on chronic dialysis. Trans Am Soc Artif Intern Organs 1991; 37:638–643.
20. Redfern AB, Zimmerman NB. Neurologic and ischemic complications of upper extremity vascular access for dialysis. J Hand Surg 1995; 20:199–204.
21. Wilbourn AJ, Furlan AJ, Hulley W, Ruschhaupt W. Ischemic monomelic neuropathy. Neurology 1983; 33: 447–451.
22. Riggs JE, Moss AH, Labosky DA, Liput JH, et al. Upper extremity ischemic monomelic neuropathy: a complication of vascular access procedures in uremic diabetic patients. Neurology 1989; 39:997–998.
23. Vincenti F, Arnaud SB, Recker R, et al. Parathyroid and bone response of the diabetic patient to uremia. Kidney Int 1984; 25:677–682.
24. Weiss RE, Reddi AH. Influence of experimental diabetes and insulin on matrix-induced cartilage and bone differentiation. Am J Physiol 1980, 238:E200–E207.
25. Andress DL, Kopp JB, Maloney NA, et al. Early deposition of aluminum in bone in diabetic patients on hemodialysis. N Engl J Med 1987; 316:292–296.
26. Diaz-Buxo JA, Burgess WP, Greenman M, et al. Visual function in diabetic patients undergoing dialysis: comparison of peritoneal had hemodialysis. Int J Artificial Organs 1984; 7:257–262.
27. Mahaffey KW, Granger CB, Toth CA, et al. Diabetic retinopathy should not be a contraindication to thrombolytic therapy for acute myocardial infarction: review of ocular hemorrhage incidence and location in the GUSTO-I trial. J Am Coll Cardiol 1997; 30:1606–1610.
28. Cheigh J, Raghavan J, Sullivan J, et al. Is insufficient dialysis a cause for high morbidity in diabetic patients. J Am Soc Nephrol 1991; 2:317.
29. Davis M, Comty C, Shapiro F. Dietary management of patients with diabetes treated by hemodialysis. J Am Diet Assoc 1979; 75:265–269.
30. Davis M, Comty C, Shapiro F. Dietary management of patients with diabetes treated by hemodialysis. J Am Diet Assoc 1979; 75:265–269.
31. Maiorca R, Vonesh EF, Cavalli PL, et al. A multicenter, selection-adjusted comparison of patient and technique survivals on CAPD and hemodialysis. Perit Dial Int 1991; 11:118–127.
32. Gokal R, Jakubowski C, Hunt L. Multicenter study of outcome of CAPD and hemodialysis patients. Nephrol Dial Transplant 1986; 1:111–114.
33. Held PJ, Port FK, Blagg CR, et al. The United States renal data systems annual data report. Am J Kidney Dis 1990; 16(suppl 2):34–43.
34. Yuan ZY, Balaskas E, Gupta A, et al. Is CAPD or hemodialysis better for diabetic patients? CAPD is more advantageous. Semin Dialysis 1992; 5:181–188.
35. Nolph KD. Continuous ambulatory peritoneal dialysis as long term treatment for end stage renal disease. Am J Kidney Dis 1991; 17:154–157.
36. Scarpioni LL, Balocchi S, Castelli A, et al. Continuous ambulatory peritoneal dialysis in diabetic patients. Contrib Nephrol 1990; 84:50–74.
37. Khanna R, Oreopoulos DG. Continuous ambulatory peritoneal dialysis in diabetics with end stage renal disease. A combined experience of 2 North American centers. In: Friedman EA, L'Esperance FA, eds. Diabetic Renal Retinal Syndrome. New York: Grune and Stratton, 1986; 363–381.
38. Rottemburg J. Peritoneal dialysis in diabetics. In: Nolph KD, ed. Peritoneal Dialysis. Boston: Martinus Nijhoff, 1985:365–379.
39. Rubin J, Oreopoulos DG, Blair RDG, et al. Chronic peritoneal dialysis in the management of diabetics with terminal renal failure. Nephron 1977; 19:265–270.
40. Moncrief JW et al. The Moncrief-Popovich catheter. A new peritoneal access technique for patients on peritoneal dialysis. ASAIO J 1993; 39:62.
41. Diaz-Buxo JA. Is continuous ambulatory peritoneal dialysis adequate long-term therapy for end-stage renal disease? A critical assessment. J Am Soc Nephrol 1992; 3:1039–1048.
42. Lin JJ, Wadhwa NK, Suh H, et al. Increased peritoneal solute transport in diabetic peritoneal dialysis patients. Adv Peritoneal Dial 1995; 11:63–66.
43. Young GA, Kopple JD, Lindholm B, et al. Nutritional assessment of chronic ambulatory peritoneal dialysis patients: an international study. Am J Kidney Dis 1991; 17:462–471.
44. Rotellar C, Black J, Winchester JF, et al. Ten years experience with continuous ambulatory peritoneal dialysis. Am J Kidney Dis 1991; 17:158–164.
45. Blumenkrantz MJ, Gahl GM, Kopple JD, et al. Protein losses during peritoneal dialysis. Kidney Int 1981; 19: 593–602.
46. Grodstein GP, Blumenkrantz MJ, Kopple JD, et al. Glucose absorption during continuous ambulatory peritoneal dialysis. Kidney Int 1981; 19:564–567.

40

Problems of Women on Dialysis

Susan S. Hou
Loyola University School of Medicine, Maywood, Illinois
Susan Grossman
St. Vincent's Medical Center of Richmond, Staten Island, New York

The care of dialysis patients has been focused first on survival and then on decreased morbidity. Rehabilitation has generally emphasized return to employment or family and community activities. Pregnancy and childbearing have been regarded as unfortunate accidents rather than as goals of treatment. Our attention to gynecological problems affecting dialysis patients has been overshadowed by attention to cardiovascular disease, infection, and other life-threatening complications of dialysis. Pregnancy in dialysis patients is still uncommon and carries a high risk for both mother and fetus. However, with the increasing length of survival of young dialysis patients and the increasing wait for transplantation, the problems associated with childbearing and contraception have become more important. The possibility and implications of conception need to be addressed with each patient. While rarely life-threatening, the problems of sexual dysfunction, dysfunctional uterine bleeding, and gynecological infections contribute to a diminished quality of life. Gynecological neoplasms are life-threatening when they occur, although they are not the most common cause of death in dialysis patients.

I. CONTRACEPTION

Early literature reported that only 10% of female dialysis patients of childbearing age menstruated (1), but a more recent report (2) indicates that the frequency of menses has increased to 42%. It is not certain how many of these women could conceive, but the risks and possibility of pregnancy and the need for contraception should be discussed with all dialysis patients of childbearing age.

Oral contraceptives offer many advantages for dialysis patients. Many dialysis patients are estrogen deficient, and women with irregular periods may be exposed to the effects of unopposed estrogen for prolonged periods of time. Estrogen deficiency is added to the many other factors that contribute to bone disease, and unopposed estrogen may increase the risk of endometrial cancer. The use of oral contraceptives would not only prevent pregnancy but would treat estrogen deficiency and allow for regular hormonal cycling. Oral contraceptives should be used with caution in hypertensive women and women at risk for thromboembolic disease. These drugs may increase the risk for lupus flares in women whose end-stage renal disease is secondary to lupus.

Mechanical methods of contraception can be used in women for whom estrogen is contraindicated. Intrauterine devices may be associated with increased uterine bleeding when patients are heparinized, and an increase in the risk of peritonitis would be expected in peritoneal dialysis patients. Other mechanical methods of birth control are acceptable in dialysis patients.

II. PREGNANCY

A. Frequency of Conception

Fertility is markedly reduced in dialysis patients. Estimates of the frequency of conception in dialysis patients range from 1.4% per year in Saudi Arabia (3) to 0.5% in the United States (4) and 0.3% in Belgium (5). The estimates from the United States and Saudi Arabia are based on surveys that covered only half the women of childbearing age treated with dialysis, while the survey from Belgium included a response from all of the dialysis units in the country. Only the report from the American National Registry for Pregnancy in Dialysis Patients (NRPDP) included a substantial number of peritoneal dialysis patients (4). Of note is that the frequency of conception in hemodialysis patients was two to three times higher than in peritoneal dialysis patients.

The reasons for the rarity of pregnancy in dialysis patients are not well understood. The hormonal changes in dialysis patients are reviewed elsewhere in this book. Nonhormonal causes of infertility have not been investigated.

It is not clear whether the difference in the frequency of conception between hemodialysis patients and CAPD patients is the result of endocrine differences or is in some way related to peritoneal dialysis itself. Recurrent peritonitis might be expected to cause tubal obstruction in peritoneal dialysis patients, but if tubal damage were a major contributor to infertility, an increase in tubal pregnancies would be expected. Few tubal pregnancies have been described in dialysis patients and none in peritoneal dialysis patients. It is possible that hypertonic dextrose damages the ovum or that the volume of fluid in the intraperitoneal space interferes with transport of the ovum from the ovary to the fallopian tubes.

Most pregnancies occur during the first few years on dialysis, but conception rates as a function of time on dialysis have not been determined. Pregnancy has occurred in women who have been on dialysis as long as 20 years. Repeat pregnancies in women who become pregnant on dialysis are not uncommon. In the 318 women whose pregnancies are recorded by the NRPDP, 8 became pregnant twice, 8 became pregnant three times, and one conceived four times (4). Although it would be expected that pregnancy would be more likely in women with regular menses, pregnancy has been reported in a woman after 9 years of amenorrhea. In contrast to dialysis patients, approximately 12% of women transplant recipients of childbearing age become pregnant.

B. Outcome of Pregnancy in Dialysis Patients

In 1980, the European Dialysis and Transplant Association reported 115 pregnancies in dialysis patients (6). Of those that were not electively terminated, only 23% resulted in surviving infants. Success rate for pregnancy in dialysis patients has improved since the EDTA report. In Saudi Arabia 30% of pregnancies resulted in surviving infants. The NRPDP recorded 222 pregnancies in women who were receiving dialysis at the time of conception. Of the 141 pregnancies that reached the second trimester, 55% resulted in surviving infants. Eighteen percent of live-born infants died in the neonatal period; 8.5% of pregnancies reaching the second trimester resulted in stillbirth, and 22% resulted in spontaneous abortion. The four induced abortions done in the second trimester were done for life-threatening maternal problems (three hypertension and one critical aortic stenosis) rather than for social reasons or anticipated problems.

C. Maternal Complications

1. Maternal Death

There have been three maternal deaths reported to the NRPDP. One death resulted from lupus cerebritis in a woman who started dialysis after conception. There were two deaths in women who conceived after starting dialysis, one as a result of hypertension and one from unknown causes. All three infants survived.

2. Hypertension

Hypertension is the most common life-threatening complication of pregnancy in dialysis patients. Of 57 case reports published in the medical literature in which blood pressure was noted in a pregnant dialysis patient, only 30% of women were normotensive throughout pregnancy (7). Sixty percent of women had blood pressures over 140/90 at some time during pregnancy, and in 25% the blood pressure exceeded 170/110. Ten percent were treated with antihypertensive medications, but blood pressure was not specified.

In cases reported to the NRPDP, approximately 80% of the 68 women for whom blood pressure measurements were available either had a blood pressure greater than 140/90 or required antihypertensive medication at some time during pregnancy (4). In over half of hypertensive pregnant dialysis patients, the blood pressure exceeds 170/110. Five of these women required intensive care unit admissions in addition to the maternal one death. Thirty-eight percent of patients who developed severe hypertension did so in the first trimester. In such cases, it was usually possible to control the blood pressure without terminating the pregnancy. Fifty percent of women with severe hypertension reached blood pressures of >170/110 in the second trimester. These cases were problematic in that preeclampsia could not be excluded and the fetus was still not viable. Three of 16 women required therapeutic abortion for hypertension. Of note, severe hypertension could be seen as late as 6 weeks postpartum.

3. Anemia

A drop in hematocrit is almost invariable in dialysis patients who become pregnant. In pregnancies reported to the NRPDP, 33% of women treated with erythropoietin and 77% of women not treated with erythropoietin required transfusion (4). Iron stores usually dropped, but there were several instances in which the hematocrit dropped despite iron saturation, which remained at acceptable levels.

D. Prematurity and Growth Restriction

Eighty-five percent of infants born to women who conceived after starting dialysis reported to the NRPDP were born before 37 weeks gestation (mean gestational age 32.4 weeks). Thirty-six percent weighed less than 1500 g at birth, and 28% were small for gestational age. Their neonatal course was complicated by respiratory distress and other complications of prematurity. Eleven of 116 live-born infants and 1 stillborn infant reported to the NRPDP had congenital anomalies (4). Eleven of 49 infants for whom follow-up data were available had long-term medical or developmental problems, most of which appeared to be the result of prematurity rather than an azotemic intrauterine environment. The mean gestational age was lower for infants who had long-term problems compared to those with normal growth and development (30.6 vs. 34.3 weeks).

III. MANAGEMENT ISSUES IN PREGNANT DIALYSIS PATIENTS

A. Preconception Counseling

Counseling of dialysis patients who are attempting pregnancy is all but impossible. The infrequency of conception makes it impossible to plan except in women who have already conceived once on dialysis. Even if a woman is actively trying to become pregnant, the likelihood of conception is low enough that changes in dialysis regimen cannot be justified. However, folic acid supplementation should be increased and good blood sugar control should be achieved in diabetic women who are attempting conception.

B. Diagnosis of Pregnancy

Pregnancy is usually diagnosed late in dialysis patients. Irregular menses are common and abdominal complaints are often attributed to other causes. A high index of suspicion is required to make the diagnosis early. Urine tests for human chorionic gonadotropin (hcg) are inaccurate even in women who have residual renal function. Small amounts of hcg are made by somatic cells, and because the hormone is partially excreted by the kidney, serum tests for β hcg are sometimes borderline or falsely positive in women who are not pregnant (8). The titers of β hcg may be higher than expected for the stage of gestation. The diagnosis and stage of gestation must be confirmed by ultrasound.

C. Management of Hypertension

Dialysis patients, particularly those on home treatment modalities, should measure their own blood pressure twice daily since severe increases in blood pressure can be abrupt. As with dialysis patients who are not pregnant, the first line of treatment is correction of volume overload. Assessment of volume status is difficult because of the expected 9 L increase in total body water during pregnancy, but cautious fluid removal should be attempted when hypertension develops. If fluid removal does not correct blood pressure, pharmacological treatment can be started. There is experience with a wide variety of antihypertensive medications in pregnancy (Table 1). Of the widely used antihypertensive drugs, only angiotensin-converting enzyme (ACE) inhibitors and, by inference, angiotensin receptor blockers are strongly contraindicated in pregnancy.

1. Angiotensin-Converting Enzyme Inhibitors

This group of drugs has been associated with oligohydramnios, which results in a number of complications. Amniotic fluid is necessary for fetal lung development, and the most serious consequence of oligohydramnios is pulmonary hypoplasia leading to neonatal death as a result of respiratory failure (9). Oligohydramnios also accounts for limb contractures in infants exposed to the drug. Direct pressure of the uterine muscle on the fetal skull is thought to result in abnormal calcification of the skull. Several instances of patent ductus have been described. This effect is

Table 1 Antihypertensive Drugs Used in Pregnancy

Drug (category)	Comments
Chronic Hypertension	
ACE inhibitors (D)	Contraindicated; 2nd and 3rd trimester use associated with pulmonary hypoplasia, hypocalvaria, renal dysplasia, neonatal anuria, contractures; no known harm in 1st trimester
α Methyl dopa (C)	Safe; 40 year use; careful developmental testing of children at ages 4 and 7; rare Coombs + hemolytic anemia, rare hepatitis
β Blockers (C)	Probably safe; fetal bradycardia, hypoglycemia, respiratory depression at birth, intrauterine growth restriction? ↓ fetal tolerance of anoxic stress
Labetolol (C)	Limited first trimester experience; less bradycardia and growth restriction than β blockers
Clonidine (C)	Probably safe; limited 1st trimester experience
Calcium channel blockers (C)	Profound ↓ BP with when used with magnesium; limited experience; reserve for severe hypertension
Hydralazine (C)	Safe; long experience with use in pregnancy; no ↑ birth defects; ineffective as a single agent
Minoxidil (C)	Very limited experience; hypertricosis and congenital anomalies in one the infant
Prazocin (C)	Limited experience; no problems noted
Thiazide diuretics (D)	↑ congenital anomalies with chlorthaldone; subnormal intravascular volume expansion, neonatal thrombocytopenia, hemolytic anemia, electrolyte abnormalities
Hypertensive Crisis	
Hydralazine (C)	Used for 40 years without serious side effects
Labetolol (C)	Shorter length of use; appears safe
Nitroprusside (C)	Fetal cyanide toxicity
Diazoxide (C)	Fatal maternal hypotension reported; limit dose to 30 mg boluses; ↓ uterine contraction; neonatal hyperglycemia

thought to be the result of the effects of ACE inhibitors on prostaglandin metabolism.

While exposure to ACE inhibitors in the second and third trimesters may have serious consequences, no ill effects have been identified as a result of first trimester exposure. Two studies, one involving 46 infants and one involving 86 infants, showed no adverse effect of exposure to ACE inhibitors in the first trimester (10). In the latter report there were four congenital anomalies, a number that was not significantly different from the expected three. Women with inadvertent first trimester exposure need not be advised to terminate the pregnancy.

There is less experience with angiotensin II receptor blockers, but it is expected that problems caused by decreased angiotensin effect will be similar to those seen in women treated with ACE inhibitors.

2. Other Antihypertensive Drugs

a. α Methyl Dopa

α Methyl dopa has been used in pregnant women for over 40 years and is still the drug of first choice for essential hypertension. Careful developmental studies have been done at 4 and 7 years of age in children exposed to the drug in utero, and no problems have been found (11).

b. β Blockers

There are several case reports of neonatal bradycardia, hypoglycemia, and respiratory depression associated with β blockers, but these problems are generally easily managed by the neonatologist (12). There are mixed data concerning whether blockers are associated with intrauterine growth restriction. There are reports of small-for-gestational-age infants of mothers treated with β blockers for diseases not usually associated with growth restriction (13). There are also data from animal models suggesting a decreased ability of the fetus to withstand anoxic stress (14). None of these problems has turned out to be a major contraindication to the use of this category of drugs in pregnant humans. Fetal bradycardia may make it difficult to interpret antenatal monitoring, which depends on changes in fetal heart rate.

c. Labetolol

Labetolol is not associated with fetal bradycardia and growth restriction and, it is widely used in preference to β blockers. Nonetheless, data on first trimester effects of the drug are still limited (10). Moreover, controlled studies have not shown it to be superior to other antihypertensive agents (15).

d. Clonidine

Clonidine is a centrally acting α_2-agonist, which has been reported in one study to have efficacy and safety similar to methyl dopa (16). In view of the limited experience with it, there is no reason to use it in preference to α methyl dopa.

e. Prazocin

No adverse effects on the fetus have been demonstrated with prazocin, but the experience with it is more limited than with labetolol, α methyl dopa, and β blockers, and it does not appear to offer any advantage. The drug can be continued in women whose blood pressure is well controlled on it at the time of conception.

f. Calcium Channel Blockers

Nifedipine, nicardipine, and verapamil have been used in severe hypertension. They do not appear to be associated with any increase in congenital anomalies when used in the first trimester. These drugs have been used for treatment of premature labor in the third trimester. Experience with diltiazem is more limited. Calcium channel blockers may potentiate the hypotensive effects and neuromuscular blockade of magnesium and the interaction should be kept in mind when the drugs are used in women with a possibility of developing preeclampsia (17,18). Because of the limited experience with all members of this group of drugs, their use is best limited to severe hypertension unresponsive to other drugs.

g. Vasodilators

Hydralazine has been used safely during pregnancy for 40 years. It is ineffective as a single oral agent but can be added to a first-line drug if the latter does not adequately control blood pressure. The more potent vasodilator, minoxidil has been associated with hypertrichosis and congenital anomalies in one case report (19). It is ineffective unless combined with a diuretic and a sympatholytic agent.

3. Drugs for Hypertensive Emergencies

a. Hydralazine

Intravenous hydralazine in doses of 5–10 mg every 20–30 minutes is the drug of first choice for hypertensive crisis in pregnancy. A single study has shown a high frequency of malignant ventricular arrhythmias in eclamptic women treated with hydralazine than in women treated with labetolol (20). Nine studies comparing hydralazine with other drugs, most often intravenous labetolol, have found no advantage of one drug regimen over another (21).

b. Labetolol

Intravenous labetolol given either as a 20 mg loading dose followed by 20 mg every 30 minutes or a 1–2 mg/min drip is the second most commonly used regimen for treating hypertensive emergencies in pregnant women. There are occasional reports of fetal bradycardia, and the newborn should be monitored for hypotension.

c. Diazoxide

There is extensive experience with the use of diazoxide in pregnancy, but the drug is now primarily of historic interest. In doses of 150–300 mg it has been associated with at least one maternal fatality from hypotension. It is also associated with decreased uterine contractions and neonatal hyperglycemia. Its only advantage is a long duration of action, which may make it useful in a woman who must be transported with minimal monitoring capability or when other drugs have failed. It should be used only in 30 mg boluses every 1–2 minutes until the desired blood pressure is reached.

D. Infections

Pregnant hemodialysis patients are probably at no more risk of infection than those who are not pregnant, but the use of antibiotics will be influenced by pregnancy. Most penicillins are safe during pregnancy. First-generation cephalosporins such as cephazolin and cephalexin are safe in pregnancy (10). Cephalosporins with a methyltetrathiazole moiety (cefoperozone, cefotetan, moxalactam, and cefamandole) are usually avoided in pregnancy because studies have shown infertility in animals (22). Sulfa drugs, such as sulfamethoxiazole, can be used in the early part of pregnancy but should be avoided in the latter part of pregnancy because there is a risk of kernicterus. Trimethoprim and trimethoprim-sulfamethoxiazole combinations are generally avoided because of the teratogenicity of folic acid antagonists. In practice, significant increases in congenital anomalies have not been noted with these drugs. The quinolone antibiotics should be avoided in pregnancy because they have been associated with weakened cartilage in young animals. Aminoglycosides should also be avoided because of their association with 8th nerve damage.

E. Peritonitis

The anatomic connection between the uterus and the intraperitoneal cavity raises the concern that peritonitis will result in intrauterine infection and vice versa. There have been few cases reported of peritonitis in pregnant CAPD patients. In three cases reported, peritonitis was followed by labor in two (23,24). One pregnancy resulted in a premature baby, who survived, and the other resulted in a stillbirth. Five additional cases of peritonitis have been reported to the NRPDP. There was only one fetal loss, which was remote from the time of peritonitis. There is one report of postpartum *Escherichia coli* peritonitis requiring removal of the peritoneal catheter resulting from ascending infection in a woman with chorioamnionitis (25).

F. Erythropoietin

There are limited but reassuring data on the use of erythropoietin during pregnancy (26). There have been no reports of teratogenicity. Since conception is not usually expected in dialysis patients, these women are generally being treated with erythropoietin and are well into the period of organogenesis when pregnancy is diagnosed. The drug has not been associated with increased difficulty controlling hypertension or with polycythemia in the infants. Dialysis patients who are not treated with erythropoietin almost always require transfusions (4). Erythropoietin requirements increase in pregnancy, and a 50–100% increase in the dose can be prescribed as soon as pregnancy is diagnosed.

G. Iron

Serum iron and ferritin usually drop during pregnancy in dialysis patients, and iron deficiency may play a role in anemia later in pregnancy. The safety of intravenous iron has not been established, but it has been widely used. There are old data indicating that iron may be transferred disproportionately to the fetus, and if intravenous iron is used, it seems prudent to give it in small doses to minimize the risk of acute iron toxicity. The outcome of pregnancy in dialysis patients treated with intravenous iron is not different from women who have not received iron.

H. Dialysis Regimens

1. Choice of Modality

When the first cases of pregnancy in peritoneal dialysis patients were reported, it appeared that the outcome was better for peritoneal dialysis patients than for hemodialysis (27). With the accumulation of more data, it has become clear that the apparent superiority of peritoneal dialysis simply reflected the overall improvement in outcome for pregnancies in dialysis patients compared to earlier reports.

There are theoretical advantages to peritoneal dialysis in that there are no rapid metabolic changes and volume removal is gradual. There may be disadvantages with difficulty maintaining adequate nutrition for pregnancy. There is no reason to switch a woman who is stable on either hemodialysis or peritoneal dialysis to another modality because of pregnancy per se. When starting dialysis during pregnancy, the usual criteria for choosing a dialysis modality can be used. Peritoneal dialysis has been successfully used in women with end-stage renal disease secondary to diabetic nephropathy. It might be relatively contraindicated in nondiabetic women who are at high risk for gestational diabetes.

2. Hemodialysis

a. Intensive Dialysis

The value of intensive dialysis (daily dialysis) in improving the outcome of pregnancy in dialysis patients has not been established, but there are theoretical reasons to support its use. Women who begin dialysis during pregnancy and have residual renal function have a better pregnancy outcome (75–80% vs. 40% infant survival) (4). It is not known whether residual excretory function or endocrine function is responsible for the better outcome, but an attempt to lower the fetal exposure to metabolic waste products seems reasonable. With daily dialysis, interdialytic weight gains are modest and the risk of hypotension with fluid removal is decreased. Polyhydramnios is common in dialysis patients. A recent report of 17 pregnancies in dialysis patients from University of São Paulo noted polyhydramnios in 17 (28). Uterine distension associated with polyhydramnios may contribute to premature labor. A high blood urea nitrogen in the fetus that has normal kidneys may cause an osmotic diuresis, which aggravates polyhydramnios. This hypothesis is supported by the observation that a urea diuresis is usual in infants born to mothers on dialysis. A report of 27 pregnancies in women in Saudi Arabia found a significantly longer dialysis time in women with successful pregnancies compared to women with unsuccessful pregnancies (12 h vs. 10 h) (3). Limited data from the NRPDP indicate that dialysis must be increased to at least 20 hours per week to achieve any improvement in outcome.

b. *Dialysis Bath*

If intensive dialysis is used, several adjustments in the dialysate composition may be necessary. Serum potassium may drop if dietary increases in potassium do not offset increased losses, and the dialysate potassium may need to be raised. With daily dialysis, hypercalcemia may occur if a bath containing 3.5 mEq/L of calcium is used, and 2.5 mEq/L is usually preferable. While potassium and calcium in the dialysate are relatively easy to adjust, bicarbonate is more problematic. The dialysate bicarbonate of 35 mEq/L is designed to offset 2 days of acid production. Daily dialysis may result in excessive bicarbonate gain. The situation is further complicated by the normal respiratory alkalosis of pregnancy in which the appropriate serum bicarbonate is 18–20 mEq/L rather than 25 mEq/L. If serious alkalosis develops, an individually formulated dialysis solution may be necessary.

c. *Anticoagulation*

In the past, recommendations have been made to minimize anticoagulant dose in pregnant women. However, the usual practice in all dialysis patients is to give the smallest amount of anticoagulation possible. An attempt at lowering heparin doses results in the same problems of clotting of the extracorporeal circuit that it does in nonpregnant patients. Although direct comparisons have not been made, clotting problems may even be increased because pregnancy is a hypercoagulable state. Heparin does not cross the placenta and is not teratogenic (29). We recommend that heparin-free dialysis be limited to women with bleeding problems. Coumadin does cross the placenta, is teratogenic in the first trimester, and may cause bleeding in the fetus in the third trimester (10). Women treated with coumadin either for recurrent access clotting or for other reasons should be switched to subcutaneous heparin in doses adequate for full anticoagulation.

3. Peritoneal Dialysis

In late pregnancy it becomes difficult for a woman to tolerate her usual exchange volume (27). Volume must be reduced and the number of exchanges increased. It may become difficult to maintain even the previous level of dialysis. To increase the amount of dialysis delivered, it is necessary to use a combination of daytime CAPD and nighttime CCPD. There is not enough data to determine whether increasing the amount of peritoneal dialysis delivered improves outcome.

I. Calcium and Phosphorus

Thirty grams of calcium are necessary for calcification of the fetal skeleton. If the patient is dialyzed on a bath containing more than 3.5 mEq/L of calcium, dialysis easily provides this amount. If she is dialyzed on a lower calcium bath, enough calcium should be absorbed from phosphate binders to provide the necessary calcium if she takes at least 2 g of calcium daily. 1,25-Dihydroxyvitamin D preparations, either oral or intravenous, are usually continued, although their effect in pregnancy is not well understood. The placenta does convert some 25-OH_2D_3 to 1,25-OH_2D_3 (30). High doses of 1,25-OH_2D_3 have been used in one patient with hypoparathyroidism without ill effects on the fetus (31).

J. Nutritional Considerations

Guidelines for nutritional care of a pregnant dialysis patient are still in a state of evolution (Table 2).

Table 2 Dietary Guidelines for Pregnant Dialysis Patients

Protein HD: 1.2 g/kg ideal body wt + 10 g/d
PD: 2.4 g/kg ideal body weight + 10 g/d
Calories: 35 kcal/kg + 300 k/cal
Sodium: 3 g/d
Potassium: 2–3 g/d
Phosphorus: 1200 mg/d
Calcium: 1–2 g as phosphate binders; 2 g/d if 2.5 mEq/L bath is used
Vitamin A and E: no supplement
Folate: 1.8 mg/d
Vitamin C: 170 mg/d
Thiamine: 3 mg/d
Riboflavin: 3.4 mg/d
Niacin: 20 mg/d
B6: 5 mg
Biotin: 600 mg
Zinc: 15 mg
Carnitine: 330 mg

1. Weight Gain

It is almost impossible to prescribe weight gain. The task confronting the health care team is usually to determine how much of observed weight gain is either pregnancy related increase in soft tissue or increased total body water appropriate for pregnancy and how much is fluid overload that should be removed with dialysis. Normal pregnancy is accompanied by an increase in total body water of approximately 9 L, most of it in the extracellular space. Fluid retention occurs to some extent in dialysis patients. A common observation early in pregnancy and occasionally a clue to the diagnosis is hypotension in response to the attempt to remove fluid. The patient should be examined carefully on a weekly basis for evidence of fluid overload, and if signs of excessive volume expansion are present, a careful attempt to remove fluid with dialysis should be made.

2. Protein and Calories

Practically, with intensive dialysis, no protein restriction is necessary during pregnancy, and provision of adequate protein and calories is frequently a problem. Supplements are often required, and several instances in which intradialytic parenteral nutrition was used have been reported (32).

3. Fluid Restriction

Daily dialysis allows for decreasing but not eliminating a fluid restriction. One goal of daily dialysis is to avoid the need to remove more than 1–2 L during a single treatment.

4. Water-Soluble Vitamins

The requirements for water-soluble vitamins increase during pregnancy, and increased frequency of dialysis increases the loss of water-soluble vitamins above the usual for dialysis patients.

Folic acid is necessary for the increased hematopoiesis that occurs during pregnancy. Preconception supplementation with 0.8 mg of folic acid has been shown to reduce the risk of neural tube defects (33). The usual renal diet is frequently low in fruits and vegetables and thus low in folate. The usual supplement for dialysis patients is 1 mg/day, and we recommend increasing the supplement to 1.8–2 mg/day.

Requirements for all vitamins are increased during pregnancy and an additional increase is required for pregnancy with additional increases required in dialysis patients. Vitamin C dose should be increased. Deficiency has been associated with neonatal scurvy.

5. Fat-Soluble Vitamins

Supplements of vitamin A are usually prescribed in normal pregnancy but should not be prescribed in pregnant dialysis patients. Excretion is decreased in dialysis patients, and it is not removed by dialysis. Very high doses of vitamin A have been associated with congenital anomalies similar to those seen with isoretinoin (34).

Standard preparations of vitamin D have little effect on dialysis patients, and their presence in vitamin preparations has little relevance.

Vitamin E supplements are not required in pregnant dialysis patients.

6. Zinc

Zinc is necessary for human reproduction, and its deficiency has been associated with teratogenesis (34). Later in pregnancy it has been associated with premature birth and atonic uterine bleeding. A supplement should be given particularly to patients taking oral iron.

IV. OBSTETRIC MANAGEMENT

Care of the pregnant dialysis and transplant patient requires close cooperation between the nephrologist and a perinatologist experienced in taking care of women with renal disease. A referral to a high-risk obstetrician should be made as soon as pregnancy is diagnosed. Because of the high frequency of severe prematurity, a level three nursery should be available.

A. Premature Labor

Prematurity is the greatest cause of morbidity and mortality in the infants of women with renal disease. There are several special considerations to bear in mind with the most commonly used treatments for premature labor. Magnesium can be used, but as in its use for preeclampsia, extreme caution must be used to avoid magnesium toxicity and respiratory depression in women with renal insufficiency (35). In dialysis patients, a loading dose can be given and supplemented after each dialysis treatment or when the magnesium level has been documented to fall below 5 mg/dL. Continuous infusion should not be used in dialysis patients.

Indomethacin has been used to treat premature labor in women with renal disease and may be especially effective in women with polyhydramnios (26). However, in women with renal insufficiency or in dialysis patients with residual renal function, there may be a loss of renal function, causing hyperkalemia and requiring initiation or increase in dialysis.

Premature labor usually occurs early enough that it is desirable to delay delivery longer than the usual 72 hours that indomethacin is used. The fetus should be monitored for any evidence of right heart strain, and the mother should be monitored for polyhydramnios.

Midtrimester losses are common in dialysis patients, and there have been a few reports of incompetent cervix. Dialysis patients should be monitored for any signs of cervical shortening or dilatation.

B. Fetal Surveillance

Because of the increased risk of stillbirth, fetal surveillance should be started as soon as there is a possibility of survival outside the mother. Because of the risk of precipitating labor, other tests should be used in preference to oxytocin challenge testing.

C. Labor and Delivery

Vaginal delivery should be the goal of management, and cesarean section should be done only for the usual obstetric indications rather than for renal disease per se. When cesarean section is done in peritoneal dialysis patients, an attempt should be made to use an extraperitoneal approach. An attempt to resume peritoneal dialysis with low-volume exchanges can be made 24 hours after operative delivery. If there is leaking from the incision, the patient should be switched to hemodialysis for 2 weeks.

D. Management Issues in the Newborn

Infants born to dialysis patients should be observed in a high-risk setting even if they appear normal. Infants of dialysis patients are born with blood urea nitrogen (BUN) and serum creatinine equal to the mother's, and following birth they experience an osmotic diuresis that results in volume contraction and electrolyte disorders unless there is careful monitoring and replacement of fluid and electrolytes.

V. DYSPAREUNIA

Some female dialysis patients may experience dyspareunia because of estrogen deficiency and resulting vaginal dryness. Dyspareunia resulting from atrophic vaginitis from low estrogen levels can be corrected by intravaginal conjugated estrogens (2–4 g daily) or oral estrogen progesterone compounds. A daily dose of 0.625 mg of conjugated estrogen and 2.5 mg of medroxyprogesterone provides enough estrogen to prevent dyspareunia. If there is breakthrough bleeding on this combination, progesterone can be increased to 5 mg. Women treated with intravaginal estrogens should receive progesterone as well because there is substantial systemic absorption.

VI. SEXUAL DYSFUNCTION

Fifty percent of female dialysis patients under the age of 55 are sexually active (2), and a majority of them experience some sexual dysfunction. They suffer from both decreased libido and decreased ability to achieve orgasm. Treatment with erythropoietin (EPO) appears to be associated with an improvement in sexual function, but most of the data collected have been in men (36). Various reasons for sexual dysfunction have been proposed, including hyperprolactinemia, gonadal dysfunction, depression, hyperparathyroidism, and change in body image.

Hyperprolactinemia is seen in 75–90% of female dialysis patients (37–39). The mean serum prolactin levels in women with sexual dysfunction are higher than in patients with normal sexual function. Treatment of hyperprolactinemia with the dopamine agonist bromergocriptine has been reported (in limited uncontrolled studies) to improve sexual function in both men and women on dialysis (40). It has not come into widespread use because hemodialysis patients are particularly susceptible to the hypotensive effects of this drug. There are no reports of its use in CAPD patients or on the use of other dopamine agonists. Bromocriptine should be started at a dose of 1.25 mg, and the first dose should be taken at night. Subsequent doses can be gradually increased. Doses of 2.5 mg bid should be adequate to suppress prolactin secretion. When correctable physical problems cannot be found, dialysis patients should be referred for sex therapy, as would patients without renal failure.

VII. HORMONE REPLACEMENT THERAPY

Holley and colleagues found that only 5% of women aged 55 or greater at the time of starting dialysis were receiving hormone replacement therapy. No firm guidelines for hormone replacement therapy have been developed in dialysis patients. Hormone replacement therapy in healthy women slightly increases the risk of breast cancer while reducing the risk of osteoporosis and heart disease. It is not known whether the risk of breast cancer would be higher in dialysis patients than in healthy women, but the risk of heart disease and bone disease are clearly increased. In the absence of specific data, these risks make treatment of postmenopausal women on dialysis with estrogen-progesterone cycling a reasonable approach. As noted, many women younger than 55 years of age have estrogen deficiency. Hormone replacement therapy is the standard of care for premenopausal women who undergo oophorectomy. Although it is not general practice, there is every reason to think that dialysis patients who are estrogen deficient should receive replacement therapy. An experienced gynecologist may have to try a number of combinations of these hormones to find a regimen that does not cause excessive bleeding.

There is limited experience with the use of other treatments for osteoporosis in dialysis patients. The use of alendronate in patients with creatinine clearance of <35 mL is not recommended by the manufacturer because of lack of experience, not because of known adverse effect. A large portion of the drug is excreted by the kidneys, and a dose adjustment would be necessary. The efficacy of alendronate in decreasing steroid-induced osteoporosis has heightened interest in its use in renal disease, and its use in dialysis patients is now an area of active investigation (41).

VIII. DYSFUNCTIONAL UTERINE BLEEDING

A. Incidence

Many women develop amenorrhea when the glomerular filtration rate falls to less than 10 mL/min. Menstruation returns in as many as 50% of premenopausal women once dialysis is started. Over half of women with end-stage renal disease (ESRD) who menstruate report hypermenorrhea (2), and 60% have irregular cycles, with similar menstrual abnormalities in hemodialysis and CAPD patients. Dysfunctional uterine bleeding is common and is of concern because it may be an early sign of endometrial cancer. Blood loss may lead to severe anemia even in women treated with EPO, although the introduction of EPO has made the management of dysfunctional uterine bleeding substantially easier.

B. Management

1. Screening for Malignancy

Management of dysfunctional uterine bleeding depends on the woman's age and on whether menses have ceased. In women >40 years of age who have had no menses for one year prior to the bleeding episode, cancer risk is high and dilatation and curettage should be performed. In women >40 years of age whose menstruation has not ceased for 1 year prior to bleeding, the cancer risk is moderate. Dilatation and curettage is not routinely necessary, and performance of several endometrial biopsies is probably sufficient to screen for malignancy. In women <40 years of age, the cancer risk is relatively small, and a yearly Pap smear is usually a sufficient screen for tumor. Women who have been exposed to immunosuppression either for treatment of their renal disease or for a transplant that has failed are at increased risk for malignancy.

2. Bloody Peritoneal Dialysate

Menstruation, ovulation, or uterine bleeding from any cause can result in bloody peritoneal fluid in peritoneal dialysis patients. There is no specific management, and treatment is rarely necessary unless there is profuse bleeding. In rare cases, frank hemoperitoneum may occur, requiring suppression of ovulation (42). An aseptic peritonitis picture during menstruation or ovulation has also been reported (43).

3. Anticoagulation

The lowest possible dosage of heparin should be used to perform hemodialysis when a woman is menstruating. Heparin-free techniques and citrate anticoagulation also are available.

4. Hormone Therapy

Recent advances in therapy have facilitated the management of dysfunctional uterine bleeding in women with end-stage renal disease.

Oral contraceptives remain the safest therapy and the first-line treatment, although they should not be used if hypertension control is a problem or if there is a history of deep vein thrombosis. There are theoretical benefits of using estrogen-progesterone combinations to prevent uterine cancer and osteoporosis.

Medroxyprogesterone acetate (Depo-Provera) can be given in a dose of 100 mg IM once a week for 4 weeks and then once a month. Because many dialysis patients have a platelet dysfunction, IM injections may result in hematoma formation. Moreover, the half-life of IM medroxyprogesterone acetate is unpredictable. Medroxyprogesterone acetate is best reserved for patients with chronic hypermenorrhea who do not respond to oral hormonal therapy. In women whose hypermenorrhea does not respond to oral contraceptives or progestins, gonadotropin-releasing hormone agonists can be used. The dosage is 7.5 mg of long-acting leuprolide acetate IM, monthly. This drug is extremely expensive. There is one report of ovarian hyperstimulation in a patient on chronic dialysis who received two doses of leuprolide acetate (44). It has been postulated that women with ESRD may be at risk for this complication because of decreased excretion of the gonadotropin-releasing hormone agonists. The use of leuprolide should be undertaken by a gynecologist familiar with the problems of patients with end-stage renal disease.

In the case of acute excessive blood loss, high-dose estrogen therapy can be used, giving 25 mg of conjugated estrogens IV every 6 hours. Bleeding usually subsides within 12 hours.

In setting of acute blood loss when bleeding time is prolonged, DDAVP can be used as it is in with other bleeding problems, in a dosage of 0.3 pg/kg in 50 mL of saline given every 4–8 hours for three to four doses.

5. Nonhormonal Treatments

a. Laser Ablation

The neodymium (Nd):YAG laser now offers a safe and effective alternative to hysterectomy. With this technique, the endometrial lining is ablated by vaporizing all three of its layers. Patients are pretreated with either danazol 200 mg four times daily for 4–6 weeks or with gonadotropin-releasing hormone agonists. The technique requires a surgeon trained and experienced in operative hysteroscopy and the use of the Nd:YAG laser. The procedure leads to permanent infertility.

b. Hysterectomy

For postmenopausal women with significant dysfunctional uterine bleeding, hysterectomy is a possible approach. The proposed operation should be carefully discussed with the patient, and concomitant medical problems and the risks of surgery should be taken into consideration. With the advent of endometrial ablation with laser, hysterectomy will now probably be reserved for women who have bleeding secondary to uterine fibroids or to other uterine or pelvic pathology that in itself warrants the surgery. Hysterectomy should be done only as a life-saving procedure in a premenopausal woman who is a candidate for renal transplantation, because the latter will frequently restore fertility.

6. Gynecological Neoplasms

a. Benign

Uterine fibroids, or leiomyomata, are extremely common, occurring in approximately 25% of women over the age of 30. There is no information about their frequency in chronic renal failure. In dialysis patients without serious comorbidities, the management of uterine fibroids is similar to the approach in women without renal failure.

b. Incidence of Malignant Tumors

Although it was previously believed that the incidence of endometrial carcinoma is increased in female dialysis patients, several recent studies suggest that breast, endometrial, and ovarian cancers are not increased in this population.

c. Screening

Guidelines for breast cancer screening are given similar to those given for the general population. Pap smears should be done yearly to screen for cervical cancer in dialysis patients. Women who have had immunosuppressive therapy, because of either previous transplantation or underlying renal disease, or women with AIDS should have PAP smears every 6 months because of the increased incidence of cervical cancer in these populations. Endometrial cancer usually presents as dysfunctional uterine bleeding, the investigation and management of which have been discussed above. Ovarian cancer usually presents with vague abdominal symptoms and later as an ovarian mass. Abdominal discomfort, nausea, and weight loss induced by ovarian cancer may initially be misinterpreted as symptoms of uremia or underdialysis. In patients on peritoneal dialysis, ovarian cancer may present as bloody peritoneal fluid, an abnormal peritoneal cell count, or a change in the color of the fluid. A high index of suspicion is necessary to detect ovarian cancer at an early and potentially curable stage.

IX. DIAGNOSTIC TESTS FOR GYNECOLOGICAL DISEASE IN DIALYSIS PATIENTS

A. Computed Tomography

Intravenous contrast infusion, if needed to perform a CT scan or angiography, is not contraindicated in a dialysis patient. Although the administration of contrast involves increasing intravascular volume and osmolality, immediate dialysis following the study can be performed if deemed necessary. A patient on peritoneal dialysis requiring an abdominal CT scan can present for the examination with dialysis fluid in the abdomen.

B. Pelvic and Abdominal Ultrasonography

The patient on peritoneal dialysis with a suspected pelvic or ovarian lesion should undergo ultrasound scanning of the involved area. In those instances where pelvic pathological changes cannot be visualized without distending the bladder, the latter can be filled via a Foley catheter. Hyponatremia will result from misguided attempts by ultrasound personnel to fill the bladder by having the patient drink water.

C. Transvaginal Ultrasound

Pelvic abnormalities can be delineated more clearly using transvaginal ultrasound because of the proximity of the probe to the pelvic organs and the relatively thin vaginal vault, which enables the use of higher sound frequencies and therefore higher resolution. On the other hand, the transabdominal probe will give a more panoramic view of the pelvis, showing the interrelationship of the major anatomic structures in the pelvic organs and their pathology. The transvaginal probe is able to furnish a more focused image of the organ of interest but permits effective imaging to no more than 7–10 cm in depth. The transvaginal ultrasound study is best done while the bladder is empty. Since many patients on dialysis are not able to fill their bladders unless a Foley catheter is placed and fluid instilled into the bladder, it makes sense to first perform a transvaginal ultrasound if the pelvic pathology is suspected and proceed to transabdominal pelvic sonogram if the information needed cannot be obtained with the transvaginal approach. CAPD patients should have the abdomen full for transabdominal ultrasound and empty for transvaginal ultrasound.

X. MANAGEMENT

The management of gynecological cancers and nonmalignant tumors in women with chronic renal failure includes surgical excisions and chemotherapy.

A. Surgery

The general approach to performing surgery in dialysis patients is discussed elsewhere. There are several additional points that pertain specifically to gynecological procedures. In patients with peritoneal catheters undergoing pelvic or abdominal operations, the catheter can be left in place unless there is bacterial contamination of the peritoneal cavity. When there is a low but measurable risk of peritoneal contamination as in a vaginal hysterectomy, 1.0 g of vancomycin hydrochloride and 1.0 g of cefoxitin can be administered prophylactically, IV, just prior to surgery. If the patient is known to be colonized with *Pseudomonas*, tobramycin 2.0 mg/kg IV should be added to the prophylactic regimen. Postoperatively, the catheter is irrigated with 500 mL of peritoneal dialysis solution three times daily to maintain patency. Irrigations are decreased to once daily when the fluid is no longer bloody. The patient can be maintained on hemodialysis for 10 days to 2 weeks before the peritoneal catheter is used again.

B. Chemotherapy

Use of chemotherapeutic agents in dialysis patients is discussed elsewhere. Chemotherapeutic agents have been given via the intraperitoneal route in patients with normal renal function who have intraabdominal tumors and occasionally in peritoneal dialysis patients. Intraperitoneal installation of chemotherapeutic agents results in local concentrations of drugs 10–20 times higher than systemic levels as well as high portal vein concentrations. Drugs that have been used intraperitoneally include 5-fluorouracil (5 FU), cisplatinum, cytarabine, and doxorubicin. 5-FU and doxyrubicin can be given in the usual doses intraperitoneally, but the dose of cisplatinum should still be reduced to 25% of the usual dose.

C. Transplantation After Curative Resection of Gynecological Neoplasms

Because immunosuppression increases the risk of tumor, most transplant centers wait 2–5 years before transplanting a patient who has had a malignancy. Early stages of cervical cancer do not contraindicate transplantation, but transplantation after treatment, thought to be curative, of other tumors must be individualized according to prognosis.

XI. GYNECOLOGICAL INFECTIONS

Female dialysis patients are subject to the same infections that occur in women without renal disease. Some changes in treatment are required because of the effect of renal failure and dialysis on drug metabolism.

Candida albicans is the most common cause of vulvovaginitis. Treatment is not affected by either renal failure of dialysis. Similarly, the treatment of nonspecific vaginitis is not changed. Metronidazole should be taken after dialysis. There have been rare cases of fungal peritonitis with torulopsis resulting from vaginal infections in peritoneal dialysis patients.

A. Chlamydia and Mycoplasma

These organisms are often the cause of nonspecific vaginitis that does not respond to metronidazole therapy. In addition, they are major causes of infertility and pelvic inflammatory disease. Treatment is to administer doxycycline 100 mg daily for 14 days. Other tetracyclines should be avoided in dialysis patients. Alternative regimens include a single 1 g dose of azithromycin, ofloxacin 150 mg daily for 7 days, or erythromycin 500 mg po qid for 14 days. Only ofloxacin and doxycycline also treat gonorrhea. Sexual partners should also be treated.

B. Genital Herpes

Oral acyclovir has been shown to shorten the intensity and duration of first-time infections with genital herpes. Acyclovir is normally excreted by the kidney and is dialyzable. When herpetic infection is severe enough to warrant use of acyclovir, the drug should be given in a reduced dosage of 200 mg po bid, with the doses scheduled in such a way that one is normally given after a dialysis session.

C. Gonorrhea

In many locations, ceftriaxone has become the initial drug of choice because of the increased incidence of penicillin-resistant gonococci. The one-time 250 mg IM dosage is not changed for dialysis patients. Treatment with penicillin follows usual dosage regimens. Probenecid, included in the usual regimen to retard renal excretion of penicillin, need not be given when treating dialysis patients. If the patient is allergic to penicillin, doxycycline in the usual dosage can be administered. Therapy of resistant strains should be guided by local information, and sensitivity results.

D. Syphilis

The treatment of syphilis is unchanged in the dialysis patient. Staff should be aware that secondary syphilis is highly contagious through blood contact. Dialysis machines should be cleaned with formaldehyde or sodium hypochlorite solution after use in a patient with secondary syphilis.

E. Human Papillomavirus

Human papillomavirus (HPV) infection has become one of the most common sexually transmitted diseases in the United States. Patients may present with venereal warts or with an abnormal Pap smear. There is no difference in therapy of this infection for dialysis patients. Women with HPV infections can be referred for transplantation but should be aware of the risk of aggravation of the disease following transplant. (Treatment of sexually transmitted hepatitis and HIV is discussed elsewhere in this volume.)

XII. CONCLUSION

With the improved survival of women treated with dialysis, our care of them should address obstetric and gynecological problems. When pregnancy occurs, it requires extreme vigilance to minimize the risk to the mother and careful management to increase the likelihood of a successful outcome. With increased understanding of the causes of infertility in women with renal failure and development of management strategies that result in healthy mothers and infants, we may reach the point of actively helping these women attempt pregnancy. Management of hormonal abnormalities, estrogen-replacement therapy, and common gynecological problems, including dysfunctional uterine bleeding, tumors, and infection, needs to be incorporated into our treatment of these women.

REFERENCES

1. Perez RJ, Lipner H, Abdulla N, Cicotto S, Abrams M. Menstrual dysfunction of patients undergoing hemodialysis. Obstet Gynecol 1978; 51:552–555.
2. Holley JL, Schmidt RJ, Bender FH, Dumler F, Schiff M. Gynecologic and reproductive issues in women on dialysis. Am J Kidney Disease 1997; 29:685–690.
3. Souqiyyeh MZ, Huraib SO, Saleh AGM, Aswad S. Pregnancy in chronic hemodialysis patients in the Kingdom of Saudi Arabia. Am J Kidney Disease 1992; 19: 235–238.
4. Okundaye IB, Abrinko P, Hou SH. A registry for pregnancy in dialysis patients. Am J Kidney Dis 1998; 31: 766–773.

5. Bagon JA, Martens J, Van Roost G, Vernaeve H, De Muylder X. Pregnancy and dialysis Am J Kidney Dis 1998; 31:756–765.
6. Registration Committee of the European Dialysis and Transplant Association. Successful pregnancies in women treated by dialysis and kidney transplantation. Br J Obstet Gynecol 1980; 87:839–845.
7. Hou SH. Pregnancy in women on haemodialysis and peritoneal dialysis. Baillière's Clin Obstet Gynaecol 1994; 8:481–500.
8. Schwartz A, Post KG, Keller F, Molzhan M. Value of human chorionic gonadotropin measurements in blood as a pregnancy test in women on maintenance hemodialysis. Nephron 1985; 39:341–343.
9. Hanssens M, Keirse MJNC, Vankelecom F, Van Assche FA. Fetal and neonatal effects of angiotensin converting enzyme inhibitors during pregnancy. Obstet Gynecol 1991; 78:128–135.
10. Briggs GG, Freeman RK, Yaffe SJ, eds. Drugs in Pregnancy and Lactation. Baltimore: Williams and Wilkins, 1994.
11. Cockburn J, Moar VA, Ounsted MK, Good FJ, Redman CWG. Final report of study on hypertension during pregnancy: the effects of specific treatment on growth and development of the children. Lancet 1982; 1:647–649.
12. Gladstone GW, Hordof A, Gersony WM. Propranolol administration during pregnancy: effects on the fetus. Pediatrics 1975; 86:962–964.
13. Pruyn SC, Phelan JP, Buchanan GC. Long term propranolol therapy in pregnancy: maternal and fetal outcome. Am J Obstet Gynecol 1979; 135:485–489.
14. Cottle MKW, Van Petten GR, van Muyden P. Maternal and fetal cardiovascular indices during fetal hypoxia due to cord compression in chronically cannulated sheep. Am J Obstet Gynecol 1983; 146:678–685.
15. Plouin PF, Breart G, Maillard F, Relier JP, Breart G, Papiernik E, the Labetalol Methyl Dopa Study Group. Comparison of antihypertensive efficacy and perinatal safety of labetalol and methyldopa in the treatment of hypertension in pregnancy: a randomized controlled trial. Br J Obstet Gynecol 1988; 95:868–876.
16. Horvath JS, Phippard A, Korda A, Henderson-Smart DJ, Child A, Tiller DJ. Clonidine hydrochloride-a safe and effective antihypertensive agent in pregnancy. Obstet Gynecol 1985; 66:634–638.
17. Waisman GD, Davis N, Davey DA, et al. Magnesium plus nifedipine: Potentiation of hypotensive effect in preeclampsia? Am J Obstet Gynecol 1988; 159:308–309.
18. Dynder SW, Cardwell MS. Neuromuscular blockade with magnesium sulfate and nifedipine. Am J Obstet Gynecol 1988; 161:35–36.
19. Kaler SG, Patrinos ME, Lambert GH, Myers TF, Karlman R, Anderson CL. Hypertrichosis and congenital anomalies associated with maternal use of minoxidil. Pediatrics 1987; 79:434–436.
20. Bhorat IE, Naidoo DP, Rout CC, Moodley J. Malignant ventricular arrhythmias in eclampsia: a comparison of labetolol with dihydralazine. Am J Obstet Gynecol 1993; 168:1292–1296.
21. Sibai BM. Drug therapy: treatment of hypertension in pregnant women. N Engl J Med 1996; 335:257–265.
22. Hedstrom S, Martens MG. Antibiotics in pregnancy. Clin Obstet Gynecol 1993; 36:886–892.
23. Jacobi P, Ohel G, Szylman P, Levit A, Lewin M, Paldi E. Continuous ambulatory peritoneal dialysis as the primary approach in the management of severe renal insufficiency in pregnancy. Obstet Gynecol 1992; 79: 808–810.
24. Gadallah MF, Ahmad B, Karubian F, Campese VM. Pregnancy in patients on chronic ambulatory peritoneal dialysis. Am J Kidney Dis 1992; 20:407–410.
25. Tison A, Lozowy C, Benjamin A, Usher R, Pritchard S. Successful pregnancy complicated by peritonitis in a 35-year-old CAPD patient. Perit Dial Int 1996; 16: S489–S491.
26. Hou SH, Orlowski J, Pahl M, Ambrose S, Hussey M, Wong D. Pregnancy in women with end stage renal disease: treatment of anemia and premature labor. Am J Dis Kidney 1993; 21:16–22.
27. Redrow M, Cherem L, Elliot J, Mangalat J, Mishler RE, Bennet WM, Lutz M, Sigala J, Byrnes J, Phillipe M, Hou S, Schon D. Dialysis in the management of pregnant patients with renal insufficiency. Medicine 1988; 67:199–208.
28. Romão JE, Luders C, Kahhale S, Pascoal IJF, Abensur H, Sabbaga E, Zugaib M, Marcondes M. Pregnancy in women on chronic dialysis. Nephron 1998; 78:416–422.
29. Ginsberg JS, Kowalchuk G, Hirsh J, Brill-Edwards P, Burrows R. Heparin therapy during pregnancy. Arch Intern Med 1989; 149:2233–2236.
30. Lester GL: Cholecalciferol and placental calcium transfer. Fed Proc 1986; 2524–2527.
31. Marx SJ, Swart EG, Hamstra AJ, DeLuca HF. Normal intrauterine development of the fetus of a woman receiving extraordinarily high doses of 1,25, dihydroxyvitamin D_3. J Clin Endocrinol Metab 1980; 51:1138–1142.
32. Brookhyser J, Wiggins K. Medical nutrition therapy in pregnancy and kidney disease. Adv Ren Replacement Ther 1998; 5:53–63.
33. Czeizel AE, Dudás I. Prevention of the first occurrence of neural tube defects by periconceptional vitamin supplementation. N Engl J Med 1992; 327:1832–1835.
34. Pitkin RM and Committee on Nutritional Status During Pregnancy and Lactation, Institute of Medicine, National Academy of Sciences, eds. Nutrition During Pregnancy, Washington, DC: National Academy Press, 1990.
35. Hussey MJ, Pombar X. Obstetric care for renal allograft recipients or for women treated with hemodialysis or

peritoneal dialysis during pregnancy. Adv Ren Replacement Ther 1998; 5:3–13.

36. Bommer J, Kugel M, Schwobel B, Ritz E, Barth HP, Seelig R. Improved sexual function during recombinant human erythropoietin therapy. Nephrol Dial Transplant 1990; 5:204–207.
37. Lim VS, Kathpalia SC, Frohman LA. Hyperprolactinemia and impaired pituitary response to suppression and stimulation in chronic renal failure: reversal after transplantation. J Clin Endocrin Metab 1979; 48:101–107.
38. Hou SH, Grossman S, Molitch ME. Hyperprolactinemia in patients with renal insufficiency and chronic renal failure requiring hemodialysis or continuous ambulatory peritoneal dialysis. Am J Kidney Dis 1985; 6: 245–249.
39. Gomez F, De La Cueva R, Wauters JP, Lemarchand-Béraud T. Endocrine abnormalities in patients undergoing long-term dialysis. Am J Med 1980; 68:522–530.
40. Muir JW, Besser GM, Edwards CRW, Rees LH, Cattell, Ackrill P, Baker LRI. Bromocriptine improves reduced libido and potency in men receiving maintenance hemodialysis. Clin Nephrol 1983; 26:308–314.
41. Saag KG, Emkey R, Schnitzer TJ, Brown JP, Hawkins F, Goemaere S, Thamsborg G, Liberman UA, Delmas PD, Malice MP, Czachur M, Daifotis AG, Glucocorticoid-Induced Osteoporosis Study Group. Alendronate for the prevention and treatment of glucocorticoid-induced osteoporosis. N Engl J Med 1998; 339:292–299.
42. Harnett JD, et al. Recurrent hemoperitoneum in women receiving continuous ambulatory peritoneal dialysis. Ann Intern Med 1987; 107:341.
43. Poole CL, et al. Aseptic peritonitis associated with menstruation and ovulation in a peritoneal dialysis patient. In Khanna R, et al., eds. Advances in Continuous Ambulatory Peritoneal Dialysis. Toronto: Peritoneal Dialysis Bulletin, 1987.
44. Hampton HL, Whitworth NS, Cowan BD. Gonadotropin-releasing hormone agonist (leuprolide acetate) induced ovarian hyperstimulation syndrome in a woman undergoing intermittent hemodialysis. Fertil Steril 1991; 55:429.
45. Nakamura Y, Yoshimura Y. Treatment of uterine heronyomias in premenopausal women with gonadotropin-releasing hormone agonists. In Pitkin RM and Scott JR, ed. Clinical Obstetrics and Gynecology 36: 9/93.

41

Complications During Plasma Exchange

André A. Kaplan
University of Connecticut Health Center, Farmington, Connecticut

I. TECHNIQUES

A. Standard Plasmapheresis

Automated plasma exchange was originally performed with centrifugation devices used in blood blanking procedures. These devices offer the advantage of allowing for selective cell removal (cytapheresis) (1). Plasma exchange can also be performed with a highly permeable filter and standard dialysis equipment, a technique often referred to as membrane plasma separation (MPS) (2). A detailed review of the available removal systems has been provided by Sowada et al. (3).

Centrifugal systems utilize G forces to separate the plasma into its different components. Separation of the plasma can be either intermittent or continuous. In the intermittent system, whole blood is collected into a receptacle (bowl) and centrifuged down to its plasma and cellular components. After separation, the cellular components are resuspended in an appropriate amount of replacement solution (e.g., albumin, fresh frozen plasma) and subsequently returned to the patient. Newer devices utilize a continuous flow system in which the whole blood is processed in an ongoing, online manner.

Separation of plasma from the blood's cellular components can also be accomplished by filtration through a highly permeable membrane. This methodology separates the blood into its cellular and noncellular components by subjecting it to sieving through a membrane whose pores allow the plasma proteins to pass but that retain the larger cellular elements within the blood path. Configuration of the semi-permeable membrane can be in a layered flat plate design (3), rolled in a tube (4), or in bundles of hollow fibers (2). The hollow fiber configuration can be used with standard dialysis equipment with the filter connected to the blood pump and pressure monitoring system while the dialysis machine is utilized in its "isolated" ultrafiltration mode, which bypasses the dialysate proportioning system.

B. Selective Plasmapheresis

Many imaginative techniques have been designed to selectively remove a particular pathogenic substance from the plasma, allowing the majority of the plasma to be returned to the patient, thus minimizing the risks of depletion coagulopathy and hypogammaglobulinemia (Table 1) (5).

Cascade filtration or double filtration plasmapheresis is a selective method of plasma fractionation in which the whole plasma separated from the cellular components is refiltered through a secondary filter with a smaller pore size in order to separate out the larger, unwanted molecules (6). This type of selective removal will limit the amount of replacement fluid required by allowing most of the smaller molecules, such as albumin (60,000 daltons), to return to the patient. This methodology has been used to selectively remove the relatively large β-lipoproteins (approximately 1 million daltons), IgM (900,000 daltons), cryoglobulins, and immune complexes.

Cryofiltration is a technique in which the removed plasma is subjected to cooling, causing certain pathogenic substances to aggregate, thus increasing their overall size and allowing for efficient secondary filtra-

Table 1 Plasmapheresis Techniques

Standard Plasmapheresis
Centrifugation
Plasma exchange
Cytapheresis
Filtration
Membrane plasma separation
Selective Plasmapheresis
Cascade filtration
Cryofiltration
Lipid apheresis
LDL immunoadsorption
Dextran binding
HELP system
Immunoadsorption
Protein A
Polymyxin B
Others

tion (7). The process can be used to selectively remove cyroglobulins and immune complexes.

Selective lipid-removal techniques are employed for the treatment of hypercholesterolemia and can limit the loss of non–lipid-containing plasma proteins and the desirable high-density lipoprotein (HDL) cholesterol. Of these, three have undergone extensive clinical trials. One is an immunoadsorbant system in which plasma is perfused over sepharose beads coated with antibodies against low-density lipoprotein (LDL) (8). Another is a dextran sulfate system by which negatively charged dextran molecules are covalently bound to the positively charged apoprotein B lipoproteins (9), and a third is known as the HELP system and involves the extracorporeal precipitation of LDL lipoproteins by negatively charged heparin (10).

C. Immunoadsorbant Techniques

There are several commercially available systems for selective immunoadsorption of a variety of targets. These systems may be designed for nonselective adsorption of immunoglobulins, such as those employing protein A, or for more selective targets, such as those mentioned above for the specific immunoadsorption of LDL cholesterol.

Protein A is a 42,000 dalton protein released from certain strains of *Staphylococcus aureus*, which can be used for the ex vivo adsorption of three of the four classes of IgG (1, 2, and 4). Binding occurs at a particular site on the heavy chain of the immunoglobulin, leaving binding sites for complement and antigens unaffected (11). These devices may work by immunomodulation, with activation of immune modulators, or by net removal of immunoglobulin.

Selective adsorption of endotoxin can be accomplished by filters impregnated with polymyxin B, an antibiotic that has the particular propensity to bind endotoxin fragments (12).

D. Anticoagulation

Regardless of the technique employed, therapeutic plasma exchange (TPE) will normally require some form of anticoagulation in order to avoid clotting within the extracorporeal circuit. For centrifugal techniques, this is often provided by citrate infusions, which bind ionized calcium in the extracorporeal circuit such that the coagulation cascade is impeded. The ionized calcium level returns towards its original level as the blood is returned to the intravascular compartment where there are substantial stores of ionized calcium and where the citrate will be metabolized to bicarbonate. Rapid infusions of citrate may exceed the patient's capability to metabolize citrate and may lead to hypocalcemia and alkalosis (see below). Membrane plasma separation, using plasma-permeable filters, commonly employs heparin anticoagulation in a manner analogous to that used for hemodialysis.

II. COMPLICATIONS OF TPE

Several reviews have outlined the potential risks of TPE (13–15), but there have been only a few large series that allow the clinician to assess the incidence of these complications (16–24). Reports from these nine series, involving more than 15,000 TPE treatments, reveal that the most common complications are citrate-induced parethesias, muscle cramps, and urticaria (Table 2) (23). Serious complications are reported at a rate of 0.025–0.2% and include life-threatening anaphylactoid reactions, which are most commonly associated with the use of plasma-containing replacement fluids (e.g., fresh frozen plasma, purified protein fraction) (25). The overall incidence of death is 0.05%, but some of these "treatment-associated" deaths were in patients with severe preexisting conditions, and the TPE treatment per se may not have been the precipitating factor.

A. Citrate-Induced Hypocalcemia

During TPE, citrate may be infused either as the anticoagulant or in the fresh frozen plasma (FFP) admin-

Table 2 Complications of Plasmapheresis

	Centrifugal system					Membrane-based system			Both
	Borberg (16)	Aufeuvre et al. (17)	Ziselman et al. (18)	Fabre et al. (19)	Rossi et al. (20)	Sprenger et al. (21)	Samtleben et al. (22)	Mokrzycki et al. (23)	Sutton et. al. (24)
No. of treatments	205	3,086	1,389	578	926	306	120	699	5,235
Adverse reactions	13%	22%	1.6%	25%	17.3%	4.2%	17.5%	9.7%	12%
Mild	0%	4.8%	0.4*	}23%	7.6%	0	5	5.4%	9%
Moderate	11.2%	16.4%	0.6%		6.5%	4.2	12.5%	2.4%	3%
Severe	2%	0.6%	0.5%	1.5%	3.1%	0	0	0.7%	0.5%
Deaths	0	0.1%	0.1%	0	0	0	0	0	0
Symptoms									
Urticaria				12%		0.7%	8.3%	2.4%	3.7%
Paresthesias	1.5%			9%	2.4%		5%	1.7%	}2.5%
Muscle cramps								0.4%	
Dizziness		15.8%							
Headaches				1%	5%			0.3%	1.2%
Nausea			0.1%	0.2%	1%			0.6%	1.5%
Hypotension			0.4%	0.5%	1.6%	2%	4.2%	1.4%	2.3%
Chest pain		0.03%	0.1%					1.3%	0.2%
Dysrhythmia				0.2%	0.7%			0.1%	0.1%
Anaphylactoid reactions	0.05%	0.03%						0.7%	0.5%
Rigors	8.8%				1.1%				
Hyperthermia	1.0%	5.3%		0.7%					
Bronchospasm					0.4%				0.1%
Seizure		0.03%							0.4%
Respiratory arrest/ Pulmonary edema		0.3%		0.2%					
Myocardial ischemia			0.1%						
Shock/MI	1.5%	0.1%	0.1%						
Metabolic alkalosis		0.03%							
DIC		0.03%							
CNS ischemia		0.03%	0.1%						
Other			0.3%		0.8%				0.8%
Hepatitis				0.7%					
Hemorrhage					0.2%				
Hypoxemia			0.1%						
Pulmonary embolism			0.1%						
Access related									
Thrombosis/hemorrhage							0.7%	0.02%	
Infection							0.3%		
Pneumothorax							0.1%		
Mechanical			0.4%	1.2%	4%	1.5%			0.08%

MI = Myocardial infarction; DIC = disseminated intravascular coagulation; CNS = central nervous system.
Source: Adapted from Ref. 23.

istered as the replacement fluid. Symptoms of citrate-induced hypocalcemia represent one of the most common complications and can occur in up to 9% of treatments (23). The incidence is highest in those treatments utilizing FFP as the replacement fluid, since this preparation is approximately 15% citrate by volume. Most often the patient will complain of perioral or distal extremity tingling or paresthesias. If severe, citrate-induced hypocalcemia may be associated with prolongation of the QT interval on electrocardiogram, thus increasing the risk of cardiac arrhythmia (26,27).

Widely used protocols suggest that citrate toxicity can be reasonably well controlled with the oral administration of calcium tablets during the procedure, reserving intravenous calcium replacement only for those who develop symptoms. Another conservative approach involves decreasing the rate of plasma exchange and decreasing the citrate to blood ratio and supplementing with heparin (24,28,29). Others have found that prophylactic replacement of intravenous calcium can significantly reduce the incidence of citrate-induced paresthesias (23,30,31). In an in-depth review of the topic, Hester et al. concluded that the incidence of citrate-induced hypocalcemic symptoms could be reduced if the citrate-infusion rate was limited to between 1.0 and 1.8 mg/kg/min (26). If symptoms occurred despite this limitation, they recommended an infusion of 10 mL of 10% calcium gluconate infused over 15 minutes approximately halfway through the procedure.

Kinetic studies have demonstrated that increases in parathyroid hormone provide an endogenous compensatory response to calcium removal during TPE (28), but patients receiving multiple treatments with albumin replacement may experience a significant loss of calcium amounting to approximately 150 mg per treatment (31). In contrast, with supplementation calcium balance can be positive.

Uhl et al. described a case of severe citrate toxicity when the citrate infusion line became disengaged from its rotary pump allowing a massive infusion of citrate into the patient (32). Seven minutes into the procedure, the patient developed signs and symptoms suggesting severe hypocalcemia, including muscle spasms, chest pain, and hypotension. Ionized calcium level was 0.64 mmol/L (normal range, 1.18–1.38 mmol/L).

B. Coagulation Abnormalities

1. "Depletion" Coagulopathy

Albumin solutions used for replacement fluid are devoid of clotting factors, and a TPE treatment with albumin as the replacement fluid will result in a depletion of all coagulation factors, including fibrinogen and antithrombin III (AT-III) (25,33,34). After a single plasma exchange, the serum levels of most of these factors will be decreased by approximately 40–60% (Table 3). Serum levels of these factors rebound in a biphasic manner, characterized by a rapid initial increase in the first 4 hours after treatment, followed by a slower increase over the next few days (23). This dual rate of recovery represents two phenomena: a reequilibration of extravascular stores with the intravascular compartment and a resynthesis of new clotting factors. Twenty-four hours after treatment, fibrinogen levels are 50% and AT-III levels are 85% of initial levels, while both factors may require 48–72 hours for complete recovery (23). Prothrombin time (PT) increases 30% and partial thromboplastin time (PTT) doubles immediately after a one plasma volume exchange (31,35). Partial thromboplastin time and thrombin time are back to normal range 4 hours postpheresis, while prothrombin time normalizes in 24 hours (25).

When multiple treatments are performed over a short period (three or more treatments per week), the depletion in clotting factors is more pronounced and may require several days for spontaneous recovery (33–35). Under these conditions, the risks of hemorrhage can be minimized by substituting between 500 and 1000 mL (2–4 units) of FFP as the replacement fluid towards the end of the procedure. This approach is most helpful in patients who are immediately post-surgery (e.g., thymectomy for myasthenia gravis), who have had a recent renal biopsy (e.g., glomerulonephritis), who have active hemoptysis (Goodpasture's syndrome or Wegener's granulomatosis), or in whom there is a desire for the immediate removal of a large-bore intravascular catheter.

Table 3 Percent Decrease in Serum Levels of Coagulation Factors After a Single Plasma Exchange

Factor	Percent
Fibrinogen	20
Prothrombin	40
Factor V	42
Factor VII	47
Factor VIII	50
Factor IX	57
Factor X	32
AT-III	42

Source: Modified from Ref. 33.

2. Thrombocytopenia

Thrombocytopenia may result from a loss of platelets in the discarded plasma, as a result of thrombosis within the plasma filter, as a consequence of heparin-induced antiplatelet antibodies, or as a result of a mild dilutional effect by the infusion of 5% albumin solution, which is relatively hyperoncotic compared to the removed plasma (36). With the older centrifugal machines such as the Haemonetics V-50 (Haemonetics, Braintree, MA), inefficient separation of the different plasmatic components resulted in platelet losses with the discarded plasma, and these treatments have been associated with decreases in platelet counts of up to 50%. The newer centrifugal devices provide more efficient separation of the plasmatic components and a more modest loss of platelets. Membrane plasma separation (MPS) can result in a 15% decrease in platelet count, possibly related to partial thrombosis within the filter (1,25,31,37). Because heparin is more commonly used as the anticoagulant, heparin-induced antiplatelet antibodies are also more likely to occur with MPS.

3. Anemia

Posttreatment decreases in hematocrit may result from hemorrhage associated with the vascular access, from substantial clotting in the extracorporeal circuit, or from treatment-related hemolysis. Initiation of treatment with a membrane plasma separator is often associated with a minimal amount of plasma tinting, which is rarely a cause for significant blood loss and can be quantified by measuring the free hemoglobin levels in the collected plasma. In most cases, plasma tinting lasts for only a few seconds; if persistent, the blood flow should be slowed in order to lower the transmembrane pressure. Hemolysis can also occur in centrifugal systems as a result of hypotonic priming solutions. Even in the absence of any extracorporeal losses or hemolysis, hematocrits may decrease by 10% after each treatment, a phenomenon that may be due to intravascular expansion related to the use of relatively hyperoncotic replacement fluids (5% albumin) (31,36,38).

4. Thrombosis

TPE treatments using albumin replacement will cause a relative depletion of all coagulation factors, including inhibitors of coagulation such as AT-III. In one report, two episodes of thrombosis were associated with a postpheresis depletion of AT-III and this deficiency may have resulted in a hypercoaguable state (39). Thrombosis has also been associated with the prolonged use of indwelling vascular catheters (23). Pulmonary embolism, cerebral ischemia, and myocardial infarction have been reported to occur in association with TPE, but the incidence is rare (0.06–0.14%) (18,40). An association with low levels of AT-III is speculative, especially since these patients will also have a concomitant depletion of "pro" coagulant factors (see above).

C. Infections

Aside from the infections related to indwelling vascular catheters, the risk of infection associated with TPE can be divided into two broad categories: those that may be the result of a posttreatment depletion of immunoglobulins, a situation most likely to occur when the replacement fluid is mostly albumin, and those that occur as a result of viral transmission from the replacement fluid, most likely to occur when the replacement fluid is fresh frozen plasma.

1. Postpheresis Infection

TPE using albumin as the replacement fluid will result in a predictable decline in levels of immunoglobulins and complement and may predispose patients to high rates of infection. One plasma volume exchange will result in a 60% reduction in serum immunoglobulin levels and a net 20% reduction in total body immunoglobulin stores (31,36). Multiple treatments over short periods, especially when associated with immunosuppressive agents, will yield more substantive decreases in immunoglobulin levels that may persist for several weeks (41,42). Although concentrations of C3 and C4 may be reduced by a series of daily treatments, because of rapid resynthesis (short half-lives), levels of these proteins rebound within several days. CH50 can be predictably lowered to about 40% of its initial value immediately after a given treatment but rebound to pretreatment values occurs within one day, and even repetitive daily treatments have a minimal effect on this parameter (41). Therapeutic plasma exchange with FFP replacement would not be expected to deplete immunoglobulin or complement levels.

The incidence of infection in patients undergoing TPE varies widely. Wing et al. compared the incidence of infection in patients with rapidly progressive glomerulonephritis (RPGN) who received standard therapy (steroids and cytotoxic agents) with or without plasma exchange (43). The apheresis-treated group had a higher occurrence of infection, but some of the control cases were taken from retrospective review and granulocytopenia was present in two of the five TPE-treated patients who developed infections, a condition that was more likely the result of the cytotoxic therapy than from the plasma exchange procedure per se. In other studies of RPGN, 9 episodes of infection were found in 34 patients treated with TPE and immunosuppression, 4 of which resulted in death (44–52). Two of these nine patients were granulocytopenic (44,50). Patients treated with TPE for myasthenia gravis appear to have a lower incidence of infection than those treated for renal disease (53–57). Of thirty-six patients with myasthenia gravis treated with TPE in addition to prednisone and azathioprine, only one patient developed an infectious complication after a mean follow-up period of 9 months (55).

There has been only one prospective, randomized trial that has attempted to disassociate the risk of infection associated with TPE and that associated with the commonly co-administered immunosuppressive medication. In this study, Pohl et al. studied 86 patients with lupus nephritis receiving cyclophosphamide and steroids, with or without TPE (58). These investigators found no increase in the rate of infection or in infection-related deaths in the apheresis-treated group. In patients treated with TPE, the infection rate was 1.22 infections per 200 weeks with three deaths, compared with 1.15 infections per 200 weeks and four deaths in the control group. Thus, in the only prospective study in which the effect of TPE could be isolated from that of drug-induced immunosuppression, treatment with TPE was not associated with any increased risk of infection.

Although the study by Pohl et al. did not find an increased risk of infection due to the addition of TPE to an already aggressive immunosuppressive regimen, there remains the possibility that immunoglobulin or complement depletion may impair a patient's ability to combat an ongoing infection. Thus, if a severe infection develops in the immediate postpheresis period, a reasonable approach would be to reconstitute normal immunoglobulin levels with a single infusion of IVIG (100–400 mg/kg intravenously) (23), similar to the replacement dose recommended in patients with hypo- or agammaglobulinemia (59,60). Because of the relatively long half-life of IgG (21 days), this approach will provide normalized immunoglobulin levels for several weeks, provided there are no further TPE treatments.

2. Risk of Viral Transmission

Risk of viral transmission during plasma exchange is directly related to replacement with FFP or other plasma-containing solutions (e.g., purified protein fraction, cryosupernatant). Albumin preparations are treated with heat and are considered to be devoid of transmissible virus (61). The same claims had been made for intravenous immunoglobulins, but an outbreak of hepatitis C from contaminated IVIG has been documented (62), promoting the initiation of new methodologies for avoiding viral transmission from IVIG preparations (63). In a review of listed complications from over 15,000 treatments, there was only one reported case of latent non-A/non-B hepatitis infection (19). Transmission of the human immunodeficiency virus (HIV) through therapeutic plasmapheresis is unlikely and would be anticipated as the result of infected FFP (64). There has been a documented case of HIV transmission to a patient treated with TPE for Guillain-Barré syndrome, but the report dates from a period in which screening for HIV-infected plasma was less well established (65). The current incidence of transfusion-acquired viral infections has declined substantially from the early 1980s and is currently estimated as 1/63,000 units for hepatitis B, 1/100,000 units for hepatitis C, 1/680,000 units for HIV, and 1/641,000 units for HTLV (66–68) (Table 4). This risk of viral transmission can be further reduced with the use of solvent detergent (SD)–treated plasma. SD-treated plasma is a cell-free, blood group–specific, coagulation-active human plasma, which has been treated in a manner to irreversibly inactivate the lipid envelope of viruses such as HIV1 and 2, HBV, and HCV and has been approved by European guidelines and the U.S. Food and Drug Administration (FDA) (69,70). Since FFP is normally provided in units of 200–300 mL, a single plasma volume exchange will involve the infusion of 10–15 units. Thus, the most compelling indication for the use of SD-treated plasma would be in a noninfected individual who is being treated for throm-

Table 4 Risk of Transfusion-Transmitted Viral Infections per Unit Transfused in the Mid-1990s

HIV	1/680,000
HCV	1/103,000
HTLV	1/641,000
HBV	1/63,000

Estimates are for the United States and assume the use of modern screening tests. Currently available solvent/detergent-treated plasma can decrease the risk of viral transmission (see text).
Source: Refs. 31–33.

botic thrombocytopenic purpura, in whom a common treatment protocol may involve multiple treatments and numerous units of FFP.

III. COMPLICATIONS RELATED TO REPLACEMENT FLUIDS

A. General Comments

In the United States, albumin is the most commonly used replacement fluid and, when compared to FFP, has the advantage of lacking viral transmission and possessing a decreased risk of anaphylactoid reactions. Disadvantages include a posttreatment coagulopathy related to the removal of clotting factors and a net loss of immunoglobulins. A 5% concentration of albumin will provide a reasonable replacement of the oncotic pressure removed with the patient's plasma (see below). Some centers prefer to dilute the albumin to approximately 3.5%, a solution that is hypo-oncotic to the plasma being removed and may render the patient more prone to hypotension. Dilution of albumin with sterile water, as opposed to saline, has been associated with hemolysis and should be avoided (71).

FFP contains all the noncellular components of normal blood and does not lead to postpheresis coagulopathy or immunoglobulin depletion. FFP is also considered essential for the treatment of thrombotic thrombocytopenic purpura (TTP) since TPE for this indication may be most useful as a means of providing a missing serum factor (72). Disadvantages include anaphylactoid reactions (most often mild, but can be life-threatening), citrate toxicity, and a small, but persistent risk of viral transmission. Because of these potential problems, FFP should be avoided except for the treatment of TTP/HUS or when hemorrhagic risks are great.

Plasma protein fraction (PPF) contains approximately 87% albumin and 13% α- and β-globulins and is easier and less costly to prepare than albumin. Although difficult to prove, the risks of anaphylactoid reaction with PPF are probably less than for that of FFP. Nonetheless, PPF has been associated with hypotensive episodes and circulatory collapse, possibly due to the presence of prekallikrein activator and bradykinin (61). As with the use of FFP, concomitant treatment with ACE inhibitors should be avoided.

B. Reactions to Protein-Containing Replacement Fluids

Reactions to plasma-containing fluids (FFP, PPF, cryosupernatant) are anaphylactoid in nature and are characterized by fever, rigors, urticaria, wheezing, and hypotension and may eventually progress to laryngospasm (73,74). This type of pulmonary distress is clearly in distinction to that of the pulmonary edema that may accompany fluid overload, in which the patient is often hypertensive and is unlikely to have associated urticaria, wheezing, and laryngospasm. In a review of several large series, the reported incidence of this type of reaction was between 0.02% and 21% (23) (Table 2). Most reactions are limited to urticaria and rigors, but the potential for life-threatening reactions is underscored by the list of 42 TPE-associated deaths compiled by Huestis, at least 30 of which were associated with FFP replacement (75). Similarly, Aufeuvre et al. reported seven deaths in 6200 treatments including nonhemodynamic pulmonary edema associated with FFP replacement (17,40). Sutton et al., in their review of over 5000 treatments from the Canadian Red Cross, reported 8 patients with severe reactions comprised of severe urticaria, itching, shortness of breath, and wheezing and noted that all 8 patients had been receiving plasma (76).

Human serum albumin consists of 96% albumin and trace amounts of α- and β-globulins, and, as opposed to FFP, anaphylactoid reactions are rare and may be associated with the formation of antibodies to polymerized albumin created by heat treatment or stabilization with sodium caprylate (61,77). Recent reports have suggested that patients taking ACE inhibitors may also been prone to an increased risk of "atypical" or hypotensive reactions to albumin (78,79).

Potential mechanisms triggering the anaphylactoid reactions described above include; (1) the presence of anti-IgA antibodies in a patient who is IgA deficient and who is receiving IgA-containing fluids (i.e. FFP, immunoglobulins); (2) contamination of the replacement fluid with bacteria, endotoxins or pyrogens; (3) the presence of a prekallikrein activator and bradykinin; and (4) the formation of antibodies to polymerized albumin (80).

C. Management

Because of the relative high incidence of these reactions, patients undergoing massive replacement with FFP (i.e. for thrombotic thrombocytopenic purpura or hemolytic uremic syndrome) are commonly pretreated with 50 mg of diphenhydramine (Benadry). In those patients who have already demonstrated a sensitivity to FFP, and in whom FFP replacement is obligatory (i.e. TTP), a successful prophylactic regimen has included 50 mg of prednisone given 13 hours, 7 hours and 1

hour before the treatment, 50 mg of diphenhydramine given 1 hour before the treatment and 25 mg of ephedrine given 1 hour before the treatment (80). Epinephrine should be available in the event of a severe life threatening reaction (laryngeal edema, etc).

IV. REACTIONS TO SELECTIVE REMOVAL TECHNIQUES

A. Protein A Columns

Protein A is a 42,000 dalton protein released from certain strains of *Staphylococcus aureus* which can be attached to sepharose, collodion charcoal, or silica and can be used for the ex vivo adsorption of three of the four classes of IgG (1, 2 and 4). The Prosorba protein A column is a single-use, nonregenerating system which is placed in series with a standard plasma exchange circuit and is FDA approved for idiopathic thrombocytopenic purpura (ITP).

Secondary effects during use of the Prosorba protein A column are common. In one large series involving 142 patients and 1306 treatments, 79% of patients experienced at least one episode of toxicity during the procedure (81). The most common side effects were fever, chills, and musculoskeletal pains, but more severe reactions, such as hypotension, were also noted. These secondary effects may result from the release of activated complement products and seem to be the basis for the recommendation that plasma perfused over the device not be reinfused into the patient at a rate exceeding 20 mL/min. For similar reasons, the device should not be used in patients who are currently taking ACE inhibitors, since these drugs block the degradation of bradykinins and may result in a severe anaphylactoid reactions as treated plasma is reinfused into the patient (78). A recent report suggests that this treatment was the cause of a systemic vasculitis (82).

B. Selective Lipid Removal

There are three conceptually different methods for the selective removal of cholesterol-containing lipoproteins. An evaluation of all three of these techniques found them to be equally biocompatible and equally efficacious in lowering LDL-associated cholesterol (83). Two reports, however, have warned of anaphylactoid reactions in patients treated with the dextran sulfate–based system in whom there was concurrent treatment with ACE inhibitors (84,85).

V. ATYPICAL REACTIONS ASSOCIATED WITH ACE INHIBITORS

Aside from their effect on the angiotensin system, ACE inhibitors will also block the degradation of bradykinins and may result in severe anaphylactoid reactions if a given apheresis procedure results in the activation of kinins or if there is a high concentration of these factors in the replacement fluid. Flushing, hypotension, abdominal cramping, and occasionally severe anaphylactoid reactions have been reported with the use of the dextran sulfate system for selective lipid removal (84,85), and in patients treated with the IMRE Prosorba column (85). A recent report describes such atypical reactions in those patients receiving albumin replacement during standard apheresis (78). In one large review, all (100%) of fourteen patients who were receiving ACE inhibitor therapy during apheresis procedures experienced atypical reactions defined as flushing or hypotension (decrease of 20 mmHg or more) (79). In contrast, only 20 (7%) of 285 patients not receiving ACE inhibitors developed atypical reactions ($p < 0.001$). The authors concluded that ACE inhibitors should be withheld for at least 24 hours before apheresis.

VI. ELECTROLYTE ABNORMALITIES

A. Hypokalemia

Five percent albumin solutions are isosmotic to plasma and contain less than 2 mEq/L of potassium (61). As a result, a 25% reduction in serum potassium levels may occur in the immediate postpheresis period (86), and there is the potential for hypokalemic arrhythmias during apheresis and in the immediate postpheresis period. Experience with hemodialysis suggests that this type of hypokalemic arrhythmia is most likely to occur in the presence of digoxin and when potassium levels approach 2 mEq/L (87). Considering the above, we follow a protocol by which we add 4 mEq/L of potassium to each liter of 5% albumin.

B. Alkalosis

Citrate, infused either as the anticoagulant or in the replacement fluid, will be metabolized to bicarbonate and can result in a substantial alkalemia. Formula B citrate solution (Fenwal, Baxter, Deerfield, IL) contains 73 mmol/L of citrate, which will yield 219 mmol/L of bicarbonate, while formula A citrate solution contains 112 mmol/L of citrate which will yield 336 mmol/L of bicarbonate. Fresh frozen plasma contains approxi-

mately 14% citrate by volume. In most patients, postpheresis bicarbonate levels are unchanged (86). In patients with renal failure, severe alkalemia may result from repeated treatments, especially when FFP is used as the replacement (88). In a most challenging situation, a patient with hemolytic uremic syndrome may require massive amounts of FFP while suffering from severe renal failure. In this case, alkalemia may necessitate frequent dialysis in order to remove the excess bicarbonate. Because of this postpheresis alkalemia, if TPE and hemodialysis are required on the same day, it is preferable to perform the TPE first in order to allow the dialysis treatment to correct the citrate-induced alkalemia.

C. Aluminum

All albumin solutions are contaminated with between 4 and 24 mmol/L of aluminum (89,90), and repetitive TPE with albumin may result in significant accumulation of aluminum. In patients with severe renal insufficiency, 60%–70% of infused aluminum is retained (90). Bone deposition of aluminum has also been reported in a patient with normal renal function (89,90).

VII. VITAMIN REMOVAL

Blood concentrations of vitamins B_{12}, B_6, A, C, and E and β-carotene have been noted to decline between 24% and 48% after a single TPE treatment, but rebound to pretreatment levels occurs within 24 hours (91). Possibly because of their large volumes of distribution as water-soluble vitamins, folate, thiamine, nicotinate, biotin, riboflavin, and pantothenate are not significantly altered by plasma exchange. The long-term effects of repetitive treatments is not known, but net removal of the protein-bound vitamin B_{12} is approximately 900 μg per treatment (31), and there is the potential for a substantial reduction in total body stores after repetitive treatments.

VIII. HYPOTENSION

The reported incidence of hypotension during TPE is 1.7% (Table 2), but the actual incidence is probably higher and dependent on its definition. Hypotension during TPE may occur for a variety of reasons, including delayed or inadequate volume replacement, vasovagal episodes, hypo-oncotic fluid replacement, anaphylaxis, cardiac arrhythmia, bradykinin reactions (e.g., reactions to ACE inhibitors), vascular access–induced external or internal hemorrhage, and cardiovascular collapse (Table 5) (these issues are discussed in detail in the previous sections). Discontinuous flow plasma exchange systems may be prone to a higher incidence of hypotensive episodes due to intermittent hypovolemia. The use of hypo-oncotic replacement solutions may also increase the risk of hypotensive events. A commonly employed preparation of replacement fluid is to dilute albumin with an electrolyte solution to achieve a concentration of 3.5% albumin. In most patients this solution is clearly hypo-oncotic to the patient's plasma and may predispose them to hypotension, even when a policy of 1:1 volume replacement is rigorously followed. An undiluted 5% albumin solution is less likely to produce a hypo-oncotic hypovolemia, except when pretreatment plasma volumes are abnormally expanded by a hyperviscosity state (Waldenstrom's macroglobulinemia).

IX. MISCELLANEOUS COMPLICATIONS

Respiratory arrest due to apnea has been reported following plasma exchange in patients who had been anesthetized with succinylcholine (40,92). Succinylcholine is an anesthetic agent that is metabolized by cholinesterase, and these apneic events were considered to be the result of abnormally low posttreatment levels of plasma cholinesterase. Cholinesterase levels are reduced by 50% immediately after a single treatment (93). Levels less than 30% of normal (approximately 1000 U/L) are likely to be associated with decreased metabolism of succinylcholine (94,95). Since FFP contains normal levels of cholinesterase, depletion of this enzyme is only expected when albumin or PPF is used as replacement. Anesthetic agents dependent on serum cholinesterase for their metabolism should be used with caution immediately post–plasma exchange, especially after a series of daily treatments. Repletion of cholinesterase with FFP may be a reasonable approach for treatments in the immediate perioperative period.

Volume-resistant hypotension, bronchospastic dyspnea, and chest pain may occur secondary to complement-mediated membrane bioincompatibility, similar to those described during hemodialysis (96). Anaphylactoid symptoms may also occur due to ethylene oxide sensitivity, which is used as a sterilizing agent (97). The incidence of filter-related leukocytopenia, thrombocytopenia, and hypo-complementemia is reduced with more biocompatible membranes, and reactions to ethylene oxide can be avoided with adequate priming of the filter (98). Severe hemolysis has occurred as a

Table 5 Potential Causes for Hypotension During TPE

Delayed or inadequate volume replacement
Vasovagal episodes
Hypo-oncotic fluid replacement
3.5% albumin solutions
Anaphylaxis
Reactions to plasma components in replacement fluids
Anti-IgA antibodies (IgA deficient patient)
Endotoxin-contaminated replacement fluid
Reactions to bioincompatible membranes
Sensitivity to ethylene oxide
Device related: Prosorba protein A column
Cardiac arrhythmia
Citrate-induced hypocalcemia
hypokalemic related (especially in patients on digitalis)
Bradykinin reactions (e.g., reactions to ACE inhibitors)
Hemorrhage
Associated with primary disease (ITP, factor VIII inhibitors)
Associated with heparin anticoagulation
Associated with vascular access
External
Internal
"Depletion" coagulopathy
Cardiovascular collapse
Pulmonary embolus
Disease-related hypotension
Guillain-Barré syndrome (autonomic dysfunction)
Waldenstrom's macroglobulinemia (rapid decrease in plasma volume)

result of inappropriately hypotonic priming solutions and from excessively high transmembrane pressure during membrane plasma separation. Chills and other symptoms of hypothermia may be experienced due to inadequately warmed replacement fluid and can be avoided by warming the replacement solutions to body temperature (Table 6).

X. DEATHS

In a review of the literature from 1983, Huestis compiled a total of 42 deaths associated with TPE (75). Of these 42, at least 30 were associated with FFP replacement, 6 were identified as occurring with albumin or PPF, while the replacement solution was uncertain in the remaining 5. The major causes of death were cardiovascular, respiratory, and anaphylactic. Unfortunately, details about these deaths and their temporal relationship to the TPE procedure were not noted. In total, Huestis calculated an estimated 3 deaths per 10,000 procedures.

In a review of 6200 treatments, Aufeuvre et al. reported a total of 7 deaths (17,40). Causes of death included nonhemodynamic pulmonary edema (FFP replacement), cardiac dysrhythmia, hemodynamic pulmonary edema, and pulmonary embolism. In an extensive review of several large series involving over 15,500 treatments, there was a total of 8 deaths, for a calculated incidence of 0.05% (23).

XI. DRUG REMOVAL

A. General Comments

When compared to what is known for hemodialysis or peritoneal dialysis (99), there is little published information regarding the removal of therapeutic agents by TPE. During plasma exchange, alterations in plasma drug levels are most dependent on the percentage of protein binding and the volume of distribution (31,100,101). Thus, a drug with a high percentage of protein binding and a relatively modest volume of distribution (<0.3 L/kg) will have the greatest likelihood of being removed by TPE. Using first-order kinetics and assuming the simplest case, the volume of plasma exchanged during a TPE treatment would have to equal 0.7 times the volume of distribution of a drug in order to remove 50% of its total body burden. Thus, a TPE treatment would have to exchange 7 L of plasma in order to remove 50% of a drug whose volume of distribution is a modest 0.15 L/kg (approximately 10 L in a 70 kg patient). As a result, even a drug with a percentage protein binding of over 90% would be minimally removed if its volume of distribution was ≥0.6 L/kg (≥42 L in a 70 kg patient). It is therefore not surprising that a 3 or 4 L TPE treatment is not commonly used for drug intoxications, despite the fact that many drugs are very highly protein bound

Drug removal information for several drugs are reviewed in the following paragraphs. Since there is a large variability in drug kinetics between individuals, it is recommended that, when possible, all daily drug dosing should be administered after the TPE treatment.

B. Specific Drugs

Indications for plasma exchange often involve the concomitant administration of steroids and immunosuppressive medication. Prednisone has a relatively large volume of distribution (1 L/kg), and despite a protein binding of between 70 and 95% neither it nor its metabolite, prednisolone, is significantly removed by plasma exchange (102). Cyclophosphamide is only

Table 6 Management Strategies to Treat and Avoid Complications of TPE

Complications	Management
Hypocalcemia	Prophylactic calcium administration (10 mL of 10% $CaCl_2$ infused over 15–30 min)
Hemorrhage	Partial FFP replacement in patients at high risk for hemorrhage; evaluate coagulation parameters before catheter removal
Sensitivity to replacement fluids	Consider diagnostic evaluation (e.g., anti-IgA antibody, anti-ethylene oxide antibody, anti-human serum albumin antibody, endotoxin assay, and bacterial cultures of replacement fluid); premedication regimen for sensitized individuals: (1) prednisone 50 mg orally 13, 7, and 1 h pretreatment, and (2) ephedrine 25 mg orally 1 h pretreatment and before pheresis
Thrombocytopenia	Consider membrane plasma separation
Volume-related hypotension	Consider continuous flow separation with matched input and output: consider increasing protein concentration of replacement fluid
Infection postpheresis	Infusion of intravenous immunoglobulin (100–400 mg/kg)
Hypokalemia	Ensure potassium concentration of 4 mmol/L in replacement solution
Membrane biocompatibility	Change membrane or consider centrifugal method of plasma separation
Hypothermia	Warm replacement fluids

Source: Adapted from Ref. 23.

12% protein bound, and its volume of distribution is relatively large (0.8 L/kg), suggesting a minimal removal by TPE (100). Azathioprine is approximately 30% protein bound, with a volume of distribution of 0.6 L/kg, and its removal would also be expected to be minor.

Most aminoglycosides have a low degree of protein binding (<5%) and a volume of distribution approximating 0.25 L/kg, thus one would not predict a substantial removal by TPE. Only 7–10% of a 100 mg dose of tobramycin was removed after two TPE treatments equaling 1700 and 2170 mL (103). Similarly, only 4–6% of body stores were removed after TPE treatments of 1725 and 2057 mL (100).

Phenytoin has a variable volume of distribution of between 0.5 and 1 L/kg and has a substantial intraerythrocytic distribution. Lui and Rubenstein reported that approximately 10% of total body stores were removed during TPE treatments of 5.6 and 6.1 L (104), suggesting that a posttreatment supplement may be required. Depending on initial serum concentrations, which varied between 8 and 17 μg/mL, the total amount removed ranged from 42 and 93 mg per treatment. Data obtained after a 3 L exchange demonstrated a net 30 mg removal (31).

Digoxin, with an enormous volume of distribution (5–8 L/kg) and a modest degree of protein binding (20–30%), is predictably unaffected by TPE (100), but removal of digibind-bound drug may be enhanced in patients with renal failure (105). Digitoxin has a greater degree of protein binding (94%), but its volume of distribution, although far less than that of digoxin (0.6 L/kg), is still too great to allow for a substantial net removal, and TPE has not been found to significantly lower its total body stores (100). Despite the modest net removal, TPE may still be useful as a treatment for intoxications since cardiac toxicity may be reduced because of the rapid lowering of serum levels (106,107).

Twenty-five percent of the active hormone thyroxine circulates in the intravascular compartment and is 99% bound to serum protein, leading to the use of TPE to treat thyroid storm when conventional methods have failed (108).

Acetylsalicylic acid is 90% protein bound and has a modest volume of distribution (0.1–0.2 L/kg), and TPE can remove substantial amounts (100). Although its large volume of distribution (2.8–4 L/kg) would suggest that net removal would be minimal, TPE has been reported to reduce the half-life of propranolol (90–96% protein bound) by approximately 75% (109). Vancomycin is only 10–50% protein bound and has a volume of distribution ranging between 0.5 and 1.1 L/kg. A one plasma volume exchange has been found to remove only 6% of total body stores, with a substantial posttreatment rebound (110).

Cisplatin is 90% protein bound and has an estimated volume of distribution of only 0.5 L/kg, suggesting that TPE may be useful in the management of cisplatin overdose. Two such cases have been reported with TPE resulting in substantial lowering of pretreatment levels from 2979 to 185 ng/mL and from 2900 to 200 ng/mL (111,112).

Theophylline is 55% protein bound and has a modest volume of distribution (0.4–0.7 L/kg), Laussen et al. reported on the use of arterio-venous and veno-venous (pumped) plasma exchange in three children with theophylline toxicity, suggesting that plasmapheresis may be useful in increasing drug clearance and decreasing its half-life (113).

REFERENCES

1. Gurland HJ, Lysaght MH, Samtleben W, Schmidt B. A comparison of centrifugal and membrane based apheresis formats. Int J Artif Organs 1984; 7:35–38.
2. Gurland HJ, Lysaght MJ, Samtleben W, Schmidt B. Comparative evaluation of filters used in membrane plasmapheresis. Nephron 1984; 36:173–182.
3. Sowada K, Malchesky PS, Nose Y. Available removal systems: state of the art. In: Nydegger UE, ed. Therapeutic Hemapheresis in the 1990s. Basel-Karger, 1990:51–113.
4. Kaplan AA, Halley SE, Reardon J, Sevigny J. One year's experience using a rotating filter for therapeutic plasma exchange. Trans Am Soc Artif Intern Organs 1989; 35:262–264.
5. Malchesky PS, Kaplan AA, Coo AP, Sadurada Y, Siami GA. Are selective macromolecule removal plasmapheresis systems useful for autoimmune diseases or hyperlipidemia? ASAIO J 1993; 39:868–872.
6. Agishi T, Kaneko I, Hasuo Y, Hayasaka Y, Sanaka T, Ota K, Abe M, Ono T, Kawai S, Yamane K. Double filtration plasmapheresis. Trans Am Soc Artif Intern Organs 1980; 26:406–409.
7. Vibert GJ, Wirtz SA, Smith JW, et al. Cryofiltration as an alternative to plasma exchange: plasma macromolecular solute removal without replacement fluids. In: Nose Y, Malchesky PS, Smith JW, eds. Plasmapheresis. Cleveland: ISAO Press, 1983:281–287.
8. Saal SD, Parker TS, Gordon BR. Removal of low-density lipoproteins in patients by extracorporeal immunoadsorption. Am J Med 1986; 80:583–589.
9. Gordon BR, Kelsey SF, Bilheimer DW, Brown DC, Dau PC, Gotto AM Jr, Illingworth DR, Jones PH, Leitman SF, Prihoda JS, et al. Treatment of refractory familial hypercholesterolemia by low density lipoprotein apheresis using an automated dextran sulfate cellulose adsorption system. Am J Cardiol 1992; 70:1010–1016.
10. Eisenhauer T, Armstrong VW Schuff-Werner P, et al. Long term clinical experience with HELP-CoA-Reductase inhibitors for maximum treatment of coronary heart disease associated with severe hypercholesterolemia. Trans Am Soc Artif Intern Organs 1989; 35: 580–583.
11. Samtleben W, Schmidt B, Gurland HJ. Ex vivo and in vivo protein A perfusion: background, basic investigations and first clinical experience. Blood Purif 1987; 5:179–192.
12. Hanasawa, K, Aoki H, Yoshioka T, Matsuda K, Tani T, Kodama M. Novel mechanical assistance in the treatment of endotoxic and septicemic shock. Am Soc Artif Intern Organs Trans 1989; 35:341–343.
13. Isbister JP. The risk/benefit equation for therapeutic plasma exchange. In: Nydegger UE, ed. Therapeutic Hemapheresis in the 1990s. Basel: Karger AG, 1990: 10–30.
14. Hazards of apheresis (editorial). Lancet 1982; 2:1025–1026.
15. Westphal RG: Complications of hemapheresis. In: Westphal RG, Kasprisin DO, eds. Current Status of Hemapheresis: Indications, Technology and Complications. Arlington, VA: American Association of Blood Banks, 1987:87–104.
16. Borberg H. Problems of plasma exchange therapy. In: Gurland HJ, Heinze V, Lee HA, eds. Therapeutic Plasma Exchange. New York: Springer-Verlag, 1980: 191–201.
17. Aufeuvre JP, Morin-Hertel F, Cohen-Solal M, Lefloch A, Baudelot J. Hazards of plasma exchange. In: Sieberth HG, ed. Plasma Exchange. Stuttgart: FK Schattauer Verlag, 1980:149–157.
18. Ziselman EM, Bongiovanni MB, Wurzel HA. The complications of therapeutic plasma exchange. Vox Sang 1984; 46:270–276.
19. Fabre M, Andreu G, Mannoni P. Some biological modifications and clinical hazards observed during plasma exchanges. In: Seiberth HG, ed. Plasma Exchange. Stuttgart: FK Schattauer Verlag, 1980:143–148.
20. Rossi PL, Cecchini L, Minichella G, De Rosa G, Alfano G, Pieralla L, Testa A, Candido A, Vittorio M, Mango G. Comparison of the side effects of therapeutic cytapheresis and those of other types of hemapheresis. Haematologica 1991; 76(suppl 1):75–80.
21. Sprenger KBG, Rasche H, Franz HE. Membrane plasma separation: complications and monitoring. Artif Organs 1984; 8:360–363.
22. Samtleben W, Hillebrand G, Krumme D, Gurland HJ. Membrane plasma separation: clinical experience with more than 120 plasma exchanges. In: Sieverth HG, ed. Plasma Exchange. Stuttgart: FK Schattauer Verlag, 1980:23–27.
23. Mokrzycki MH, Kaplan AA. Therapeutic plasma exchange: complications and management. Am J Kidney Dis 1994; 23:817–827.
24. Sutton DMC, Nair RC, Rock G, and the Canadian Apheresis Study Group. Complications of plasma exchange. Transfusion 1989; 29:124–127.
25. Flaum MA, Cuneo RA, Appelbaum FR, Disseroth AB, Engel WK, Gralnick HR. The hemostatic imbalance of plasma exchange transfusion. Blood 1979; 54:694–702.

26. Hester JP, McCullough J, Mishler JM, Szymanski IO. Dosage regimens for citrate anticoagulants. J Clin Apheresis 1983; 1:149–157.
27. Olson PR, Cox C, McCullough J. Laboratory and clinical effects of the infusion of ACD solution during platelet-pheresis. Vox Sang 1977; 33:79–87.
28. Silberstein LE, Naryshkin S, Haddad JJ, Strauss JF. Calcium homeostasis during therapeutic plasma exchange. Transfusion 1986; 26:151–155.
29. Huestis DW. Complications of therapeutic apheresis. In: Pinada AA, Valbonesis M, Diggs JC, eds. Therapeutic Hemapheresis. Milan: Wichtig Editore, 1986: 179–186.
30. Buskard NA, Varghese Z, Wills MR. Correction of hypocalcemic symptoms during plasma exchange. Lancet 1976; 2:344–345.
31. Kaplan AA, Halley SE. Plasma exchange with a rotating filter. Kidney Int 1990; 38:160–166.
32. Uhl L, Maillet S, King S, Kruskall MS. Unexpected citrate toxicity and severe hypocalcemia during apheresis. Transfusion 1997; 37:1063–1065.
33. Chrinside A, Urbaniak SJ, Prowse CV, Keller AJ. Coagulation abnormalities following intensive plasma exchange on the cell separator. Br J Haematol 1981; 48:627–634.
34. Gelabert A, Puig L, Maragall S, Monteagudo J, Castillo R. Coagulation alterations during massive plasmapheresis. In: Sieverth HG, ed. Plasma Exchange. Stuttgart: FK Schattauer Verlag, 1980:71–75.
35. Kaplan AA. Therapeutic plasma exchange for the nephrologist: Semin Dial 1995; 8:294–298.
36. Chopek M, McCullough J. Protein and biochemical changes during plasma exchange. In: Ulmas J, Berkman E, eds. Therapeutic Hemapheresis: A Technical Workshop. Washington, DC: American Association of Blood Banks, 1980:13–52.
37. Keller AJ, Chirnside A, Urbaniak SJ. Coagulation abnormalities produced by plasma exchange on the cell separator with special reference to fibrinogen and platelet levels. Br J Haematol 1979; 42:593–603.
38. Wood L, Jacobs P. The effect of serial therapeutic plasmapheresis on platelet count, coagulation factors plasma immunoglobulin and complement levels. J Clin Apheresis 1986; 3:124–128.
39. Sultan Y, Bussel A, Maisonneuve P, Sitty X, Gajdos P. Potential danger of thrombosis after plasma exchange in the treatment of patients with immune disease. Transfusion 1979; 19:588–593.
40. Aufeuvre JP, Mortin-Hertel F, Cohen-Solal M, Lefloch A, Baudelot J. Clinical tolerance and hazards of plasma exchanges: a study of 6200 plasma exchanges in 1033 patients. In: Beyer JH, Burgerg H, Fuchs C, Nagel GA, eds. Plasmapheresis in Immunology and Oncology. Basel: Karger, 1982:65–77.
41. Keller AJ, Urbaniak SJ. Intensive plasma exchange on the cell separator. Effects on serum immunoglobulins and complement components. Br J Haematol 1978; 38:531–540.
42. Kaplan AA. Towards a rational prescription of plasma exchange: The kinetics of immunoglobulin removal (editorial). Semin Dial 1992; 5:227–229.
43. Wing EJ, Bruns FJ, Fraley DS, Segel DP, Adler S. Infectious complications with plasmapheresis in rapidly progressively glomerulonephritis. JAMA 1980; 244:2423–2426.
44. Lockwood CM, Pinching AJ, Sweny PM, Rees AJ, Pussell B, Uff J, Peters DK. Plasma exchange and immunosuppression in the treatment of fulminating immune-complex crescentic nephritis. Lancet 1977; 1: 63–67.
45. Rossen RD, Hersh EM, Sharp JT, McCredie KB, Gyorkey F, Suki WN, Eknoyan G, Reisberg MA. Effect of plasma exchange on circulating immune complexes and antibody formation in patients treated with cyclophosphamide and prednisone. Am J Med 1977; 63:674–682.
46. Lockwood CM, Pearson TA, Rees AJ, Evans DJ, Peters DK, Wilson CB. Immunosuppression and plasma-exchange in the treatment of Goodpasture's syndrome. 1976; Lancet 1:711–715.
47. Johnson JP, Whitman W, Briggs WA, Wilson CB. Plasmapheresis and immunosuppressive agents in antibasement membrane antibody-induced Goodpasture's syndrome. Am J Med 1978; 64:354–359.
48. Depner TA, Chafin ME, Wilson CB, Gulyassy PF. Plasmapheresis for severe Goodpasture's syndrome (abstr). Kidney Int 1976; 8:409.
49. Lang CH, Brown DC, Staley N, Johnson G, Ma KQ, Border WA, Dalmasso AP. Goodpasture's syndrome treated with immunosuppression and plasma exchange. Arch Intern Med 1977; 137:1076–1078.
50. Rosenblatt SG, Knight W, Bannayan GA, Wilson CB, Stein JH. Treatment of Goodpasture's syndrome with plasmapheresis. Am J Med 1979; 66:689–696.
51. Walker RG, Dapice AJF, Becker GJ, Kincaid-Smith P, Craswell PW. Plasmapheresis in Goodpasture's syndrome with renal failure. Med J Aust 1979; 1:875–879.
52. McKenzie PE, Taylor AE, Woodroffe AJ, Seymour AE, Chan YL, Clarkson AR. Plasmapheresis in glomerulonephritis. Clin Nephrol 1979; 12:97–108.
53. Pinching AJ, Peters DK, Davis JN. Remission of myasthenia gravis following plasma-exchange. Lancet 1976; 2:1373–1376.
54. Dau PC, Lindstrom JM, Cassel CK, Denys EH, Shev EE, Spitter LE. Plasmapheresis and immunosuppressive drug therapy in myasthenia gravis. N Engl J Med 1977; 297:1134–1140.
55. Behan PO, Shakir RA, Simpson JA, Burnett AK, Allan TL, Haase G. Plasma-exchange combined with immunosuppressive therapy in myasthenia gravis. Lancet 1979; 2:438–440.

56. Newsom-Davis J, Wilson SG, Vincent A, Ward CD. Long-term effects of repeated plasma exchange in myasthenia gravis. Lancet 1979; 1:464–468.
57. Winklestein A, Volkin RL, Starz TW, Maxwell NG, Spero JA. The effects of plasma exchange on immunologic factors (abstr). Clin Res 1979; 27:691.
58. Pohl MA, Lan SP, Berl T, and the Lupus Nephritis Collaborative Study Group. Plasmapheresis does not increase the risk for infection in immunosuppressed patients with severe lupus nephritis. Ann Intern Med 1991; 114:924–929.
59. Consensus on IVIG. Lancet 1990; 1:470–472.
60. Haas A. Use of intravenous immunoglobulin in immunoregulatory disorders. Ann Intern Med 1987; 107: 367–382.
61. Finlayson JS. Albumin products. Semin Thromb Hemost 1980; 6:85–120.
62. Bjoro K, Froland SS, Yun Z, Samdal HH, Haaland T. Hepatitis C infection in patients with primary hypogammaglobulinemia after treatment with contaminated immune globulin. N Engl J Med 1994; 331:1607–1611.
63. Schiff RI. Transmission of viral infections through intravenous immune globulin (editorial). N Engl J Med 1994; 331:1649–1650.
64. Kiprov D, Simpson D, Romanick-Schmiedl S, Lippert R, Spira T, Busch D. Risk of AIDS-related virus (human immunodeficiency virus) transmission through apheresis procedures. J Clin Apheresis 1987; 3:143–146.
65. Boucher CA, de Gans J, van Oers R, Danner S, Goudsmit J. Transmission of HIV and AIDS by plasmapheresis for Guillain-Barré syndrome. Clin Neurol Neurosurg 1988; 90:235–236.
66. Lackritz EM, Satten GA, Aberle-Grasse J, Dodd RY, Raimondi VP, Janssen RS, et al. Estimated risk of transmission of the human immunodeficiency virus by screened blood in the United States. N Engl J Med 1995; 333:1721–1725.
67. Schreiber GB, Busch MP, Kleinman SH, Korelitz JJ. The risk of transfusion-transmitted virus invections. The Retrovirus Epidemiology Donor Study. N Engl J Med 1996; 334:1685–1690.
68. AuBuchon JP, Birkmeyer JD, Busch MP. Safety of the blood supply in the United States: Opportunities and Controversies. Ann Intern Med 1997; 127:904–909.
69. Biesert L, Suhartono H. Solvent/detergent treatment of human plasma—a very robust method for virus inactivation. Validated virus safety of OCTAPLAS. Vox Sang 1998; 74(suppl 1):207–212.
70. Klein HG, Dodd RY, Dzik WH, Luban NL, Ness PM, Pisciotto P, Schiff PD, Snyder EL. Current status of solvent/detergent-treated frozen plasma. Transfusion 1998; 38:102–107.
71. Steinmuller DR. A dangerous error in the dilution of 25 percent albumin (letter). N Eng J Med 1998; 338: 1226–1227.
72. Rock GA, Shumak KH, Buskard NA, Blanchette VS, Kelton JG, Nair RC, Spasoff RA, and the Canadian Apheresis Study Group. Comparison of plasma exchange with plasma infusion in the treatment of TTP. N Engl J Med 1991; 325:393–397.
73. Ring J, Messmer K. Incidence and severity of anaphylactoid reactions to colloid volume substitutes. Lancet 1977; 1:466–469.
74. Bambauer R, Jutzler GA, Albrecht D, Keller HE, Kohler M. Indications of plasmapheresis and selection of different substitution solutions. Biomater Artif Cells Artif Organs 1989; 17:9–27.
75. Huestis DW. Mortality in therapeutic haemapheresis (letter). Lancet 1983; 1:1043.
76. Sutton DMC, Nair R, Rock G, and the Canadian Apheresis Study Group. Complications of plasma exchange. Transfusion 1989; 29:124–127.
77. Stafford CT, Lobel SA, Fruge BC, Moffitt JE, Hoff RG, Fadel HE. Anaphylaxis to human serum albumin. Ann Allergy 1988; 61:85–88.
78. Brecher ME, Owen HG, Collins ML. Apheresis and ACE inhibitors (letter). Transfusion 1993; 33:963–964.
79. Owen HG, Brecher ME. Atypical reactions associated with use of angiotensin-converting enzyme inhibitors and apheresis. Transfusion 1994; 34:891–894.
80. Apter AJ, Kaplan AA. An approach to immunologic reactions with plasma exchange. J Allergy Clin Immunol 1992; 90:119–124.
81. Snyder Jr HW, Henry DH, Messerschmidt GL, et al. Minimal toxicity during protein A immunoadsorption treatment of malignant disease: an outpatient therapy. J Clin Apheresis 1991; 6:1–10.
82. Case presentation. N Engl J Med 1994; 331:792–799.
83. Schaumann D, Olbricht CJ, Welp M, et al. Extracorporeal removal of LDL-cholesterol: prospective evaluation of effectivity, selectivity and biocompatibility (abstr). J Am Soc Nephrol 1992; 3:392.
84. Olbricht CJ, Schauman D, Fisher D. Anaphylactoid reactions, LDL apheresis with dextran sulphate and ACE inhibitors. Lancet 1992; 3:908–909.
85. Kroon AA, Mol MJTM, Stalenhoff APH. ACE inhibitors and LDL-apheresis with dextran sulphate adsorption. Lancet 1992; 340:1476.
86. Orlin JB, Berkman EM. Partial plasma exchange using albumin replacement: removal and recovery of normal plasma constituents. Blood 1980; 56:1055–1059.
87. Morrison G, Michelson EL, Brown S, Morganroth J. Mechanism and prevention of cardiac arrhythmias in chronic hemodialysis patients. Kidney Int 1980; 17: 811–819.
88. Pearl RG, Rosenthal MH. Metabolic alkalosis due to plasmapheresis. Am J Med 1985; 79:391–393.
89. Mousson C, Charhon SA, Ammar M, Accominotti M, Rifle G. Aluminum bone deposits in normal renal function patients after long-term treatment by plasma exchange. Int J Artif Organs 1989; 23:664–667.

90. Milliner DS, Shinaberger JH, Shurman P, Coburn JW. Inadvertent aluminum administration during plasma exchange due to aluminum contamination of albumin replacement solutions. N Engl J Med 1985; 312:165–167.
91. Reddi A, Frank O, DeAngelis B, Jain R, Bashruddin I, Lasker N, Baker H. Vitamin status in patients undergoing single or multiple plasmapheresis. J Am Coll Nutr 1987; 6:485–489.
92. MacDonald R, Robinson A. Suxamethonium apnea associated with plasmapheresis. Anaesthesia 1980; 35: 198–201.
93. Wood GJ, Hall GM. Plasmapheresis and plasma cholinesterase. Br J Anaesth 1978; 50:945–948.
94. Bowen RA. Anaesthesia in operations for the relief of hypertension. Anaesthesia 1960; 15:3–10.
95. McCaul K, Robinson GD. Suxamethonium extension by tetrahydroaminoacrine. Br J Anaesth 1962; 34: 536–542.
96. Jorstad S. Biocompatibility of different hemodialysis and plasmapheresis membranes. Blood Purif 1987; 5: 123–137.
97. Nicholls AJ, Platts MM. Anaphylactoid reactions due to haemodialysis, haemofiltration or membrane plasma separation. BMJ 1982; 285:1607–1609.
98. Aeschbacher B, Haeverli A, Nydegger UE. Donor safety and plasma quality in automated plasmapheresis. Vox Sang 1989; 57:104–111.
99. Bennet WM, Aronoff GR, Golper TA, Morrison G, Singer I, Brater DC. Drug Prescribing in Renal Failure. 2nd ed. Philadelphia: American College of Physicians, 1991.
100. Sketris IS, Parker WA, Jones JV. Effect of plasma exchange on drug removal. In: Valbonesi M, Pineda AA, Biggs JC, eds. Therapeutic Hemapheresis. Milan: Wichtig Editore, 1986:15–20.
101. Jones JV. The effect of plasmapheresis on therapeutic drugs. Dial Transplant 1985; 14:225–226.
102. Stigelman WH, Henry DH, Talbert RL, Townsend RJ. Removal of prednisone and prednisolone by plasma exchange. Clin Pharmacol 1984; 3:402–407.
103. Appelgate R, Schwartz D, Bennett WM. Removal of tobramycin during plasma exchange therapy. Ann Intern Med 1981; 94:820–821.
104. Liu E, Rubenstein M. Phenytoin removal by plasmapheresis in thrombotic thrombocytopenic purpura. Clin Pharmacol Ther 1982; 31:762–765.
105. Rabetoy GM, Price CA, Findlay JW, Sailstad JM. Treatment of digoxin intoxication in a renal failure patient with digoxin-specific antibody fragments and plasmapheresis. Am J Nephrol 1990; 10:518–521.
106. Peters U, Risler T, Grabenese B. Digitoxin elimination by plasma separation. In: Sieberth HG, ed. Plasma Exchange: Plasmapheresis-Plasmaseparation. Stuttgart: FK Schattauer Verlag, 1980:365–368.
107. Arsac Ph, Barret L, Chenais F, Debru JL, Faure J. Digitoxin intoxication treated by plasma exchange. In: Sieberth HG, ed. Plasma Exchange: Plasmapheresis-Plasmaseparation. Stuttgart: FK Schattauer Verlag, 1980:369–371.
108. Ashkar FS, Katims RB, Smoak WM, Gilson AJ. Thyroid storm treatment with blood exchange and plasmapheresis. J Am Med Assoc 1979; 214:1275–1279.
109. Talbert RL, Wong YY, Duncan DB. Propranolol plasma concentrations and plasmapheresis. Drug Intell Clin Phram 1981; 15:993–996.
110. McClellan SD, Whitaker CH, Friedberg RC. Removal of vancomycin during plasmapheresis. Ann Pharmacother 1997; 31:1132–1136.
111. Jung HK, Lee J, Lee SN. A case of massive cisplatin overdose managed by plasmapheresis. Korean J Intern Med 1995; 10:150–154.
112. Chu G, Mantin R, Shen YM, Baskett G, Sussman H. Massive cisplatin overdose by accidental substitution for carboplatin. Toxicity and management. Cancer 1993; 72:3707–3714.
113. Laussen P, Shann F, Butt W, Tibballs J. Use of plasmapheresis in acute theophylline toxicity. Crit Care Med 1991; 19:288–290.

42

Economic Issues in Dialysis: Influence on Dialysis-Related Complications in the Managed-Care Era

Theodore I. Steinman
Beth Israel Deaconess Medical Center and Harvard Medical School, Boston, Massachusetts

I. INTRODUCTION

Economic issues in dialysis must be reviewed in context of the overall changes occurring in our health care system. Increasing and complex pressures in our present economic environment have wrought changes far beyond our expectations. Medical advances have led to decreased hospitalizations and less "need" for hospitals, a situation that reflects better care. On the other hand, lower total income for hospitals (after salaries, benefits, and supplies) results in less money available to pay for teaching medical and nursing students, for unrecovered costs of biomedical research, for the training of tomorrow's doctors and other providers of care, and for the care of those for whom there is no payer. The goal of everyone involved in medicine is to maintain superior quality of care (that has become our standard) while attempting to decrease the costs of care. Financial pressures have assisted the formation of systems of care where the economies of scale and efficiencies of providing care can best be achieved. Collaboration is necessary to strengthen our delivery system in this era of shrinking health-care dollars. The public is entitled to readily available health care of the highest quality at the most reasonable cost. Medicine must never compromise its fundamental obligation of care of patients and the overall health of those we serve, regardless of their ability to pay.

II. THE BASIS FOR THE GROWTH OF MANAGED CARE

When Medicare and Medicaid were enacted in 1965, it was anticipated that successive national legislation would result in universal health insurance coverage within one or, at the most, two decades. The federal actuaries estimated in those early days that total outlays for Medicare in 1990 would come to $10 billion, a far cry from the staggering $180 billion total, which was reached in 1996 (1). No one was able to predict the explosive rise of national health-care total expenditures from $41 billion in 1965 to $1 trillion in 1996, and there is an expected doubling of total expenditures to exceed $2 trillion dollars by the year 2007 or shortly thereafter (2). The growth of managed care was fostered by dramatic increases in national health-care spending since the passage of Medicare and Medicaid. In 1965 just under 6% of the gross domestic product (GNP) was expended on health care, and this had risen to almost 14% by 1997 (2). The significant growth in dollar expenditures is but a part in a much larger transformation in health-care spending patterns.

Private health insurance accounted for approximately 25% of the national total of $41 billion in 1965. Federal, state, and local governments accounted for 25% of the total, and the remaining 50% represented out-of-pocket outlays by consumers (3). Consumer out-of-pocket share for health-care expenditures has declined progressively to a current value of around 18%, and the public has paid little attention to their declining total financial commitment to expenditures. The government (primarily federal) is now contributing about two thirds of the increased spending. Private health insurance now pays only about 15% of the total health-care expenditures, and indemnity insurance is rapidly falling as a percentage of the financial pie. These major shifts reflect the steep rise of inpatient hospital care costs, and most of these costs were covered by added spending by government and employers. It is not surprising that most of the population with good private or public health insurance coverage had little concern with steeply climbing health-care expenditures. Only to a minor degree (approximately 20%) do personal out-of-pocket payments become a financial factor. With this anomalous financing arrangement, the model for a competitive marketplace has only limited applicability. This becomes ever more important based on the fact that governmental budgets, insurance, and charity continue to provide access at some level to all persons irrespective of their ability to pay (4).

Fiscal discipline virtually disappeared from the health-care marketplace during the first two decades of Medicare when the principal payers—employers, private health insurance, and government—tended to honor, with few or no questions, all bills submitted for reimbursement by providers. It was not until the mid-1980s that Medicare began to pay closer attention to dollar costs. At the same time employers and private health insurance plans looked toward managed care plans to moderate their annual increases in premium costs. Medicare shifted from a cost-plus reimbursement for hospital inpatient care to a prospective payment system. It took until the early 1990s for the market to fully respond to these developments with large-scale deceleration in employers' annual contribution to premium increases. In contrast, Medicare outlays continue to rise at an annual rate of around 10% (1).

Examination of the health-care system infrastructure leads one to focus on:

1. Delivery of health-care services (hospitals, dialysis clinics, physicians, and other health personnel)
2. Health education
3. Biomedical research

III. MANAGED CARE TODAY

In the early to mid-1990s, the annual expenditure data gave some credence to the advocates of greater reliance on the competitive marketplace. For-profit managed care organizations (MCOs) expanded rapidly, and their medical loss ratio during the 1980s was often in the 70–75% range, which meant that they were able to extract 25–30 cents of every premium dollar for marketing, expansion, and profits (including high salaries for management) (5). Shifting potential enrollees from fee-for-service to managed care can generate a one-time cost savings of 10–15%, but future profits may become more elusive. In 1994–95 over 90% of for-profit managed care plans were profitable; in 1996–97 less than 40% have turned a profit (6).

Equity investors helped generate the shift from fee-for-service into for-profit health maintenance organizations (HMOs) since the capital they invested helped spur the expansion in HMO enrollments. A downturn in the stock market would make it difficult for heavily indebted for-profit MCOs to survive.

Most of the healthy population have already enrolled in managed care plans, and it will be more difficult for the for-profit companies to maintain a favorable bottom line in face of the increasing trend toward direct contracting between payers and providers, direct negotiating with Medicare by provider-sponsored organizations, and the establishment by the teaching hospitals, large academic health centers, and other types of health-care systems to launch independent HMOs or enter into partnerships with established HMOs.

HMOs will now be forced to enroll patients with established chronic illnesses, and it is evident that MCOs have little experience in caring for people with end-stage renal disease (ESRD). It is evident that MCOs/HMOs have only a superficial idea of the true cost of caring for a patient with ESRD, and this will set the stage for a radical transformation in the health-care delivery system. Some of the role of the acute care hospital will be progressively peripheralized (7). Most patients will require treatment in clinics, at home, and in specialized ambulatory centers. This chronically ill population will require access to nurses and other mid-level personnel for follow-up and ongoing care. Patients will need to accept increased personal responsibility for their own care and well-being. There will need to be a reliance on advice and reinforcement from membership in support groups. Patients' care will need to be directed by a management team headed by the physician, who will in turn direct a considerable number of associates and assistants. The nonphysician personnel will actually provide many of the services that the patient requires. This model is already well established in the dialysis population, and therefore the nephrology community is well positioned to readily adapt to changes wrought by MCOs/HMOs. The following (4) summarizes the trends that characterize the U.S. health-care agenda:

No great urgency to take action to provide health-care coverage for all the population.

An initial preference to enlarge the scale and scope of the competitive marketplace to extend its control over the financing and delivery of health-care services. Vigorous counterefforts via new federal and state legislation will be the response to limit the degree of managerial freedom previously available to managed care plans.

New federal legislation reducing the numbers of present and prospective Medicaid enrollees and encouraging parallel actions by the states to contain their future outlays for Medicaid.

Agreement among the political leadership to support the Balanced Budget Act of 1997, which mandates a substantial reduction in Medicare outlays in future years. The Senate initiative to raise the age for Medicare eligibility failed, as did the income-adjusted premium rates for Medicare B.

Modest changes in regulations governing private health-care insurance aimed at facilitating continued coverage for workers changing jobs and new federal funding to facilitate coverage for large numbers of low-income children.

With this overall backdrop, we will now focus on economic issues specific to dialysis units.

IV. FINANCES RELATED TO DIALYSIS

Financial management of the entire dialysis process requires expertise that evades most nephrologists. Expert help is needed for the vast majority of nephrologists to help define all issues of cost, tracking funds management, and assistance with contract negotiations. Financial departments of the large dialysis chains generally have systems in place to provide the above assistance. However, the issue of tracking funds management varies from dialysis chain to dialysis chain. True costs of any system, especially in a hospital setting, is difficult to understand and follow under the best circumstances (8).

The issue of cost-effectiveness of test-treatment strategies needs to be understood by the nephrologist (9). In the era of cost containment, physicians need reliable data about specific interventions. A necessary learning step for nephrologists is how to interpret economic analyses and estimate their own costs of implementing recommended interventions. With the care of the dialysis patient moving towards national guidelines that can be outlined in algorithms of care, the nephrologist must understand the cost implications of each step in an algorithm (10,11). This is a critical component of any contract negotiations. Every component of care must have a cost analysis performed so that maximum utilization of limited financial resources is employed.

Estimates of costs without substantiating data will create problems. This is especially true in the hospital setting, where it is difficult to fully understand true costs in contrast to filed charges. Data on expenditures, start-up costs, and general overhead are frequently neglected when examining the bottom line. There is a need for cost data and a standardized protocol so that missing data can be detected. A bridge between care delivery and economic analysis is a necessary link (12).

More than half of the dialysis provided in the United States to the ESRD population is done by three vertically integrated mega-providers: Fresenius Medical Care (FMC), Gambro Healthcare, and Total Renal Care. Other organizations are attempting to impact the marketplace and become large-scale providers (e.g., Renal Care Group), and their presence in the marketplace is being felt. The publicized rationale for consolidation of dialysis units is to obtain economics of scale; eliminating duplicity does reduce administrative overhead. These large national chains have definitely changed the delivery of care. Data management has improved, but the doctor-patient interaction has suffered. In many cases, the doctor-patient relationship has become a nurse-patient or staff-patient relationship, a reflection of decreased physician presence in the dialysis unit. The patient has often become a pawn in the "return-on-investment" game that results from selling of individually owned dialysis units to one of the national companies (13). Economic vitality must never be confused with quality of care as viewed from an outcome standpoint or patient satisfaction as determined by surveys (e.g., Kidney Disease Quality of Life questionnaire—see below).

Increasing regulation of the dialysis industry has occurred in a profound fashion over the past two decades, and this is a consequence of government experiences with escalating costs beyond anticipated projections. The cost increase is related more to providing care for more patients rather than to an increase in cost per patient. In fact, the per-patient costs have declined in real dollars over the past 20 years, but the government never really fully anticipated the large number of patients who would be candidates for ESRD therapy. A composite rate-payment schedule for dialysis has led to cost control as a major factor in patient care. Declines in reimbursement have led the dialysis industry to seek individuals skilled in business management to help run medical operations. Larger organizations negotiate better pricing for supplies. Vertically integrated organizations internally supply their own equipment and disposables. Such an internal supply line apparently results in cost savings since the marketing and distribution costs can be virtually eliminated. Such economic factors can sometimes result in the patient being "lost in the system."

Financial compensation for nephrologists has dramatically changed in the past few years. A fee-for-service reimbursement mechanisms is coming to a close in most parts of the country and will probably almost totally disappear within the next few years. Capitation for global services is being progressively employed as a method of payment, the attempt being to encourage routine care that can be captured with a global fee. A modified fee-for-service reimbursement mechanism may be utilized for circumstances defined as extraordinary (14). Nephrology services reimbursement can potentially be carved out from a payer/HMO/MCO as a new method for reimbursement (15). Advantages of a financial single specialty carve-out include the following:

1. Payer can transfer risk to the physician group.
2. It is easier to negotiate a single-speciality carveout with the payer than a global capitation contract for a random population (for all services to be delivered).
3. Carveouts can increase practice volume and thus physician income, assuming that the reimbursement is adequate.
4. Participating single-specialty independent practice associations (IPAs) can get exclusive contracts with the payer.
5. The physician must closely observe his/her practice efficiency.
6. Long-term relationship between physician and payer is cemented if the physician group is the first in the market and your group's performance has become known to the payers.
7. A contract with multispecialty IPAs means access to more of the premium dollar because of a demonstrated track record with payers.

There must be detailed explanations of how bonuses will be allocated within the physician group. It is critical not to provide vague details that are open to misinterpretation. In a managed care capitated environment, physicians should be eligible for incentive pay based on improved outcomes, open access to care, and patient satisfaction results (16,17). Reimbursement incentives should never be tied to cost savings generated by denial of services. Later in this chapter the issue of reimbursement for physicians based on outcomes is explained further.

An information booklet must be kept in a dialysis unit detailing issues of financial concern involving the patient (18). Evaluation and management services that should be delivered to the patient as part of the monthly capitation payment (MCP) need to be clearly stated in written form for patients to understand. This is a critical reminder to physicians of their responsibilities to the patient. For physicians themselves there must be a similar booklet that notes the required documentation for every level of service. Physicians need to know how billing is done within Medicare and other insurer regulations. This booklet will need to be updated because of the rapid changes that are occurring in the area of reimbursement. The steady shift of segments of the population from a fee-for-service to a capitated environment mandates constant physician information updating.

There is a demonstrated need to avoid unnecessary tests and treatment when viewed in the context of quality-adjusted life-year (QALY) (9). Physicians will need to understand the issues of sensitivity analysis when viewing such QALY, which relates to the value of a specific strategy (test or treatment) as viewed by the general public (e.g., how much should society pay for an intervention when considering the benefit to the patient and society?).

V. DEMOGRAPHICS AND EXPENDITURES RELATED TO DIALYSIS

The percent change in Medicare payments for ESRD services have been declining more than the decline in the medical Consumer Price Index (CPI), the bottom line being that reimbursement for ESRD care has not been keeping pace with medical inflation. While there is still an increase in the medical CPI, it is declining as compared to previous years. Since 1983 the payment rates for ESRD services have remained essentially the same. With the government attempting to control overall expenditures, measured in both actual and inflation-adjusted dollars, reimbursement for dialysis care (the composite rate) has dramatically declined. Despite the cost per patient being less today as compared to 1983,

Table 1 Distribution of Medicare Payments for ESRD Patients per Year (1995) at Risk

Medical supply	$1007	
Laboratory	$ 927	60% of total
Nephrologist	$2177	
Ambulance	$ 912	
Internal medicine	$ 727	
General surgery	$ 634	22% of total
Radiology	$ 424	
Cardiology	$ 310	
Urology	$<200	
Other		18% of total

Medicare pays 80% of allowed charges. Breakdown of where payments go for services delivered and the percentage of total payments per group.
Source: HCFA; USRDS, 1997.

ESRD total expenditures is now approaching $14 billion. While ESRD comprises only 0.5% of the Medicare population, expenditures for this group amount to 5.5% of the Medicare budget. There has been a 40% growth in the number of dialysis facilities since 1990, increasing from 2200 to approximately 3000.

Expenditures for hospital inpatient care and dialysis outpatient care are almost equal. Spending per patient varies significantly depending on modality of dialysis, patient age, number of co-morbid conditions, and diabetic status. Payments to nephrologists are a small portion (approximately 7%) of total patient costs, but the nephrologist receives the largest proportion of physician provider payments (as appropriate) (see Tables 1 and 2). The change in Medicare payments as reflected by an annualized percent increase is noted on Table 3. While the percent increase appears large, the actual total dollars represents a small increase that is below that of the adjusted medical CPI. Another factor in the total increase in expenditures is a decline in the adjusted annual mortality rates (19). In 1989 the U.S. Renal Data System (USRDS) noted a 24.0% adjusted annual mortality rate. By 1996 this had declined to 22.3%. Therefore, with fewer patients dying, the costs of care for an expanding patient population have increased overall. Table 4 provides an estimate of the total ESRD costs for 1995 as analyzed in the 1997 USRDS Annual Report.

In an attempt to control costs in face of a movement towards managed care, the Health Care Financing Administration (HCFA) has undertaken a Medicare Capitation Demonstration Project. The goal is to determine if cost savings can be achieved and quality of care improved in a capitated environment for patients with chronic illness. ESRD is an obvious disease entity to be studied because the boundaries of the illness are readily defined. Table 5 provides the HCFA reimbursement schedules based on patient age and diabetic status. This payment is for yearly global services and encompasses all resources needed by the patient, including physician care in both the inpatient and out-

Table 2 Medicare MCP Payments by Specialty per Patient per Year (1995) at Risk

		% Change
Total payments	$1615	10.3
Nephrologist	$1284	11.2
Internal medicine	$ 250	7.5
Multispecialty	$ 57	7.9
Urology	$ 7	−3.3
General practice	$ 4	13.5
Emergency medicine	$ 4	3.8
Other	$ 4	6.9

MCP = Monthly capitation payment.
Payment schedule as distribution pieces of the pie for outpatient services only. Percentage change in payments from 1991 to 1995.
Source: HCFA; USRDS, 1997.

Table 3 Increase in Medicare Payments by Source of Claim, 1991–1995

Source	Annualized percent increase
Hospital	14
Dialysis unit	13
Physician/Supplier	12
Other distribution	28
Transportation	
Medications	
Home health services	

Source: HCFA; USRDS, 1997.

Table 4 1995 Medicare Component and Total Expenditures for the ESRD Population

Total spending	$13.06 billion
Non-Medicare component	
MSP: Employer Group Health Plans	
Patient out-of pocket obligations	
HMO payments	
Organ donor acquisition	
Medicare expenses	$ 9.74 billion

MSP = Medicare secondary payor.
Source: USRDS, 1997.

Table 5 Medicare Capitation Demonstration Payment[a]

Diagnosis	Age (y)	Payment/year
Nondiabetic	<65	$3970
Nondiabetic	>65	$4968
Diabetes mellitus	<65	$4938
Diabetes mellitus	>65	$5684

[a]Per patient reimbursement based on diagnosis and age of patient. There is a small geographic adjustment to the payment based on location. This payment is for global services, including both inpatient and outpatient venues.
Source: HCFA.

patient setting. When examining the current costs (Table 6), the goal of the physician is to maintain quality of care in a cost-effective delivery system.

VI. FINANCIAL IMPLICATIONS OF VASCULAR ACCESS

Access complications are a major cause of morbidity and mortality in the ESRD population. The most common causes for hospitalization relate to access (thrombosis, local infections, septicemia, etc.). Total expenditures for maintaining vascular access in the United States are now approaching $1 billion per year, and this translates to $6.7–$7.9 thousand per patient per year (19). These costs represent only the tip of the iceberg, since problems derive both directly and indirectly from access complications. Vascular access can be divided into three types: tunneled-cuffed catheters (TCC), prosthetic bridge grafts (PBG), and arterio-venous fistulas (AVF). Each of these has the potential for complications to varying degrees. Since the introduction of TCCs in the 1980s, this modality of access has gained a major role in the marketplace. Of all new hemodialysis patients, 18.9% were being dialyzed with TCCs 60 days after starting dialysis (20). Despite the increasing popularity of TCCs, complications include problems with initial placement, inadequate dialysis, thrombosis, and catheter-related infections (21).

Over 20 years ago PBGs (e.g., polytetrafluoroethylene, PTFE) were introduced and offered a valuable addition to access in patients whose native vessels did not support development of a fistula. Unfortunately, these grafts, which now are the dominant access, are particularly prone to problems, especially venous stenosis and thrombosis. These problems of venous stenosis and thrombosis occur at a rate of approximately 1–1.5 times per patient per year (21), resulting in cumulative patency rates of PBGs in most centers of only 55–75% at one year and 50–60% at 2 years. However, the number of procedures per graft are much greater than the 1- to 1.5-fold rate of venous stenosis and thrombosis. In New England, there are approximately 4 procedures per graft per patient per year in contrast to 5.9 procedures per graft per patient per year in the western United States and 4.9 procedures per graft per patient per year in the Far West (22). Some of the increased use of grafts may be explained by delayed referral to the nephrologist (see below). Therefore, the cost implications of PBGs are enormous.

Although the AVF does have some disadvantages, it is the best possible vascular access for hemodialysis. The issues of venous stenosis, infection, and vascular steal syndrome are noted, but at a lower incidence when compared to the PBG. Despite its obvious advantages, the relative number of AVFs being created has been decreasing. Patients starting dialysis in 1990 had a 70% greater chance of having a PBG created than an AVF as compared to 1986. In 1996, only 17.9% of hemodialysis patients were using an AVF 60 days after the initiation of therapy. The overall complication rate for PBGs is twice as high as that for AVFs. Specifically, PBGs have 6 times the rate of thrombosis and 10 times the rate of infection as AVFs (21,22).

Appropriate access creation before the initiation of dialysis is the single area that could generate the most cost savings while improving the quality of care. The type of access has the potential to generate cost savings. PBGs are much more expensive to create and to maintain as compared to AVF. Table 7 shows that Med-

Table 6 Medicare Payments for ESRD per Patient Year at Risk[a]

Type of patient	Cost
All ESRD	$38,000
Dialysis	$45,000
Hemodialysis	$46,000
CAPD/CCPD/APD	$41,000
Other[b]	$53,000
Transplantation[c]	$16,000

CAPD = Continuous ambulatory peritoneal dialysis; CCPD = continuous cycling peritoneal dialysis; APD = automated peritoneal dialysis.
[a]For all ages, including diabetics and nondiabetics, 1991–1995 (intent-to-treat analysis).
[b]Medicare covered medications, ambulance transportation, home health services.
[c]Functioning transplant at 1/1/91 and new transplants thereafter; no censoring at graft failure.
Source: USRDS, 1997.

Table 7 1994 Demographics and Costs of Fistulas Versus Grafts in the ESRD Population

	Fistulas	Grafts
Age (y)	56 years	60 years
% Females	37%	58%
% Black	33%	47%
% Diabetic	21%	27%
% PVD #	23%	30%
Medicare spending[a]	$41,000	$46,000

PVD = Peripheral vascular disease.
[a]Medicare spending is per year at risk for ESRD. In 1994 the cost savings for placing a fistula vs. a graft was $5183/patient/year when adjusting for demographics, co-morbid conditions, and region of the country.
Source: HCFA; USRDS, 1997.

icare spending is $41,000 per year per patient at risk for ESRD when a fistula is in place and $46,000 when PBG is the primary access. This table shows the 1994 demographics and costs of AVFs versus PBGs, the analysis being done by patient age, percent females, percent blacks, percent diabetics, and percent of patients with peripheral vascular disease.

Regional variations in spending per ESRD patient per year at risk were noted in the Dialysis Outcome Practice Pattern Study (DOPPS), with New England doing a better job when compared to other parts of the country with regard to placement of AVF over PBG. Table 8 notes the type of permanent access currently being used by the prevalent ESRD population (19). Grafts are three times more likely to be the type of permanent access as compared to fistulas. Examination of the incident population shows a steady drop in the use of fistulas. The Dialysis Outcome Practice Pattern Study suggests that $5183 per patient can be saved if a fistula is used in place of a graft (1994 data adjusted for demographics, co-morbid conditions, and region of the country). If the patient lives for more than one year, the savings are decreased to $3620 since some patients will die during the year. This explains the difference between $5183 and $3620. Fistulas are 60% less likely to fail as compared to grafts (23). Woods and colleagues (24) noted the relative risk (RR) of access failure by age. The RR of access failure increases by 40% over 10 years. Patients >65 years of age with fistulas have an RR of 0.76 as compared to grafts (fistulas are 24% less likely to fail as compared to grafts for this segment of the ESRD population). The RR of access failure for a patient with an AVF, compared with a patient of the same age with a PBG, was 67% lower at the age of 40 years, 54% lower at 50 years, and 24% lower at 65 years.

Table 8 Vascular Access for ESRD

Access type	Percentage
Arterio-venous fistulas	22
Prosthetic grafts	63
Tunneled-cuffed catheters (as permanent access)	15

Tunneled-cuffed catheters in this table relate to permanent use for access and are independent of temporary access.
Source: USRDS, 1997.

Thirty-eight percent of hemodialysis patients had AVFs in 1986–1987. This figure dropped to 18% a decade later, 1996–1997. There has been a 12-fold increase in the number of tunnelled-cuffed catheters used over the past decades. PBGs as the first permanent vascular access are 2.2 times more likely to be in place as compared to AVFs. As dialysis time progresses (at 60 days after initiation of hemodialysis) PBGs are placed 2.8 times more frequently than are AVFs. Ongoing education is needed since 22% of nephrologists surveyed throughout the country thought that PBGs were better than AVFs (25). Measures to decrease vascular access morbidity among hemodialysis patients should include reversing the current trend toward increased use of PBGs, particularly in patients younger than 65 years.

A potential solution to the access issue may come about with a global capitation payment for ESRD services. A model to promote the increased utilization of fistulas would include a subcapitation of the access surgeon. Paying the surgeon a one-time fee, no matter how many times the patient requires an access, would stimulate individuals to do the most cost-effective procedure (e.g., fistula creation). Surgeons should be paid well for their talent, but the one-time fee per patient has the possibility of generating savings. In our institution, the surgeon must call the nephrologist before access creation if a fistula cannot be performed. This approach stimulates the surgeon to think about the issue and gets their buy-in to the appropriate use of fistulas. This may be a factor in explaining why the northeast section of the United States has a greater percentage of AVFs as compared to PBGs. Having a fistula in place at the start of hemodialysis improves the quality of life (26). The Kidney Disease Quality of Life (KDQOL) instrument was designed in 1994 and represents a long-form assessment of physical functioning, role limitations caused by physical health problems, role limitations caused by emotional problems, social functioning, emotional well-being, pain, energy/fatigue, general health perceptions, symptoms/problems, effects of kidney disease on daily life, burden of kidney disease, cognitive function, work status, sexual function, quality of social interaction, social support, dialysis staff encouragement, and patient satisfaction. An 80-item short form (KDQOL-SF) has now replaced the 134-item long form and is now being used in the dialysis setting (27,28).

VII. COSTS OF LATE REFERRAL TO NEPHROLOGISTS

Factors that relate to the choice of access are frequently beyond the nephrologist's control. Delayed referral of chronic renal failure patients to renal specialists has been described as a factor in the prevalence of comorbid conditions and an increased morbidity and early mortality of ESRD patients commencing renal replacement therapy (29). Early intervention may retard the progression of chronic renal failure as well as lead to the most appropriate placement of a proper access.

A series of studies have compared early referral (ER) to late referral (LR) to nephrologists, and all have demonstrated a higher mortality in the first 12–24 months for the LR group. Khan and colleagues (30) demonstrated that 2-year patient survival with ER was 59% compared to only 25% with LR. Also, Campbell et al. found a one-year mortality of 39% in urgent referrals (<1 month), 19% in intermediate referrals (1–4 months), but only 6% in ER (>4 months) before initiation of dialysis (31). Even after correcting for age and gender with matched controls, Innes and colleagues noted a median survival of only 2.6 months for patients who had started on dialysis within a month after referral (32).

Prolonged hospitalization at the initiation of dialysis is associated with higher costs, and this directly relates to the timing of referral. In one study, the total number of hospital days was 9.07 in ER compared to 30.24 for LR (33). This study by Muirhead et al. demonstrated large differences in costs related to the initiation of renal replacement therapy for ER ($4,980) as compared to LR ($23,633). In another study by Jungers and colleagues in France, the total savings in French francs incurred during the first year with ER were dramatic as compared to LR (34). Similar cost savings are noted when permanent vascular access is planned early and therefore done as an outpatient procedure. When access is placed late, invariably during the hospitalization at initiation of dialysis, the cost of hospitalization due to hemodialysis access placement was $10,557 (35). In this study by Garella, the cost of access related to ER was only $2,900. Despite these published studies noting higher costs, reports from the USRDS 1996 Annual Data Report (20) showed that only 43.9% of patients had a permanent access placed or attempted 30 days before the onset of ESRD. Similar data were obtained from Wave 2 of the Dialysis Morbidity and Mortality Study (DMMS) in the United States (36) indicating as follows: 31% of patients have late detection of kidney disease (<3 months before the start of ESRD) and therefore the issue of access is an emergency, and 38% of patients received a late referral to the nephrologist (<3 months before the initiation of dialysis) despite the diagnosis of chronic renal failure being established. No attempted permanent vascular access at the start of dialysis was noted in 56% of patients, and it is this portion of the patient pool that could generate the most cost savings (37,38). Vascular access issues are potentially amenable to change, especially with the advent of managed care and case management intervention.

A 1993 National Institutes of Health (NIH) consensus conference noted that 70–75% of patients in the United States with ESRD were not referred to a nephrologist until immediately before initiation of dialysis (29). Ifudu and colleagues noted that in a New York City inner-city dialysis unit between 1990 and 1994, only 43% of patients received pre-ESRD care from a nephrologist as compared to 45% receiving care from a nonnephrologist (39). Twelve percent of the eventual dialysis population received no medical care before ESRD, and this necessitated a 100% use of temporary access for this group of patients. When nephrology care was given more than 3 months before the initiation of dialysis, 64% of the patient population had a fistula as their type of vascular access. Internal medicine care (without nephrology input) resulted in only 11% of patients having a fistula that could be used for the first hemodialysis treatment.

Education programs are the potential key to success and should be part of any dedicated ESRD clinic. Employment can be maintained to a greater degree if education is instituted before the start of dialysis. A study by Rasgon and colleagues (40) demonstrated that 46.7% of blue-collar workers who received pre-ESRD education intervention continued working after initiation of dialysis. In contrast, a control group of similar workers who did not receive education intervention had a continued employment of only 23.5%. Predialysis interventions increase illness-related knowledge and can extend the predialysis interval (41,42). Intense education has substantial benefits, even leading to a delay in the need for renal replacement therapy. The current practice pattern indicates a need for change in our current system of care for patients with chronic renal failure. Education for the patient and communication between physicians is a critical step. The nonnephrologist must be educated to appreciate the implications of early referral, and the nephrologist must do a better job in transmitting this information to their colleagues.

Consensus guidelines must be established by the nephrology community on the timing of referral for chronic renal failure patients, and wide dissemination of these guidelines must be provided to internists, general practitioners, and family practitioners. The ultimate goal is that early referral will provide a better clinical condition at the initiation of renal replacement therapy. In particular, improved nutritional status, improved biochemical parameters, reduced hospitalization, and reduced risk of death would be the beneficial result of ER (43,44). Adequate planning of chronic access for peritoneal dialysis and/or hemodialysis is a consequence of ER and thus avoids the need for temporary acute catheters and their associated complications (45). Enrollment of chronic renal failure patients in pre-ESRD classes would lead to a better understanding of their kidney disease and therefore change the chronic renal failure patient from a passive caretaker into an active care participant.

There is an association between the amount of residual renal function at initiation of dialysis and subsequent outcomes. Early intervention is cost-effective with regards to improved morbidity and mortality. When residual renal function exists at initiation of renal replacement therapy, the total number of hospital days is 10.6. When there is no residual renal function when dialysis starts, then hospitalization is estimated to be 25 days (46,47). Having patients enter the system earlier will allow preservation of residual renal function. When dialysis is started the long-term benefits are noted: the longer the duration of pre-ESRD care, the longer the survival (48,49). In addition, there is an association between residual renal function at initiation of renal replacement therapy and concurrent nutritional status. A spontaneous decrease in dietary protein intake is noted with a decline in glomerular filtration rate (50). Malnutrition, adverse lipid profile, and unsuccessful adaptation to a high protein intake (necessitated once dialysis starts) are consequences of not having access to a nephrologist early in the course. Survival outcomes are correlated with the serum albumin at the initiation of hemodialysis. At initiation of dialysis, nutritional status as measured by serum albumin predicts survival: there is a 64% 2-year survival if the serum albumin is less than 3.5 g/dL compared to an 85% survival if the serum albumin is greater than 4.0 mg/dL (51). This all speaks to the cost-effectiveness of having the patients in the nephrology pipeline at an early stage of renal failure. At the start of dialysis, major risk factors for death include left ventricular hypertrophy as well as hypoalbuminemia. Both of these problems are medically approachable, and the management of these issues is covered in other chapters. Paying attention to detail in the chronic renal failure population will lead to overall better results and cost-effectiveness. While it may cost more to get the patient into the system earlier, cost savings 2–3 years after initiation of dialysis are documented (52).

VIII. GERIATRIC ISSUES AND THE COST IMPLICATIONS IN ESRD

The older the patient becomes, the more expensive the care. A rise in total expenditures is not surprising. As stated previously, Medicare payments for all patients on dialysis (considering all ages) is $38,000 per year (Table 6). For the ESRD patient >75 years of age, the expenditures rise to almost $60,000 per patient per year. The relative difference between the patient with diabetes mellitus and the nondiabetic gets smaller with increasing age. Table 9 shows the cost differential in the age range of 0–19 years being $12,000 per patient per year between the diabetic and nondiabetic. This figure falls to $6000 per year for the patient ≥75 years of age with diabetes as compared to the nondiabetic. When making decisions about initiating, withholding,

Table 9 Relative Difference in Costs per Year of ESRD Care for Diabetics and Nondiabetics[a]

Age (yr)	Diabetic	Nondiabetic
0–19	$34,000	$22,000
≥75	$54,000	$48,000

[a]Age ranges 0–19 years compared to ≥75 years. The cost differential falls from $12,000 to $6000 between the lowest and highest age ranges.
Source: HCFA; USRDS, 1997.

or terminating dialysis in the elderly, several important points must be considered (53):

The elderly are a heterogeneous group united by chronological, but not necessarily biological, age. Biological age has a variable expression depending on the pace of aging as well as the impact of co-morbid conditions, whose number and severity increases with age.

When analyzing the results of renal replacement therapy, the importance of quality survival supersedes absolute survival. The goal of renal replacement therapy in the elderly is to add life to years and not simply years to life. While there may be little disagreement as to the definition of quality of life, the yardstick for its measurement has been elusive.

Funding for the elderly population is noted specifically in Tables 5 and 9. Despite complex co-morbid and psychosocial conditions, survival and quality of life in the elderly patient on hemodialysis is frequently acceptable since 82% of elderly patients are maintained on center hemodialysis (54). Five-year patient survival in the elderly age range is between 20 and 40%. Vascular access problems are particularly important for the elderly and contribute to significant morbidity as well as adding cost to the system. Cardiovascular complications also require special attention since they complicate the issues of intradialytic hypotension, malnutrition, inadequate dialysis, increased incidence of infections, and gastrointestinal bleeding and are a factor in withdrawal from dialysis (55). Table 10 outlines issues noted in a hemodialysis patient population with a mean age of 75 years and multiple co-morbidities at initiation of dialysis. Despite these co-morbidities most of these patients were doing well.

Table 10 Dialysis in the Elderly

Co-morbid conditions	
Diabetes	17.2%
Coronary heart disease	35%
Cerebrovascular disease	10%
Chronic obstructive pulmonary disease	18%
Peripheral vascular disease	22%
Survival	
3 years	47%
5 years	22%
Quality of life indicators	
Social contacts	90%
Spent time outdoors	86%
Ranked high on Karnovsky scale	73% with scale >80%

Mean age of 75 years. Percentage of co-morbid conditions in this population and their percent survival at 3 and 5 years after initiation of renal replacement therapy. Measures of quality of life indicate a high degree of positive functioning; 40% of this age group perceived their health to be better than 70-year-old subjects, while only 25% regarded their health as worse.
Source: Refs. 54, 55.

IX. COMPLICATIONS OF DIALYSIS AND COST IMPLICATIONS

Access infection frequently leads to septicemia, graft thrombosis, septic emboli, and increased morbidity/mortality from these complications. *Staphylococcus aureus* is the most common organism associated with graft infections, especially the initial infection. For individuals who have repeated *Staphylococcus* infections, prophylaxis is a potentially cost-effective approach. If there are repeated infections, then nasal cultures should be done to determine if the patient is a carrier for *S. aureus*. If such nasal cultures are positive, then a prophylactic regimen can lead to cost savings. Several different modalities have been tried for *S. aureus* prophylaxis, including the following:

1. Mupirocin ointment to nares b.i.d × 5 days each months. Also apply at the exit site in case of a tunneled-cuffed catheter.
2. Trimethoprim-sulfamethoxazole three times per week.
3. Rifampin 600 mg per day × 5 days every 3 months.

It is difficult to provide if one modality of prophylaxis is better than another. However, a systematic approach should be tried.

Vancomycin-resistant enterococcus (VRE) is becoming a major problem around the country. In CAPD patients there is a very high death rate from patients who develop VRE peritonitis (56). Attempts have been made to employ other modalities of therapy. Synercid has been shown to be effective against VRE. The following approach to VRE infections is recommended:

1. Do not use vancomycin prophylactically.
2. Discourage vancomycin use because of familiarity with this drug and ease of dosing.
3. Reserve vancomycin for the circumstance where it is specifically needed.

4. Try cefazolin 20 mg/kg IV as an empiric alternative to vancomycin for infections with enterococci.

The Centers for Disease Control and Prevention (CDC) is always updating its VRE guidelines. They should be contacted if there are any questions in doubt.

The repeated use of vancomycin is now being associated with the first signs of vancomycin-resistant, methicillin-resistant *S. aureus* (MRSA). Our major standby for MRSA was vancomycin, but resistant isolates are now becoming noted. If this antibiotic is used on an ongoing basis, then we can expect an increased prevalence of vancomycin-resistant MRSA. The cost implications of such are enormous. The percentage of dialysis centers treating more than one patient with VRE doubled from 1995 to 1996, going from 11.5% in 1995 to 21.3% in 1996 (57). The highest percentage of units reporting VRE cases were government-owned (Veterans Administration) (32%), followed by nonprofit (28.8%) and for-profit units (17.3%). Dialysis patients have represented up to 22% of hospitalized patients infected or colonized with VRE. Hemodialysis or peritoneal dialysis was noted to be an independent risk factor for VRE bacteremia.

Dialysis infection precautions are another area that have major financial implications for dialysis. Hepatitis C infections are potentially the most costly on a long-term basis to the dialysis population. While routine screening of patients or staff for hepatitis C antibody is not necessary for purposes of infection control, dialysis centers may wish to conduct serological surveys of their patient populations to determine the prevalence of the antibody in their dialysis center (58). Determining the duration of hepatitis C virus infections is helpful in predicting outcome: the longer the duration of infection, the more likelihood the clinical consequences of liver disease. In addition, the age of the patient makes a difference: the younger the patient at the time of infection, the greater the number of years at risk. Cirrhosis, chronic active hepatitis and death are linearly associated with a younger age of onset of hepatitis C infections. As the area of information grows about hepatitis C, it is important to do viral genotype (which may have implications for prognosis). Measuring the viral load of hepatitis C RNA by polymerase chain reaction (PCR) is another necessary step in assessment of the patient because of the potential implications of treatment with interferon. Each of these infections are covered in more detail in other chapters, but the issue of the financial implications of these problems should be known to the physicians and dialysis administrators. The overall incidence of hepatitis C in 1996 was reported to be 0.4% among patients, the same percentage as noted among staff. In 1996, 44% of centers tested patients for anti-HCV, and the prevalence of anti-HCV at these centers was 10.1% (58). Anti-HCV prevalence ranged from 5.2 to 16.1% among ESRD networks. Networks with higher anti-HCV prevalence rates were more likely to test their patients for anti-HCV.

Personal protective equipment (PPE) is defined as equipment that protects workers from contact with potentially infectious materials. This equipment must be used when there is potential for bloodborne pathogens, and dialysis is the classical example (59). The financial costs of not using such PPE are enormous, and the potential for litigation and closure of the unit exists. Under normal work conditions, protective equipment must not allow potentially infectious materials to contact clothes, undergarments, skin, or mucous membranes. Workers must be trained to use equipment properly, and the protective equipment must be appropriate for the task. It is critical that the equipment remain free of physical flaws that could compromise safety. A critical issue is making sure that gloves fit properly. Attention to detail will save a large amount of money downstream. The medical director of a dialysis unit is ultimately responsible for adherence to CDC guidelines. Any deviation leaves the facility and staff vulnerable.

X. DEALING WITH THE MANAGED CARE ENVIRONMENT

Medical management programs must be standardized across the entire nephrology community. A common approach will allow the maximum benefit of continuous quality improvement (CQI) programs when they are initiated to improve patient care. Although the gameboard might look different in this new world of managed care, the game pieces remain the same. To be effective in managed care is to provide quality medical care of high value. The skill sets that we bring to the organization are those that have made us succeed in the past; these same skill sets enable us to be successful as we move forward. All physicians, nurses, and ancillary staff must be knowledgeably involved in the process if we are to succeed in managed care. Managed care education is a key factor to success, and we must not waste our efforts in an unremitting barrage of criticism (since managed care will not disappear).

Capitation will be the reimbursement mechanism to health-care providers as the major way of controlling costs. It is predicted that more than 90% of the working U.S. population will receive its health insurance through managed care within the next decade (14). Currently, managed care has had little experience with capitation payments for chronically ill patients who consume large financial and physical resources. The ESRD population represents a vulnerable group of patients, and their care could potentially be compromised in a capitated environment. Nephrologists will need to serve as advocates for ESRD patients through a mechanism of quality care driven by a CQI model. Cost-effective delivery of care will occur as nephrologists join together to form Independent Practice Associations (IPAs).

The unique level of care necessary to maintain the health of the typical renal patient via the ESRD program requires an understanding of the political realities of budgetary constraints in both the public and private sectors (60). Government agencies, health-care institutions, insurance companies, and MCOs are now setting the rules for health care, rendering physicians' authority and patients' rights increasingly irrelevant (61). Patients and physicians are aligned together in the era of managed care, and the professional ethics of physicians are potentially a barrier to insurance companies, MCOs, and other health-care payors.

Cost-effective medicine is a permanent part of our landscape, and physicians must buy into the processes that dictate effective utilization of limited financial resources. Fighting managed care at every step will be a losing battle, and it is our responsibility to take the lead in health-care delivery by admitting that we are dealing with finite resources. A disease-management approach would work well with ESRD and may be an effective alternative to the current health-care delivery system. A case-management approach would support the nephrologist in his/her role as the principal caregiver for the patient with progressive renal failure and ESRD. A healthier patient reaching ESRD due to improved management will cost less because of reduced hospitalization and lower mortality rates (62).

Quality needs to be defined and measured via a mechanism that can be easily understood and replicated anywhere in the world. Quality is measured in terms of excellence of outcomes, patient satisfaction, and appropriate use of resources. Quality cannot be translated directly into reducing length of hospital stays, and centers of excellence cannot be defined as institutional organizations that have negotiated the lowest cost package from the insurer. The cost-containment aspect of quality can focus on reducing inappropriate health services and avoiding preventable adverse events. Physicians can cut costs and improve quality by addressing these two above issues.

Quality can be measured in terms of structure, process, and outcomes (63). The structure of care is defined by:

1. System characteristics
2. Provider characteristics
3. Patient characteristics

The process of care is defined by:

1. Technical issues
2. Interpersonal style

Outcome is measured by:

1. Clinical endpoints
2. Functional status
3. General well-being
4. Patient satisfaction

The Medical Outcomes Study conceptual framework can address the three issues of structure, process, and outcome (64).

XI. FINANCIAL CONCERNS FOR NEPHROLOGY IN A CAPITATED/ MANAGED CARE ENVIRONMENT

Since capitated payments for ESRD patients will be based on a per patient per month reimbursement, regardless of the services delivered, it is critical to know every component of cost delivered to the ESRD patient and who controls the flow of dollars. Therefore, it is incumbent on nephrologists to form a subspecialty Independent Practice Association (a nephrology IPA) because no individual, group practice, or academic division has the sophistication to handle the intricate cost accounting. Broad participation by academic and practice-based nephrologists in such an IPA within a state region will create an opportunity with HMOs/ MCOs based on knowing total cost and the value of ESRD care (65). There must be a financial incentive available to enhance outcomes. What currently exists in the MCO market is financial reward for saving dollars. Less care delivered leads to savings in the short term while resulting in increased long-term costs because of a diminished prophylactic approach to care. This is absolutely wrong and shameful.

Financial incentives must be based on improved outcomes. The nephrology community must set the standards of care and the desired goals. We need to monitor ourselves, and our colleagues will demand the highest care from us and themselves. Bonus payments should only be based on improved outcomes. Outcomes in this situation mean not only morbidity and mortality, but can be measured by nutritional status (serum albumin), dialysis clearance (Kt/V), management of anemia (level of hematocrit), iron status, and management of renal osteodystrophy (calcium, phosphorus, PTH values, etc.). The nephrology community will decide what markers will denote quality of care, and reimbursement for improved outcomes will follow. The model must be clear and easily understood by every participant in the system. When finances are on the table, disagreement can easily occur unless the ground rules are explicit. Fewer complications should be translated into improved reimbursement. Local networks are essential for success in implementing global capitation. Working within your defined nephrology community will enhance dialogue and trust (because you know each other). As soon as decisions are made by individuals who are strangers, mistrust will occur.

XII. UNDERSTANDING THE REIMBURSEMENT SYSTEM CHANGE

Since reimbursement is in an astonishing flux with the advent of managed care and capitated contracts, nephrologists need to understand financial systems. Complementing clinical acumen with an understanding of finances will facilitate negotiations. The individual nephrologist will not be able to accumulate the necessary information to do effective contract negotiations of their own accord. Medical entrepreneurs will be a necessary addition for appropriate contract negotiations, otherwise reimbursement may be inadequate (66).

How do nephrologists obtain adequate information to financially protect themselves? There are a plethora of courses and seminars currently being offered about managed care and capitation. To date most of these offerings have been a hodgepodge of topics with the "take-home" message being that we are in a rapidly changing environment and the nephrologist needs to "understand the system." As stated above, the hope for the future is through collaborative efforts that are organized through single-specialty IPAs. Nephrologists need to join organizations within their own state, since any contract negotiations with Medicaid have to be within state boundaries. However, a regionwide or statewide IPA can be part of a larger network (and the establishment of those are now in process).

Extension of the Medicare Secondary Payor (MSP) from 18 to 30 months, effective August 1997, will create a large financial impact on HMOs/MCOs. Such organizations barely understand the impact of this legislation to date since the number of ESRD patients in any one insurance organization is relatively small. Since HMOs/MCOs have virtually no experience with the financing of ESRD care, their cost structuring currently exists in a near-vacuum. Current premiums charged by HMOs/MCOs are based mainly on a healthy population and will not be adequate to cover costs generated by a chronically ill segment of their patient pool who will become fully incorporated into the cost structure. It is evident that premiums charged will need to be increased or companies will be in deficit spending in short order. Only the largest organizations with a million or more covered lives can absorb the costs of the ESRD patient without raising premiums. This cost factor will invariably lead to more consolidation of HMOs/MCOs.

As stated in an earlier section, the HCFA Capitation Demonstration Project has now been launched. While it is important to obtain results from this study, I do not believe that adequate information will be forthcoming in a sufficient period of time to impact the marketplace. Market forces driven by organizations already launched into the managed care arena will produce data well before the Demonstration Project results are available. The bottom line is that health care for the chronically ill costs money and someone needs to pay the bill. Patients will need to pay more for their health care coverage unless all of us pay. We could rapidly develop into a two-tiered or multitiered system (those of means will get coverage and those without will not receive adequate coverage). Therefore, some innovative strategies must be employed to appropriately finance care for the chronically ill. This may eventuate in some form of a national health insurance.

XIII. COST IMPLICATIONS OF STAFFING

The issue of employee turnover in the dialysis unit is a hidden cost that is rarely factored in the overall expenditures. Significant factors implicated in staff turnover include the following:

1. Variables in organizational structure
2. Employee characteristics
3. Needs and values
4. Nature of tasks performed

Motivational factors need to be included in the overall scheme of employee satisfaction. No quantitative or qualitative research could be found on the potential causes of turnover in freestanding dialysis clinics. Staff turnover of a for-profit dialysis company over a year has been noted in one report (67). The effect of turnover and retention is a major issue since the U.S. Department of Labor estimates that it costs a company up to one third of a new hire's annual salary to replace an employee (68). Turnover drains profits and adversely affects the overall efficiency of an organization. Tangible costs include recruitment, selection, training of new personnel, advertising expenses, and the manpower expense related to the hiring process. It has been estimated that the cost of replacing personnel in a dialysis unit is $5,000–$6,000 per employee (67).

Intangible costs include the increased workload experienced by employees to maintain the level of services during staff shortages, low morale, reduced productivity, and a negative organization image. Understanding the relational causes of turnover and the strategies used to minimize it may be of significant value to renal administrators. Major reasons for employees leaving relate to job satisfaction and job opportunity. Unless there is a motivational aspect to the position in the dialysis unit, there will be increased turnover. The relative strength of the goal achievement motive is directly related to the lowest unfilled need, which serves as the primary motivator of behavior. The hierarchical structure of needs from the lowest to the highest are as follows:

1. Physiological—in organizational settings physiological needs are satisfied by adequate wages and comfortable work settings. If these needs are not satisfied, the organization is dominated by the physiological needs and all others are pushed into the background.
2. Safety—needs include security, stability, freedom from fear, and the need for structure and limits. Security needs are satisfied in the workplace by job continuity, a grievance system, and adequate employee benefits.
3. The feeling of belonging—there is a need to develop close associations with other persons, and this is satisfied by social interaction among employees and teamwork.
4. Esteem—needs include ego fulfillment in terms of prestige received from within and from outside the organization. If self-esteem is satisfied, the end result is feelings of self-confidence, worth, and adequacy.
5. Accomplishments—there is a need for a sense for self-fulfillment and accomplishment through personal growth and development. Unmet needs create a tension within people that leads them to behave in ways that reduce the tension and restore internal equilibrium (69).

In the dialysis setting, the leadership (physicians, nurse managers, administrators) must pay attention to job satisfaction, growth, and appropriate motivation. If we are aware of the issues that lead to a high turnover in employees, there can be an eventual positive result. The patient is the true beneficiary of longevity in the workplace. If employees do terminate, especially on a voluntary basis, there should be an exit interview and completion of a questionnaire, which should be returned to a higher authority outside the dialysis unit to maintain anonymity. Issues to be addressed in any questionnaire about satisfaction in the workplace must include work schedule, direct supervisor, benefits, job duties, orientation on initiating the job, physical work environment, ongoing training, workload, communication, advancement opportunities, and salary. If we can identify any recurring pattern, it may help future employees. Managing employee turnover is of critical importance to organizations, especially for issues related to quality of care and patient comfort. Identifying causative factors through data collection offers a basis for developing strategies to reduce turnover.

XIV. SUMMARY

The role of the entire health-care team is to maximize quality of care and maintain patient satisfaction. In the era of ever-growing managed care, cost-effective delivery of care mandates that all members of the team address the issue of accountability. First and foremost we are accountable to patients, second of all to colleagues in the workplace, and then to the payors. The patient remains the center of the hub at all times, and all efforts must be directed towards our goal of quality of care to maintain quality of life. Financial implications are part of every one of our test-treatment strategies. Being aware of our fiscal responsibility as a complement to our patient responsibility will be a mandate for all in the immediate future.

REFERENCES

1. Congressional Budget Office. Reducing the Deficit: Spending and Revenue Options. Washington, DC: Government Printing Office, 1997:298.

2. Congressional Budget Office. The Economic and Budget Outlook, 1998–2007. Washington, DC: Government Printing Office, 1997;126.
3. Altman SH, Wallack SS. Health care spending: Can the United States control it? In: Altman S, Reinhardt U, eds. Strategic Choices for a Changing Health Care System. Chicago: Health Administration Press; 1996.
4. Ginzberg E. The changing US health care agenda, JAMA 1998; 279:501–504.
5. Source Book of Health Insurance Data, 1996. Washington, DC: Health Insurance Association of America, 1997.
6. Patients, Profits and Health System Change: A Wall Street Perspective. Washington, DC: Center for Studying Health System Change, May 1997. Issue Brief No. 9.
7. Ginzberg E. Tomorrow's Hospital: A Look to the Twenty-First Century. New Haven, CT: Yale University Press, 1996.
8. Steinman TI. Administrational and organizational aspects of dialysis. In: Malluche H, Sawaya P, eds. Updated Textbook of Clinical Nephrology, Dialysis and Transplantation. Desenhofen, Germany: Dustri-Verlag Publishing Co., 1998.
9. Nichol G, Dennis DT, Steere AC, Lightfoot R, Wells G, Shea B, Tugwell P. Test-treatment strategies for patients suspected of having Lyme disease: a cost-effectiveness analysis. Ann Int Med 1998; 123:37–48.
10. Schriger DL, Baraff LJ, Rogers WH, Cretin S. Implementation of clinical guidelines using a computer charting system. JAMA 1997; 278:1585—1590.
11. Granata AV, Hillman AL. Competing practice guidelines: using cost-effectiveness analysis to make optional decisions. Ann Int Med 1998; 128:56–63.
12. Balas AE, Kretschmer R, Gnann W, West DA, Boren SA, Centor RM, Nerlich M, Gupta M, West TD, Soderstrom NS. Interpreting cost analysis of clinical intervention. JAMA 1998; 279:54–57.
13. Coutts L. Consolidation and the future of renal care. Nephrol News Issues 1998; 12:47.
14. Steinman TI. Managed care, capitation and the future of nephrology. J Am Soc Nephrol 1997; 8:1618–1623.
15. Gallop E. Carveouts: A specialist's dream. Phys Managed Care Rep 1998; 6:5–6.
16. Schmittdiel J, Selby JV, Grumbach K, Quesenberry CP. Choice of a personal physician and patient satisfaction in a health maintenance organization. JAMA 1997; 278: 1596–1599.
17. Longo DR, Land G, Schramm W, Fraas J, Hoskins B, Howell V. Consumer reports in health care. Do they make a difference in patient care? JAMA 1997; 278: 1579–1584.
18. Hall MA, Berenson RA. Ethical practice in managed care: a dose of realism. Ann Int Med 1998; 12837–12848.
19. USRDS 1997 Annual Data Report. National Institutes of Health, National Institute of Diabetes and Digestive and Kidney Diseases. Bethesda, MD: U.S. Renal Data System, April 1997.
20. USRDS 1996 Annual Data Report. National Institutes of Health, National Institute of Diabetes and Digestive and Kidney Diseases. Bethesda, MD: U.S. Renal Data System, April 1996.
21. Beathard GA. Complications of vascular access. Early diagnosis and treatment. Proceedings, National Kidney Foundation Spring Clinical Nephrology Meetings, March 26–29, 1998, Nashville, TN, pp. 62–63.
22. Chertow GM. Grafts vs fistulas for hemodialysis patients: Equal access for all? JAMA 1996; 276:1343–1344.
23. NIH Consensus Statement: Morbidity and mortality of dialysis. Ann Intern Med 1994; 121:62–70.
24. Woods JD, Turenne MN, Strawderman RL, Young EW, Hirth RA, Port FK, Held PJ. Am J Kidney Dis 1997; 30:50–57.
25. Held PJ. Personal communication.
26. Obrador GT, Pereira BJG. Early referral to the nephrologist and timely initiation of renal replacement therapy: a paradigm shift in the management of patients with chronic renal failure. Am J Kidney Dis 1998; 31:398–417.
27. Hays RD, Kallich JD, Mapes DL, Coons SJ, Carter WB. Development of the Kidney Disease Quality of Life (KDQOL) Instrument. Qual Life Res 1994; 3:329–338.
28. Hays RD, Kallich JD, Mapes DL, Coons SJ, Amin N, Carter WB. Kidney Disease Quality of Life Short Form (KDQOL-SF), Version 1.3. A Manual for Use and Scoring. P-7994. Santa Monica, CA: RAND, 1997.
29. NIH Consensus Statement: Morbidity and mortality of dialysis. Ann Intern Med 1994; 121:62–70.
30. Khan IH, Catto GR, Neil E, MacLeod AM. Death during the first 90 days of dialysis: a case-control study. Am J Kidney Dis 1995; 25:276–280.
31. Campbell JD, Ewignan B, Hosokawa M, Van Stone JC. The timing of referral of patients with end-stage renal disease. Dial Transplant 1989; 18:660–686.
32. Innes A, Rowe PA, Burden RP, Morgan AG. Early deaths on renal replacement therapy: the need for early nephrological referral. Nephrol Dial Transplant 1992; 7:467–471.
33. Muirhead N, Blyndal K. Potential cost savings of planned dialysis start (abstr). J Am Soc Nephrol 1995; 6:553.
34. Jungers P, Zingraff J, Page B, Albouze G, Hannedouche T, Man NK. Detrimental effects of late referral in patients with chronic renal failure: a case-control study. Kidney Int 1993; 43:S170–S173.
35. Garella S. The cost of dialysis in the USA. Nephrol Dial Transplant 1997; 12:10–21.
36. Hirth RA, Turenne MN, Woods JD, Young EW, Port FK, Pauly MV, Held PJ. Predictors of type of vascular access in hemodialysis patients. JAMA 1996; 276: 1303–1308.

37. Sesso R, Belasco AG. Late diagnosis of chronic renal failure and mortality in maintenance dialysis. Nephrol Dial Transplant 1996; 11:2417–2420.
38. Eadington DW, Craig KJ, Winney RJ. Late referral for RRT: Still a common cause of avoidable morbidity (abstr). Nephrol Dial Transplant 1994; 9:1686.
39. Ifudu O, Dawood M, Homel P, Friedman EA. Excess morbidity in patients starting uremia therapy without prior care by a nephrologist. Am J Kidney Dis 1996; 28:841–845.
40. Rasgon S, Schwankovsky L, James-Rogers A, Widrow L, Glick J, Butts E. An intervention for employment maintenance among blue-collar workers with end-stage renal disease. Am J Kidney Dis 1993; 22:402–412.
41. Rettig R. The social contract and the treatment of permanent kidney failure. JAMA 1996; 275:1123–1126.
42. Friedman EA. End-stage renal disease therapy: an American success story. JAMA 1996; 275:1118–1122.
43. Khan IH, Catto GRD, Edward N, MacLeod AM. Chronic renal failure: factors influencing nephrology referral. Q J Med 1994; 87:559–564.
44. Mendelssohn DC, Singer PA. Referral for dialysis in Ontario. Arch Intern Med 1995; 155:2473–2478.
45. Hood SA, Schillo B, Beane E, Rozas V, Sondheimer JH, and Members of the Michigan Renal Plan Task Force of the Michigan Public Health Institute. An analysis of the adequacy of preparation for end-stage renal disease care in Michigan. ASAIOJ 1995; 41:M422–M426.
46. Bonomini V, Albertazzi A, Vangelista A, Bortolotti GC, Stefoni S, Scolari MP. Residual renal function and effective rehabilitation in chronic dialysis. Nephron 1976; 16:89–99.
47. Bonomini V, Feletti C, Scolari MP, Stefoni S. Benefits of early initiation of dialysis. Kidney Int 1985; 28:S57–S59.
48. Lysaght MJ, Vonesh EF, Gotch F, Ibels L, Keen M, Lindholm B, Nolph DK, Pollock CA, Prowant B, Farrell PC. The influence of dialysis treatment modality on the decline of remaining renal function. ASAIO Trans 1991; 37:598–604.
49. Bonomini V, Baldrati L, Stefoni S. Comparative cost/benefit analysis in early and late dialysis. Nephron 1983; 33:1–4.
50. Ikizler A, Greene J, Wingard R, Parker R, Hakim RH. Spontaneous dietary protein intake during progression of chronic renal failure. J Am Soc Nephrol 1995; 6: 1386–1391.
51. Hakim RM, Lazarus JM. Initiation of dialysis. J Am Soc Nephrol 1995; 6:1319–1328.
52. Obrador G, Ruthazer R, Port F, Held P, Pereira B. Trends in residual renal function (RRF) at the initiation of dialysis in the U.S. ESRD population (abstr). J Am Soc Nephrol 1997; 8:145.
53. Ismail N. Clinical challenges with the care of the geriatric ESRD patient: dialysis. Proceedings, National Kidney Foundation, Spring Clinical Nephrology Meeting, March 26–29, 1998, Nashville, Tennessee, pp. 119–122.
54. Ismail N. Renal replacement therapy in the elderly: an old problem with young solutions. Nephrol Dial Transplant 1997; 12:873–876.
55. Latos DL. Chronic dialysis in patients over age 65. J Am Soc Nephrol 1996; 7:637–646.
56. Troidle L, Kliger AS, Gorban-Brennan M, Fekrig M, Golden M. Nine episodes of CPD-associated peritonitis with vancomycin resistant enterococci. Kidney Int 1996; 50:1368–1372.
57. Editorial. Number of centers reporting VRE cases in 1996 doubled. Nephrol News Issues 1998; 12:43–44.
58. Masuko K, Mitsui T, Iwano K, Yamazaki C, Okuda K, Meguro T, Murayama N, Inoue T, Tsuda F, Okamoto H, Miyakawa Y, Mayumi M. Infection with hepatitis GB virus C in patients on maintenance hemodialysis. N Engl J Med 1996; 334:1485–1490.
59. Peacock E. Dialysis infection precautions. Proceedings, National Kidney Foundation Spring Clinical Nephrology Meetings, March 26–29, 1998, Nashville, TN, pp. 189–192.
60. Renal Physicians Association/American Society of Nephrology: Position Paper on Managed Care and Nephrology. Washington, DC, December 9, 1995.
61. Kerr EA, Mittman BS, Hays RD, Leake B, Brooke RH. Quality assurance in capitated physician groups: Where is emphasis? JAMA 1996; 276:1236–1239.
62. Steinman TI. The dialysis facility of the future: the financial and social environment. Semin Nephrol 1997; 17:298–305.
63. Retting RA, Sadler JH, Meyer KB, Wasson JH, Parkerson GR Jr, Kantz B, Hays RD, Patrick DL. Assessing health and quality of life outcomes in dialysis: a report on an Institute of Medicine workshop. Am J Kidney Dis 1997; 30:140–155.
64. Tarlov AR, Ware JE Jr, Greenfield S, Nelson EC, Perrin E, Zubkoff M. The Medical Outcomes Study: an application of methods for monitoring the results of medical care. JAMA 1989; 262:925–930.
65. Steinman TI. HCFA capitation payments and nephrology manpower projections: How will primary care of ESRD by nephrologists be affected? Semin Dial 1997; 10:318–323.
66. Steinman TI. How nephrologists can understand the reimbursement system change. Nephrol News Issues. In press.
67. Bednar B, McMullen N. A retrospective analysis of employee turnover in a healthcare setting. Nephrol News Issues 1998; 12:35–39.
68. White G. Employee turnover: the hidden drain. Hum Resources Focus 1995; 15–17.
69. Mobley WH. Intermediate linkages in the relationship between job satisfaction and employee turnover. J Appl Psychol 1997; 62:237–240.

43

Economic Issues, Referral Patterns, and Choice of Treatment Modality of End-Stage Renal Disease in Europe

Norbert Lameire
University Hospital of Gent and University of Gent, Gent, Belgium

Wim Van Biesen
University Hospital of Gent, Gent, Belgium

Maria E. Wiedemann
Baxter Deutschland GmbH, Unterschleissheim, Germany

I. INTRODUCTION

The first part of this chapter will provide a short description of the various European health-care systems, focusing on the health-care economics, health-care reforms, and their influence on health-care provision and outcome in general. These different systems create divergent backgrounds for the therapy of end-stage renal disease (ESRD). In the second part, the differences in the provision of the several dialysis modalities in some of the European countries will be described. The third part of the chapter will discuss the various European funding systems and reimbursement strategies for dialysis. Finally, the last part will summarize some recent data on referral patterns of ESRD patients in Europe and their impact on choice of dialysis modality and patient outcome.

Data published by the Organization for Economic Co-operation and Development (OECD), the World Health Organization (WHO), and official country registries have been used for this comparative analysis. In addition, documents from the different funding agencies from the various countries and, in limited cases, from additional specific surveys have been consulted. The following countries have been selected for this review: United Kingdom, France, Germany, Sweden, Norway, Finland, Denmark, Belgium, the Netherlands, Switzerland, Austria, Italy, and Spain. Data from the United States, Canada, and Japan have been included for comparative purposes. Since a great number of countries are covered in this review, graphical presentation of the data was necessary.

II. EUROPEAN HEALTH-CARE SYSTEMS

According to WHO, the health-care systems present in different countries are strongly influenced by the underlying norms and values prevailing in the respective societies. Like other human service systems, health-care services often reflect deeply rooted social and cultural expectations of the citizenry. Although these fundamental values are generated outside the formal structure of the health-care system, they often define its overall character and capacity. Health-care systems are therefore different all over the world and are strongly influenced by each nation's unique history, traditions, and political system. This has led to different institutions and a high variation in the type of social contracts between the citizens and their respective governments.

In some societies, health care is viewed as a predominantly social or collective good from which all citizens belonging to that society should benefit, no matter what individual curative or preventive care is needed. A principle related to this view is that of solidarity, where the cost of care is intentionally cross-subsidized from the young to the old, from the rich to the poor, and from the healthy to the diseased.

Other societies, more influenced by the market-oriented thinking of the 1980s, increasingly perceive health care as a commodity to be bought and sold on the open market. These marketing incentives possibly allow more dynamic and more efficient health-care services and a more efficient control of growth in health-care expenditure. This concept of health services as a market commodity is for the moment not prevailing in Europe.

Today, three main models of health care based on the source of their funding can be distinguished: the Beveridge Model, the Bismarck Model and the Private Insurance Model.

In the Beveridge Model, funding is mainly based on taxation and is characterized by a centrally organized National Health Service where the services are provided by mainly public health providers (hospitals, community doctors). In this model, health-care budgets compete with other spending priorities. The countries falling under this model are the United Kingdom, Italy, Spain, Sweden, Denmark, Norway, Finland, and Canada.

The Bismarck Model is mainly funded by a premium-financed social/mandatory insurance and is mainly found in countries like Germany, France, Austria, Switzerland, and Benelux. Japan also has a premium-based mandatory insurance fund system. This model results in a mix of private and public providers and allows more flexible spending on health care.

In the Private Insurance Model, funding of the system is based on premiums voluntarily paid into private insurance companies and in its pure form exists practically only in the United States. In this system the funding is predominantly private, with the exception of social care through Medicare and Medicaid. The great majority of the providers in this model belong to the private sector.

In this chapter, the models mentioned above will be referred to using the terms "public," "mix," and "private," respectively. All health-care systems are aiming at "perfection," i.e., they try to achieve an optimal mixture of access to health care, quality of care, and cost-efficiency. Only the latter aspect of cost-efficiency will be briefly discussed here.

The efficiency of a given health-care system for providing equity/access and quality of care can be measured as the cost of the system, calculated either as a percentage of the gross national product (GNP), spent on health care, or even better for comparison expressed as expenditures for health care in "purchasing power parities," defined as the equivalent amount of U.S. dollars spent per head of population per year.

Figure 1 shows the calculations of the cost of health care expenses for the year 1994 in the three groups of countries. Between \$971 and \$2010 per head is spent on health care in "public" countries, which is much less than the amount spent by the "mix" countries. The latter spend from \$1484 to \$2294 per year per head of population.

Despite the lowest rate of access to health care (with only 85% of the population covered by either Medicare and Medicaid or by private insurance) and the lowest quality performance (based on the number of life-years lost or the number of stillbirths), the United States spends \$3498 per year on health care, 3.5 times more than is spent by Spain, for example. Consequently, the amount of money spent on health care in a given system is in itself not an indicator of its quality, but is more related to differences in provider structures in the systems. "Public" countries tend in general to spend less money on health care compared to "mix" and "private" countries, but this does not seem to be associated with differences in quality outcomes.

Two important questions can be raised: (1) Will the increase in quality requirements stimulated by the development of new health technologies and the growing quantitative needs due to the increasing age of the populations lead to ever-growing costs in the future? (2) How will the governments in various countries respond to these new challenges? The elderly population has already considerably increased in all countries included in this review.

Taken together with the high life expectancy in virtually all countries, some realistic calculations on the growth of the costs of health care can be made. According to calculations made in 1993 by the National European Research Associates (NERA), most countries will reach a level of health care cost of 10–11% of their GNP; it is predicted in the United States to reach more than 15% of the GNP in the year 2000.

It is interesting to note that health care expenses have grown over the past 50 years because of and/or in spite of several health-care reforms. After World War II, a first major wave of reforms focused on equity, creating access to health care for everybody. Hospital care was seen as the main provider. The second wave of reforms in the 1970s tried to improve quality by focusing more on prevention and primary care. An increase in the quality of ambulatory care was emphasized in an effort to curb growing hospital expenses.

Today, further reforms are necessary because of uncontrolled increases in cost. The increasing need to care

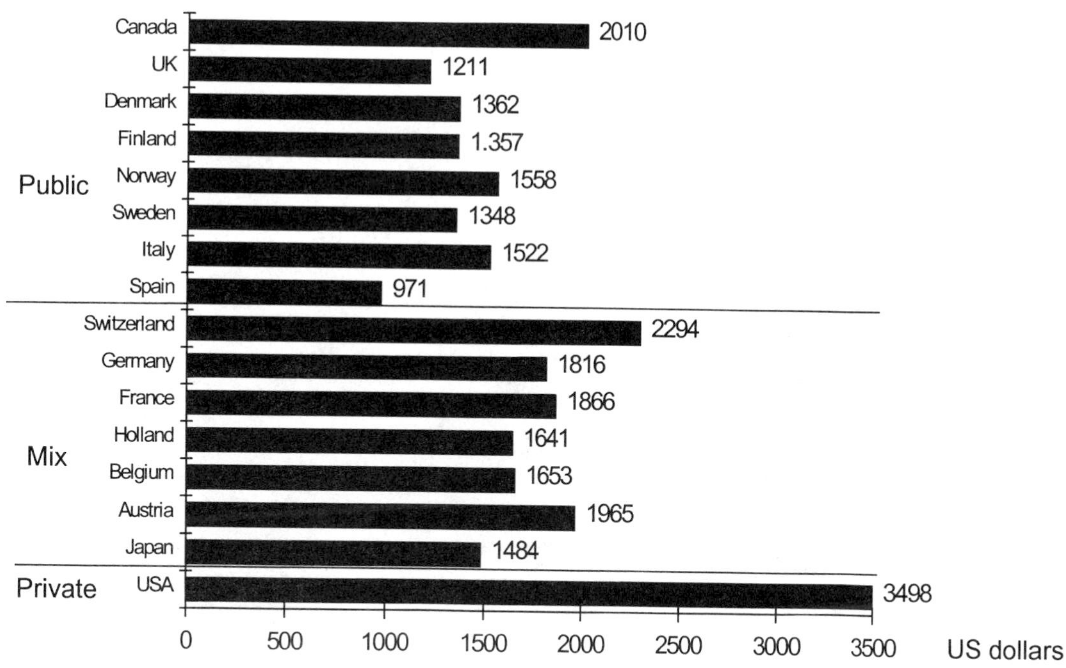

Fig. 1 Health-care expenses in U.S. dollars for the year 1994 in the "public," "mix," and "private" countries, expressed as "purchasing power parities."

for a growing elderly population, the development of new technologies and improved care in general in the face of a growing economic constraint create a number of dilemmas for all governments. It is thus not surprising that all current reform efforts are centered around cost and cost control.

The principle of solidarity and the assurance of quality in health care, more specifically in the fast-growing segment of chronic diseases, such as ESRD, may be questioned in the future.

III. ESRD THERAPIES

Three treatment modalities in various forms and at various sites are available for patients with ESRD: kidney transplantation (Tx), hemodialysis (HD), and peritoneal dialysis (PD). Although the great majority of the patients are potential candidates for renal transplantation, the shortage of donors will probably not be solved in the near future and the need for chronic dialysis will even become greater. This part of the chapter therefore focuses on dialysis. For discussion of the access to health care in the specific and expensive segment of therapy of ESRD, the grouping of the countries according to their predominant health-care system (see above) will be used.

It is interesting to note that of the "public" health-care providers, Italy and Spain allow a high share of "private" dialysis providers, while of the "mix" health care providers, the Netherlands and Switzerland restrict dialysis to public providers. Consequently, a regrouping of the countries based on the type of dialysis provider model ("public," "mixed," or "private") is necessary.

"Public" countries include now the Netherlands, Switzerland, the United Kingdom, Norway, Finland, Sweden, Denmark, and Canada. "Mix" countries consist of Germany, Austria, Belgium, France, Italy, and Spain. "Private" countries include the United States and Japan.

Since there is no single indicator of access to ESRD treatments, substitute indicators such as prevalence, take-on rate, proportion of patients living with a kidney transplant, share of home-care/peritoneal dialysis patients, and growth of the number of ESRD patients will be used.

A. Prevalence

Prevalence is defined as the total number of ESRD patients treated per million population (pmp) for 1994/1995 year end. As can be noted from Figure 2, in "public" countries the prevalence ranges from 412 to 575

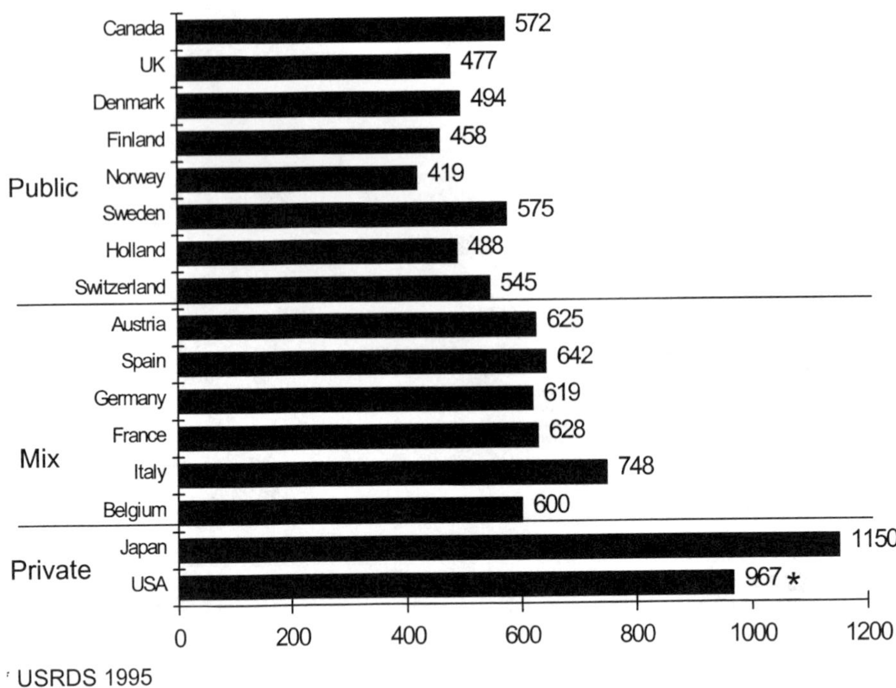

Fig. 2 Prevalence of treated ESRD patients per million population in 1994/1995, based on data from several national registries, EDTA data, USRDS.

pmp and is in general lower than in "mix" countries, where it ranges from 600 to 748 pmp. The highest prevalence is found in "private" countries," with 1150 in Japan and 967 pmp in the United States, respectively.

B. Number of Patients Accepted

Take-on rate is defined as the number of new patients per million population taken into a ESRD program in 1995. Figure 3 shows the take-on rates of various countries, ranging from 60 to 104 pmp in "public" countries, 94 to 125 pmp in "mix" countries, and 194 to 253 pmp in "private" countries.

C. Share of Transplanted Patients

A further indicator for access to ESRD patient care is the share of kidney transplant patients as a percentage of total ESRD patients. Figure 4 indicates a considerably higher share of transplanted patients in "public" versus "mix" and "private" countries. In "public" countries the range of transplanted patients extends from 45 to 81%. In "mix" countries the range is from 20 to 48%. The U.S. patient share is 27.2%, whereas the Japanese share is 0.3% with practically no transplant program.

D. Share of Home-Care/Peritoneal Dialysis Patients

Figure 5 demonstrates the total share of home dialysis patients (including PD) and PD as a percentage of the total number of dialysis patients. There is a clear difference in the share of home treatments within the three dialysis provider systems: in "public" countries a range of 20–52% of patients (average ~ 30%) are treated with home therapies (HD and PD). In "mix" countries, this share of home therapy ranges from 9 to 17%, and in "private" countries it ranges between 6% in Japan and 17% in the United States. PD predominates as home-care treatment in all countries.

A comparison between the share of PD patients within each "provider type" of dialysis within each country reveals that the higher the share of "public"

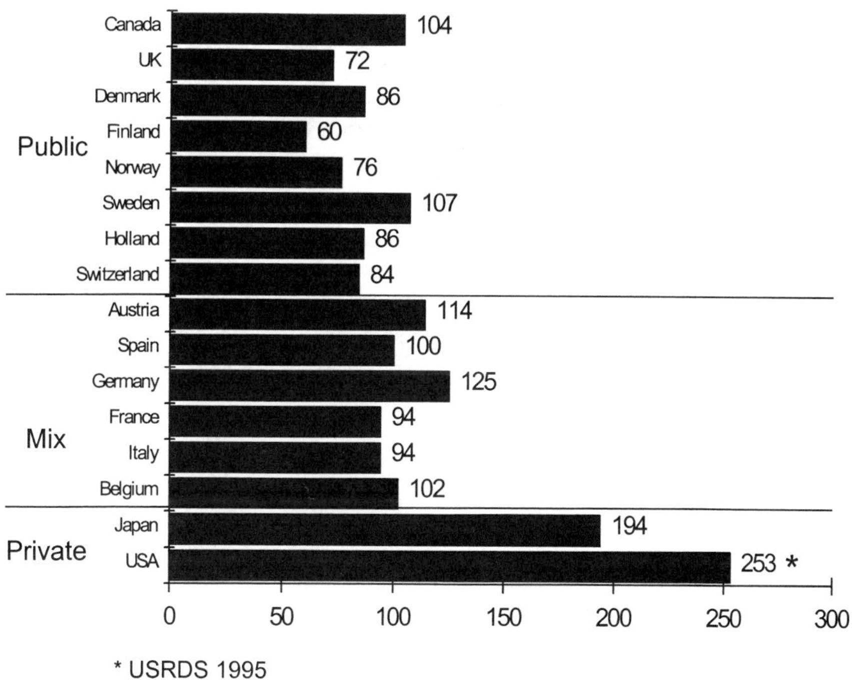

Fig. 3 Take on rate of new patients in an ESRD program per million population in 1995, based on data from several national registries and the USRDS.

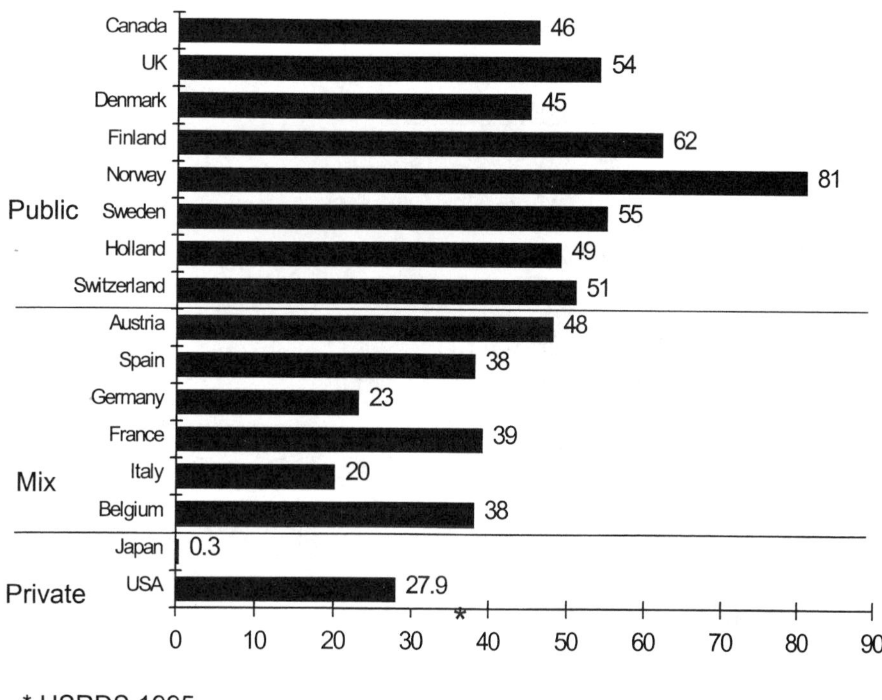

Fig. 4 Share of transplanted patients in percentage of total number of ESRD patients per million population in 1995.

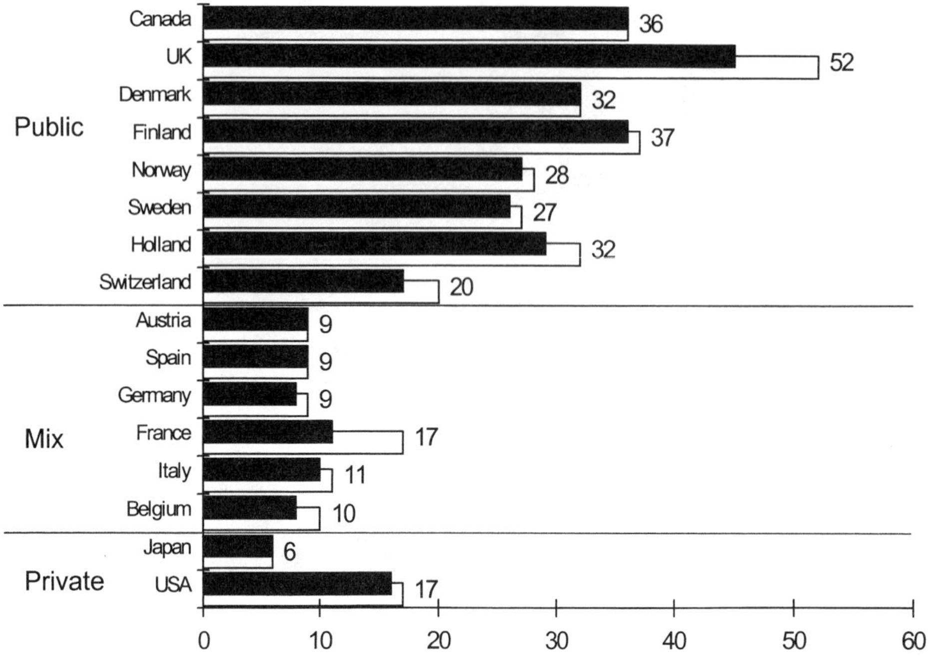

Fig. 5 Share of home dialysis (open bars) and peritoneal dialysis (closed bars) as percentage of total dialysis patients.

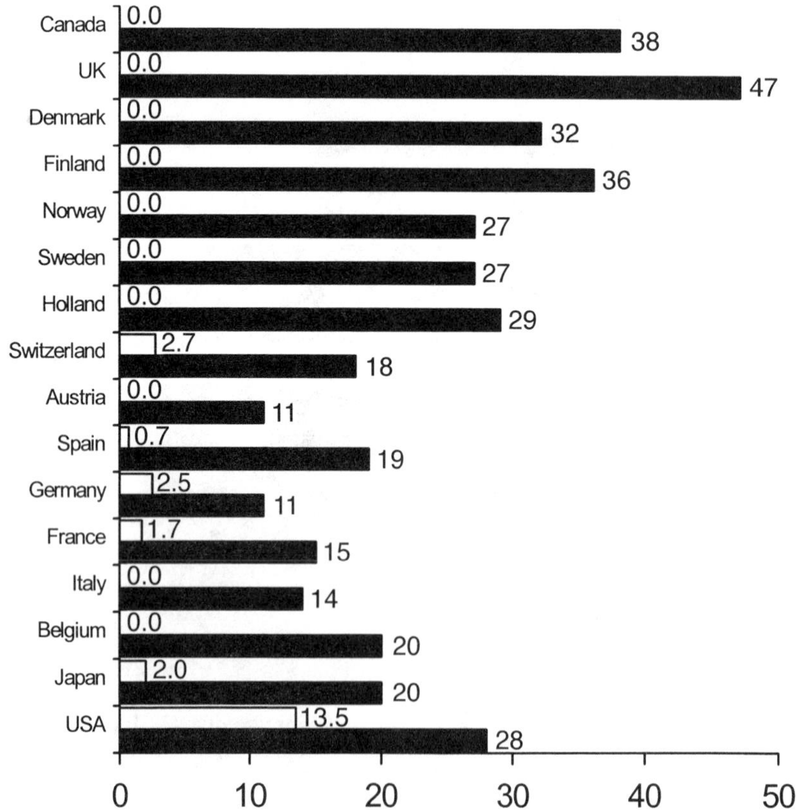

Fig. 6 PD utilization in public (closed bars) and in private (open bars) dialysis provider segments in different countries, based on several registries and Baxter Europe data system.

provision, the higher the utilization of PD. Figure 6 shows the main reason for these differences: with the exception of the United States, "private" providers have an extremely low share of PD in contrast to public providers regardless of their health-care system: of all dialysis patients, on average about 1.5% (range 0–13%) are treated with PD in the private sector, whereas public providers of all countries have a PD utilization rate of about 30% (range 11–47%).

E. Growth in ESRD Patients

Figure 7 shows the evolution of the increase in patient take-on rates from 1994 to 1995. There is a higher growth rate in the "public" countries (4–8.3%) compared to "mix" countries (4–6.3%), but the highest growth rates are observed in the "private" countries (United States and Japan).

F. Conclusions

Three main conclusions from this analysis of access to ESRD therapies can be made:

1. There are lower prevalences and take-on rates of ESRD patients in "public" countries. This can be explained by an overall lower dialysis capacity, including a lower number of physicians involved in ESRD patient care and a lower number of hemodialysis stations per million population.

   Because of a lack of published data, some telephone surveys in selected countries revealed major differences in the number of physicians available for ESRD care (e.g., UK-4 physicians pmp, Germany-23 pmp, Italy-66 pmp). "Public" countries have fewer physicians than "mix" countries and many fewer than "private" countries. This correlates with the overall number of physicians in a given country (doctors per 10,000 population): UK 16.1, Germany, 32.8, Italy 51.9. Also the number of dialysis chairs pmp differs between "public," "mix," and "private" countries: they range from 45 to 88 pmp in "public" countries, 55 to 152 pmp in "mix" countries, to a much high capacity in "private" countries (Japan 468 chairs pmp; United States 144 chairs pmp).
2. There is a much higher share of transplantation and home care, especially PD, in "public" countries.

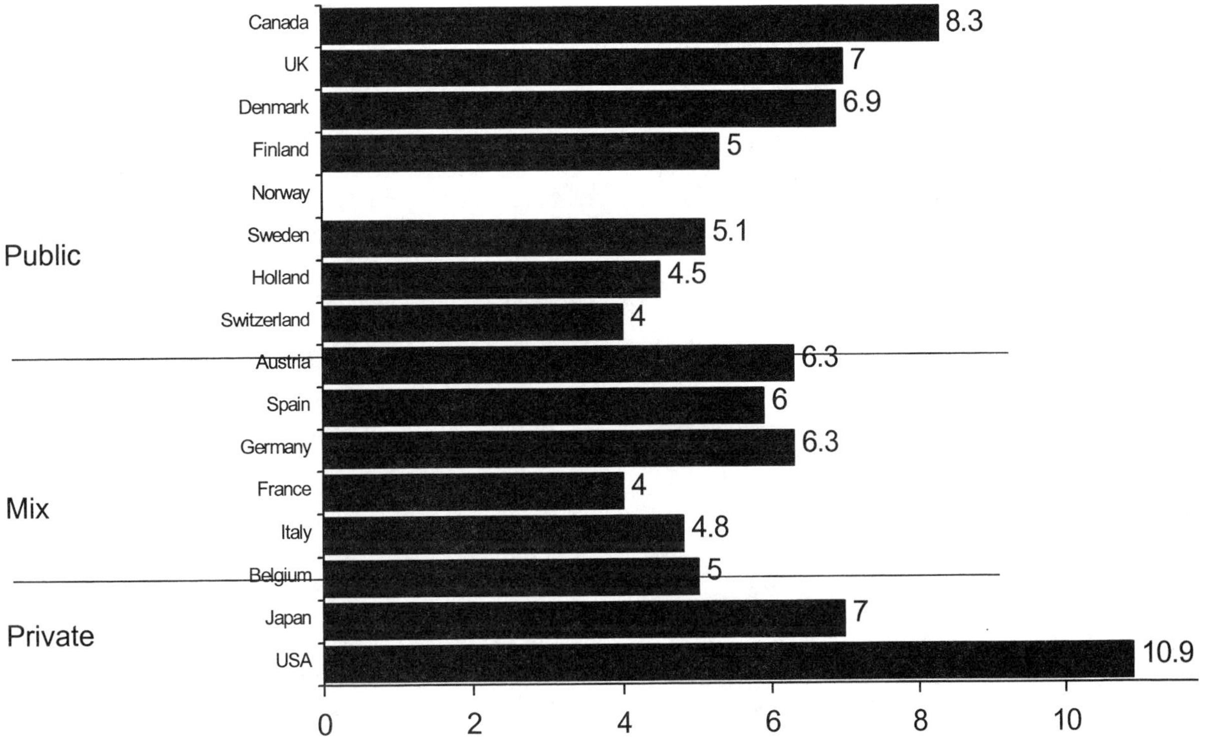

Fig. 7 Percent increase in treated ESRD patients in 1995, based on several registries and Baxter Europe database.

3. The requirements for ESRD treatments—although considerable—have by far not reached their limit. There are unmet needs in "public" countries today. But in general, needs will increase in the future due to a growing elderly population and higher life expectancy. It will be a major task for health policymakers to allow these patients to obtain equal access and quality ESRD care in the future. Governments will have to use the right funding and reimbursement strategies in a cost-constraint health-care environment.

G. Evolution of RRT in Central and Eastern Europe

The conditions of RRT were rather poor in the countries located in central and eastern Europe belonging to the so-called "socialist bloc." However, due to the political and socioeconomic changes that took place at the end of the 1980s and beginning of the 1990s together with the introduction of open-market economies in at least some of these countries, the availibility of dialysis and renal transplantation has greatly increased. According to a recently published special survey the number of hemodialysis units increased by 56% and the number of centers performing peritoneal dialysis increased by 296% during the period 1990–1996. The number of treated patients on hemodialysis and peritoneal dialysis increased by 78% and 306%, respectively. The introduction of modern hemodialysis machines and a wider choice of different dialyzers and concentrates allowed greater individualization of dialysis procedures; the latter together with the introduction of erythropoietin notably increased both quality of life and treatment outcome.

IV. ECONOMIC ISSUES OF ESRD TREATMENT

In view of the overall cost-containment approach in health care, the correct assessment of cost of the various ESRD treatment modalities and the funding possibilities will become the major issue for both health policy makers and providers in the immediate future. A growing number of ESRD patients will have to be provided with the most appropriate therapy from a medical, quality of life, and economic point of view.

In the following, some economic issues of dialysis therapy—a small but rather expensive segment within the total health-care sector—will be discussed. The data are based on published data from funding authorities, mainly for the year 1995. Some adjustments and calculations were made by the authors to make the data comparable, such as annualization of costs or fees, assuming a HD treatment of 156 sessions per year and PD performed during 365 days. Because kidney transplantation is not only the best quality treatment providing the best quality of life but also the most economic therapy, we will not discuss in detail cost assessment of transplantation.

The term "cost" will be used mainly for countries with global hospital budgets where the true cost of dialysis treatments was calculated. The term "reimbursement" is used when there are specific treatment rates/prices to be paid. These treatment rates are not necessarily identical to the real costs.

Treatment categories involved are related to treatment sites [HD-hospital treatment, HD-in-center treatment, HD limited care (LC), home HD] and treatment modalities [HD, PD, and automated PD (APD)]. For CAPD, a double bag system was applied. The cost elements within each treatment category of dialysis include treatment cost (all supplies and services and overhead costs), doctor's or center fee, training costs (if separately funded), patients' cost (if separately funded), erythropoietin prescriptions, and extra reimbursement for transportation.

A. General Differences in Funding and Reimbursement

Because of the variety of health-care systems, funding and reimbursement are different from country to country. In "public" systems (e.g., Canada, United Kingdom, northern European countries) there is nearly always a global budget for dialysis within a hospital. This is true also for the public segments within countries with mixed public and private providers (Spain, Italy, France, Germany, Austria). Treatment-specific rates ("reimbursement" rates) for dialysis are reimbursed in all "private" segments and "mix" countries. Within those treatment-specific rates, a variety of fees, e.g., doctors fee, fees for centers, for patients or nurses, or for training, exist. In case of home PD, a doctors fee is not always paid, and PD supplies are sometimes covered through nonhospital drug/supply budgets (e.g., northern Europe, Austria, Switzerland). In the United States one composite rate for dialysis (DRG = diagnostic related group) is paid, regardless of the type of dialysis modality.

B. Comparison of Annual Cost/Reimbursement per Patient/Modality in Selected European Countries

For each "type" of country as defined above, an example of the annual cost/reimbursement per dialysis modality will be given.

1. The United Kingdom

The United Kingdom will serve as an example of countries funded through a global hospital budget. In this country, this budget is negotiated between government purchasing administrations and providers (hospital trusts, GP fundholders). The cost can differ between the various providers. Figure 8 shows the cost per patient per year. It reveals a major cost advantage for PD therapies, mainly because of considerable lower personnel expenses. It can be calculated that, like in most northern European countries and Canada, almost two CAPD patients could be treated at the same cost as one patient in center HD.

2. Germany

Germany can be considered as an example of a country with "mixed public and private" providers. Figure 9 shows that the highest reimbursement is paid for in-hospital HD, followed by in-center HD (mainly private practices or nonprofit associations), and finally by limited care HD. Home HD and twinbag PD occur at nearly at the same level but far below the level of center treatments. APD therapies are reimbursed nearly at the same level as limited care HD. Of the total reimbursement, the doctor receives a lower fee for home patients than for center patients. Erythropoietin and transportation costs are reimbursed out of different budgets outside the dialysis funding and affect insurance funds but not the providers. These reimbursements are much higher for HD than for PD.

3. Belgium

Figure 10 shows the reimbursement per year up to 1995 and the recent increase for PD since 1996. Major differences in reimbursements for hospital HD are noted depending on the "type" of hospital providing the dialysis. Although the reimbursement per dialysis session is the same, the reimbursement per session for the hospital is different; for example, a university hospital receives a higher reimbursement than a nonuniversity hospital. Recently, the reimbursement for PD has been increased, and the reimbursement for in-center HD has been linked to the number of patients treated in a nonhospital environment (e.g., limited care or home). The

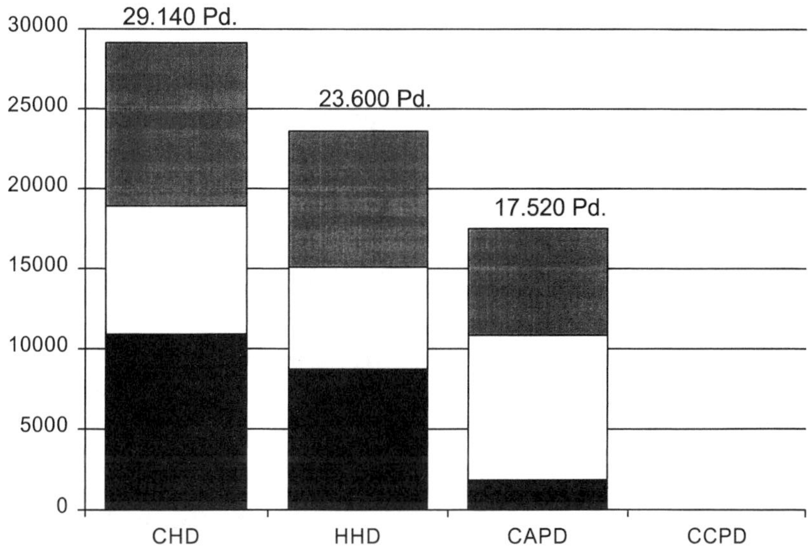

Fig. 8 Annual cost of each dialysis modality per patient in the UK, based on Review of Renal Services, 1994. Hatched bars: Overhead costs; white bars: supply costs; black bars: staff costs.

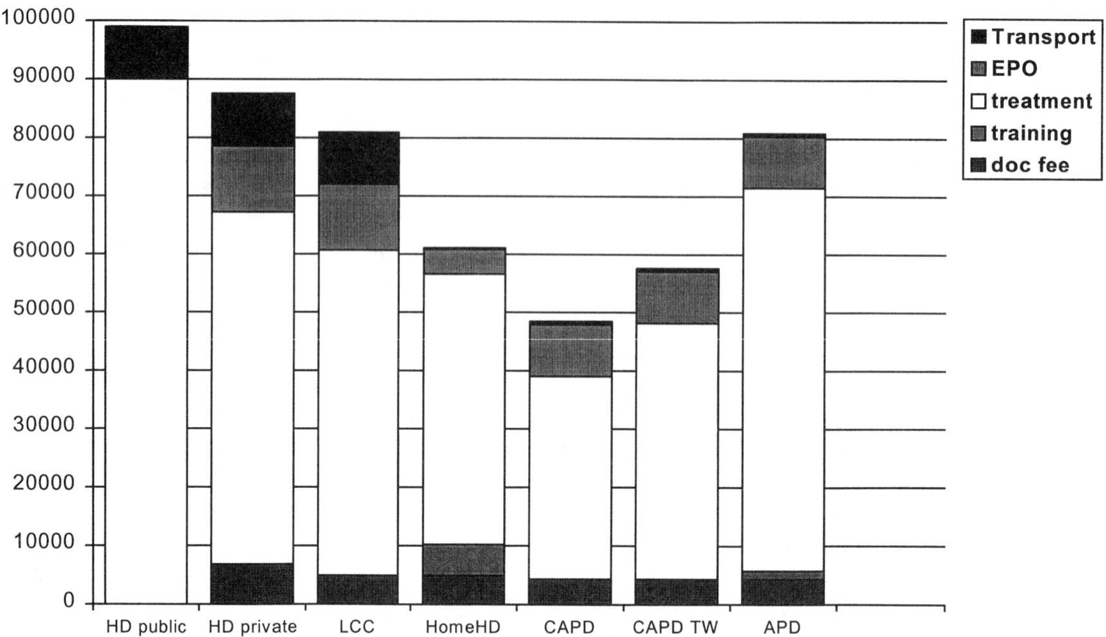

Fig. 9 Reimbursement per year in German marks for several dialysis modalities in Germany (1994–1995).

impact of this change in reimbursement policy on the distribution of dialysis patients is not yet known.

4. France

Figure 11 shows the cost/reimbursement data for France, which is the European country with the greatest difference in reimbursement between PD and hemodialysis. No doctor's fee is paid for treating PD patients.

C. Differences in Cost Structure Between In-center Hemodialyis and CAPD

Reimbursement and cost curves in the various countries are not very different from each other, irrespective of the individual health-care system. The distribution of treatment modalities in the various countries may therefore be linked to other aspects besides reimbursement.

In the following, the cost structure of the two main dialysis modalities, in-center HD and CAPD, will be briefly analyzed. Figure 12 shows data from the Baxter Consulting Cost Study performed in 17 hospitals and free-standing centers in the United States. Emphasis has been put not on the absolute cost in dollars per therapy, but on the distribution of key cost elements, like supplies, labor cost, and structural/overhead costs. The latter are the fixed cost elements, independent of the number of patients, and should be separated from the variable costs for supplies, drugs, etc., which are only spent for active patient use. As can be noted, the total cost of HD is 30% higher than that of CAPD. This is due to the considerably higher fixed costs, such as labor and overhead costs, based on the equipment and building structure for the dialysis centers (34%). These fixed costs amount to 77% of the total cost, whereas the variable costs, like disposables, drugs, and other supplies, share 23%. Note that in absolute figures the variable costs in HD are lower than those of CAPD. Although CAPD has in general a lower total cost, the distribution of costs is different. The highest cost element (66%) is the variable supply cost, whereas the labor and the overhead costs are only 24% and 10%, respectively. The fixed cost includes the backup, training, and both emergency and regular controls of the home patients in the center.

D. Impact of Dialysis Cost on Total Health-Care Systems Expenditure

Table 1 illustrates the relative share of dialysis cost within total health-care expenditure in the limited number of countries where data are available. A considerable amount of total health-care expenditure (0.7–1.8%) is spent for ESRD therapy in a relatively small segment of the population.

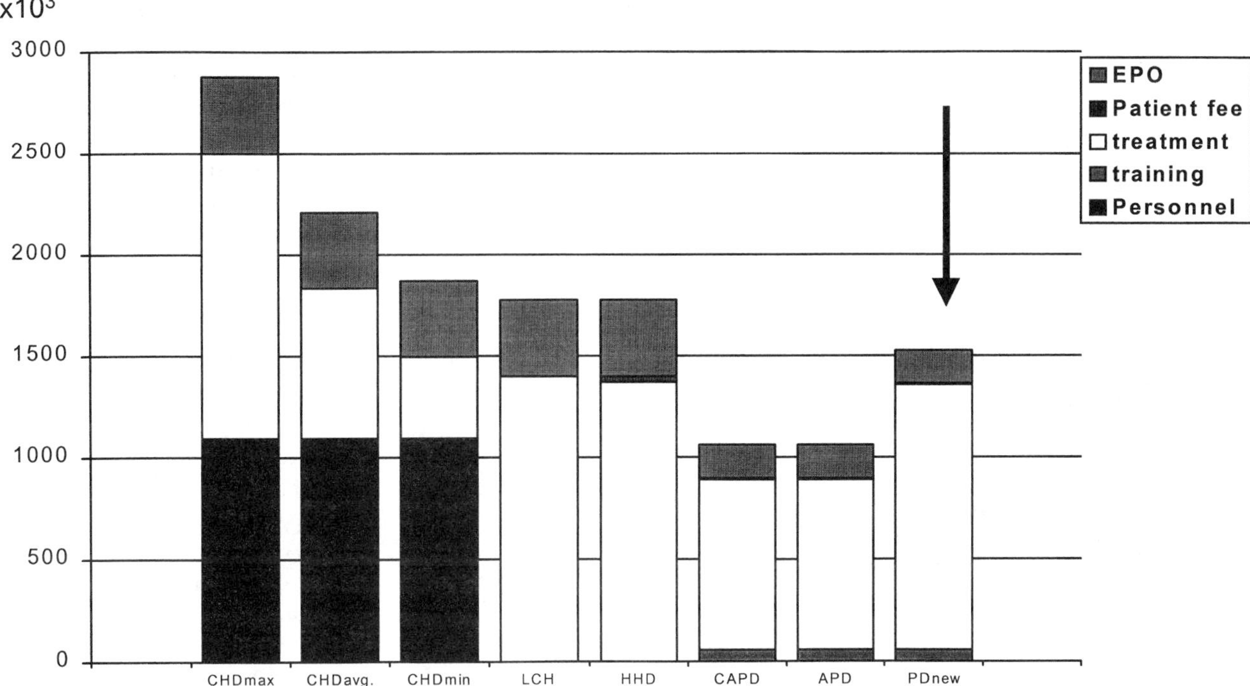

Fig. 10 Reimbursement per year in Belgian francs in 1996.

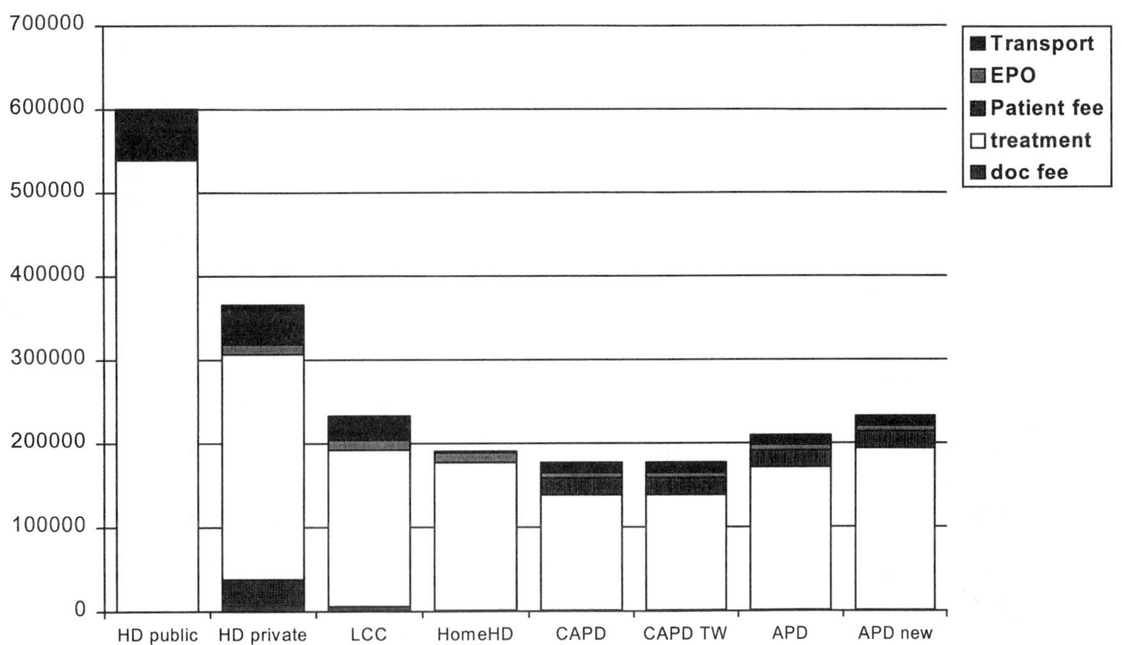

Fig. 11 Reimbursement per year in French francs in 1996.

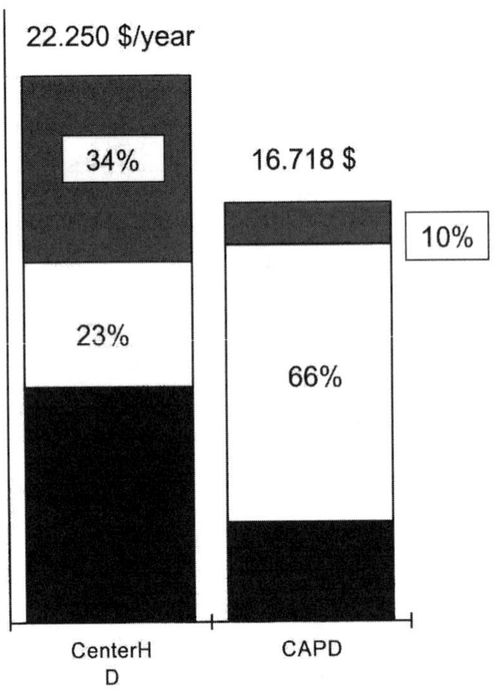

Fig. 12 Cost structure differences between in-center hemodialysis and CAPD. Hatched bars: Overhead costs; white bars: supplies costs; black bars: personnel costs.

E. Summary

Different health-care systems have different funding and reimbursement procedures for dialysis modalities. "Public" countries have various cost levels, depending on the treatment modality, within their global budget, and the real costs of individual modalities are not always known. On the other hand, "mix" countries show a variety of treatment rates related to the variety of modalities. It is interesting to see that these treatment rates are very similar to the cost patterns.

Table 1 Total Dialysis Cost, Share of Health Care, and Share of Population, 1994

Country	Cost in total billion local currency	% of health-care cost	% of population
United Kingdom	300 Million Pd.	0.7	0.022
Switzerland	130 Million SF	1.0	0.03
Germany	3000 Million DM	1.3	0.05
France	7000 Million FF	1.5	0.035
Italy	2000 Billion Lira	1.5	0.06
Belgium	6800 Million BF	1.8	0.037

Some European governments (e.g., Belgium), pressed by the existing limited funding resources, are nowadays discussing the introduction of new reimbursement policies to create incentives for home treatment. One may, however, assume that decision making is only partly driven by reimbursement rates and will be more influenced by the inherent differences in the cost structure of a given modality. On one hand, the high fixed costs and investments for HD and, on the other, the high variable costs and low labor and investment costs for home PD should be considered. This considerable difference in the cost structures of the two modalities creates above all a different view between providers and health-care authorities.

At present, CAPD is a less expensive modality than HD and offers some interesting savings potential. In addition, CAPD offers the opportunity to increase the total patient number without the need for major additional investments or new fixed costs. These considerations could at least partly explain the high utilization rate of PD in the "public" countries and in the "public" segment of "mix" countries. However, the current emphasis on increasing the delivered PD dose and the growing use of the more expensive automated forms of PD will make the reimbursement advantages of PD in the future minimal.

Providers in "private" centers are driven more by the microeconomic aspects. It is important from a business perspective to maximize the utilization of every HD station to offset the high fixed costs and maximize the profits. Consequently, the decision making is very much depending on the providers perspective, being either public or private, having either limited or over-hemocapacity, or having personally invested into dialysis stations as a private provider.

The future funding for ESRD treatment with the constant growth of patients will depend on a health-care policy taking all aspects discussed in this chapter into account. New creative managed care systems accompanied by quality guidelines will have to be evaluated and tested in many countries.

V. IMPACT OF REFERRAL PATTERN OF EUROPEAN ESRD PATIENTS TO NEPHROLOGISTS

Education of ESRD patients about the available dialysis options should start as early as possible and is, to a certain extent, dependent on the pattern of referral of

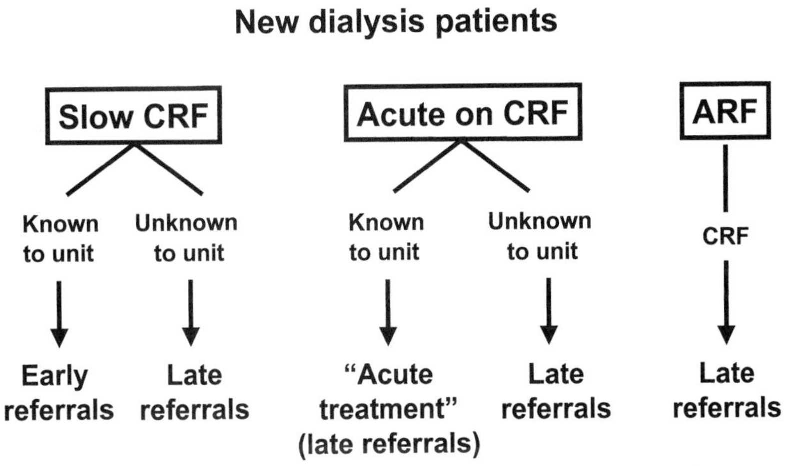

New dialysis patients

Slow CRF: Known to unit → Early referrals; Unknown to unit → Late referrals

Acute on CRF: Known to unit → "Acute treatment" (late referrals); Unknown to unit → Late referrals

ARF → CRF → Late referrals

Fig. 13 Flow of ESRD patients and referral pattern to the renal unit.

the chronic renal failure patient by the primary care physician or nonnephrological specialist to the renal dialysis unit. According to studies in Sweden (1) and a recent hypothesis using the Danish National Registry Report on Dialysis and Transplantation 1995, approximately 70% of ESRD patients who have the opportunity to receive adequate education on treatment options select peritoneal dialysis. In contrast, if , because of late referral, no education about the different dialysis modalities was possible, the patient is almost always started on hemodialysis in an emergency. The patient often remains on this form of therapy because no option for change in modality is provided.

Late referral occurs in approximately 20–50% of ESRD patients (3–6), and according to an earlier U.S. (4) and more recent French (5) and Swiss studies (7), an improvement in this referral pattern over the years has not been observed. The percentage of late referrals remained constant over the years 1983–1988 at the University of Missouri (4) and during the years 1990–1995 at the Necker Hospital in Paris (5). In a follow-up survey at the University of Missouri (8), an absence of firm guidelines for referral and lack of good communication between primary care providers and nephrologists were recognized as emergent needs.

Not only does late referral affect the lack of choice between dialysis modalities, but, according to several studies it also determines to a certain extent the outcome of these patients. Because of the greater morbidity, the initial duration of hospitalization is longer, with important consequences for the cost of therapy. Both earlier (9) and more recent reports (6,10–14) suggest that late referral to a nephrologist might contribute to early deaths on renal replacement therapy.

In a recent analysis of the impact on patient mortality in late versus early referral in Sao Paulo, the 6-month patient survival was 87% in the early referral and 69% in the late referral group. Despite the fact that in the late referral group the hazard ratio of mortality was 2.77 times that of the early referrals, in a multivariate analysis, time of referral was not associated with higher mortality risk (11). Early mortality, which was 12% in a large U.S. renal unit, was associated with coexisting diseases and hypoalbuminemia as well as with presentation with advanced renal failure (12).

A. Preliminary European Survey

Because relatively few data are available on the actual flow of predialysis patients and the referral pattern in most European countries, we organized a mailed survey to 14 European dialysis centers to gather information on the number of new ESRD patients admitted for dialysis in 1993–1995, the referral pattern of the patients, and the selection of the mode of dialysis (15). These 14 centers were selected because of their longstanding interest in and knowledge of the issues involved in the ESRD modality selection. Furthermore, the nephrologists in these centers are also known to have no bias towards either peritoneal or hemodialysis.

The definitions used in the survey were rather simple and straightforward. Early referral was applied to an ESRD patient known in the renal unit for at least 1 month and to whom the different modes of dialysis were sufficiently explained. Late referral was applied to a patient admitted for dialysis in an emergency, who therefore was not offered sufficient information. In both categories, the number of patients, the dialysis modality, and the eventual change of modality after the initial hospitalization period were noted. In the late referral group, one or two hemodialysis sessions were sometimes performed in an emergency via central venous catheter (e.g., over a weekend), followed by a start of peritoneal dialysis within 2–3 days of admission. These patients were considered as initially treated by peritoneal dialysis.

Table 2 summarizes the number of patients, some of the demographic characteristics, the number of diabetic patients, and the distribution in either early and late referrals in these 14 centers. A total number of 2236 ESRD patients were taken into dialysis between 1993 to 1995. The mean age was 57.3 years and the male-to-female ratio was 1.5:1. The percentage of diabetics was 17%. Overall, 1653 early and 583 late referrals, as defined above, were reported. This represents an overall late referral rate of 26%.

A rather high variability between the individual centers was noted, with the late referral patients ranging from as high as 51% in Brussels (Hopital Brugmann) to as low as 14% in Leicester and Berlin. Striking differences in referral pattern between centers in a same country were noted, such as between Leicester and Manchester in the United Kingdom and between Vicenza and Brescia in Italy, respectively.

Figures 14 and 15 show the distribution of the two dialysis modalities (hemodialysis and peritoneal dialysis) in the early referral (Fig. 14) and the late referral (Fig. 15) patients. Assuming that these patients have been offered some education about dialysis modalities, again a strikingly high variability in the applied dialysis strategies between centers, even in the same country, is observed. The admittance of these patients to a peritoneal dialysis program varies from as high as 94% in Manchester to as low as 15% in Brugge. Part of this variability can be explained by local circumstances, such as a lack of sufficient hemodialysis posts in Manchester, for example.

It is remarkable to note the different policy between the two French centers: early referral patients are taken on peritoneal dialysis at a rate of 73% in Colmar and only 29% in Caen. The interpretation of the results in the late referrals is more problematic, since some unexpected data were obtained. Although in the majority of the centers hemodialysis was applied in a greater percentage of these patients, in some centers like Thessaloniki, Colmar, Manchester, and Gent patients may at onset be treated in an emergency with one to three hemodialysis sessions and afterwards be transferred to peritoneal dialysis. In our unit, if a rapid evaluation of the medical, social, and psychological situation in such a patient leads to the conclusion by both the medical and nursing staff and the family that chronic hemodialysis is not suitable, that patient will receive a peritoneal dialysis catheter and be started on an in-hospital CAPD program. Such a decision can be reached in a few days after admission.

B. European/Flemish Survey

One survey (16,17) evaluated the impact of late referral of ESRD patients on the choice of dialysis modality and on morbidity and mortality. Duration of initial hos-

Table 2 Absolute Number of ESRD Patients Admitted Between 1993 and 1995

City	Total	Age	M/F	Nondiabetic	Diabetic	Early referrals	Late referrals
Gent	122	58.2	64/58	97	25	91	31
Manchester	238	—	142/96	205	33	148	90
Amsterdam	94	57.1	55/39	80	14	75	19
Colmar	129	58.9	79/50	103	26	86	43
Leicester	457	56.7	294/163	371	86	392	65
Berlin	119	—	69/50	91	28	102	17
Madrid	160	—	77/83	128	32	136	24
Thessaloniki	93	60.26	57/36	67	26	58	35
Caen	111	59.4	72/39	97	14	85	26
Brugge	93	57.87	53/40	69	24	75	18
Brescia	153	61	98/55	123	30	137	16
Brussels	98	55.33	65/33	82	16	48	50
Vicenza	113	55.17	75/38	89	24	76	37
Vienna	256	55	144/142	—	—	144	112
Total	2236	57.72	1344/892	1602	378	1653	583

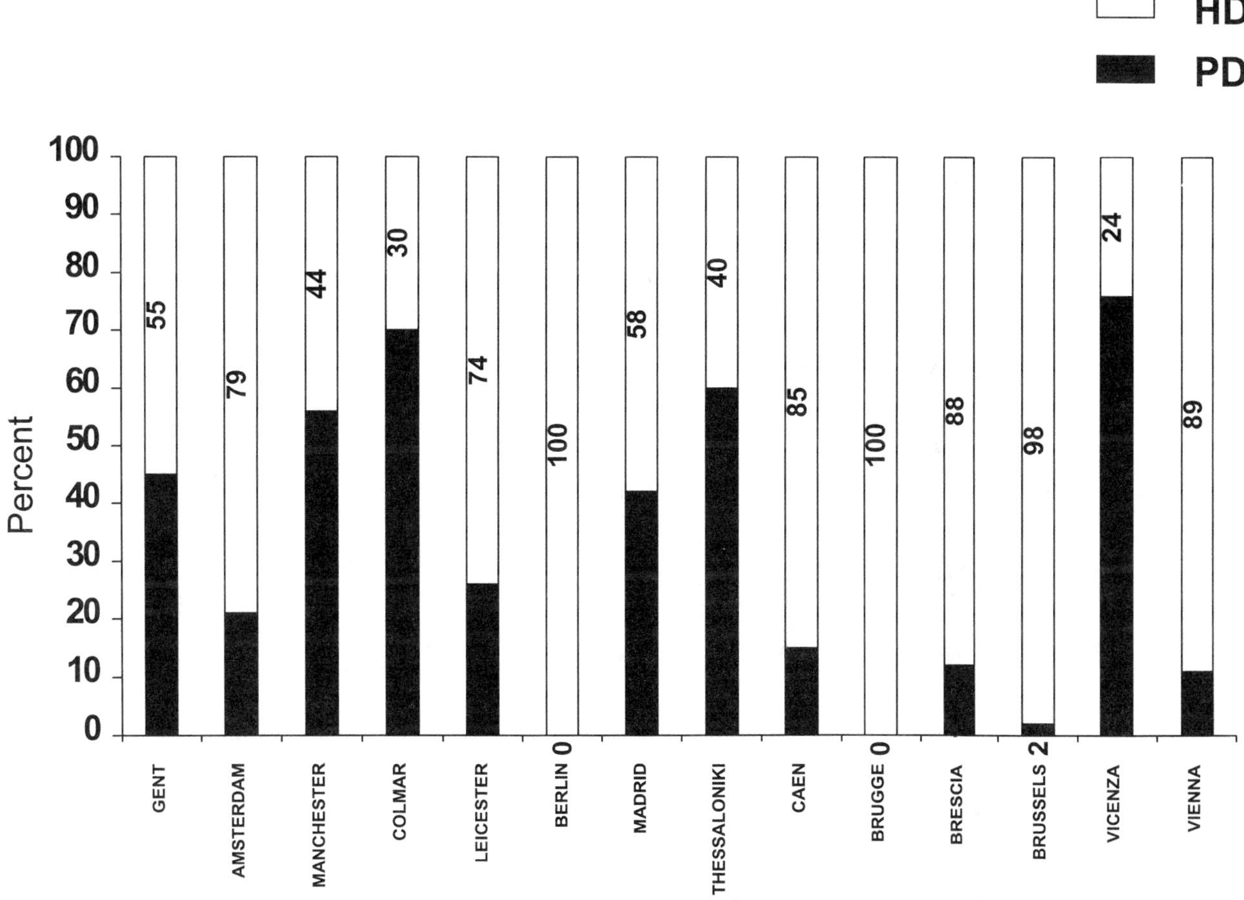

Fig. 14 Distribution of dialysis modalities in early referral patients.

pitalization was used as parameter, since hospitalization costs account for more than 40% of the ESRD treatment budget (18,19).

Since by definition timely initiation dialysis is impossible in late referral patients, the consequences of late referral for the concept of "early" or "healthy start" were evaluated. A retrospective analysis was performed using a questionnaire sent to 18 nephrology units in seven European countries. Patients who started RRT between January 1, 1996, and December 31, 1997, were included in this study. Eight nephrological units that are part of a quality surveillance group in Flanders comprising 331 patients completed an extended questionnaire, while 10 other European centers, comprising 450 patients, completed a limited version of the questionnaire. All the participating centers provide both hemodialysis and peritoneal dialysis. The variables and the results of the limited and of the extended questionnaire are given in Tables 2 and 3, respectively. In the extended questionnaire the specialty of the referring physician (general internal medicine, general practitioner, endocrinologist, cardiologist, urologist) and the status of the patient one year after the start of RRT (death, transplanted, still on dialysis, recovery of renal function) were registered.

As shown in Table 3, of a total of 781 patients 65% were early referrals and 35% were late referrals. There was a slight predominance of males (57% vs. 43%). About one in three patients in the total group was started on PD. Late referral patients started relatively more often on HD than early referral patients (77% vs. 51%, $p < 0.001$).

The creatinine clearance at first visit to the renal unit was higher in the early than the late referral patients (28.1 ± 23.4 vs. 6.9 ± 8.8 mL/min, $p < 0.001$); in contrast, the creatinine clearance at the start of RRT was not different (7.6 ± 3.9 vs. 7.1 ± 4.6 mL/min, $p = 0.18$) between both groups. The number of hospitalization days at the start of RRT was significantly lower in the early compared to the late referral patients (15.1

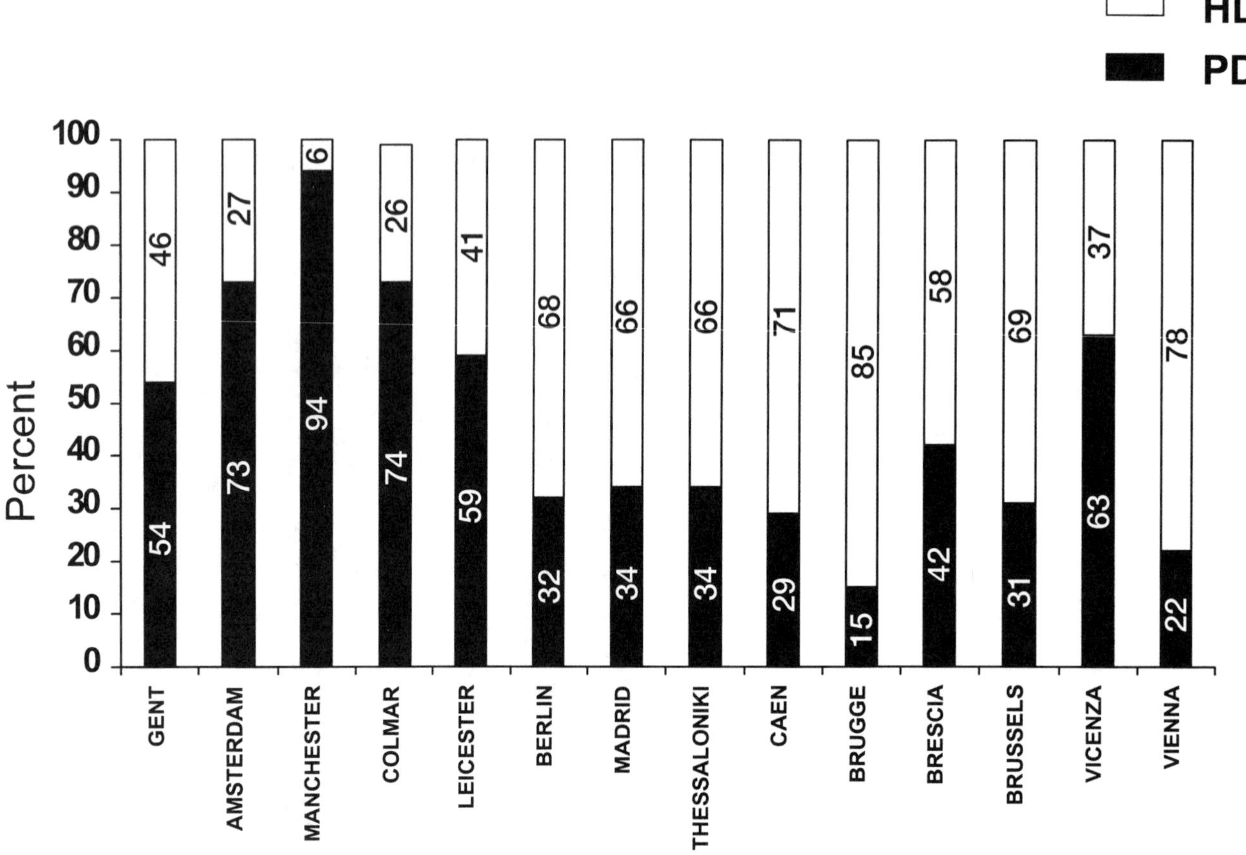

Fig. 15 Distribution of dialysis modalities in late referral patients.

Table 3 Demographic Parameters in the Total Group and in Late- and Early-Referral Patients in the European Survey

Parameter	Total group (n = 781)	Late referral (n = 271)	Early referral (n = 510)	p-Value
M/F	57%/43%	57%/43%	57%/43%	0.97
PD/HD	33%/67%	23%/77%	49%/51%	<0.001
C_{cr} first (mL/min)	21.7 ± 22.3	6.9 ± 8.8	28.1 ± 23.4	<0.001
Residual C_{cr} (mL/min)	7.4 ± 4.2	7.1 ± 4.6	7.6 ± 3.9	0.18
Hospitalization at start RRT (days)	19.3 ± 19.8	27.8 ± 23.7	15.1 ± 16.0	<0.001
Age (years)	61.1 ± 15.7	62.1 ± 16.3	60.5 ± 15.5	0.2
No. of antihypertensive drugs	1.5 ± 1.0	1.4 ± 1.1	1.5 ± 1.0	0.4
Diastolic BP (mmHg)	83.3 ± 16.1	85.2 ± 19.5	82.4 ± 14.4	0.13
Pulmonary edema (Y/N)	21%/79%	31%/69%	17%/83%	0.003
Uremic symptoms (Y/N)	71%/29%	83%/17%	66%/34%	0.001

HD, Hemodialysis; C_{cr}, creatinine clearance; RRT, renal replacement therapy; Y, yes; N, no.

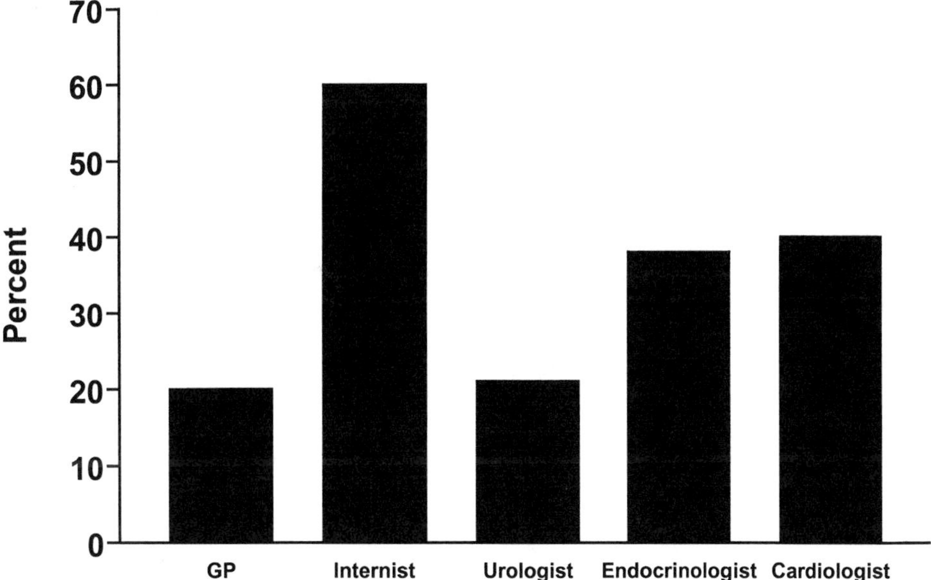

Fig. 16 Specialty of referring physicians of late referral patients in Flanders as a percentage of the absolute number of patients referred in that category.

± 16.0 vs. 27.8 ± 23.7 days, $p < 0.001$). There were no differences in age, diastolic blood pressure, or number of antihypertensive drugs between early and late referral patients. More patients did not receive antihypertensive medication in the late referral group (28.6% vs. 15.5%, $p = 0.004$); diastolic blood pressure in the patients not taking antihypertensive drugs was higher in the late referral patients (83.5 ± 15.8 vs. 74.4 ± 15.0 mmHg, $p = 0.03$), whereas in patients taking antihypertensive medication no difference (86.8 ± 13.9 vs. 84.1 ± 13.9 mmHg, $p = 0.6$) was found (Fig. 2).

The prevalence at start of RRT of uremic symptoms (82.8% vs. 17.2%) and pulmonary edema (31.2% vs. 17.2%, $p = 0.003$) was higher in the late referral patients. The results for the variables of the extended Flemish survey are shown in Table 3. The biochemical parameters in both patient groups, including hematocrit, serum parathormone, serum bicarbonate, and serum albumin levels at start of dialysis, were not different.

At start of RRT, the residual creatinine clearance was 10–15 mL/min in only 18% of the patients, 5–10 mL/min in 54% of the patients, and <5 mL/min in 34% of the patients. These percentages were comparable in early and late referral patients. One year after the start of RRT, the number of deaths was higher (26.7% vs. 16.4%, $p = 0.07$) and the number of transplanted patients lower (4.7% vs. 17.5%, $p = 0.02$) in the late referrals.

The specialty of the physician referring the patient to the nephrologist is displayed in Figure 16. The largest number of patients is referred by the general practitioner, but the percentage of late referrals in this specialty is lower than for the other specialties. The absolute number of patients coming from general internists, endocrinologists, cardiologists, and urologists is lower, but the fraction of late referrals is higher in these specialties than for the general practitioners.

Acces for the first hemodialysis was an arteriovenous fistula in only 7% and 51% of late and early referral patients, respectively. The creatinine clearance at the start of RRT was significantly higher (9.5 ± 3.6 vs. 7.0 ± 3.5 mL/min, $p = 0.001$) in the patients who survived compared to those who died during the first year of RRT.

C. Discussion of Survey Results

Although the optimal moment of initiation of RRT is still debated, there is evidence that a "too late" start has detrimental and partly irreversible consequences for the outcome of the patient (14,20–23). It is conceivable that, besides the attention given to a number of secondary medical complications during the pre-ESRD phase, such as anemia (24,25), left ventricular hypertrophy (26), hyperparathyroidism (27), and malnutrition (28), nonmedical factors such as education of pre-ESRD patients may also exert a positive impact on their prognosis (1).

Between 25 and 30% of ESRD patients are referred to the nephrologist less than one month before the start of dialysis. The reason for the late referral of chronic renal failure patients to the nephrologist is not clear. One explanation may be the insidious evolution of chronic renal failure in the majority of patients (Figure 13). In some patients, renal insufficiency only becomes obvious with the appearance of frank uremic symptoms leading to consultation with a physician. This type of late referral can only be avoided by regular screening of renal function in otherwise asymptomatic patients, which is economically unrealistic.

Other patients may have consulted a nonnephrologist but are referred to the nephrologist too late; this can occur for a variety of reasons. The referring physician may not be aware of the severity of the disease or the importance of adequate pre-ESRD care. It has also been suggested that the medical plethora in some of the European countries might play an important role in the problem of late referral (29).

It is also possible that some late referral patients are in fact hidden nonreferrals. Khan et al. (30) in the United Kingdom, and Mendelssohn et al. (31) in Canada found that a substantial number of ESRD patients was not referred, the number increasing with age and comorbid conditions. This suggests that many physicians probably decide for themselves whether RRT should or should not be used in a patient with certain comorbid conditions without asking the advice of an nephrologist (4, 32).

A recent study from Italy (33) found that the trend for late referral was higher in elderly patients; it is therefore difficult to foresee the possible expansion of the dialytic pool in elderly patients. Some of these seriously ill or old patients may still appear in a dialysis unit where RRT is started in an attempt to improve their general condition. In some of these patients RRT is indeed futile, explaining the relative high number of deaths due to withdrawal of dialysis in this category, as shown by Innes et al. (10).

For other patients however, a timely start of RRT could have prevented the further deterioration of their general condition. Correct education of the whole medical community on the actual status and outcome of RRT could prevent such errors. It is remarkable that the problem of late referral has been known for years without any apparent change in referral policy (3,9,21,34–36).

In another group of patients, ESRD is the consequence of a sudden and unexpected deterioration of a preexisting mild or moderate renal insufficiency. This deterioration is frequently the result of iatrogenic diagnostic or therapeutic procedures. That this may be an important cause for late referral is suggested by our observation that the highest percentage of late referral patients comes from general internists and cardiologists (Fig. 16). Screening of renal function in patients at risk and consulting a nephrologist before certain high-risk investigations are planned or medications are started can have great preventive value. In this context, the nephrologist should develop guidelines on the prevention of deterioration of renal function in high risk patients.

Finally, some patients suffering from severe acute renal failure do not recover and remain dialysis dependent. This type of patient was excluded from this analysis because the prognosis is generally poor due to the severe underlying pathology.

The proportion of patients opting for peritoneal dialysis is higher in the early referrals. It is clear from Table 2 that the reasons to start RRT are different in the early and late referral patients, the latter often arriving in an emergency situation. In such cases an urgent hemodialysis session results in a prompt correction of the clinical status of the patient. Moreover, motivating a patient to start with PD takes time and persuasive power from the dialysis team and confidence and comprehension from the patient, which are often absent in the late referral patient. The impact of intensive education and information on modality choice has been demonstrated (1,37).

In agreement with the results of other studies (10,30,37), late referral in our survey clearly had a negative impact on the morbidity and mortality of ESRD patients, as demonstrated by a longer duration of hospitalization at start of RRT, a lower number of successfully transplanted patients, and a higher mortality during the first year of treatment. Although there was apparently no difference in diastolic blood pressure or number of antihypertensive drugs taken between early and late referrals in this study, the incidence of untreated hypertension was much higher in the late referrals. In the group taking antihypertensive drugs, however, diastolic bloodpressure was not different between early and late referrals.

Late referral also has important economical consequences. First, there is the prolonged need for hospitalization at the start of RRT, which substantially increases the costs of ESRD treatment (4,18,19). Second, there is the lower take-on rate for transplantation and the preferential choice for HD, both also resulting in increased cost of an ESRD program.

Levin et al. (38) performed a limited economical analysis to assess the cost/benefit of a pre-ESRD treatment-education program. Even with inclusion of all the costs of the teaching program, there was still a major economic benefit in favor of the program. Other studies have demonstrated that in well-prepared ESRD patients, the rate of employment is higher (39).

There was no difference in creatinine clearance at start of RRT between early and late referral patients. It is remarkable to note that there were no differences in serum creatinine or residual renal creatinine clearances, either mean or median values, at initiation of dialysis between the different patient groups. Similar results have been found by Halabi et al. (7). In contrast, the group in Valenciennes showed that serum creatinine was higher (10.34 vs. 8.21 mg/dL) and creatinine clearance calculated with the Cockroft and Gault formula was lower (7.08 vs. 9.03 mL/min) in late referrals compared to early referred patients (40). Jungers et al. (6) found a slightly lower calculated creatinine clearance in the patients with delayed referral.

The mean creatinine clearance at the start of RRT was 7.4 (4.1 mL/min in our study), far below the values of 10–15 mL/min recommended by the "healthy start" DOQI guidelines (41). Although Slingeneyer (37) found a higher creatinine clearance at start of dialysis in the early referrals, only 1.7 and 4.6% of late and early referrals, respectively, were started at a creatinine clearance greater than 12 mL/min. At first glance, the referral pattern seems thus not to have a great effect on the "healthy start" concept. However, this is partly due to the low number of the early referral patients who started according the DOQI guidelines. The "healthy start" concept and the DOQI guidelines were only formulated at the end of this study period. It is thus conceivable that their acceptance and application by nephrologists will only become widespread after some time. Furthermore, it appeared that in some of the centers participating in this survey, budget restrictions made early start impossible, even in early referred and well-prepared patients. The fact that creatinine clearance at start of RRT was lower in the patients who died compared to those who survived during the first year of RRT is in favor of the concept of early start. Urea kinetic modeling has recently been used to predict the optimum timing of commencement of dialysis (23), and the Kt/V urea at the start of dialysis was inversely correlated with the hospital admission rate and with the number of inpatient days during the first 6 months after the start of dialysis. These findings suggest thus that patients may well benefit from the earlier commencement of dialysis, perhaps at a time when their Kt/Vurea has declined to the point at which CAPD would be considered inadequate.

An important fact to note is that the degree of renal dysfunction, whether it is judged by serum creatinine or creatinine clearance, or for that matter by residual Kt/V urea, is not the direct cause for initiation of dialysis in almost one third of ESRD patients. In late referral patients, urgent dialysis is performed mostly for serious overfilling, sometimes at residual creatinine clearances well above 15 mL/min. It appears, however, that, probably due to induced ultrafiltration, the residual renal function rapidly falls to very low levels, necessitating the continuation of dialysis. Second, substantial efforts in continuing education on management and referral policy of preterminal renal failure patients should be focused in the future not only on general practitioners, but also on other specialists of internal medicine, notably general internists and cardiologists.

The question can be raised whether these efforts should not take priority over those for earlier start of dialysis, otherwise at least one third of the patients will continue to be admitted in an emergency situation. It is this latter category of patients that to a large extent determines the early outcome in dialysis, which will probably be less affected by initiating dialysis earlier in patients who are already under adequate nephrological care.

In conclusion, one in three ESRD patients is still a late referral patient. Late referral has consequences for the choice of dialysis modality, the general outcome of the patient, and the cost of ESRD treatment. Establishment and widespread dissemination of adequate and clear guidelines for general practitioners and non-nephrological specialists on when and how to refer patients to a nephrologist, information about the importance of close nephrological follow-up, and development of educational programs for chronic renal failure patients are urgently needed.

BIBLIOGRAPHY

General Health Care

WHO, European Healthcare Reforms, Analysis of Current Strategies, Copenhagen, 1996.

Altenstetter C, Björkman JW, eds. Health Policy Reform, National Variations and Globalization, London, 1996.

OECD in Figures, Statistics on the Member Countries, 1996 Edition.

OECD 1993, Facts and Trends, Health Policy Studies N. 3.

NERA, Financing Healthcare with Particular Reference to Medicines, Vol. 1, Summary and Overview, London, May 1993.

Schneider M, et al. Gesundheitssysteme im Vergleich, Basys, Ausgabe 1994.

ESRD in General

Lindholm B, Bergström J, Economical Structure and Organisation of ESRD Therapies in Different Countries, EDTA 1987, Abstract ISPD, 1987.

Valderrabano F, Berthoux F, Jones EHP, Mehls O on behalf of the EDTA-ERA Registry. Report on management of renal failure in Europe, XXV, 1994. Nephrol Dial Transplant 11 (suppl 1): 2–21, 1996.

Data by Country

Austria

Österreichische Gesellschaft für Nephrologie, Österreichisches Dialyseregister, 1995.

Reimbursement Data: PD Informationsveranstaltung, Wien, 1995 (Hörl, Nayer, Meisl).

Belgium

OECD Health Policy Studies No. 2, Chapter 3, page 31. Reform of the Healthcare System in Belgium, Paris, 1992.

IRC 2000: Le livre Blanc de la Nephrologie, Societe de la Nephologie-Sanesco, September 1995, page 43 data on patients.

Gheyle D, Jegers M, Matthus P, Kostenvergelijking . . . Continue Ambulante Peritoneale Dialyse en Centrumhemodialyse, Gezondheiszorg, 50, Nr. 12, 1994.

Ministere des Affaires Sociales de la Sante Public, reglement, modifiant.

Canada

Baxter Market Survey, Canada, 1994, 1995.

C.O.R.R. Canadian Replacement Registry, 1996 (1994 data).

Denmark

Dansk Nefrologisk Selskab, Danish National Registry, Report on Dialysis and Tranplantation in Denmark, 1995.

Eastern Europe

Rutkowski B, Ciocalteu A, Djukanovic L, Kiss I, Kovac A, Krivoshiev S, Kveder R, Polenakovic M, Puretic Z, Stanaityte M, Tareyeva I, Teplan V, CEE Advisory Board in Chronic Renal Failure, and Zavitz F. Evolution of renal replacement therapy in central and eastern Europe 7 years after political and economical liberation. Nephrol Dial Transplant 1998; 13:860–864.

Finland

Finnish Registry for Kidney Diseases, Annual Report, 1994.

France

'IGAS: Enquete sur la Dialyse, Code mission SA/AC/AP 940041, Rapport n.94.092, Septembre 1994, pp. 9,13,14,17,23,24,29,30.

Tarif de dialyse juillet 1993 CNAM, CRAM.

Avenant N. 14, a la Convention Intervenue le 22 aout 1990, Annexe III a la Dialyse Peritoneale.

Convention -Type pour la dialyse a domicile.

IRC 2000, Livre blanc de la Nephrologie, 1995, pp. 28,43,54.

Germany

QuasiNiere, 1995, in EDTA Registry, Report on Management of Renal Failure, 1996.

KfH Jahresbericht 1994.

QuaSi-Niere in der Dialysepatient 3/95, s. 21–22.

Reimbursement: EBM Kapitel F V. Nephrologie (Dialyse), 790–793, Stand 1995.

Nebel, die Kosten der Nierenersatztherapie, Referat 14.5.1995, Dresden.

Holland

Renine, Registratie Nierfunktievervanging Nederland, Nr. 3 Augustus 1995, De Charro.

Reimbursement: COTG Central Orgaan Tarleven Gezondheidszorg.

Tarieven Nierfunctievervangende Therapie per 1 Januari, 1995.

Bijlage bij circulaire PS/ at/ 1 /95/ 11c COTG code.

Italy

OECD, the Reform of Healthcare Systems Healthpolicy Studies, No. 5, Paris, 1994, Chapter 13 on Italy.

ISIS Numero Speciale 50 dic. 1992.

ANED (Associazione Nazionale Emodializzati), 1991, updated to 1995.

Piano Sanitario Nazionale, Azione Programmativa C. 3 Assistenza Ai Nefropatici cronici, 1991.

Reimbursement: R. Testa in Notiziario A. L.E. Numero Speciale, Supplemento, La Dialisi, Milano, 1992.

Nomenclatore Tariffario (La Nuova Tariffa si Riferisce ad una singola Prestazione) (Codice 39.95–39.95.9 + 54.98.1- 54.98.2

Japan

ISDT (Japanese Registry) 1995.

Baxter data, 1996.

Norway

National Nephrology Association Norway.

Spain

Catalan Register (RMRC), 1994, Evolucio de la insufficiencia renal terminal tractada a Catalunya.

IRC 2000 /EDTA Registry 1993.

Sociedad Espanola de Nefrologia, Comite de Registro, Alicante, Septembre 1994.

Baxter Spain update, 1995.

Reimbursement: BOE num. 52 Jueves 29 Febrero 1996 3.8:-3.10 tarifas maximas por session de tratamiento, tarifas maximas por dia de tratamiento 1996, suplementos.

Proyecto de Orden del Ministerio de Sanitad y consumo . . . con entidades.

Sweden

National Nephrology Association.

Svenskt Register för Aktiv Uremivärd.

Switzerland

EDTA Registry 1994, Vol. 11, 1996, Supplement 1.

SVK Geschäftsbereichte 1993, 1994.

Secretariat FMH Bern

SVK, Tarifvereinbarung für Hämodialysen, Peritonealdialyse und Nierentransplantationen, Vereinbarung mit VESKA, Jan. 1991.

United Kingdom

Review of Renal Services, July and Nov. 1994, NHS Executive.

Baxter UK survey, 1995.

United States

Nephrology Resource directory Lexington, KY.

HCFA numbers 1994.

Medicare average rates ($130 per dialysis treatment).

Excerpts from the USRDS 1997 Annual Report. Am J Kidney Dis 1997; 30(suppl 1).

REFERENCES

1. Ahlmen J, Carlsson L, Schonborg C. Well-informed patients with end-stage renal disease prefer peritoneal dialysis to hemodialysis. Perit Dial Int 1993; 13(suppl 2): S196–S198.
2. Danish National Registry Report on Dialysis and Transplantation in Denmark 1995. The Danish Society of Nephrology, 1996.
3. Ratcliffe PJ, Phillips RE, Oliver DO. Late referral for maintenance dialysis. Br Med J 1984; 288:441–443.
4. Campbell JD, Ewigman B, Hosokawa M, Van Stone JC. The timing of referral of patients with end-stage renal disease. Dial Transplant 1989; 18:660–686.
5. Jungers P. Late referral to maintenance dialysis: detrimental consequences. Nephrol Dial Transplant 1993; 8: 1089–1093.

6. Jungers P, Shkiri H, Zingraff J, Muller S, Fumeron C, Giatras I, Touam M, Nguyen AT, Man NK, Grünfeld JP. Bénéfices d'une prise en charge néphrologique précoce de l'insuffisance rénale chronique. Soc Néphrol, Toulouse, October 2–3, 1997, Abstract 5.
7. Halabi G, Monnerat C, Teta D, Wauters JP. Le transfert tardif au néphrologue pour dialyse chronique: une pratique en augmentation. Soc Néphrologie, Toulouse, October 2–3, 1977, Abstract 161.
8. Nolph GB. What findings should prompt primary care physicians to refer to nephrologists? Presentation at Alberta Nephrology Days, April 27–28, 1996.
9. Jungers P, Zingraff J, Page B, Albouze G, Hannedouche T, Man NK. Detrimental effects of late referral in patients with chronic renal failure: a case-control study. Kidney Int 1993; 43 (suppl 41):S170–S173.
10. Innes A, Rowe PA, Burden RP, Morgan AG. Early deaths on renal replacement therapy: the need for early nephrological referral. Nephrol Dial Transplant 1992; 7:467–471.
11. Sesso R, Belasco AG. Late diagnosis of chronic renal failure and mortality on maintenance dialysis. Nephrol Dial Transplant 1996; 11:2417–2420.
12. Khan IK, Catto GRD, Edward N, Mac Leod AM. Death during the first 90 days of dialysis: a case control study. Am J Kidney Dis 1995; 25:276–280.
13. Ifudu O, Dawood M, Homel P, Friedman EA. Excess morbidity in patients starting uremia therapy without prior care by a nephrologist. Am J Kidney Dis 1996; 28:841–845.
14. Ellis PA, Reddy V, Bari N, Cairns HS. Late referral of end-stage renal failure. QJ Med 1998; 91:727–732.
15. Lameire N, Van Biesen W, Dombros N, Dratwa M, Faller B, Gahl G, Gokal R, Krediet R, LaGreca G,. Maiorca R, Matthys E, Ryckelynck J, Selgas R, Walls J. The referral pattern of patients with ESRD is a determinant in the choice of dialysis modality. Perit Dial Int 1997; 17(suppl 2):S161–S166.
16. Van Biesen W and the LOK group nephrology. Het verwijzingspatroon in Oost- en West-Vlaanderen van patienten met terminale nierinsufficientie. Tijdschr Geneesk 1998; 54:1615–1621.
17. Van Biesen W, Wiedemann M, Lameire N. ESRD treatment: a European perspective. J Am Soc Nephrol 1998; 9:555–562.
18. Garella S. The costs of dialysis in the USA. Nephrol Dial Transplant 1997; 12(suppl 1):10–21.
19. Jacobs C. The costs of dialysis treatments for patients with end stage renal disease in France. Nephrol Dial Transplant 1997; 12(suppl 1):29–32.
20. Hakim R, Lazarus J. Initiation of dialysis. J Am Soc Nephrol 1995; 6:1319–1328.
21. Kjellstrand C, Hylander B, Collins A. Mortality on dialysis: on the influence of early start, patient characteristics, and transplantation and acceptance rates. Am J Kidney Dis 1990; 15:483–490.
22. Bonomini V, Feletti C, Scolari M, Stefoni S. Benefits of early initiation of dialysis. Kidney Int 1985; 28(suppl 17):S57–S59.
23. Tattersall J, Greenwood R, Farrington K. Urea kinetics and when to commence dialysis. Am J Nephrol 1995; 15:283–289.
24. Valderrabano F. Recombinant erythropoetin: 10 years of clinical experience. Nephrol Dial Transplant 1997; 12(suppl 1):2–9.
25. Revicki D, Brown R, Feeny D, Henry D, Teehan B, Rudnick M, Benz R. Health related quality of life associated with recombinant human erythropoetin therapy for predialysis chronic renal disease patients. Am J Kidney Dis 1995; 25:548–554.
26. Levin A, Singer J, Thompson C, Ross H, Lewis M. Prevalent left ventricular hypertrophy in the predialysis population: identifying opportunities for intervention. Am J Kidney Dis 1996; 27:347–354.
27. Gonzalez E, Martin K. Renal osteodystrophy: pathogenesis and management. Nephrol Dial Transplant 1995: 10(suppl 3):13–21.
28. Schulman G, Hakim RM: Improving outcomes in chronic hemodialysis patients: Should dialysis be initiated earlier? Sem Dial 1996; 9:225–229.
29. Wauters JP, Leski M. Insuffisance rénale chronique et pléthore médicale. Méd Hyg 1995; 53:379.
30. Khan I, Catto G, Edward N, McLeod A. Chronic renal failure: factors influencing nephrology referral. Q J Med 1994; 87:559–564.
31. Mendelssohn DC, Toh Kua B, Singer PA. Referral for dialysis in Ontario. Arch Int Med 1995; 155:2473–2478.
32. Sesso R, Fernandes P, Ançao M, Drummond M, Draibe S, Sigulem D, Ajzen H. Acceptance for chronic dialysis treatment: insufficient and unequal. Nephrol Dial Transplant 1996; 11:982–986.
33. Buniva C, Marcielo A, Ciuffreda L, Iadarola AM, Ferro M, Bechis F, Piccoli GB, Malcangi U. Referral to nephrologist: analysis on 740 outpatients follow-up. 34th Congress of the ERA-EDTA, September 1997, Geneva (abstract).
34. Hood S, Sondheimer J. Impact of pre-ESRD management on dialysis outcomes: a review. Sem Dial 1998; 11:175–180.
35. Obrador G, Pereira B. Early referral to the nephrologist and timely initiation of renal replacement therapy: a paradigm shift in the management of patients with chronic renal failure. Am J Kidney Dis 1998; 31:398–417.
36. Ismail N, Neyra R, Hakim R. The medical and economical advantages of early referral of chronic renal failure patients to renal specialists. Nephrol Dial Transplant 1998; 13:246–250.
37. Slingeneyer A. Multicenter study on patient referral to dialysis (abstr). Perit Dial Int 1998; 18:136.
38. Levin A, Lewis M, Mortiboy P, Faber S, Hare I, Porter

E, Mendelssohn D. Multidisciplinary predialysis programs: quantification and limitations of their impact on patient outcomes in two Canadian settings. Am J Kidney Dis 1997; 29(4): 533–540.

39. Rasgon S, James R, Chemleski B, Ledezma M, Mercado L, Besario M, Trivedi J, Miller M, Dee L, Pryor L, Yeoh H. Maintenance of employment on dialysis. Adv Ren Replac Ther 1997; 4:152–159.

40. LemaitreV, Gobert P, Bridoux F, Glowacki F, Provot F, Vanhille Ph. Début de dialyse au cours de l'insuffisance chronique terminale: 134 patients de 1994 à 1996. Soc Néphrol, Toulouse, October 2–3, 1997, Abstract 60, p. 5.

41. The National Kidney Foundation Dialysis Outcomes Quality Initiative (NKF-DOQI). Am J Kidney Dis 1997; 30 (suppl 2, 3).

44

Dialysis Delivery in Canada: Can Systemic Shortcomings Cause Complications?

David C. Mendelssohn
St. Michael's Hospital and University of Toronto, Toronto, Ontario, Canada

I. INTRODUCTION

The hypothesis that underlies this chapter is that shortcomings in dialysis system design, and not only intrinsic issues related to technology, patients, and/or providers, can cause complications of dialysis. At least five problems may be attributed to dialysis system issues, including nonreferral, late referral, modality mismatching, late initiation of dialysis, and reduced quality of dialysis (Table 1).

This chapter will describe dialysis delivery in Canada. While it is not my intent to be parochial, it is my opinion that many of the systemic issues recently identified within this Canadian context are also in operation in other jurisdictions, as all countries struggle with the universal dilemma of providing this expensive therapy to the expanding population that requires it. Specifics may be different from country to country, but the common issues and problems are greater than the differences.

Canada's government-sponsored, single-payer health-care system is its most highly valued social program and is the fundamental defining feature of the nation. Many foreign observers are impressed that quality indicators show very good results in Canada compared to the United States despite a much smaller percentage of gross domestic product (GDP) spent on health care (9.2% vs. 14.2% in 1996). However, as fiscal problems deepen, this percentage of GDP has been in decline for 4 consecutive years, from a peak level of 10.2% in 1992 (1). Whereas Canada was the second highest spender on health care as a percentage of GDP among Organization for Economic Cooperation and Development (OECD) countries in the early 1990s, its rank had fallen to fifth by 1995 (behind the United States, Germany, France, and Switzerland) (2) (Table 2). As a result, many critics are becoming increasingly concerned that the Canadian health-care system is no longer stable and is not sustainable in its current form.

Problems in dialysis delivery are one high-profile example of how the Canadian health-care system can fall short of expectations. This chapter will examine the general aspects of the Canadian health-care system, consider aspects of the dialysis-delivery system, such as access, quality, and modality distribution, consider whether dialysis-related complications can be a result of systemic, rather than patient, provider, or technology-specific issues, and finally extend these arguments beyond Canada.

The medical systems in all Canadian provinces are not identical, but much commonality exists. This chapter will focus to a large extent upon the recent problems in Ontario, Canada's most populous province, with 11 million inhabitants and a health-care budget of $17.7 billion.

II. CANADIAN HEALTH CARE

In 1867, at the time of the birth of the Canadian nation, it was decided that important jurisdictions should be federally controlled. Health care was not well developed and therefore was given, through the British

Table 1 Complications of Dialysis that May Result from Health-Care System Deficiencies

Nonreferral (rationing)
Late referral for dialysis
Modality mismatching
Late initiation of dialysis
Decreased quality of dialysis

Late initiation may or may not be secondary to late referral to a nephrologist.

North America Act, to the provinces to administer. As a result, the federal government in Ottawa can influence provincial health policy in only two ways.

First, it can use legislative authority, as it did in the late 1960s with the introduction of the enormously popular universal, single-payer, government-sponsored health insurance scheme (Medicare). Another important example of this mechanism was the Canada Health Act of 1985 (3), which enshrines the five fundamental conditions that must guide provincial health policy if federal financial support is to be delivered to a province: (a) universal coverage, (b) accessibility, (c) portability, (d) comprehensiveness, and (e) public funding and administration.

The second lever deployed by the federal government to influence provincial health policy involves transfer payments. Ottawa transfers federally collected tax dollars to the provinces for the funding of health care. If conditions in the Canada Health Act are not met, Ottawa can withhold payments. However, the amount of these transfer payments is decreasing with time. When Medicare was conceived, the intent was that 50% of provincial health funding would come from the federal government in Ottawa. This had progressively decreased to 33% by 1994 (4). Provinces are feeling increasingly burdened by what they perceive to be more and more unrealistic federal requirements and are also more inclined to challenge them as the financial lever that controls them is eroded.

Table 2 Total Health-Care Expenditure as a Percent of Gross Domestic Product, by Year, Selected OECD Countries

Country	1993	1996
United States	14.3	14.2
Germany	10.1	10.5
Switzerland	9.5	9.8
France	9.4	9.6
Canada	10.2	9.2

Source: OECD Health Data, 1997.

At the provincial level, health care is the single largest public expenditure, consuming about a third of a province's budget. There is a perception in government that health-care spending is out of control. In fact, when Medicare began in the early 1970s, it was predicted by some that an open-ended system, with no control of consumers or providers, would eventually bankrupt the government. By the early 1990s, provincial governments had indeed run up huge public debt and decided that public spending must be scaled back. Of course, health care became a major target. Nonetheless, the public's seemingly insatiable demand for instantly accessible, high-quality, high-technology medicine continues, as does the popularity of Canadian-style Medicare. As might be predicted, major service-delivery problems have become increasingly apparent.

Canada's health-care system has always functioned well in the area of availability of primary care providers. Roughly 50% of physicians are general and family doctors, a much higher percentage than in the United States. Access to specialist care is only through referral and is constrained in many sectors by centralization of technology and waiting lists. Elective, high-technology procedures like hip and knee replacements (5), coronary artery bypass grafting (6), and radiotherapy for cancer (7) are available much less quickly in Canada than in the United States.

Unlike in the United States, market forces do not operate directly to cause expansion of service availability in Canada. Because of the Canada Health Act (public administration and public funding), virtually all allocation decisions are made by government officials. Although they may seek advice from providers and hospitals, they are not bound by this. With a global cap on health-care spending in Ontario over the past 5 years, program expansion has been determined by a process of competitive lobbying for resources. Expansion of one program means redistribution of money from other areas of health-care spending. Especially for high-cost programs, the incentive for government to act may be absent, and bureaucratic inertia can be difficult to overcome. For that matter, the same lobbying occurs within each hospital. Each hospital is given a global budget to provide services, with programs like dialysis competing with all others for adequate funds. Occasionally a problem becomes a public issue, which is generally followed by Ministry announcements of expansion. Recent examples in Ontario include oncology services, cardiovascular surgery, and dialysis.

III. DIALYSIS IN CANADA

Canada has a very well-developed dialysis-delivery system. By global standards, access is reasonable compared to most other western nations, and quality is quite high. Canada's end-stage renal disease (ESRD) patients have benefited from universal government funding, incentives for providers that do not cause them to limit the quality of treatment for fear of erosion of personal profit, and dominance of university-based dialysis and transplantation programs. Notwithstanding the considerable merits of Canada's system, which I readily acknowledge, this chapter will focus primarily upon its shortcomings. To do so, I will discuss problems in Canada's largest province, Ontario, and especially in its largest city, Toronto, with a regional population of approximately 4.5 million people.

IV. DIALYSIS IN ONTARIO

A. Access to Dialysis

Problems in the delivery of dialysis care in Ontario, and especially in Toronto, are well documented (8). Two areas that merit special consideration are the problems of nonreferral and late referral. In the next few paragraphs, I will demonstrate first that dialysis planning has not always kept up with known needs based on historical trends of growth of ESRD patients. Next, I will show that over and above the known need, there is a very large unmet need related to patients with ESRD who are not referred to ESRD centers in Ontario and most likely in the rest of Canada. Finally, I will discuss the problem of late referral. Together, these problems highlight that access to dialysis in Canada is less than ideal.

In the early 1990s, nephrologists in the Toronto region perceived that chronically inadequate resources for dialysis had reached a critical level and that patient care was being compromised. When numerous meetings with the Ministry of Health and Hospitals proved fruitless in obtaining a response, a deliberate campaign in the scientific literature (8–10) and lay press (11,12) was embarked upon to highlight concerns.

In this regard, we published in the *Canadian Medical Association Journal* a descriptive analysis of data reported to the Toronto Region Dialysis Registry between 1981 and 1992 (8). All 504 existing patients enrolled in dialysis programs in 1981, and all 3794 new patients entering the programs from 1982 to 1992 were included. The objective of the study was to analyze trends in the demand for and supply of dialysis in the Toronto region and to determine if anticipated dialysis expansion would be sufficient to provide for the projected growth of the dialysis population.

From 1981 to 1992, the number of dialysis patients in the metropolitan Toronto region grew from 504 to 1422 patients, an increase of 182.1%. The average rate of growth was 9.8% per year. Of the total increment of 733 patients from 1981 to 1991, 344 (47%) were over 65 years of age, nonetheless the average crude mortality rate had remained constant at 13.8–17.3% per year. The transplantation rate declined from a peak of 20.2% in 1982 to 7.8% in 1992. Since 1981, the Toronto region had a much higher ratio of both total dialysis patients per hemodialysis (HD) station and HD patients per HD station than the rest of Ontario or the rest of Canada. The Toronto region HD utilization index (reflecting actual treatments relative to treatments budgeted) was 100.8% in 1991 and 102% in 1992, with a range in individual hospitals from 98 to 124% (with 85% considered optimal). We concluded that the growth of the dialysis population of metropolitan Toronto had caused a critical shortage of resources (Fig. 1). This trend was attributed mainly to a fall in transplant rate and an increase in the number of elderly patients entering dialysis programs, combined with insufficient funding for expansion of facilities. Continuation of this trend was expected to limit universal access to this expensive but life-sustaining therapy.

Other components of this dialysis crisis campaign included a letter to the editor of the *New England Journal of Medicine* (9), and an article in *Contemporary Dialysis and Nephrology* (10). Simultaneously, two articles written for public consumption were published opposite the editorial page in the national newspaper, *The Globe and Mail* (11), and in the largest local newspaper, *The Toronto Star* (12).

Finally, the then provincial opposition political party took the issue to a legislative committee for study. Detailed local and provincial planning committees were struck (13–16). All reports documented inadequate dialysis planning and argued for a proactive approach. The formation of a standing provincial committee comprising government, providers, and patients was recommended to jointly comanage this complex problem. While some dialysis expansion did come about, it has been a classic example of too little, too late. The Ontario Ministry of Health has rejected the joint comanagement model. Most recently, the Ministry of Health

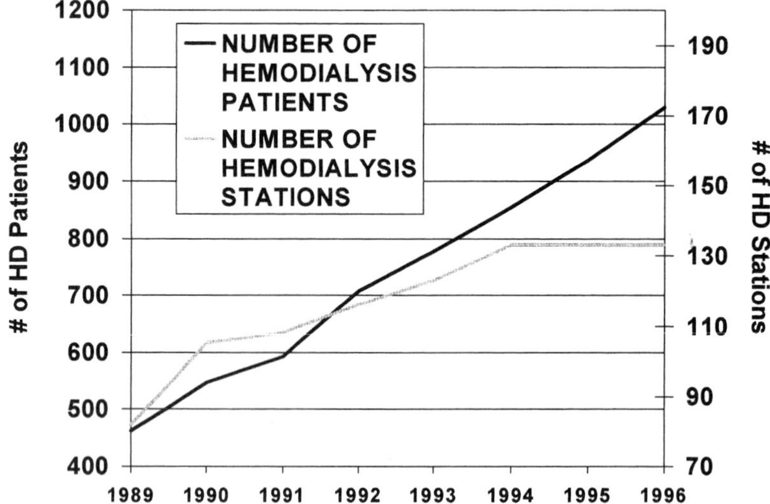

Fig. 1 In 1994, the Toronto region HD patient projections (black line) were expected to far exceed the plans for expansion of HD capacity (gray line). (From Ref. 8.)

has delayed decisions while it argues with hospitals about repatriation of funds from existing programs to new ones when patients transfer and about other issues of integration and hospital restructuring. Hemodialysis overcrowding in the Toronto region continues.

Notwithstanding the overcrowding in some regions, dialysis still expands by roughly 10% per year in Canada and in Ontario, as in other western societies (17). However, the incidence rate of ESRD (104.1 per million in 1996) is only 40% of the U.S. rate (262 per million in 1995) (17,18) (Fig. 2). This large difference suggests that while the Canadian system struggles to provide adequate resources for known patients, based on predictable historical trends, there is, in addition, a very large unmet need as well.

There is deep concern on the part of the Canadian nephrology community that patients who might benefit from dialysis are not receiving it. Evidence to support this is mainly indirect. For example, there are wide variations in incidence rates between, and even within, provinces (17) (Fig. 3). Manitoba has the highest rate of ESRD at 157.5 new patients per million population in 1995, while British Columbia has the lowest (89.6) (17). The Ontario rate is 108.6, but a 1992 report showed that the Ottawa-Kingston region of Eastern Ontario had the highest rate (130.5), while The Hamilton-Kitchener area had the lowest rate (77.8) (19). It seems unlikely that population differences account for these large differences.

It has also been pointed out that the curve of incidence rates of ESRD versus time shows a unique plateauing in recent years in Canada, while all other jurisdictions show a continuing upwards trend (20) (Fig. 4). For example, the national rate was 100.2 per million in 1992, 101 in 1993, 105.1 in 1994, and 104.4 in 1995. It is argued that only if the true need were being met would the ESRD incidence rate plateau. By this measure, it would appear that there is still an unmet need even in the United States and Japan, while the Canadian plateau is inappropriate and indicates that rationing of dialysis therapy is occurring. It is of interest that the U.S. rate of increase has been less steep during the past 2 years (18).

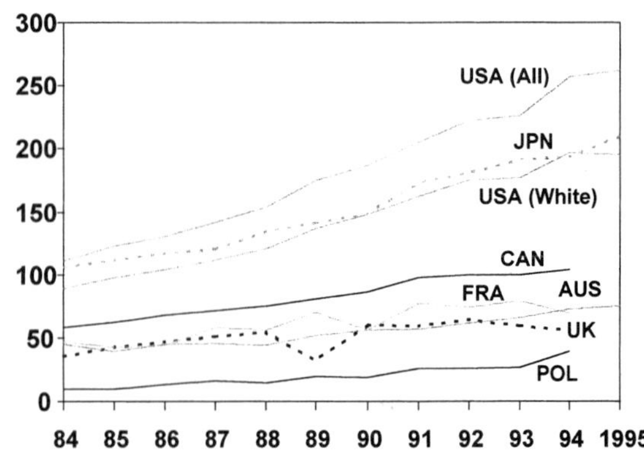

Fig. 2 Treated ESRD Incidence Rate for Selected Countries, 1984–1995. (From Ref. 18.)

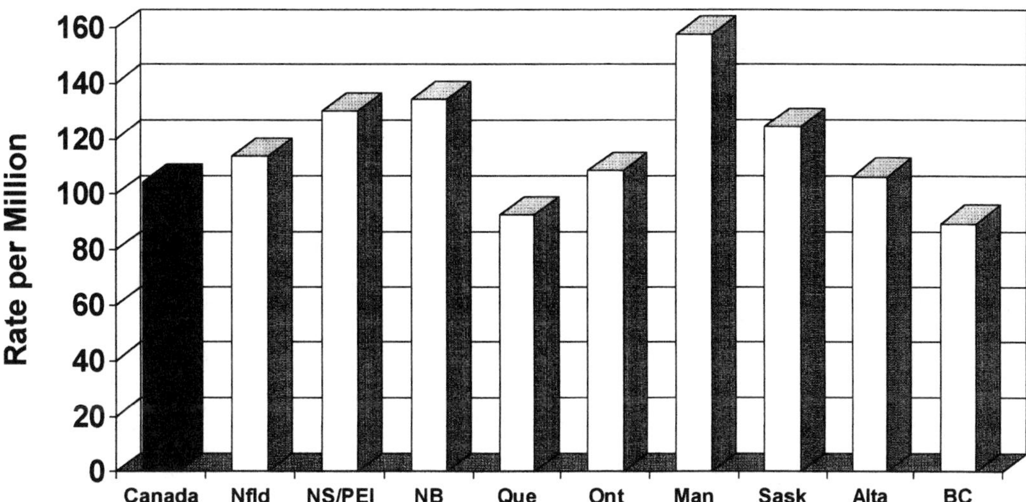

Fig. 3 Interprovincial variation in incidence rates of ESRD, Canada, 1995. (Data from CORR Annual Report, 1997.)

Another line of reasoning suggesting unmet need indicates that there is a large gender difference in ESRD treatment rates. For example, for new patients aged 45–64, the male rate is 630 per million, while the female rate is 400 (17). In contrast, in the United States there is only a small male predominance (18). It would seem that some Canadian women are disadvantaged in accessing therapy for ESRD.

The final line of evidence involves international comparisons of ESRD incidence rates, which shows that Canada's incidence rate is much less than that of the United States and Japan and is also less than Germany, Spain, and Israel (18). There are three possible explanations for this. First, it is possible that the Canadian population has a truly lower incidence of ESRD than the U.S. population. However, this seems unlikely because the health status of the two populations does not appear to be strikingly different. There is a similar rate of other major diseases and a similar pattern of causes of ESRD, with diabetic kidney disease and glomerulonephritis being the two most common etiologies. Second, it is possible that more Canadian nephrologists withhold dialysis from potential patients with ESRD than their American counterparts. Again, this issue has been studied and does not appear to be the case (21). Finally, it is possible that patients who might benefit are not referred to ESRD treatment centers by primary care physicians and/or community-based internists.

We recently published the results of a study designed to determine patterns of referral to nephrologists (by family physicians and community internists) of patients with kidney disease in Ontario (22). A random sample of 1924 members of the Ontario Medical Association, Sections on General and Family Practice and Internal Medicine, received a mailed survey instrument. Of 1778 eligible respondents, responses were received from 728 physicians (40.9%). The survey questionnaire was designed to elicit both actual patterns of practice and attitudes of nonnephrologist physicians who care for and possibly refer renal patients. A hypothetical question about a patient with various age and comorbid features revealed that physicians were less likely to refer for dialysis as age and comorbidity increased (Table 3). In response to the direct question: "In the past 3 years, did you care for a patient who, after due consideration, died of renal failure without referral for dialysis?" 14.2% of family physicians and 44.6% of internists said yes. Overall, 67.4% of respon-

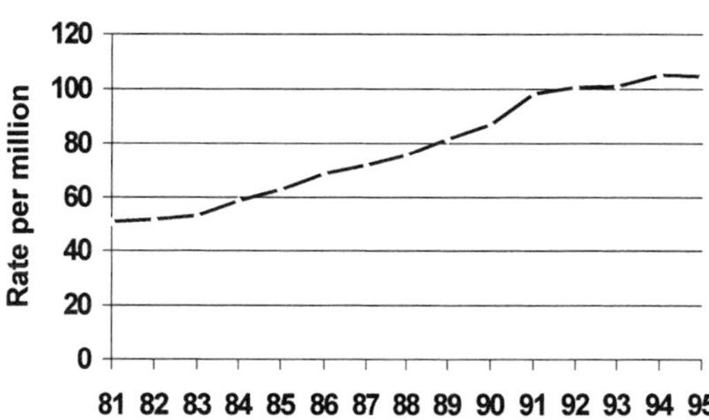

Fig. 4 Incidence rate of ESRD in Canada, 1981–1995. Note the plateau from approximately 1991 to 1995. (Data from CORR Annual Report, 1997.)

Table 3 Effect of Age and Comorbidity on Nonreferral for Dialysis in Ontario[a]

Comorbidity	25 y	50 y	70 y	85 y
Otherwise healthy	0	0	4.8	34.1
Schizophrenic	2.5	4.8	26.8	—
IQ < 70	12.8	19.0	43.8	—
Diabetic	0	0.4	12.9	55.9
Myeloma	—	—	36.2	—
Mild dementia	—	—	24.4	—
Severe dementia	—	—	81.4	—

[a]Respondents were asked "Consider the following patients with renal failure. What would you do about the dialysis?" Choices were "eligible for dialysis," refer to nephrologist," or "ineligible for dialysis, no referral." Answers, of 728 family physicians and internists, reflect percent nonreferral.
Source: Ref. 22.

dents strongly or somewhat agree that rationing of dialysis was occurring at the time of the survey. These results suggest that nonreferral for dialysis occurs in Ontario and is influenced by both age and coexisting disease. Given that modern dialysis can be applied effectively to almost all patients, this raises the concern that patients who might benefit are not being referred to dialysis centers. This referral pattern is likely part of the explanation for the gap in incidence rates between Canada and the United States.

It is of interest to note that a Toronto area dialysis planning study published in January 1995 agreed that the incidence rate of ESRD ought to approach the rate seen in the United States (14). Because implementation of such a high target would be expensive, the Ontario Ministry of Health asked that another estimate of demand be performed. These consultants did not consider potential unmet need and generated much lower estimates of demand (23). The original Toronto report was never given credence by the government. A more recent provincial report was more pragmatic in its suggested approach, arguing that whatever target is chosen will be arbitrary and that, therefore, an information system be engaged that could determine if supply-demand mismatching was occurring and allow for upwards or downwards adjustment, if necessary (16). This approach has also been rejected by government.

One final problem leading to suboptimal treatment is late referral of patients approaching ESRD. In the survey of Ontario physicians described above, we showed that patients with microscopic hematuria (79.2%), proteinuria (69.5%), and creatinine in the 120–150 μmol/L range (84.3%) were generally not referred to nephrologists by family physicians (22). At creatinine levels between 151 and 300 μmol/L, 27.8% would still not refer. Only when the creatinine level was above 301 μmol/L would almost all refer to a nephrologist. This raises a concern that many patients with potentially serious, and possibly reversible, renal diseases are not referred until substantial irreversible scarring has occurred and that measures to slow the rate of progression towards ESRD may not be implemented.

Age and comorbidity are once again known factors associated with late referral. Late referral has the potential to lead to (a) progression of the comorbid diseases that begin in the predialysis stage (e.g., left ventricular hypertrophy, renal osteodystrophy), (b) acceleration of onset of ESRD, (c) worsened patient survival, (d) more frequent use of temporary vascular access devices, (e) less use of native AV fistulae, (f) a suboptimal biochemical, physical, and psychological state on initiation of dialysis, (g) worse vocational outcomes, and (h) increased health-care costs. It is of interest to note that late referral has been documented not only in Canada (22), but also in Europe and America (24–31).

In summary, it appears that the Canadian dialysis-delivery system does not provide accessible dialysis therapy to all who might benefit. Nonreferral leads to death from ESRD, while late referral and insufficient HD resources may, in addition, lead to morbidity and reduced quality of life.

B. Quality of Dialysis

While access to dialysis has been problematic, it has been the general feeling of Canadian nephrologists that quality of dialysis has been quite good, at least until now. Again, many reasons are apparent. First, physicians may not own facilities and are not subject to direct pressure to compromise quality for the sake of higher profit. Second, dialysis is largely university based, although community-based dialysis is increasing in many provinces.

Unfortunately, there are no national data reporting delivered dose of dialysis. The Canadian Organ Replacement Registry (CORR) does report fairly loose data on dose prescribed (17). For HD in 1995, the minimum number of hours was reported as 2 in 3.7% of centers, 3 in 74.1% of centers, and 4 in 21.0% of centers. Urea kinetic modeling was used to determine dialysis prescription by 80% of centers in 1995 and had gone up in each of the 3 years it was tracked. In terms of frequency of monitoring patients with urea kinetics,

64.5% of centers report this is done monthly, with the rest reporting it every 3 (29%) or 6 months (6.5%). Finally, target Kt/V is reported as >1.4 in 30% of centers, 1.2–1.4 in 55% of centers, and 1.0–1.2 in 11% of centers.

For CAPD, 90.8% of patients were reported to be receiving four exchanges per day, while 5.6% and 3.7% received 5 and 3 exchanges per day, respectively. Fluid volume per exchange was reported to be 1.5 L in 5.8% of patients, 2.0 L in 82.8%, 2.5 L in 10.9%, and 3.0 L in 0.4%.

Further indication that quality of dialysis is reasonably high in Canada at present is that reuse is not widespread (11/84 hospitals report reuse nationwide) and Registered Nursing (RN) labor dominates. Standardized mortality rates nationwide are 134 per 1000 patient years of follow-up from 1990 to 1994. This is much less than the American experience (232 per 1000 patient-years in 1992). In the CANUSA study, the risk of death in CAPD patients prospectively followed in American centers was 90% higher than that for Canadian centers and was not explained by known differences in comorbidity or demographics (32,33). It is reasonable to suspect that this difference in mortality between Canada and the United States is largely a reflection of quality of dialysis, but it may also be partly explained on the basis of subtle differences in case mix.

The Toronto region maintains its own dialysis registry, and reliable data pertaining to dialysis dose delivered are available from there (34). Note that roughly 17% of Canada's ESRD patients are dialyzed in the Toronto region, but whether or not the Toronto experience reflects system performance nationwide is not known.

On December 31, 1996, there were 1253 patients on hemodialysis in the Toronto region. Adequacy data were reported for 1005 (80%). The mean urea-reduction ratio (URR) was 69%; 73% of patients had a URR > 65% (Fig. 5). Mean serum albumin was 39 g/L; mean hemoglobin was 108 g/L. Erythropoeitin was used by 88% of hemodialysis patients. There were 799 patients on peritoneal dialysis (PD), and data were provided to the registry for 602 patients (75%). Mean albumin was 36 g/L, mean hemoglobin was 111 g/L, and 72% of PD patients were on erythropoeitin. Adequacy data were also collected for PD patients but have not yet been analyzed.

In Ontario there is now concern that fiscal pressure will lead to changes in the quality of delivered dialysis. Hospitals are struggling with severe economic constraints, and a Health System Restructuring Commission is recommending closure of many existing facilities all over the province. Downsizing and mergers to prevent outright closure are commonplace. The Wellesley Hospital in Toronto, with a large dialysis program serving 225 patients, was closed in 1998.

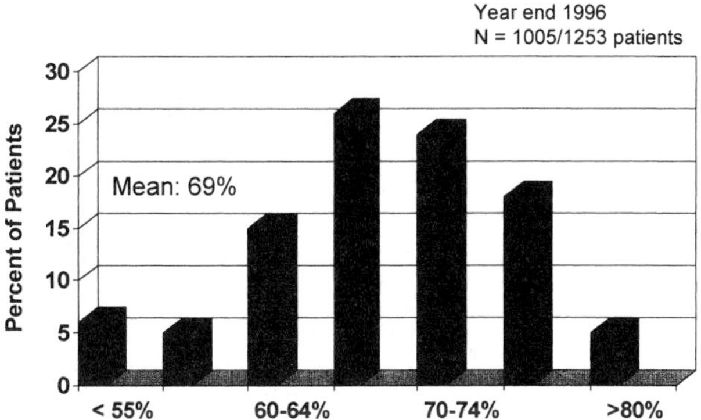

Fig. 5 Frequency distribution of urea reduction ratio in the Toronto region, hemodialysis patients, 1996. (From Ref. 34.)

In this context, there is a trend to put pressure on nephrologists to implement reuse of dialyzers. At The Toronto Hospital, the largest Canadian academic teaching hospital and site of the largest dialysis population (600 patients), reuse has been ongoing for several years, and recently nursing staffing changes were implemented to adjust the skill mix and reduce RNs. This was necessary so that the hospital could cut $1,000,000 from the hemodialysis budget without treating fewer patients. Finally, the Ministry is encouraging independent health facilities (IHFs), including large American companies, to compete with the hospital sector for future dialysis expansion. Fresenius Medical Care (formerly National Medical Care) of Massachusetts is part of a group that has been awarded a license for IHFs in Eastern Ontario. Issues of integration and quality assurance are of some concern.

C. Modality Distribution

The Canadian dialysis-delivery system utilizes PD to a greater extent (34%) than most other relatively prosperous western nations (17) (Fig. 6). Only the United Kingdom, with a lower incidence rate of ESRD and a lower per capita GDP, utilizes more (18). In contrast, PD makes up only 17% of the total in the United States, a country with a higher incidence rate of ESRD and higher per capita GDP (18). Within Canada there are large variations between provinces. New Brunswick (47.4%), has the highest provincial usage of PD, while Quebec (28.8%) has the lowest (17).

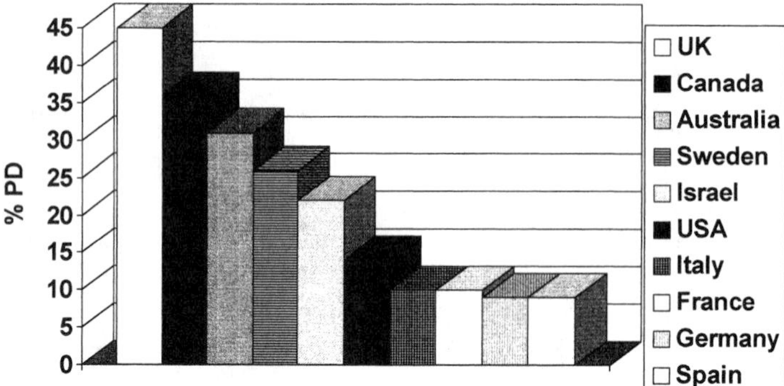

Fig. 6 International comparisons of percent utilization of CAPD/CCPD. (From Ref. 18.)

Even within provinces, large regional differences are seen. For example, hemodialysis resource constraints are well documented in the Toronto region, a factor that certainly impacts on the high prevalence of PD there. For example, Toronto has fewer HD stations per million population than the rest of Ontario or the rest of Canada, has a higher ratio of HD patients per station, has 50% of its prevelent patients on PD, and starts 68% of its incident patients on PD (35) (Fig. 7). The Toronto Region Dialysis Registry tracks a hemodialysis overcrowding summary statistic that expresses actual treatments divided by funded capacity. This varied between 101% and 104% from 1991 to 1994; in 1995 it was 109% (A. Chery, personal communication).

Of course the optimal mix of modalities has not been defined. For example, there is no consistently accepted survival advantage of hemodialysis or peritoneal dialysis, while cost of hospital-based methods are roughly double that of home-based therapy (36,37). Canadian nephrologists are supportive of the notion of maximizing the use of cost-effective, home-based modalities but believe that while these modalities should be encouraged, they should not be made mandatory (38).

While it is perceived by physicians that lack of hemodialysis resources in some regions of Canada may lead to excessive reliance on CAPD and has compromised ideal patient care (8), the perspective of the provincial government payer is different. While patient outcomes are important, they are often competing with mounting concern about the apparent epidemic of new cases of ESRD, with its attendant ever-escalating cost.

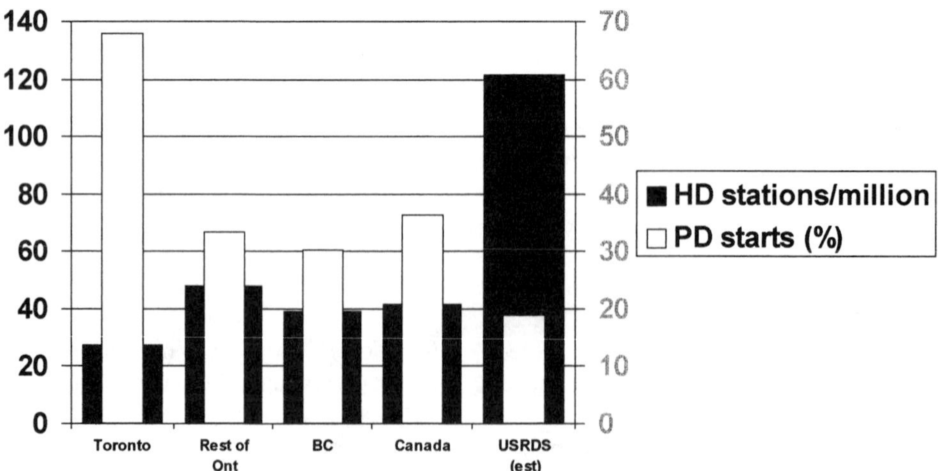

Fig. 7 The number of HD stations per million population (solid bars) and the percentage of PD starts (open bars) in 1993. Toronto, the rest of Ontario, BC, Canada, and the United States are compared. Toronto was severely constrained with respect to HD station availability, resulting in many more patients commencing PD as initial therapy. (From Ref. 35.)

Increased use of the more cost-effective forms of dialysis is a priority, especially because outcomes are apparently equivalent.

Because of the lack of information available and the difficulties associated with designing an experimental study, we surveyed by mail questionnaire all physicians belonging to the Canadian Society of Nephrology (39). This yields information about "expert opinions," which might become a gold standard until better data become available. Preliminary results based on the 143 of 233 (61.4%) Canadian nephrologists who responded to the three mailings report that decisions about modality are based most strongly on patient preference, followed by quality of life, morbidity, mortality, and rehabilitation. When asked about the current relative utilization of each modality, nephrologists felt that hospital-based HD is slightly overutilized, CAPD is about right, while cycler PD, community-based full care, self-care, and home HD are underutilized. A hypothetical question about optimal distribution to maximize survival revealed that a type of HD should constitute 62.8% of the modality mix, with more emphasis on cycler PD (14.9%), community-based full care HD (13.8%), self-care HD (14.5%), and home HD (9.0%) than is current practice (Table 4).

These preliminary results suggest that the current national average 66:34% HD:PD ratio is reasonable but could be modified within each modality to a more community-based system. By extension, they suggest that Canadian nephrologists believe that regions like Toronto, where this ratio is skewed, are suboptimally designed. It appears that nephrologists are sensitive to cost-effective alternatives but believe strongly in patient choice and a balanced ESRD-delivery system. Whether this kind of information will be accepted by government planners and lead to better dialysis system design is not yet known.

Table 4 Optimum Modality Distribution[a]

	Survival, wellness, and quality of life	Cost-effectiveness	CORR 1995
Hospital-based HD	25.5	17.9	52.3
Community-based full-care HD	13.8	11.9	—
Community-based self-care HD	14.5	16.1	11.5
Home HD	9.0	11.9	2.1
CAPD	21.5	29.7	27.8
Cycler PD	14.9	11.9	4.8
IPD	1.2	1.0	0.8

[a]Respondents were asked "You are asked to design a regional dialysis network for a state or province of 10 million people, with a typical case mix. You are not to have ownership of a facility, only to advise government planners. All patients expected to benefit would be offerred dialysis (no rationing). Based on your opinion about maximizing the outcomes as indicated, what mix of modalities would you suggest? Please assign a percent value to each modality, such that each column total equals 100%." The table shows the responses from 143 Canadian nephrologists. The last column represents the 1995 Canadian distribution.

V. CAN DIALYSIS COMPLICATIONS BE CAUSED BY SYSTEMIC SHORTCOMINGS?

The premise that underlies this chapter is that shortcomings in dialysis system design can cause dialysis complications. In the preceding few pages, I have tried to describe the problems that exist within the Canadian health-care and dialysis-delivery systems. Most of the arguments that I have advanced are empirical or quantitative and have been (or will be) published.

To link these shortcomings to adverse patient outcomes is problematic, because to my knowledge there is not a well-developed literature in this area. Where such information is available, I will refer to it. In general, however, I will use arguments that are intuitive and obvious to most practicing nephrologists, supplemented by real anecdotes from our experiences at The Toronto Hospital.

In the recent past, attention has begun to focus on predialysis care and efficient entry of patients into ESRD programs. For example, a recent publication by the U.S. National Institutes of Health Consensus Conference on the Morbidity and Mortality of Dialysis states that an important goal is early referral to a multidisciplinary renal team (40). In this way, interventions may be initiated that will allow for the timely, elective creation of a dialysis-access device (AV fistula, graft, or peritoneal dialysis catheter insertion) and prevent the catastrophic commencement of dialysis, with subsequent prolonged hospital stay. Because all of this predialysis care can be accomplished either as an outpatient service or with day surgery, there is a potential to save substantial precious health-care resources.

A recent Canadian publication contrasted two predialysis programs (35). At St. Pauls Hospital in Vancouver, the clinic was successful in showing that predialysis clinic patients had better homeostatic parameters, less use of temporary dialysis access, and less consumption of hospital resources compared to patients who received usual care. However, a program at the Toronto Hospital was less successful. While predialysis access was created in 89% of patients who went through the clinic, the percent of patients who started dialysis as an outpatient was not increased as intended (Fig. 8). This was attributed to hemodialysis resource constraints, which preclude elective, outpatient initiation of dialysis.

At TTH, hemodialysis positions for chronic outpatients are frequently not available. In this circumstance, the practice is to wait for uremic symptoms to occur and then to admit these patients to inpatient beds so that dialysis can be initiated in positions normally reserved for acute problems. This can lead to an admission of up to a month, and sometimes more. The negative consequences for the patient are obvious, and ironically, the system as a whole is handicapped in many ways as well.

In 1993, even this option became saturated. Because all other local dialysis hospitals were similarly full and could not treat new ESRD patients, several patients required transfer to hospitals outside the Toronto region for dialysis (8). These centers were as far away as Kingston and London, Ontario, more than 200 km away. One frail 75-year-old man commuted for several winter months 75 km to Oshawa to receive hemodialysis.

Excessive reliance on PD in Toronto has been known to cause patients to be started on PD who are not considered to be good candidates. In this circumstance, there is the occasional pleasant surprise, and a patient does better than could have been predicted.

> An 83-year-old woman with cancer of the lung, who lives alone, was seen in predialysis clinic in January 1992. She was described by the renal coordinator as "horrified" when PD was described and said that she could not imagine doing it. Because of HD resource constraints, PD was recommended nonetheless. Peer support convinced her to start PD while she was put on the HD waiting list. She was trained in February 1992 on a UV flash system with home-care support. Eventually, a live-in nanny was employed as well. To date (September 1997) the patient has had five episodes of peritonitis, with four treated at home, and is doing well. In October 1994 she requested coming off the HD waiting list.

Often, however, such a good outcome is not the case.

> A 55-year-old man had diabetes, two previous myocardial infarctions with grade 4 left ventricular function, peripheral vascular disease with amputations of several toes, retinopathy, and neuropathy. He had a history of alcohol abuse and noncompliance. He was admitted to a community hospital without hemodialysis capability with renal failure and was started on PD. Within one month he developed an umbilical hernia, which was repaired with replacement of the PD catheter. Three months later he was transferred to TTH for CAPD training. However, he had a catheter leak and was managed with IPD for 2 months. CAPD training was given despite concerns that the patient could not succeed because of a lack of insight, hostility, and lack of social support. Training took a considerable length of time. He was angry with caregivers, whom he blamed for his failure to thrive. He was transferred to HD 2

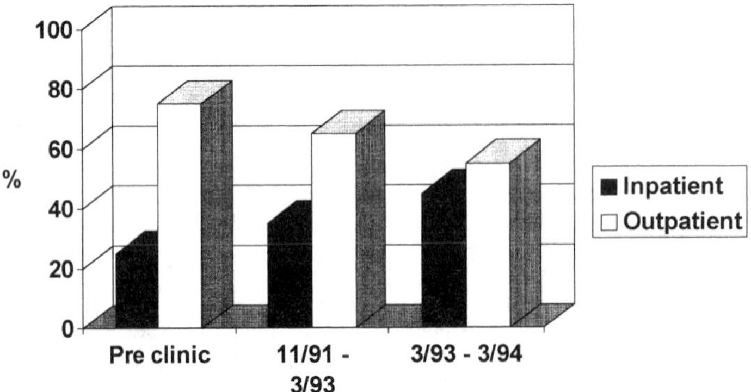

Fig. 8 Status of patients at the onset of dialysis at TTH: comparison of inpatient and outpatient dialysis starts prior to and two periods after the establishment of a predialysis clinic. Note that there was a progressive decline in outpatient starts, coinciding with a lack of HD resources. (From Ref. 35.)

months later because of ultrafiltration problems and failure to cope. He survived on HD for almost 2 years but required frequent and prolonged hospitalizations for his various medical problems.

Most nephrologists agree that it is not wise to force patients to do home or self-care dialysis against their wishes. It is quite easy for such patients to resist being trained or to sabotage their own treatment. Even if well motivated, it is usually possible to predict that a patient is in a very marginal social situation or has a high likelihood of failure for other reasons.

While there are sound economic arguments in favor of encouraging patients to choose home-based or self-care therapies for ESRD, it is also well known that the selection of a wrong modality can be costly and cancel some or all the cost savings associated with a less expensive initial modality selection. Prichard has argued that a treatment modality change includes a set of start-up costs, which makes the most cost-effective therapy in almost all cases a therapy that can be successfully maintained (37). The case above illustrates this concept dramatically.

Prichard has also shown that among patients medically eligible for either HD or PD allowed to choose freely among dialysis modalities, 50% will choose home-based or self-care methods (41). This important observation deserves further comment. First, Canadian nephrologists agree that patient choice is the most important single factor in modality selection (39). However, it is difficult for any provider to provide information about competing modalities without introducing elements of bias. For example, by playing up the more liberal diet and painless exchanges of PD compared to the restrictions and painful needling of HD, it is easy to influence choice in favor of PD. Conversely, by emphasizing efficiency of small solute removal and technique survival, it is possible to influence choice in favor of HD. Second, what should be done if a patient selects a method that is clearly inferior or contraindicated, given their comorbidities and social circumstances? Just because 50% will choose home or self-care does not mean that this percentage will lead to optimal patient outcomes.

A 45-year-old woman had IDDM, retinopathy, neuropathy, and hearing deficit. She was a poorly controlled diabetic with a history of noncompliance. After renal education, she was overwhelmed and had many questions about not starting dialysis. Finally, she decided that the night cycler was the only acceptable treatment choice. Eventually, a PD catheter was inserted. Within one month it was clear that the patient was not compliant with either her medications or her dialysis regime. She requested a change to CAPD. She skipped her appointment with the transplant team. She was lost to follow-up for 4 months. She was upset about her health problems, social isolation, and treatment burden. Psychiatry was involved because of occasional suicidal ideation, but it was felt she was not clinically depressed. Sixteen months after starting PD she was failing because of noncompliance and uremic symptoms. She transferred to HD at her request. Two months later she was found dead at home. Suicide was suspected.

When it is not easy to transfer patients from PD to HD, complications are managed differently as well. For example, refractory peritonitis is treated with intermittent PD instead of early catheter removal and transfer to HD. When catheter removal is indicated, it is common to simultaneously reimplant a new catheter or to wait 4–6 weeks and then reimplant. In this way, HD is used only temporarily. Even frequently relapsing peritonitis might not be switched to HD because of considerations related to HD resources. Similarly, complications of PD such as inadequate dialysis, yeast peritonitis, hernias, scrotal leaks, and pleuro-peritoneal fistulas are often managed with modifications of, rather than interruption of, PD. Finally, with increased attention to adequacy of peritoneal dialysis (32), it seems likely that the requirement to switch to HD because of inadequate dialysis might increase, putting further strain on the system. The CORR database has some important insights to this potential problem. In 1982, 1.9% of CAPD failures were due to inadequate dialysis; this percentage had increased to 11.3% in 1995 (even prior to publication of the CANUSA study).

While HD resource constraints cause clinical innovation and, in some cases, successful reintroduction of PD, there are many circumstances in which such therapeutic trials have failed and have served only to prolong or increase morbidity. It seems likely attempting to maintain patients on PD who ought to be switched is not cost-effective if prolonged or repeated hospital admissions are required and /or if a switch to HD is ultimately required.

VI. WHAT IS BEING DONE IN CANADA?

There are only 250–300 nephrologists in Canada, almost all of whom are members of the Canadian Society of Nephrology. There is no other national organization (analogous to the Renal Physicians Association) that concerns itself with advocacy and political activity. The CSN has undergone a significant metamorphosis in recent years, as the dialysis dilemma worsens. Historically, its function has been limited to delivering an annual scientific meeting and interacting with the Royal College of Physicians and Surgeons, the national specialist accreditation body, concerning educational issues.

At the annual general meeting in 1995, the CSN formed a Professional and Public Policy Committee. This committee also deals with human resources, guidelines, and economic issues. While still early in its evolution, this committee has already catalyzed a CSN policy document "Principles of ESRD Care," that sets out general official CSN policy on diverse issues such as rationing, resources, modality selection, and transplantation (38). The focus is on provision of ethical, cost-effective, and optimum patient care. The document is intended to educate and inform policymakers, and other stakeholders, and to form the basis for the development of a consistent, proactive renal care system in each province.

The CSN Professional and Public Policy Committee is currently involved in two important guideline development projects. First, it is developing a Canadian version of dialysis clinical practice guidelines, using NKF/DOQI guidelines for dialysis as a starting point. Second, it is finalizing referral guidelines for elevated creatinine for use by family physicians and community internists. The goal is to have patients referred early and to allow all competent patients who might benefit and who choose dialysis to receive it. Future projects include an academic analysis of the true incidence of ESRD in Canada. The CSN is also building linkages to other important stakeholders such as the Kidney Foundation. Hopefully, these activities will allow the CSN to be a strong advocate for an accessible, high-quality ESRD delivery system for the new millennium.

VII. LOOKING BEYOND CANADA

In order to support the hypothesis that systemic problems lead to dialysis complications, I have focused on the problems in Canada's dialysis-delivery system. At first glance, this may not seem relevant to the situation in other nations. I will now argue that these issues are indeed generalizable. All payers must struggle with a similar dialysis dilemma—how to provide high-quality, accessible ESRD therapy within overall paradigms of cost containment. For example, a review of 11 industrialized nations showed that financial and/or reimbursement factors stood out as the most important factor in ESRD treatment modality distribution in nearly every country or region studied and is a complex one, involving physicians and facilities, each having different financial interests (42).

Canada stacks up fairly well on a global scale with respect to dialysis provision. I will arbitrarily divide the world nations into four groups in order to compare their situation to Canada's. They are (a) third world nations, (b) poorer industrialized nations, (c) similar industrialized nations, and (d) the United States and Japan.

Third world nations cannot afford to provide dialysis to their citizens. In general, dialysis is provided privately, and therefore only to the wealthy. Access is quite limited, and death from ESRD is the usual course.

Poorer industrialized nations like Mexico also face issues of accessibility. Cost-containment strategies (overt or covert) work in the first instance on limiting access to treatment and second on promoting use of less expensive modalities. Rates of treatment of ESRD are less than in Canada. Often these nations rely even more heavily on PD than Canada does, and complications related to inadequate access to HD would be even more important. In theory, if resource constraints are severe, there may also be pressure to provide suboptimal quality of PD or HD even to stable chronic patients.

Most western nations have rates of ESRD similar to Canada's. Most also use more HD than Canada. Quality indicators in some of these nations show longer hemodialysis treatment times, infrequent reuse of dialyzers, and better survival than reported from North America.

Finally, let us consider briefly dialysis in the United States. Treatment rates are very high, given the open-ended entitlement program that exists, so that access to dialysis is excellent (43). Late referral to dialysis centers remains a problem and might grow worse in the growing managed care environment (29). There is severe pressure to contain cost through limiting the reimbursement rate per treatment. This, combined with physician ownership of many facilities, creates perverse incentives to provide suboptimal treatment quality (44). Some critics believe this is the root cause of the poor survival rates in the United States. The United States also has 83% of its prevalent dialysis patients on HD and only 17% on PD. It is interesting to speculate that this reliance on HD might be excessive in some regions, limiting patient choice and constraining patients to treatment regimes that might limit their independence and compromise their lifestyle. While it is unusual to require PD as a back-up for temporary problems on HD, it is occasionally a valuable, life-saving option when a patient runs out of vascular access sites. If PD resources are not available, these patients could experience premature death.

VIII. CONCLUSIONS

Canada's single-payer, government-sponsored health insurance system has been a noble social experiment. Despite its considerable merits, it is now facing severe fiscal problems.

Dialysis has always been at the center of the debate between cost containment on the one hand and access and quality on the other. Access to dialysis has been limited in Canada compared to the United States, but quality of care has been good. However, fiscal pressures may lead Canadian dialysis provider institutions and physicians to consider incorporating some of the cost-containing solutions that have generated controversy when applied widely in the United States. These might include increased dialyzer reuse and a shift to less expensive labor to replace registered nurses. Nephrologists will need to be vigilant in monitoring quality indicators and outcomes to ensure that these practices, if implemented, do not impact adversely on patient care.

Economic and political forces impact profoundly on ESRD treatment modality selection in Canada, just as they do in other countries. In the final analysis, the conclusion is the same as has been reached many times before: optimal treatment requires sufficient resources. If resources do not permit selection of optimal therapy for each and every patient, then it can be anticipated that problems will be encountered.

The growth rate of ESRD therapy is an anomaly in the fiscally challenged health-care environment of the late 1990s. It will be an ongoing challenge for patients and providers to secure the resources necessary for accessible, high-quality therapy, respecting patient choice of modality when appropriate. Physicians have always had a critical advocacy role for their patients. Emotion-based advocacy was useful in 1972, for example, when nephrologists in the United States succeeded in persuading Congress to create the open-ended entitlement to Medicare for ESRD therapy that has allowed wonderful access to dialysis care in that country. However, I believe that emotion-based advocacy will increasingly need to be complemented by empirical evidence.

In this regard, a considerable challenge exists for the nephrology community to study, in a much more comprehensive way than we have so far, issues of accessibility, quality, cost-effectiveness, modality selection, and links of these parameters to clinical outcomes. Outcome analysis must not be limited to survival and hospitalization but must include quality of life and rehabilitation. Finally, proactive dialysis planning and effective, efficient system design are essential ingredients in providing optimal patient care and must involve nephrologist input. Only in this way will our advocacy efforts for patients and their families be rewarded.

ACKNOWLEDGMENTS

I would like to thank Sharon Izatt and Maggie Chu from the Home Peritoneal Dialysis Unit of the Toronto Hospital, who both reviewed a preliminary version of this manuscript, offered suggestions, and provided the illustrative case vignettes.

REFERENCES

1. Health Canada 1997: National Health Expenditures in Canada 1975–1996 Fact Sheets, Policy and Consultation Branch, Ottawa.
2. OECD Health Data, 1997.
3. Canada Health Act, R.S.C., 1985.
4. Health Canada 1996: National Health Expenditures in Canada 1975–1994, Full Report. Policy and Consultation Branch, Ottawa, January 1996.
5. Coyte P, Wright J, Hawker G, Bombardier C, et al. Waiting times for knee replacement surgery in the United States and Ontario. NEJM 1994; 331:1068–1071.
6. Canadian Cardiac Care Network of Ontario. Data Driven Decision Making Report, Vol. 1, No. 1, 1996.
7. MacKillop W, Zhou Y, Quirt C. A Comparison of Delays in the Treatment of Cancer with Radiation in Canada and the United States. Int J Radiat Oncol Biol Phys 1995; 32(2):531–539.
8. Mendelssohn DC, Chery A, for The Toronto Region Dialysis Committee. Dialysis Utilization in the Toronto Region from 1981–1992. Can Med Assoc J 1994; 150: 1099–1105.
9. Mendelssohn DC, Skorecki KL, Cardella CJ. Health care in Canada and the United States. N Engl J Med 1993; 329:965.
10. Mendelssohn DC, Kriger F, Winchester J. A comparison of dialysis in the United States and Canada. Contemp Dial Nephrol 1993; 14:27–31.

11. Mendelssohn DC, Skorecki KL, Cardella CJ, Thimm A. Dialysis in Toronto: a crisis in waiting. The Globe and Mail 1993; Oct. 8:A27.
12. Mendelssohn D, Roscoe J, McCready W. Public deserves straight talk on growing dialysis crisis. The Toronto Star 1994; March 2:A21.
13. Report of the Working Group on Renal Services, Toronto, Ontario, January 1995.
14. Final Report of the Steering Committee of the Central East Region Dialysis Planning Study, Ontario, January 1995.
15. Ontario Legislative Assembly, Standing Committee on Social Development, Dialysis Treatment in Ontario, 1994.
16. Report of the Ontario Renal Services Advisory Committee, January 1996.
17. Annual Report 1997, Vol. 1: Dialysis and Renal Transplantation, Canadian Organ Replacement Register, Canadian Institute for Health Information, Ottawa, Ontario, March 1997.
18. U.S. Renal Data System, USRDS 1997 Annual Data Report, The National Institutes of Health, National Institute of Diabetes and Digestive and Kidney Diseases, Bethesda, MD, April 1997.
19. Canadian Organ Replacement Register, 1992 Ontario Report, Canadian Institute for Health Information, Don Mills, Ontario, March 1994.
20. Kjellstrand CM, Moody H. Hemodialysis in Canada: a first class medical crisis. CMAJ 1994; 150:1067–1071.
21. Mackenzie JK. Decisions for dialysis: a survey of Canadian dialysis directors. Clin Inv Med 1993; 16 (suppl):B107.
22. Mendelssohn DC, Kua BT, Singer PA. Referral for dialysis in Ontario. Arch Int Med 1995; 155:2473–2478.
23. Sinclair Decision support. Quantitative Study of Demand for Renal Dialysis in Ontario, June 1995.
24. Eadington DW. Delayed referral for dialysis: higher morbidity and higher costs. Semin Dial 1995; 8:258–260.
25. Ratcliffe PJ, Phillips RE, Oliver DO. Late referral for maintenance dialysis. Br Med J 1984; 288:441–443.
26. Innes A, Rowe PA, Burden RP, Morgan AG. Early deaths on renal replacement therapy: the need for early nephrological referral. Nephrol Dial Transplant 1992; 7:467–471.
27. Campbell JD, Ewigman B, Hosokawa M, Van Stone JC. The timing of referral of patients with end-stage renal disease. Dial Transplant 1989; 18(12):660–668.
28. Jungers P, Zingraff J, Page B, Albouze G, Chauveau P, Page B, Hannedouche T, Man N-K. Late referral to maintenance dialysis: detrimental consequences. Nephrol Dial Transplant 1993; 8:1089–1093.
29. Ifudu O, Dawood M, Homel P, Friedman EA. Excess morbidity in patients starting uremia without prior care by a nephrologist. Am J Kidney Dis 1996; 28:841–845.
30. Eadington DW, Craig KJ, Winney RJ. Comorbidity and biochemical indices modulate the impact of late referral on survival on RRT (abstr). Nephrol Dial Transplant 1994; 9:960.
31. Khan IH, Catto N, Edward N, MacLeod AM. Chronic renal failure: factors influencing nephrology referral. Q J Med 1994; 87:559–564.
32. Churchill DN, Taylor DW, Keshaviah PR, for the CANADA-USA Peritoneal Dialysis Study Group. Adequacy of dialysis and nutrition in continuous peritoneal dialysis: association with clinical outcomes. J Am Soc Nephrol 1996; 7:198–207.
33. Churchill DN, Thorpe KE, Vonesh EF, et al. Lower probability of patient survival with continuouos peritoneal dialysis in the United States compared with Canada. J Am Soc Nephrol 1997; 8:965–971.
34. Toronto Region Dialysis Registry. Indicators of Adequacy of Treatment, 1996, Toronto, 1997.
35. Levin A, Lewis M, Mortiboy P, Faber S, Hare I, Porter E, Mendelssohn DC. Multidisciplinary predialysis programs: quantification and limitations of their impact on patient outcomes in two Canadian settings. Am J Kidney Dis 1997; 29:533–540.
36. Goeree R, Manalich J, Grootendorst P, et al. Cost analysis of dialysis treatments for end stage renal disease. Clin Inv Med 1995; 18:455–464.
37. Prichard SS. The costs of dialysis in Canada. Nephrol Dial Transplant 1997; 12(Suppl 1):22–24.
38. Mendelssohn DC, for the CSN Professional and Public Policy Committee. Principles of end stage renal disease care. Ann RCPSC 1997; 30:271–273.
39. Mendelssohn DC, Jung B, Blake P, Mehta R. Attitudes of North American nephrologists towards dialysis modality selection: 1) Canadian results. JASN 1997; 8: 222A.
40. NIH Consensus Statement—Morbidity and Mortality of Dialysis. Ann Int Med 1994; 121:62–70.
41. Prichard SS. Treatment modality selection in 150 consecutive patients starting ESRD therapy. Perit Dial Int 1996; 16:69–72.
42. Nissenson AR, Pritchard SS, Cheng IKP, et al. Nonmedical factors that impact on ESRD modality selection. Kidney Int 1993; 43(S40):S120–S127.
43. Inglehart JK. The American health care system: the end stage renal disease program. N Engl J Med 1993; 328: 366–371.
44. Klahr S. Anemia, dialysis, and dollars. NEJM 1996; 334:461–462.

45

Outcomes and Intermodality Transfers in Patients on Renal Replacement Therapy in Canada and Europe

Peter G. Blake*
University of Western Ontario, Ontario, Canada

Wim Van Biesen**
University Hospital of Gent, Gent, Belgium

Norbert Lameire**
University Hospital of Gent and University of Gent, Gent, Belgium

Rosario Maiorca**
University and Civil Hospital, Brescia, Italy

PART I: IN CANADA

I. INTRODUCTION

The Canadian system for delivering renal replacement therapy (RRT) to patients with end-stage renal disease (ESRD) is potentially of more than local interest for a number of reasons. First, the quality and completeness of data collection achieved by the Canadian Organ Replacement Register (CORR) is very good by international standards and so the resulting database allows questions concerning the demographics and clinical outcomes of ESRD patients to be addressed and answered in a way that has not often been possible in other countries (1). Second, the geographic and cultural proximity to the United States makes Canada a natural control for trends identified in the much larger U.S. ESRD population and so helps the observer to distinguish between trends that are specific to one country only and those that may have broader relevance. Third, the Canadian health-care system is an interesting mix of public and private elements, which might be expected to influence acceptance rates for RRT in contrasting ways. Thus, there are fee-for-service payments to nephrologists for the care of ESRD patients, and these might be expected to act as an incentive to initiate more patients on RRT. However, almost all RRT is provided through publicly funded hospitals, and, given public spending constraints, this might be expected to limit growth in acceptance rates.

II. DELIVERY OF RRT IN CANADA

A brief description of RRT services in Canada is appropriate before looking at comparative outcomes between different RRT modalities. In Canada, health care is administered on a provincial basis within the constraints of the guiding principles of the Canada Health Act, which mandates universal coverage and access as well as predominantly public funding and administration. Almost all RRT is delivered via a relatively small number of large, publicly funded hospitals, the majority of which are affiliated with universities. These RRT programs are funded out of hospital global budgets although in some provinces supplemental direct dedicated funding is made available for chronic dialysis because of the high cost and life-sustaining nature of

*Part I in Canada.
**Part II in Europe.

the treatment and because of the apparent relentless growth in demand for it.

In general, it costs Canadian hospitals significantly less to maintain ESRD patients on peritoneal dialysis (PD) as compared to hemodialysis (HD), and because HD expansion also tends to require more initial capital input, both government and hospitals have been inclined to support substantial use of PD (2,3). Thus, in Canada over the past decade, about 40% of new patients have been on PD by day 90 after initiation of RRT, and overall about 35% of prevalent dialysis patients are maintained on this modality (1). Most HD is provided via hospital-based "in-center" units, but a significant minority of more stable patients are treated in self-care units with lower staff-to-patient ratios. There has also been a recent increase in the numbers treated in small satellite units, but home HD remains little used. There has been controversy over the high proportion of patients doing PD in the larger Canadian cities where government-funded HD expansion has had particular difficulty keeping up with population growth (3). Accordingly, there has been a perception that, in some centers, patients have been directed to PD without being given any real choice in terms of modality selection. Recently, in response to these criticisms, HD capacity has been significantly expanded and there has been greater decentralization of HD into small communities. This has contributed to a fall in the proportion of dialysis patients doing PD to about 30% in 1997 (1,4) (Fig. 1).

As already mentioned, the majority of dialysis is delivered via teaching hospitals, and therefore most Canadian nephrologists have an academic appointment and have teaching and research commitments in addition to clinical responsibilities. Nephrological care of RRT patients is remunerated on a fee-for-service basis by single-payer, provincial health plans and, in all provinces, these have tended to pay substantially more for the medical care of in-center HD patients compared to that of PD and self-care HD patients (2,5). Thus, there is an incentive to physicians to maintain more patients on in-center HD, while there is an incentive to hospitals and governments to maintain more on PD. The relatively high proportion of patients on PD would suggest that the former incentive has, in practice, generally been more powerful than the latter. Recently, the largest province, Ontario, has switched to a modality-independent capitation fee for physician care of all chronic dialysis patients, but it is too early to judge if this will affect modality distribution.

Acceptance rates for RRT are relatively low in Canada at about 120 per million population per annum, compared to over 260 per million in the United States. This discrepancy has been hotly debated and is partly accounted for by the absence of a large black population with a high incidence of ESRD in Canada (6,7). However, even the Caucasian incidence rate in Canada is 50% lower than that in the United States and is more like that seen in western Europe. It has been argued that this reflects the almost inevitable rationing of treatment that occurs in a single-payer, publicly funded and publicly delivered health-care system, but there are probably other factors, including geographical distance constraints for many potential patients outside larger cities. An alternative, more palatable explanation is that there may be a lower incidence of ESRD related to better primary health care, but this is unproven. The ongoing growth in incidence rates suggests that there is still substantial ongoing unmet need, however (7).

Renal transplantation rates in Canada run at about 30 per million per year and, unlike ESRD incidence rates, have not changed appreciably in the past decade

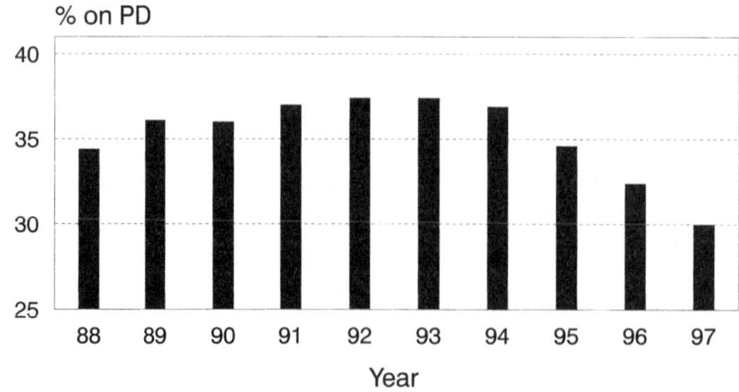

Fig. 1 Changes with time in percentage of Canadian prevalent chronic dialysis patients being maintained on PD. (Adapted from Ref. 1.)

so that waiting lists have become increasingly long (1). Again, this transplant rate is similar to that in northern European countries and is about a third less than that in the United States. While cadaveric transplant rates have stayed the same or even fallen, the use of living donors, both related and unrelated, has increased significantly in recent years. There is no doubt that in Canada, as elsewhere, transplantation is the least costly treatment for ESRD, but its use has been limited by lack of donors and also by the lack of suitability of the majority of contemporary dialysis patients for surgery and immunosuppression because of age and comorbidity (8).

Against this background there are a number of key questions that need to be addressed. One is how outcomes for patients in general are changing with time and how they compare to those in the United States and elsewhere. Another is how the high proportion of patients on PD do relative to those on HD and how this compares with the situation in other countries. Implicit in this question is the issue of whether a policy of high PD usage as is practiced in many countries with predominantly publicly delivered health-care systems is consistent with good patient outcomes as compared to countries where HD is more dominant. A third issue is whether transplantation leads to better survival than staying on dialysis.

III. OUTCOMES OF DIALYSIS

A. Mortality

Uncorrected one-year mortality rates for new patients initiating RRT in Canada measured from the time of first treatment fell steadily over the course of a decade, from 19.5% in the cohort of 1986 to 15.5% in the cohort of 1996 (1,9). This improvement occurred despite a rise in acceptance rates for RRT from 70 to 110 per million over this period and a consequent steady increase in the mean age of incident patients over the same period from 52 to 58 years of age (Table 1) (1). Similarly, during that time the proportion of patients with diabetes mellitus rose from 30 to 38% and the proportion whose ESRD is actually attributed to diabetes rose from 23 to 28% (Table 1) (1).

The same trend towards improved survival is even more apparent when mortality rates are adjusted for age, gender, race, and province using a Poisson regression model. For HD and PD there were decreases of 23 and 36%, respectively, in the adjusted relative risk of mortality between the cohorts that started dialysis in the period 1981–1984 and the cohort that started in the period 1993–1996 (Table 2). In PD, in particular, the decline in adjusted mortality was marked in patients both above and below age 65 (Table 3).

These one-year mortality rates are intermediate between those reported in the United States and those in Europe and Japan (10). However, if the first 90 days on RRT are omitted, as is the practice with U.S. registry data, the mortality rate falls to 10.7%, which is quite similar to values in Europe (10). Of course, when these comparisons are being made, it is only fair to point out that the high U.S. mortality rates may partly reflect the much higher acceptance rates for RRT in that country compared to Canada and Europe and the much higher transplant rates compared to Japan. Both of these differences likely lead to a significantly older and frailer ESRD population in the United States. This is likely a major factor underlying the recently reported excess mortality in U.S. PD patients compared to their Canadian counterparts (11). Mortality was over 90%

Table 1 Trends in Acceptance Rates, Mean Age, and Prevalence of DM in Incident Canadian RRT Patients, 1988–1996

Year	Acceptance rate per million population	Average age of incident patients	% of incident patients with DM
1988	72.7	54	29.6
1989	77.6	55	29.2
1990	82.7	55	29.1
1991	93.9	56	31.4
1992	96.3	56	31.4
1993	100.3	57	33.0
1994	105.7	58	34.7
1995	108.8	58	35.0
1996	110.9	59	37.9

Source: Adapted from Ref. 1.

Table 2 Adjusted Mortality Rate Ratios in Successive Cohorts of Canadian HD and PD Patients, 1981–1996[a]

Cohort	HD	PD
1981–1984	1.00	1.00
1985–1988	0.94	0.88
1989–1992	0.90	0.71
1993–1996	0.77	0.64

[a]Using risk ratio of 1.0 for mortality on each modality in the period 1981–1984.
Source: Adapted from Ref. 9.

Table 3 Adjusted Mortality Rates per 100 Patient-Years in Successive Cohorts of Canadian PD Patients, Classified by Age, 1981–1996

Cohort	Age 45–64	Age 65+
1981–1984	20.5	39.4
1985–1988	17.8	34.9
1989–1992	15.4	28.5
1993–1996	13.1	27.0

Source: Adapted from Ref. 9.

higher in the United States and this difference persisted even after correction for demographics, comorbidity, and indices of adequacy and nutrition, may relate to a number of factors, but there has to be a suspicion that the degree of unmeasured comorbidity may be much greater in a country with such high acceptance and transplant rates as are found in the United States.

B. HD Versus PD

The relatively high proportion of ESRD patients doing PD in Canada as well as the completeness of data collection by CORR makes the country particularly suitable for studying comparative outcomes between HD and PD. As already mentioned, this important issue has been to some extent politicized in Canada because of widely expressed concerns that PD, in at least some regions of the country, has been excessively used in unsuitable patients because of a shortage of government-funded HD spots due to fiscal constraints on health-care spending.

When PD and HD were first compared using CORR data in 1987, there was no significant difference in patient survival using an intention-to-treat analysis with censoring at the time of a permanent modality switch (12). These data were consistent with those in a variety of studies from the United States and Europe in the late 1980s and early 1990s which showed generally equivalent patient survival on the two modalities (13–16). Technique survival was, of course, notably less with PD, but as this did not appear to be affecting patient survival and as PD was less expensive, the policy of high PD usage appeared appropriate (12). In 1995, however, the U.S. registry, using a prevalent analysis, found a significantly higher mortality rate in U.S. PD patients in general, compared to their HD counterparts (17). This excess risk in PD was estimated at 19% overall and was particularly marked in older patients, diabetics, and females. This study appeared during a period when concern was being expressed in Canada about undue fiscal pressures to direct patients to PD and also at the same time as the publication of the Canada-USA (CANUSA) study, which gave rise to questions about the adequacy of delivered clearances on PD (6,18). Against this background, there was questioning of the high use of PD in Canada, and the publication of CORR data in 1997 showing superior outcomes on PD, as compared to HD, caused some surprise and perhaps some confusion (19).

Before considering the CORR data in more detail and why it apparently differs so much from the U.S. data, consideration has to be given to some of the pitfalls of studies comparing outcomes on the two modalities (20,21). First, registry-based comparisons are not randomized controlled trials, and so, for comparisons to be legitimate, corrections have to be made for demographic, comorbid, and other differences between patients on the two modalities. Factors such as age, sex, race, presence or absence of diabetes, and center size are relatively easy to deal with, but comorbidity and associated functional status are much more problematic and sufficiently detailed information to measure them reliably will not typically be found in a registry. Thus, the U.S. registry data on which the 1995 study by Bloembergen et al. was based had no correction for comorbidity, and even the 1997 CORR data had only a count of the number of comorbid conditions with no information as to their severity or as to how they impact on functional status, factors known to have an important impact on survival (17,19,22).

A second issue that is clearly critical is the type of analysis being done. Typically this is based either on intention to treat or on the treatment actually received. A pure intention-to-treat analysis assigns patients to the modality they are using at the initiation of dialysis or, more often, at 90 days after initiation, as it may take some time to make a definitive modality selection. All subsequent events are assigned to that initial modality, even if the patient subsequently switches or is transplanted. As switches from PD to HD are much more common than those in the opposite direction, both cohorts will eventually comprise predominantly HD and transplant patients, and so the analysis will increasingly tend to obscure any survival benefit for either modality. This can be dealt with by modifying the analysis to censor patients who are transplanted or who switch modalities. This modification of intention to treat is criticized, however, because it excludes deaths that occur in patients shortly after a modality switch, which perhaps should be attributed to the original modality. Thus, as PD-to-HD switches are more common, this censoring may underestimate adverse outcomes on PD. This can be dealt with by having a "grace period" of 30, 60, 90, or 120 days after a switch during which deaths are not censored but rather attributed to the initial modality. While this type of analysis is widely used, it also presents problems. If the grace period is too short, there will be a bias in favor of the initial modality if the second modality is truly superior. However, if the grace period is too long there may be a bias in favor of the second modality if the initial modality is truly superior. A typical compromise is to use 60 days, but it may be better still to test a variety of time periods and see how much the final result is altered.

When a treatment-received analysis is done, switches are an even bigger issue, as deaths at some stage subsequent to the switch will have to be attributed to the new modality rather than just censored. Thus, the potential for obscuring a true treatment difference is even greater.

With either type of analysis, the time at which patients enter the analysis is also important. Patients who present late for RRT tend to be sicker and also tend to be treated with HD. These patients may have a high early mortality rate and so the inclusion of patient data from the early weeks of dialysis may bias the analysis against HD (19). Typically, data from the first 90 days are excluded, in part to get around this problem but also because a significant number of patients who plan to do PD spend some initial time on HD. If data from a longer initial period is omitted, as was the policy with the U.S. registry analysis published in 1995, there is the potential to bias the analysis against PD because it is during this early period, when residual renal function is maximal, that PD may be most beneficial (17,19). For the same reason, a prevalent patient-based analysis will tend to make HD look relatively better, and an incident-based one will have the opposite effect.

A third issue that should be kept in mind is that many of the statistical methods used to do these analyses, such as the Cox proportional hazards model, presume that possible risk factors for mortality such as diabetic status, comorbidity, and modality confer proportional risks that remain constant with time (23). This presumption is not always justified, however, and clearly in the case of modality is not appropriate because PD, relative to HD, performs better in the first 3 years, compared to years 4 and 5 (19,24,25).

The CORR study published in 1997 made a comprehensive attempt to deal with these pitfalls by correcting for the number of comorbid conditions, by redoing the HD-versus-PD comparison using both treatment-received and intention-to-treat methodologies, and by varying both the time of initiation of analysis and the duration of postswitch grace periods (19). It thus could reasonably be said to be the most methodologically sophisticated analysis to address this issue in any country to date. The study comprised almost all of the over 10,000 incident patients in Canada in the period 1990–1994. In the treatment-received analysis, corrected mortality rates were found to be significantly lower on PD than on HD with a relative risk of 0.73 for all patients on PD compared to 1.00 for those on HD. Subgroup analysis showed that the advantage for PD was greatest in nondiabetics and in younger diabetics but less in older diabetics, where the trend in favor of PD did not achieve statistical significance (Table 4). In the intention-to-treat analysis, the advantage for PD did not reach significance in the original publication, but when 1995 data were added in a more recent publication, increasing the number of patients to over 14,000, statistical significance was achieved in the group as a whole and was greatest in nondiabetics less than 65 years of age (26) (Table 4).

On closer analysis, it becomes apparent that the advantage of PD over HD in both analyses is concentrated in the first 2–3 years after the initiation of treatment (Fig. 2). This raises the issue of whether PD, in the early years of ESRD, is an inherently superior therapy or whether the difference is due to unmeasured or undetected baseline comorbidity differences between patients on the two modalities. Just as in the United States, there is a suggestion in recent studies of a tendency for comorbidity to be greater in HD patients in Canada (27,28). The CORR study attempted to deal with this by correcting for diabetic status and for the number of major comorbid condition as well as for age, sex, and center size but did not take into account the

Table 4 Mortality Rate Ratios for PD Relative to HD (where HD Is 1.00) in Canadian Patients Initiating RRT, 1990–1995, Using Treatment-Received and Intention-to-Treat Methodologies

	Treatment-received method, relative risk (95% CI)	Intention-to-treat method, hazard risk (95% CI)
All	0.73 (0.69, 0.77)[a]	0.93 (0.87, 0.99)[a]
Non-DM <65 yrs	0.53 (0.46, 0.60)[a]	0.84 (0.87, 0.99)[a]
Non-DM >65 yrs	0.75 (0.65, 0.86)[a]	0.95 (0.86, 1.05)
DM <65 yrs	0.76 (0.65, 0.83)[a]	0.90 (0.82, 1.10)
DM >65 yrs	0.88 (0.75, 1.04)	1.04 (0.87, 1.24)

[a]95% Confidence Intervals do not cross 1.0 and so observation is significant at $p < 0.05$.
Source: Adapted from Ref. 26.

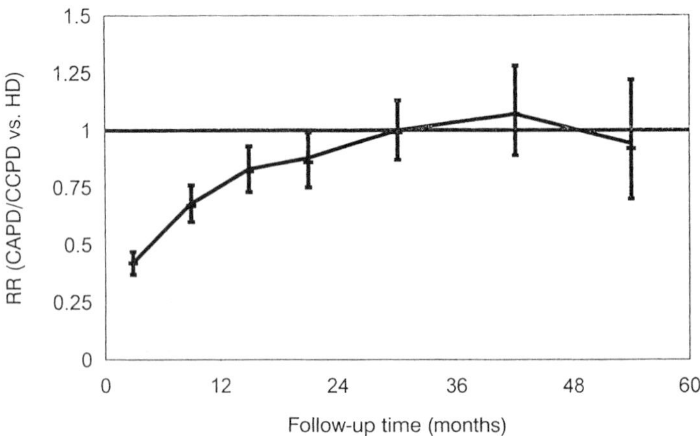

Fig. 2 Mortality rates for PD relative to HD by follow-up interval, adjusted for age, primary renal diagnosis, and comorbid conditions and estimated using Poisson regression. (From Ref. 26.)

severity, as distinct from the number, of comorbid conditions (19). It is arguable, however, whether comorbidity alone can explain all the apparent superiority of PD in Canada. Is it possible that PD is inherently superior in the early years of ESRD? One plausible explanation might be the apparently better preservation on PD of residual renal function during this time (29). Recent studies have emphasized the strong association of residual function with patient survival in PD patients (18,30).

It is particularly interesting that the results of these analyses are not significantly affected by varying the way modality switches are dealt with. Thus, censoring at transplantation or at 30, 90, or 120 days, instead of at 60 days, postswitch does not alter the results appreciably (19). However, varying the time after initiation of dialysis at which patients enter the analysis has a strong impact. Thus, omitting the first 90 days from the treatment-received analysis causes the advantage for PD to lose statistical significance, and including the first 90 days in the intention-to-treat analysis increases the significance of the advantage for PD (19,26). The powerful influence that these early weeks after initiation have on the outcome of the analysis would tend to suggest that there is an early unmeasured excess of comorbidity on HD, consistent with the tendency of late or fulminant ESRD presentations to be, by their nature, directed to that modality. In support of this interpretation is the fact that the 1995 U.S. analysis that showed such poor results with PD used a methodology that excluded patients from the analysis for an average of 12 months postinitiation of dialysis, thus omitting a key proportion of the period when PD performs best relative to HD (18). When this methodology was changed in subsequent cohorts to include incident patients from 90 days after initiation of dialysis, the apparent benefit for HD lost its statistical significance (31). This suggests that some of the apparently strong differences in relative outcomes on the two modalities between Canada and the United States are methodological rather than real (11). The issue of how the early months on RRT are analyzed is obviously important, but it is unclear if it alone explains all the apparently better results with PD in Canada (11,31).

Two recent studies clarify these issues further. Collins et al. studied over 116,000 U.S. incident patients from 1994 to 1996 using an intention-to-treat analysis with censoring after a period of grace of 60 days post–modality switch (32). They found that in nondiabetic patients there was a significantly higher risk of mortality on HD, while in older female diabetics there was a significantly higher risk on PD. For younger and for male diabetics, there was no significant difference. These more contemporary results are thus quite similar to the recent CORR results, again suggesting that most of the difference between the United States and Canada in relative outcomes on PD was methodological rather than real (17,19,31).

Also, Murphy et al. have recently reported a cohort of 822 Canadian patients at 11 centers followed prospectively for up to 3 years from their time of initiation of dialysis in 1993 and 1994 (28). These patients, half of whom were on PD at 90 days after initiation, had very detailed data on comorbidity collected. Unadjusted risk of mortality was lower on PD, but there was no difference between survival on the two modalities, either overall or in any subgroup, once comorbidity was adjusted for.

The relative merits of HD and PD in terms of patient survival will not be definitively answered without a randomized controlled trial, but the feasibility of such a trial is questionable. In the absence of a definitive study, some conclusions can be drawn, however. The evidence suggests strongly that patient survival on PD in Canada is at least as good as that on HD and that the difference between relative outcomes in Canada and the United States may have been overstated. Given the lower cost of PD in Canada, it seems reasonable to conclude that the policy of high PD usage followed over the past two decades has been cost-effective, at least as far as survival is concerned. Furthermore, these analyses mainly deal with the period prior to the recent dramatic changes in PD prescription practices, and these might be expected to reduce PD mortality rates significantly (4,9).

C. Technique Failure on PD

The above findings on patient survival on PD mainly pertain to the first 2–4 years of dialysis, partly because most of the studies are relatively recent but also because only a minority of PD patients continue on the modality after that time. Much of this patient loss relates to death and transplantation, which are at least as likely to occur on HD, but a significant proportion is, of course, due to technique failure (TF), which continues to be much more common on PD (1). It could be argued that while TF in PD is undesirable, it need not be seen as a critical problem for the modality if its rate is relatively stable and if, as has been suggested, overall patient survival is as good as, or better than, on HD. However, there is little doubt that many of the causes of TF are potentially life-threatening and expensive as well as unpleasant for the patient. Thus, if the causes of TF could be more successfully managed, PD could be an even more cost-effective treatment for ESRD.

This raises the issue of whether TF rates are changing in PD. A number of forces that might be altering TF rates need to be considered. Peritonitis is generally the most common single cause of TF, but peritonitis rates have been decreasing over the past decade, mainly due to better PD technology, and this might be expected to reduce TF (34–36). More recently, there has been heightened awareness of the problem of inadequate clearances on PD, and since about 1994 prescriptions have changed markedly with greater use of larger-volume dwells and of automated PD (4,37,38). This too might be expected to lessen TF rates, although the trend may be too recent for much effect to be apparent yet. In contrast, the greater availability of HD facilities in many Canadian centers in recent years has made modality switching for sociomedical reasons, such as increasing age and frailty and "burnout," more feasible, and this may show up as an increase in TF rates, emphasizing that TF can be a difficult endpoint to evaluate. Has there been a change in the pattern of TF in recent years, and is there any evidence that the high PD usage in Canada has been associated with excessive or increasing TF?

Special cohort studies to look at TF on PD are being done using the CORR database but have not yet been published. However, certain conclusions can be drawn from annual CORR reports (1) (Table 5). First, if TF is defined as any switch from PD to HD and if the

Table 5 Changes in Numbers, TF Rates, and Causes of TF for Canadian PD Patients, 1988–1995

Year	Prevalent patients at start of year	Incident patients during year	Total PD patients during year	Number of TF	% TF	% of TF due to peritonitis	% of TF due to inadequate PD
1988	1665	775	2440	284	11.6	30.6	5.3
1989	1763	835	2598	294	11.3	30.9	7.5
1990	2014	894	2908	322	11.1	32.0	7.8
1991	2188	1081	3269	334	10.2	24.3	10.2
1992	2521	1148	3669	373	10.2	24.9	11.8
1993	2826	1191	4017	441	11.0	26.3	18.6
1994	3091	1232	4323	608	14.1	24.3	24.2
1995	3353	1127	4480	627	14.0	15.6	25.7
1996	3394	UK[a]	UK	658	UK	15.7	25.7

[a]UK = unknown (data not available).
Source: Adapted from Ref. 1.

denominator is taken as the sum of prevalent patients at the start of the year plus incident patients during the year, then the rate of TF stayed between 10–12% per annum between 1998 and 1993 and then rose a little to 14% in 1994 and 1995, the two most recent years for which information is available (1). This recent rise in TF may not be significant, but it perhaps reflects the expansion in HD capacity that occurred in the period concerned. The fact that TF has been relatively stable at a time when comorbidity and age are increasing and when mortality is falling is probably a relative success anyway. However, it could also be argued that the absence of a decreasing rate of TF during a period of technological advance is disappointing. Again, it should be pointed out that the available data are likely still too early to detect any improvement in TF or survival consequent upon the very recent changes that have been occurring in PD prescription practices (4).

If we look more closely at individual causes of TF, some interesting trends are apparent. TF due to peritonitis has fallen from over 30% of all causes, in the period 1988–1990, to about 25% in the period 1991–1994 and to 15–16% in 1995 and 1996 (Table 5). In contrast, inadequate dialysis as a stated cause of TF has risen from only 5% in 1988 to 10% in 1991 and 25% in 1995 and 1996 (1). This dramatic increase likely represents an increased awareness of the issue of inadequate dialysis rather than a true growth in the prevalence of the problem. The increase in overall TF rate in 1995 and 1996 can be totally attributed to an increase in this category and suggests that physicians are more aware of this complication and more willing and able to transfer patients to HD when they diagnose it. All this suggests not that PD is being less well practiced but that the expectations have risen as a result of all the recent attention given to adequacy of clearances (18,37,38).

III. DIALYSIS VERSUS TRANSPLANTATION

It is widely accepted that renal transplantation improves quality of life and is less costly than treatment with chronic dialysis (8). The issue of whether renal transplantation actually improves survival, relative to dialysis, has been somewhat controversial, however. A recent U.S. study appeared to show that survival was improved by renal transplantation (39). This study compared patients who had received a transplant with those who had not, despite being on the waiting list. The rationale was that patients on the waiting list who did not receive a transplant were a more appropriate control group for those who were transplanted than were dialysis patients in general. Similar findings have also recently been reported from Germany (40). This issue has now been addressed in the Canadian context by Rabbat et al. (41). The database used was all 5241 patients who initiated RRT between 1990 and 1995 in the province of Ontario. Of these patients, just over 1100 were wait-listed for renal transplant and just over 700 actually received a graft in the period concerned. A time-dependent Cox nonproportional hazards model was applied, using as a reference point the time interval from the date of wait listing to the time of transplantation, with adjustment for age, gender, race, and cause of ESRD. Compared to the mortality rate during this period, the relative risk of dying in the first 30 days after transplantation was 2.91 (95% confidence interval 1.34–6.32), and this was highly significant (41). In patients surviving more than one year after transplantation, however, the relative risk decreased to 0.25 (95% confidence interval 0.14–0.42). This long-term benefit was particularly notable in patients whose primary disease was glomerulonephritis or diabetes. The overall conclusion was that patients who receive a renal transplant have a higher early mortality risk but ultimately have a net survival advantage compared to dialysis patients who are wait-listed but not transplanted (41). As with the studies comparing dialysis modalities or outcomes in different countries, there is a concern in these studies that patients who are wait-listed but do not receive a transplant may represent a more high-risk subgroup than those who do receive a transplant. The rationale here is that all patients on a transplant list are not necessarily treated equally and that physicians may exhibit subtle biases towards giving scarce organs to healthier recipients. Furthermore, the sicker patients on the list may not be called for transplant because of intercurrent medical problems or may be more often on hold and so less likely to receive a graft. This excess risk might not be detected in an analysis, such as this one, that did not have sufficient information to correct in detail for functional status and number and severity of comorbid conditions. It should also be pointed out that the comparison is complicated by the fact that the relative risks of dialysis and transplantation are not proportionate, being excessive for transplant in the early postoperative period and for dialysis subsequently. Nevertheless, the relative risks associated with transplantation for greater than one year are strikingly low relative to those on dialysis, both in the Canadian analysis and in those from elsewhere (39–41). While there will always be controversy about this issue, the balance of evidence would seem to suggest that transplantation improves survival.

IV. CONCLUSION

The Canadian model for delivery of RRT in conjunction with the CORR allows some critical questions concerning cost-effective management of ESRD to be addressed, with potential implications for other jurisdictions also. While registry analyses can never be as definitive as well-constructed randomized controlled trials, some general conclusions can be drawn. A policy of high PD utilization, as practiced in Canada, appears to be both cost-effective and consistent with excellent and still improving survival rates. In particular, there is no evidence that PD is intrinsically inferior to HD in terms of patient survival, and, as used in Canada, there is at least some suggestion that it is superior in first few years of RRT. Notwithstanding this, PD is still associated with significant TF, and this does not appear to be falling despite recent technological advance. It remains unclear whether major improvements in technique survival in PD can be achieved or whether the main role of the modality will be to act as a transitional therapy for the first 2–4 years of RRT. Either way, the modality would appear to have a significant role to play in terms of delivery of cost-effective RRT.

Transplantation remains the most desirable form of RRT, in terms of quality of life, cost-effectiveness, and, it appears, patient survival. A strategy to optimize the role of transplant is thus ideal, but, unfortunately, scarcity of donors and the relatively modest improvements in long-term graft survival rates have limited this option.

Finally, the importance of good data collection in monitoring the effectiveness of any system of delivering RRT cannot be overstated. Not only does the data collection need to be comprehensive and accurate, but the questions that it is used to answer must be incisive and relevant and there must be an awareness of the multitude of potential confounders.

REFERENCES

1. Annual Report 1998, Vol. 1. Dialysis and Renal Transplantation, Canadian Organ Replacement Register. Ottawa, ON: Canadian Institute for Health Information, March 1998.
2. Prichard SS. The cost of dialysis. Adv in Perit Dial 1988; 4:66–69.
3. Mendelssohn DC, Chery A. Dialysis utilization in the Toronto region from 1981–1992. Can Med Assoc J 1994; 150:1099–1105.
4. Blake PG, Bloembergen WE, Fenton SSA. Changes in the demographics and prescription of peritoneal dialysis during the past decade. Am J Kidney Dis 1998; 32(suppl 4):344–351.
5. Nissenson AR, Prichard SS, Cheng IKP, et al. Nonmedical factors that impact on ESRD modality selection. Kidney Int 1993; 43:S120–S127.
6. Mendelssohn DC, Kreiger F, Winchester J. A comparison of dialysis in the US and Canada. Contemp Dial Neph 1993; 20:27–31.
7. Mendelssohn DC, Kua BT, Singer PA. Referral for dialysis in Ontario. Arch Int Med 1995; 155:2473–2478.
8. Laupacis A, Keown P, Pus N, et al. A study of the quality of life and cost-utility of renal transplantation. Kidney Int 1996; 50:235–242.
9. Moran JE. Changes in the dose of peritoneal dialysis: Have these independently affected outcomes? Am J Kidney Dis 1998; 32(suppl 4):552–557.
10. U.S. Renal Data System, USRDS 1997 Annual Data Report. National Institutes of Health, National Institute of Diabetes and Digestive and Kidney Diseases. Bethesda, MD. April 1997. IV. The USRDS Dialysis Morbidity and Mortality Study: Wave 2. Am J Kidney Dis 1997; 30(suppl 1): S67–S85.
11. Churchill ND, Thorpe KE, Vonesh EF, Keshaviah PR. Lower probability of patient survival with continuous peritoneal dialysis in the United States compared with Canada. J Am Soc Nephrol 1997; 8:965–971.
12. Posen G, Arbus G, Hutchison T, Jeffery J. Survival comparison of adult non-diabetic patients treated with either hemodialysis or CAPD for end-stage renal failure. Perit Dial Bull 1987; 7:78–79.
13. Burton PR, Walls J. Selection adjusted comparison of life expectancy of patients on continuous ambulatory peritoneal dialysis, haemodialysis and renal transplantation. Lancet 1987; 1:1115–1119.
14. Serkes KD, Blagg CR, Nolph KD, Vonesh EF, Shapiro F. Comparison of patient and technique survival in continuous ambulatory peritoneal dialysis (CAPD) and hemodialysis: a multicenter study. Perit Dial Int 1990; 10: 15–19.
15. Maiorca R, Vonesh EF, Cavilli P, et al. A multicenter, selection adjusted comparison of patient and technique survivals on CAPD and hemodialysis. Perit Dial Int 1991; 11:118–127.
16. Held PJ, Port FK, Turenne MN, et al. Continuous ambulatory peritoneal dialysis and hemodialysis: comparison of patient mortality with adjustment for comorbid conditions. Kidney Int 1994; 5:1163–1169.
17. Bloembergen WE, Port FK, Mauger EA, Wolfe RA. A comparison of mortality between patients treated with hemodialysis and peritoneal dialysis. J Am Soc Nephrol 1995; 6:177–183.

18. Churchill DN, Taylor DW, Keshavian PR. Adequacy of dialysis and nutrition in continuous peritoneal dialysis: association with clinical outcomes. J Am Soc Nephrol 1996; 7:198–207.
19. Fenton SSA, Schaubel DE, Desmeules M, et al. Hemodialysis versus peritoneal dialysis: a comparison of adjusted mortality rates. Am J Kidney Dis 1997; 30: 334–342.
20. Port KF, Wolfe RA, Bloembergen WE, Held PJ, Young EW. A study of outcomes for CAPD versus hemodialysis patients. Perit Dial Int 1996; 16:628–633.
21. Blake PG. Do mortality rates differ between hemodialysis and CAPD? A look at the Canadian vs U.S. data. Dial Transplant 1996; 25:75–100.
22. Burton H, Kline S, Lindsay R, Heidenheim A. The relationship of depression to survival in chronic renal failure. Psychosom Med 1986; 48:261–269.
23. Cox DR. Regression models and life tables. J R Stat Soc Series B 1971; 34:187–220.
24. Foley RN, Parfrey PS, Kent GM. Early and late mortality in ESRD: hazards of the Cox model. J Am Soc Nephrol 1997; 8:A1303.
25. Foley RN, Murphy SW, Barrett BJ, et al. Mortality risk in ESRD: an evolving process. J Am Soc Nephrol 1998; 9:A1062.
26. Schaubel DE, Morrison HI, Fenton SSA. Comparing mortality rates on CAPD/CCPD and hemodialysis. The Canadian Experience: Fact or Fiction? Perit Dial Int 1998; 18:478–484.
27. Held PJ, Bloembergen WE, Young EW, et al. A comparison of patients initiating hemodialysis and peritoneal dialysis in the US. J Am Soc Nephrol 1997; 8: 219A.
28. Murphy SE, Foley RN, Barrett BJ, et al. Comparative mortality of hemodialysis and peritoneal dialysis in Canada. J Am Soc Nephrol 1998; 9:A1208.
29. Lysaght MJ, Vonesh EF, Gotch F, et al. The influence of dialysis treatment modality on the decline of remaining renal function. ASAIO Trans 1991; 37:598–604.
30. Blake PG. A critique of the Canada/USA (CANUSA) peritoneal dialysis study. Perit Dial Int 1996; 16:243–245.
31. Vonesh EF, Moran J. Mortality in end-stage renal disease: A reassessment of differences between patients treated with hemodialysis and peritoneal dialysis. J Am Soc Nephrol 1999; 10:354–365.
32. Collins AJ, Hao W, Xia H, et al. Mortality risks of peritoneal and hemodialysis. Am J Kidney Dis 1999; 34:1065–1074.
33. Jindal KK, Hirsch DJ. Excellent technique survival on home peritoneal dialysis: results of a regional program. Perit Dial Int 1994; 14:324–326.
34. Kiernan L, Kliger A, Gorban-Brennan N, Juergensen P, Finkelstein F. Comparison of continuous ambulatory peritoneal dialysis-related infections with different Y-tubing exchange systems. J Am Soc Nephrol 1995; 5: 1835–1838.
35. Dasgupta MK, Fox S, Gagnon D, Bettcher K, Ulan RA. Significant reduction of peritonitis rate by the use of twin-bag system in a Canadian regional CAPD program. Adv Perit Dial 1991; 11:223–226.
36. Blake PG, Burkart JM, Churchill DN, et al. Recommended clinical practices for maximizing peritoneal dialysis clearances. Perit Dial Int 1996; 16:448–456.
37. NKF DOQI PD Adequacy Work Group. NKF DOQI clinical practice guidelines for adequacy of peritoneal dialysis. Am J Kidney Dis 1997; 30:67–136.
38. Port FK, Wolfe RA, Mauger EA, Berling DP, Jiang K. Comparison of survival probabilities for dialysis patients vs cadaveric renal transplant recipients. JAMA 1994; 15:1339–1343.
39. Wolfe RA, Ashby VB, Milford EL, et al. Comparison of mortality in all patients on dialysis, patients on dialysis awaiting transplantation, and recipients of a first cadaveric transplant. N Engl J Med 1999; 341:1725–1731.
40. Rabbat CG, Thorpe KE, Russell JD, Churchill DN. Comparison of mortality risk between wait-listed dialysis patients and recipients of cadaveric first renal transplants in Ontario. J Am Soc Nephrol 1998; 9:A3532.

PART II: IN EUROPE

I. INTRODUCTION

Although the life expectancy of patients with end-stage renal disease (ESRD) has improved over the last decades, it is still below that of the general population. Basically, an ESRD patient and his or her treating physician can select among four different modalities: renal transplantation, conventional hemodialysis (HD), high-flux hemodialysis, and peritoneal dialysis (PD). The question whether short treatment at high efficiency (high-flux HD) is as effective as a longer treatment at standard clearance is beyond the scope of this chapter and will not be addressed.

Since most centers in Europe can offer both PD and HD, the choice of an appropriate renal replacement therapy (RRT) is influenced by a number of medical and nonmedical factors (1). It is obvious that for the patients, total survival and quality of life are among the most influential factors. Many studies comparing outcomes of PD and HD are available, with seemingly conflicting results. All these studies differ, however, in methodology, and their interpretation is difficult (2). A basic understanding of the statistical methods used for survival analysis and their pitfalls is crucial for a correct interpretation and will therefore be provided in the first part of this section. It should be clear that not only the outcome of one single RRT modality is of importance, but rather the outcome of a treatment flowchart, as many patients are transferred from one modality to another. Therefore, data on technique failure and the underlying mechanisms and the outcome after transfer are of importance and will be discussed. Because renal transplantation is the ultimate treatment modality for many patients, outcomes after transplantation will be discussed in the light of the preceding dialysis modality. Finally, the benefits of an "integrated-care" approach to ESRD patients will be addressed (3).

II. STUDIES COMPARING HD AND PD DIALYSIS IN EUROPE

European data on take-on rate of patients on dialysis, utilization of different dialysis modalities, and the impact of socio-economic factors are discussed in Chapter 43. Studies comparing outcome of patients on PD and HD in Europe are listed in Table 1. The overall conclusion is that survival rates on PD and HD are comparable. It is, however, of note that the utilization of PD in Europe varies from country to country and from center to center (16). All of the centers participating in the studies mentioned in Table 1 have a high number of PD patients. This is of importance since center experience is one of the determinants of survival (15,19,37).

All of these studies included incident patients. Although some of them corrected for differences in comorbidity, no study corrected for differences in delivered dialysis dose. Maiorca and Cancarini (4) and Maiorca et al. (5) reported that survival for patients on PD or on HD was similar, even if inadequate dialysis (defined as Kt/V urea < 1 per treatment for HD and Kt/V urea < 1.7 per week for PD) was accounted for. However, in most studies the majority of PD patients were on an 8 L/day schedule, which is currently considered a "minimum" dose. Since measurements of adequacy and adaptation of delivered dose were earlier common practice in HD, it is conceivable that the incidence of underdialysis was higher in the PD than in the HD patients. Time of referral of patients to the renal unit and patient compliance were also not accounted for in any of the studies in Table 1, although they may be important factors.

In the study of Van Biesen et al. (3), intention-to-treat survival in PD and HD patients was comparable, with a 50% survival of 72 months (Fig. 1).

Until now, no randomized controlled studies of PD versus HD have been performed, and thus no hard data favoring one dialysis method over another are at present available. There is, however, enough evidence in the present literature to claim that survival outcomes in PD and HD are at least comparable in centers experienced in both methods. Recent data obtained in Canada suggest that survival in the first 2–3 years after start of RRT might even be better in PD (18).

III. TECHNIQUE FAILURE AND REASONS

Due to the nature of the technique itself and to the high patient involvement, it is not surprising that in most

Table 1 Outcomes of European Patients on PD and HD

Number of patients included	Years of follow-up	Relative risk of death	Comments	Ref.
281 HD; 297 PD	1981–1993	PD = HD	Correction for comorbidity; to 1986 HD pts on acetate dialysis	4–7
371 HD; 373 PD	1981–1996	PD = HD	Extension of previous studies; subanalysis of pts from 1991–1996 showed similar results	8
83647 HD; 11336 PD	1981–1984	PD = HD	No correction for comorbidity	9
329 HD; 610 PD	1983–1985	PD = HD	No correction for comorbidity	10, 11
842 HD; 272 PD	1984–1988	PD = HD		12
1296	1986–1987	PD >HD		13
276 HD; 158 PD	1974–1985	PD = HD	Diabetes not included in comorbidity	14
968 HD; 660 PD	1985–1989	PD = HD		15
223 HD; 194 PD	1978–1996	PD = HD	Intention-to-treat analysis	3

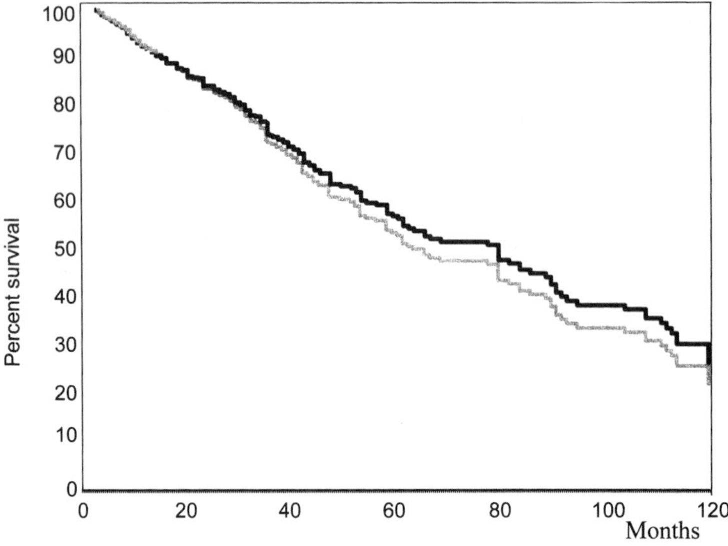

Fig. 1 Intention-to-treat survival analysis of ESRD patients at the University Hospital Gent. Dotted line: PD patients; full line: HD patients; p = NS.

studies technique failure is higher in PD than in HD (3,4–6,8,10). Differences in technique failure are influenced by the experience and the propensity of a given center to change modality when faced with clinical or technical problems. At the end of the follow-up period in a study of Maiorca et al. (7), 8 out of 281 HD patients had changed modality versus 54 out of 297 PD patients ($p < 0.001$). Peritonitis (37%) and patient or partner choice (37%) were the most important reasons for drop-out in the PD patients, and intradialytic hypotension (63%) and vascular access problems (37%) were the major reasons in the HD patients. These authors also analyzed technique success, whereby death and transfer to another modality were considered as final events and all other reasons for stopping the technique were censored. Compared to HD, technique success was worse for PD, but this difference decreased with increasing age of the patients. Surprisingly, the causes of drop-out did not differ significantly with age. Another remarkable finding was that patient drop-out was higher in the period 1987–1992 than in an earlier period (1981–1986) and this despite accrued experience. Patient choice as underlying cause of drop-out increased from 21.5 to 57.5% of transferred patients. It is thus conceivable that increasing attention to adequacy targets and the accompanying use of more complicated and demanding dialysis schedules have a negative impact on technique success. In the studies of Van Biesen et al. (3,19), technique success after 3 years was 61% and 48% in HD and PD patients, respectively. Age (relative risk increasing 3% per year older than 56 years of age, $p < 0.001$) had a negative impact on technique success. Diabetes mellitus had a negative impact on technique success in the HD patients (relative risk 1.6, $p < 0.001$) but not in the PD group (relative risk 1.3, $p > 0.05$); this result is possibly due to the higher drop-out from HD for reasons of vascular access problems in diabetic patients.

IV. REASONS FOR TRANSFER TO ANOTHER MODALITY

Table 2 lists the major reasons for modality transfer in two European centers, Brescia and Gent. The reasons

Table 2 Reasons for Transferring Patients from Dialysis Modalities, Gent and Brescia

Transfers PD ⇒ HD	
Peritonitis/Exit site infection	48%
Patient/Partner choice	26%
Ultrafiltration/Adequacy problems	20%
Leakage or hernia	6%
Transfers HD ⇒ PD	
Vascular access problems	33%
Cardiovascular problems	34%
Blood pressure problems	16%
Personal choice	15%
Relapsing hemorrhage	2%

for transfer from PD to HD are merely PD-related problems that can be solved by transferring the patient to HD. In contrast, cardiovascular problems that are not solved by transferring the patients are the most frequent reasons for shifting HD patients to PD. In a study by Gokal et al. (11), age had no influence, but smoking was related to transfer from PD to HD; the underlying explanation of this observation is, however, unclear. It was calculated in the same study that temporary transfer from PD to HD was necessary in up to 0.4 occasions with a mean duration of 19.4 days per patient year. Data concerning temporary transfer from HD to PD because of access problems were not provided. In the study of Gentil et al. (12), technique survival was shorter for PD than for HD ($p < 0.001$). Age older than 60 years and diabetes had a negative impact on technique survival (relative risk of 2.3, $p < 0.01$, and 4, $p < 0.004$, respectively). Woodrow et al. (20) found a technique survival of 93, 73, and 63% at 1, 3, and 5 years, respectively, after start of CAPD. The CAPD system used (Y-system or not) did not influence technique survival, although peritonitis rates were lower in the patients on the Y-set system.

V. OUTCOME AFTER TRANSFER TO ANOTHER MODALITY

Although studies describing outcomes after transfer from one modality to another can give useful information about the most beneficial sequence of treatment modalities, such studies are scarce. In a prospective study of Singh et al. (21), outcome of patients who were transferred from HD to PD was described. All transfers were because of free choice of the patients, but total follow-up after transfer was only 6 months in 26 patients and 1 year in 20 patients. Before transfer to PD, patients were on HD for a median of 38 months (range 3–312). After 6 months, 14 of the original 40 patients had dropped out of the study: 9 because of inadequate treatment, 1 because of death, 3 because of mental deterioration, and 1 because of lost follow-up. Nutritional parameters tended to decline during the time on PD, and Kt/V urea became inadequate in an important number of patients. All patients, irrespective of residual renal function or body weight, were on a PD dose of 8 L/day. The authors conclude that it is dangerous to transfer patients from HD to PD without adapting the dialysis dose to adequacy parameters. Although no data on residual renal function in this study are provided, it can be assumed that most of these patients must have lost their renal function at the moment of their transfer as their median stay on HD was more than 3 years (22). It is now well accepted that adequacy parameters are difficult to obtain in patients without residual renal function (23).

Canaud and Mion (24) also describe a decline in total Kt/Vurea and in nutritional parameters after transfer from HD to PD. After an increase in mortality rate during the first 6 months after transfer, mortality rates abruptly decreased and patient survival became excellent. This temporary increase in mortality during the first 6-month period after transfer from PD to HD was also observed in the study by Woodrow et al. (20). A too-late transfer from PD to HD can explain these observations. Davies et al. (25) also found that patients who were transferred from PD to HD because of "failure to thrive" on PD had a very poor survival, probably because of prolonged underdialysis and/or malnutrition.

A close follow-up of adequacy and nutritional status and a timely transfer to HD when needed is thus mandatory. Patient outcome may be greatly improved by a more rapid change of dialysis modality in patients with recurrent and/or severe peritonitis or in those in whom PD is unable to produce adequate dialysis.

In the study of Van Biesen et al. (3), intention-to-treat analysis demonstrated a better survival in the patients who were transferred from PD to HD compared to those remaining on PD (log rank, $p < 0.01$), with a median expected survival time of 95.7 months in the transferred patients versus only 35.5 months in the patients remaining on PD. For patients starting on HD, however, there was no difference in outcome whether they were transferred to PD or remained on HD (log rank, $p = 0.17$), with mean expected survival times of 56.4 and 49.9 months, respectively. It has to be stressed that in this center, smooth transfer between dialysis modalities is the rule, which may at least in part explain these results.

From Gent and Brescia, the survival of 111 patients starting on PD and transferred to HD afterwards and 56 patients started on HD and transferred to PD were evaluated. The data were corrected for age and presence of diabetes mellitus. Age at start of RRT was not different between the two groups (57.6 ± 15.2 years vs. 54.7 ± 13.4 years, respectively, $p = 0.21$), and the prevalence of diabetes was equal (20 vs. 11 patients, respectively, $p = 0.8$). A Cox regression analysis was performed, the results of which are summarized in Table 3.

Survival of patients starting on PD and transferred to HD was better than of those starting on HD and transferred to PD (log rank, $p = 0.02$). Figure 2 also

Table 3 Results of Cox Regression Analysis

	Relative risk	T-value	p-Value
Diabetes mellitus	1.95	2.5	0.02
Age (per year >55)	1.03	3.7	0.001
PD as first modality	0.52	−2.9	0.01

demonstrates that, after transfer, the mortality rate of patients transferred from HD to PD declines, whereas the mortality rate of patients from PD to HD remains unchanged. This observation can again be explained by the importance of the residual renal function and by the difference in the reasons for transfer (Table 2). That keeping patients too long on PD can have disastrous consequences is shown in Figure 3, which represents the survival after 4 years for patients who remained on their initial modality. It is clear that mortality rate in this subgroup of patients was higher in the PD patients compared to the HD patients. It is interesting to note that the increase in mortality coincides with the decline in residual renal function (25).

VI. OUTCOME AFTER RENAL TRANSPLANTATION

For ESRD patients, renal transplantation offers increased rehabilitation, freedom from dialysis, correction of anemia and of other uremia-related diseases such as renal osteodystrophy. A successful transplantation greatly improves quality of life and is cost-effective in the long run (26). There is, however, a price to pay, with increased risk of infections, development of hyperglycemia and malignancies, and corticoid-induced osteoporosis and avascular necrosis, all complications of the necessary immunosuppressive therapy. These complications may even be associated with a greater mortality risk in the early posttransplant period. Since all available dialysis modalities should aim at a good preparation for transplantation, the impact of a given modality on outcome after transplantation will be briefly discussed. Cosio et al. (27) analyzed long-term outcome of 523 patients receiving a kidney transplant in the period 1984–1991. After a follow-up of 84 ± 14 months, 28% had died and 23% had lost their grafts. Older age, diabetes, smoking, and length of time on dialysis before transplantation correlated with reduced patient survival in a multivariate analysis. The dialysis modality itself had no influence on long-term outcome. In an extensive review of all studies comparing long-term outcome after transplantation, Maiorca et al. (28) found no differences in survival of patients transplanted either from HD or PD.

At the Gent transplant center survival after transplantation was better for patients who started RRT on PD than those who started on HD. Three out of the 53 patients who initially started on PD and 12 out of the 44 patients who initially started with HD died after transplantation during the observation period ($p < 0.01$), which was equal in both groups (57.8 ± 37.6 vs. 56.2 ± 45.3 months, NS). However, HD patients were longer on RRT before transplantation than PD patients (32.1 ± 27.8 months vs. 24.1 ± 19 months, $p = 0.001$), and this might have affected their outcomes.

The incidence of early graft dysfunction was higher in patients coming from HD compared to patients transplanted from PD (29,30). A recent study (30) comprising 234 transplanted patients (117 HD, 117 PD) calculated a delayed graft function in 23.1% of PD versus 50.4% of HD patients ($p < 0.001$). A multivariate model with cold ischemia time ($p < 0.001$), PD as pretransplant dialysis modality ($p = 0.01$), urinary volume during the first 24 hours after transplantation ($p = 0.001$), body weight gain during the first 72 hours ($p = 0.05$) and fluid load ($p = 0.01$) resulted in an R^2 of 0.32 ($p < 0.001$) (31). Using Cox regression analysis, the relative risk for a prolonged T1/2 Screat was increased with 4% per hour cold ischemia time ($p = 0.01$) and with 1% per kg body weight gain ($p = 0.02$); fluid load administered after renal transplantation decreased the relative risk with 5% per liter ($p < 0.001$), and PD as pretransplant dialysis modality favorably modified the relative risk by a factor 1.6 ($p = 0.01$). Many studies (for review see Ref. 32) suggest that delayed graft function negatively influences the long-term outcome of the graft.

VII. CONCEPT OF INTEGRATED CARE FOR ESRD

The slower decline of residual renal function, the preservation of vascular access sites, the incidence of technique failure, the better outcome after transfer from PD to HD as compared to transfer from HD to PD, and the similar to even better results after renal transplantation all point in favor of the "integrated-care" approach. In this concept, timely referred ESRD patients are first started on PD, transferred to HD when needed, and transplanted whenever possible. In this approach, all different types of RRT are offered by the same team, giving the patient a feeling of safety and comfort because he or she is familiar with all team members. This

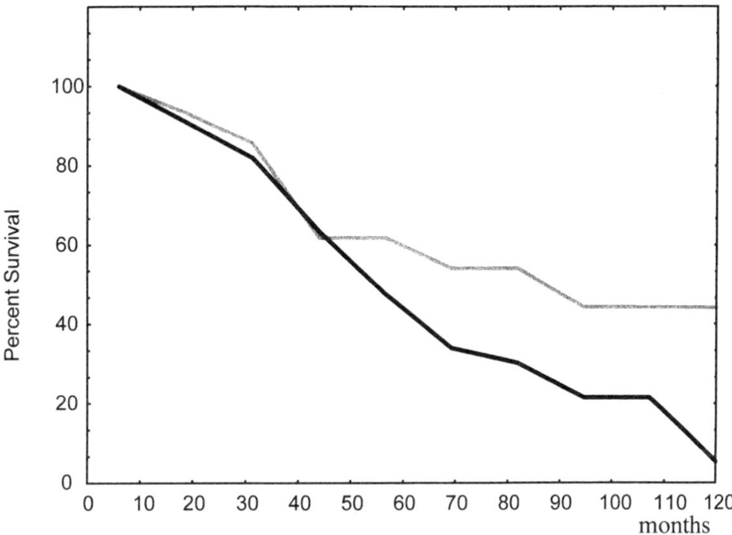

Fig. 2 Survival of patients (UH Gent) transferred from HD to PD (full line) versus patients transferred from PD to HD (dotted line); $p = 0.02$.

approach also guarantees a back-up with another dialysis modality, which is sometimes necessary. Gokal et al. (11), for example, found a total of 106 occasions of temporary need for HD in 338 CAPD patients during a follow-up period of 2 years. In analysis of patient survival over the period 1978–1996 (3), it was found that patients who were treated with such a model of integrated care had a better outcome than the other patients (Fig. 5). Admittedly, this was a retrospective study and the number of patients was rather small; therefore, confirmation of these results in a larger patient population is needed.

It can be argued that the analysis of integrated care as shown in Figure 5 can be criticized on statistical grounds as no correction was made for the (obligatory) time on PD in the integrated-care group. This problem cannot be adequately solved by using other statistical methodology and can in fact only be addressed by a randomized prospective study. However, when analysis was done of matched trios of 1 integrated-care patient with 2 HD patients who had been at least as long on HD as their "match" was on PD, a survival advantage was still present in the integrated-care patients (Fig. 4).

An integrated-care approach of ESRD patients makes sure that all possible RRTs, when applied in a logical sequence, are optimally used for each patient. By starting ESRD patients on PD, vascular access possibilities, still the Achilles heel of hemodialysis (33–35), can be preserved longer. Moreover, since most of the reasons for transfer of PD to HD are predictable, there is in general enough time to create an arteriovenous fistula. The implementation of an integrated-care approach with PD as first dialysis modality can also be an answer to the ever-increasing number of ESRD patients.

VIII. ADDENDUM. IMPACT OF METHODOLOGY AND STATISTICS ON SURVIVAL RESULTS

Analysis of survival data requires the use of special statistical methods, since not all patients will have died at the end of a given observation period. In these patients, the total survival time is not known, and therefore the data of these patients cannot be used in "classical" statistical methods (36). For example, if a patient starts on PD 36 months before the end of the observation period, all one can say is that this patient's survival on PD was more than 36 months, since no data on his "real" survival are available. Techniques for survival data analysis such as Kaplan-Meier or Cox regression have been developed to analyze this type of "censored" information. It should, however, be realized that the results become less reliable as the ratio of censored to uncensored cases increases.

Calculation of a Kaplan-Meier curve is relatively simple and is provided in most statistical packages. Basic to this method is the fact that the survival function S(t), being the probability of being alive at a moment

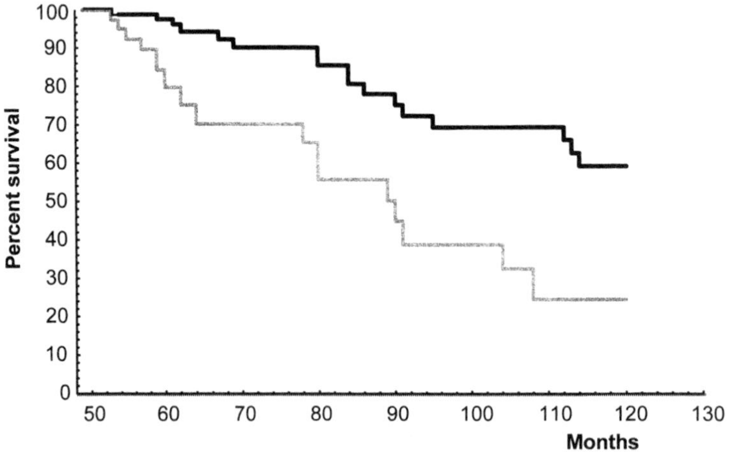

Fig. 3 Survival of patients (UH Gent) maintained on PD (dotted line) or HD (full line) for more than 48 months; $p = 0.01$. Number of surviving patients at 48 months is taken at 100%.

ti, can be expressed as the product of the probabilities of surviving to time point t(i-x), under the condition that one has survived to time point t(i-x-1) [notation S(t(i-x)/t(i-x-1)]. At any time point, S (t/t-1) can be estimated from the ratio of the number of patients, n, who survive a certain time interval to the total number of patients, N, who entered that interval. This also indicates that deviation from reality is greatest in the longest survival times, because less patients become available to provide reliable estimations.

In a Cox regression model, corrections can be made for different comorbidity factors. The Cox model assumes that independent variables are related to survival time by a multiplicative effect on the hazard function, HO (t), being the underlying "basic" hazard equal to all participants. The relation can thus mathematically be expressed as

$$h(t) = HO\ (t)eb1X1 + b2X2 + \cdots bnXn \qquad (1)$$

where bi is the regression coefficient for the comorbid condition Xi. Unfortunately, HO (t) is unknown, and only the relative risk, being the ratio of the hazards of two different subjects, can be calculated. If this is done, and the two subjects differ only for one comorbid con-

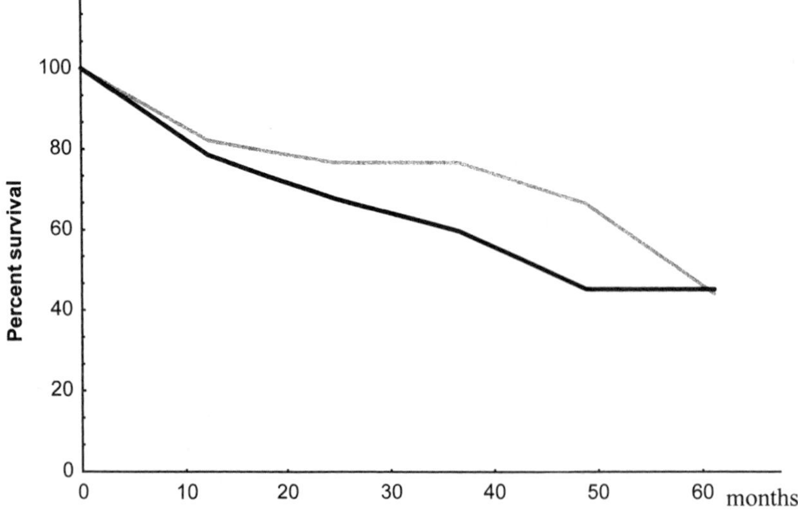

Fig. 4 Survival of patients (UH Gent) who were treated with "integrated care" (dotted line) compared to the survival of patients who were started and remained on hemodialysis. The two groups of patients were "matched" for the same duration of time of dialysis before the inclusion in the survival study.

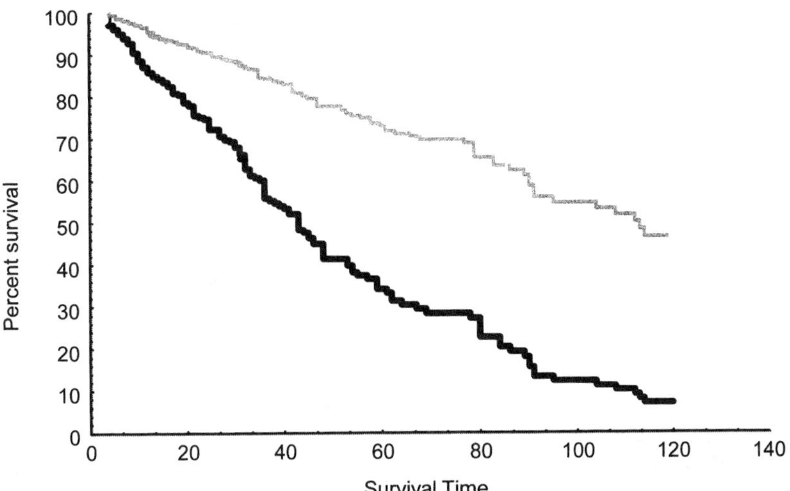

Fig. 5 Differences in ESRD patient survival (hemodialysis and peritoneal dialysis patients at the Gent University Hospital) according to the Cox regression analysis; risk factors are considered to be absent (dotted line) or are taken at the median (full line). Both curves represent the same patient population.

dition XI, Eq. (1) then becomes hl/(t)/h2(t) = ebi(Xi1-Xi2). This number is then the relative risk for subject 1 compared to subject 2. It should, however, be stressed that the curves that result from a Cox regression analysis are merely the results of "predictive calculations" rather than a reflection of reality. Results can, for example, be presented with all comorbidity factors entered as absent, and the resulting curve will show seemingly better results compared to a curve where comorbid conditions are taken as the mean. Figure 5 illustrates this important point. Another point is that patients can be included as "incident," i.e., patients who start new on ESRD treatment, or as "prevalent," i.e., patients who were already on ESRD treatment for some time (Fig. 6). In the latter case, patients who start RRT and die during the inclusion window are excluded from the study. Therefore, this type of analysis favorizes the method with the highest initial mortality. The use of "incident" or "prevalent" patients can give very different results, as shown by Vonesh and Moran (37).

Another important point is the period of time considered as "survival time." In a first modality survival

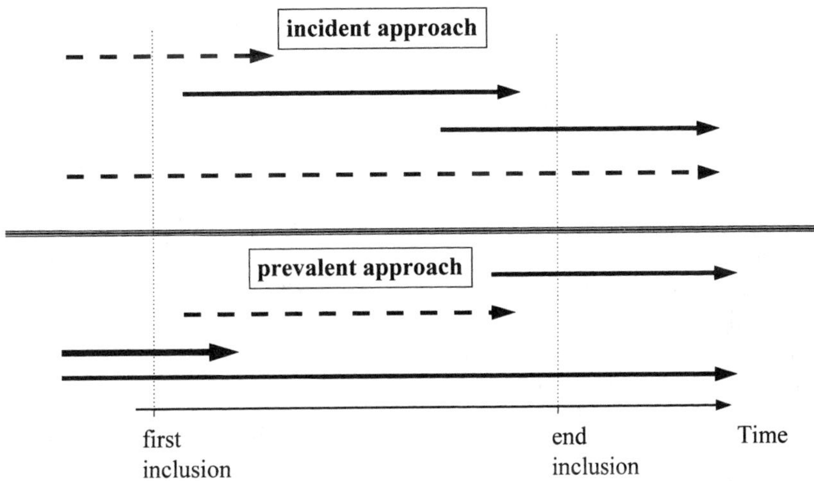

Fig. 6 Illustration of the differences between incident versus prevalent patient inclusion approach. Patients included in the analysis (full lines); patients not included in the analysis (dotted lines).

analysis, survival time is considered as the time on the initial RRT. Only death is considered as the final event, and patients are censored by transfer to another dialysis modality, at transplantation, loss of follow-up, or at the end of observation. In the intention-to-treat survival analysis, survival time is considered as the sum of the time on HD and the time on PD. Death is considered as the final event, and patients are censored at the moment of transplantation, at loss of follow-up, or at the end of the observation, but not when they are transferred from one dialysis modality to another.

The two previous analyses consider only the time on RRT and exclude the time after transplantation. These analyses are thus applicable to all patients whether they are on the waiting list or not. For patients not on the waiting list, the intention-to-treat analysis gives their life expectancy. For patients on the waiting list, it shows their probability to survive until a renal graft becomes available.

In the total survival analysis, survival time is considered as the total time on PD, on HD, and after transplantation. Technique success is defined as the probability of having a patient alive on his initial modality. Death and change of modality are considered as final events, and patients are censored at the moment of transplantation or at the end of follow-up. Another way to calculate technique survival is to censor patients at death, the underlying reasoning being that technique survival would have been longer if the patient had not died. In this type of analysis, only real technique failures are accounted as endpoints. It is obvious that the results of such an analysis are more flattering than those of technique success, where death is also considered as technique failure.

Most survival analyses use the first modality survival approach. It is, however, clear that this "survival" does not reflect clinical reality, as most ESRD patients are treated successfully with different treatment modalities. Therefore, total survival time and intention-to-treat modality survival are of more interest for the individual patient (3).

Besides all these considerations, it should be appreciated that all statistical methods have their own shortcomings (38,39): it is virtually impossible to include all important comorbid conditions and to exclude those that are meaningless. For example, in survival of dialysis patients it is very difficult to account for delivered dialysis dose, declining residual renal function, patient compliance, center experience, and all other factors known to have an impact on patient outcome. In addition, an evaluation of the severity of the condition is often very difficult to make. Congestive heart failure or diabetes mellitus are, for example, difficult to grade. In most studies a patient who has had diabetes for 3 years is given the same risk as a patient who has suffered for 20 years, while the cardiovascular damage caused by the disease can be very different. Mortality comparisons should thus be viewed with caution, especially regarding the type of comorbid conditions included and the way the severity of the comorbidity is scored. All these may cause unequal distribution of risk factors between different populations.

A last point with regard to the correct interpretation of Cox proportional hazards results (and for other methods of assessing relative risks as well) is that, from a clinical point of view, the relative risk for mortality can only be interpreted if the real mortality is known. When the relative mortality risk of group A to group B is 2 and if the real mortality risk in group B is 1/10,000, the real mortality risk will be 2/10,000 in group A. This can be a statistically significant difference but is from a clinical point of view quite meaningless. In this regard, it is also of note that studies with a low number of patients are subject to false-negative results (i.e., no statistically significant difference is found while in reality there is one), while in studies with large patient numbers, false-positive results can emerge (i.e., statistically significant differences are present without clinical meaning).

In conclusion, the interpretation of papers analyzing survival comparisons should be done with attention paid to the methodological biases and their implications, realizing, however, that a "perfect" comparison is nearly impossible.

REFERENCES

1. Nissenson A, Prichard S, Cheng I, Gokal R, Kubota M, Maiorca R. Non-medical factors that have impact on ESRD modality selection. Kidney Int 1993; 43:S120–S127.
2. Port F, Wolfe R, Bloembergen W, Held P, Young E. The study of outcomes for CAPD versus hemodialysis patients. Perit Dial Int 1996; 16:628–633.
3. Van Biesen W, Vanholder R, Veys N, Dhondt A, Lameire N. An evaluation of survival of ESRD patients: peritoneal dialysis or hemodialysis: is that the question?
4. Maiorca R, Cancarini G. Outcome of peritoneal dialysis: comparative studies. In: Gokal R, Nolph K, eds. The Textbook of Peritoneal Dialysis. Dordrecht: Kluwer Academic Publishers, 1994:699–734.
5. Maiorca, Vonesh E, Cavalli P, De Vecchi A, Giangrande A, La Greca G, Scarpioni L, Bragantini L., Cancarini G, Cantaluppi A, Castelnovo C, Castiglioni A, Poisetti P, Viglino G. A multicenter, selection-adjusted compar-

ison of patient and technique survivals on CAPD and hemodialysis. Perit Dial Int 1991; 11:118–127.
6. Maiorca R, Brunori G, Zubani R, Cancarini C, Manili L, Camerini C, Movilli E, Pola A, d'Avolio G, Gelatti U. Predictive value of dialysis adequacy and nutritional indices for mortality and morbidity in CAPD and HD patients. A longitudinal study. Nephrol Dial Transplant 1995; 10:2295–2305.
7. Maiorca R, Cancarini G, Zubani R, Camerini C, Manili L, Brunori G, Movilli E. CAPD viability: a long-term comparison with hemodialysis. Perit Dial Int 1996; 16: 276–287.
8. Cancarini G, Brunori G, Zani R, Zubani R, Pola A, Sandrini M, Zein H, Maiorca R. Long-term outcome of peritoneal dialysis. Perit Dial Int 1997; 17(suppl 2): S115–S118.
9. Survival on renal replacement therapy: data from the EDTA registry. Nephrol Dial Transplant 1988; 2:109–122.
10. Gokal R, King J, Bogle S, Marsh F, Oliver D, Jakubowski C, Hunt L, Baillod R, Ogg C, Ward M. Outcome on continuous ambulatory peritoneal dialysis and hemodialysis: 4 year analysis of a prospective multicentre study. Lancet 1987; 2:1105–1109.
11. Gokal R, Baillod R, Bogle S, Hunt L, Jakubowski C, Marsh F, Ogg C, Oliver D, Ward M, Wilkinson R. Multi-center study on outcome of treatment in patients on continuous ambulatory peritoneal dialysis and haemodialysis. Nephrol Dia Transplant 1987; 2:172–178.
12. Gentil M, Carriazo A, Pavon M, Rosado M, Castillo D, Ramos B, Algarra R, Tejuca F, Banasco P, Milan J. Comparison of survival in continuous ambulatory peritoneal dialysis and hospital hemodialysis: a multicentric study. Nephrol Dial Transplant 1991; 6:444–451.
13. Marcelli D, Stannard D, Conte F, Held P, Locatelli F, Port F. ESRD patient mortality with adjustment for comorbid conditions in Lombardy versus the United States. Kidney Int 1996; 50:1013–1018.
14. Burton P, Walls J. Selection-adjusted comparison of life-expectancy of patients on continuous ambulatory peritoneal dialysis, haemodialysis, and renal transplantation. Lancet 1987; 1:1115–1119.
15. Lupo A, Tarchini R, Cancarini G, Catizone L, Cocchi R, De Vecchi A, Viglino G, Salomone M, Segoloni G, Giangrande A. Long-term outcome in continuous ambulatory peritoneal dialysis: a 10 year survey by the Italian cooperative peritoneal dialysis study group. Am J Kidney Dis 1994; 24:826–837.
16. Lameire N, Van Biesen W, Dombros N, Dratwa M, Faller B, Gahl G, Gokal R, Krediet R, La Greca G, Maiorca R, Matthys E, Ryckelynck J, Selgas R, Walls J. The referral pattern of patients with ESRD is a determinant in the choice of dialysis modality. Perit Dial Int 1997; 17(suppl 2):S161–S166.
17. Khan I. Survival on renal replacement therapy in Europe: Is there a "center-effect"? Nephrol Dial Transplant 1996; 11:300–307.
18. Fenton S, Schaubel D, Desmeules M, Morrison H, Mao Y, Copleston P, Jeffery J, Kjellstrand C. Hemodialysis versus peritoneal dialysis: a comparison of adjusted mortality rates. Am J Kidney Dis 1997; 30:334–342.
19. Van Biesen W, Dequidt C, Vijt D, Vanholder R, Lameire N. Analysis of the reasons for transfers between hemodialysis and peritoneal dialysis and their effect on survivals. Adv Perit Dial 1998; 14:90–94.
20. Woodrow G, Turney J, Brownjohn A. Technique failure in peritoneal dialysis and its impact on patient survival. Perit Dial Int 1997; 17:360–364.
21. Singh S, Yium J, Macon E, Clark E, Schaffer D, Teschan P. Multicenter study of change in dialysis therapy-maintenance hemodialysis to continuous ambulatory peritoneal dialysis. Am J Kidney Dis 1992; 19:246–251.
22. Lameire N, Vanholder R, Vijt D, Lambert MC, Ringoir S. A longitudinal five year survey of urea kinetic parameters in CAPD patients. Kidney Int 1992; 42:426–432.
23. Lameire N, Van Biesen W. The impact of residual renal function on the adequacy of peritoneal dialysis. Perit Dial Int 1997; 17(suppl 2):S102–S110.
24. Canaud B, Mion C. Place de la dialyse péritoneale continue ambulatoire au sein d'un programme de traitement de l'insuffisance rénale chronique. Problèmes posés par les transferts de DPCA en transplantation ou en hémodialyse. Néphrologie 1995; 16:129–135.
25. Davies S, Phillips L, Griffiths A, Russel L, Naish P, Russel G. What really happens to people on long-term peritoneal dialysis? Kidney Int 1998; 54:2207–2217.
26. Suthanthiran M, Strom T. Renal transplantation. N Engl J Med 1994; 331:365–376.
27. Cosio F, Alamir A, Yim S, Pesavento T, Falkenhain M, Henry M, Elkhammas E, Davies E, Bumgardner G, Ferguson R. Patient survival after renal transplantation: the impact of dialysis pre-transplant. Kidney Int 1998; 53:767–772.
28. Maiorca R, Sandrini S, Cancarini G, Camerini C, Scolari F, Cristinelli L, Filippini M. Kidney transplantation in peritoneal dialysis patients. Perit Dial Int 1994; 14(suppl 3):162–167.
29. Perez-Fontan M, Carmona A, Falcon T, Moncalian J, Oliver J, Valdes F. Renal transplantation in patients undergoing chronic peritoneal dialysis. Perit Dial Int 1996; 16:48–51.
30. Vanholder R, Van Loo A, Heering P, Van Biesen W, Lambert MC, Hesse U, Van Der Vennet M, Grabensee B, Lameire N. Reduced incidence of acute renal graft failure in patients treated with peritoneal dialysis compared to hemodialysis. Am J Kidney Dis 1999; 33:934–940.
31. Van Biesen W, Vanholder R, Van Loo A, Lameire N. Immediate posttransplant outcome is better in peritoneal dialysis than in hemodialysis patients. Transplantation 1999.

32. Samaniego M, Baldwin WM, Sanfilippo F. Delayed graft function: immediate and late impact. Curr Opin Nephrol Hypert 1997; 6:533–537.
33. Bell D, Rosenthal J. Arteriovenous graft life in chronic hemodialysis. A need for prolongation. Arch Surg 1988; 123:1169.
34. Windus D. Permanent vascular access: a nephrologist's view. Am J Kidney Dis 1993; 21:457–471.
35. Hakim R, Himmelfarb J. Hemodialysis access failure: a call to action. Kidney Int 1998; 54:1029–1040.
36. Lagakos S. Statistical analysis of survival data. In: Bailar J, Mosteller F, eds. Medical Uses of Statistics. 2d ed. Boston: NEJM Books, 1992:281–291.
37. Vonesh E, Moran J. Further comparisons of mortality between hemodialysis and peritoneal dialysis (abstr). Perit Dial Int 1998; 18(suppl 1):S56.
38. Nolph K. Why are reported relative mortality risks for CAPD and HD so variable? (inadequacies of the Cox proportional hazards model). Perit Dial Int 1996; 16: 15–18.
39. Vonesh E. Relative risks can be risky. Perit Dial Int 1993; 13:5–9.

46

The Approach to Dialysis in Developing Countries

V. Jha and Kirpal S. Chugh
Postgraduate Institute of Medical Education and Research, Chandigarh, India
Sumant Chugh
Boston Medical Center, Boston, Massachusetts

I. INTRODUCTION

The 1995 World Bank annual development report (1) divided all countries into three income groups on the basis of annual per capita gross national product (GNP): high (per capita GNP equivalent to $9,386 or higher), middle (GNP equivalent to more than $765 but less than $9,386), and low (GNP less than $765). The low and middle income countries have been collectively grouped under the head of "developing countries," signifying that people in these countries have a lower standard of living with access to fewer goods and services. Currently there are about 125 developing countries with populations of over 1 million, with a total population of more than 4.7 billion. Of these, 1.5 billion live in the middle-income countries whereas the rest, 3.2 billion, reside in low-income countries. More than 1.3 billion people live on less than $1 a day and another 2 billion are only slightly better off. Most of this population lives on the Asian and African continents (except certain Middle East and far eastern countries) and in east European and South American countries. In contrast, the developed (high-income) countries, concentrated in North America and western Europe, include 25 countries each with a population of 1 million or more and a combined population of about 0.9 billion, constituting less than one sixth of the world's population.

Whereas the high-income group countries have industrial economies, the developing countries depend mainly upon agriculture and natural resources as the source of income. There are large disparities in the socioeconomic structures of various countries included in this heterogeneous group. For example, in 1995 the 10 largest countries—Argentina, Brazil, China, India, Indonesia, Mexico, Pakistan, Russia, Thailand, and Turkey—accounted for 59% of the developing world's GNP. By contrast, sub-Saharan Africa accounted for 10.4% of the world population but only 1.1% of the world GNP. Over the last decade, the economy as well as the social indices have improved rapidly in some regions. The average infant mortality rates (IMR) for low- and middle-income countries have halved from 105 per 1000 live births in 1970 to 52 in 1995. This average, however, masks regional disparities. The IMR remains above 90 in sub-Saharan Africa and 70 in southern Asia. Primary school enrollments have actually declined in some African countries.

Great disparities are encountered in the demographic, racial, ethnic, cultural, and behavioral patterns of people living in these countries, and these are reflected in the health-care–delivery systems. In contrast to the industrialized nations, where health care is for the most part universally available, a vast population of people living in developing countries do not have access to even the basic amenities like sanitation and safe drinking water.

Most of the developing world has a two-tier health-care–delivery system (2). The patients do not have to pay for medical advice, basic investigations, and treatment, but they must pay for disposables and drugs in the government-run, nonprofit hospitals. On the other hand, a large number of private hospitals are run for profit where the patient has to pay for all services.

II. DIALYSIS FACILITIES

The number of centers providing regular dialysis varies from 1.5 per million population (pmp) in the United Kingdom to 20.3 pmp in Japan (3). These units are both hospital-based or minimal care (free-standing) units located in metropolitan and nonmetropolitan areas. The exact number of dialysis units in various developing countries is not known. Available data show that the number varies greatly in different countries (Fig. 1). In some countries, like Brazil (3.3 pmp) (4) and Uruguay (9.03 pmp) (5), dialysis facilities are comparable to those available in the developed world, whereas in others, like Algeria (0.8 pmp) (6) and China (0.2 pmp) (7), the facilities are meager. Zimbabwe, with a population of 11 million, has only two dialysis centers. We conducted a survey of dialysis units in India that revealed that there are only about 0.2 dialysis centers pmp (8). About 68% of these centers are in the private sector and are accessible only to upper-income patients. Most of the dialysis centers have only two to four dialysis stations, grossly insufficient for the number of patients needing such facilities. Moreover, a majority of the population of the developing countries lives in remote rural areas where dialysis facilities are not available. As a result, patients and their families have to travel long distances and in many instances have to be relocated, with resultant loss of livelihood.

III. CHRONIC RENAL FAILURE

The exact number of patients with chronic renal failure requiring renal replacement therapy in the developing world is not known. Unlike the developed world, most developing countries lack renal registries that could provide guidelines for health-care providers and funding agencies. Most of the available data, including those from the most populous countries, China and India, reflect a collection of experiences of individual physicians and not the situation in its totality.

The reported annual incidence of end-stage renal disease (ESRD) patients shows a wide variation ranging from as low as 13 pmp in Paraguay to as high as 250 in the Dominican Republic (4–9). In 1993, the average incidence rate reported by the Latin American Registry was 33.3 pmp (9), far less than that reported by the more established registries in the United States and Europe. Barsoum (10) reported an incidence rate of 200 per million in the Egyptian population. "Guesstimates" from the rest of the world put the incidence as 100–200 pmp (8). The reasons are likely to be differences in racial composition, environmental conditions, and criteria used for diagnosis. It is also evident that a vast majority of these patients die without receiving any form of dialysis. The acceptance rates on dialysis are about 80 ppm in Egypt (10), 20 ppm in Malaysia (11), 5–8 pmp in India (8) and China (7), and even lower in many other countries (Fig. 2).

The mean age of ESRD patients requiring dialysis in most developing countries is much lower than in industrial countries, varying between 32 and 42 years in most countries of the Indian subcontinent (12–15) and even lower (about 25 years) in parts of black Africa

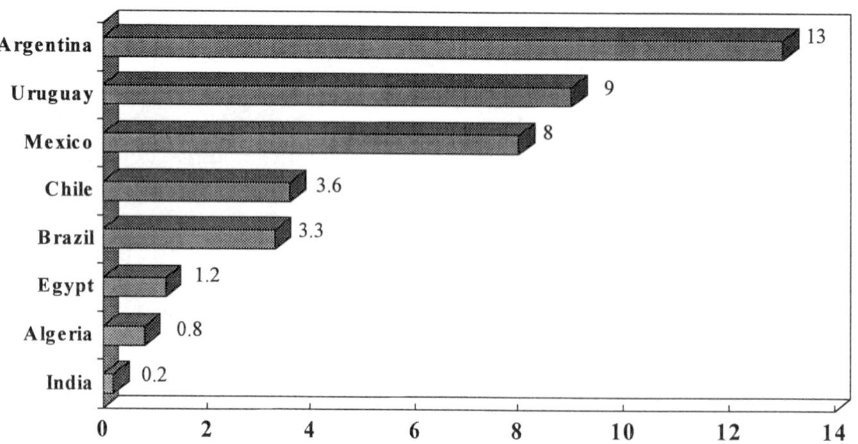

Fig. 1 Number of dialysis units per million population in selected countries.

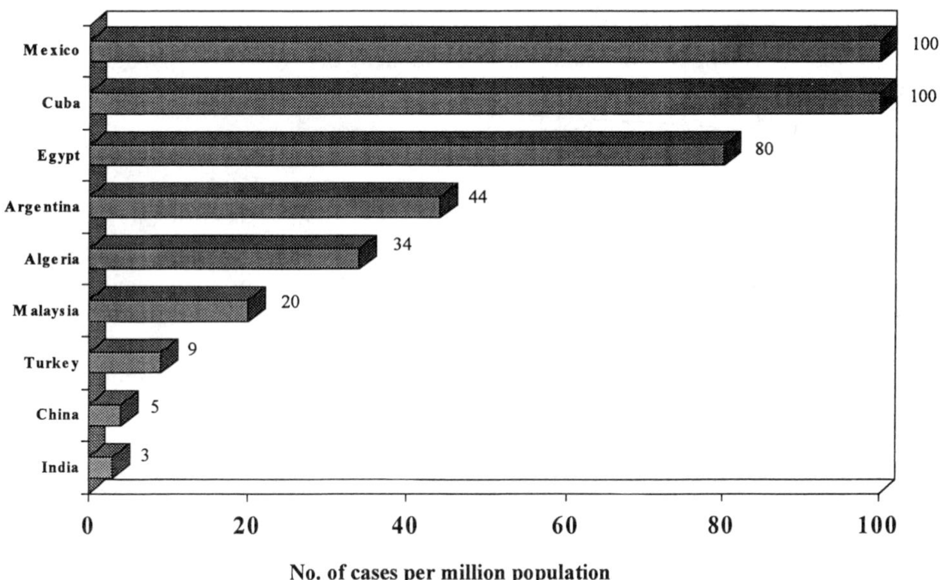

Fig. 2 Acceptance rates for ESRD therapy in developing countries.

(M.S. Abdullah, personal communication). This difference has resulted from an increase in the lifespan in affluent countries, with more and more of the surviving older population developing renal failure. The other possible reasons for the difference could be the delay in detecting renal disease and failure to institute timely preventive measures in patients with progressive renal disease, resulting in a faster deterioration of renal function and progression to ESRD in the younger population. In our center, over 70% of patients had sought specialist advice for the first time only after their serum creatinine had risen to >6 mg/dL. Late referrals also lead to a faster progression of co-morbid conditions, increase the cost of therapy, and worsen the overall patient survival. Predialysis care is almost nonexistent outside a few selected institutions.

The relative prevalence of various primary renal diseases amount patients with ESRD is highly variable in different countries. Chronic glomerulonephritis continues to top the list of causes of ESRD (Table 1) throughout most of the developing world (12,16). In patients over 40 years of age, diabetic nephropathy is the most frequent cause of ESRD (36.5%) and chronic glomerulonephritis and hypertensive nephrosclerosis occur

Table 1 Etiology of ESRD in the Indian Population

Disease	Public sector (government-funded) hospital[a] (%)	Private sector hospital[b] (%)
Chronic glomerulonephritis	36.64	21.18
Diabetic nephropathy	23.84	30.29
Hypertensive nephrosclerosis	13.47	10.09
Chronic interstitial nephritis	14.35	23.09
ADPKD	3.53	2.27
Multisystem	2.87	
Unknown	3.76	
Chronic pyelonephritis		9.45
Others	1.54	3.57

[a]From Ref. 12.
[b]From Ref. 13.

with almost equal frequency. In one report from a private hospital in south India, which mainly caters to high-income patients, diabetic nephropathy and chronic interstitial nephritis were reported to be the most frequent causes of ESRD (13). Certain geographic regions have a high incidence of renal stone disease, and obstructive uropathy forms an important cause of ESRD in these areas.

ESRD treatment facilities are not available uniformly to all sections of the society in many south Asian countries. Women, elderly persons, and small children often bear the brunt of such discrimination. On the other hand, no distinction is made in relation to sex, age, or race in Latin American nations with relatively well-developed ESRD programs (16).

A. Equipment

Because of economic constraints, many developing countries continue to use equipment that is considered outdated and obsolete in the western world. Although some centers have modern dialysis machines with volumetric ultrafiltration control and microprocessor-based controls with provision for bicarbonate dialysis, most units continue to use old and refurbished machines that have been received as donations. Since spare parts are not easily available and are expensive and dialysis technicians are a rare breed, once a machine breaks down, it remains out of action for long periods of time. Because of these constraints, dialysis continues to be carried out with older machines with central delivery systems using acetate buffer, and only limited facilities are available for individualizing the dialysis to suit the needs of a patient. In some developing countries, changes in the government policies have allowed improvement in the availability and quality of dialysis therapy.

Similrly, despite the increasing use of newer bicompatible membranes in the rest of the world, membranes made of cuprophane are still being used extensively in the developing world. In order to reduce the cost of dialysis, dialyzer reuse is practiced routinely. Reuse is more prevalent in private units with intent to increase the profits. In the advanced countries, the cleaning of dialyzers for reuse is done with automatic machines, and strict criteria laid down by the Association for Advancement of Medical Instrumentation are followed to ensure freedom from bacterial and pyrogenic contamination and maintenance of fiber bundle volume. In contrast, dialyzers are usually reprocessed manually in the developing countries and no attempt is made to measure the level of contaminants or the fiber bundle volume. This results in delivery of inadequate dialysis, frequent occurrence of pyrogenic reactions, and even sepsis following dialysis (16).

B. Cost

The annual dialysis costs are less than $10,000 in Brazil, India, China, and Egypt and about $13,000 in Uruguay and the Philippines, mainly because of the lower salaries paid to the staff and the low cost of consumables (8). However, there is a vast disparity in the ways dialysis is funded in different countries. Long-term maintenance dialysis remains out of reach for most people in low- or middle-income level countries and mass-based maintenance dialysis programs are almost nonexistent. In recent years, increase in government funding for dialysis has allowed coverage of the entire population in some South American countries like Brazil and Uruguay (4,5). However, in most of the developing world, dialysis is inextricably linked to transplant programs, and only those scheduled to undergo renal transplantation are accommodated in the government-funded dialysis programs (2). In some cases, treatment expenses are partly reimbursed by the employers. Therefore, most patients on long-term maintenance dialysis are either government employees who are covered under the medical reimbursement rules or a small proportion of those owning private businesses. The economic aspects of dialysis in India are listed in Table 2.

C. Dialysis Prescription

Because of the economic constraints in the developing countries, most patients receive their first dialysis when they are in a state of advanced uremia and have already developed complications like hyperkalemia, severe acidosis, pericarditis, or encephalopathy (8). The serum creatinine levels in the majority are over 15 mg% at the time of initiation of dialysis, corresponding to a GFR of <2 mL/min. Moreover, in the developed world, the dialysis prescription is guided by urea kinetic modeling, and most patients receive 4–5 hours of dialysis three times a week. The most prevalent practice in the developing countries is to give two 3- to 4-hour sessions of hemodialysis (HD) every week. The dialysis time often has to be cut short to accommodate more patients. The decision on frequency of dialysis is often based on patient symptomatology and financial considerations. Dialysis frequency is increased only if the patient develops complications like pericarditis, encephalopathy, or hyperkalemia. It is not an uncommon practice for patients to gradually reduce the frequency

Table 2 Economic Aspects of Dialysis in India[a]

	($) U.S.
Costs in government-funded hospitals	
Creation of native AV fistula	25
Prosthetic graft	80
Hemodialysis (twice a week)	1,500–2,000[b]
Costs in private hospitals	
Creation of native AV fistula	80
Prosthetic graft	200
Hemodialysis (twice a week)	4,000–5,000[b]
Continuous ambulatory peritoneal dialysis costs	
O set	4,800[b]
Y set	7,200[b]
Double-bag set	10,000[b]

[a]Total population: 940 million; per capita GNP: $340; budgeted health-care expenditure: $6 per year.
[b]Annual expenditure.

of dialysis because of financial reasons, leading ultimately to discontinuation of dialysis or death from complications of underdialysis.

Data on the adequacy of such dialysis schedules are not available. Some nephrologists believe that a satisfactory Kt/V and TACurea can be achieved in Indian ESRD patients by two 4-hour dialysis sessions/week (17). This has been attributed to the lower protein content of the diet with consequent lower generation of uremic toxins and to smaller body weight. This assumption, however, needs to be tested in rigorous clinical trials. It is our experience that most patients continue to suffer from uremic symptoms on such dialysis schedules and long-term survivors are few and far between. However, the situation seems to be improving steadily in countries where the governments have earmarked separate funds for dialysis. In Uruguay, the mortality rate decreased from 235 per 1000 patient-years in 1981 to 88 per 1000 patient-years in 1991 (5). A similar improvement was observed in the 1990s in many eastern European countries following the collapse of the socialist regimes (18,19).

D. Infections in HD Patients

A combination of poor living conditions, inadequate dialysis, malnutrition, hypoalbuminemia, and frequent blood transfusions makes dialysis patients prone to a variety of bacterial, viral, and fungal infections. Some of these are specific to the tropical region. Infection remains one of the most important causes of morbidity and mortality in these patients (20). According to a recent report of the Latin American Registry (9), infections were responsible for 40.2 deaths per 1000 patient-years, second only to cardiac causes (57.5/1000 patient-years). Data from a private hospital in India show that cardiac causes and infections were responsible for 33% and 22% of all deaths, respectively, in patients on HD (21). The infection rate is higher in government-funded hospitals, which cater to patients from the low-socioeconomic group.

Bacterial infections encountered among patients on maintenance HD are generally due to *Staphylococcus aureus* or gram-negative bacilli. The common sources are the respiratory tract and vascular access sites, commensurate with the increased use of subclavian and jugular catheters to secure temporary vascular access, the incidence of catheter-related *S. aureus* infection has risen in recent years. Hot and humid climate and poor hygienic conditions predispose to the development of such infections. In our own center one episode of catheter-related sepsis is observed every 3.2 patient-weeks. *S. aureus* constitutes over 60% of culture isolates. Thirty-five percent of the isolates are resistant to commonly used antibiotics, including methicillin. In rare instances this may lead to the development of right-sided endocarditis. Patients with pulmonary infections often present late with features of septicemia and/or respiratory failure. Besides the increased mortality and morbidity, need for expensive antibiotics increases the overall cost of treatment.

E. Tuberculosis

A number of developing countries are endemic for tuberculosis with tuberculin skin positivity rates of over 50%. Dialysis patients are especially susceptible to this infection because of the impairment in cell-mediated immunity. The incidence of tuberculosis in dialysis patients has been reported to vary between 4 and 9% in Indonesia (22), Saudi Arabia and United Arab Emirates (23), China (24), Poland (25), and Bangladesh (14), and over 10–15% in India (8) and 24% in Turkey (26). The majority of patients present within 1 year of initiation of dialysis. Lung is the primary site of involvement in 50–70% and lymph nodes in 5–22% of patients. Urinary and gastrointestinal tracts are less frequently involved. A common mode of presentation is with pyrexia of unknown etiology. Demonstration of mycobacteria is generally difficult and unrewarding. The role of the Mantoux test in establishing the diagnosis is doubtful because of a high positivity rate in the general population and also because defective cell-mediated immunity (CMI) can render it falsely negative in uremics. The positivity is as low as 6–20% in uremics with tuberculosis (24). Indirect tests include demonstration of raised levels of adenosine deaminase, anti-PPD-IgG by ELISA, and mycobacterial DNA by polymerase chain reaction in blood and pleural, pericardial, ascitic, or crebrospinal fluids. In many cases, the diagnosis is established retrospectively after observing a good therapeutic response to antitubercular agents. Appropriate therapy consists of administration of at least two bactericidal agents—isoniazid (INH) and rifampicin—for 12 months to ensure complete eradication of the disease. We have observed recurrence in about 25% of patients who receive only a short (6-month) course of chemotherapy. The dose of ethambutol needs to be reduced by 65% since it is excreted predominantly through the kidney. Establishing the diagnosis is particularly important because of the increased risk of dissemination when these patients receive immunosuppressive drugs following renal transplantation.

An increase in the incidence of tuberculosis in the developing world is being apprehended because of the impending AIDS epidemic. A primary INH resistance rate of 45–60% has been reported from some parts of India (27). INH prophylaxis, commonly practiced in the west, is unlikely to be successful and may paradoxically lead to an increase in infection with multidrug-resistant mycobacteria. Currently, the role of genetic factors in the development of tuberculosis is being postulated. John et al. (28) examined the frequency of various HLA-A and B antigens among South Indian patients who developed tuberculosis while on dialysis or following renal transplantation and compared them with a control population. HLA-A68 (subtype 28) was more frequent among patients who developed tuberculosis, and the relative risk of development of tuberculosis was 2.2 in those with this specificity. Studies in nonuremic Caucasian and African American populations with tuberculosis have shown that HLA-B 8 occurs with greater frequency in the former group and B15 in the latter.

F. Hepatitis

Viral hepatitis is among the most common viral infections encountered in dialysis patients. Unlike in nonuremics, the virus does not get cleared after infection in a vast majority of patients. Chronic liver disease may develop in an indolent fashion and transaminasemia is often absent or transient. In western countries effective screening of patients and blood products for the hepatitis viruses, strict isolation practices, reduction in requirement of blood transfusions with regular use of erythropoietin, and universal hepatitis B virus (HBV) vaccination programs have led to a substantial decline in the incidence viral hepatitis in the dialysis population.

Only limited data are available on the incidence and prevalence of HBV and hepatitis C virus (HCV) infections in the developing countries. Even among the developing countries, significant variation has been reported in the prevalence of hepatitis B surface antigen positivity. In certain countries like Taiwan, the prevalence is as high as 25–30% in the general population, whereas in India it varies from 3 to 5% in the general population and 6 to 30% in dialysis patients (29–31). In addition to patients who are already infected with the virus at the time of initiation of dialysis, a large number become infected while on dialysis. In a study of 283 patients over a 3-year period, Thomas et al. (30) found HBV positivity in 11% of patients at the time of entry into the dialysis program and another 31% became positive after initially testing negative. This high transmission rate was thought to be related to transfusion of blood inadequately screened for hepatitis B and improper isolation of positive patients. Because of an inadequate number of machines, many units do not use separate machines for HBV-positive individuals, and even where machines are marked for these cases, cross-contamination occurs through inadequately trained staff handling such patients and sharing of disposables. In recent years, the practice of HBV vaccination for all CRF patients and dialysis staff has gained wide acceptance and has substantially brought down the positivity rate. It is well known that an adequate antibody response is seen only in a relatively small proportion of uremic individuals and the titers tend to fall with passage of time. Although periodic monitoring of the titers and administration of booster doses is recommended, the facilities to measure antibody levels are scarce and therefore the exact seroconversion rates are largely unknown. In studies from India, the conversion rates vary from 16 to 60% (31,32). A number of strategies have been employed to improve the conversion rates. These include intradermal administration of the vaccine and use of GM-CSF as adjuvant (32,33). Not only did these measures lead to higher conversion rates, but the titers reached protective levels earlier and remain elevated for longer periods of time.

The course of hepatitis B infection in the dialysis population has not been well studied in the developing countries. In a study by Jha et al. (33), 8 of 11 HBsAg-positive dialysis patients died over a 3-year period, 50% from liver failure. This contradicts reports from the western literature in which HBV positivity in the dialysis population is considered to be benign. According to these authors, uncontrolled uremia due to inadequate dialysis could be responsible for the altered course of hepatitis and increased mortality. The incidence of hepatitis B infection has been shown to be much higher in those who did not develop protective antibody levels compared to those who did (34).

In recent years, HCV has emerged as the primary cause of viral hepatitis in patients on regular dialysis therapy. In contrast to the general population, blood transfusion does not appear to be the most important source of this infection in the uremics. This infection assumes a greater significance than HBV because of the nonavailability of a vaccine. The prevalence of anti-HCV positivity varies between 16 and 82% using different types of assays (35–39). The serotypes reported from the developing countries are different from those seen in the advanced countries. The predominant genotypes reported are 1a, 1b, 2a, and 3a from Brazil (4) and 1a, 1b, and 4 from Saudi Arabia (39).

As with HBV infection, a large proportion of patients who are initially HCV negative seroconvert while on dialysis. The conversion rate was as high as 15% per year in Taiwan (38). Even though the Centers for Disease Control (CDC) does not recommend isolation of anti-HCV-positive patients in dialysis units, the seroconversion rate was reduced from 8% per year to zero by isolating these patients in the Dialysis Unit of the University of Sao Paulo, Brazil, over an 18-month period (4). In several countries blood products are not routinely screened for HCV. In view of such compelling data, strict enforcement of screening and infection-control measures for prevention of transmission of HCV infection in dialysis patients must be instituted until an effective vaccine becomes available.

Data on the prevalence of recently discovered hepatitis GB virus are not available from the developing world.

G. Human Immunodeficiency Virus

HIV infection has not yet become a major problem in the dialysis population in the developing countries. No data are available on the magnitude of this problem from African countries with high HIV positivity rates. The reported prevalence of this infection in dialysis units varies from 0.5 to 2% (40). In most cases transfusion of unscreened blood or transplantation of contaminated graft transmits the infection. As of today, most dialysis units are not equipped to take care of HIV-positive patients because of a lack of screening programs and disposables. Because of the prevailing socioeconomic and cultural practices, these patients either discontinue dialysis on their own or are refused further care by the dialysis units.

The World Health Organization (WHO) has anticipated a shift in the center of the AIDS pandemic to Asia in the next few years, and the figure of HIV-infected individual is likely to rise from 4 million at present to over 20 million. With such an exponential growth in the numbers of HIV-positive individuals, it is only a matter of time that such patients would develop ESRD and require dialysis.

IV. WATER TREATMENT FOR DIALYSIS

In most developing countries, facilities for water purification are either not available or are inadequate. In some areas where the water supply is deficient or irregular, dialysis is carried out using water transported by tankers. Replacement of spent filters and cartridges is carried out infrequently. This exposes the patients to substantial risk of exposure to a number of contaminants.

A bizarre accident in a large 131-patient dialysis unit in the city of Caruaru in northeastern Brazil resulted in the death of 50 dialysis patients (41). All patients dialyzed during a 4-day period in February 1996 using water from tank trucks developed visual disturbances, nausea, and vomiting after dialysis. Over the next 4 months, 50 patients died of liver failure despite being transferred to other dialysis units. Investigations by the local health authorities in association with the CDC revealed that water used for dialysis had been contaminated by a toxin named "microcystin-LR" produced by an algae of the family Cyanobacteriaceae. Water samples from the lake from which the water was taken as well as the truck and dialysis filters were positive for microcystin. The toxin was also detected in the liver tissue of the affected patients. Investigations also revealed that the filters and cartridges in the water-treatment plant had not been replaced on stipulated dates, allowing the contaminated water to come in contact with the dialysis membrane. The dialysis unit was subsequently closed down.

V. BONE DISEASE

Three distinct features characterize the renal bone disease seen among dialysis patients in developing countries. First, conditions like vesico-ureteric reflux and distal renal tubular acidosis remain undiagnosed for long periods, leading to development of renal rickets and growth retardation. Such patients often present for the first time with gross bony abnormalities. Coexistent protein-energy malnutrition may further compound this problem. Second, calcitriol therapy is not available to a majority of patients due to its high cost. The mainstay of treatment in these cases remains the cheaper but much less effective ergocalciferol. Third, inadequate treatment of water used for dialysis, continuing use of aluminum-containing phosphate binders, lack of facilities to perform aluminum assays, and nonavailability of appropriate measures has led to a high incidence of aluminum-related bone disease in many areas. In a multicenter study of 782 iliac crest bone biopsies (see Ref. 4), osteitis fibrosa was observed in 31%, mixed bone disease in 22%, adynamic bone disease in 22%, and osteomalacia in 25%. Significant staining for aluminum was noted in 60% of cases, Interestingly, hypercalcemia was noted in only 9% of cases, indicating a combination of malnutrition and inadequate vitamin D therapy.

VI. NUTRITION

Malnutrition is rampant in most parts of the developing world. The reported frequency of malnutrition among ESRD patients in developing countries ranges from 42 to 77% (42–44). In one study (44) 77% of patients were hypoalbuminemic, and in another (42) the average serum albumin was 2.39 g/dL at the time of entry into the dialysis program. Delay in initiation and delivery of inadequate dialysis and imposition of protein restriction in patients who are already on a deficient diet contribute to this problem. In a study in Indian ESRD patients, Sharma et al. (42) found the average daily energy intake to be 1014 kcal with a protein intake of 0.34 g/kg body weight. Both these figures are far below the recommended dietary intake. Some patients accustomed to a vegetarian diet with a low protein content find it very hard to change their dietary habits in order to improve the dietary protein intake. Beheray et al. (45) found that the intake remained low despite adequate dialysis and strict dietary counseling. The resultant protein-energy malnutrition leads to a decrease in cell-mediated immunity, increases the incidence of infections and septicemias, and prevents development of adequate antibody response to various vaccines.

VII. CONTINUOUS AMBULATORY PERITONEAL DIALYSIS

Continuous ambulatory peritoneal dialysis (CAPD) is gradually becoming the preferred form of dialysis in countries with limited resources. Nissenson et al. (46) observed that countries with fixed annual health-care allocations to hospitals or regions have a higher CAPD use because of its cost-effectiveness. An increasing proportion of patients are now being initiated on CAPD compared to hemodialysis in countries like the United Kingdom, Australia, and New Zealand where government-funded hospitals provide dialysis services. Since the procedure does not require expensive equipment and after the initial training period the patient no longer requires regular visits to the dialysis center, CAPD offers greater independence and mobility as well as a better quality of life compared to patients on hemodialysis. These qualities make CAPD the ideally suited form of dialysis for patients in the developing world.

CAPD utilization, however, varies greatly among various developing nations (Fig. 3). Whereas 50–90% of dialysis patients are on CAPD in some South American countries (47), its use in other developing countries is much less common. In contrast to the advanced nations, the cost of chronic peritoneal dialysis is two to four times higher than that of HD in developing countries. The main reason for this is the lack of indigenous facilities to manufacture PD fluid with a consequent need to import the bags. One notable exception is Mexico, which has factories to manufacture PD fluid (16). The low cost of therapy there has allowed it to have the highest proportion of patients in the world on this form of therapy.

Good long-term survival, however, is yet to be reported from CAPD patients in the developing coun-

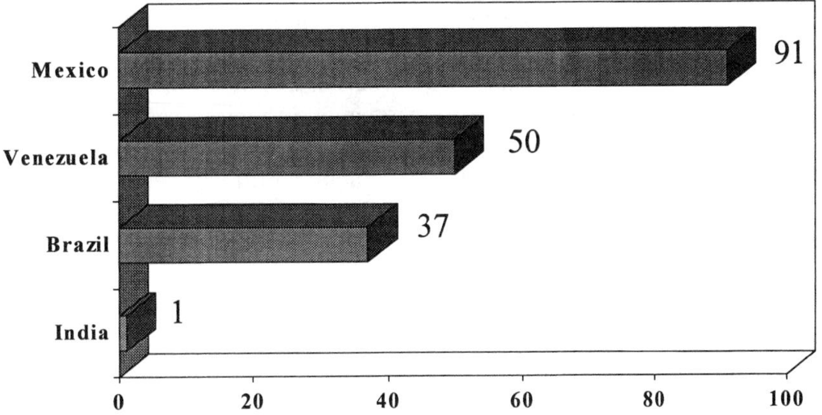

Fig. 3 Proportion of patients on CAPD in some developing countries.

tries. In a study of 132 South African patients, Zent et al. (48) recorded mean patient survival to be 17.3 months. The peritonitis rates were high and showed a strong association with black race and poor socioeconomic status of patients. El Matri et al. (49) reported a peritonitis rate of 1.8 per patient year in Tunisia. In a study from Belgium (49), where African ESRD patients often seek treatment because of lack of facilities in their own countries, very poor results were reported in terms of follow-up and compliance. Patients often did not report until they developed a major complication. Survival was less than 2 years in 85% of over 7500 cases in Mexico, which has the largest CAPD program among the developing nations (16). The factors that have contributed significantly to the dismal success rates of CAPD in developing countries are (a) uneducated and poorly compliant patients, (b) hot and humid climate and poor hygienic conditions, increasing the risk of infections, (c) poor patient training, and (d) lack of adequately trained social workers, dedicated nurses, and dietitians.

The higher cost of CAPD is the major deterring factor to this procedure gaining popularity in India. Presently, there are fewer than 500 patients on CAPD in India. Financial constraints force a significant proportion of these patients to reduce the number of exchanges or to reuse the transfer sets, leading to inadequate dialysis and increased incidence of infections. Most patients are on three exchanges per day, and cycler-assisted peritoneal dialysis is practiced rarely. Limited data are available on the adequacy of this form of dialysis. In a study of 55 patients, Abraham et al. (50) found the weekly combined renal and peritoneal creatinine clearances to be 70 L at the time of initiation of dialysis. However, a significant proportion of this appears to be contributed by the residual renal function, and as this dwindles with time, the efficacy of dialysis is likely to decrease. The patients, however, refuse to increase the dialysis dose because of resource constraints, leading to reappearance of uremic symptoms and eventually increased mortality. It is therefore obvious that in developing countries good results can be achieved only in selected patients who have enough resources and can strictly adhere to the basic principles of asepsis.

VIII. SPECIAL SITUATIONS

A. Acute Renal Failure

Acute renal failure (ARF) constitutes the most common nephrological emergency encountered by physicians in the developing world. There are significant differences between the spectrum of ARF encountered in the developing and developed countries. The improvement in the standard of living and universal health care has almost completely eradicated community-acquired ARF from the advanced countries. ARF is seen mainly in hospitalized elderly individuals with multisystem involvement following extensive surgery and in the intensive care setting. On the other hand, ARF frequently develops secondary to diarrheal diseases, tropical infections like falciparum malaria, leptospirosis, snake bite, intravascular hemolysis, and obstetric accidents throughout the developing world (51). The problem is compounded by the lack of adequate medical staff at the primary care level to intervene at the stage when the renal failure is still preventable with appropriate measures. By the time patients reach referral hospitals, most are in a state of advanced uremia with superadded complications like infections and gastrointestinal bleeding. Because of the reversible nature of this ailment, most patients with ARF are accepted for dialysis in all government and private hospitals, unlike patients with chronic renal failure. In many centers, ARF patients constitute as many as 50% of all patients on dialysis. Temporary vascular access in these patients is gained either by intermittent femoral catheterization or by subclavian or internal jugular catheterization. Many centers still depend upon creation of an arteriovenous shunt to gain vascular access.

Acute cortical necrosis, the most catastrophic form of ARF, constitutes a significant proportion of cases. The incidence declined from 7.2% in the 1970s and 1980s to 3.6% in the 1990s (52), but these patients still constitute a significant burden on the dialysis unit because of the long duration during which they require dialysis. Over 50% of these cases are seen following obstetric accidents. The condition can now be diagnosed reliably by its characteristic appearances on CT scan so that both the patient and the treating physicians can become aware of the need for long-term management.

B. Acute Peritoneal Dialysis

Intermittent peritoneal dialysis (PD) using a rigid catheter over a pointed stylet is frequently used for management of acute renal failure in many parts of the developing world. Patients usually receive 20–40 cycles of dialysis, each cycle lasting for one hour. Although this method is slow and not ideal for rapid correction of fluid overload or life-threatening hyperkalemia or metabolic acidosis, it is the only one available in the majority of the small hospitals. In these situations, acute PD may serve as a life-saving measure and is often helpful in gaining time till the patient can be transferred to a center where HD facilities are available. It has the added advantage of not requiring trained personnel and can be set up even in small hospitals located in remote places. However, this form of dialysis cannot be done if a patient has undergone recent abdominal surgery, has paralytic ileus, or has severe pulmonary edema where the dialysate volume may further compromise the respiration.

C. Continuous Renal Replacement Therapies

Over the last decade, various modes of continuous renal replacement therapy (CRRT) like arteriovenous or venovenous hemofiltration or hemodiafiltration have been utilized to treat critically ill patients with ARF, especially those in the ICU. This modality has many advantages over traditional HD in that it can be carried out in hypotensive patients, produces less hemodynamic instability, and allows removal of unlimited amounts of fluid, which permits administration of parenteral nutrition. Specialized machines that regulate the ultrafiltration and replacement fluid volumes and anticoagulation, obviating the need for constant monitoring by the staff, have become available in the developed countries. This treatment modality, however, is currently being practiced in a very small number of centers in the developing countries (53). The filters used for hemofiltration (HF) are 10 times more expensive than used for HD. In the absence of hemofiltration machines, the procedure requires very close monitoring to ensure proper anticoagulation and avoid excessive ultrafiltration. This makes the procedure manpower-intensive and puts an added load on an already stressed workforce. In most instances, a venovenous procedure is performed with the help of a pump, anticoagulation is administered intermittently, and the rate of ultrafiltration (UF) is adjusted manually by changing the height of the UF column or rate of infusion of replacement fluid. The replacement fluid used is either Ringer's lactate or normal saline, to which small amounts of sodium bicarbonate and calcium chloride are added.

D. Dialysis in Children

Children with acute and chronic renal failure in need of dialysis present unique problems to nephrologists in developing countries. ARF in the neonatal period most frequently follows birth asphyxia or sepsis and is at a later age most likely due to hemolytic uremic syndrome, diarrheal diseases, or septicemia. Special small surface area dialyzers and tubings with smaller priming volume are not available in most countries, and therefore hemodialysis is usually not possible in infants or small children. As a result, most patients are managed by intermittent peritoneal dialysis. Gaining access to the peritoneal cavity is a problem in small babies, and a variety of devices have been tried, including plastic IV cannulas and femoral catheters for hemodialysis. CAPD is not possible in this age group due to non-availability of suitable equipment and small-volume CAPD bags.

In conclusion, the approach to dialysis in developing countries is overwhelmingly influenced by the prevailing political and socioeconomic conditions. A vast majority of the population cannot derive the benefit of modern dialysis therapy of the standard practiced in the developed world. In recent years, active support of dialysis programs by some governments has led to substantial improvement in the quality and quantity of dialysis being provided in a number of countries. However, in the majority of developing countries, inadequate dialysis, frequent infections, and malnutrition continue to be prevalent among the patient population.

REFERENCES

1. Annual Development Report 1995. Washington, DC: The World Bank, 1995.
2. Chugh KS, Jha V. Differences in the care of ESRD patients worldwide: required resources and future outlook. Kidney Int 1995; 48:S7–S13.
3. D'Amico G. Comparability of the different registries on renal replacement therapy. Am J Kidney Dis 1995; 25:113–118.
4. Noronha IL, Schor N, Coelho SN, Jorgetti V, Romao Jr. FE, Zatz R, Burdmann EA. Nephrology, dialysis and transplantation in Brazil. Nephrol Dial Transplant 1997; 12:2234–2243.
5. Fernandez JM, Schwedt E, Ambrosoni P, Gonzalez F, Mazzuchi N. Eleven years of chronic hemodialysis in Uruguay: Mortality time course. Kidney Int 1995; 47: 1721–1725.
6. Salah H. An overview of renal replacement therapy in Algeria. Saudi J Kidney Dis Transplant 1994; 5:190–192.
7. Li L. End stage renal disease in China. Kidney Int 1996; 49:287–301.
8. Jha V, Chugh KS. Dialysis in developing countries: priorities and obstacles. Nephrology 1996; 2:65–72.
9. Mazzuchi N, Schwedt E, Fernandez JM, Cusumano AM, Ancao MS, Poblete H, Saldana-Arevalo M, Espinosa NR, Centurion C, Castillo H, Gonzalez F, Milanes CL, Infante M, Ariza M. Latin American registry of dialysis and renal transplantation: 1993 annual dialysis data report. Nephrol Dial Transplant 1997; 12: 2521–2527.
10. Barsoum RS. The Egyptian transplant experience. Transplant Proc 1992; 24:2417–2420.
11. Lim TO, Lim YN, Tan CC, Lee DG, Morad Z. Malaysian dialysis and transplant registry report. Nephrology 1998; 4:123–126.
12. Sakhuja V, Jha V, Ghosh AK, Ahmed S, Saha TK. Chronic renal failure in India. Nephrol Dial Transplant 1994, 9:871–872.
13. Mani MK. The management of end-stage renal disease in India. Artif Organs 1997; 22:182–186.
14. Rashid HU, Ahmed S, Rahman M, Hasan M, Noor Y, Mosaddeque M. Experience of hemodialysis in Bangladesh. In: Abstract Book, First International Congress on Dialysis in the Developing Countries, Singapore, November 2–5, 1994.
15. Kumar H, Alan F, Naqvi SA. Experience of hemodialysis at a kidney center. J Pak Med Assoc 1992; 42: 234–236.
16. Trevino-Becerra A. Development of artificial organs to treat chronic renal failure in Latin America. Artif Organs 1997; 22:174–176.
17. Desai JD, Shah BV, Sirsat KA. Urea kinetics: a guide to dialysis prescription (abstr). Indian J Nephrol 1991; 1:41.
18. Rutkowski B, Puka J, Lao M, Baczyk K, Chrzanowski W, Kokot F, Ksiazek A, Nartowicz E, Poplawski A, Sulowicz W, Scewcyzk Z. Renal replacement therapy in an era of socio-economic changes-report from the Polish registry. Nephrol Dial Transplant 1997; 12: 1105–1108.
19. Rutkowski B, Ciocalteu A, Djukanovic L, et al. Treatment of end-stage renal disease in central and eastern Europe: overview of current status and future needs. Artif Organs 1997; 22:187–191.
20. Jain S, Chugh KS. Morbidity and mortality burden of infections and infestations in chronic maintenance dialysis patients in developing countries. Proceedings of the First International Congress on Dialysis in the Developing Countries, Singapore, November 2–5, 1994.
21. Shah BV, Nair S, Sirsat RA, Ingle AV. Outcome of end stage renal disease: experience at a private hospital. Ind J Nephrol 1992; 2:151–154.
22. Roesli RMA, Soedarsono S, Soedarsono W. Patient to patient insurance system. A system to help hemodialysis patients in Indonesia. In: Abstract Book, First International Congress on Dialysis in the Developing Countries, Singapore, November 2–5, 1994.
23. Pingle A, Shakuntala RV, Chowdhry Y, Menon J, Pingle S. Presentation, treatment and outcome of tuberculosis in an oriental population with end-stage renal disease. In: Abstract Book, First International Congress on Dialysis in the Developing Countries, Singapore, November 2–5, 1994.
24. Zhang X, Hou F, Wei D. Tuberculosis in chronic renal failure patients with or without renal replacement therapy. Chung Hua Nei Ko Tsa Chih 1995; 34:666–669.
25. Sulima-Gillow A, Rutkowski B, Kustosz J, Zdrojewski Z. Tuberculosis—an increasing risk for patients treated with long-term hemodialysis. Pol Arch Med Wewn 1994; 92:251–259.
26. Cengiz K. Increased incidence of tuberculosis in patients undergoing hemodialysis. Nephron 1996; 73: 421–424.
27. Vasanth Kumari R, Jagannath K, Rajasekaran S. Bacteriological status and prevalence of drug resistance in district tuberculosis centers in Tamil Nadu. Lung India 1993; 9:27–31.
28. John GT, Murugesam K, Jayaseelam L, Pulimood RB, Jacob CK, Shastry JCM. HLA phenotypes in Asians developing tuberculosis on dialysis or after renal transplantation (letter). Natl Med J India 1995; 8:144.

29. Malhotra KK, Prabhakar S, Sharma RK, Dash SC, Singh RN. Hepatitis B in a hemodialysis unit in New Delhi. J Assoc Phys India 1985; 33:216–217.
30. Thomas P, Kirubakaran MG, Jacob CK, Srinivasa NS, Hariharan S, John JT, Shastry JCM. Hepatitis B infection in a dialysis unit in South India. J Assoc Phys India 1987; 35:284–285.
31. Kher V, Krishnamurthy G. Strategies against hepatitis B virus infection in renal failure patients: when, why and how? Ind J Nephrol 1996; 6:137–141.
32. Anandh V, Dhanraj P, Nayyar V, Ballal HS. GM-CSF as an adjuvant to hepatitis B vaccination in hemodialysis patients. A preliminary report. Ind J Nephrol 1997; 7:109–111.
33. Jha R, Kher V, Naik S, Elhence R, Gupta A, Sharma RK. Hepatitis B associated liver disease in dialysis patients: role of vaccination. J Nephrol 1994; 6:98–102.
34. Krishnamurthy G, Kher V, Naki S. Increased incidence of hepatitis B virus infection among HBsAg vaccine low responder chronic renal failure patients on maintenance hemodialysis. Ind J Hematol Blood Trans 1994; 12:2–6.
35. Salunkhe PM, Naik SR, Semwal SN, Naik S, Kher V. Prevalence of antibodies to hepatitis C virus in HBsAg negative hemodialysis patients. Indian J Gastroenterol, 1992; 11:164–165.
36. Gunaydin M, Bedir A, Akpolat T, Kuku I, Pekbay A, Esen S, Ozyilkan E, Arik N, Cengiz K. Prevalence of serum HCV-RNA among hemodialysis patients in Turkey. Infection 1997; 25:307–309.
37. Abdelnour GE, Matar GM, Sharara HM, Abdelnoor AM. Detection of anti-hepatitis C-virus antibodies and hepatitis C-virus RNA in Lebanese hemodialysis patients. Eur J Epidemiol 1997; 13:863–867.
38. Huang CC. Hepatitis in patients with end-stage renal disease. J Gastroenterol Hepatol 1997; 12:S236–S241.
39. Bosmans JL, Nouwen EJ, Behets G, Gorteman K, Huraib SO, Shaheen FA, Maertens G, Verpooten GA, Elseviers MM, de Broe ME. Prevalence and clinical expression of HCV-genotypes in haemodialysis-patients of two geographically remote countries: Belgium and Saudi-Arabia. Clin Nephrol 1997; 47:256–262.
40. Sakhuja V, Sud K, Maitra S, Jha V, Sehgal S, Chugh KS. Prevalence of HIV infection in a dialysis unit. Ind J Nephrol 1994; 4:42–44.
41. Jochimsen EM, Carmichael WW, An J, Cardo DM, Cookson ST, Holmes CEM, de C. Antunes MG, de Melo Filho DA, Lyra TM, Barreto VST, Azevedo SMFO, Jarvis WR. Liver failure and death after exposure to microcystins at a hemodialysis center in Brazil. N Engl J Med 1998; 338:873–878.
42. Sharma AK, Arora M, Gupta HP, Gupta R, Makkad PK. Energy intake and nutritional status in patients with end-stage renal disease. Ind J Nephrol 1997; 7:97–99.
43. Roesma J. Renal nutritional problems in Indonesia: a study in two capital cities. In: Chugh KS, ed. Asian Nephrology. New Delhi: Oxford University Press, 1993:656–661.
44. Saxena S, Jayraj PM, Mittal R, Shukla P, Agarwal SK, Tiwari SC, Dash SC. Clinical and laboratory features of patients with chronic renal failure at the start of dialysis in North India. Ind J Nephrol 1995; 5:4–8.
45. Beheray SS, Shah BV. Dietary protein intake in Indian patients with chronic renal failure. Ind J Nephrol 1996; 6:19–21.
46. Nissenson AR, Prichard SB, Cheng IKP, Gokal R, Kubota M, Maiorca R, Reilla MC, Rottembourg J, Steward JH. Non-medical factors that impact on ESRD modality selection. Kidney Int 1993; 43(suppl 40):S120–S127.
47. Santiago-Delpin EA, Cangiano JL. Renal disease and dialysis in Latin America. Transplant Proc 1991; 23: 1851–1854.
48. Zent R, Myers JE, Donald D, Rayner BL. Continuous ambulatory peritoneal dialysis: an option in the developing world. Perit Dial Int 1994; 14:48–51.
49. El Matri A, ben Abdullah T, Kechrid C, Ben Maiz H, Ben Ayed H. Continuous ambulatory peritoneal dialysis in Tunisia. Nephrologie 1990; 11:153–156.
50. Abraham G, Bhaskaran S, Soundarajan P, Ravi R, Nitya S, Padma G, Jayanthi V. Continuous ambulatory peritoneal dialysis. J Assoc Phys India 1996; 44:599–601.
51. Chugh KS, Sitprija V, Jha V. Acute renal failure in the tropical countries. In: Davison AM, Cameron JS, Grunfeld J-P, Kerr DNS, Ritz E, Winearls CG, eds. Oxford Textbook of Nephrology. 2d ed. Oxford: Oxford University Press, 1998:1714–1734.
52. Chugh KS, Jha V, Sakhuja V, Joshi K. Acute renal cortical necrosis—a study of 113 patients. Renal Failure 1994; 16:37–47.
53. Malakar D, Thomas PP, Jacob CK, Shastry JCM. Continuous renal replacement therapy in critically ill patients with renal failure. J Assoc Phys India 1993; 14: 335–336.

47

The Environmental Aspects of Dialysis

Rita De Smet
University Hospital, Gent, Belgium

Norbert Fraeyman
Heyman Institute, Gent, Belgium

Nicholas Andrew Hoenich and Peter George Blain
University of Newcastle-upon-Tyne, United Kingdom

I. INTRODUCTION

Hemodialysis and peritoneal dialysis are the most widely used modalities of treatment of patients with acute or chronic renal failure, with transplantation as the ultimate goal. Both dialysis and renal transplantation therapy make extensive use of disposable materials. The use of these materials yields easy access to either the general circulation or the peritoneal cavity under sterile conditions. Disposables are also extensively used in different other clinical applications. Those materials are mostly synthetic polymers. Their widespread use is attributed to their ease of manufacturing into the final product or its component, their ability to make the material into a variety of devices, and their relatively low production costs. The choice of the appropriate material is generally determined by economical, practical, and patient-related factors. After use, many of these items are discarded and are considered as medical waste. For dialysis treatments, this consists of dialyzers, intravenous fluid administration sets and bags, dressings, syringes, dialysis tubing sets, and concentrate containers. In addition, dialysis waste consists of glass, metal needles, and cardboard. The packaging materials are from the individual item as well as from the bulk supply packaging. Hemodialysis and peritoneal dialysis originate also liquid waste from body fluids and the used dialysis fluids.

The majority of the solid waste is burned in municipal or medical waste incinerators. It is well known that during the incineration of waste, a large number of toxic compounds are formed and are emitted into the environment. Among these compounds, dioxins have received most attention. Dioxins enter into the environment via the stack emission and ashes of the incinerator and are globally distributed.

Today, concern about the environment has become part of the political agenda in developed countries, and concerns about global warming, acid rain, the depletion of the ozone layer, and the greenhouse effect are no longer a minority interest.

II. DEFINITION OF MEDICAL WASTE

In the United Kingdom, the Controlled Waste Regulations (1992) define medical waste as follows:

1. Any waste that consists in a whole or in part of human or animal tissue, blood or other body fluids, excretions, drugs or pharmaceutical products, in swabs or dressings or syringes, needles, or other sharp instruments. This waste may be hazardous to any person coming in contact with it unless rendered safe.
2. Any other waste arising from clinical nursing, dental, veterinary, pharmaceutical or similar practice, investigation, treatment, care, teaching or research, or the collection of blood for transfusion, being waste that may cause infection to any person coming into contact with it.

Such waste may further be subcategorized into five groups:

Group A: soiled surgical dressings, swabs, and all other contaminated waste from treatment areas, material other than linen from cases of infectious disease and all human tissues, animal carcasses and tissues from laboratories, and all related swabs and dressings
Group B: discarded syringes, needles, broken glass, and other sharp objects
Group C: laboratory and postmortem waste
Group D: pharmaceutical and chemical waste
Group E: used disposable items

Belgium catalogs waste, following the directives of the European Community, in four categories: household waste, industrial waste, particular waste, and dangerous waste. Medical waste is defined as a particular waste and includes all kinds of waste, irrespective of the origin, the presence or the composition arising from medical or veterinary treatment, including laboratory and postmortem waste.

Medical waste is subdivided into nonrisk medical waste and risk medical waste. *Nonrisk medical waste* is waste that presents no particular risk for those coming in contact with it. Its origin but not its composition is comparable with household waste. Glass, paper, and cardboard are collected separately from other nonrisk medical waste. *Risk medical waste* is waste with a certain risk of bacterial or viral infection, poisoning, or injury for the manipulator or that requires special treatment for esthetic reasons.

III. MATERIALS FOR MEDICAL DEVICES

The importance of polymers in daily life is beyond doubt. Proteins, carbohydrates, nucleic acids, rubber, and resins are natural polymers, while plastics and synthetic fibers are synthesized from organic chemicals.

Plastic materials are made from oil or gas; monomers are formed after cracking processes and are subsequently polymerized. Polymers are manufactured by several consecutive chemical and mixing processes of monomers, catalyzers, solvents, and additives followed by mechanical procedures to obtain products with specific properties. During fabrication, additives such as antioxidants, plasticizers, fillers, and stabilizers are supplemented to maintain or improve the characteristics of the polymer. Additives can be anchored to the basic polymer; plasticizers are blended with the polymer and will not bind chemically. Chemical compounds can migrate to the surface of the polymer to change the surface properties. Each polymer has its own particular advantages, and for each application an ideal polymer is required to guarantee an optimum performance.

The polymers are produced as raw material. These materials coming from the suppliers are used as such or are compounded or converted by the device and/or packaging industry. Most frequently raw materials for these industrial sectors are polypropylene (PP), polyethylene (PE), polyvinyl chloride (PVC), polystyrene (PS), polycarbonate (PC), and polyurethane (PU) (1). Such materials are used extensively in a variety of clin-

Table 1 Commonly Used Polymeric Materials in Clinical Application

Polymer	Application
Polyvinylchloride	Blood and solution bags, surgical packaging, IV sets, dialysis devices, catheter bottles, general tubing, cannulae
Polyethylene	Pharmaceutical bottles, extension sets, catheters, flexible containers
Polypropylene	Burette chambers, connectors, syringes, packaging material, containers
Polycarbonate	Rigid moldings
Polyamide (nylon)	Packaging materials, molded components
Polyethyleneterephthalate	Mesh
Polyurethane	Catheters, tubing, components, potting compound
Ethyl vinyl acetate	Infusion bags, tubing
Polyester ether	High-pressure tubings, surgical products
Silicone	Catheters, tubing set components
Polystyrene	Culture flasks, vacuum bottles, packaging

ical applications, as shown in Table 1. In addition, silicone and natural or synthetic rubber are also used.

The consumption of medical plastic disposables is increasing. This higher need is attributed to the need to prevent infections, hygienic reasons, and its easy usage. The annual growth between 1994 and 2000 in medical plastics over the whole world is estimated to be 6.38% (2); in the United States demand will reach 1423 million kg in the year 2000. PVC will remain important, and its production will reach 424 million kg in the year 2000 due to the versatile processing and low costs for the production of the polymer. PP production is expected to increase by 3% annually to 232 million kg in the year 2000 (3).

Nowadays, developments in the medical device industry tend to stress quality. Properties such as the decomposition of the material after sterilization, biocompatibility, cytotoxicity, and pyrogenocity are tested to current international standards and guidelines. An important segment in the medical sector is the packaging industry. The package provides information and instructions concerning the products and guarantees the characteristics, performances and the purposes of devices during transport and storage, with the recycling symbol indicating the method of waste disposal.

The high needs and demands of plastics in medicine load the environment with increasing amounts of medical waste products. The impact of used materials on waste production and its resulting environmental pollution was up to now not a major concern of the medical sector; however, new polymers that are less pollutant are today produced by the industry and find their application in medicine.

A. Dialyzers, Blood Tubings, Fluid Bags, CAPD Bags, Connectors, and Containers

Four countries—France, Germany, Japan, and the United States—produce the membranes used in renal replacement therapy. The membranes are either cellulosic or synthetic polymers (Fig. 1). The former include regenerated cellulose (with Cuprophan), modified cellulose membranes with cellulose diacetate (CA) cellulose triacetate (CTA), and synthetically modified cel-

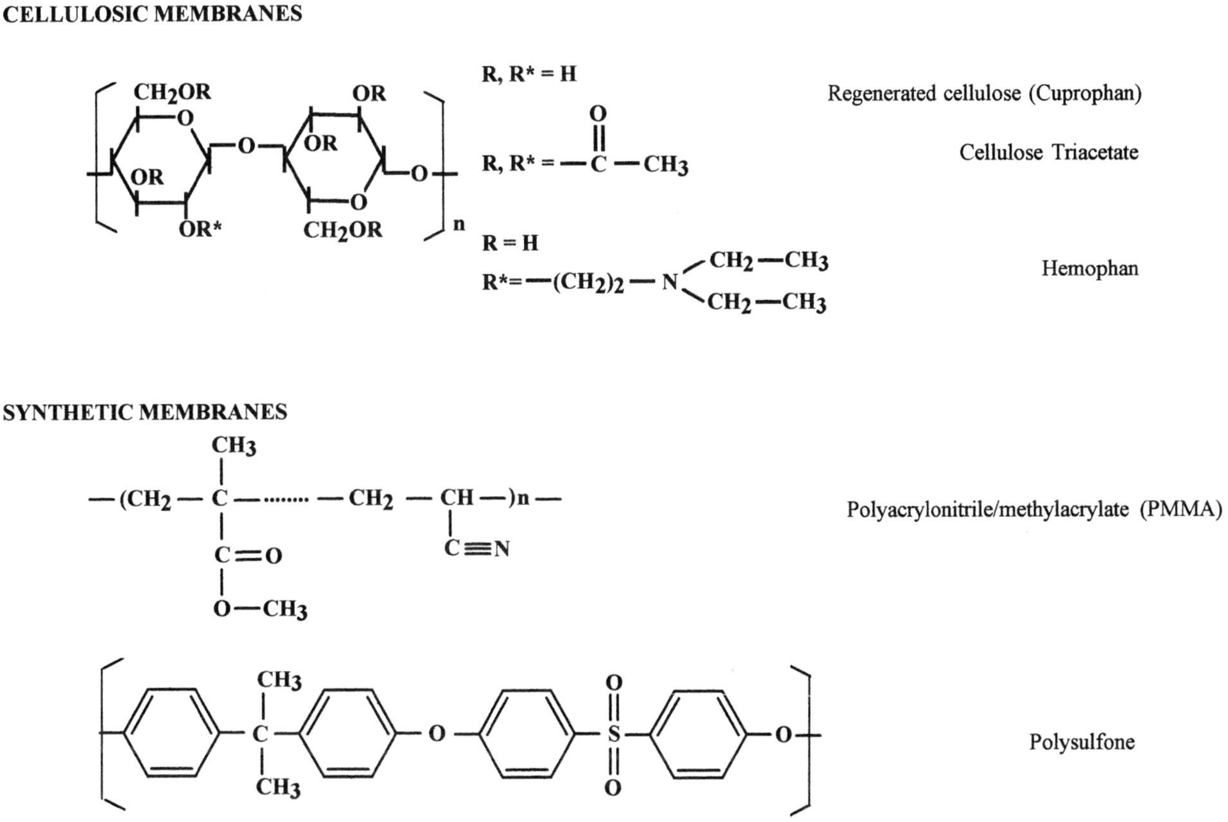

CELLULOSIC MEMBRANES

CH2OR, OR, O, OR, O, OR, O, OR*, CH2OR, n

R, R* = H — Regenerated cellulose (Cuprophan)

$R, R^* = -\overset{O}{\overset{\|}{C}}-CH_3$ — Cellulose Triacetate

R = H
$R^* = -(CH_2)_2-N(CH_2-CH_3)_2$ — Hemophan

SYNTHETIC MEMBRANES

$-(CH_2-C(CH_3)(C{=}O\,O{-}CH_3)-\cdots\cdots-CH_2-CH(C{\equiv}N)-)_n-$ — Polyacrylonitrile/methylacrylate (PMMA)

CH3, C, CH3, O, O, S, O, O, n — Polysulfone

Fig. 1 Chemical structures of cellulosic and synthetic hemodialysis membranes.

lulose, Hemophan and synthetically modified cellulose (SMC). The latter group include polysulfone (PSu), polyamide (PA), polyacrylonitrile/methylacrylate (PMMA), and polyacrylonitrile AN69 (PAN) (4). The hemodialyzer contains a membrane housed in PC casing or potted in PU. The sealing around the header manifolds is generally of silicone rubber (SIR).

Different technical or chemical procedures are necessary to make polymers suitable for dialysis membranes. The membranes must be biocompatible and give an adequate dialyzer clearance; to achieve this, cellulose membranes are, for example, modified with acetate (5) and swelling agents are used to form the pores. Residuals of the production process such as solvents, catalyzers, or particles have to be nonhazardous or nontoxic to patients. However, the cytotoxicity of residual substances in the rinse solutions of dialyzers was demonstrated on isolated mitochondria (6), and a loss of polyethyleneglycol (PEG) from polysulfone membranes after reuse with oxidizing agents as hypochlorite and peracetic acid was shown (7).

Medical tubing such as bloodlines for hemodialysis and bags with physiological solutions or CAPD solutions are mostly made of PVC. The production of PVC is cheap; the basic components are sodium chloride and ethylene, and the monomer vinylchloride contains a chloride atom on alternate carbon atoms (Fig. 2). PVC is rigid, and in order to be used in a flexible sheet or tubular form, the polymer needs to be blended with heat stabilizers (heavy metals) and plasticizers. The addition of a plasticizer weakens the PVC chain interactions, which allows increased interchain flexibility. The dominant additive is plasticizer, accounting for up to 40% of the bulk of the final material. The most commonly used plasticizer is di-(2-ethylhexyl)-phthalate (DEHP) (Fig. 2), the clinical impact of which will be discussed later. The choice of additives to be used in the manufacturing of medical grade PVC compared to those used for general purpose applications such as building products is limited. Table 2 illustrates the formulation of PVC for medical applications based upon European Pharmacopoeia guidelines. PVC has been used for many years, and the fact that plasticizers migrate into the blood, dialysate, or CAPD effluent is well known (8).

More recently, alternative polymers such as polyolefins (POs) became available, and these will gradually replace the PVC CAPD bags. Polyolefins are hydro-

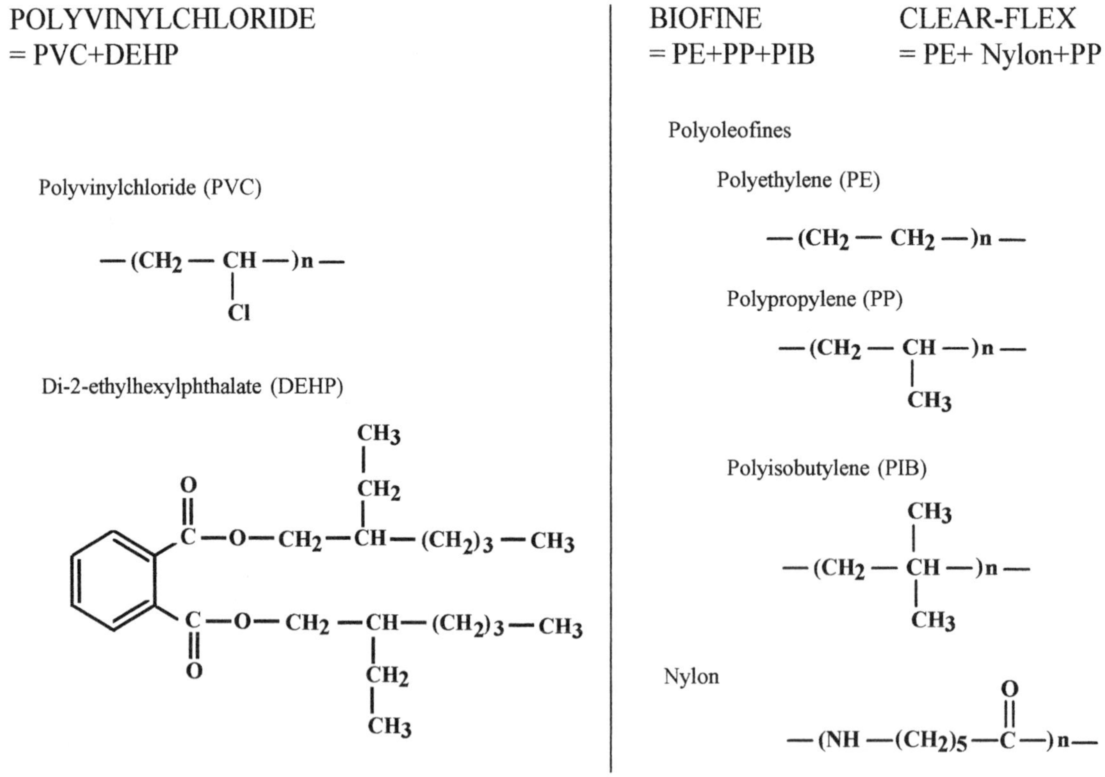

POLYVINYLCHLORIDE
= PVC+DEHP

Polyvinylchloride (PVC)

$$-(CH_2-\underset{\displaystyle Cl}{\underset{|}{CH}}-)n-$$

Di-2-ethylhexylphthalate (DEHP)

$$C_6H_4\left[\overset{O}{\overset{\|}{C}}-O-CH_2-\overset{CH_3-CH_2}{CH}-(CH_2)_3-CH_3\right]_2$$

BIOFINE
= PE+PP+PIB

CLEAR-FLEX
= PE+ Nylon+PP

Polyoleofines

Polyethylene (PE)

$$-(CH_2-CH_2-)n-$$

Polypropylene (PP)

$$-(CH_2-\underset{\displaystyle CH_3}{\underset{|}{CH}}-)n-$$

Polyisobutylene (PIB)

$$-(CH_2-\overset{\displaystyle CH_3}{\overset{|}{\underset{\displaystyle CH_3}{\underset{|}{CH}}}}-)n-$$

Nylon

$$-(NH-(CH_2)_5-\overset{O}{\overset{\|}{C}}-)n-$$

Fig. 2 Chemical structures of PVC, DEHP, Biofine, and Clear-Flex.

Table 2 Components of Medical Grade PVC Used in the Manufacture of Blood Bags and Tubing Sets

Polyvinylchloride	≅55%
Plasticizer	≅40%
N,N-diacylethylenediamine	~1%
Linseed oil or epoxy soya oil	10%
Calcium/Zinc stearate	~1%
Zinc octanoate	~1%

carbons (C_2H_{2n}) and contain no chloride atoms. In this material, flexibility is achieved by specific three-dimensional configuration of the carbon atoms and not by the addition of a plasticizer (Fresenius, personal communication). To this polymer family of polyolefins belong PP, high-density polyethylene (HDPE), low-density polyethylene (LDPE), and polyisobutylene (PIB) (Fig. 2). Biofine^R (Fresenius Medical Care, Bad Homburg, Germany) is a PO film 100–150 μm thick and is built up of seven layers. Semi-rigid PE is inert and is used for solution containers. Clear-flex^R (Baxter, Nivelles, Belgium) is a three-layer polymer of polyethylene, nylon, and polypropylene. The inner layer of PE comes in direct contact with the dialysis fluid, the nylon forms a barrier to gas, while the PP reduces the permeability to water (9). The POs have improved biocompatibility and do not affect leukocyte function as compared to conventional PVC bags (10).

In addition, extracorporeal circuit components may also contain a number of natural or synthetic rubbers, silicone, polyurethane, polyesters such as polyethyleneterephthalate (PET) used in meshes, PAs, or nylons and polycarbonate (PC).

B. Glass

Although glass bottles for infusion fluids are no longer used in western Europe and the United States, glass still constitutes an important fraction of medical waste. Because glass is inert, ampules or vials are frequently utilized for drugs in solution since glass is usually more compatible for medication than PVC. Adsorption of drugs to the glass wall is almost negligible; hence no change in concentration during storage will occur. However, mini plasco-vials of PE with drugs in solution (E. Braun Melsungen AG, Melsungen, Germany) gradually are replacing the glass vials.

C. Metals

The amount of metals in medical devices is low. Presterilized dialyzers, in particular those sterilized by γ-irradiation, use aluminum bags. According to the European Pharmacopoeia, less than 1% zinc octanoate and less than 1% calcium or zinc stearate may be added as stabilizers to PVC during the production of tubings and bags (11). Needles for access to the patient's circulation as well as for blood sampling are manufactured from medical-grade stainless steel containing 70% iron, 18% chromium, 9% nickel, 1.5% manganese, 0.10% cobalt, 0.05% molybdenum, and 0.01% tungsten (12). Trace amounts of heavy metals such as lead are also present in paper and cardboard (13).

D. Packaging

Medical products and devices are packed for transport. The packaging cardboard and bags of paper and/or polyethylene or metal foil keep the individual device sterile until use and protect the material against damage. The packaging also provides the user information about the product name, application, product code, lot number, sterilization technique and sterilization date, expiration date, and CE mark (14). With the advent of the European Directive on packaging, the recycling mark is also included.

IV. WASTE GENERATION

Within the European Community 2.5 billion tons* of waste are annually generated by households and industry and thus require disposal. About half of the waste is agricultural in origin and accounts, together with domestic waste, for around 114 million tons (4% of total waste). Approximately 7% of solid waste is of plastic origin. A wide variety of plastics ranging from low- and high-density polyethylene, polypropylene, polystyrene, as well as PVC are discarded in waste. Such plastics originate not only from medical applications but also from industry, construction, and domestic sources.

The type and nature of medical waste in the context of general waste production needs to be considered. Medical waste represents less than 1% by weight of all waste generated. Hospitals, laboratories, doctors' offices, as well as patients in their home produce medical waste. A breakdown of the waste produced by a typical district 900-bed general hospital in the United King-

*One metric ton = 1000 kg.

Table 3 Waste Generation Within the Hospital of Royal Victoria Infirmary, Newcastle Upon Tyne

	Domestic waste (%)	Medical waste (%)
Outpatients	2	2
Pharmacy	2	7
Accident and emergency	4	7
X-ray	2	2
Intensive therapy unit	2	6
Operating theaters	4	12
Laboratories	5	6
Wards	63	63
Administration	16	—

Source: Ref. 46.

dom, the Royal Victoria Infirmary in Newcastle upon Tyne, is shown in Table 3. The average medical waste generated per bed per annum is 0.59 tons, however, considerable variations in this figure are known to exist. In contrast, the Freiburg University Hospital with 1900 beds generates only 0.026 tons per bed per annum of medical waste. This difference can be explained by introduction in 1991 of the "green dot" system, requiring rigorous sorting of waste at the point of origin.

In comparison, within the city of Newcastle upon Tyne, 121,000 households generate 118,000 tons of waste per annum, or 0.975 tons (975 kg) per household. The paper and card content of this waste is 0.34 tons (35%), while the plastic content is 0.058 tons (6%), and glass accounts for a further 0.078 tons (8%).

A. Solid Waste

Hemodialysis and CAPD techniques preferentially use disposables in order to minimize the risk of infection and contamination. The disposables are safe for patients, doctors, and nurses; they are easy to handle and are not expensive. Dialysis equipment consumes 8% of the global disposable medical device (Fresenius, personal communication).

During 1997 the renal division of the University Hospital of Gent treated 77 end-stage renal disease patients with hemodialysis. These patients underwent 12,000 hemodialysis treatment sessions with polysulfone, Hemophan, and cellulose triacetate membranes. The additional dialysis material consisted of polycarbonate, polyurethane, PVC, Pivipol, acrylonitrile-butadienestyrene (ABS), polyester, polypropylene, rubber, silicone, latex, vinyl, Teflon, glass, stainless steel, cotton, and adhesives. The packaging materials were cardboard, bags of aluminum, polyethylene, and polyethyleneterephthalate.

The solid waste at the hemodialysis center is collected as follows:

1. Risk medical waste: dialyzers, tubings and needles, wound dressing and glass contaminated with biological fluids
2. Nonrisk medical waste: medical noncontaminated disposables as bags of substitution fluid, packaging materials, containers
3. Household waste: paper, packaging materials, cardboard, plastics
4. Noncontaminated glass: bottles, ampules, vials

The solid waste generated by one hemodialysis patient amounted to 2.8 kg per treatment or 437 kg of waste per annum. This is comparable with the waste of 476 kg of one habitant of the city of Gent (Table 4). The total amount of solid waste produced by the hemodialysis center is ±34,000 kg a year; this is ≈2.5% of the total hospital waste. All the waste, except noncontaminated glass, is burned in a licensed incinerator. The incineration of medical risk waste costs about $2/kg, which is 10 times more expensive than for the incineration of medical nonrisk and household waste, since extra precautions are required during its handling.

In addition, in 1997 41 patients were treated by home peritoneal dialysis. Peritoneal dialysis treatments amounted to 8295 peritoneal treatment days at home and 707 days in the hospital. Most patients performed four exchanges per day except those using the home cycler system. The polymers used in the large majority of the bags are PVC (Twin-bag) or Clear-flex^R. A minority of patients use Stay-Safe equipment, which is completely PVC-free. The sterile parts are packed in an outer wrapping foil. All the materials are transported and supplied in cardboard. For patients treated by CAPD, waste generation was calculated by weighing the empty bags. In the hospital, the CAPD bags, all the consumables, and cardboard were discarded as nonrisk medical waste, except when a patient suffered from peritonitis. At home, the patients discarded the used CAPD bags, tubing, and packaging via their domestic combustible waste. The cardboard was collected separately and recycled.

For a CAPD patient the total solid waste generated per day is 1.69 kg (Table 4). Extrapolation indicates that the annual waste generated by these patients amounts to 15,000 kg. The vast amount of waste is an additional problem for the CAPD patient treated at home; CAPD treatments result in an additional 600 kg

Table 4 Solid Waste of One Hemodialysis Session (1 HD Patient) and Four CAPD Sessions (1 CAPD Patient) at the University Hospital Gent and of One Inhabitant of the City of Gent

	Solid waste (kg)		
	HD patient, 1 dialysis	CAPD patient, 1 day	City inhabitant, 1 day
Risk medical waste			
Plastics	1.43		
Glass, needles, dressing	0.08	0.04	
Nonrisk medical waste			
Plastics	0.37	1.15	
Household waste			
Plastics	0.25		0.52
Cardboard/paper	0.57	0.50	0.23
Glass (noncontaminated)	0.10		0.07
Other waste			
Garden and vegetables			0.20
Metals			0.03
Other			0.25
Total	2.80	1.69	1.30

Solid waste produced in 1 year: HD patient—437 kg: CAPD patient—617 kg; city inhabitant—475 kg.

waste per annum besides normal domestic waste. The patient needs sufficient space for sorting and storing the waste, and in addition the city collects taxes for waste collection.

Taken together, these examples illustrate that dialysis centers and CAPD patients at home produce a considerable quantity of waste and consequently contribute to environmental pollution caused by incineration of this waste. Plastics are more prevalent in dialysis waste than in normal domestic waste, and these materials may contribute to the formation of dioxins upon combustion (see below).

B. Liquid Waste

The fluid waste generated during 1997 by the hemodialysis center of the University Hospital of Gent amount to 3.8 million liters of dialysis fluid containing 156,000 liters of concentrate. In addition, sterilizing fluids accounted for a further 2,160 liters and was made up of 560 liters of 10% acetic acid, 1,200 liters of hypochloride, and 250 liters of Citrosteril and 150 liters of Dialox, two commercial disinfectants. In addition, fluid waste generated from the CAPD patients was further 72,000 liters, more than 90% being combined with waste from the patient's home.

Plasticizers are not chemically bound to polymers and leach out of PVC in the dialysate and than appear into the environment. The dialysate from hemodialysis patients and CAPD effluents contains plasticizers, mostly DEHP and the derivatives mono-2-ethylphthalate, 2-ethylhexanol, and phthalic acid. DEHP has been detected in air, water, soil, and food and is incorporated in the body (15).

V. SOLID AND LIQUID WASTE DISPOSAL

Solid waste is disposed either via landfill sites or via incineration. Within Europe it has been estimated that 70% of the waste produced is disposed via landfill sites; however, there are major national variations, with, for example, only 10% of waste disposed via this route in Switzerland. The waste disposed of in landfill sites is predominantly domestic in nature, although some of this waste originates from hospitals.

Incineration remains the most common method of disposal of medical waste. Indeed, the volume of highly contaminated ashes or physicochemical contaminants from gas-cleaning systems which is disposed of in landfills is reduced to less than 10% of the original weight of waste. Incineration may be undertaken onsite, i.e., in the hospital, or it may be transported to an off-site facility. Both are unpopular in the communities in which they located, particularly if waste is imported from other areas. Within the United Kingdom many hospitals have their own incinerators for the disposal of medical waste. The Environmental Protection Act governs the burning of waste in incinerators and its discharge into the atmosphere. The regulations make provision for the implementation of the European Council Directive 94/67/EC on the incineration of hazardous waste be ensuring that all incineration processes are controlled by the Environmental Protection Act 1990.

Germany has modern two-stage incineration plants, such as the one in Kiel, which handles all medical waste from the Schleswig-Holstein region. In other parts of Germany, municipal incinerators have been modified to allow the disposal of medical waste. Currently much of the disposal of medical waste originating from hospitals is contracted out, as in Belgium. In these countries private contractors remove and transport the waste to the incinerator. Contracting out, while simplifying the disposal process, may involve considerable expense; the contract price in the United Kingdom for such removal in 1997 ranged between \$288 and \$512 per ton.

Prior to incineration, medical waste that is considered infectious may undergo specific treatment, such as autoclaving. This technique could also be used to treat medical waste for disposal via a landfill site, but since there is no bulk reduction this technique is rarely used.

As a rule the aqueous waste generated from renal replacement therapy is discharged into the sewer system without further treatment. The sewage system in metropolitan areas may, however, not only handle waste water but also rain water. Under conditions of heavy rainfall the plant capacity may be exceeded, with untreated sewage being discharged directly into the receiving stream or the sea. It is generally assumed that the aqueous waste originating from the treatment of patients with renal failure is noninfectious.

The solid waste from hemodialysis and CAPD consists mostly of plastic materials and cardboard. The polymer materials are composed of carbon (C), hydrogen (H), oxygen (O), sulfur (S), and nitrogen (N); only PVC contains chlorine (Cl) atoms (Figs. 1,2). Cardboard is an organic material and contains low quantities of heavy metals.

During incineration the waste is essentially oxidized since incineration is carried out at approximately 10% oxygen. Incineration potentially destroys organic materials including pathogens found in medical waste. A complete incineration of the plastics generates carbon dioxide (CO_2), water (H_2O), hydrochloric acid (HCl), sulfur oxides (SO_x), and nitrogen oxides (NO_x).

Combustion in a municipal or medical incinerator is nearly always incomplete, and in addition to oxides and acids, hazardous compounds are formed, including carbon mono-oxide (CO), polycyclic hydrocarbons (PAHs), polychlorinated dibenzodioxins (PCDDs), and polychlorinated dibenzofurans (PCDFs) (16,17). These chemical reaction products enter the environment via stack emissions and ashes and are globally distributed. Humans and animals have direct contact by inhalation and intake of contaminated food (Fig. 3). It is clear that these chemicals contribute to environmental pollution and represent a health risk for the general population.

In the atmosphere, hydrochloric acid, sulfur oxides, and nitrogen oxides, become respectively, H_2SO_4 and HNO_3 and contribute to the formation of acid rain.

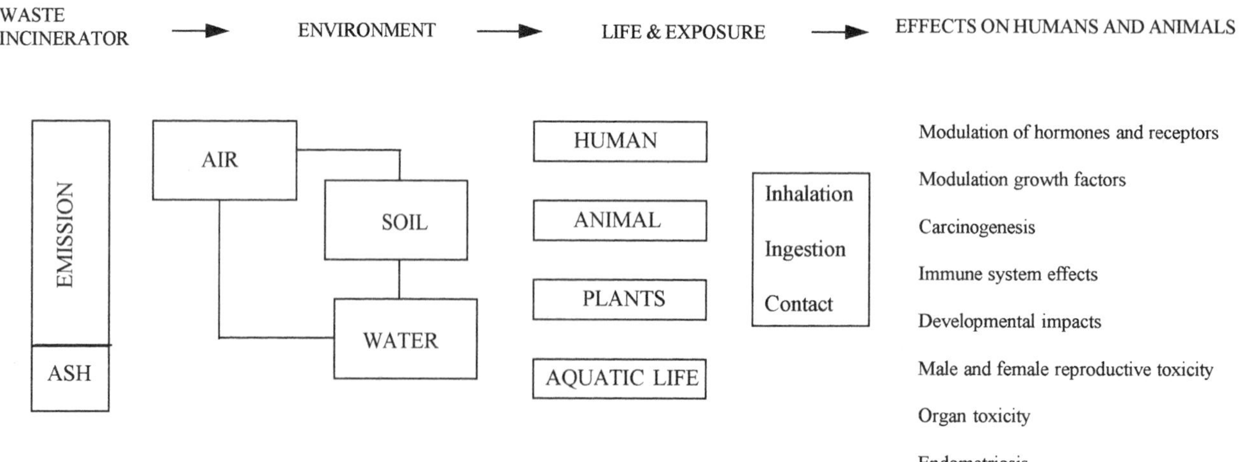

Fig. 3 Schematic representation of global distribution of pollutants from waste incineration and effects on humans and animals.

PAHs are recognized carcinogens, and the polychlorinated dibenzodioxins and dibenzofurans are considered the most toxic pollutants of waste incinerators (see below) (18–20).

Heavy metals are also present in solid waste (cardboard and PVC), needles, and metallized foils. Following combustion, the inorganic complex residue containing the metals leaves the incinerators as bottom ash and fly ash while a small quantity is also discharged into the atmosphere in the form of vapors or fumes.

VI. ENVIRONMENTAL AND HEALTH ISSUES

Medical waste is an important source of dioxins due to the extensive consumption of PVC in the medical sector (16). The presence of chlorine in PVC, the increased consumption of this polymer, together with the pollution of dioxins and the assumed health risk, has evidently resulted in the hypothesis that PVC is the ultimate cause of all problems. However, according to current scientific knowledge it is clear that this explanation is too simple. It should also be pointed out that the production of toxic compounds also arises from the incineration of fossil fuels, from the production of organic chemicals, and from the emission of exhaust from motor vehicles.

Harrad (21) in the United Kingdom estimated that annual environmental loading from the stack emission was about as 10.9 kg from municipal waste incinerators, 7.7 kg from industrial emissions, 5.1 kg from domestic emissions, 1.7 kg from the production of organic chemicals, and 0.7 kg from motor vehicle exhaust. The contribution from medical waste incineration was estimated to be 1.7 kg.

A. Polychlorinated Dibenzodioxins and Polychlorinated Dibenzofurans

1. Origin

Dioxins are formed as products of incomplete combustion involving chlorinated compounds, such as chlorine-bleached paper and PVC. Dioxins are the common name for the whole group of PCDDs and PCDFs. Dioxins were first identified in the emissions of municipal incinerators in the Netherlands in 1977. Some years later they were also detected in the flue gas and the fly ash of solid waste incinerators in other European countries, North America, and Japan (22).

The toxic compounds are formed at the low temperatures (<600°C) in the postcombustion zone of the incinerator during the cooling down of combustion gases. When the gases from the combustion chamber are cooled down, the fly ash (residue particles) in these gases acts as an active catalytic surface for the formations of dioxins. Metals such as copper and iron on the fly ash catalyze these reactions (23).

Excess oxygen and low furnace temperature yield high PCDD/Fs. Chlorine, copper, sodium, potassium, and zinc have a positive correlation with dioxin concentrations, whereas HCl, SO_x, and NO_x do not (24).

The three basic ingredients needed for dioxin formation are an organic material, a chlorine source, and a metallic catalyst in processes with relative low temperature (25). Other sources of dioxins are the combustion of oil, coal, lignite, and wood, other incineration processes, chemical production of chlorophenols, chlorobenzenes and dyes, pulp bleaching in the paper and metal industries, and traffic (24).

2. Characteristics

Dioxins are a group of tricyclic aromatic compounds substituted with one to eight chlorine atoms. Chlorinated dioxins are derivatives of dibenzo-*p*-dioxin. Depending on the precursors and the locations of chlorine substitution, different congeners are formed. Polychlorinated dibenzofurans are chlorine-substituted derivatives of dibenzofuran (Fig. 4). They have similar physical and chemical properties. These compounds are stable, highly hydrophobic, and lipophilic (25,26).

Identification and determination of the concentration of polychlorinated dioxins and furans in gas, fly ash of waste incinerators, and biological and environmental samples are performed with gas chromatography-mass spectrometry (GC-MS) after a series of complex and difficult sample treatments (22,27). Reliable analyses of dioxins are necessary to obtain data on emission and transport of dioxins and to correlate possible health effects with that data. To harmonize the determination methods on the mass concentration of dioxins in atmospheric emissions, two approaches used. The first approach is the use of certified Standard Reference Materials issued by the National Institute of Standards and Technology (28); the second involves the directives of the European Community concerning sampling, extraction, and sample clean-up identification and quantification (29).

3. Toxicity

A varying number of chlorine atoms may occupy the positions on the cyclic structure giving rise to 135 variants of PCDF and 75 variants of PCDD. Of the 210 total variants, 17 are considered most toxic (the "dirty 17") (30).

It must be mentioned that 2,3,7,8-tetrachlorodibenzo-*p*-dioxin (TCDD) was emitted following an industrial accident in Seveso, Italy (30). It is accepted practice to compare the relative toxicity of dioxins to that of 2,3,7,8-TCDD in terms of their "toxic equivalent factor." The concentration on dioxins in a sample is expressed as the sum of the individual concentrations of the dioxins multiplied by their individual toxic equivalent, or TEQ (29,30) (Fig. 4).

The most toxic dioxin is 2,3,7,8-TCDD, a compound fatal in a single, very-low-level dose to certain species such as the hamster but at the same time having no effect on dogs. Humans and animals have direct or indirect contact with dioxins via inhalation and the food chain, especially through the consumption of fat-containing foods such as milk, meat, and fish, Additionally, dioxins are also present in soils and vegetation. Dioxins are persistent in human tissues, with estimated half-lives ranging between 5 and 10 years. The levels of dioxins in the environment and the food chain were studied by de Jong et al. (22), who showed that in the Netherlands the daily intake ranges between 30 and 70 pg TEQ, the bulk of the intake originating from milk and fat. These intakes are within the tolerable limits for dioxins (0.006–100 pg of 2,3,7,8-TCDD) as set by the World Health Organization.

To control dioxin pollution, three emission indicators are evaluated: the concentration of dioxins in the atmosphere in fg/m^3, dioxin depositions in ng TEQ/m^2, and the dioxin concentrations in cow's milk in pg TEQ/g fat. The dioxin concentration in fat of cow's milk in the northern part of Belgium (Flanders) was 1.4 pg TEQ dioxin/g fat in 1997 (30). In the Netherlands, 382 g TEQ/yr of dioxins were emitted into the air by municipal incinerators, whereas the traffic emitted 7 g TEQ/yr of dioxins in 1991 (24).

The effect of dioxins on humans is controversial, although it has been proposed that they have hormone-active properties. Dioxins cross the cell membranes and bind to a receptor in the cytoplasm. They act through

POLYCHLORINATED DIBENZODIOXINS

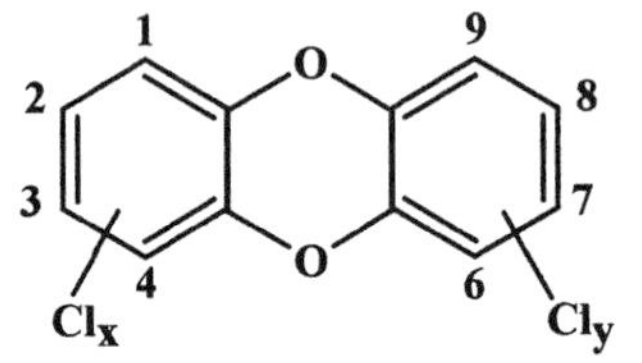

POLYCHLORINATED DIBENZOFURANS

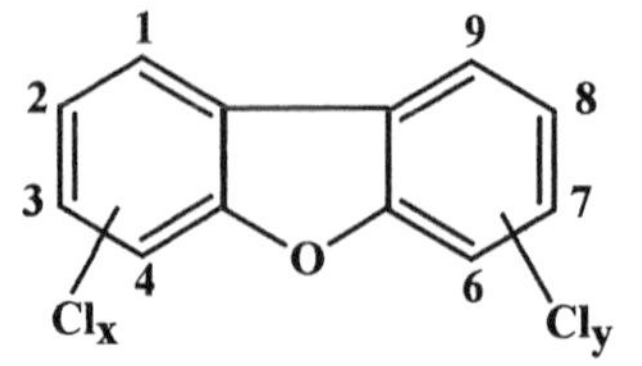

Compound		Toxic equivalent fator (TEQ)
2,3,7,8-Tetrachlorodibenzodioxin	TCCD	1
1,2,3,7,8-Pentachlorodibenzodioxin	P$_e$CDD	0.5
1,2,3,4,7,8-Hexachlorodibenzodioxin	H$_x$CDD	0.1
1,2,3,7,8,9-Hexachlorodibenzodioxin	H$_x$CDD	0.1
1,2,3,6,7,8-Hexachlorodibenzodioxin	H$_x$CDD	0.1
1,2,3,4,6,7,8-Heptachlorodibenzodioxin	H$_p$CDD	0.01
Octachloordibenzodioxin	OCDD	0.001
2,3,7,8-Tetrachlorodibenzofuran	TCCF	0.1
2,3,4,7,8-Pentachlorodibenzofuran	PeCDF	0.5
1,2,3,7,8-Pentachlorodibenzofuran	PeCDF	0.05
1,2,3,4,7,8-Hexachlorodibenzofuran	HxCDF	0.1
1,2,3,7,8,9-Hexachlorodibenzofuran	HxCDF	0.1
1,2,3,6,7,8-Hexachlorodibenzofuran	HxCDF	0.1
2,3,4,6,7,8-Hexachlorodibenzofuran	HxCDF	0.1
1,2,3,4,6,7,8-Heptachlorodibenzofuran	HpCDF	0.01
1,2,3,4,6,8,9-Heptachlorodibenzofuran	HpCDF	0.01
Octachlorodibenzofuran	OCDF	0.001

Fig. 4 Chemical structures of polychlorinated dibenzodioxins and polychlorinated dibenzofurans. The toxic equivalent factor is given for the 17 dioxins; 2,3,7,8-tetrachlorodibenzodioxin (TCDD) has TEQ = 1, the other related compounds have a TEQ between 0.5 and 0.001.

a ligand-activated transcription factor, termed the dioxin or aryl hydrocarbon receptor (Ahr), which acts in concert with another structurally related protein—the aryl hydrocarbon nuclear translocator (Arnt). The formed complex is transported to the nucleus and is involved with different biological functions. Dioxins have been related to developmental and reproductive toxicities, dermal toxicity, endocrine effects, hepatotoxicity, carcinogenesis, and the induction of diverse phase I and phase II drug-metabolizing enzymes. Many toxic effects such as endometriosis and the reproductive and developmental problems observed in wildlife populations appear to be related to TCDD-like congeners (Fig. 3) (16,26,31,32).

B. Heavy Metals

The chemical and physical characteristics of inorganic residues in the ashes and emissions of incinerators are different from the metals in the waste, due to chemical reactions at high temperatures in the presence of oxygen, chlorine, fluorine, and sulfur. For example in the presence of hydrogen chloride, lead chloride ($PbCl_2$) is formed. The reaction products are more soluble in water and can be toxic and affect health. The biological effects of the emission of heavy metals in the environment were first monitored by the use of mosses (33). Heavy-metal uptake takes place through the surface of the plants and vegetables. The metal content was analyzed with inductively coupled plasma atomic emission spectroscopy (ICP-AES) and atomic adsorption spectrometry (AAS). Heavy metals and their reaction products from dialysis materials are only a minor part of the pollution produced by the heavy metal industries and by vehicle exhaust emissions.

C. Plasticizers

As already discussed, a substantial element of the medical waste generated during renal replacement therapy consists of polyvinylchloride. PVC has attracted considerable environmental attention since its manufacture consumes some 30% of the world production of chlorine. Vinyl chloride monomer is a potent carcinogen. Other environmental issues of concern include emissions during production, the use of heavy metals as stabilizers, the migration of plasticizers, and the emission of hydrogen chloride and dioxin during incineration. The most commonly used plasticizer is DEHP. The plasticizer is also used in many nonmedical products, and as a consequence, this compound has been detected in the environment (34). DEHP is a clear oily liquid, which is highly fat soluble but poorly water soluble. It is not bound to the PVC and readily migrates within and out of the matrix when in contact with protein-containing solutions such as blood or fluids used for parenteral nutrition. This migration is influenced by a variety of factors, including temperature, the amount of free surface phthalate on the inner walls of the tubing, the amount of phthalate that moves from the bulk of the material to the inner surface by diffusion, the solubility of phthalate in the perfusate, and the mechanical stress to the material (e.g., caused by blood pumps in the extracorporeal circuit).

Early clinical concerns regarding plasticizers were focused on their release from blood storage bags (35–39). Plasticizer kinetics in extracorporeal circulatory procedures has also received attention (40). For patients receiving regular dialysis therapy, the results in the literature show a considerable variability; Nassberger et al. (39) estimate the release per treatment to range between 7.7 and 8.4 mg, while Kevy and Jacobson (40) found much larger releases (32–90 mg/dialysis). In a more recent study by Ljunnggren (41), the amount of DEHP extracted from blood tubing sets over a 6-hour period ranged between 52 and 73 mg.

The clinical consequences of repeated plasticizer exposure in patients being treated for end-stage renal disease have not been fully elucidated. Mettang et al. (42) failed to demonstrate a relationship between the amount of plasticizer present and the intensity of pruritus; however, their studies showed that postdialysis concentrations in serum of DEHP as well as its major derivatives, mono-2-ethylhexyl phtalate (MEHP) and phthalic acid, were elevated. The same group also studied the kinetics of DEHP and its derivatives in patients receiving CAPD treatment (8). The results indicate that patients on CAPD are regularly exposed to considerable amounts of phthalic ester derivatives and that MEHP appears to be absorbed across the peritoneal membrane.

D. Ethylene Oxide

Ethylene oxide gas remains the most widely used mode of sterilization for medical disposables, and concerns about environmental and health problems for the patients related to the release of ethylene oxide have been expressed. As a consequence, manufacturers are increasingly turning to less polluting alternative sterilization methods such as steam and γ-irradiation.

VII. REDUCTION OF ENVIRONMENTAL POLLUTION AND STRATEGY FOR THE SAFE AND ECONOMIC MANAGEMENT OF WASTE

The increased awareness of environmental pollution by stack emissions has led to monitoring such emissions on a national and global scale including via the U.S. space shuttle program and the Mir mission. The latter has measured the distribution of carbon monoxide and nitric oxide in the free troposphere. Control of emissions by legislation has also been introduced. For example, the U.S. Environmental Protection Agency (EPA) has issued rules to control emissions from solid waste incineration plants. These rules govern both municipal and medical waste incinerators. With respect to the latter, the EPA estimates that in the United States the regulation will affect about 2400 incinerators. The result will be a reduction in the emissions of dioxins, lead, cadmium, mercury, etc. of more than 25 tons per annum. Furthermore, reduction of particulate matter, carbon monoxide, and hydrogen chloride will be over 7000 tons as a consequence of the application of the rules.

Minimization of waste may be achieved through any process or activity that avoids, eliminates, or reduces the waste at its source. Methods include the following:

1. Reduce the amount of packaging: The volume and weight of any packaging should be decreased to a minimum to maintain the quality of the device. A reduction could involve dealing with cardboard necessary for packaging as indicated by the recently introduced Packaging and Packaging Waste Directive. The full implementation of the Packaging Waste Directive will eventually lead to a redesigning of packaging allowing its reuse.
2. Organization of pick-up and removal services: The introduction of packaging levies such as those that already exist in France and Germany could be used to underwrite schemes for the collection of packaging waste. Alternatively, reduction of waste may be achieved by the introduction of new technologies such as the Bicart[R] (Gambro AB, Sweden) cartridge constructed of polypropylene for bicarbonate powder used in the production of dialysis fluid, which can be recycled after use.
3. Sorting of waste at the source: The correct implementation of a waste strategy requires sorting of different types of waste: clinical and domestic waste, glass, and paper. Such an approach reduces the cost since the disposal of medical waste is more expensive than the disposal of domestic waste. The sorting of waste at the source requires extra space, which may not be readily available. The placing of medical waste in domestic waste bags must be avoided, since this would not only endanger health but also leads to prosecution. Sorting at the source is clearly an important measure. Within the United Kingdom, this approach is still in its infancy. However, a pilot study in Scotland during 1996 showed that the introduction of waste sorting at the point of production led to a 30% reduction in medical waste (43). Whether individual renal units or hospitals will adopt this approach will depend largely on the costs of implementing such a measure as well as on future regulatory changes.
4. Recycling plastics: Recycling of medical plastics can partially reduce the incineration of waste, as only nonmedical risk materials can be used. Recycling of tubings or CAPD bags can only provide materials of lower quality and purity than the original polymer. Recycling cardboard, paper, and glass is environmentally more advantageous than recycling PVC.
5. Reuse of dialyzers: Historically, hospitals use supplies and equipment that are cleaned and sterilized between uses. Today products for single use have replaced many such items. The reprocessing of materials raises a number of technical, economic, ethical, and legal issues. Within the United Kingdom reuse is not widespread. The Medical Device Agency (MDA) bulletin DB 9501 clearly outlines the responsibilities of the user and the reprocessor and suggests that reuse of single-use devices should only be undertaken if stringent requirements are met to ensure that the reprocessed item is safe and retains its integrity. In contrast, in the United States 77% of the renal units reuse the dialysis membranes, with the average number of reuses being 14 (44). Reuse of membranes reduces not only the number of units handled and disposed of but also reduces the amount of packaging materials. Before reuse, great care should be given to remove as much as possible the clotted blood, fibrin, and deposited proteins remaining at the end of treatment and restoring the device to its original condition. The device

is then further disinfected and stored until the next use, at which time the disinfecting fluid is removed. Historically disinfection was undertaken with formaldehyde (HCHO). The use of formaldehyde was associated with a number of problems; at air levels above 0.13 ppm formaldehyde is an irritant, and the threshold limit for long-term exposure is 3 ppm. Prolonged exposure to formaldehyde has been associated with asthma and contact dermatitis. Repeated exposure of patients' blood to trace amounts of formaldehyde has, on the other hand, been responsible for the production of antibodies to the N antigen of the red cell surface MN antigen system (45). The most commonly used reagent used in the reprocessing of dialyzers is Renalin^R, in which the active disinfection components are hydrogen peroxide and peracetic acid. Glutaraldehyde-based solutions have also been used for reprocessing; the environmental exposure limits for glutaraldehyde are 0.2 ppm. The fluids used to clean and sterilize dialyzers during reprocessing are disposed of via domestic drains. Aldehydes decompose to formic acid. Hydrogen peroxide and acetic acid in themselves are harmless in the environment, but peracetic acid reacts with bleach (hypochlorite) to form hydrochloric acid. The mixture of the two compounds is a strong oxidizing agent, which may damage metal drains and pipes either within the renal unit or in the hospital.

6. Replacement of PVC by materials giving less dioxin pollution: PVC and the subsequent exposure of peritoneal dialysis fluid to plasticizers may be minimized by use of alternative materials, such as polyoleofins, for CAPD bags. Similarly, the PVC bloodlines may be replaced by polyurethane. However, chlorine is present in many sources other than PVC, so that removal of PVC will have a rather modest impact on dioxin emission.
7. Better control by governments of emissions and ashes of waste incinerators and improvement in the combustion of waste incinerators: The emission and formation of dioxins in waste incinerators can be reduced by (23): (a) complexation of metals with ethylenediaminetetraacetic acid (EDTA) inhibits the forming of dioxins, (b) Addition of basic compounds such as potassium hydroxide (KOH) and disodium carbonate (Na_2Co_3) to change the acidity of the fly ash to inhibit the formation of dioxins, (c) cleaning of the flue gas to remove the PCDD/PCDFs that are already formed, and (d) using filter systems that work at higher or lower temperatures than the optimum temperatures for the formation of PCDD/PCDFs.
8. Electrical energy from the heat generated from incinerators: Because medical waste is largely incinerated, this provides a potential energy source. Although the incineration of waste, particularly that containing plastics, has been a problem in the past, the introduction of legislation to control emissions and the construction of new incinerators offers the possibility of the generation of heat from this source. Domestic waste is already sorted and selectively burned in many cities. For example, in the city of Newcastle upon Tyne, 54% of the waste generated from domestic households is burned. This provides 2,000,000 British thermal units (BtU) of energy per annum as well as 15,000 megawatts of electricity, which is fed into the National Grid and for which the city is paid. The Department of Environment estimates that the potential energy available from the incineration of medical waste is equivalent to the incineration of 0.2 million tons of coal.
9. Biodegradable polymers: The application of biodegradable polymers in medicine are hitherto limited to implantable devices, where elimination of the device is necessary. The materials most frequently used are copolymers of lactic acid and glycolic acid. Degradable polymers for disposals and their packaging are not manufactured. Research is necessary to develop new materials and to study degradation processes in particular conditions. It is evident that degradable polymers should reduce the amount of combustible waste and thus decrease environmental pollution.

VIII. CONCLUSION

In the 1980s and 1990s the quality of the devices and materials were central in the evolution of medical technology, resulting in improved health care. This was realized by the invention of new synthetic materials, by the introduction of disposable medical devices, by better-controlled production processes, and by scientific and clinical research on the performance of new materials.

In the treatment of renal failure bioincompatibility was a major problem caused by cellulose membranes. Recently, the industry produced new materials and modified the cellulose membranes, and new synthetic membranes became available.

Plasticizers in PVC of bags and tubings leak out the polymeric material into the blood of patients. New plasticizer-free polymers are now manufactured. Meanwhile the consumption of synthetic materials resulted in enormous amounts of waste, causing damage to human health and the environment. Waste incineration products (e.g., dioxins) contaminate the environment, persist in the food chain, and are toxic to and slowly damage living organisms.

The time has come to find a balance between the environment, industry, and the economy. New materials should be evaluated not only on their biocompatibility, but also on their environmental impact at the different stages of their production and as waste. Research on the effects of pollution on health and teaching medical students and health professionals the dangers of environmental pollution are of great importance. It is the responsibility and the task of governments, industries, and consumers of medical devices to protect the environment and to guarantee the quality of life on earth in this millennium.

REFERENCES

1. Pearson LS. The 1995 medical device technology raw materials survey. Med Device Technol 1995; (Sept):38–41.
2. The Freedonia Group Inc., Cleveland Ohio. Medical plastics, the shape of things to come. Med Device Technol 1996; (Sept):34.
3. The Freedonia Group Inc., Cleveland Ohio. Medical plastics. Med Device Technol 1997; (Jan/Feb):38–29.
4. Klinkman H, Vienken. Membranes for dialysis. J Nephrol Dial Transplant 1995; 10(suppl 3):39–45.
5. Masuda T, Fukui K. Cellulose triacetate as membrane material. In: LaGreca G, Ronco C, eds. Cellulose Triacetate Evaluation of a Dialysis Membrane. Milan: Wichtig, 1994:9–20.
6. Tabouy LJ, Chauvet-Monges AMT, Brunet PJ, Braguet DL, Garcia PA, Berland YF, Crevat AD. In vitro mitochondrial test to assess haemodialyser biocompatibility. Nephrol Dial Transplant 1997; 12:1635–1639.
7. Krautzig S, Manhiout A, Koch KM, Lemke HD. Reuse with oxidizing agents leads to a loss of polyvinylpyrrolidone from polysulfone membranes. Blood Purif 1994; 12:176.
8. Mettang T, Thomas S, Kiefer T, Fischer FP, Kuhlmann U, Wodarz R, Rettenmeir AW. The fate of leached di-(2-ethylhexyl)phthalate in patients undergoing CAPD treatment. Perit Dial Int 1996; 16:58–62.
9. Carozzi S, Nasini MG, Schelotto C, Caviglia PM, Santoni O, Pietrucci A. A biocompatibility study on peritoneal dialysis solution bags for CAPD. Adv Perit Dial 1993; 9:138–142.
10. Fischer FP, Passlick-Deetjen J, Kirchgessner J, Kuhlmann U, Mettang T. Polyolefin-containing CAPD bags and PMO function. Nephrology 1997; 3(suppl 1):S407.
11. Blass CR. PVC as a biomedical polymer-plasticizer and stabilizer toxicity. Med Device Technol 1992; (April): 32–40.
12. Versieck, Cornelis R. Trace Elements in Human Plasma or Serum. Boca Raton, FL: CRC Press, 1989.
13. Hasselriis F, Licata A. Analysis of heavy metal emission data from municipal waste combustion. J Hazardous Mater 1996; 47:77–102.
14. Kreuzer M. Spreading the message: the significance of CE-marking. Med Device Technol 1998; (May):38–39.
15. Mettang T, Fischer FP, Dunst R, Kuhlmann U, Rettenmeier AW. Plasticizers in renal failure: aspects of metabolism and toxicity. Perit Dial Int 1997; 17(suppl 2): S31–36.
16. Thornton J, McCally M, Orris P, Weinberg J. Dioxin and medical waste incinerators. Public Health Rep 1996; 111:299–313.
17. Tong HY, Monson SJ, Gross ML, Huang LQ. Monobromopolychlorodibenzo-p-dioxins and dibenzofurans in municipal waste incinerator flyash. Anal Chem 1991; 63:2697–2705.
18. Schlatter C. Environmental pollution and human health. Sci Total Environ 1994; 143:93–101.
19. Kang JJ, Fang HW. Polycyclic aromatic hydrocarbons inhibit the activity of acetylchlolinesterase purified from electric eel. Biochem Biophys Res Comm 1997; 238:367–369.
20. Perera FP. Environment and cancer: Who are susceptible? Science 1997; 278:1068–1073.
21. Harrad SJ, Jones KC. A source inventory and budget for chlorinated dioxins and furans in the United Kingdom environment. Sci Total Environ 1992; 126(1–2): 89–107.
22. de Jong AP, Liem AK, Hoogerbrugge R. Study of polychlorinated dibenzodioxins and furans from municipal waste incinerator emissions in The Netherlands: analytical methods and levels in the environment and human food chain. J Chromatogr 1993; 643:91–106.
23. Addink R, Paulus RH, Olie K. Prevention of polychlorinated dibenzo-p-dioxins/dibenzofurans formation on municipal waste incinerator fly-ash using nitrogen and sulfur compounds. Environ Sci Technol 1996; 30: 2350–2354.
24. Olie K, Addink R, Schoonenboom M. Metals as catalysts during the formation and decomposition of chlorinated dioxins and furans in incineration processes. J Air Waste Manage Assoc 1998; 48:101–105.

25. Buser HR, Rappe C, Bergqvist PA. Analysis of polychlorinated dibenzofurans, dioxins and related compounds in environmental samples. Environ Health Perspect 1985; 60:293–302.
26. Watts RJ. Hazardous Wastes: Sources, Pathways, Receptors. New York: John Wiley, 1997:116–119.
27. Huang LQ, Tong HY, Donnelly JR. Characterization of dibromopolychlorodibenzo-p-dioxins and dibromopolychlorobenzo-furans in municipal waste incinerator flyash using gas chromatography/mass spectrometry. Anal Chem 1992; 64:1034–1040.
28. Alvarez R. Standard reference materials for dioxins and other environmental pollutants. Sci Total Environ 1991; 104:1–7.
29. Publikatieblad van de Europese Gemeenschappen (Publications from the European Communities), Nr.L 113/11, April 1997.
30. Vlaanse Milieumaatschappij. Milieu- en natuurrapport Vlaanderen: thema's. Leuven-Apeldoorn: Mira-T, 1998: 60–67.
31. Safe S. Polychlorinated biphenyls (PCBs), dibenzo-p-dioxins (PCDDs), dibenzofurans (PCDFs), and related compounds: environmental and mechanistic considerations which support the development of toxic equivalency factors (TEFs). Crit Rev Toxicol 1990; 21(1): 51–88.
32. Koninckx PR, Braet P, Kennedy SH, Barlow DH. Dioxin pollution and endometriosis in Belgium. Hum Reprod 1994; 9:1001–1002.
33. Markert B, Herpin U, Siewers U, Berlekamp J, Lieth H. The German heavy metal survey by means of mosses. Sci Total Environ 1996; 182:159–168.
34. Bauer MJ, Herrmann R. Estimation of the environmental contamination by phthalic acid esters leaching from household wastes. Sci Total Environ 1997; 208(1–2): 49–57.
35. Baker RW. Diethylhexyl phthalate as a factor in blood transfusion and haemodialysis. Toxicology 1978; 9(4): 319–329.
36. Smistad G, Waaler T. Migration of plastic additives from soft polyvinyl chloride bags into normal saline and glucose infusions. Acta Pharm Nord 1989; 1(5): 287–290.
37. Rubin RJ, Ness PM. What price progress? An update on vinyl plastic blood bags. Transfusion 1989; 29:358–361.
38. Kicheva YI, Kostov VD, Chichovska M. In-vitro and in-vivo studies of the effect of the concentration of plasticizer di(2-ethylhexyl) phthalate on the blood compatibility of plasticized poly(vinyl chloride) drain tubes. Biomaterials 1995; 16(7):575–579.
39. Nassberger L, Arbin A. Ostelius J. Exposure of patients to phthalates from polyvinyl chloride tubes and bags during dialysis. Nephron 1987; 45(4):286–290.
40. Kevy SV, Jacobson MS. Hepatic effects of phthalate plasticizer leaks from poly (vinyl chloride) bags following transfusion. Environ Health Perspect 1982; 45: 57–64.
41. Ljunnggren L. Plasticizer migration from blood lines in hemodialysis. Artif Organs 1984; 8:99–102.
42. Mettang T, Thomas S, Kiefer T, Fischer FP, Kuhlmann U, Wodarz R, et al. Uraemic pruritus and exposure to di-(2-ethylhexyl) phthalate (DEHP) in haemodialysis patients. Nephrol Dial Transplant 1996; 11(12):2439–2443.
43. Mallick NP, Jones E, Selwood N. The European (European Dialysis and Transplantation Association-European Renal Association) Registry. Am J Kidney Dis 1995; 25(1):176–187.
44. U.S. Renal Data System, USRDS 1997 Annual Data Report. Bethesda, MD: National Institutes of Health, National Institute of Diabetes and Digestive and Kidney Diseases, 1997.
45. Klein E. Effects of disinfectants in renal dialysis patients. Environ Health Perspec 1986; 69:45–47.
46. Getting Sorted: The Safe and Economic Management of Hospital Waste. London: Audit Commission Publications, Her Majesty's Stationery Office, 1997.

48

Perioperative Anesthetic Management of the High-Risk Renal Patient

William C. Wilson and Ravindra L. Mehta
University of California, San Diego, San Diego, California

I. INTRODUCTION

This chapter reviews the perioperative anesthetic considerations for management of the high-risk renal patient. The fundamental principles emphasized include (a) avoidance of acute renal failure (ARF) in patients at risk (due either to preexisting disease or to the nature of the operative procedure) and (b) limitation of uremia-related complications in patients with known preexisting chronic renal failure (CRF) or insufficiency. For patients with CRF, emphasis is placed upon recognition of the major pathophysiological changes, understanding the effects of renal failure on drug kinetics, and avoidance of techniques that may jeopardize residual renal function (1).

II. PREOPERATIVE EVALUATION

Appropriate perioperative management for high-risk patients depends on identifying and minimizing important risk factors for complications and quickly treating problems when they occur. Accordingly, the first step is to identify the patient at high risk for ARF and to evaluate those with preexisting CRF in terms of systemic manifestations frequently encountered.

A. Identification of the Patient at High Risk for ARF

In a recent meta-analysis of preoperative risk factors for postoperative renal failure (involving 28 studies and 10,865 patients), preexisting renal disease emerges as the most important preoperative risk factor for the development of postoperative ARF (2). Unfortunately, few studies use the same criteria for ARF, and there is a lack of consistent criteria for establishing risk factors. Furthermore, the literature provides little quantitative information concerning the degree of risk associated with most risk factors. However, certain systemic diseases, several known nephrotoxic drugs, and certain surgical procedures or conditions are associated with an increased risk of renal failure (Table 1).

B. Preoperative Considerations for the CRF Patient

1. Neurological

Several neurological and psychological considerations are common to patients with CRF. These patients are chronically fatigued, may be depressed and lethargic, have a decreased seizure threshold, and may have muscular irritability and autonomic and peripheral neuropathies. The possibilities of drug interactions regarding any antidepressants and the effects of perioperative medications upon seizure threshold must be considered. For example, etomidate lowers the seizure threshold, may promote hypertension, and should be avoided unless the patient is hemodynamically unstable, in which case etomidate becomes the induction drug of choice. Enflurane should be avoided in renal failure patients for seizure threshold issues (as well as fluoride-induced

Table 1 Risk Factors for Perioperative Acute Renal Failure

Category	Disorder/drug/procedure/comments
Preexisting Renal Insufficiency	↓'d GFR, ↓'d renal reserve
Systemic diseases with renal effects	Congestive heart failure
	Diabetes
	Liver failure, jaundice
	Peripheral vascular disease
	Polycystic kidney disease
	Renovascular hypertension
	Rheumatoid arthritis
	Scleroderma
	SLE
	Wegener's granulomatosis
Nephrotoxic drug exposure	Acetominophen (usually with hepatotoxicity)
	Allopurinol
	Aminoglycosides (proximal tubule necrosis)
	Amphotericin B (GN and ATN)
	Asparaginase
	Cephalosporins (especially with aminoglycosides)
	Cisplatin (ATN)
	Cyclosporin-A
	I.V. contrast (oliguria within 24 h)
	Methotrexate
	NSAIDs (especially phenacetin, indomethacin, ibuprofen, naproxen)
	Nitrosoureas
	Penicillins (interstitial nephritis)
Procedures associated with ARF	Biliary surgery
	Burns
	Cardiac surgery
	Genitourinary/Obstetric
	Transplant
	Trauma
	Vascular surgery (especially suprarenal x-clamp)
Intra-op hypovolemia Intra-op hypotension	Prolonged hypotension or hypovolemia can cause ARF in normal patients and exacerbates the renal effects of all the above conditions.

↓'d = Decreased; GFR = glomerular filtration rate; SLE = systemic lupus erethematosis; GN = glomerulonephritis; ATN = acute tubular necrosis; I.V. = intravenous; NSAIDS = nonsteroidal antiinflammatory drugs; ARF = acute renal failure; X-clamp = cross clamp.

renal toxicity) unless no other potent vapors are available, as may occur in certain foreign countries.

2. Cardiovascular

Cardiovascular complications are common in patients with CRF.

Hypertension is present in the majority of patients with CRF for a variety of reasons: (a) increased activity of the renin-angiotensin-aldosterone (RAA) system, (b) sequelae of systemic disease causing CRF (diabetes mellitus, systemic lupus, scleroderma, etc.), as outlined in Table 2, or (c) fluid overload. Intravascular volume overload may also lead to congestive heart failure (CHF). Prys-Roberts (3) demonstrated that hypertensive patients manifest increased hemodynamic lability (higher highs and lower lows) compared to normotensive patients, thus blood pressure control with drugs and preoperative dialysis is recommended. Hypotension during induction may occur following overaggressive preoperative dialysis and consequent intravascular depletion.

Pericarditis and pericardial effusions are common in end-stage renal disease (ESRD) and can contribute to myocardial irritability and failure. Uremic cardiomyopathy is multifactorial in etiology, developing from a combination of chronic fluid overload, hypertension, uremic toxins, and atherosclerotic coronary artery dis-

Table 2 Anesthetic Considerations and Preventative Measures for Systemic Diseases Associated with CRF

Systemic disease	Anesthetic implication(s)	Preventative measures
Preexisting renal insufficiency (↓'d GFR)	Fluid overload/Volume depletion	Ensure euvolumeia, Maintain adequate MAP
	Hypertension	
	Decreased renal reserve	Avoid nephrotoxins
	↓'d clearance & ↑'d drug bioavailability	↓ drug dose and ↑ interval
Diabetes	Difficult laryngoscopy	Awake intubation
	Gastroparesis	Full stomach precautions
	HTN	Maintain MAP
	CAD	5 Lead ECG
	PVD	Consider A-line, PAC
	Hyperglycemia	Glucose control
Rheumatoid arthritis	Difficult laryngoscopy	Awake intubation
	↓'d FRC, pleural effusions	Maintain ↑'d FIO_2/PEEP
	CAD	5 Lead ECG
	Steroid dependency	Periop. corticosteroids
	Joint limitation	Careful positioning
Scleroderma	Difficult laryngoscopy	Awake intubation
	Myocardial fibrosis	Avoid myocardial depressants
	Conduction problems	5 Lead ECG
	Gastroesophageal reflux	Full stomach precautions
SLE	↓'d FRC, pleural effusions	Maintain ↑'d FIO_2/PEEP
	Steroid dependency	Periop. corticosteroids
	↓'d seizure threshold	Avoid abrupt ↓'d (sedative)
	Post-op infections	Antibiotics, pulmonary care
Wegener's	Difficult laryngoscopy	Awake intubation
	Pulmonary involvement	Maintain adequate FIO_2/PEEP

↓'d = Decreased; ↑'d = increased; MAP = mean arterial blood pressure; HTN = systemic hypertension; CAD = coronary artery disease; PVD = peripheral vascular disease; ECG = electrocardiogram; A-line = arterial catheter; PAC = pulmonary arterial catheter; FRC = functional residual capacity; FIO_2 = fractional inspired oxygen concentration; PEEP = positive end expiratory pressure.

ease, as well as from many of the systemic diseases that cause CRF to develop, such as scleroderma, systemic lupus erythematosus, and rheumatoid arthritis.

Left ventricular hypertrophy, diastolic dysfunction, dilated cardiomyopathies, and diminished responsiveness to alpha and beta receptors due to autonomic dysfunction can all contribute to diminished responsiveness to acute hemodynamic changes (4). Thus ESRD patients should be carefully evaluated preoperatively with regard to cardiovascular disease. Evidence of ischemia should be evaluated with either thallium persantine or dobutamine echocardiogram preoperatively. Furthermore, these patients should be monitored intraoperatively with a 12 lead electrocardiogram (ECG) for detection of ischemic and/or electrolyte-mediated electrophysiological abnormalities. Because of diastolic dysfunction, fluid bolus tolerated by a normal individual may lead to ventricular dilation and congestive heart failure. Thus, CRF patients should receive intraarterial and central venous pressure (CVP) monitoring for large body weights with expected fluid shifts. Patients with preoperative evidence of failure or known LVEF < 35%, pulmonary hypertension, should also be monitored with a transesophageal echo (TEE) and pulmonary artery catheter (PAC).

3. Airway and Pulmonary

Airway difficulties are not unusual in patients with CRF. However, most of the airway considerations relevant to CRF patients originate as sequelae of systemic diseases responsible for causing the CRF, such as rheumatoid arthritis or diabetes (Table 2). Indeed, Hogan et al. (5) found that difficult laryngoscopy occurred in only 2.7% of renal transplant recipients without diabetes and in 32% of those with long-standing diabetes.

Table 3 Airway Complications to Avoid in Renal Failure Patients

Complication	Reasons Risk ↑'d with CRF	Anesthetic Principles
Failure to intubate and/or ventilate	Many diseases causing CRF are associated with intubation difficulty	Evaluate airway, if predictably difficult, intubate awake
Perioperative hypoxemia	CRF patients suffer from ↓'d FRC, ↑'d Qs/Qt, ↑'d V/Q mismatch, anemia, and ↑'d VO_2 All these factors ⇒ hypoxemia	Preoxygenation (100% O_2) with a properly fitting face mask will ↑ the PAO_2, PaO_2, @ ↑ induction. ↑ FIO & PEEP will ↑ intraop PaO_2
Esophageal intubation	An ↑'d incidence of esophageal intubation occurs with difficult airways; DA can be associated with CRF; esophageal intubation must always be considered and avoided	Esophageal intubation is a problem of recognition, not commission; ETTs placed electively or emergently must be verified with end-tidal CO_2, fiberoptic bronchoscopy, etc.
Aspiration	Aspiration risk is ↑'d in CRF patients due to gastroparesis, ↑'d acidity and volume of gastric contents, and ↑'d rate of reflux	Cricoid pressure should be applied to all CRF patients undergoing an IV induction; patients with known difficult airways should be intubated awake
Hemodynamic compromise	Postdialysis hypovolemia, cardiomyopathy, ↑$[K^+]$, ↓$[Ca^{2+}]$, ↑'d response to induction drugs, ↓'d response to α & β agonists	Consider CRF patients dry until proven otherwise; start an IV, use ↓ doses of hypnotics, have fluids and pressors handy prior to ETT

PAO_2 = Partial pressure of oxygen; ETT = endotracheal tube; RSI = rapid sequence intubation; TTJV = transtracheal jet ventilation; C-spine = cervical spine.

Table 3 summarizes the airway complications and anesthetic considerations frequently encountered in CRF patients.

The primary mechanism for difficult laryngoscopy in diabetic CRF patients is the diabetic "stiff joint syndrome," which is characterized by decreased cervical spine flexibility and especially decreased mobility at the atlanto-occipital (A-O) joint (6).

The principal airway manifestations of rheumatoid arthritis include cricoarytenoid joint and temperomandibular joint (TMJ) arthritis and limitation of cervical spine mobility (ankylosis) (7). Because there is paradoxical hypermobility at the A-O joint, most of the neck motion is forced to hinge at this fulcrum, leading to an increased risk of cervical spine injury during direct laryngoscopy. The cricoarytenoid joint involvement in diabetic renal failure patients may present with hoarseness, stridor, or difficult intubation due to decreased vocal cord mobility and inability to pass a standard-sized endotracheal tube (ETT). Successful intubation frequently requires use of a fiberoptic bronchoscopic and a small ETT in awake, topicalized, patients (8).

Wegener's granulomatosis involves both renal and pulmonary manifestations. The important difficult airway considerations involve tracheal malacia and stenosis. Wegener's patients frequently present to the operating room (OR) for laser bronchoscopy and/or airway stent placement. However, some may present for other procedures, such as renal transplant, without any previously recognized airway concerns. The characteristic saddle nose deformity (due to Wegener's-induced cartilage destruction) is an important diagnostic feature, which should alert the anesthesiologist of the likelihood of Wegener's-associated airway issues.

Scleroderma patients have thickened inelastic skin and decreased neck range of motion. Scleroderma patients have been known to present to the OR with an unexpected difficult airway. Indeed, despite an entirely normal preoperative airway examination (except for decreased neck range of motion), scleroderma patients may be impossible to intubate using conventional techniques (9).

Difficult airway can also result from complications of life-saving therapy necessary to treat the specific conditions associated with renal failure (e.g., chemotherapy for head and neck cancer, chronically ventilated burn, or trauma patients). Additional discussion regarding these and other pathological or anatomical conditions associated with difficult airways may be found in a recent review by Wilson and Benumof (10).

Pulmonary considerations include pleural effusions

and pulmonary edema (hypoalbuminemia, fluid overload, congestive heart failure). Additionally, CRF patients, particularly those on peritoneal dialysis (PD), may have decreased functional residual capacity (FRC) and are thus at increased risk of atelectasis and increased right-to-left shunt. Additional factors which impair gas exchange include pulmonary edema due to reduced water excretion, decreased serum albumin, and heart failure. In the case of PD patients, lung volume is diminished by the PD fluid. These patients should have their PD fluid drained immediately prior to entering the OR. Additionally, chest infections are more common in CRF patients (partially due to reduced immunity).

4. Fluids, Solutes (Electrolytes and Metabolites), pH

The fundamental problem resulting from ARF and CRF is an inability to regulate the internal milieu, including fluids, solutes (albumin, electrolytes, BUN, creatinine, and other waste products) as well as acid-base balance.

In ARF, oliguria typically persists for 10–20 days, occasionally as long as 30–45 days. During this period dialysis will be required every 2–3 days. During the diuretic phase, 5–6 L of urine are made daily, and management focuses upon replacing fluid and electrolyte losses. The urine specific gravity is typically 1.010 (isosthenuric) at this time as the kidney is unable to dilute or concentrate. However, if the patient survives, renal function usually returns toward normal over time.

If dialysis is not undertaken during the acute phase, several deleterious changes will occur:

1. There will continue to be a progressive rise in blood urea nitrogen (BUN) creatinine, uric acid, magnesium, phosphate, sulfate, polypeptides, and organic acids.
2. Potassium will rise 0.3–3.0 mEq/L/day, unless there are concomitant gastrointestinal (GI) losses (diarrhea or vomiting). The potassium rise is greatest in muscular patients or those suffering from rhabdomyolysis, trauma, or burns. The hyperkalemia will cause peaked T waves on ECG, then progress to wide complex QRS and eventually electromechanical dissociation (EMD) or ventricular fibrillation (V-Fib) arrest. Unfortunately, serum calcium is typically decreased, and this further exacerbates the electrophysiological changes.
3. A decrease in serum proteins, especially albumin, along with hyponatremia and anemia will exacerbate the propensity toward fluid leaving the capillary membranes causing pulmonary edema and also tend to decrease the volume of distribution of protein-bound drugs (i.e., increase the free fraction available to act pharmacologically).
4. The increased inorganic acids (phosphate, sulfate) and organic acids lead to a combined anion gap/nonanion gap metabolic acidosis.
5. Increased products of metabolism, urea, hypermagnesemia contribute to decreased alertness and prolongation of neuromuscular blockade.

Reduced clearance of renally excreted aminoglycoside antibiotics, metabolic acidosis, and hypocalcemia are additional conditions that tend to prolong neuromuscular blockade in CRF patients. The characteristic electrolyte and acid-base changes seen with CRF are shown in Table 4.

Elective surgery should be delayed until dialysis is completed for patients suffering from the fluid or solute changes reviewed above. In patients on CRRT, this may be continued in the OR during long procedures. However, a nurse or technician with expertise in CRRT must be available to manage this during the operation, with the anesthesiologist and nephrologist collaborating on therapeutic goals.

5. Gastrointestinal

GI considerations include increased gastric emptying time, as well as a propensity for nausea and vomiting.

Table 4 Anesthetic Implications of Electrolyte and Acid-Base Changes Associated with CRF

GFR <50%	Nonanion gap metabolic acidosis Inadequate $NaHCO_3$ reabsorption
GRF <30%	Mixed gap, nonanion gap metabolic acidosis Retention of fixed acids ($SO_4^=$, $PO_4^=$)
GFR <15–30%	Hyperkalemia Inability to excrete dietary load of potassium Hypocalcemia Phosphate retention and inadequate activation of vitamin D Hypermagneseumia

Hypermagnesiumea, hypocalcemia, and metabolis acidosis potentiate the effects of nondepolarizing NMBs
Chronic hyperphosphatemis leads to atherosclerosis, disruption of the cardiac conduction pathways
Patients with GFR <15% but also on CVVHD may have hypophosphatemia

CRF = Chronic renal failure; GFR = glomerular filtration rate; NMB = neuromuscular blocking drugs; CVVHD = continuous venoveno hemodialysis.

Thus, metoclopramide, cisapride, or other gastropropulsive drugs may be of benefit as premedications. Cisapride is chemically similar to metoclopramide but lacks the central nervous system–depressant and antidopaminergic effects that can occur with metoclopramide. Cisapride has been associated with Q-T interval prolongation and Torsade de pointes, particularly when used in combination with other drugs that inhibit its clearance (e.g., erythromycin) (11).

Additionally, cricoid pressure should be applied and a rapid sequence or modified rapid sequence induction should be considered whenever airway intubation is required. However, if the patient is known to have a difficult airway, or significant risk factors for difficult intubation, an awake intubation should be planned (12).

Other GI considerations include hiccoughs, which may persist even during general anesthesia, necessitating neuromuscular blockade for cases that require complete lack of movement (e.g., neurosurgical procedures). There is also a tendency toward GI ulceration with the possibility of GI bleeding. Prophylaxis with H_2 blockade should commence at least 30 minutes prior to induction of anesthesia.

Finally, drug-related and viral hepatitis (types C and B predominantly) as well as hemosiderosis may lead to chronic hepatic congestion. Universal precautions should be observed, and hepatotoxins must be avoided in these patients as well.

6. Endocrine Disease

Endocrine manifestations of CRF include activation of the renin-angiotension, aldosterone pathways leading to hypertension. Additionally, secondary hyperparathyroidism occurs leading to demineralization of bone calcium stores and the potential for pathological fractures, especially in end-stage patients who have not received calcium supplements. Be careful when moving and positioning these patients. Additional endocrine abnormalities include carbohydrate intolerance, hyperuricemia, and adrenal insufficiency.

7. Bleeding Tendency (Platelet Defect)

Uremic patients have a tendency to bleed due to a platelet factor deficiency, von Willebrand's component of factor VIII (vWF). Although thrombocytopenea does occur in CRF, the platelet count is usually in the normal range but the bleeding time is prolonged. Desmopressin acetate (dDAVP) 0.03 μg/kg IV slowly over 30 minutes will improve bleeding time by inducing the release of vWF from storage sites on the vascular endothelium. Onset occurs at 0.5–1 hour, and duration is 8 hours. However, a period of 1–3 days must elapse before a second dose will have a similar effect. Alternatively, conjugated estrogen 3 mg/kg IV divided over 5 daily doses is efficacious prior to major operations and may have a persistent effect for 2–3 weeks.

Frequent dialysis will also improve bleeding time (13). Similarly, administration of packed red blood cells (PRBCs) and administration of erythropoietin have both demonstrated improvement in reversing uremia-induced bleeding time prolongation.

8. Anemia

CRF is associated with an anemia of chronic disease which is multifactorial in origin. Decreased erythropoietin, as well as decreased RBC lifespan (hemolysis from RBC membrane fragility), intrinsic marrow suppression (partly resulting from decreased iron, folate, vitamin B_{12}, and B_6), and chronic hyperparathyroid-induced marrow fibrosis all contribute to the anemia. Not surprisingly, given the multifactorial nature of the anemia associated with CRF, hemotological laboratory findings include a normochromic normocytic profile with hematocrit ranging between 20 and 25%.

Anemia decreases the oxygen-carrying capacity of blood. The chief compensation invoked to increase the oxygen delivery (DO_2) in CRF patients is increased cardiac output. Additionally, metabolic acidosis and increased 2,3-diphosphoglycerate facilitate oxygen offloading to the tissues (i.e., rightward shift in the oxyhemoglobin disassociation curve). Beware of conditions that impair these compensatory mechanisms (i.e., myocardial depression, alkalosis, hypothermia, hypophosphatemia—as may occur with CVVHD).

C. Evaluation of Preoperative Volume Status

A quick evaluation of the patient's volume status can be made by palpating the peripheral pulse, blood pressure, heart rate, presence of orthostatic hypotension, skin color and turgor, and quality of mucous membranes. However, many patients with ESRD are hypertensive and may have strong peripheral pulses, despite recent dialysis, and relative intravascular depletion. Thus, even in the setting of a robust preoperative hemodynamic evaluation, induction drug dosages should be modified and titrated to hemodynamic response.

D. Review of Available Lab Data

The chest radiograph and ECG should be thoroughly reviewed by the anesthesiologist prior to planning the anesthetic care. The presence of pleural effusions, cardiomegaly, etc. are frequently encountered in renal failure patients and can complicate care. Similarly, ECG evidence of myocardial ischemia may trigger need for further evaluation or increased preoperative medical management and intraoperative monitoring. Serum potassium should be 5.0 mmol/L or less. Values above 5.5 mmol/L should be addressed prior to induction of anesthesia. Close coordination among the surgeon, anesthesiologist, and nephrologist promotes optimum preparation of the patient. If necessary, dialysis should be performed prior to the surgery and anticoagulation should be avoided or a minimal amount of heparin should be used.

E. Informed Consent

After a thorough review of the history, physical, and laboratory data, an assessment of risk factors relating to patient and procedural issues can be made. The anesthesiologist is obligated to discuss the risk of anesthesia, and the surgeon likewise discusses the operative risks with the patient prior to surgery. Sufficient information must be provided to allow the patient or his or her surrogate to make an informed decision regarding the plans, risks, and alternate forms of therapy. It is often helpful for the nephrologist to be present when the discussion for surgery is done as the patient usually has had a long-term relationship with the nephrologist and it can make the process somewhat easier.

III. PREPARATION FOR ANESTHESIA AND SURGERY

Much of the preparation for surgery may have already transpired during the initial preoperative evaluation. However, the anesthesiologist may assume care for the patient during any stage of the evaluation process and must verify that all of the important work performed up until that point has been done correctly, including a survey of airway, breathing, circulation, IV access, laboratory data monitoring, and positioning issues.

A. Establishing or Maintaining a Definitive Airway

Plans for establishing or confirming a definitive airway are a first priority. Because of several issues common to renal insufficiency (increased incidence of delayed gastric emptying), a consideration of a rapid sequence induction of anesthesia is generally indicated. However, patients with anatomical, pathological, or historical indicators of difficult intubation (see Sec. II.B) should have their trachea intubated awake (i.e., difficult airway considerations should be prioritized higher than aspiration considerations). Indeed, Ovassapian et al. (13) intubated the tracheas of 108 consecutive patients at high risk for aspiration using an awake fiberoptic technique without a single case of aspiration.

B. Intravenous Access

Fragility of vessels requires careful and gentle manipulation while placing peripheral IVs and arterial lines in CRF patients. At least one moderately large-bore (16g) peripheral IV must be established for ESRD patients at risk of significant blood loss to ensure hydration. Avoid arterial or venous cannulation in the same extremity as an arterial-venous (A-V) fistula. Central venous access should be considered in patients with poor peripheral veins. The right atrial pressure can serve as a measure of intravascular volume in CRF patients. However, consideration should be made for placement of an internal jugular vein (9fr) catheter-introducer for placement of a PA catheter in patients with congestive heart failure or pulmonary artery hypertension.

C. Monitoring the High-Risk Renal Patient

Monitoring for patients with renal failure includes standard American Society of Anesthesiologists (ASA) monitoring, as well as arterial and central venous access. Ability to monitor exhaled gas CO_2 concentration is useful for ensuring adequacy of ventilation. Urine output may be nonexistent, thus TEE CVP and/or Swan-Ganz catheter may be necessary.

1. Monitoring and Preservation of Residual Renal Function

A clinically accurate measure of renal preservation and function does not exist. Decreased urine output and rising serum BUN and creatinine are the standard indicators for the development of worsening ARF. Creatinine (which is nether secreted nor reabsorbed to any appreciable amount in patients with normal renal function) is a good inverse measure of GFR. However, creatinine elevations occur after the renal insult has occurred and only reflect the degree of renal insufficiency once a steady state is achieved. Indeed, a doubling of serum creatinine generally represents a 50% decrease in GFR at steady state. However, creatinine may double from 0.8 to 1.6 in a 24-hour period in a patient with essentially zero GFR because it takes that long for creatinine to accumulate in the blood. Serial determination of creatinine clearance is currently the most sensitive test for predicting the onset of perioperative renal dysfunction; however, the test is not practical for measuring renal function under OR conditions (14). The ability to measure intrarenal blood flow distribution may ultimately improve our predictive and diagnostic abilities to assess perioperative ARF. However, methodological constraints limit its use at this time.

2. Monitoring Intraoperative Volume Status

Systolic pressure variation (SPV) is a technique for gauging intravascular volume status, which we find very useful in renal failure patients. Arterial blood pressure has long been known to decrease with positive pressure ventilation. SPV is a method of quantifying these changes. Perel has shown in both animal experiments and clinical studies that SPV directly correlates with intravascular depletion (15,16). Indeed, when the systolic pressure (delta down component) decreases by more than 10 mmHg in patients ventilated with 10–15 cc/kg, these patients are clinically volume underresuscitated (see Fig. 1).

D. Positioning for Patients with Renal Failure

1. Protection of Arterial-Venous Fistula

CRF patients possessing an A-V fistula for dialysis access should be examined preoperatively for the presence of a bruit and or thrill. The A-V fistula characteristics should be documented in the preoperative evaluation note. During the anesthetic, the A-V fistula should be reexamined every 30 minutes throughout the case to ensure patency. The continued presence (or abrupt absence) of a bruit or thrill should be chronicled in the anesthetic record. Additionally, IVs, tourniquets, and blood pressure cuffs should be relegated to the contralateral extremity in order to promote A-V fistula patency.

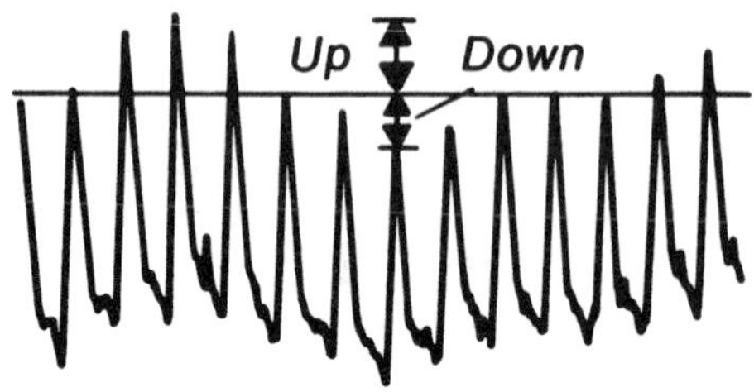

Fig. 1 The Systolic Arterial Pressure Variation (SPV) can be used as a measure of ventricular responsiveness to volume. A decrease in LV preload (either from hypovolemia, or absence of atrial augmentation) will be manifest by an increase in the Δ Down component of the SPV curve. (From Ref. 15, used with permission.)

2. Gentle Manipulation and Positioning of Anesthetized ESRD Patients

Anesthetized ESRD patients must be gently manipulated during positioning because the decreased mineralization of bone calcium (due to secondary hyperparathyroidism) increases the risk that pathological fractures may occur during positioning. Additionally, the skin and vessels of ESRD patients are fragile, partly due to uremic factors and partially due to the side effects of corticosteroids, which may be used for systemic diseases causing CRF or as immunosuppressive therapy following renal transplantation. The supine position with arms extended away from the body and supported upon arm boards provides for excellent venous and arterial access intraoperatively. However, certain procedures (e.g., coronary artery bypass grafting) require that the arms be tucked close to the patient's side, promoting improved surgical access. Padding of dependent body parts is required to minimize hypoperfusion/pressure-induced tissue ischemia.

IV. INTRAOPERATIVE ANESTHETIC MANAGEMENT

The goals for anesthetic management for patients with renal failure are shown in Table 5. Besides physiological stability, analgesia and amnesia should be ensured once the patient's hemodynamic status is demonstrated to be stable enough to tolerate anesthetics.

A. Pharmacological Considerations in the Renal Failure Patient

Renal failure causes several physiological changes that have pharmacokinetic and pharmacodynamic interaction on administered drugs. Pharmacokinetic effects describe how the drug concentration in the body may be altered because of renal failure, whereas pharmacodynamic effects describe how a given concentration of drug in the blood may have increased or decreased potency due to factors associated with ESRD.

The pharmacokinetics of a drug are determined by the volume of distribution (Vd) and the clearance of the active drug (and active metabolites). The volume

Table 5 Goals for General Anesthesia for High-Risk Patients

1. Reestablish and/or maintain normal hemodynamics
   a. For hypotension, fluids first, then vasopressors
   b. For hypertensives, preop BP control (esp. w/β-blockade)
   c. Frequent evaluation of base deficit, hct., Uo (unless anephric)
   d. Titration of additional anesthetics if robust BP
2. Maximize surgical exposure and minimize tissue edema
   a. Limit fluids according to needs
   b. Limit blood loss by allowing anesthetic catch-up
   c. Muscle relaxation should be optimized (frequent small doses)
   d. NGT or OGT to empty stomach and decompress bowel
   e. Avoid N_2O, (if necessary, use only briefly)
3. Limit hypothermia
   a. Monitor core temperature
   b. Warm fluid
   c. Keep patient covered and room warm
4. Help limit blood loss and coagulopathy
   a. Encourage surgeon to stop and pack if blood loss excessive
   b. Frequently monitor hct, ionized Ca^{2+}, plt and coag studies
   c. Provide calcium PRN large citrated product administration
5. Limit complications to other systems
   a. Monitor ICP, maintain CPP > 70
   b. Monitor PIP, be vigilant for PTX
   c. Measure urine output
   d. Monitor peripheral pulses
6. Preserve vascular access sites
   a. Save veins on nondominant hand (if no access in place)
   b. Monitor and maintain patency of vascular access (fistulae/graft)
   c. Avoid use of tunneled or nontunneled access catheters

Hct = Hematocrit; Uo = urine output; BP = blood pressure; NGT = nasogastric tube; OGT = orogastric tube; N_2O = nitrous oxide; Ca^{2+} = calcium; ICT = intracranial pressure; CPP = cerebral perfusion pressure; PIP = peak inspiratory pressure; PTX = pneumothorax.

of distribution can be calculated by dividing the intravenous drug dose (in milligrams) by the plasma concentration (mg/mL). The volume of distribution is decreased for most anesthetic drugs in renal failure patients, meaning that there is a greater fraction of active drug for any mg amount of drug administered. The clearance of water-soluble drugs (e.g., many neuromuscular blocking drugs and reversal agents) occurs predominantly via the kidney and is thus prolonged. However, most drugs are lipid soluble in the active phase, become metabolized by the liver to charged species, and are then excreted by the kidneys. Most drugs used during anesthesia have a decreased clearance in renal failure, thus they are present longer in the body than usual.

The pharmacodynamics of most drugs in renal failure are also altered in such a way that a given concentration of drug has a greater than normal effect at the receptor site. Indeed, the MAC for inhaled drugs is decreased. In general, drug dosages in renal failure patients should be decreased by 20–50%.

B. Induction of General Anesthesia in Renal Failure Patients

Hypotension can occur at induction by direct myocardial depression and vasodilation from the drugs, suppression of endogenous catecholamines, as well as the initiation of positive pressure ventilation. Patients at high risk for developing postoperative renal failure (diabetes, peripheral vascular disease, coronary artery disease, polycystic kidney disease) or hypotension (trauma, pump failure, intravascular depletion, sepsis, and other vasodilated states) must be judiciously monitored to ensure maintenance of blood pressure at induction and beyond.

1. Induction of Anesthesia (General Considerations)

It has been frequently said that more soldiers were killed during World War II by thiopental than by bullets. Indeed, Halford wrote a compelling negative critique of pentothal following the Pearl Harbor experience (17). However, in the same edition of *Anesthesiology*, Adams and Gray present a case (with an accompanying editorial) clarifying that it is not necessarily the drug but rather the *dose* that is lethal to the hemodynamically unstable patients (18).

Thiopental and propofol should be avoided for induction in unstable renal failure patients. These patients best tolerate etomidate (0.2 mg/kg) (Table 6). Indeed, even ketamine, which is known to have indirect sympathomimetic properties, may promote hypotension in hypovolemic patients (because of ketamine's direct myocardial depressant effects) (19).

2. Specific Induction Drugs

Etomidate is an imidazole derivative that provides remarkable hemodynamic stability in critically ill pa-

Table 6 Induction Drugs, Sedatives, and Analgesics for High-Risk CRF Patients

	IV Dose	Metabolite	Comments
Induction Drug			
Propofol	0.25–0.5 mg/kg For non-CRF patients: 2 mg/kg	Hepatic and pulmonary metabolism	Although propofol has numerous benefits when administered to elective patients and is satisfactory for stable CRF patients, it is relatively contraindicated in the hypovolemic CRF patient
Thiopental	0.5–1 mg/kg For non-CRF patients: 4 mg/kg	Hepatic metabolism	Although the standard induction dose of thiopental is 4.0 mg/dL, in the CRF patient, less is appropriate; if hemodynamically unstable, much less (dose-dependent myocardial depression and systemic vasodilation)
Etomidate	0.2 mg/kg	Renal cleared and hepatic metabolism	Induction drug of choice for hemodynamically unstable CRF patients; multiple doses may worsen acidosis and cause adrenal suppression
Ketamine	1–2 mg/kg	Norketamine	Larger doses release endogenous catecholamines leading to hypertension and tachycardia; however, ketamine causes direct myocardial depression, which will cause hypotension in hypovolemic CRF patients (already maximal sympathetic output)
Sedative			
Midazolam	0.05 mg/kg	1-Hydroxy midazolam	Rarely used for induction, mainly used as a sedative
Diazepam	0.05 mg/kg	Oxazepam	Rarely used for induction, mainly used as a sedative
Analgesic			
MSO_4	0.1 mg/kg	Morphine-6 glucuronide	Analgesic doses provided; induction doses are 1–5 mg/kg and associated with significant histamine release
Fentanyl	2 μ/kg	Hepatic metabolism	Analgesic dose provided at left; induction doses are 25 μg/kg
Meperidine	1 mg/kg	Normeperidine	Normeperidine causes seizures; meperidine is not an induction drug.

tients. In stable patients with ischemic heart disease and valvular disease, etomidate does not cause significant alteration in hemodynamic parameters (20). However, etomidate like any drug that causes loss of consciousness, can lead (indirectly) to hypotension in patients who are maintaining their cardiovascular system via a high resting catecholamine state. In repeat doses etomidate can cause adrenal suppression. Etomidate, like valium, is dissolved in propylene glycol, which is irritating to veins (pain, phlebitis). Furthermore, the propylene glycol can lead to significant metabolic acidosis and renal failure if administered as an infusion or as multiple induction dose equivalents for prolonged periods.

Etomidate is metabolized primarily in the liver, with the majority of metabolites excreted via kidneys (85%) and bile (13%), and only 2% is excreted unchanged (21). The standard induction dose is 0.2–0.3 mg/kg IV. Specific guidelines for dosage adjustments for patients with renal impairment have not been developed and are probably unnecessary. However, prolonged infusions in CRF patients are contraindicated due to the propylene glycol–mediated metabolic acidosis.

Ketamine, a phencyclidine derivative, is a unique

disassociative anesthetic that produces amnesia and intense analgesia. Ketamine interacts with at least three receptor types: (a) antagonist at *N*-methyl D-aspartate (NMDA) receptors responding to L-glutamate, (b) opioid agonist at μ receptors (analgesia) and κ receptors (dysphoria), (c) CNS muscarinic receptor antagonist. The standard induction dose for ketamine is 2–5 mg/kg IV, or 5–10 mg/kg IM. When very small doses of ketamine (0.5–2 mg/kg) are used, respiration and airway reflexes usually remain intact. Larger doses may trigger release of endogenous catecholamines, often leading to hypertension and tachycardia. However, ketamine is a direct myocardial depressant. Cardiomyopathic or hypovolemic CRF patients, like other hemodynamically unstable patients, may have a high baseline endogenous sympathetic tone. In these patients, the myocardial depressant properties of ketamine prevail and severe hypotension may occur. Ketamine is a bronchial smooth muscle relaxant (22), making it suitable for use in asthmatic patients. Recovery from ketamine can be associated with hallucinations.

Ketamine is metabolized in the liver by the microsomal enzymes to metabolites, which are then altered to the glucuronid form and excreted into the urine. Specific guidelines for dosage adjustments in renal impairment have not been developed, as no dosage adjustments are needed for infrequent intermittent administrations. However, prolonged infusions are not recommended as the metabolites are 90% renally excreted.

Thiopental is a derivative of barbituric acid. Sodium thiopental is the standard intravenous induction drug used by many anesthesiologists. The standard induction dose in stable patients is 4–6 mg/kg. The induction dose in hemodynamically unstable patients must be significantly decreased (i.e., 0.5–0.25 mg/kg in some patients with CHF). The induction dose of thiopental should be decreased in ESRD patients because of the lower volume of distribution. The major side effects of thiopental are dose-dependent depression of respiration and hypotension secondary to a combination of cardiac depression and systemic vasodilation. Hypotension with thiopental and other induction agents can be life-threatening in volume-depleted ESRD patients.

Propofol, an alkylphenol derivative, is a relatively new hypnotic agent that appears to have several advantages over thiopental for certain procedures (23). Emergence from brief anesthetics with propofol is extremely rapid because it is cleared more rapidly from the brain than thiopental. This is due to propofol's larger volume of distribution and high clearance from the blood (clearance actually exceeds hepatic blood flow). Propofol has some intrinsic antiemetic properties, and patients frequently emerge from anesthesia hungry and euphoric. Another benefit of propofol is its recently recognized intrinsic bronchodilator affects.

Despite these benefits, propofol is relatively contraindicated in hemodynamically unstable CRF patients. The hemodynamic side effects of propofol are similar to those of thiopental. Propofol causes irritation and discomfort during intravenous administration. This is reduced by administration it into larger veins and following pretreatment with intravenous lidocaine (0.5 mg/kg) or fentanyl (2 μ/kg).

Propofol is metabolized in the liver by conjugation to inactive glucuronide and sulfate metabolites and eventually excreted via the kidneys. The clearance of propofol exceeds estimated hepatic blood flow, suggesting extrahepatic routes of metabolism. The elimination half-life of 3–12 hours is the result of slow release of propofol from fat stores, but this is clinically insignificant. In normal patients, about 70% of a single dose is excreted renally in 24 hours (90% in 5 days). The kinetics of propofol are minimally affected by chronic hepatic or renal disease. However, for hemodynamic considerations, the induction dose of propofol (like pentothal) should be decreased in CRF patients.

Midazolam is a short-acting benzodiazepine used for anxiolysis and amnesia, as a premedication and during conscious sedation, monitored anesthetic care cases, and rarely as an induction agent. Midazolam has an induction time similar to pentothol. However, its prolonged recovery time and significantly higher cost limit midazolam's use as an induction drug compared to pentothal. Midazolam's mechanism of action is mediated by binding to, and potentiating, the inhibitory neurotransmitter gamma-aminobutyric acid (GABA). Midazolam has twice the affinity for GABA benzodiazepine receptors than does diazepam.

Midazolam is primarily metabolized via the liver to alpha-hydroxymidazolam, which is equipotent to midazolam. Other, less pharmacologically active metabolites (1-hydroxymidazolam and 1,4 hydroxylmidazolam) are produced in small amounts (<5% of the dose is metabolized) and are conjugated by the liver with subsequent renal excretion.

Although the half-life of midazolam is not markedly prolonged in patients with CRF, the renally excreted metabolites will accumulate, and the peak levels of midazolam can be higher in these patients. Additionally, CRF patients can experience hemodynamic instability during induction and prolonged recovery from anesthesia. Furthermore, prolonged recovery times following continuous infusion of midazolam for sedation have been reported in intensive care unit (ICU) patients with renal impairment.

Diazepam is a long-acting benzodiazepine. Because diazepam is the most rapidly absorbed benzodiazepine following an oral dose, it is used orally for the short-term management of anxiety disorders and acute alcohol withdrawal, as a skeletal muscle relaxant, and by anesthesiologists as a premedication providing anxiolysis and amnesia. However, diazepam's long duration of action limits its usefulness for conscious sedation, and monitored anesthetic care cases. In the ICU, diazepam is used mainly as a prophylactic or treatment for alcohol withdrawal, whereas midazolam, ativan, and propofol are favored as sedation medications owing to their shorter duration of action.

The half-life of diazepam is 30–60 hours. Metabolism of diazepam is primarily hepatic and involves demethylation and 3-hydroxylation. Diazepam is primarily metabolized to one major active metabolite (desmethyldiazepam) with a half-life of 30–100 hours. However, two minor active metabolites are also formed: temazepam (3-hydroxydiazepam) and oxazepam (3-hydroxy-*N*-diazepam), with half-lives of 9.5–12 and 5–15 hours, respectively. At therapeutic doses, desmethyldiazepam is found in plasma at concentrations equivalent to those of diazepam. Oxazepam and temazepam plasma concentrations are usually undetectable. All three metabolites are subsequently glucuronidated and excreted in the urine. Thus, diazepam dosage must be decreased for CRF patients on the basis of degree of renal impairment and clinical response.

3. Opiates (Morphine, Fentanyl, Meperidine)

a. Morphine

Morphine is derived as an alkaloid extract from the unripened seed capsules of the opium poppy, *Papaver somniferum*. It was first isolated in 1803 and is the prototype of the opiate agonists. Today, the poppy plant is still the source of the drug because synthesis of morphine is difficult. Morphine is the prototypical opiate analgesic used for the relief of moderate to severe acute and chronic pain, preoperative sedation, and as a supplement to anesthesia. Morphine is the drug of choice for pain associated with myocardial infarction and cancer. Morphine, as well as other opioids, can produce feelings of euphoria, well-being, and tranquility, subjecting them to potential abuse.

Metabolism of morphine occurs primarily in the liver but also may occur in the brain and kidneys. Morphine is conjugated with glucuronic acid to form 3-glucuronide (50%), 6-glucuronide (5–15%), and 3,6-glucuronide and other minor metabolites. Morphine 3-glucuronide antagonizes morphine and may cause hyperalgesia and myoclonus occasionally seen with high-dose morphine therapy. In addition, the 3-glucuronide metabolite may be important in the development of tolerance to morphine. Morphine 6-glucuronide is a more potent analgesic than morphine and contributes to morphine's clinical activity. With chronic dosing of morphine, the glucuronide metabolites accumulate in concentrations greater than that of morphine. Excretion occurs predominantly in the urine and bile as the morphine 3-glucuronide and 6-glucuronide metabolites. In patients with renal dysfunction, accumulation of the morphine 3-glucuronide and 6-glucuronide occurs at an excellerated pace, leading to prolonged serum levels and increased toxicity. Thus, morphine dosage should be modified to prevent accumulation of the metabolites and their effects.

b. Fentanyl

Fentanyl is a lipid-soluble opiate with an analgesic potency approximately 100 times greater than morphine (10 mg morphine = 100 μg fentanyl = 75 mg meperidine). The alpha elimination curve for fentanyl is significantly more rapid than for morphine and meperidine. However, the beta-elimination curve for fentanyl is similar to that for morphine and meperadine. Thus, for normal patients small doses of fentanyl (50–250 μg) have a short clinical duration (30–45 min), whereas larger doses (>1000 μg) last as long as morphine (3–4 h). Fentanyl is used to aid induction and maintenance of general anesthesia and to supplement regional and spinal analgesia.

Drug accumulation or prolonged duration of action with fentanyl can occur in patients with renal impairment. Patients with ESRD require close monitoring, decreased dose, and less frequent dosing intervals to avoid overdosing. Patients with less renal impairment should receive doses modified depending on clinical response and degree of renal impairment.

c. Meperidine

Meperidine is a synthetic opiate belonging to the phenylpiperidine class. Outside the United States meperidine is known as pethidine; in the United States it is known as demerol. Other members of this group include diphenoxylate and loperamide, agents commonly used to treat diarrhea, as well as the extremely potent analgesics fentanyl, alfentanil, and sufentanil. Meperidine is recommended for relief of moderate to severe pain but also has the unique ability to interrupt postoperative shivering (24) and shaking chills induced by amphotericin B (25). Meperidine is metabolized to normeperidine, a compound capable of inducing seizures when it accumulates. Thus meperidine is not a good choice for the chronic treatment of pain or prolonged use in ESRD patients (increased risk of seizures due to accumulation of normeperidine). If necessary to provide to a patient with renal insufficiency, the following adjustments are recommended:

CrCl > 50 mL/min: no dosage adjustment needed
CrCl 10–50 mL/min: reduce recommended dose by 25%
CrCl < 10 mL/min: reduce recommended dose by 50%

B. Maintenance of General Anesthesia in Renal Failure Patients

Sedative and amnestic drugs should be titrated as blood pressure allows, because hemodynamically unstable patients receiving only oxygen and neuromuscular relaxants may have recall if they survive (26). Anesthesia can be maintained with inhalational vapors or intravenous drugs such as propofol, and opioid supplementation is frequently appropriate.

1. Intravenous Anesthetics

All of the induction drugs mentioned above can be used for IV maintenance. However, repeated doses or prolonged infusions of certain drugs are not recommended in CRF patients. For example, etomidate in repeated doses may cause adrenal suppression. Furthermore, propylene glycol, the diluent used with etomidate, can cause a severe metabolic acidosis, which would undoubtedly be more profound in renal failure patients. Prolonged infusions of ketamine and barbiturates may lead to prolonged emergence in renal failure patients. In contrast, infusion of propofol are compatible with rapid emergence (27). Finally, there is no particular requirement for total IV anesthesia for patients with renal failure, and most inhaled drugs are less expensive and equally satisfactory anesthetics.

2. Volatile Anesthetics

All volatile anesthetics produce dose-dependent depression of myocardial contractility. Desflurane, isoflurane, and sevoflurane maintain cardiac output better than enflurane or halothane (mainly through a peripheral vasodilation effect), whereas halothane maintains blood pressure better at the same MAC level of either isoflurane or enflurane (28). The only volatile anesthetic drug proven to cause direct renal injury is the fluoride-related nephrotoxicity of methoxyflurane (29) (Table 7). However, enflurane and sevoflurane are best avoided due to a theoretical potential for renal injury.

Jaundice and liver failure are significant independent risk factors for perioperative renal failure. As such, hepatotoxic compounds should be avoided in patients

Table 7 Inhaled Drugs and CRF

Drug (FDA Approval)	MAC (%)	Comments
Halothane (1956)	0.77	Greater decrease in hepatic blood flow than other inhaled drugs; however, not necessarily contraindicated in CRF or renal insufficiency
Methoxyflurane (1959)	0.16	*Absolutely contraindicated in renal insufficiency*; releases large amounts of nephrotoxic F^- ion over a long time; no longer used in United States
Enflurane (1972)	1.7	Chemical isomer of isoflurane, provides excellent skeletal muscle relaxation; however, releases nephrotoxic F^- ion; also, CNS excitation, occasionally promoting seizures; therefore, *relatively contraindicated in renal insufficiency*
Isoflurane (1981)	1.1	Lower blood solubility allows for a more rapid change in anesthetic depth than with enflurane or halothane; however, less rapid than Des or Sevo
Desflurane (1993)	6.0	Very low blood:gas partition coefficient, but pungency obviates use during inhaled induction; cardiovascular effects similar to isoflurane; useful at end of case to facilitate rapid extubation conditions
Sevoflurane (1995)	1.7	*Relatively contraindicated in renal insufficiency*; 1995 FDA warning not to use <2 L/min flow, 1.25 MAC × 8 hr in 2 L/min flow in volunteers led to proteinuria and PCT and DCT injury

MAC = Minimum alveolar concentration; FDA = Federal Drug Administration; esp. = especially; F^- = fluoride; CNS = central nervous system; Des. = desflurane; Sevo. = sevoflurane; PCT = proximal convoluted tubule; DCT = distal convoluted tubule.

with renal insufficiency or at high risk of such. Halothane was initially associated with the development of fulminant hepatitis. The National Halothane Study, conducted in the mid-1960s, found that halothane was not associated with any type of hepatic injury more frequently than any other anesthetic drug (30). However, renal insufficiency patients with preexisting liver disease or hepatic injury constitute a special group. Halothane is known to decrease hepatic blood flow to a far greater degree than any other inhaled drug. Because, isoflurane increases hepatic artery blood flow at both 1 and 2 MAC, it is, in the author's opinion, the maintenance drug of choice for renal insufficiency patients with liver dysfunction (31). Additionally, halothane is arrhythmogenic in higher concentrations particularly in the setting of concomitant hypercarbia and high-dose epinephrine (as may occasionally occur in spontaneously ventilating renal failure patients). Thus it is best to avoid halothane in unstable patients with renal insufficiency because hepatic blood flow may already be compromised by hypotension and/or ischemia.

Sevoflurane is the newest commercially available inhaled anesthetic. Sevoflurane was first developed as a rapid induction and emergence agent due to its insolubility. However, its primary utility has been in smooth, rapid inhaled induction of anesthesia due to its low pungency (well-tolerated) and high potency. Additionally, recovery from anesthesia has been shown to proceed even faster with desflurane than with sevoflurane (32). However, due to the possibility of renal toxicity resulting from sevoflurane, it is best avoided in the setting of renal impairment. Sevoflurane reacts with carbon dioxide absorbents to produce Compound A (CH2F-O-C[=CF2][CF3]). Because of concern about the potential nephrotoxicity of Compound A, sevoflurane was not released in the United States until 1995 (4 years after release in Japan). The current package insert warning recommends the use of fresh gas flow rates of 2 L/min. Despite this concern, sevoflurane has been used safely since 1991 in Japan, without significant nephrotoxicity. Furthermore, although nephrotoxicity was demonstrated in rats, several investigators have been unable to detect significant renal injury following low flow sevoflurane in humans (33,34).

Recently, more sensitive tests of renal injury have demonstrated Compound A–associated renal injury. Indeed, Eger et al. demonstrated that 1.25 MAC sevoflurane plus Compound A produced dose-related injury to glomeruli (i.e., nephrotic range proteinuria) and tubules (i.e., glucosuria and urinary excretion of alpha-glutathione-S-transferase) (35).

In clinical settings with high potential for renal impairment, such as hypotension or toxin exposure (e.g., aminoglycosides, contrast media, rhabdomyolysis) or during anesthesia for severe burns or critically ill patients, sevoflurane is best avoided.

3. Nitrous Oxide

The routine use of nitrous oxide (N_2O) is best avoided in situations involving bowel obstruction and the serious potential of closed space gas accumulation (pneumocephalus, pneumothorax, etc.), however it is otherwise satisfactorily tolerated in renal failure patients. N_2O has the propensity to preferentially fill gas-containing structures (such as pneumothorax, pneumocephaly, and obstructed bowel) and thus causes these structures to expand. This occurs because the blood:gas partition coefficient of N_2O (0.47) is 34 times greater than that of nitrogen (0.014). Thus, the capacity of the blood to bring nitrous oxide to the gas-containing structures is greater than the capacity of the blood to remove nitrogen. N_2O can support combustion and should be avoided if the cautery is used near any distended segment of bowel that contains gas. N_2O can be used during the last 15–30 minutes to promote rapid awakening and regaining of protective reflexes. However, in patients so ill or severely injured that postoperative extubation is not anticipated, there is no benefit to the use of N_2O. Furthermore, when there is a risk of pneumocephalus or pneumothorax, N_2O should be avoided.

C. Neuromuscular Blockade

Neuromuscular blockade (NMB) is required for most intraabdominal neurosurgical, and cardiothoracic surgical cases. In these situations, muscle relaxation facilities exposure or prevents inadvertent patient movement, which could be life-threatening, and thus NMB must be profound. Additionally, patients with ARDS may require NMB to facilitate mechanical ventilation in the ICU and in the OR. When renal insufficiency is present, NMB drugs that are predominantly renally cleared should be avoided (Table 8).

Atracurium and *cis*-atracurium are the only two NMB drugs with durations of action that are not prolonged in renal failure patients. Both atracurium and *cis*-atracurium are metabolized by serum esterases and spontaneous Hofmann elimination to produce laudanosine. The metabolite laudanosine produces seizures in animals and may promote CNS excitatory activity in humans. Because *cis*-atracurium is three times more potent than atracurium and lower doses are required,

Table 8 Comparative Pharmacology of Neuromuscular Blocking Drugs and the Effect of Renal Failure on Duration of Action

	Succinylcholine	Mivacurium	Atracurium Cis-atra	Vecuronium	Rocuronium	Pancuronium	Gallamine
NMB type	Depolarizing	Nondepolarizing	Nondepolarizing	Nondepolarizing	Nondepolarizing	Nondepolarizing	Nondepolarizing
Intubating dose 2X ED_{95} (Mg/Kg)	1–2	0.15	0.4–0.5 0.1 (Cis-atra)	0.1	0.6	0.1	1.0
Time till onset (min)	1–1.5	2.5–4	3–5	3–5	1–2	3–5	3–5
Duration in normal (min)	5–10	10–20	20–30	25–35	35–45	40–70	40–70
Prolongation in RF patient	Minimal	Minimal	None	Minimal	Minimal	Significant	Exceedingly significant
Renal excretion (% unchanged)	Insignificant	Insignificant	Insignificant	15–20	15–25	70–80	95
Biliary excretion (% unchanged)	Insignificant	Insignificant	Insignificant	40–60	50–70	5–10	0
Hepatic metab. (% Degraded)	Insignificant	Insignificant	Insignificant	20–30	10–20	10–30	Insignificant
Hydrolysis in plasma (%)	100 Enzymatic	100 Enzymatic	Spontaneous and enzymatic	No	No	No	No
Histamine release	Minimal	Minimal	Moderate Min (Cis-atra)	None	None	None	None
Utility in renal failure	OK unless $[K^+]$ high	OK	OK unless hypotensive	Slight increased duration	Slight increased duration	Significant and unpredictable increased duration	*Contraindicated* in RF due to increased duration

2X ED_{95} is the normal intubating dose. In emergency situations, the intubating dose of rocuronium can be doubled to increase onset and bring intubating conditions close to that provided by succinylcholine. Cis-atra = *cis*-atracurium, an isomer of atracurium that is three–four times more potent, with less histamine release. Both atricurium and *cis*-atra are metabolized via spontaneous and enzymatic methods.

the corresponding laudanosine concentrations following *cis*-atracurium are one-third those that would be expected following an equipotent dose of atracurium. Additionally, *cis*-atracurium releases less histamine than atracurium and is the best choice for renal failure patients. Additionally, the duration of action of vecuronium is only slightly prolonged and has significant benefits in patients with renal failure (36). Major histamine releasers (e.g., atracurium, curare, metubine) should be avoided during induction in hemodynamically unstable patients (37).

D. Regional Anesthesia and Renal Failure

Neuraxial anesthesia (spinal or epidural) is contraindicated in hemodynamically unstable renal failure patients because it is impractical (patient may not be able to assume the lateral or sitting position for drug placement), takes time to set up, and can result in several common deleterious side effects (sympathectomy-mediated hypotension) and complications (decreased GFR, local anesthetic-induced seizures, total spinal anesthesia, or cardiac arrest). Indeed, in World War I neuraxial blockade was frequently employed, causing Admiral Sir Gordon Taylor to proclaim spinal anesthesia to be "the best form of euthanasia" he knew for war injuries. Furthermore, renal failure itself presents several significant limitations to the use of neuroxial anesthesia (Table 9).

Uremic bleeding is a real concern, which is heightened when contemplating placing a large needle in the epidural or subarachnoid spaces with the theoretical possibility of hematoma formation. The primary platelet dysfunction of uremia is reversed with frequent dialysis (38). When the bleeding time and coagulation profile are normal, neuroaxial blockade should not be avoided on the basis of uremia-related platelet dysfunction.

The addition of small amounts of epinephrine to the local anesthetic solutions (e.g., lidocaine) used for epidural anesthesia is best avoided in uremic patients because the combination of acidosis, hyperkalemia, and elevated catacholamines increase the risk of cardiac dysrhythmias. Furthermore, acidosis decreases the central nervous system threshold for seizures following local anesthetics, thus doses must be carefully titrated to avoid toxicity. These considerations also pertain to local anesthetic and catacholamine administration during topicalization of the airway for awake intubation techniques.

However, regional anesthesia in stable patients with renal insufficiency, or otherwise at risk for renal failure (diabetics, patients with peripheral vascular disease), may be an excellent option. Indeed, regional anesthesia

Table 9 Limitations to Use of Regional Techniques in High Risk Renal Failure Patients

Problem/Limitation	Consequences and Implications	Comments and Tips
Bleeding Tendency	May cause epidural hematoma or spinal cord compression	Frequent dialysis may limit RF induced defect
Sympathetic Block	Hypotension and Bradycardia especially problematic in patients with concomitant autonomic dysfunction	Prehydration and prophylactic vasopressor administration can abate or attenuate these undesired effects (dose titrated to effect)
Decreased Duration	Increased cardiac output is likely etiology of early washout of local anesthetic from epidural space and other regional depots (i.e. brachial plexus)	Continuous techniques (both epidural and axillary block) can mitigate against the increased washout phenomena. Subarachnoid blocks (spinals) are not effected by this phenomena.
Uremic or Diabetic Neuropathy	Renal failure patients with neuropathies are relative contraindications to regional techniques, which may be incorrectly blamed for any exacerbation in condition	Selected use in patients with clear indications is acceptable. Careful pre-op examination and documentation of neurologic function is mandatory for these patients
Uremia Associated Acidosis	Can decrease the seizure threshold	Limit the dose and duration especially in RF patients with uremia or a history of seizures

avoids the administration of drugs with altered activity in renal failure such as muscle relaxants, their antagonists, narcotics, benzodiazepines, etc.

Brachial plexus block is the anesthesia of choice for placement or revision of arterio-venous fistula for dialytic access. However, it should be recognized that the duration of brachial plexus blockade may be decreased by as much as 38% on renal failure patients, as reported by Bromage and Gertel (39). The decreased duration in renal failure patients has been attributed to the increased cardiac output (compensation for anemia) and thus faster tissue washout of the local anesthetic from the brachial plexus.

V. ADJUNCTIVE CONSIDERATIONS FOR THE HIGH-RISK RENAL PATIENT UNDERGOING ANESTHESIA

A. Fluid Management

Patients with renal failure more often than not present to the OR with total body fluid overload and frequently intravascular overload as well, whereas intravascular volume depletion and hypotension play a critical role in morbidity and mortality of acute tubular necrosis associated with anesthesia and surgery. Because urine output is a poor indicator of intravascular volume status in the patient with renal failure or renal insufficiency, central venous or transesophageal echo monitoring is needed to gauge intravascular status.

1. Fluid Administration

Many authors recommend against administration of lactated Ringer's in renal failure patients due to the potassium content. However, the authors believe that lactated Ringer's should not be avoided a priori, as there are only 4 mEq/L of potassium (the same as normal blood), whereas there are normally approximately 4500 mEq of potassium in the body of a 70 kg patient. Thus the total added potassium is negligible. On the other hand, if the patient is hyperkalemic (or at risk due to severe acidosis, rhabdomyolysis, etc.), potassium-containing solutions (lactated Ringer's) should be avoided. If unsure, use normal saline, but be reminded that large quantities of normal saline will exacerbate the hyperchloremic metabolic acidosis associated with acute tubular necrosis.

2. Administration of Human Recombinant Erythropoietin

Because of chronic anemia, preoperative self-donation of autologous blood is usually contraindicated. Preoperative administration of erythropoietin can increase the red cell mass. However, this expensive option should be initiated at least 6 weeks prior to surgery, as it takes 2–3 weeks for significant red blood cell mass (or count) increases, and the extra 3 weeks allow autologous self-donation of two to three units of blood (one unit per week for 3 weeks preoperatively).

3. Readministration of Salvaged Blood from the Operative Field

The use of salvaged blood should be considered for every patient with uremic anemia undergoing surgical procedures with increased risk for significant blood loss. Indeed, several investigators have recently demonstrated the safety and efficacy of retransfusing salvaged blood, even in the setting of intraabdominal trauma (40). Laparoscopy used to collect the blood is becoming a particularly powerful technique (41). For noncontaminated intraabdominal blood involving liver, spleen or retroperitoneal injury, thoracic, or extremity injuries, cell saver technique is considered standard practice.

4. Dopamine or Diuretics to Promote Urine Production

Patients with normal renal function or significant renal reserve preoperatively may have a decrease in urine output intraoperatively. After insuring that the Foley catheter is in the bladder and unobstructed, one must ensure adequate intravascular volume and that the blood pressure for renal perfusion. Once these maneuvers are accomplished, consideration is given to administration of urine-producing drugs.

Dopamine infused in low "renal" doses (2–3 μg/kg/min) is known to promote diuresis and renal blood flow in normal patients. However, dopamine has not been shown to avert the onset of or ameliorate the course of ARF in the OR or in critically ill patients (42). Generally, diuretics and dopamine solely for promotion of diuresis should be avoided in order to ensure that pressure and intravascular volume are adequate. However, certain patients (e.g., lung transplant, pneumonectomy) do not tolerate excessive extravascular water, and thus low-dose dopamine as a diuretic in ventilated, euvolemic patients is warranted. Similarly, conventional diuretics can be used to achieve the same goal.

In patients with ARF or CRF nonresponsive to diuretics and/or dopamine, continuous renal replacement therapy (CRRT) should be contemplated for fluid and solute control in the OR.

B. Acid-Base Management

Acid-base status measured via arterial blood gas sampling and the derived base deficit is frequently abnormal in patients with renal failure. The metabolic acidosis is initially nongap due to HCO_3^- losses. However, over time phosphates and sulfates accumulate, causing a mixed-gap, nongap metabolic acidosis. The metabolic acidosis causes a decreased myocardial response to both endogenous and exogenous catecholamines. However, the oxyhemoglobin disassociation curve is shifted rightward by acidosis, thereby improving oxygen delivery to tissues.

C. Antibiotics and Perioperative Renal Failure

Preoperative antibiotics are frequently employed. Certain antibiotics (e.g., aminoglycosides and vancomycin) have nephrotoxic potential. Additionally, most antibiotics are water soluble and cleared by the kidney and require significant dosage adjustments to avoid severe overdose (aminoglycosides, vancomycin).

Extremity and orthopedic operations are typically covered with a first-generation cephalosporine such as cefazolin. However, open fractures may require addition of an aminoglycoside. Patients with intraabdominal abscesses require broad-spectrum coverage of both gram-positive and gram-negative bacteria (e.g., anaerobes and enterobacteriacea) for these procedures Cefoxitin alone may be as efficacious as clindamycin and tobramycin, or the classic cocktail of ampicillin, gentamicin, and flagyl may be used.

A single preoperative dose of an appropriate antibiotic is adequate prophylaxis for fresh contaminated wounds resulting from penetrating and blunt injuries. Postoperative antibiotics should be reserved for delayed operations (>12 hours postinjury) and for enteric perforations. For surgical cases associated with massive transfusion requirements, antibiotics should be repeated more frequently than in the patient with minimal hemorrhage. However, patients with renal insufficiency have decreased clearance of many antibiotics requiring a decrease in dosage or increase in interval. Optimal duration of treatment under these circumstances is not well established (43).

D. Thermal Management

Hypothermia is a major co-morbid condition that may occur during surgery, and every effort should be made to avoid development of this condition. Pharmacological paralysis prevents normal heat-production mechanisms (shivering), and vasodilating anesthetic agents prevent heat-conservation mechanisms (vasoconstriction). Hypothermia may exacerbate existing platelet defects and prolong the coagulation process. Additionally, hypothermia promotes platelet sequestration, reduces drug metabolism, and induces vasoconstriction. Hypothermia and acidosis combined reflect a decrease in cardiac output and tissue perfusion, thus counteracting an important compensatory mechanism of the patient with renal failure. The hypothermic myocardium is susceptible to ectopy, especially ventricular dysrhythmias. Many studies have identified hypothermia as a factor associated with increased morbidity and mortality in severely injured patients (44). Furthermore, moderate hypothermia (35.5–34.5°C) is neuroprotective and may be tolerated in certain conditions (i.e., no clinical manifestations of bleeding) (45).

Although hypothermia in renal failure per se has not been rigorously studied, a critical, yet frequently overlooked area is the cooling effect of the replacement fluid and dialysate in patients on CRRT. It is now well recognized that there is a significant drop in core temperature if the solutions are not heated (46–48). It is recommended that replacement solutions and dialysate be heated prior to infusion. This is easily achieved with the newer CRRT systems, which have a heater inline, but requires an external heater to be placed in line for the nonintegrated systems.

VI. POSTOPERATIVE CONSIDERATIONS

Postoperative ICU considerations relevant to renal protection include close control of fluid, solute and acid-base status, monitoring for and prevention of bleeding and shock, coagulopathy, and special conditions that can further impair renal reserve (abdominal compartment syndrome, sepsis, MOSF, additional toxin exposure such as aminoglycosides, radiocontrast). Additionally, drug dosages should be modified as described above and nutritional repletion begun early. Three areas require special mention: the need to ensure adequate postoperative oxygenation, ventilation (including treatment of hyperkalemia, abdominal compartment syndrome), and the issues of wound healing and infection.

A. Oxygenation and Ventilation Assured, Beware of Recurization

Following major surgical procedures in high-risk renal patients can be associated with impaired oxygenation (decreased FRC, hypoventilation, right-to-left shunting from atelectesis, fluid overload, leaky capillaries, etc.). Hypoventilation can occur from residual anesthetic concentration (inhaled or intravenous), uremic toxins, as well as residual neuromuscular blockade, or "recurization." Because hypoventilation can occur and renal patients have other pulmonary considerations, oxygen must be supplied postoperatively for the first day postextubation.

Recurization is a phenomenon that occurs when the concentration of neuromuscular blocking drug available to bind at the neuromuscular junction paradoxically increases. This phenomenon is likely to occur when long-acting renally cleared drugs (e.g., pavulon, metubine) are reversed by a short-acting cholinesterase inhibitor (e.g., tensilon). To protect the patient from the recurization phenomenon, use short-acting drugs with minimal renal clearance and avoid reversal drugs until the patient has a complete train of four on neuromuscular blockade monitor, and use longer-acting cholinesterase inhibitors such as physostigmine.

B. Avoiding Large Doses of Analgesics with Renal Clearance

Because of the propensity for hypoventilation and hypoxia, postoperative analgesia must be carefully titrated. Opiate-derived analgesics should be used sparingly. Morphine is metabolized to morphine 6-glucuronide (renally cleared), which has analgesic and respiratory-depressant properties, which can accumulate in patients with renal failure. Demerol should be avoided because its chief metabolite nor-meperidine accumulates in patients with renal failure and can promote seizures. The opiate-based analgesic of choice in patients with renal failure is fentanyl. Because 100 μg of fentanyl is equivalent to 10 mg of morphine, or 75 mg of demerol, fentanyl should be titrated carefully.

C. Aggressive Treatment of Hyperkalemia

Hyperkalemia can become significant in the first 24 hours postoperative as a combination of factors may be operative, such as excess mobilization from injured or necrotic tissue and bank blood administration. Intermittent techniques can rapidly lower potassium, however, CRRT is the ideal mode of postoperative fluid and solute control in the unstable patient. The choice of anticoagulant (heparin, citrate, or no anticoagulant) for CRRT should be based upon the pathophysiology to avoid complications related to dialysis. If dialysis requiring heparin is planned for postoperative fluid and solute balance, efforts should be made to wait 24 hours postoperatively as dialysis may further lower platelet count and the heparin may promote or exacerbate postoperative bleeding.

D. Abdominal Compartment Syndrome

Abdominal compartment syndrome is a condition with particular relevance to renal function. Abdominal compartment syndrome results from increased intraabdominal pressure (IAP), usually due to bowel and interstitial tissue edema following laparotomy in patients with shock and massive fluid resuscitation (49). The increased IAP results in impairment of circulation, decreased tissue perfusion, and renal as well as other organ dysfunction (cardiovascular, gut, pulmonary) (50). The tense abdomen leads to increased peak airway pressures, hypercarbia, and oliguria. Decreased thoracic venous return, with decreased cardiac output and decreased renal function due to hypoperfusion, are components of the syndrome. Additionally, increased IAP causes decreased tidal volume, increased ventilatory pressures, and increased atelectasis. Increased IAP can also cause venous hypertension and elevate ICP.

Abdominal compartment pressures may be monitored by attaching an indwelling Foley catheter to a pressure transducer, leveled to the symphysis pubis (51). Pressures greater than 20–25 mmHg require decompression (52). Normal postoperative abdominal pressure is 0–5 mmHg water. At pressures greater than 10 mmHg hepatic arterial blood flow decreases, at 15 mmHg cardiovascular changes occur, at 15–20 mmHg oliguria occurs, with anuria occurring at pressures between 20 and 40 mmHg (53).

These patients require emergency decompressive laparotomy to relieve the symptoms. However, opening the abdomen results in a rapid decrease in IAP with a resultant reperfusion syndrome that can lead to hypotension and intractable asystole unless proper preparation occurs. Indeed, Morris described asystole following decompression in 4 of 16 patients who underwent rapid decompression (54).

Preparation for decompression of abdominal compartment syndrome involves maneuvers similar to those taken immediately prior to clamp removal during a thoracic aortic aneurysm repair: (a) intravascular volume is increased, (b) dopamine or other inotropes and vasopressors are in line and running, and (c) acidosis (if severe) is treated with sodium bicarbonate. Be ready to increase minute ventilation (but also be prepared to transiently decrease PEEP and driving pressure). The increased minute ventilation will be necessary to eliminate CO_2 (neutralize lactate emanating from gut and increased CO_2 from administered bicarbonate). Calcium chloride is administered to protect against increased potassium that is washed out from the gut. Calcium is also useful to bolster the transient hypocalcemia following sodium bicarbonate administration. Morris et al. (54) recommend 2 L of normal saline, with 50 g mannitol and 50 mEq sodium bicarbonate per L, prior to abdominal wall release.

E. Impaired Wound Healing and Infection

Wound healing is impaired in renal failure patients partly due to uremia, but also secondary to systemic diseases causing CRF (diabetes, CHF, etc.) as well as treatment for systemic diseases (e.g., steroid therapy). These same factors increase the risk of postoperative infections. Thus, all intraoperative procedures must be performed with strict sterility, and postoperative technique must also be meticulous. Nutrition is another important element in the fight against infection and in the promotion of wound healing. Enteral nutrition should be started immediately postoperative unless specifically contraindicated (pancreatitis, perforated viscus, small bowel obstruction).

VII. SUMMARY

The ESRD patient requires several unique considerations to prevent and manage complications related to anesthesia and surgery. An understanding of the pathophysiology of the underlying disease and the requirements for adequate anesthesia and preparation for surgery are key to avoiding adverse outcomes. Provided a systematic approach is followed, the perioperative and operative management of the ESRD patient can be simplified.

REFERENCES

1. Cranshaw J, Holland D. Anaesthesia for patients with renal impairment. Br J Hosp Med 1996; 55(4):171–175.
2. Novis BK, Roizen MF, Aronson S, Thisted RA. Association of preoperative risk factors with postoperative acute renal failure. Anesth Analg, 1994; 78(1): 143–149.
3. Prys-Roberts C. Anaesthesia and hypertension. Br J Anaesth 1984; 56:711–724.
4. Foley RN, Parfrey PS, Harnett, et al. Clinical and echocardiographic cardiovascular disease in patients starting end stage renal disease therapy; prevalence, association and progress. Kidney Int 1995; 47:186.
5. Hogan K, Rusy D, Springman SR. Difficult laryngoscopy and diabetes mellitus. Anesth Analg 1998; 67: 1162–1165.
6. Salzarulo HH, Taylor LA. Diabetic "stiff joint syndrome" as a cause of difficult endotracheal intubation. Anesthesiology 1986; 64:366.
7. Khanam T. Anesthetic risks of rheumatoid arthritis. Br J Hosp Med 1994; 52:320–325.
8. Wilson WC. Emergency airway management. In: Brown D, ed. Cardiac Intensive Care. Philadelphia: W.B. Saunders, 1998:705–734.
9. Kanter GJ, Barash PG. Undiagnosed scleroderma in a patient with a difficult airway. Yale J Bio Med 1998; 71:31–33.
10. Wilson WC, Benumof JL. Pathophysiology, evaluation and treatment of the difficult airway. In: Breen PH, Barash P, eds. Anesthesiology Clinics of North America. Philadelphia: W.B. Saunders, 1998:29–75.
11. Wysowski DK, Bacsanyi J. Cisapride and fatal arrhythmia. N Engl J Med 1996; 335:290–291.
12. Wilson WC. Application of the ASA difficult airway algorithm. In: Hanowell LH, Waldron R, eds. Airway Management. Philadelphia: Lippincott-Raven Press, 1996:119–130.
13. Stewart JH, Castaldi PA. Uremic bleeding: a reversible platelet defect corrected by dialysis. Q J Med 1967; 143:409.

13a. Ovassapian A, Krejcie TC, Yelich SJ, et al. Awake fiberoptic intubation in the patient at high risk for aspiration. Br J Anaesth 1989; 62:13.

14. Kellen M, Aronson S, Roizen MF, Barnard J, Thisted RA. Predictive and diagnostic tests of renal failure: a review. Anesth Analg 1994; 78(1):134–142.
15. Perel A, Pizov R, Cotev S. The systolic pressure variation is a sensitive indicator of hypovolemia in ventilated dogs subjected to graded hemorrhage. Anesthesiology, 1987; 67:498–502.
16. Pizov R, Segal E, Kaplan L, et al. Determinants of systolic pressure variation in patients ventilated after vascular surgery. J Cardiotharac Vasc Anesth 1995; 9(5):547–551.
17. Halford FJ. A critique of intravenous anesthesia in war surgery. Anesthesiology, 1943; 4:67–69.
18. Adams RC, Gray HK. Intravenous anesthesia with pentothal sodium in the case of gunshot wound associated with or accompanying severe traumatic shock and loss of blood: report of a case. Anesthesiology 1943; 4:70–73.
19. Weiskopf RB, Bogetz MS, Roizen MF, Reid IA. Cardiovascular and metabolic sequelae of including anesthesia with ketamine or thiopental in hypovolemic swine. Anesthesiology 1984; 60:214.
20. Gooding JM, Weng J, Smith RA, et al. Cardiovascular and pulmonary responses following etomidate induc-

tion of anesthesia in patients with demonstrated cardiac disease. Anesth Analg 1979; 58:40.
21. Nimmo WS, Miller M. Pharmacology of etomidate. Contempt Anesth Pract 1983; 7:83.
22. Sarma VJ. Use of ketamine in acute severe asthma. Acta Anaesthesiol Scand 1992; 36:106.
23. Sebel PS, Lowden JD. Propofol: a new intravenous anesthetic. Anesthesiology 1989; 71:260–277.
24. Pauca AL, Savage RT, Simpson S, et al. Effect of pethidine, fentanyl and morphine on post-operative shivering in man. Acta Anaesthiol Scand 1984; 28:138–143.
25. Burks LC, Aisner J, Fortner CL, et al. Meperidine for the treatment of shaking chills and fever. Arch Intern Med 1980; 140:483–484.
26. Bogetz MS, Katz JA. Recall of surgery for major trauma. Anesthesiology 1984; 61:6–9.
27. Sebel PS, Lowden JD. Propofol: a new intravenous anesthetic. Anesthesiology 1989; 71:260–277.
28. Scheller MS. New volatile anesthetics: desflurane and sevoflurane. Semin Anesthesia 1992; 11;114–122.
29. Burchardi H, Kaczmarczyk G. The effect of anaesthesia on renal function. Eur J Anaesthesiol 1994; 11(3): 163–168.
30. Bunker JP, Forrest WH, Mosteller F, eds. The National Halothane Study; A Study of the Possible Association Between Halothane Anesthesia and Postoperative Hepatic Necrosis. Washington, DC: U.S. Government Printing Office, 1969.
31. Therlin L, Andreen M, Inestedt L. Effect of controlled halothane anesthesia on splanchnic blood flow and cardiac output in the dog. Acta Anaesthiol Scand 1975; 19:146.
32. Eger EI 2nd, Bowland T, Ionescu P, Laster MJ, Fang Z, Gong D, Sonner J, Weiskopf RB. Recovery and kinetic characteristics of desflurane and sevoflurane in volunteers after 8-h exposure, including kinetics of degradation products. Anesthesiology 1997; 87(3): 517–526.
33. Bito H, Ikeuchi Y, Ikeda K. Effects of low-flow sevoflurane anesthesia and low-flow isoflurane anesthesia. Anesthesiology 1997; 86:1231–1237.
34. Kharasch ED, Frink EJ Jr, Zager R, Bowdle TA, Artru A, Nogami WM. Assessment of low-flow sevoflurane and isoflurane effects on renal function using sensitive markers of tubular toxicity. Anesthesiology 1997; 86(6):1238–1253.
35. Eger EI, Gong D, Koblin DD, Bowland T, Ionescu P, Laster MJ, Weiskopf RB. Dose-related biochemical markers of renal injury after sevoflurane versus desflurane anesthesia in volunteers. Anesth Analg 1997; 85(5):1154–1163.
36. Hunter JM. Muscle relaxants in renal disease. Acta Anaesthesiol Scand Suppl 1994; 102:2–5.
37. Wilson WC, Anesthesia for colorectal surgery. In, Block GE, Moosa AR, eds. Operative Colorectal Surgery. Philadelphia: W.B. Saunders, 1994:107–126.
38. Rabiner SF, Drake RF. Platelet function as an indicator of adequate dialysis. Kidney Int 1975; 7:S144.
39. Bromage PR, Gertel M. Bracheal plexus anesthesia in chronic renal failure. Anesthesiology 1972; 36:488–493.
40. Smith LA, Barker DE, Burns RP. Autotransfusion utilization in abdominal trauma. Am Surg 1997; 63(1): 47–49.
41. Zantut LF, Machado MA, Volpe P, Poggetti RS, Birolini D. Autotransfusion with laparoscopically salvaged blood in trauma: report on 21 cases. Surg Laparosc Endosc 1996; 6(1);46–48.
42. Cottee DB, Saul WP. Is renal dose dopamine protective or therapeutic? Crit Care Clin 1996; 12(3):687–695.
43. Hirshberg A, Mattox KL. Duration of antibiotic treatment in surgical infections of the abdomen. Penetrating abdominal trauma. Eur J Surg Suppl 1996; 576: 56–58.
44. Ham AA, Coveler LA. Anesthetic considerations in damage control surgery. Surg Clin North Am 1997; 77(4):909–920.
45. Marion DW, Penrod LE, Kelsey SF, et al. Treatment of traumatic brain injury with moderate hypothermia. N Engl J Med 1997; 336:540–546.
46. Yagi N, Leblanc M, Sakai K, et al. Cooling effect of continuous renal replacement therapy in critically ill patients. Am J Kidney Dis 1998; 32(6):1023–1030.
47. Matamis D, Tsagourias M, Koletsos K, et al. Influence of continuous haemofiltration-related hypothermia on haemodynamic variables and gas exchange in septic patients. Inten Care Med 1994; 20(6):431–436.
48. van Kuijk WH, Hillion D, Savoiu C, et al. Critical role of the extracorporeal blood temperature in the hemodynamic response during hemofiltration. J Am Soc Nephrol 1997; 6:949–955.
49. Reeves ST, Pinosky ML, Byrne TK, Norcross ED. Abdominal compartment syndrome. Can J Anaesth 1997; 44(3):308–312.
50. Wilson WC, et al. Anesthesia for abdominal trauma. In Grande CM, Smith CE, eds. Anesthesiology Clinics of North America. Philadelphia: WB Saunders, 1999; 17(1):27–75.
51. Iberti TJ, Kelly KM, et al. A simple technique to accurately determine intra-abdominal pressure. Crit Care Med 1987; 15:1140.
52. Kron IL, Harman PK, Nolan SP. The measurement of intra-abdominal pressure as a criteria for abdominal re-exploration. Ann Surg 1984; 199:28.
53. Schein M, Wittmann DH, Aprahamian CC, Condon RE. The abdominal compartment syndrome: the physiological and clinical consequences of elevated intra-abdominal pressure. J Am Coll Surg 1995; 180:745–753.
54. Morris JA Jr, Eddy VA, Blinman TA, et al. The staged celiotomy for trauma. Issues in unpacking and reconstruction. Ann Surg 1993; 217:576–586.

Index

About the Editors

NORBERT LAMEIRE is Chairman of the Department of Internal Medicine, Chief of the Renal Division, University Hospital, and Professor of Medicine, University of Gent, Belgium. The author, coauthor, editor, or coeditor of numerous articles and scientific papers related to renal function, Dr. Lameire is a subject editor and deputy editor-in-chief of *Nephrology, Dialysis, and Transplantation*; editor-in-chief of *Acta Clinica Belgica*; and is a European Coordinator of the Task Force for Disaster Relief and council member of the International Society of Nephrology. He received the M.D. (1965) and Ph.D. (1970) degrees from the University of Gent, Gent, Belgium.

RAVINDRA L. MEHTA is Associate Professor of Medicine in the Division of Nephrology at the University of California, San Diego. An expert in dialytic management of acute renal failure with continuous renal replacement techniques (CRRT), Dr. Mehta is the U.S. coordinator of the Task Force for Disaster Relief of the International Society of Nephrology Commission on Acute Renal Failure; section editor for *Blood Purification*; a member of the editorial board of *Advances in Renal Replacement Therapy*; and the author or coauthor of numerous scientific articles, papers, and book chapters. He received the M.B.B.S. degree (1976) from the Government Medical School in Amritsar, India, and the M.D. (1979) and D.M (1981) degrees from the Post Graduate Institute of Medical Education and Research, Chandigarh, India.